CONTENTS

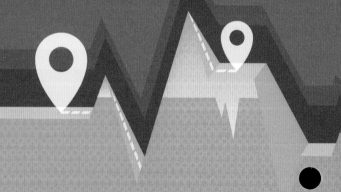

PRIORITIES IN
CRITICAL CARE NURSING

NINTH EDITION

PRIORITIES IN
CRITICAL CARE NURSING

Linda D. Urden
DNSc, RN, CNS, NE-BC, FAAN
Professor
Hahn School of Nursing and
   Health Science and Beyster
   Institute for Nursing Research
University of San Diego
San Diego, California

Kathleen M. Stacy
PhD, RN, APRN-CNS, CCNS, FCNS
Critical Care Clinical Nurse Specialist
Clinical Professor
Hahn School of Nursing and Health Science
University of San Diego
San Diego, California

Mary E. Lough
PhD, RN, CCNS, FCCM, FAHA, FCNS, FAAN
Nurse Scientist
Clinical Nurse Specialist
Stanford Health Care;
Clinical Assistant Professor
Stanford University
Stanford, California

Associate Editor

Kimberly Sanchez
PhD, RN, CCRN-K, ACCNS-AG
Clinical Nurse Specialist
Keck Medical Center of USC
Los Angeles, California

ELSEVIER

Elsevier
3251 Riverport Lane
St. Louis, Missouri 63043

PRIORITIES IN CRITICAL CARE NURSING, NINTH EDITION

ISBN: 978-0-323-80981-8

Notice

Practitioners and researchers must always rely on their own experience and knowledge in evaluating and using any information, methods, compounds or experiments described herein. Because of rapid advances in the medical sciences, in particular, independent verification of diagnoses and drug dosages should be made. To the fullest extent of the law, no responsibility is assumed by Elsevier, authors, editors or contributors for any injury and/or damage to persons or property as a matter of products liability, negligence or otherwise, or from any use or operation of any methods, products, instructions, or ideas contained in the material herein.

Previous editions copyrighted 2020, 2016, 2012, and 2009.

Executive Content Strategist: Lee Henderson
Director, Content Development: Ellen Wurm-Cutter
Senior Content Development Specialist: Kathleen Nahm
Publishing Services Manager: Deepthi Unni
Senior Project Manager: Kamatchi Madhavan
Design Direction: Ryan Cook

Printed in India
Last digit is the print number: 9   8   7   6   5   4   3   2   1

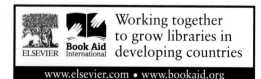

Sarah J. Berger, MS, RN, ACCNS-AG, CCRN
Clinical Nurse Specialist
Critical Care
University of California San Francisco
    Health
San Francisco, California
*Chapter 10, Cardiovascular Clinical
    Assessment and Diagnostic Procedures*

Janine Wong Berta, MS, RD-AP, CNSC
Instructor
Nutrition, Food Science, and Packaging
San Jose State University
San Jose, California;
Clinical Nutrition Supervisor
Clinical Nutrition
Stanford Health Care
Palo Alto, California
*Chapter 5, Nutritional Alterations and
    Management*

Darlene M. Burke, PhD, MS, MA, RN, CCRN-K, CNE
Associate Faculty
Nursing & Allied Health
MiraCosta College
Oceanside, California;
Consultant/Owner
Professional Source Nurse Consulting
Carlsbad, California
*Chapter 16, Neurologic Clinical Assessment
    and Diagnostic Procedures*

Jacqueline Fitzgerald Close, PhD, APRN
Retired
San Diego, California
*Chapter 20, Gastrointestinal Clinical
    Assessment and Diagnostic Procedures*
*Chapter 21, Gastrointestinal Disorders and
    Therapeutic Management*

Joni L. Dirks, MSN, NPD-BC, CCRN-K
Program Manager
Providence Nursing Institute
Providence St. Joseph Health
Spokane, Washington
*Chapter 12, Cardiovascular Therapeutic
    Management*

Caroline Etland, PhD, RN, CNS, ACHPN
Associate Professor
Kaye M. Woltman and Melisa R. McGuire
    Palliative Care Fellow
Hahn School of Nursing and Health
    Science
University of San Diego
San Diego, California

Céline Gélinas, PhD, RN
Professor
Ingram School of Nursing
McGill University;
Researcher
Centre for Nursing Research and Lady
    Davis Institute for Medical Research
Jewish General Hospital
Montreal, Quebec, Canada
Chapter 7, Pain and Pain Management

Kelly K. Dineen, BSN, JD, PhD
Professor of Law & Professor of Medical
    Humanities (secondary)
School of Law
Creighton University
Omaha, Nebraska
Chapter 2, Ethical and Legal Issues

Julie-Kathryn Graham, PhD, APRN, ACCNS-AG
Assistant Professor
School of Nursing
San Diego State University
San Diego, California;
Clinical Nurse Specialist
Education, Research and Professional
    Practice
Sharp Chula Vista Medical Center
Chula Vista, California
*Chapter 26, Shock, Sepsis, and Multiple
    Organ Dysfunction Syndrome*

Natalie B. de Haas-Rowland, MSN, RN, CCNS, CCRN-CSC-CMC
Clinical Nurse Specialist
Keck Medical Center of USC
Los Angeles, California
Chapter 3, Facilitating Care Transitions

Margaret Jordan Halter, PhD, APRN
Editor
*Foundations of Psychiatric-Mental Health
    Nursing*
Manual of Psychiatric Nursing Care
Elsevier Inc.
St. Louis, Missouri;
Former Associate Dean
Nursing
Ashland University
Mansfield, Ohio;
Former Clinical Nurse Specialist
Medical Staff
Cleveland Clinic Akron General
Akron, Ohio
*Chapter 4, Psychosocial and Spiritual
    Considerations*

Annette Haynes, MS, RN, CCRN, CCNS
Cardiovascular Clinical Nurse Specialist
Stanford Health Care, California
Chapter 11, Cardiovascular Disorders

Patricia Henry, MSN, RN, FNP-BC, CCNS, CCRN
Clinical Nurse Specialist
Nursing Professional Practice
Stanford Health Care
Palo Alto, California
Chapter 11, Cardiovascular Disorders

Misty Jenkins, MSN, APRN, ACNP-BC
Acute Care Nurse Practitioner
Pulmonary Critical Care Medicine
Ochsner Health
New Orleans, Louisiana
Chapter 6, The Older Adult

Amy Larsen, MS, RN, ACCNS-AG, CCRN, SCRN
Critical Care Clinical Nurse Specialist
Center for Nursing Excellence and
    Innovation
University of California San Francisco
    Health
San Francisco, California
*Chapter 10, Cardiovascular Clinical
    Assessment and Diagnostic Procedures*

Mary E. Lough, PhD, RN, CCNS, FCCM, FAHA, FCNS, FAAN
Nurse Scientist
Clinical Nurse Specialist
Stanford Health Care;
Clinical Assistant Professor
Stanford University
Stanford, California
Chapter 8, Sedation and Delirium Management
Chapter 10, Cardiovascular Clinical Assessment and Diagnostic Procedures
Chapter 22, Endocrine Clinical Assessment and Diagnostic Procedures
Chapter 23, Endocrine Disorders and Therapeutic Management

Eugene E. Mondor, MN, BScN, RN, CNS, CNCC(C)
Clinical Nurse Specialist
Adult Critical Care
Royal Alexandra Hospital
Edmonton, Alberta, Canada
Chapter 24, Trauma

Robyn A. Myers, MSN, RN, CPNP
Pediatric Nurse Practitioner
Pediatric General Surgery
St. Louis Children's Hospital
St. Louis, Missouri
Chapter 25, Burns

Kimberly Sanchez, PhD, RN, CCRN-K, ACCNS-AG
Clinical Nurse Specialist
Keck Medical Center of USC
Los Angeles, California
Chapter 3, Facilitating Care Transitions
Chapter 18, Kidney Clinical Assessment and Diagnostic Procedures
Chapter 19, Kidney Disorders and Therapeutic Management

Cass Piper Sandoval, MS, RN, CCNS
Clinical Nurse Specialist, Adult Critical Care
Center for Nursing Excellence and Innovation
University of California San Francisco Health
San Francisco, California
Chapter 10, Cardiovascular Clinical Assessment and Diagnostic Procedures

Carrie J. Scotto, PhD, RN
Assistant Professor
School of Nursing
Ursuline College
Pepper Pike, Ohio
Chapter 4, Psychosocial and Spiritual Considerations

Jennifer Seigel, RN, CPNP, CWCN
Pediatric Nurse Practitioner
Pediatric Surgery
St. Louis Children's Hospital
St. Louis, Missouri
Chapter 25, Burns

Kathleen M. Stacy, PhD, RN, APRN-CNS, CCNS, FCNS
Critical Care Clinical Nurse Specialist
Clinical Professor
Hahn School of Nursing and Health Science
University of San Diego
San Diego, California
Chapter 13, Pulmonary Clinical Assessment and Diagnostic Procedures
Chapter 14, Pulmonary Disorders
Chapter 15, Pulmonary Therapeutic Management
Chapter 17, Neurologic Disorders and Therapeutic Management

Carol Ann Suarez, MSN, APRN, ACNS-BC, FNP, PHN
Clinical Faculty
Health and Human Services—Nursing
California State University San Marcos
San Marcos, California;
Clinical Nurse Specialist
Quality and Patient Safety
Palomar Health
Escondido, California
Chapter 27, Hematologic and Oncologic Emergencies

Linda D. Urden, DNSc, RN, CNS, NE-BC, FAAN
Professor
Hahn School of Nursing and Health Science and Beyster Institute for Nursing Research
University of San Diego
San Diego, California
Chapter 1, Caring for the Critically Ill Patient

Julie M. Waters, MSN, RN, CCRN
Professional Development Specialist
Cardiovascular Intensive Care Unit
Providence Sacred Heart Medical Center
Spokane, Washington
Chapter 12, Cardiovascular Therapeutic Management

Carrie M. Wilson, MSN, RN, CPNP, WCC
Washington University
Pediatric Surgery
St. Louis, Missouri;
Pediatric Nurse Practitioner
Pediatric Surgery
St. Louis Children's Hospital
St. Louis, Missouri
Chapter 25, Burns

Kathrine Anne Winnie, DNP, RN
Clinical Nurse Specialist
Department of Nursing Professional Development & Nursing Excellence
Keck Hospital of USC
Los Angeles, California
Chapter 3, Facilitating Care Transitions

Fiona Winterbottom, MSN, DNP, RN
Clinical Nurse Specialist
Critical Care Medicine
Ochsner Health
New Orleans, Louisiana
Chapter 6, The Older Adult

REVIEWER

James Graves, PharmD
University of Missouri Health Center
Columbia, Missouri

To all front-line dedicated, professional, critical care nurses who continue to provide expert care for patients in these most challenging times and to student nurses who will be assuming professional roles in a health care environment calling for unprecedented devotion and commitment for all that you do.

LDU & KMS & MEL & KS

We are grateful to the many students, nurses, and educators who made the first eight editions of *Priorities in Critical Care Nursing* successful. The emphasis in this book continues to be on priorities for the critical care nurse. We believe that prioritizing conditions and issues will assist critical care nurses in quickly assessing and intervening in the most efficient and effective manner.

With this edition, we welcome aboard a *new Associate Editor*, Kimberly Sanchez, PhD, RN, CCRN-K, ACCNS-AG! She is a critical care clinical nurse specialist at Keck Medical Center, University of Southern California. Dr. Sanchez is also co-author of Chapter 3, *Facilitating Care Transitions*.

ORGANIZATION

The book comprises nine major units, with three appendices. The chapter content of Unit I, *Foundations in Critical Care Nursing*, forms the basis of practice, regardless of the physiologic alterations of the critically ill patient. Although chapters in the book may be studied in any sequence, we recommend that Chapter 1, "Caring for the Critically Ill Patient," be studied first, because it clarifies the major assumptions on which the entirety of the book is based. Chapter 2, "Ethical and Legal Issues," delineates theories and strategies for dealing with the ethical dilemmas that arise daily in critical care and provides a base of information to help the critical care nurse be cognizant of practice issues that may have legal implications. Chapter 3, "Facilitating Care Transitions," is a new chapter that provides information regarding the crucial step of patient movement across care settings, procedural departments, and discharge to various sites. Hand-off communication and procedures are discussed, along with important patient and family education principles.

Unit 2, *Common Problems in Critical Care*, examines potential critical care practice problems. Chapter 4, "Psychosocial and Spiritual Considerations" (new chapter title), examines the theoretic basis and nursing process for alterations in self-concept, spiritual practices, and coping. Chapter 5, "Nutritional Alterations and Management" (new title), examines the nutrition needs of critically ill patients and provides specific recommendations for different disorders. Chapter 6, "The Older Adult" (new title), addresses the needs of critically ill older adult patients in the critical care unit. The concepts of pain and pain management in critically ill patients are discussed in Chapter 7, "Pain and Pain Management." Sedation, agitation, and delirium are described in Chapter 8, "Sedation, Agitation, and Delirium Management" (new title). Chapter 9, "Palliative and End-of-Life Care" (new title), delineates special needs for dealing with end-of-life and palliative care.

Unit 3, *Cardiovascular Alterations*, and Unit 4, *Pulmonary Alterations*, are each organized according to the three-chapter format of Clinical Assessment and Diagnostic Procedures, Disorders, and Therapeutic Management. Unit 5, *Neurological Alterations*; Unit 6, *Kidney Alterations*; Unit 7, *Gastrointestinal Alterations*; and Unit 8, *Endocrine Alterations*, are each organized according to the two-chapter format of Clinical Assessment and Diagnostic Procedures and Disorders and Therapeutic Management.

Unit 9, *Multisystem Alterations*, addresses disorders that affect multiple body systems and necessitate discussion as a separate category:

Trauma; Burns; Shock, Sepsis, and Multiple Organ Dysfunction Syndrome; and Hematological Disorders and Oncological Emergencies.

Appendix A, *Patient Care Management Plans*, contains the core of critical care nursing practice in a nursing process format: signs and symptoms, outcome criteria, and nursing interventions. The Patient Care Management Plans are referenced throughout the book within the *Priority Patient Care Management* boxes. Appendix B, *Physiologic Formulas for Critical Care*, features common hemodynamic and oxygenation formulas and other calculations presented in easily understood terms. Appendix C, *Laboratory Values*, lists the most common laboratory tests listed in Système International Units.

EVIDENCE-BASED PRACTICE AND RESEARCH

The power of research-based critical care practice has been incorporated into nursing interventions. To foster critical thinking and decision making, a boxed menu of priority patient problems complete with specific etiologic or related factors accompanies each medical disorder and major medical treatment discussion and directs the learner to the section of the book where appropriate patient management is detailed.

NINTH EDITION CONTINUING FEATURES

In keeping with the emphasis on priorities in critical care, *Priority Patient Care Management* boxes list the most urgent patient problems to be addressed. To facilitate student learning, the *Patient Care Management Plans* (Appendix A) incorporate patient problems, etiologic or related factors, clinical manifestations, and interventions with rationales. These *Plans of Care* are cross-referenced throughout the book. **QSEN** boxes that alert the nurse to special evidence-based considerations to specific practices and interventions that ensure safe patient care and best outcomes.

SPECIAL FEATURES IN THIS EDITION

- **QSEN** boxes—A variety of additional **QSEN** boxes have been added to this edition. These boxes highlight quality and safety issues that are key to the care of critically ill patients. Boxes devoted to this material are identified with the **QSEN** icon and address the following issues:
  - Patient-Centered Care
  - Teamwork and Collaboration
  - Evidence-Based Practice
  - Quality Improvement
  - Safety (replaces Patient Safety Alert box)
  - Informatics
- **Pharmacologic Management** tables outline common medications, along with any special considerations, used in treatment of the different disorders presented in the text.
  Priority Patient and Family Education boxes list the special topics that should be taught where key content is a priority for educating patients and families.
- **Data Collection** boxes contain information that should be included as part of the patient's history.

- **Priority Patient Care Management** boxes display the diagnoses associated with particular disorders in a summary format with references to the corresponding patient care management plans in Appendix A.

NEW TO THIS EDITION

- Expanded Internet references, which guide the reader to additional resources on chapter content, in **QSEN**: *Informatics* boxes.
- Chapter 3, "Facilitating Care Transitions," provides guidance for critical care nurses to ensure patient safety through all phases and locations of care transitions to other departments and discharge; it also includes patient and family education.
- There is a greater emphasis on the psychosocial and spiritual well-being of critical care patients; this includes renaming Chapter 4 "Psychosocial and Spiritual Considerations."
- Nutritional considerations for each disorder are cross-referenced to the *Nutritional Alterations and Management* chapter.
- Canadian/SI units are included to promote international understanding of common laboratory values with a new *Common Laboratory Values* Appendix.
- The International Council of Nurses (ICN) Cultural Competence for Nurses box is integrated with a discussion of the importance of awareness and appropriate actions for nurses interacting with members of the health care team and patients and families.
- **QSEN**: Informatics boxes have been expanded to include a discussion of all disorders.
- Two new Patient Care Management Plans, "Stress Overload" and "Impaired Spiritual Status," have been added for this edition.
- Another new feature to this edition is "Trending Priorities in Health Care." The intent of this feature is to identify societal and other issues facing health care today that are important to understand when providing care and services to critically ill hospitalized patients. It offers a context from which to consider factors when planning care. Topics include (but are not limited to): addiction, homelessness, mental health issues, limited English proficiencies, healing health environments. These vignettes are intended to create discussion among students and faculty for entering the care environment and planning individualized care.

EVOLVE RESOURCES FOR *CRITICAL CARE NURSING*

We are pleased to offer additional new and updated resources for students and instructors on our companion site, Evolve Resources for *Priorities in Critical Care Nursing.*

Student Resources

Student Resources are available at http://evolve.elsevier.com/Urden/priorities/ and include the following:

- Case Studies
- Next-Generation NCLEX® Examination (NGN)—Style Single-Episode Case Studies
- Self-assessment opportunities, including:
  - NCLEX® Review Questions
  - CCRN® Review Questions
  - PCCN® Review Questions
- Audio Glossary
- A selection of assessment animations and video clips for specific chapters
- Selected critical care skills from Elsevier's Clinical Skills Critical Care Collection

Instructor Resources

Instructor Resources, available at http://evolve.elsevier.com/Urden/priorities/, provide a variety of aids to enhance instruction. Instructors have access to all of the Student Resources listed above, as well as the following:

- TEACH for Nurses—detailed lesson plans that offer:
  - List of all student and instructor chapter resources
  - Teaching Strategies that present a chapter outline, content highlights, and learning activities
  - New Case Study for select chapters
  - Answers to the Student Resource Case Studies provided for select chapters
- Test Bank of approximately 600 questions
- PowerPoint presentations by chapter, including lecture notes on most slides and audience response questions
- Image Collection containing all images from the text
- Next-Generation NCLEX® Examination (NGN)—Style Case Studies for Critical Care Nursing
- Next-Generation NCLEX® Examination (NGN)—Style Single-Episode Case Studies

Priorities in Critical Care Nursing, Ninth Edition, represents our continued commitment to bringing you the best in all things a textbook can offer: the best and brightest in contributing and consulting authors, the latest in scientific research, a logical organizational format that exercises diagnostic reasoning skills, and artwork that enhances student learning. We pledge our continued commitment to excellence in critical care education.

Linda D. Urden
Kathleen M. Stacy
Mary E. Lough
Kimberly Sanchez

ACKNOWLEDGMENTS

The talent, hard work, and inspiration of many people have produced the Ninth Edition of *Priorities in Critical Care Nursing.* We appreciate the assistance of the editorial team that worked with us on this edition: Lee Henderson and Kathleen Nahm. We are also grateful to our project manager, Kamatchi Madhavan, for her scrupulous attention to detail.

1

Caring for the Critically Ill Patient

Linda D. Urden

CONTEMPORARY CRITICAL CARE

Modern critical care is provided to patients by an interprofessional team of health care providers who have in-depth education and expertise in the specialty field of critical care. The team consists of physician intensivists, specialty physicians, nurses, advanced practice nurses (APNs) such as clinical nurse specialists (CNSs) and nurse practitioners (NPs), and other specialty clinicians: pharmacists, respiratory therapy practitioners, other specialized therapists, social workers, and clergy.

Critical care patients are at high risk for actual or potential life-threatening health problems. Critical care is provided in specialized units or departments, and importance is placed on the continuum of care, with an efficient and as seamless as possible transition of care from one setting to another (see Chapter 3).

A new feature for this book is "Trending Priorities in Health Care." The intent of these topical discussions is to highlight societal trends and issues inherent in society that effect health care as it is delivered throughout various sites and geographical settings. The discussions are placed in boxes, with references and resources, and will occur throughout the book. Examples include limited English proficiency (LEP), homelessness, and external disaster preparedness.

CRITICAL CARE NURSING ROLES

Registered Nurses

Nurses provide and contribute to the care of critically ill patients in a variety of roles. The most prevalent role for the professional registered nurse (RN) is that of direct care provider. The American Association of Critical-Care Nurses (AACN) has delineated role responsibilities that are important for acute care and critical care nurses (Box 1.1).[1]

Expanded-Role Nursing Positions

Nurses in expanded-role nursing positions interact with critical care patients, families, and the health care team. Other nurse clinicians, such as patient educators, cardiac rehabilitation specialists, diabetes educators, nurse informaticists, care coordinators, and infection control specialists, also contribute to care. The specific types of expanded-role nursing positions are determined by patient needs and individual organizational resources.

Advanced Practice Nurses

APNs have met educational and clinical requirements beyond the basic nursing educational requirements for all nurses. The most commonly seen APNs in critical care areas are the CNS and the NP or acute care nurse practitioner (ACNP). APNs have a broad depth of knowledge and expertise in their specialty area and manage complex clinical and systems issues. The organizational system and existing resources of an institution determine what roles may be needed and how the roles function.

CNSs serve in specialty roles that use their clinical, teaching, research, leadership, and consultative abilities. They work in direct clinical roles and systems or administrative roles and in various other settings in the health care system.

NPs and ACNPs manage direct clinical care of a group of patients and have various levels of prescriptive authority, depending on the state and practice area in which they work. They also provide care consistency, interact with families, plan for patient discharge, and provide teaching to patients, families, and other members of the health care team.[2]

CRITICAL CARE NURSING PROFESSIONAL ACCOUNTABILITY

American Association of Critical-Care Nurses (AACN)

The nursing specialty organization most closely associated with critical care nurses is the AACN. Created in 1969, it is the world's largest specialty nursing organization. AACN is focused on "creating a health care system driven by the needs of patients and their families, where acute and critical care nurses make their optimal contribution."[3]

AACN serves its members through a national organization and many local chapters. The top priority of the organization is education of critical care nurses via national, regional, local, and online opportunities. AACN publishes numerous materials, journals, evidence-based practice (EBP) summaries, practice alerts, linkages between critical care nurses, and job postings related to the specialty. It also provides multiple clinical tools to support critical care patient and nursing practice. AACN is at the forefront of setting professional standards of care.

BOX 1.1 Acute and Critical Care Nursing

The American Association of Critical Care Nurses (AACN) defines acute and critical care nursing as the specialty that manages human responses to actual or potential life-threatening problems. Nurses rely on a body of specialized knowledge, skills, and abilities to:

- Restore, support, promote, and maintain the physiologic and psychosocial stability of patients of all ages across the life span
- Assimilate and prioritize information in order to take immediate and decisive evidence-based, patient-focused action
- Anticipate and respond with confidence and adapt to rapidly changing patient conditions
- Respond to the unique needs of patients and families coping with unanticipated treatment as well as quality-of-life and end-of-life decisions
- Establish and maintain safe, respectful, healing, and caring environments
- Recognize the fiscal responsibility of nurses working in a resources intensive-driven environment
- Use health care interventions designed to restore, rehabilitate, cure, maintain, or palliate for patients of all ages across the life span

From American Association of Critical-Care Nurses. *AACN Scope and Standards for Acute and Critical Care Nursing Practice.* Aliso Viejo, CA: AACN; 2015.

Certification

The *AACN Certification Corporation* was created in the 1970s and is a separate company that develops and administers many critical care specialty certification examinations for RNs. There are numerous certification examination options for RNs.[4] There are also certifications for APNs.

According to the Certification Corporation, certification is considered one method to maintain high quality of care and to protect consumers of care and services: "Achieving board certification demonstrates to patients, employers, and the public that a nurse's knowledge reflects national standards and a deep commitment to patient safety."[5]

Certification has been associated with positive outcomes in three areas: patient, for example, less need for mechanical ventilation, lower rates of complication; nurse, for example, workplace empowerment, improved knowledge, and skills; and organizational, for example, intent to leave the organization, nurse turnover.[6]

EVIDENCE-BASED NURSING PRACTICE

Multiple changes and increased health care costs have led to an increased presence of managed care, pay for performance, and regulations with punitive financial actions toward health care organizations that do not meet established thresholds.

This has resulted in a greater emphasis on demonstrating the effectiveness of treatments and practices on outcomes. It has become essential for nurses to use the best data available to make patient care decisions and carry out appropriate nursing interventions. The content of this book is research-based, with the most current, cutting-edge research abstracted and placed throughout the chapters as appropriate to topical discussions.

AACN has promulgated several EBP summaries in the form of a *Practice Alert.* These alerts are directives that can be used as a quick reference for practice areas. They are succinct, supported by evidence, and address both nursing and multidisciplinary activities. Each alert is organized into five areas and includes scope and impact of the problem, expected outcome, supporting evidence, implementation/organizational support for the practice, and references.[7] Examples of practice alerts are listed in Box 1.2.

BOX 1.2 Evidence-Based Practice

AACN Practice Alert Examples
- Initial and Ongoing Verification of Feeding Tube Placement in Adults (updated January 29, 2020)
- Assessing Pain in Critically Ill Adults (December 1, 2018)
- Assessment and Management of Delirium Across the Life Span (updated October 1, 2018)
- Accurate Dysrhythmia Monitoring in Adults (updated May 2018)
- Ensuring Accurate S-T Segment Monitoring (updated May 17, 2018)
- Prevention of Aspiration in Adults (updated May 17, 2018)
- Managing Alarms in Acute Care Across the Life Span (April 3, 2018)

AACN, American Association of Critical Care Nurses.

DIAGNOSIS AND PATIENT CARE MANAGEMENT

It is crucial that nurses document their observations and diagnosis of patient conditions, and the interventions that they carry out to address these issues. In order to accomplish this, there must be a consistent methodology that includes common terms that will provide classifications across a variety of patient conditions and settings.

International Classification for Nursing Practice (ICNP)

The classification that is used for this book to document nursing patient care management is the ICNP is a collaborative project coordinated under the International Council of Nurses (ICN). There are three elements of ICNP: (1) nursing phenomena, sometimes referred to as nursing diagnosis; (2) nursing interventions; and (3) nursing outcomes.[8]

The tools are intended to be useful at the point of care and do not replace nursing clinical judgment and decision making.[9,10] Priority Patient Care Management boxes that reflect related patient conditions are found throughout the book and are designated with the ⊚ icon.

Algorithms

It is essential that nurses are skillful in clinical reasoning and clinical judgment to address the complexities of health care. An algorithm is a tool that includes data such as physiologic values, symptomology, definitions of conditions, and lists of possible related disorders. This facilitates nurses in quickly assimilating multiple data points to design the most evidence-based, accurate, and timely plan of care. Algorithms are found throughout this book (see Fig. 23.2).

HOLISTIC CRITICAL CARE NURSING

Caring

The priority in critical care is using technology and treatments necessary for maintaining stability in the physiologic functioning of the patient. Keeping the *care* in nursing care is one of our biggest challenges.

The caring aspect between nurses and patients is most fundamental to the relationship and to the health care experience. Holistic care focuses on patient's uniqueness, human integrity, and stresses that the body, the mind, and the spirit are interdependent and inseparable. All aspects need to be considered in planning and delivering care.

Patient-Centered Critical Care

The differences between nurses' and patients' perceptions of caring point to the importance of establishing individualized care that recognizes the uniqueness of each patient's preferences, condition, and physiologic and psychosocial status.

TRENDING PRIORITIES IN HEALTHCARE

Caring for LGBTQ+ Patients

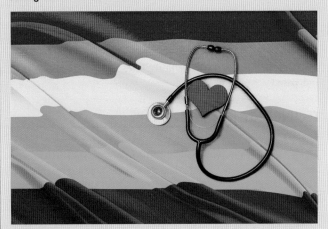

iStock.com/leolintang.

Sexual and gender minorities are a National Institutes of Health—designated health disparity population in the United States.[1] Understanding sexual orientation and gender identity is an important first step in providing care for the lesbian, gay, bisexual, transgender, queer, and all other identities (LGBTQ+) community.[2] Information on sexual orientation and gender identity assists with patient-centered care and provides organizational data on populations served, similar to other demographic information.[2] The use of chosen names and pronouns in personal interactions with the LGBTQ+ community also promotes inclusivity and patient-centered care.[2]

Sexual Orientation

Sexual orientation is one's physical and emotional attraction to others.[2] One's sexual orientation may be identified by the following:
- Straight or heterosexual—men physically and emotionally attracted to women and vice versa[2]
- Homosexual—individual physically and emotionally attracted to the same gender[2]
- Gay—individual physically and emotionally attracted to the same gender, usually referring to men[2]
- Lesbian—women physically and emotionally attracted to women[2]
- Bisexual—individual physically and emotionally attracted to the same and different gender[2]
- Something else—individual who identifies as something other than the categories provided, for example, asexual and pansexual[2]
- Unknown—individual who does not know their sexual orientation[2]

Gender Identity

Gender identity is one's inner sense of being male, female, or something else.[2] Gender identity should not be confused with sex assigned at birth.[2] Information about sex assigned at birth may further stratify males who do not select transgender male upon data collection episodes (e.g., a patient selection of male for gender and female for sex assigned at birth would inform health care workers the patient is a transgender male).[2]
- Male—individual assigned male at birth who has a male gender identity, but also inclusive of transgender male (see below)[2]
- Female—individual assigned female at birth who has a female gender identity, but also inclusive of transgender female (see below)[2]
- Transgender male—individual assigned female at birth who has a male gender identity[2]
- Transgender female—individual assigned male at birth who has a female gender identity[2]
- Something else—individual who identifies as something other than the categories provided, like nonbinary, gender diverse, and gender fluid[2]

Pronouns

Pronouns are words used when referring to an individual and not using their name.[2] Pronouns include he/him/his, she/her/hers, they/them/theirs, and ze/hir/hirs (pronounced zee, hear, hears and used for nonbinary gender identities).[2]

For additional information about the LGBTQ+ community, check out the following websites:
- Centers for Medicare & Medicaid Services LGBT Partners—https://www.cms.gov/Outreach-and-Education/Outreach/Partnerships/LGBT
- GLAAD—https://www.glaad.org/resourcelist
- National LGBTQIA+ Health Education Center—https://www.lgbtqiahealtheducation.org/
- The Joint Commission LGBT Field Guide—https://www.jointcommission.org/lgbt/

References

1. National Institutes of Health. https://www.nimhd.nih.gov/about/overview/. Accessed October 17, 2021.
2. National LGBT Health Education Center. *Ready, Set, Go! A Guide for Collecting Data on Sexual Orientation and Gender Identity.* Updated 2020. https://www.lgbtqiahealtheducation.org/wp-content/uploads/2018/03/TFIE-47_Updates-2020-to-Ready-Set-Go-publication_6.29.20.pdf. Updated 2020. Accessed October 17, 2021.

An important aspect in the care delivery to and recovery of critically ill patients is the personal support of family members and significant others. The value of patient-centered and family-centered care should not be underestimated.

It is important for families to be included in care decisions and to be encouraged to participate in the care of the patient as appropriate to the patient's personal needs and physiologic stability. This important aspect is represented in the Quality and Safety Education for Nurses (QSEN): Patient-Centered Care boxes throughout the book.

Cultural Care

Cultural diversity is defined as "the awareness of the presence of differences among members of a social group or units."[11] Diversity includes not only ethnic sensitivity but also sensitivity and openness to differences in lifestyles, opinions, values, and beliefs.

Cultural competency is defined as "a developmental process in which one achieves increasing levels of awareness, knowledge, and

skills along a continuum, improving one's capacity to work and communicate effectively in cross-cultural situations."[12] It must be supported with policies, procedures, and dedicated resources. If this competency is not present, miscommunication, lack of understanding regarding health information, and treatments may negatively affect outcomes.[12]

Cultural competence is one way to ensure that individual differences related to culture are incorporated into the plan of care. Interventions must be tailored to the uniqueness of each patient and family. See Box 1.3 for nursing practice cultural competencies.[13]

COMPLEMENTARY AND ALTERNATIVE THERAPIES

Complementary therapies offer patients, families, and health care providers additional options to assist with healing and recovery.

The two terms *alternative* and *complementary* have been in the mainstream for several years. *Alternative* denotes that a specific therapy is an option or alternative to what is considered conventional treatment of a condition or state. The term *complementary* was proposed to describe therapies that can be used to complement or support conventional treatments.

AACN has published guidelines for consideration by the critical care nurse when implementing complementary therapies in the critical care patient care areas.[14,15]

Guided Imagery

One well-studied complementary therapy is guided imagery, a mind-body strategy that is frequently used to decrease stress, pain, and anxiety. Additional benefits of guided imagery are (1) decreased side effects, (2) decreased length of stay, (3) reduced hospital costs, (4) enhanced sleep, and (5) increased patient satisfaction.[16] The patient's involvement in the process offers a sense of empowerment and accomplishment and motivates self-care.

Massage

A comprehensive review of the literature revealed that the most common effect of massage was reduction in anxiety, with additional reports of a significant decrease in tension. There was also a positive physiologic response to massage in the areas of decreased respiratory and heart rates and decreased pain.[17]

Animal-Assisted Therapy

The use of animals has increased as an adjunct to healing in the care of patients of all ages in various settings. In the acute care setting, animals are brought in to provide additional solace and comfort for patients who are critically or terminally ill. Fish aquariums are used in patient areas and family areas because they humanize the surroundings.

Scientific evidence indicates that animal-assisted therapy results in positive patient outcomes in the areas of attention, mobility and orientation, improved communication, and mood in patients.[18–20]

Music Therapy

Music therapy is the clinical and evidence-based use of music interventions to accomplish individualized goals within a therapeutic relationship to address physical, emotional, cognitive, and social needs. It is administered by a credentialed professional who has completed an approved music therapy program. It includes creating, singing, and moving and/or listening to music.[21]

Research has demonstrated music therapy effectiveness using music therapy in communication, overall physical rehabilitation, movement, motivation, support for patients and families, and an outlet for expression of feelings.[22,23]

One study reported that patients with mechanical ventilation who listened to music had reduced anxiety, systolic blood pressure, and respiratory rate.[22] Another study reported significant decreases in respiratory rate, heart rate, and self-reported anxiety and pain.[23]

TECHNOLOGY IN CRITICAL CARE

Technology can augment or add value to the work.[24] An example of augmentation is the evolving electronic health record (EHR) that was originally designed to capture data for clinical decision making and to increase the efficiency of health care providers. A newer phenomenon has been identified that is related to technology. The concept of *alarm fatigue* is discussed in Box 1.4.

The *ANA Core Principles on Connected Health* has published 13 principles as a guide to health care professionals who use connected health technologies to provide quality care.[25] AACN has promulgated *TeleICU Nursing Practice Recommendations* that are organized into essential elements for (1) tele-ICU nurses, (2) tele-ICU nurse leaders, (3) tele-ICU nurses and nurse leaders, and (4) tele-ICU health care organizations.[26]

An opportunity for critical care nurses is working in a role that encompasses the tele-ICU (also termed *telehealth*). Tele-ICU is defined as "a collaborative interprofessional care model focusing on critically ill patients that is enabled by leveraging audio, video, data, and other technologies."[26] It links experts in critical care with clinicians at the care delivery site.

INTERPROFESSIONAL COLLABORATIVE PRACTICE

Collaboration and partnerships have been shown to increase quality of care and services while containing or decreasing costs.[27–32] The Interprofessional Education Collaborative (IPEC) updated the *Core Competencies for Interprofessional Collaborative Practice* in 2016.

IPEC sponsors included associations of nursing, dentistry, medicine, osteopathy, public health, and pharmacy. Their goal was to establish a set of competencies to serve as a framework for professional socialization of health care professionals.

They also intended to assess the relevance of the competencies and develop an action plan for implementation.[33] These competencies are especially important as we move forward with health care refinancing, quality initiatives, and explore innovative care delivery models using the skill sets of all health care providers in the most effective and efficient manner. Box 1.5 delineates the four interprofessional collaborative core competencies.[33]

INTERDISCIPLINARY CARE MANAGEMENT TOOLS

Many quality improvement tools are available to the interdisciplinary team for managing care. The three evidence-based tools addressed in this chapter are clinical algorithm, practice guideline, and protocol. All these tools may be embedded in the EHR.

Algorithm

An *algorithm* is a stepwise decision-making flowchart for a specific care process or processes. Algorithms guide the clinician through the

QSEN BOX 1.4   Safety

Alarm Fatigue

There continues to be an evolution of technologies to monitor, diagnose, and support therapies in the treatment of critically ill persons. Most of the modalities have both visual and auditory warnings to alert clinicians when there are deviations outside of desired parameters.

Alarm fatigue has been identified as a condition when "clinicians experience high exposure to medical device alarms, causing alarm desensitization and leading to missed alarms or delayed response."[1] This condition, occurring especially among nurses, has been identified as an important patient safety with reports, literature summaries, and recommendations to manage alarm fatigue.[1-4]

There are several contributors to alarm fatigue[4]:

- Artifacts in the ECG waveform may be caused by poor lead preparation, problems with adhesive placement and replacement, improper care and maintenance of lead wires and cables
- Alarm settings, limits, and delays (some related to factory default settings)
- Alarm settings are based on clinical population versus individual patient
- Lack of proper staff education regarding electrode placement, default alarm limits and delays, and basing alarm settings on individual patients
- Lack of patient/family education regarding necessity for alarms (and not to silence or change the alarm limits themselves)

Management related to these issues then should be directed toward resolution, for example, staff education regarding proper skin preparation and lead placement; individualizing alarm settings specific to each patient condition, patient/family education.

Additional resources related to addressing technologies and safety issues include the following:

- htpps://www.aami.org—Association for the Advancement of Medical Instrumentation (AAMI)
- htpps://www.ecri.org—Emergency Care Research Institute (ECRI)
- htpps://www.jointcommisssion.org—The Joint Commission (TJC)
- htpps://www.psnet@ahrq.gov—Patient Safety Network (PSNet)

References

1. Woo M, Bacon O. Alarm fatigue. In: Hall KK, Shoemaker-Hunt S, Hoffman L, et al, eds. *Making healthcare safer III: a critical analysis of existing and emerging patient safety practices*. Agency for Healthcare Research and Quality (US); 2020. https://www.ncbi.nim.nih.gov/books/NBK555522/?report=printable. Accessed September 21, 2021.
2. National Association of Clinical Nurse Specialists. Alarm fatigue: strategies to safely manage clinical alarms and prevent alarm fatigue. 2013–2014. https://www.nacns.org/resources/toolkits-and-reports/alarm-fatigue-toolkit/. Accessed September 22, 2021.
3. Pelter MM, Drew BJ. Patient Safety Network. Harm from alarm fatigue. https://psnet.ahrq.gov/web-mm/harn-alarm-fatigue. December 1, 2015.
4. Jacques S, Williams EA. Patient Safety Network. Reducing the safety hazards of monitor alert and alarm fatigue. https://psnet.ahrq.gov/perspective/reducing-safety-hazards-monitor-alert-and-alarm-fatugue. Accessed September 21, 2021.

AHRQ.gov/sites/default/files/wysiwyg/research/findings/making-healthcare-safer/mhs3/alarm-fatigue-1.pdf

"if, then" decision-making process, addressing patient responses to particular treatments.

Well-known examples of algorithms are the advanced cardiac life support algorithms published by the American Heart Association. Weaning, medication selection, medication titration, individual practitioner variance, and appropriate patient placement algorithms have been developed to give practitioners additional standardized decision-making abilities.

Practice Guideline

A *practice guideline* is usually created by an expert panel and developed by a professional organization (e.g., AACN, Society of Critical Care Medicine [SCCM], American College of Cardiology), and government agencies (e.g., Agency for Health Care Research and Quality). Practice guidelines are generally written in text prose style rather than in the flowchart format of algorithms. They recommend future research and development of tools to translate research findings into practice.[34]

Although not a guideline per se, another interdisciplinary team derived from five professional organizations (including AACN and SCCM) created a policy statement, *Responding to Requests for Potentially Inappropriate Treatment in Intensive Care Units*. This document provided recommendations for potential disagreements in the critical care unit regarding inappropriate treatments.[35]

Protocol

A *protocol* is a common tool in research studies. Protocols are more directive and rigid than guidelines, and providers are not supposed to vary from a protocol. Patients are screened carefully for specific entry criteria before being started on a protocol. There are many national research protocols, such as for cancer and chemotherapy studies. Protocols are helpful when built-in alerts signal the provider to potentially serious problems.

Order Set

An *order set* consists of provider orders that are used to expedite the order process after a standard has been validated through analytic review of practice and research. Order sets complement and increase compliance with existing practice standards. They can also be used to

QSEN BOX 1.5   Teamwork and Collaboration

Core Competencies for Interprofessional Collaborative Practice

Values/Ethics for Interprofessional Practice
- Work with individuals of other professions to maintain a climate of mutual respect and shared values.

Roles/Responsibilities for Collaborative Practice
- Use the knowledge of one's own role and the role of other professions to appropriately assess and address the health care needs of patients and populations served.

Interprofessional Communication
- Communicate with patients, families, communities, and other health professionals in a responsive and responsible manner that supports a team approach to maintaining health and treatment of disease.

Interprofessional Teamwork and Team-Based Care
- Apply relationship-building values and principles of team dynamics to perform effectively in different team roles to plan and deliver patient-/population-centered care that is safe, timely, efficient, effective, and equitable.

represent an algorithm or protocol in order format. All are embedded within the EHR for easy access and retrieval.

QUALITY, SAFETY, AND REGULATORY ISSUES IN CRITICAL CARE

In the critical care environment, patients are particularly vulnerable because of their compromised physiologic status, multiple technologic and pharmacologic interventions, and multiple care providers who frequently work at a fast pace. It is essential that care delivery processes that minimize the opportunity for errors are designed and that a "safety culture" rather than a "blame culture" is created.[36] Health care outcomes are now transparent, easily accessed, and publicly reported. It is critical that nurses are accountable for their care, collect, monitor and analyze quality data, and participate in review and follow-up on outcomes.[37]

Quality and Safety Issues

Patient safety is a major focus of attention by health care consumers, providers of care, administrators of health care institutions, and payors.

The definition of medical errors and approaches to resolving patient safety issues often differs among nurses, physicians, administrators, and other health care providers. Subsequently through its use of expert panels, the Institute of Medicine (IOM) has published numerous reports related to quality, safety, and the patient care environment.

Medication administration is one of the most error-prone nursing interventions for critical care nurses.[38] Many medication errors are related to system failures, with distraction as a major factor. Various interventions have been created to decrease medication errors.

When an injury or inappropriate care occurs, it is crucial that health care professionals promptly explain how the injury or mistake occurred and the short-term or long-term effects on the patient and family.

The patient and family should be informed that the factors involved in the injury will be investigated so that steps can be taken to reduce or prevent the likelihood of similar injury to other patients.

Quality and Safety Regulations

There are numerous regulations governing health care, including local, state, national, Medicare/Medicaid, and payer requirements. *The Joint Commission (TJC)* is an independent, not-for-profit organization. Its goal is to evaluate these health care entities using their pre-established standards of performance to ensure that high levels of care are provided in these entities. It establishes National Patient Safety Goals (NPSGs) annually[39] that are to be implemented in health care organizations (Box 1.6).

The *Safe Medical Devices Act* requires that hospitals report serious or potentially serious device-related injuries or illness of patients or employees to the manufacturer of the device and to the US Food and Drug Administration (FDA) if a death has occurred. In addition, implantable devices must be documented and tracked.[40] The reporting serves as an early warning system so that the FDA can obtain information on device problems. Failure to comply with the act results in civil action.

The FDA requires that a drug company place a boxed warning on the labeling of a prescription drug or in literature describing it. This boxed warning (also known as a "*black box warning*") indicates that the drug carries a significant risk of serious or life-threatening adverse effects.[41]

BOX 1.6 Safety QSEN

2021 Hospital National Patient Safety Goals
- Identify patients correctly.
- Improve staff communication.
- Use medications safely.
- Use alarms safely.
- Prevent infection.
- Identify patient safety risks.
- Prevent mistakes in surgery.

From The Joint Commission. *National Patient Safety Goals Effective January 1, 2021.* Hospital Accreditation Program. Oak Brook Terrace, IL: The Joint Commission; 2020.

Examples include warfarin, celecoxib (Celebrex), rosiglitazone (Avandia), and ciprofloxacin (Cipro). Alerts are published as soon as a drug is found to meet the criteria. Providers are to use caution when prescribing the medications and to consider alternative medications that have fewer adverse effects.

QUALITY AND SAFETY RESOURCES

The Institute for Safe Medication Practices (ISMP) is a not-for-profit organization dedicated to medication error prevention and safe medication use. It has numerous tools to assist care providers, including newsletters, education programs, safety alerts, consulting, patient education materials, and error-reporting systems. One newsletter is devoted specifically to nurses. It offers a very comprehensive array of tools.[42]

The *Institute for Healthcare Improvement (IHI)* is an interdisciplinary organization focused on quality that also offers many tools and resources, including educational materials, conferences, case studies, publications, white papers, and quality measure tools. IHI developed the "bundle" concept, which consists of EBPs on specific high-risk quality issues as determined by a multidisciplinary group. IHI publishes many bundles, such as central line, ventilator, and sepsis bundles.[43]

The *National Quality Forum* is another not-for-profit organization that facilitates consensus building with multiple partners to establish national priorities and goals for performance improvement. They also establish common definitions and consistent measurement. In addition, their goal is that all health care providers and stakeholders are educated regarding quality, priorities, and outcomes.[44]

The *Healthcare Information and Management Systems Society (HIMSS)* is an interdisciplinary organization focused on patient safety and quality of care. This organization specifically focuses on integration of patient safety tools and practices to enhance communication, quality, efficiency, productivity, and clinical support systems.[45]

The *National Database of Nursing Quality Indicators (NDNQI)* is a national quality database devoted entirely to nursing. The database provides ongoing nurse-sensitive indicator consultation and research-based expertise. It is the only nursing national quality measurement program that provides hospitals with unit-level quality performance comparison reports.[46]

The *Quality in Safety and Education (QSEN)* project established standards for educating RNs at the baccalaureate and master's levels of academic education. In this model, knowledge, skills, and attitudes were created so that nurses would be able to continuously improve the quality and safety of the health care systems for which they work. There are six major categories that delineate knowledge, skills, and

---

QSEN

BOX 1.7   Competencies

Patient-Centered Care
- Recognize the patient or designee as the source of control and full partner in providing compassionate and coordinated care based on respect for patient's preferences, values, and needs.

Teamwork and Collaboration
- Function effectively within nursing and interprofessional teams, fostering open communication, mutual respect, and shared decision making to achieve quality patient care.

Evidence-Based Practice
- Integrate best current evidence with clinical expertise and patient/family preferences and values for delivery of optimal health care.

Quality Improvement
- Use data to monitor the outcomes of care processes and use improvement methods to design and test changes to continuously improve the quality and safety of health care systems.

Safety
- Minimizes risk of harm to patients and providers through both system effectiveness and individual performance.

Informatics
- Use information and technology to communicate, manage knowledge, mitigate error, and support decision making.

From Cronenwett L, Sherwood G, Barnsteiner J, et al. Quality and safety education for nurses. *Nursing Outlook.* 2007;55(3):122.

QSEN

BOX 1.8   Internet Resources

Critical Care Nursing Practice
- Agency for Healthcare Research and Quality (AHRQ): https://www.ahrq.gov
- AHRQ Patient Safety Network (PSNet): https://www.psnet.ahrq.gov/about-psnet
- AHRQ Rapid Response Systems: https://psnet.ahrq.gov/primer/rapid-response-systems
- American Association of Critical-Care Nurses (AACN): https://www.aacn.org
- Healthcare Information and Management Systems Society (HIMSS): https://www.himss.org
- Institute for Healthcare Improvement (IHI): http://www.ihi.org
- IHI Rapid Response Teams: http://www.ihi.org/Topics/RapidResponseTeams/Pages/default.aspx
- International Society for Rapid Response Systems: https://rapidresponsesystems.org
- Interprofessional Education Collaborative (IPEC): https://www.ipecollaborative.org
- Institute for Safe Medication Practices (ISMP): https://www.ismp.org
- Medline Plus: Health Information in Multiple Languages: https://medlineplus.gov/languages/languages.html
- National Academy of Medicine: https://nam.edu/
- National Database of Nursing Quality Indicators (NDNQI): Pressganey.com/resources/program-summary/ndnqi-solution-summary
- National Quality Forum (NQF): htpps://qualityforum.org/about NQF
- National Library of Medicine (NLM): https://medlineplus.gov/spanish/
- Quality and Safety Education for Nurses (QSEN): https://qsen.org/
- Society of Critical Care Medicine (SCCM): www.sccm.org
- The Joint Commission (TJC): https://www.jointcommission.org/
- US Food & Drug Administration (FDA): https://www.fda.gov/

All sites accessed September 14, 2021.

---

attitudes for each section (see Box 1.7).[47] Boxes that address all of the QSEN competencies are presented throughout the book; the QSEN icon **QSEN** appears in these boxes. Box 1.8, **QSEN** Informatics, lists the web addresses of all the quality, safety, and regulatory resources mentioned in this chapter. Refer to Table 1.1 and to Box 1.9 **QSEN** Teamwork and Collaboration, which describes rapid response teams, a key interdisciplinary practice.

HEALTHY WORK ENVIRONMENT

The health care environment is stressful; increasing challenges in the areas of financial constraints, regulatory requirements, consumer scrutiny, quickly changing technologies and treatment regimens, and workforce diversity contribute daily to conflicts and difficulties. In this environment, it is essential to offer support for health care providers that can mitigate these challenges and ensure a healthy place to work.

There is an increasing amount of evidence that unhealthy work environments lead to medical errors, suboptimal safety monitoring, ineffective communication among health care providers, and increased conflict and stress among care providers.

AACN has formulated standards for establishing and sustaining a healthy work environment (HWE).[48] The intent of the standards is to promote creation of environments that have a positive impact on nursing and patient outcomes. Evidence-based and relationship-centered principles were used to create the standards of professional performance. A summary of the six standards is provided in Box 1.10. Fig. 1.1 illustrates the interdependence of each standard and the ultimate impact on optimal patient outcomes and clinical excellence.

Halm reported that appropriate staffing and HWEs were associated with better patient outcomes (e.g., fewer falls, fewer complications, lower mortality, fewer surgical site infections, and fewer catheter-associated urinary tract infections) and better nurse outcomes (e.g., higher quality of care and safety ratings, less job dissatisfaction and burnout, and decreased intention to leave their jobs).[49] Findings from a 2018 critical care nurse environment study indicate that there continues to be a positive relationship between HWEs and both patient and nurse outcomes.

TABLE 1.1 CRISIS Criteria for RRT Activation

Circulatory	• HR < 50BPM or > 120 BPM • Sys BP <90 mmHG or > 180 mmHG • MAP <60 mmHG • Acute onset of chest pain • Sudden loss of large blood volume
Respiratory	• RR <8 breaths/min or >26 breaths/min • 02 sat <92% despite 02 administration • Airway compromise (stridor) • Shortness of breath/dyspnea • Labored breathing
Intuition	• Subjective feeling that something is not right
Significant neurologic change	• Altered mental status • Agitation • Seizure • Decrease in Glasgow Coma Scale ≥2
Intervention	• Requiring a higher level of care (i.e., cardioversion) • Resulting in upgrade in level of care (e.g. patient requiring intensive care and is on the medical surgical unit)
Sepsis (Levy and Fink et al., 2001)	• SIRS + Source of Infection • HR >90BPM (e.g. Pneumonia, surgical site) • RR >20 breaths/min or Paco2 <32 mmHG • Temperature >38 °C or <36 °C • WBC >12,000 mU/L or <4,000 mU/L

Note: This should be based on acceptable parameters per organization.

BP, Blood pressure; *BPM,* beats per minute; *°C,* Degrees in Celsius; *HR,* heart rate; *MAP,* mean arterial pressure; *mU/L,* Milliunits per liter; *O₂,* oxygen; *RRT,* rapid response team; *sat,* saturation; *sys,* systolic.

Mitchell Levy, Mitchell Fink, et al. 2001. SCCM/ESICM/ACCP/ATS/SIS International Sepsis Definitions Conference. *Crit Care Med.* 2003;31(4):1250–1256. https://doi.org/10.1097/01.CCM.0000050454.01978.3B.

Used with permission from Ricardo Padilla, PhD, RN, CCRN. September 2022.

QSEN

BOX 1.9 Teamwork and Collaboration

Rapid Response Teams (RRT)

Inpatients often show signs of clinical deterioration for several hours prior to arrest, and more than 20,000 annual cases of in-hospital arrest could be prevented if clinical deterioration can be detected early on.[3–5] It is critical that nurses play an integral part in the identification and intervention should clinical deterioration arise. Early identification of deterioration can trigger appropriate management, thereby reducing the need for higher acuity care, reducing length of hospitalization and admission costs, thus improving survival.[6]

The RRT is composed of a multidisciplinary team that extends critical care services throughout the hospital in the noncritical care setting.[2–11] The most common model of the RRT is a critical care nurse-led model, with some models including physicians, respiratory therapists,[12] and advanced practice providers such as nurse practitioners[13] and clinical nurse specialists (CNSs).[14] These advanced-trained critical care clinicians aim at early identification and management of clinical deterioration averting cardiopulmonary arrest or unintended transfer to the critical care unit.

Many RRTs have emergency standing orders or protocols, so it is important to understand the level of intervention they can provide. Examples of standing orders that RRTs can initiate include establishing emergent intravenous access, administration of medications such as naloxone for oversedation, and even laboratory and diagnostic orders such as electrolytes, arterial blood gases, chest x-ray, and electrocardiograms.[17]

Ricardo Padilla, PhD, RN, CCRN
Quality and Patient Safety Specialist, Loma Linda University Medical Center Murrieta
Assistant Clinical Professor, University of San Diego Hahn School of Nursing

References

1. National Institute for Health and Clinical Excellence. *Acutely ill patients in hospital: recognition of and response to acute illness in adults in hospital.* London, England: National Institute for Health and Clinical Excellence; 2007.
2. Padilla RM, Mayo AM. Patient survival and length of stay associated with delayed rapid response system activation. *Crit Care Nurs Q.* 2019;42(3):235–245. https://doi.org/10.1097/CNQ.0000000000000264.
3. Smith GB, Prytherch DR, Schmidt P, et al. Hospital-wide physiological surveillance: a new approach to the early identification and management of the sick patient. *Resuscitation.* 2006;71(1):19–28.
4. Beaumont K, Luettel D, Thomson R. Deterioration in hospital patients: early signs and appropriate actions. *Nurs Stand.* 2008;23(1):43–48.
5. Padilla RM, Urden LD, Stacy KM. Nurses' perceptions of barriers to rapid response system activation: a systematic review. *Dimens Crit Care Nurs.* 2018;37(5):259–271.
6. Vincent JL, Einav S, Pearse R, et al. Improving detection of patient deterioration in the general hospital war environment. *Eur J Anaesthesiol.* 2018;35(5):325–333. https://doi.org/10.1097/EJA.0000000000000798.
7. Stolldorf DP, Jones CB. Deployment of rapid response teams by 31 hospitals in a statewide collaborative. *Jt Comm J Qual Patient Saf.* 2015;41(4):186–191. https://doi.org/10.1016/s1553-7250(15)41024-4.
8. Kohn LT, Corrigan J, Donaldson MS. *To Err Is Human: Building a Safer Health System.* Washington, DC: National Academy Press; 2000.
9. Institute of Medicine. *Crossing the Quality Chasm: A New Health System for the 21st Century.* Washington, DC: National Academy Press; 2001.
10. Berwick DM, Calkins DR, McCannon CJ, Hackbarth AD. The 100,000 lives campaign: setting a goal and a deadline for improving health care quality. *J Am Med Assoc.* 2006;295(3):324–327. https://doi.org/10.1001/jama.295.3.324.
11. International Society for Rapid Response Systems. About rapid response systems: making hospitals safer. https://rapidresponsesystems.org/?page_id=1074. Accessed January 2020.
12. Agency for Healthcare Research and Quality. Rapid response systems. https://psnet.ahrq.gov/primer/rapid-response-systems. Accessed January 2020.
13. Morse KJ, Warshawsky D, Moore JM, Pecora DC. A new role for the ACNP: the rapid response team leader. *Crit Care Nurs Q.* 2006;29(2):137–146.
14. Jenkins SD, Lindsey PL. Clinical nurse specialists as leaders in rapid response. *Clin Nurse Spec.* 2010;24(1):24–30. https://doi.org/10.1097/NUR.0b013e3181c4abe9.
15. Devita MA, Bellomo R, Hillman K, et al. Findings of the first consensus conference on medical emergency teams. *Crit Care Med.* 2006;34(9):2463–2478.
16. Bellomo R, Goldsmith D, Uchino S, et al. Prospective controlled trial of effect of medical emergency team on postoperative morbidity and mortality rates. *Crit Care Med.* 2004;32(4):916–921.
17. Institute for Healthcare Improvement. Rapid response team sample order set. *institute for clinical systems improvement.* http://www.ihi.org/resources/Pages/Tools/RapidResponseTeamSampleOrderSet.aspx. Accessed February 2020.
18. Good VS, Kirkwood PL. Advanced critical care nursing. In: *Unit 1: The Evolving Critical Care Environment.* 2nd ed. St Louis: Elsevier; 2017.

TRENDING PRIORITIES IN HEALTHCARE

Bullying in Nursing

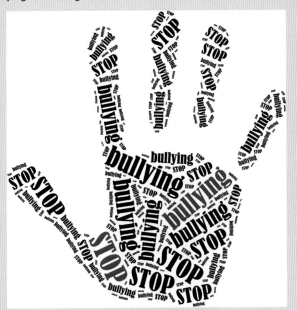

iStock/S-S-S.

Bullying in nursing is not a new phenomenon and has been present for decades. It has been identified around the world in all practice settings and specialties including academia. Bullying is defined as "… unwanted harmful actions intended to humiliate, offend, and cause distress in the recipient…including actions that harm, undermine, and degrade. Bullying actions present serious safety and health concerns, and they can cause lasting physical and psychologic difficulties for the targets."[1] Frequently there is abuse of power that can demoralize the target who feels defenseless.[1]

In bullying situations, communication of crucial information, lack of appropriate provider communication, and lack of collaborative decision making may lead to medical errors and poor patient outcomes.[2] Persons who are bullied may be less likely to act or speak up when medical errors occur.[3] In a recent systematic review[4] regarding the impact of bullying on nursing errors, researchers reported four areas: (1) work environment, (2) individual-level connections between bullying and nursing practice errors, (3) barriers to communication, and (4) communication impairment. Researchers in Australia determined that bullying has continued over the past four decades and has changed only in relation to context and that the role of nurse managers is essential in managing bullying.[5]

Bullying actions may include hostile remarks, verbal attacks, intimidations, withholding of support, threats, and taunts.[1] They may come from the top down (employer to employee), bottom up (employee to employer), or horizontally (employee to employee).[1] The following are psychosocial consequences of negative interactions and bullying identified by Italian researchers[6]:

- anxiety
- sleep disorders
- chronic fatigue, exhaustion
- apathy
- headaches
- depression
- excessive food consumption; reduced appetite
- intentional absence from work
- increased consumption of tobacco, alcohol, drugs

AACN has published a position statement[7] regarding zero tolerance for bullying in which they recommend actions for nurses to take regarding bullying:

1. Communicate respectfully, online and in person
2. Hold self and other accountable for unacceptable behavior
3. Seek solutions as a team
4. Develop a mentoring system among peers, supervisors, physicians
5. Contribute to building healthy work environments
6. Participate in interprofessional committees to develop policies and strategies for abuse prevention

References

1. American Nurses Association. *Position statement on incivility, bullying, workplace violence*; 2015. https://www.nursingworld.org/practice-policy/nursing-excellence/official-position-statements/id/incivility-bullying-and-workplace-violence/. Accessed October 18, 2021.
2. Nicotera AM, Mahon MM. Between rocks and hard places: exploring the impact of structural divergence in the nursing workplace. *Manag Commun Q.* 2013;27(1):90—120.
3. Wilson BL, Phelps C. Horizontal hostility: a threat to patient safety. *JONA's Healthc Law, Ethics, Regul.* 2013;15(1):51—57.
4. Johnson AH, Benham-Hutchins M. The influence of bullying on nursing practice errors: a systematic review. *AORN J.* 2020;111(2):199—210.
5. Hartin P, Birks M, Lindsay D. Bullying in nursing: how has it changed over 4 decades? *J Nurs Manag.* 2020;28:1619—1626.
6. Bambi S, Guazzini A, Piredda M, Lucchini A, Grazia De Marinis M, Rasero L. Negative interactions among nurses: an explorative study on lateral violence and working in nursing work settings. *J Nurs Manag.* 2019;27:749—757.
7. American Association of Critical-Care Nurses. AACN position statement: zero tolerance for bullying, incivility, and verbal abuse. https://www.aacn.org/policy-and-adcovacy/aacn-position-statement-zero-tolerance. Accessed October 18, 2021.

BOX 1.10   Healthy Work Environment Standards

Standard I: Skilled Communication
Nurses must be as proficient in communication skills as they are in clinical skills.

Standard II: True Collaboration
Nurses must be relentless in pursuing and fostering true collaboration.

Standard III: Effective Decision Making
Nurses must be valued and committed partners in making policy, directing and evaluating clinical care, and leading organizational operations.

Standard IV: Appropriate Staffing
Staffing must ensure the effective match between patient needs and nurse competencies.

Standard V: Meaningful Recognition
Nurses must be recognized and must recognize others for the value each brings to the work of the organization.

Standard VI: Authentic Leadership
Nurse leaders must fully embrace the imperative of a healthy work environment, authentically live it, and engage others in its achievement.

From American Association of Critical-Care Nurses (AACN). *Standards for Establishing and Sustaining Healthy Work Environments. A Journey to Excellence.* 2nd ed. Aliso Viejo, CA: AACN; 2016.

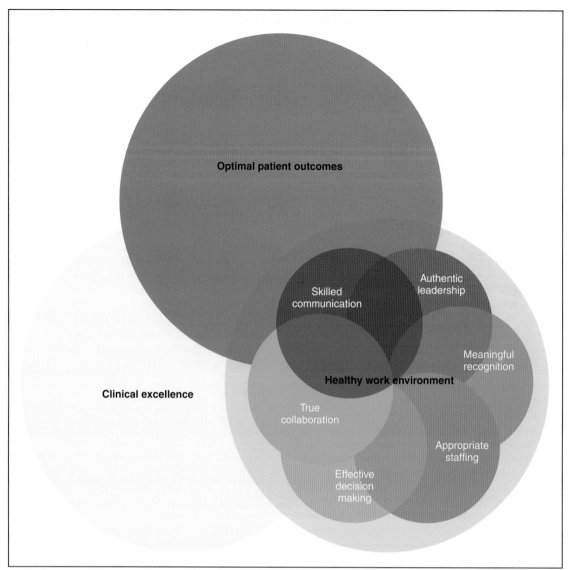

Fig. 1.1 Interdependence of Healthy Work Environment, Clinical Excellence, and Optimal Patient Outcomes. (From American Association of Critical-Care Nurses. *Standards for Establishing and Sustaining Healthy Work Environments.* 2nd ed. Aliso Viejo, CA: AACN; 2016.)

REFERENCES

1. American Association of Critical-Care Nurses. AACN scope and standards for acute and critical care nursing practice. http://www.aacn.org. Accessed September 23, 2021.
2. American Association of Critical-Care Nurses. http://www.aacn.org. Accessed March 28, 2022.
3. American Association of Critical-Care Nurses. http://aacn.org/certification-get-certified. Accessed September 23, 2021.
4. American Association of Critical-Care Nurses. Board certification. http://www.aacn.org/certification?tab=First-Time%20certification. Accessed September 23, 2021.
5. American Association of Critical-Care Nurses. Value of certification. http://www.aacn.org/certification/value-of-certification-resource-center. Accessed September 23, 2021.
6. Halm MA. Specialty certification: a path to improving outcomes. *Am J Crit Care.* 2021;30(2):156–160.
7. American Association of Critical-Care Nurses. Practice alert: prevention of CAUTI in adults. http://www.aacn.org/clinical-resources/practice-alerts/prevention-of-cauti-in-adults. Accessed September 23, 2021.
8. International Classification for Nursing Practice (ICNP). About ICNP. http://ICN.CH/what-we-do/projects/ehealth-icnp/about-ICNP. Accessed September 23, 2021.
9. International Classification for Nursing Practice (ICNP). *Nursing intervention statements,* 2019 https://www.icn.org.
10. Warren JJ, Coenen A. *International classification for nursing practice (ICNP): most-frequently asked questions*; 1998. https://www.ncbi.nlm.nih.gov/pmc/articles/PMC61310/.
11. Darnell LK, Hickson SV. Cultural competent patient-centered nursing care. *Nurs Clin North Am.* 2015;50:95–108.
12. ThinkCulturalHealth.hhs.gov. Accessed March 28, 2022.
13. International Council of Nurses. Position statement: cultural and linguistic competence. https://www.ICN.ch. Accessed March 28, 2022.
14. Kramlich D. Strategies for acute and critical care nurses implementing complementary therapies requested by patients and family members. *Crit Care Nurse.* 2016;36(6):52–58.
15. Kramlich D. Complementary health practitioners in the acute and critical care setting: nursing considerations. *Crit Care Nurse.* 2017;37(3):60–65.
16. Tusek DL, Cwynar RE. Strategies for implementing guided imagery program to enhance patient experience. *AACN Clin Issues.* 2000;11(1):68.

17. Richards KC, Gibson R, Overton-McCoy AL. Effects of massage in acute and critical care. *AACN Clin Issues.* 2000;11(1):77.

18. McKenney C, Johnson R. Unleash the healing power of pet therapy. *Am Nurse Today.* 2008;3(5):29.

19. Cole K, Fawlinski A. Animal-assisted therapy: the human-animal bond. *AACN Clin Issues.* 2000;11(1):139.

20. Miller J. Therapy animals: infection prevention, safety and impact on patients and staff. *Am Assoc Crit Care Nurse.* https://www.AACN.org/blog/therapy-animals-infection-prevention-safety-and-impact-on-patients-and-staff. Accessed September 23, 2021.

21. American Music Therapy Association. *Definition and Quotes about music therapy.* American Music Therapy Association; 2000. https://www.musictherapy.org/about/quotes/?print=y.

22. Bradt J, Dileo C, Grocke D. Music interventions for mechanically ventilated patients. *Cochrane Database Syst Rev.* 2014;12:CD006902.

23. Golino AJ, Leone R, Gollenberg A, et al. Impact of an active music therapy intervention on intensive care patients. *Am J Crit Care.* 2019;38(1):48.

24. Harrington L. Going digital: what does it really mean for nursing? *AACN Adv Crit Care.* 2016;27(4):358.

25. American Nurses Association. ANA core principles on connected health. https://www.nursingworld.org. Accessed September 23, 2021.

26. American Association of Critical-Care Nurses. AACN teleICU nursing practice: an expert consensus statement supporting high acuity, progressive and critical care. https://www.AACN.org. Accessed September 23, 2021.

27. Wheelan SA, Burchill CN, Tilin F. The link between teamwork and patients' outcomes in intensive care units. *Am J Crit Care.* 2003;12(6):527.

28. Boyle DK, Kochinda C. Enhancing collaborative communication of nurse and physician leadership in two intensive care units. *J Nurs Adm.* 2004;34(2):60.

29. Falise JP. True collaboration: interdisciplinary rounds in nonteaching hospitals—it can be done. *AACN Adv Crit Care.* 2007;18(4):346.

30. Golanowski M, Beaudry D, Kurz L, Laffey WJ, Hook ML. Interdisciplinary shared decision-making—taking shared governance to the next level. *Nurs Adm Q.* 2007;31(4):341.

31. Reina ML, Reina DS, Rushton CH. Trust: the foundation for team collaboration and healthy work environments. *AACN Adv Crit Care.* 2007;18(2):103.

32. Manojlovich M, Antonakos C. Satisfaction of intensive care unit nurses with nurse-physician communication. *J Nurs Adm.* 2008;38(5):237.

33. Interprofessional Education Collaborative Expert Panel. *Core Competencies for Interprofessional Collaborative Practice: Report of an Expert Panel.* Washington, DC: Interprofessional Education Collaborative; 2011. Updated 2016.

34. Davidson JE, Aslakson RA, Long AC, et al. Guidelines for family-centered care in the neonatal, pediatric and adult ICU. *Crit Care Med.* 2017;45(1):103.

35. Bosslet GT, Pope TM, Rubenfeld GD, et al. An official ATS/AACN/ACCP/ESICM/SCCM policy statement: responding to requests for potentially inappropriate treatment in intensive care units. *Am J Respir Crit Care Med.* 2015;191(11):1318.

36. The Joint Commission. Behaviors that undermine a culture of safety. *Sentinel event alert.* https://www.jointcommission.org/setinel_event.aspx. Accessed September 23, 2021.

37. Easter K, Tamburri LM. Understanding patient safety and quality outcome data. *Crit Care Nurse.* 2020;38(6):58–66.

38. Henneman EA, Gawlinski A, Blank FS, Henneman PL, Jordan D, McKenzie JB. Strategies used by critical care nurses to identify, interrupt, and correct medical errors. *Am J Crit Care.* 2010;19(6):500.

39. The Joint Commission. 2021 Hospital national patient safety goals. http://www.jointcommission.org. Accessed September 20, 2021.

40. Medical Device Reporting. http://www.rqmplus.com/services/regulatory-affairs/clinical-evaluation-plans/report-cer. Accessed September 23, 2021.

41. US Food and Drug Administration. Warnings for industry: warnings and precautions, contraindications, and boxed warning sections of labeling for human prescriptive drug and biological products-content and format. https://www.fda.gov/regulatory-information/search-fda-guidance-documents/warnings-and-precautions-contraindications-and-boxed-warning-sections-labeling-human-prescription. October 2011.

42. Institute for Safe Medication Practices. About ISMP. http://www.ISMP.org. Accessed September 20, 2021.

43. Institute for Healthcare Improvement. Using bundles to improve health care quality. http://www.ihi.org. Accessed September 23, 2021.

44. National Quality Forum. About NQF. http://www.NQF.org. Accessed September 23, 2021.

45. Healthcare Information and Management Systems Society. Patient safety and quality outcomes. http://www.HIMSS.org. Accessed September 23, 2021.

46. American Nurses Association (ANA). National database nursing quality indicators (NDNQI). http://www.nursingworld.org. Accessed September 23, 2021.

47. Quality Safety Education for Nurses Institute. Quality and safety education for nurses. http://www.QSEN.org. Accessed September 23, 2021.

48. American Association of Critical-Care Nurses. *AACN standards for establishing and sustaining healthy work environments. A journey to Excellence.* 2nd ed. http://www.aacn.org. Accessed September 23, 2021.

49. Halm M. The influence of appropriate staffing and healthy work environments on patient and nurse outcomes. *Am J Crit Care.* 2019;28(2):152.

2

Ethical and Legal Issues

Kelly K. Dineen and Linda D. Urden

MORALS

Morals are traditions of belief about right or wrong human behavior. Informed by individual and group values, morality consists of standards of conduct that include moral principles, rules, virtues, rights, and responsibilities. Moral norms form the basis for right action and provide a framework for the evaluation of behavior through a system of ethics.[1,2]

ETHICS

Ethics is a generic term for the reasoned inquiry and understanding of a moral life, in other words, a systematic examination of morality. Different theories or systems of ethics identify which moral norms (or rules) should be used and prioritized to evaluate whether conduct is ethical.[1,2]

Applied Ethics

Health care ethics is the attempt to use moral norms to evaluate conduct and to resolve particular ethical problems in context.[1] The extreme situations at the end of life or beginning of life garner most of the attention around health care ethics; however, day-to-day nursing decisions and actions also implicate ethics.[3]

Nursing Implications

Day-to-day nursing decisions fall within the realm of ethics if they:
1. pertain to things within the nurse's control
2. will show respect or fail to show respect for patients (or their loved ones)[4]

Therefore most nursing decisions and interactions with patients fall within the realm of ethics. Most of the time, there is a right thing to do, and it can be done without conflict or resulting harm.

The most common ethical problems identified by nurses involve end-of-life care, conflicts with physicians, organizational restraints, conflicts with patients' families, and conflicts between required interventions and patients' privacy and dignity.[3]

ETHICAL PROBLEMS

Ethical problems (also called *ethical* or *moral dilemmas*) occur only when there is some conflict surrounding an ethical decision.[4] An ethical problem exists if a person is morally obligated or appears to be obligated to two or more conflicting potential courses of action. The result is that both something right and something wrong will occur.[1,5]

NURSES AND MORAL DISTRESS

Nurses work in a system in constant flux. As the most constant health professional presence at the bedside, critical care nurses navigate the complexities in health care in a high-stakes, high-stress environment while also managing:
1. Frontline patient care, including emergency situations
2. Increasingly innovative and highly technical care delivery
3. Financial and staffing constraints
4. Emotional and behavioral responses from patients and families, coworkers, and themselves

These direct care, organizational, and structural pressures amplify a complex moral environment with frequent ethical dilemmas.[3,6]

Moral Distress

Moral distress is widely discussed in the literature as a serious problem for nurses.[7-12] Moral distress was first described by Jameton as distress that occurs when the nurse knows the correct thing to do but is prevented from acting on it.[6]

The nurse knows the ethically appropriate action but feels unable to act consistently with that course or acts inconsistently, and therefore unethically, because of one or more barriers.[4,12] High levels of moral distress are often a signal of unit or system-wide issues.[7,13]

Two Moral Distress Components

The first, initial distress, occurs contemporaneously with the situation creating the distress; the second, reactive distress, includes lingering feelings about one's failure to act and is associated with long-term consequences to the nurse.[7] Consequences are significant, including compassion fatigue and burnout.

In critical care, moral distress arises most frequently from use of technology at the end of life, particularly when its use is seen as medically nonbeneficial (or futile). It also occurs when surrogate decision makers refuse consent for care that nurses perceive as in the patient's best interest or when nurses have difficulty accessing resources to reduce patient suffering.

Significant emotional and physical stress and resulting feelings of loss of personal integrity, as well as professional dissatisfaction, are common in the reactive distress phase of moral distress.

Over time, relationships with coworkers and patients, as well as quality of care, are negatively affected. Personal relationships and family life may also be negatively affected; nurses experiencing moral distress may resign their position or even leave the profession.[13]

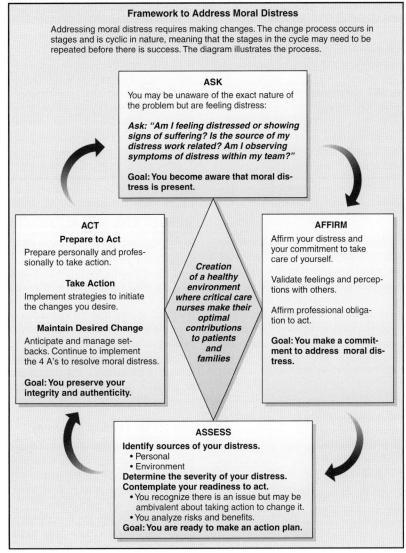

Framework to Address Moral Distress

Addressing moral distress requires making changes. The change process occurs in stages and is cyclic in nature, meaning that the stages in the cycle may need to be repeated before there is success. The diagram illustrates the process.

ASK

You may be unaware of the exact nature of the problem but are feeling distress:

Ask: "Am I feeling distressed or showing signs of suffering? Is the source of my distress work related? Am I observing symptoms of distress within my team?"

Goal: You become aware that moral distress is present.

ACT

Prepare to Act

Prepare personally and professionally to take action.

Take Action

Implement strategies to initiate the changes you desire.

Maintain Desired Change

Anticipate and manage setbacks. Continue to implement the 4 A's to resolve moral distress.

Goal: You preserve your integrity and authenticity.

Creation of a healthy environment where critical care nurses make their optimal contributions to patients and families

AFFIRM

Affirm your distress and your commitment to take care of yourself.

Validate feelings and perceptions with others.

Affirm professional obligation to act.

Goal: You make a commitment to address moral distress.

ASSESS

Identify sources of your distress.
 • Personal
 • Environment
Determine the severity of your distress.
Contemplate your readiness to act.
 • You recognize there is an issue but may be ambivalent about taking action to change it.
 • You analyze risks and benefits.
Goal: You are ready to make an action plan.

Fig. 2.1 The American Association of Critical-Care Nurses' "4 A's to Rise Above Moral Distress." (From American Association of Critical-Care Nurses. Position statement: moral distress. Aliso Viejo, CA: AACN; 2004.)

Tool to Address and Resolve Moral Distress

The *4 A's to Rise Above Moral Distress* model (Fig. 2.1) approach has been previously endorsed by the American Association of Critical-Care Nurses (AACN). The model asserts that changes must be made in order to address moral distress. Four components must be addressed:
1. Ask—why one is feeling distressed and to what is it related
2. Affirm—the distress and make a commitment to oneself, validating with others
3. Assess—sources of distress and determine the severity of it
4. Act—preparing, taking action, and maintaining the desired change
    Successful trajectory through the model leads to optimal contributions to patients and families.

Moral Resilience

Moral resilience is defined by Rushton as "the capacity of an individual to sustain or restore their integrity in response to moral complexity, confusion, distress, or setbacks."[7] The capacity to develop and improve

moral resilience has been identified as critical to reducing moral distress and enhancing ethical competence.[14,15]

    The American Nurses Association (ANA) provides an excellent overview of the concept in *A Call to Action: Exploring Moral Resilience Toward a Culture of Ethical Practice.*[13] Nurses who are morally resilient likely feel empowered to exercise moral courage, and moral courage may prevent moral distress in the first instance.[16]

    Box 2.1 contains a list of actions that nurses can take individually to address moral distress and build moral resilience.

VIRTUES

Virtues are habits of character or learned behaviors that predispose individuals to behave ethically.[1] In addition to courage, the virtues commonly expected of nurses include knowledge, wisdom, patience, compassion, and honesty. In contrast to personality traits or actions, virtues focus on the nurse's character or ways of being as a moral person.[16,17]

BOX 2.1 Recommendations to Foster Individual Moral Resilience

Individual Nurse's Actions

1. Adopt American Nurses Association (ANA)'s Healthy Nurse Healthy Nation strategies to support your general well-being as a foundation for cultivating moral resilience.
2. Read, review, and implement the *ANA Code of Ethics for Nurses With Interpretive Statements* to gain knowledge and strengthen ethical competence.
3. Seek opportunities to learn how to recognize, analyze, and take ethically grounded action in response to ethical complexity, disagreement, or conflict.
4. Cultivate self-awareness in order to recognize and respond to your symptoms of moral suffering, including moral distress.
5. Pursue educational opportunities to cultivate mindfulness, ethical competence, and moral resilience.
6. Develop your personal plan to support well-being and build moral resilience.
7. Become involved and initiate workplace efforts to address the root causes of moral distress and other forms of moral suffering.
8. Develop and practice skills in communication, mindfulness, conflict transformation, and interprofessional collaboration.
9. Identify and use personal resources within your organization or community, such as ethics committees, peer-to-peer support, debriefing sessions, counseling, and employee assistance programs.

From American Nurses Association. A call to action: exploring moral resilience toward a culture of ethical practice. https://www.nursingworld.org/~4907b6/globalassets/docs/ana/ana-call-to-action-exploring-moral-resilience-final.pdf. Accessed September 15, 2019.

Humility is an often overlooked but critical virtue for all health care professionals. The virtue of humility encompasses several other practices, including self-knowledge, reflection and perspective taking, and intellectual honesty (admitting what you do not know and seeking help).[18]

The virtue of caring may be of particular importance for nursing; some have distinguished between caring *about* the patient and caring *for* the patient as two kinds of embodied virtues in nursing.[19] Practicing these virtues can better prepare nurses to act in an ethically appropriate and professional manner.

ETHICAL PRINCIPLES

As mentioned previously, moral norms (or rules) form the basis of ethics. In health care, certain principles—descriptive and prescriptive rules that provide a basis for ethical reasoning and actions—are common norms applied when analyzing ethical issues.[19] These norms create nurses' obligations and corresponding patients' rights. Four principles most commonly appealed to are:

1. respect for persons/autonomy
2. beneficence
3. nonmaleficence
4. justice

These principles are used in this chapter and explained in Table 2.1.

If an action comports with one or more principles and does not conflict with any other principle, there is no ethical problem. For example, providing comfort through positioning or massage to a patient corresponds to beneficence. As long as that is done with the

patient's permission and there is no risk associated with the actions, there is no conflict.

When principles do conflict, the nurse and other stakeholders must carefully justify privileging one principle over another. Justification requires those involved to carefully describe the reasons for their actions and specify why the individual circumstances in the context of the patient's situation warrant overriding one or more principles in favor of others.[1]

For example, there are often classic conflicts between autonomy (honoring the patient's wishes) and beneficence (advancing the course of action most likely to medically benefit the patient). Justification would include an analysis in context.

Respect for Persons/Autonomy

The principle of *respect* for persons requires nurses to respect the patient's inherent dignity and capacity for rational choice; this includes the obligation to honor the patient's right to *autonomy*, which is the right to determine what is done to or for them without coercion or undue interference from others.[1,20]

Autonomy is also the foundation of the legal and ethical requirement of informed consent and includes the right of patients with decision-making capacity to refuse some or all treatments.[1,20]

Decision-making capacity requires that the patient possesses a set of values and goals, is able to understand the nature of the illness or injury, is able to reason through available treatment options and consequences of each (including doing nothing), and can communicate choice. Decision-making capacity is a fluid concept and can fluctuate based on health status.[2,20]

TABLE 2.1 Ethical Principles in Critical Care

Principle	Definition	Example Nursing Obligations	Patient Rights
Respect for persons/ autonomy	Respect for the inherent and unconditional dignity of persons and to freely exercise choice about what happens to them	Truth-telling; provision of complete, accurate, and understandable information; timely communication; maintaining privacy and confidentiality; self-reflection to minimize bias	Self-determination; privacy; confidentiality
Beneficence	Promoting and maximizing benefit	Competent practice; advocacy for patient safety; acting for best interest of the patient	Appropriate, evidence-based care; effective care
Nonmaleficence	Avoiding and minimizing harm	Careful practice; self-reflection to minimize errors	Safe care and treatment
Justice	Equitable distribution of benefits and burdens and scarce resources	Advocacy for equitable public policy in health care; self-reflection and advocacy to minimize disparities in care	Access to care; equitable care

Promoting autonomous decision making is a crucial and sometimes difficult responsibility of critical care nurses. Patients in critical care may lack decision-making capacity because of their illness or injury. Capacity may also fluctuate during treatment.

When a patient lacks capacity, decisions are made by surrogate decision makers—typically family, friends, or others who have been named as the preferred decision maker by the patient or as designated by state laws. One exception to the need for informed consent is in emergency situations. The emergency treatment exception is limited, and every effort should be made by the critical care nurse to keep the surrogate decision maker informed as soon as possible.

Surrogate decision makers are required by law to make the decision that the patient would have made if he or she were able to; this is called the *substituted judgment standard*. This means surrogates should not choose based on their own personal preferences but instead based on their knowledge of the patient's values and preferences.

Patients and families must have all the relevant information and the ability to understand and weigh options before they can make a decision that is consistent with the patient's values. Only when that is not possible should surrogates make decisions based on the patient's best interest.[1,2,20] Nurses frequently advocate for the patient, and by extension the surrogate decision maker, with other members of the health care team.

Confidentiality of patient information and *privacy* in patient interactions must be protected and honored by health care providers out of respect for persons. Confidentiality relates to information or data, whereas privacy relates to the person (i.e., privacy is what a patient expects in a clinical encounter; confidentiality is how the information from the clinical encounter is treated).

Confidentiality requires that patient information may be shared only with individuals involved in the care of the patient. Exceptions to this occur only if maintaining confidentiality seriously jeopardizes the welfare of others. These exceptions are usually reflected in state or federal laws, such as mandatory reporting laws.[2]

Privacy is closely aligned with confidentiality of patient information but relates to the person. Nurses must minimize violations of patient privacy by ensuring that doors and curtains are closed during interactions and taking extra steps to keep the patient covered during procedures.

Beneficence and Nonmaleficence

The ethical principles of beneficence and nonmaleficence require actions that maximize good and minimize harm to the patient, often in a delicate balance. The principle of *beneficence* presupposes compassion and requires the promotion of others' well-being through positive action and the desire to do good.[1,17]

In contrast, *nonmaleficence* dictates that nurses prevent and minimize harm and correct harmful situations.[17] Benefits must be maximized, and harms must be minimized. In critical care practice, every decision to act or not to act carries the serious potential for harm even though the intent is to benefit the patient. Thoughtfulness and care are necessary in defining and balancing benefit and harm in terms of both immediate and long-term goals for the patient.

Justice

The principle of *justice* means that there is an equitable distribution of social benefits and the limited resource of organs for transplant. Another is access to health care, which is an issue of social justice, although it is not a constitutional right in the United States. Countless studies have demonstrated the negative impact of the system of care delivery on the health status of US residents.

The *Patient Protection and Affordable Care Act*[21] attempted to improve the just distribution of health care access by increasing the availability of health insurance for many Americans. At the same time, escalating health care costs, expanded technologies, an aging population, and a scarcity of health care personnel in some settings make the issue of health care allocation more complex.

Conflicting Principles

Conflict between principles is common and usually does not lead to an ethical problem. For example, suppose a patient is unconscious and needs emergency surgery for suspected peritonitis secondary to appendicitis and rupture. Surgery does harm to the patient and carries the potential for further harm to the patient in terms of risks; however, the benefits of surgery outweigh the need to avoid harm because of the known general clinical effectiveness of the intervention and the lack of reasonable, less harmful alternatives. In addition, the potential for further harm in the absence of surgical intervention is very high in terms of sepsis and possible death.

On balance, surgery honors beneficence. Because the patient is unconscious and cannot consent, autonomy is overridden. However, this is justified because time is of the essence, and delay would increase the likelihood of harm in this particular situation. It is justifiable to override autonomy in this situation because of the competing reality of death in a patient with a treatable condition. This is an ethical resolution of conflicting principles.

Principles can also be resolved in an unethical way. Two common examples of the unethical resolution of conflicting principles are paternalism and continuation of nonbeneficial care (medical futility).

Paternalism

Paternalism is an example of an unethical resolution of conflicting principles of beneficence and autonomy. Paternalism exists when the nurse or physician makes a decision for the patient without consulting the patient or by disregarding the patient's preferences.

Paternalism still creeps in, albeit more covertly, in many health care situations. Fast-paced and high-pressure health care environments may lead less thoughtful providers to impose their recommendations on patients implicitly or explicitly.

Medical Futility

The concept of *medical futility* is difficult to define, and disputes have resulted in various discussions and proposed criteria to predict outcomes of care.[22–26] Futile care generally means there would be no useful results of health care interventions. Medical futility has been defined in countless ways; many prefer the terms *medically ineffective* or *nonbeneficial care*.[23]

TRENDING PRIORITIES IN HEALTHCARE

Limited English Proficiency

DoYOU
SPEAK...

iStock.com/S-S-S

Communication between patients and the health care team is essential for creating a trusting relationship, improving the patient experience, and ensuring quality health care. While communication with the health care team can be challenging for many patients, patients with limited English proficiency (LEP) are increasingly disadvantaged. A patient is considered to have LEP if English is not their primary language and they have a limited ability to read, write, speak, and understand English. Patients with LEP experience frustration with the health care system, increased medical errors, and poorer quality health care.[1]

In 1995 the US Department of Health and Human Services Office of Minority Health established the Center for Linguistic and Cultural Competence in Health Care (CLCCHC). Subsequently, the National Culturally and Linguistically Appropriate Services (CLAS) Standards were developed in 2000 and revised in 2013 to improve health care quality and eliminate health care disparities. Four of these standards specifically address communication and language assistance for the patient with LEP[2]:

- Offer language assistance to patients who have LEP or other communication needs to facilitate timely access to all health care and services at no cost to them.
- Inform all patients of the availability of language assistance services in their preferred language, clearly, verbally, and in writing.
- Ensure the competence of individuals providing language assistance, avoiding the use of untrained individuals or minors as interpreters.
- Provide easy-to-understand print and multimedia materials and signage in the languages commonly used by the patients in the service area.

Unfortunately, many health care organizations are struggling to meet these standards. To start, health care organizations need to collect baseline data regarding language and interpreter preferences. One suggestion is to track interpreter needs and use in the electronic record, so it is easily extractable.[3] It is crucial that health care organizations develop programs to meet the needs of the patients they serve.

References

1. Yeheskel A, Rawal S. Exploring the 'patient experience' of individuals with limited English proficiency: a scoping review. *J Immigr Minor Health.* 2019;21(4):853–878.
2. US Department of Health and Human Services Office of Minority Health. *National CLAS standards*; 2018. https://minorityhealth.hhs.gov/omh/browse.aspx?lvl=2&lvlid=53.
3. Taira BR, Kim K, Mody N. Hospital and health system-level interventions to improve care for limited English proficiency patients: a systematic review. *Jt Comm J Qual Patient Saf.* 2019;45(6):446–458.

In general, *futility* means that the treatments, especially aggressive critical care, do not meet the underlying goals of care (i.e., the treatment is harming the patient in some way without countervailing justification, such as benefit for the patient's overall condition). This usually occurs when there is a conflict between beneficence, nonmaleficence, and sometimes autonomy.

In critical care, futility is most often discussed in the context of end-of-life interventions. This is a pervasive ethical problem in the United States. According to Hofmann and Schneiderman,[26] "death is not necessarily a medical failure; a bad death is not only a medical failure, but also an ethical breakdown."

Too many people in the United States experience a bad death. In general, providers fail to discuss death with patients, fail to refer to programs such as hospice or even palliative care appropriately, and persist in aggressively treating patients in high-tech settings far past the appropriate time.

Moral distress is extremely common among nurses who feel compelled to provide continued, painful, invasive care that will not benefit the patient or is contrary to the patient's wishes.[24,25] Critical care nurses are on the forefront of this reality and can educate patients and families about options, clarify the realities associated with coding patients, and work with health care colleagues to foster thoughtfulness about the goals of care.

PROFESSIONAL NURSING ETHICS AND THE NURSING CODE OF ETHICS

A professional ethic forms the framework for any profession and is based on three elements:[27]
1. the professional code of ethics,
2. the purpose of the profession, and
3. the standards of practice of the professional.

The code of ethics developed by the profession is the delineation of its values and relationships with and among members of the profession and society. The professional standards describe specifics of practice in various settings and subspecialties. Nursing professionals must stay consistent with their values and ethics and ensure that the ethical environment is maintained wherever nursing care and services are performed.[18,27,28]

The nursing code of ethics contains statements and directives for ethical nursing behavior.[28] The *ANA Code of Ethics for Nurses*[18] provides the major source of ethical guidance for the nursing profession. The nine statements of the code are presented in Box 2.2. Further delineation of each of the provisions along with in-depth discussion and examples of application can be found on the ANA website, https://www.nursingworld.org/practice-policy/nursing-excellence/ethics/code-of-ethics-for-nurses/.

Situational and Organizational Ethical Decision Making in Critical Care

As discussed earlier, the critical care nurse encounters ethical issues on a daily basis. Pavlish et al.[29] studied nurses involved in ethical problems, their early indicators and risk factors, nurse actions, and outcomes. From this study, they derived risk factors for patients, families, health care providers, and health care organizations. Additionally, they described several early indicators for ethical dilemmas (Box 2.3). Research has indicated that screening critically ill patients periodically may help identify ethical conflicts earlier.[30]

Responding to individual ethical issues is not enough; there must be a proactive program with a systematic approach to address ethical situations.[31,32] Preventive programs should identify, prioritize, and address concerns about ethics at an organizational level. Over time, measurable outcomes should demonstrate reduced disparities between current practices and ideal practices.[33]

Neglect of ethical problems or inadequate processes or resolution at the individual or systems level results in harm to more than patients; this often results in poor staff morale, moral distress, increased operational and legal costs, negative public relations, and loss of trust in the profession. Because nurses are on the frontline of health care ethics, especially in the critical care setting, they have a unique and essential role in the resolution of ethical problems. Box 2.4 lists intranet resources related to ethics.

Framework for Resolving Ethical Problems

Ethical problems are ubiquitous in critical care and often related to conflicts surrounding the use of technology, including the withdrawal of technology. Ethical problems in critical care occur when there is:
1. conflict between the right action and the ability to take it,
2. uncertainty about the right action, or
3. conflict about which of several right actions is most ethical.[4]

BOX 2.3 Early Indicators for Ethical Dilemmas

- Signs of patient suffering (prolonged, unrelieved pain)
- Signs of unrealistic expectations (unwavering belief in patient recovery)
- Signs of nurses' moral distress (believe treatment not helpful, causes suffering)
- Signs of conflict (disagreement, different opinions)
- Signs of poor communication (avoidance of end of life and other difficult topics)
- Signs of ethics violations (disrespect for autonomy, disregard of right to information)

From Pavlish CL, Hellyer JH, Brown-Saltzman K, Miers AG, Squire K. Screening situations for risk of ethical conflicts: a pilot study. *Am J Crit Care*. 2015;24:13.

BOX 2.4 Informatics QSEN

Internet Resources: Ethical Issues
American Journal of Bioethics: www.bioethics.net
- Bioethics news and blog
American Nurses Association (ANA): www.nursingworld.org
- Ethics and Human Rights Issues: www.nursingworld.org/practice-policy/nursing-excellence/ethics/
- Code of Ethics for Nurses: www.nursingworld.org/practice-policy/nursing-excellence/ethics/code-of-ethics-for-nurses/
American Society for Bioethics and the Humanities (ASBH): www.asbh.org
Catholic Health Care Association of the United States: www.chausa.org/ethics/overview
The Hastings Center: www.thehastingscenter.org
United States Department of Veterans Affairs National Center for Ethics in Health Care: www.ethics.va.gov

---

Dealing with an ethical problem effectively requires the individuals involved to pause, expand group consciousness about the issue, validate assumptions, look for patterns of thoughts or behaviors, and facilitate reflection and inquiry before making any decision.[33,34]

To facilitate the ethical decision-making process, a model or framework should be used. The Stakeholders-Facts-Norms-Options

---

BOX 2.2 American Nurses Association Code of Ethics for Nurses

1. The nurse practices with compassion and respect for the inherent dignity, worth, and unique attributes of every person.
2. The nurse's primary commitment is to the patient, whether an individual, family, group, community, or population.
3. The nurse promotes, advocates for, and protects the rights, health, and safety of the patient.
4. The nurse has authority, accountability, and responsibility for nursing practice; makes decisions; and takes action consistent with the obligations to promote health and provide optimal care.
5. The nurse owes the same duties to self as to others, including the responsibility to promote health and safety, preserve wholeness of character and integrity, maintain competence, and continue personal and professional growth.
6. The nurse, through individual and collective effort, establishes, maintains, and improves the ethical environment of the work setting and conditions of employment that are conducive to safe, quality health care.
7. The nurse, in all roles and settings, advances the profession through research and scholarly inquiry, professional standards development, and the policy generation of both nursing and health policy.
8. The nurse collaborates with other health professionals and the public to protect human rights, promote health diplomacy, and reduce health disparities.
9. The profession of nursing, collectively through its professional organizations, must articulate nursing values, maintain the integrity of the profession, and integrate principles of social justice into nursing and health policy.

From American Nurses Association. *Code of Ethics for Nurses*. Washington, DC: ANA; 2015.

(SFNO) model is provided in the next section, because it is easy to remember and useful both for individual patient dilemmas and for examining organizational dilemmas.

SFNO Model for Deliberation of Ethical Problems

SFNO[4] is an easily memorized acronym that stands for:
1. stakeholders
2. facts
3. norms
4. options

Using this model, the nurse would first identify the ethical question; for example, should the ventilator be withdrawn from a patient? Thereafter the nurse should use the SFNO model as an organizing device that allows the nurse (and health care team) to ensure that important considerations are identified, and that group deliberation is facilitated by use of a framework. Box 2.5 provides a useful guide to use of the SFNO model.

To illustrate the use of this model, consider the following straightforward example. An older-adult woman with chronic obstructive pulmonary disease (COPD) is on a ventilator, receiving artificial nutrition through a gastric tube, intravenous fluids, and antibiotics for pneumonia. The patient does not have capacity and does not have an advance directive.

The patient's only child, an adult daughter, approaches the team and says the patient would not want to remain on the ventilator and requests that it be withdrawn. The treating physician believes that after the pneumonia is treated, it may be possible to wean the patient from the ventilator. The initial question is whether withdrawing the ventilator is ethically appropriate.

Stakeholders

Stakeholders include the following:
- The patient
- The patient's adult daughter
- Extended family
- Nurses
- Other health care team members
- The health system
- Other similarly situated patients are more remote stakeholders

Facts

Many facts are not *immediately available*, including, but are not limited to:
- Whether there are other relevant stakeholders in terms of family members or loved ones
- The underlying severity of the COPD
- The degree to which the patient has previously expressed her wishes to her daughter and in what context
- Information about the patient that reveals her likes, dislikes, and values
- The patient's prognosis if the pneumonia is treated
- The degree to which the patient is in pain or is suffering
- The likelihood of suffering both with continued ventilation and if the ventilation is withdrawn
- The time in which evidence of improvement from the pneumonia is expected
- The anticipated likelihood of successfully weaning the patient from the ventilator
- The underlying cognitive status of the patient
- The likelihood that the patient will be able to engage in activities that are consistent with her values if treatment is continued

Norms

Norms include the following:
- Respect for persons means that the patient's autonomous decisions should be honored; however, we do not yet know to what extent the request is an expression of the wishes of the patient or of the daughter.
- Beneficence requires the caregivers to maximize benefit.

QSEN | **BOX 2.5   Patient-Centered Care**

SFNO Approach to Case Analysis

Stakeholders
- Who has a stake in the decision being made? Why?
- Who will be significantly affected by the decision made? Why? Please be specific.
- Are there reasons to give priority to one stakeholder over another?

Facts
1. What additional facts are necessary to inform your decision-making process?
2. What factual issues might generate disagreement?
3. What facts are relevant to a solution?

Norms
- What ethical principles, norms, or values are at stake?
- Which do you think are relevant, and which might appear to conflict or generate disagreement?

Options
- Consider a wide variety of alternatives. Resist the urge to quickly reach a recommendation.
- What actions or policies deserve serious consideration?

- Explore the values behind the alternatives (cognitive dissonance and perspective taking foster ethical and professional development).
- Explore the processes and strategies that can improve decision making. Compensatory strategies for professional decision making include seeking help, managing emotions, anticipating consequences (including short-term and long-term consequences), recognizing rules and context, and testing your assumptions and motives.
- Narrow the options to arrive at a few ethically acceptable options.
- If the ethical ideal is not possible, what compromise solutions are most attractive?
- Justification criteria may be helpful in explaining your reasons for selecting one or two options as superior:
  - *Necessity:* Is it necessary to infringe on the values or norms under consideration to achieve the intended goal?
  - *Effectiveness:* Will the action be effective in achieving the desired goal?
  - *Proportionality:* Is the desired goal important enough to justify overriding another principle or value?
  - *Least infringement:* Is the policy or action designed to minimize the infringement of the principle or value that conflicts with it?
  - *Proper process:* Has the decision been made using proper processes?

Adapted from DuBois JM. Solving ethical problems: analyzing ethics cases and justifying decision. In: *Ethics in Mental Health Research.* Oxford: Oxford University Press; 2008; Volpe RL, et al, eds. Guidance for facilitators and facilitation guide. In: *Exploring Integrity in Medicine: The Bander Center for Medical Business Ethics Casebook,* 2nd ed. St. Louis: Saint Louis University; 2017.

- Nonmaleficence requires the caregivers to minimize harm.
- The extent to which the current treatments honor these norms depends on the specific answers to the above-listed facts.
- Conversely, if information becomes available that the patient clearly expresses a wish to not be on a ventilator under any circumstance, respect for persons may trump beneficence.

Options for Care

- The team could do nothing (i.e., maintain the ventilation).
- The team could also begin weaning the ventilator but continue the other treatments.
- If improvement from the pneumonia is expected after a few additional days of intravenous antibiotics, the team could work with the daughter to reach agreement to postpone removal for a few days and reassess the situation.
- Mediating options are always worth exploring and often offer additional time to collect the information identified as necessary.
- The team could also explore withdrawal of all but comfort care measures if that is consistent with the patient's previously expressed wishes or the patient's values.

Strategies for the Promotion of Ethical Decision Making

The complexity of health care and ethical dilemmas encountered frequently in clinical practice demand the establishment of expertise in clinical ethics and mechanisms and processes for resolution.

The field of clinical ethics (also known as *health care ethics* or *bioethics*) arose directly from dilemmas in critical care situations in the past many years. Clinical ethics is now an established, interdisciplinary profession, and hospitals almost always have resources available to assist with mitigation and resolution of ethical problems.

Institutional Ethicists, Ethics Committees, and Ethics Consultation Services

Almost every hospital has an Institutional Ethics Committee (IEC), and many have ethics consultation services or individual professional ethicists assigned to hospitals. IECs arose as a response to ethical and legal dilemmas in the 1960s and 1970s.

In some states, law requires such sources, and they are strongly encouraged, mandated, or legislated as part of the requirement that hospitals have mechanisms for addressing ethics issues in patient care.

Institutional Ethicists and Consultants, and Consultation Services

Ethics consultations can provide the various stakeholders involved with an informed "outside" perspective and use professional expertise to assist with resolution. Recommendations issued in response to ethics consultations are generally guidance rather than mandates.

Institutional Ethics Committees

IECs were originally envisioned to provide education and foster ethical approaches to systemic and organizational issues. IECs still function this way at some facilities when individual ethicists or consultation services exist to assist providers and families at the bedside with ethical dilemmas. At others, IECs serve primarily as consultation services to assist with individual ethical problems.

Many facilities have specialized or subdivided IECs based on clinical service. Regardless of the person, service, or committee involved, every hospital should have one or more ways to assist with ethical problems at the bedside (ethics consultations).

Ethics Rounds and Conferences

At hospitals with individual ethicists or consultation services, ethicists often round with other providers on each patient in critical care. In the absence of this more structured approach, nurses may consider developing a regular method of conducting ethics rounds with the assistance of their facility's ethicist or a member of the IEC.

Ethics rounds can increase early identification of risk factors for emerging ethical problems and allow for proactive resolution. An individual patient ethics conference may be scheduled to include appropriate stakeholders or a multidisciplinary group to discuss unit issues.[34,35]

LEGAL ISSUES

The practice of nursing is influenced by and sometimes governed by the law. This influence extends far beyond malpractice. Legal systems operate at the local, state, and federal levels and affect health care in a range of matters, from a lawsuit between private parties to enforcement actions brought by government agencies against individuals or health systems.

Generally speaking, the law is concerned with minimum standards rather than best practices or even ethical practice. In other words, practice that meets legal criteria is often far less than what meets ethical criteria or criteria for best practices. Nursing licensure is one example; licensure is a legal tool to protect the public that indicates only that a nurse has demonstrated the minimum basic competencies to practice as an entry-level nurse. Licensure does not set best practice.

This chapter highlights some of the laws and legal systems that figure prominently in nursing practice, including:

1. Administrative law—illustrated by the regulation of the profession by state boards of nursing (BONs)
2. Tort law—illustrated through negligence lawsuits against nurses for their actions or inactions
3. Constitutional law—illustrated through a discussion of the legal rights of patients to make decisions to accept or refuse treatment
4. Federal and state health care statutory laws—illustrated through self-determination laws and select federal laws

Administrative Law: Professional Regulation

Functions of Boards of Nursing

The regulation of nursing practice is intended to protect the health and safety of state citizens by:

1. Regulating the conditions of licensure
2. Regulating the scope of practice
3. Establishing a framework of standards of nursing practice
4. Removing incompetent or unsafe practitioners through disciplinary actions
5. Prohibiting unlicensed persons from providing services reserved for licensed individuals

In addition, the regulation of nursing can enhance the professional status and the public's trust of nurses.

Scope of Practice. BONs maintain expectations for and limits of nursing practice in each state through the licensure of nurses and through challenges to non-nurses engaged in professional activities that intrude on the nursing scope of practice. *Scope of practice* generally refers to the broad range of activities that nurses perform and manage in the delivery of care that "require education and training consistent with professional standards commensurate with the RN's education, demonstrated competencies, and experience."[36]

Scope of practice is framed broadly to account for the many professional nursing settings and roles and also to account for activities that are reserved for professional nurses and activities that may be delegated with appropriate supervision.

Scope of practice provisions are also intended to prevent unlicensed professionals from providing services that are reserved to licensed professionals (see Box 2.6, Scope of RN Practice).

Standards of Practice. BONs also typically develop state standards of nursing practice through rulemaking. These standards of practice—*Nurse Practice Acts* (NPAs)—communicate the expectations of safe and effective nursing practice within the scope of practice. State standards of practice also assist BONs in evaluating the ongoing practice of nursing. Thus, to fully understand the expectations for and limitations of nursing in a particular state, it is necessary to review both the NPA and the regulations (also known as *rules*) of the BON.

Specialty Nurse Standards of Practice. In addition to standards developed by BONs, many specialty nursing organizations have developed standards of practice. The BON standards establish broad expectations of safety and efficacy, whereas *specialty standards* are more targeted and aimed at fostering excellence in the specialized field.

An example of specialty standards are those developed by the AACN.[37] Specialty standards are helpful in establishing and measuring

---

BOX 2.6 **Scope of RN Practice**

Model Nursing Act (Model Statutory Law)
The practice of registered nursing shall include:
1. Providing comprehensive nursing assessment of the health status of patients.
2. Collaborating with health care team to develop and coordinate an integrated patient-centered health care plan.
3. Developing the comprehensive patient-centered health care plan, including (a) establishing nursing diagnoses, (b) setting goals to meet identified health care needs, and (c) prescribing nursing interventions.
4. Implementing nursing care through the execution of independent nursing strategies and the provision of regimens requested, ordered, or prescribed by authorized health care providers.
5. Evaluating responses to interventions and the effectiveness of the plan of care.
6. Designing and implementing teaching plans based on patient needs.
7. Delegating and assigning nursing interventions to implement the plan of care.
8. Providing for the maintenance of safe and effective nursing care rendered directly or indirectly.
9. Advocating the best interest of patients.
10. Communicating and collaborating with other health care providers in the management of health care and the implementation of the total health care regimen within and across care settings.
11. Managing, supervising, and evaluating the practice of nursing.
12. Teaching the theory and practice of nursing.
13. Participating in development of health care policies, procedures, and systems.
14. Wearing identification that clearly identifies the nurse as an RN when providing direct patient care, unless wearing identification creates a safety or health risk for either the nurse or the patient.
15. Other acts that require education and training consistent with professional standards as prescribed by the BON and commensurate with the RN's education, demonstrated competencies, and experience.

BON, State board of nursing; *RN,* registered nurse.
Modified from National Council of the State Boards of Nursing (NCSBN). *NCSBN Model Act.* Chicago, IL: NCSBN; 2012, updated 2014.

---

quality care and often reflect a consensus opinion of experts in the particular specialty of appropriate nursing care (see Box 2.7, Standards of Care for Acute and Critical Care Nursing).

Standard of Care. The extent to which specialty standards are introduced in a legal context varies widely from state to state. Of note, the legal term, *standard of care*, is not the same as the standards of practice.

In some cases, specialty standards of practice or care have been introduced in court to help establish a legal standard of care, but not all courts will consider these. The legal standard of care and the use of specialty standards are discussed further in the following section on tort law.

TORT LAW: NEGLIGENCE AND PROFESSIONAL MALPRACTICE, INTENTIONAL TORTS

Many civil lawsuits for injuries fall under the legal heading of torts. *Torts* are civil lawsuits based on negligent actions or inactions or intentional acts, such as assault, battery, or defamation. For the lay public, the standard for behavior for negligence is based on *reasonableness*, or what a *reasonably prudent person* would do under the circumstances. This is also known as *ordinary negligence*.

In a professional capacity, individuals are judged based on their professional standard of care. Nurses caring for acutely and critically ill patients may be alleged to have acted or failed to act in a manner inconsistent with the professional standard of care as part of a lawsuit that focuses in whole or in part on the alleged failure. This is *professional malpractice or negligence law* applied to professional behavior.

There are many types of cases based in tort law, but this chapter focuses on negligence and professional malpractice and the intentional torts of assault and battery.

Ordinary Negligence

Generally, the standard for *negligence* is failing to act as a reasonably prudent person would under the circumstances or acting in a way a reasonably prudent person would not act under the circumstances. There are four criteria or elements for all negligence cases:
1. duty to another person (Duty)
2. breach of that duty (Breach)
3. that caused (Causation)
4. harm to the person that has monetary value (Harm).

All four elements must be satisfied for a case to go forward. These cases are referred to as *professional negligence* or *professional malpractice*.

Professional Malpractice

Although negligence claims may apply to anyone, malpractice requires the alleged wrongdoer to have special standing as a professional. In civil cases alleging wrongdoing by health care professionals, the terms *malpractice* and professional *negligence* are used interchangeably.

Malpractice is a negligence action applied to a professional. If a nurse's actions or inactions are inconsistent with the standard of care, causing harm to the patient, the nurse (and usually the nurse's employer) is subject to liability in professional negligence (meaning they may be ordered to pay the patient for that harm).

Recent research findings indicate that malpractice claims involving critical care nurses are separate from others in emergency or perioperative areas. Intensive care location and permanent injury increased

BOX 2.7 Standards of Care for Acute and Critical Care Nursing

Standard 1: Assessment

The nurse obtains comprehensive data pertinent to the situation and/or patient's health.

Competencies

- Collects data from the patient, family, other health care providers, and the community, as appropriate, to develop a holistic picture of the patient's needs or conditions
- Prioritizes data collection based on patient characteristics related to the immediate condition and anticipated needs
- Uses valid evidence-based assessment techniques, instruments, and tools
- Documents relevant data in a clear and retrievable format

Standard 2: Diagnosis

The nurse analyzes and synthesizes data from the assessment in determining diagnoses or conditions relevant to care.

Competencies

- Derives diagnoses and relevant conditions from the assessment data
- Validates diagnoses with the patient, family, and other health care providers
- Documents diagnoses and relevant conditions in a clear and retrievable format

Standard 3: Outcomes Identification

The nurse identifies optimal outcomes for the patient.

Competencies

- Identifies outcomes from assessments and diagnoses in collaboration with the patient, family, and interprofessional team
- Identifies preferences and values in formulating appropriate outcomes that meet diversity and cultural needs in collaboration with the patient, family, and interprofessional team
- Considers associated risks, benefits, best available evidence, clinical expertise, and essential costs when formulating outcomes, to avoid placing unnecessary financial burdens on the patient and/or family
- Modifies outcomes based on changes in a patient's condition or situation
- Documents identified outcomes as measurable goals in a clear and retrievable format

Standard 4: Planning

The nurse caring for the patient develops a plan that prescribes strategies and alternatives to attain outcomes.

Competencies

- Uses clinical judgment and inquiry in developing an individualized plan using best evidence
- Collaborates with the patient, family, and interprofessional team to develop the plan
- Establishes priorities and continuity of care within the plan (transfer of information/handoffs)
- Includes strategies for health promotion/education and prevention of complications or injury
- Considers associated risks, benefits, best evidence, clinical expertise, resources, and cost when developing the plan
- Documents and provides handoff of the plan in a clear and retrievable manner

Standard 5: Implementation

The nurse caring for the patient implements the plan.

Competencies

- Employs strategies to promote and maintain a safe environment
- Coordinates implementation of the plan with the patient, family, and interprofessional team
- Intervenes to prevent and minimize complications and alleviate suffering
- Facilitates learning for patients, families, and the community
- Provides age and developmentally appropriate care with respect to diversity
- Documents implementation in a clear and retrievable format

Standard 6: Evaluation

The nurse evaluates processes and progress toward attainment of goals and outcomes.

Competencies

- Conducts systematic and ongoing evaluations using evidence-based techniques, tools, and instruments
- Collaborates with the patient, family, and interprofessional team in the evaluation process
- Revises the assessment, diagnoses, outcomes identification, plan, and interventions based on information gained during the evaluation process
- Documents the results of evaluations in a clear and retrievable format

Modified from American Association of Critical-Care Nurses. *AACN Scope and Standards for Progressive and Critical Care Nursing Practice.* Aliso Viejo, CA: AACN; 2019.

the risk of payments awarded. Researchers concluded that focusing on skin integrity and patient monitoring could lessen severe harm to patients.[38]

Just as in ordinary negligence, the person bringing the lawsuit (plaintiff) must prove the *elements of negligence.* In the health care context, the patient-plaintiffs (person[s] bringing the lawsuit) must prove that:

1. the nurse had a duty to care for the patient;
2. the nurse breached that duty by deviating from the standard of care; and
3. the breach actually caused the harm that would not have occurred in the absence of negligence.

The legal standard of care for nurses is established by expert testimony of a nurse in a similar area of practice and is generally "the care

that an ordinarily prudent *nurse* would perform under the same circumstances."[39]

In the case of specialized nurses, the standard of care is measured against the "learning, care, and skill normally possessed and exercised by practitioners of that specialty under the same or similar circumstances."[40] The standard of care determination focuses more on accepted practice of competent nurses rather than best practice of excellent nurses (which may be reflected in some specialty standards of practice). In addition to expert testimony, courts may rely on multiple types of evidence to establish the standard of care.

Duty

Duty to the injured party is the first element of a malpractice case and is established through the existence of the nurse-patient relationship.

Nurses assume a *duty* to the patient to provide care that is consistent with the standard of care when the nurse-patient relationship is established.

Case law recognizes the nurse-patient relationship as a separate and distinct relationship from the doctor-patient relationship[41] and as a prerequisite for determining whether a nurse owes the patient a duty to provide care in accordance with the requisite standard of care.

If a nurse shows that he or she (1) was not assigned to that particular patient on the date that the negligence allegedly occurred or (2) was not working on the day or at the time the negligence allegedly occurred, there was no relationship and therefore no duty. Because no duty is imposed on the nurse, negligence allegations will fail.[42]

Breach

Breach is the failure to act consistently within applicable standards of care. For a nurse to be found negligent, the patient-plaintiff must establish that the nurse had a *duty* to provide care and that the nurse failed to provide care consistent with those standards.

Moreover, the nurse's failure, or breach, *must have caused the damages* about which the patient-plaintiff seeks redress. A breach of duty does not exist if the standard of care is met.

Harm Caused by the Breach

Patient-plaintiffs must prove that the nurse breached his or her duty to the patient and that the breach caused the patient to sustain injuries or damages for which he or she seeks monetary remuneration.

Causation of the harm is a pivotal element in civil cases filed against nurses. If patient-plaintiffs fail to establish that some act or omission directly resulted in the harm or if something else can be shown to have caused the harm, recovery will be denied.

Damages

The fourth element of negligence is damages. *Damages* are the monetary value or cost of the injury suffered. For liability to be imposed against a nurse caring for an acutely or critically ill patient, that patient must prove that something the nurse did or failed to do was inconsistent with the standard of care and that the inconsistency caused harm or injury that has a monetary value.

Patient-plaintiffs in a malpractice case can usually point to additional medical bills associated with their injuries to satisfy this element.

The number of nurses being named defendants in these cases is increasing, and this is especially true for advanced practice nurses. Nurses caring for acutely and critically ill patients need to carefully consider whether to purchase professional liability insurance and, if so, the amount and type of coverage that is needed.

Most institutions will provide some level of malpractice insurance coverage for nurses, but the amount and circumstances under which each nurse is covered are important considerations. In addition, institutional policies will generally not cover actions against nurses brought by the state BON.

Professional Malpractice and the Nursing Process

Malpractice claims may be premised on care delivered at any point from the moment a nurse-patient relationship is established to patient discharge. What constitutes reasonable care has been the focus of many cases filed against health care professionals and the hospitals in which they practice.

If the nurse reasonably executes every component of the nursing process in accordance with the requisite standard of care, reasonable care will have been provided. However, if the nurse fails with regard to a single component of the nursing process, care provided to an acutely

or critically ill patient may be deemed insufficient, unreasonable, and negligent.

The following are examples of malpractice resulting from failures in particular stages of the nursing process.

Assessment Failure: Failure to Assess and Analyze the Level of Care Needed by the Patient

Nurses caring for acutely and critically ill patients have a duty to assess and analyze the level of care needed by their patients. Where a nurse allegedly fails to fulfill this responsibility, liability for negligence may be threatened.

To withstand allegations of failure to assess and analyze, it is important for nurses not only to assess and analyze the level of care needed by patients but also to document their assessment findings and all actions taken to properly care for patients.

Failure to assess and analyze the situation and to document the assessment findings, the interventions, and the patient's response to those interventions exposes the nurse and the hospital to liability for negligence.

Assessment Failure: Failure to Assess and Clarify the Patient's Condition

Nurses are responsible for obtaining appropriate and complete information on a patient's condition upon assuming care, adequately assessing the patient, and clarifying and reporting any discrepancies.

Planning Failure: Failure to Appropriately Diagnose

Nurses caring for acutely and critically ill patients must plan effective courses of treatment. Such a course of treatment depends on a proper diagnosis. Historically, cases of failure to diagnose have been filed against physicians, rather than nurses.

However, nurses who diagnose patient conditions may find themselves the target of a failure to diagnose a case and need to be aware that liability may be imposed if the plan of care is based on an erroneous diagnosis.

Implementation Failure: Failure to Communicate Patient Findings in a Timely Manner

Nurses spend more time with patients than do any other health care professionals, and this is especially true for nurses caring for acutely and critically ill patients. As a result, these nurses are in the best position to promptly detect changes in a patient's condition. However, detection is only the first step.

Nurses caring for acutely and critically ill patients must promptly communicate troublesome patient findings. Failure to properly communicate patient findings can be devastating for patients and can be the reason that patients file malpractice causes of action.

Implementation Failure: Failure to Take Appropriate Action

Cases from across the United States continue to affirm that it is the nurse's responsibility to take affirmative action when action is indicated. Nursing staff should have recognized the emergency nature of the situation and taken proper steps to notify the attending physician.

Failure to take appropriate action in cases involving acutely and critically ill patients has included not only issues regarding physician notification but also failure to follow physician orders,[43,44] failure to properly treat,[45] and failure to appropriately administer medication.[45-47]

To avoid allegations of failure to take appropriate action, nurses caring for acutely and critically ill patients need to recognize signs and symptoms of complications and patient compromise.

Implementation Failure: Failure to Document

Nurses caring for acutely and critically ill patients are required not only to take appropriate action but also to accurately document their findings, interventions performed, and patients' response to interventions.

Failure to thoroughly and accurately document any aspect of care gives rise to negligence causes of action.

Implementation Failure: Failure to Preserve Patient Privacy

Nurses have a legal duty to preserve patient privacy and confidentiality. State and federal statutes and case law affirm this duty. In addition, the actions of nurses could expose their employers to severe penalties from the federal government for violations of federal laws, such as the Health Insurance Portability and Accountability Act.[48]

Nurses can ensure that the privacy of acutely and critically ill patients is protected by following patient directives and institutional policies and procedures, which should comply with state privacy laws and federal laws.

Nurses must also avoid any discussions about specific patients with anyone except other health care professionals involved in the patient's care in nonpublic settings. Discussions about specific patients are never appropriate in public areas, such as elevators, cafeterias, gift shops, and parking lots.

Evaluation Failure: Failure to Act as a Patient Advocate

From admission to discharge, nurses have a duty to act as a patient advocate. For nurses caring for acutely and critically ill patients, this duty imposes the responsibility to evaluate the care that is being given to patients.

Courts continue to hold that all nurses, including nurses caring for acutely and critically ill patients, have a nondelegable duty to act as patient advocate. Failure to act as patient advocate exposes the nurse and the hospital to substantial liability and, more importantly, exposes patients to life-altering and life-ending complications that could have been avoided.

Advocating for the patient means taking concerns up the chain of command. Simply documenting concerns is insufficient to protect the nurse from liability.

Wrongful Death

Wrongful death cases are a variation of negligence action in which the harm is the death of the individual. For families and health care professionals, wrongful death cases are among the most traumatic. In these cases, the life-and-death nature of the health care experience is exposed.

In reviewing these kinds of cases, one learns that what is at issue is rarely the use, misuse, or malfunction of sophisticated, cutting-edge technology or the miscalculation of a complex formula. On the contrary, a review of wrongful death cases suggests that the alleged failures at issue are typically foundational matters of patient care and critical thinking.

To avoid wrongful death liability, it is imperative that nurses caring for acutely and critically ill patients remain vigilant, recognize the signs and symptoms of complications and compromise, and take affirmative action to advocate for the best interest of the patient.

Assault and Battery

Assault and battery are examples of *intentional torts* (rather than negligence actions) that are frequently brought against health care providers. Although they are often used together, they are actually two separate torts.[49] *Assault* is any intentional act that creates imminent apprehension of harmful or offensive contact with the plaintiff. With assault, no actual contact is necessary.

Battery is any intentional act that brings about actual harmful or offensive contact with the plaintiff. *Harmful* means physical harm, whereas *offensive* means contact that a reasonable person would consider offensive under the circumstances.

In health care cases, patient consent is a defense to these claims. Consent can be general or limited in scope. *Assault* may be alleged if a patient was aware that he or she was going to be touched in a manner not authorized by informed consent. For example, the act of telling a patient that he or she will be restrained may be assault.

Battery occurs if the health care professional touches the patient in an unauthorized manner. The act of restraining a patient without consent is battery. Another defense to assault and battery is an *emergency situation*. Thus cutting a patient's throat to create an emergency tracheostomy to create an airway may be justified, whereas cutting a patient's neck on the wrong side in opposition to the informed consent may be battery.

CONSTITUTIONAL LAW: PATIENT DECISION MAKING

Patient autonomy or self-determination is a patient right guaranteed by state law and the US Constitution under the 14th Amendment. The right of competent adult patients to refuse treatment is well established.

This right has evolved from the laws of informed consent, the laws of assault and battery (the right to be free from fear of harm and unwanted touching), and historic legal rights granted to individuals to say what is done with their own bodies.

The US Supreme Court described this as the right to "possession and control of his own person, free from all restraint or interference of others, unless by clear and unquestionable authority of law."[50]

Patients With Decision-Making Capacity

Decision-making capacity means a person has the ability to:
1. take in and understand information,
2. process the information in accordance with his or her own personal values and goals,
3. make a decision based on the information, and
4. communicate the decision.

A person does not lack decision-making capacity merely because the decision is at odds with what others would decide or even if it seems foolish.[51] A person with decision-making capacity is often described as *having capacity* or as *competent*.

In the health care setting, a *competent adult* patient has the right to refuse even life-sustaining treatment for any reason, without regard for that individual's motivations.

Patients Without Decision-Making Capacity

Patients *without decision-making capacity* include individuals who were previously competent (individuals who reached adulthood but lost competence because of illness or injury), individuals who were never competent (individuals born with severe to profound cognitive disabilities), individuals who are not yet competent (primarily children younger than the age of majority), and individuals with fluctuating competence (e.g., individuals with cyclic disorders, such as the manic phase of bipolar disorder, that can seriously impair decision making).

The law allows for others to stand in their place as surrogate decision makers. The law also imposes standards of judgment for surrogate decision makers to guide and evaluate decisions.

Numerous legal mechanisms exist that can simplify at least the legal issues surrounding decision making for patients without decision-making capacity. There are state laws that may specify categories of individuals who may make decisions for patients who have lost capacity (often called *statutory surrogates*). State probate laws allow for appointment of a guardian to make some or all decisions for individuals who have more sustained loss of capacity.

Adults who have capacity can plan for decisions and appoint decision makers to direct their future care through advance directives (statements of wishes in future situations or the appointment of a future decision maker in the event they should lose capacity).

These include, but are not limited to, *living wills, individual directives, and durable powers of attorney*. The legal requirements and analyses are more stringent for decisions that may directly affect life, including decisions to forgo or withdraw treatment at the end of life.

Never and Not Yet Competent Patients

Competent adults can refuse treatment for any reason, even if others believe it is in opposition to their best interests. However, for patients who are not yet competent (i.e., children) and the patients who were never competent, the law imposes a best interest standard.

The standard is self-explanatory; parents and legal guardians of children have a legal obligation to make informed decisions based on the best interests of the patient.

Previously Competent Patients

Most legal decisions involve decisions to withdraw or forgo life-sustaining treatment in patients without decisional capacity and who have not specified their wishes before losing capacity.

In addition to affirming the states' ability to set high evidence standards in favor of preserving life, court cases established that in the absence of specific directions from the patient, surrogate decision makers should make a *substituted judgment* standard. This means that decision makers must base their decisions on the patient's known preferences and values before they lost capacity and use their best judgment in deciding what the patient would have wanted (in light of those values and preferences).

There are a wide variety of state law—based procedures for individuals with decision-making capacity to direct their future care through documents and the appointment of surrogate decision makers in the event they should lose capacity. Each state has resources on the available options for residents.

Advance Directives

Patients themselves can provide clear direction by preparing statements (usually required to be in writing) in advance that specify their wishes. *Advance directive* is a generic term meaning all statements of future health care wishes in the event of incapacity. These statements include the living will and the durable power of attorney for health care.

A *living will* specifies that if certain circumstances occur, such as terminal illness, the patient will decline specific treatments, such as cardiopulmonary resuscitation and mechanical ventilation.

It has proven to be of limited value, because it does not cover all treatments; for example, in some states, nutritional support may not be declined through a living will.

Living wills are more useful if the patient has a life-limiting condition and can use the living will to express their wishes in light of the anticipated course of their foundation.

Advance directives vary by state but are generally legally binding documents that allow individuals to specify a variety of preferences, including naming people they want to serve as their decision makers, particular treatments they want to avoid, and circumstances in which they wish to avoid them.

The *durable power of attorney for health care* is a directive through which a patient designates an "agent," someone who will make decisions for the patient if the patient becomes unable to do so. The agent is obligated to use the patient's values and preferences to make the decision the patient would make if he or she were able to do so. This is perhaps the most useful tool if the agent is selected carefully and understands the associated responsibilities.

Once a patient creates an advance directive in his or her own state, other states will honor it under the full faith and credit doctrine. Nurses may care for critically ill patients in one state who have executed an advance directive in another. The fact that it was drafted in another state does not negate its validity.

The Patient Self-Determination Act of 1990 is an example of a federal statute that affects practice.[52] The Act was a response to medicine's ability to keep people alive with advanced technology and the decision-making difficulties that arose in response. It was designed to encourage competent patients to consider what they would want in the event of serious illness and to encourage them to complete advance directives.

The Act requires most health care institutions to provide patients at the time of admission written information of their rights under state law to make medical decisions, including the right to refuse treatment and the right to formulate advance directives.

The Act also makes it illegal for a facility to require advance directives or discriminate against patients based on their advance directive or lack thereof. Providers must have written policies and procedures:

1. to inform all adult patients at initiation of treatment of their right to execute an advance directive and of the provider's policies on the implementation of that right;
2. to document in the medical record whether an individual has executed an advance directive;
3. *not* to condition care and treatment or otherwise discriminate on the basis of whether a patient has executed an advance directive;
4. to comply with state laws on advance directives; and
5. to provide information and education to staff and the community on advance directives.

Futile (or Nonbeneficial) Treatment

Especially in critical care, nurses face situations in which continued aggressive treatment is extremely unlikely to benefit the patient. This may mean that supportive care and comfort are the best actions for the patient's well-being. All critical care nurses will observe and deliver care at some point that feels useless, unnecessary, and even harmful and painful to the patient.

Nurses play an incredibly valuable role in the health care team by advocating for the best interest of the patient in a holistic way. Nurses may be responsible for reminding the team of the "big picture" and the need to provide quality of life and compassionate care to the patient.

Many providers have reported feeling obligated to continue treating patients in the absence of any reasonable chance of improvement. There is no legal obligation to provide care that is not, in the provider's judgment, reasonably calculated to improve the patient's condition or symptoms.

To deal with these situations, most institutions have futility policies for discontinuing futile or nonbeneficial care. Some states have laws to deal with these situations designed to facilitate communication between the providers and patients, with procedures for resolution.

Orders Not to Resuscitate (DNR)

Do not resuscitate (DNR) orders are perhaps the oldest form of effectuating patient's wishes to refuse future medical treatment. As part of some institutional futility policies, unilateral DNR orders (meaning ordered by the physician without the agreement of the patient) are permitted but should be rarely used. Furthermore, state laws vary as to the permissibility of the practice.

Policies that address orders to withhold or withdraw treatment should exist in all critical care units, and nurses should be familiar with those policies. The DNR policies should include:

1. patient diagnosis
2. prognosis
3. consent if competent
4. the surrogate decision maker's consent if the patient is not competent
5. documentation of any conflict with advance directives or family member opinion
6. a second practitioner's concurrence for DNR orders if required
7. periodic review
8. exact treatments should be specific and clear

Other orders to withhold or withdraw treatment may involve any intervention, including mechanical ventilation, oxygen, intravenous vasoactive agents or other medications, serial laboratory tests, imaging tests, pulmonary artery catheters, and other invasive monitoring. The legal and ethical implications of these orders for each patient must be carefully considered.

Hospital policies should exist to guide the withdrawal of care in light of state and federal legal constraints. In addition, hospital ethicists and ethics committees can play a valuable role to providers negotiating the complexities of these decisions.

Brain Death

Since 2013 new legal issues surrounding brain death have emerged that have relevance for critical care nurses. Patients are legally dead by the *irreversible cessation* of either (1) the cardiopulmonary system or (2) the entire brain, including the brainstem. Death is pronounced in accordance with acceptable medical standards.[53]

Typically, the determination of death by neurologic criteria is done in accordance with hospital policy and follows the guidelines set out by the American Academy of Neurology.[54] Once testing consistent with brain death is confirmed, the patient is declared dead and either the patient is prepared for the allocation of organs or all mechanical support is removed because they are *legally dead*. This is *not* the same thing as withdrawal of care for terminally ill, but still alive, patients.

There are a number of government and private organization websites with excellent information on health care law (Box 2.8).

QSEN | BOX 2.8 **Informatics**

Internet Resources: Legal Issues
- American Association of Nurse Attorneys: www.TAANA.org
- American College of Legal Medicine: www.ACLM.org
- American Health Care Lawyers Association: www.healthlawyers.org
- American Society of Law and Medicine: www.ASLME.org
- Health Care Law Resources and Information: www.findlaw.org
- Health and Human Resources: www.HHS.gov

REFERENCES

1. Beachump TL, Childress JF. *Principles of Biomedical Ethics*. 5th ed. Oxford: Oxford University Press; 2001.
2. Furrow F, Greaney T, Johnson S, Jost T, Schwartz R. *Bioethics: Health Care Law and Ethics*. 8th ed. Eagan MN: West Publishing; 2018.
3. Rainer J, Schneider JK, Lorenz RA. Ethical dilemmas in nursing: an integrative review. *J Clin Nurs*. 2018;27:19–20.
4. DuBois JA. *Framework for Analyzing Ethics Cases. Ethics in Mental Health Research*. New York: Oxford Press; 2008. www.sites.google.com/a/narrativebioethics.com/emhr/home.
5. Purtilo RB, Doherty RF. *Ethical Decisions in the Health Professions*. 5th ed. St. Louis: Saunders; 2011.
6. Jameton A. *Nursing Practice: The Ethical Issues*. Englewood Cliffs, NJ: Prentice-Hall; 1984.
7. Rushton CH, Caldwell M, Kurtz MCE. Moral distress: a catalyst in building moral resilience. *Am J Nurs*. 2016;116(7):40–49.
8. Hiler CA, Hickman RL Jr, Reimer AP, Wilson K. Predictors of moral distress in a US sample of critical care nurses. *Am J Crit Care*. 2018;27(1):59–66.
9. Altaker KW, Howie-Esquivel J, Cataldo JK. Relationships among palliative care, ethical climate, empowerment, and moral distress in intensive care unit nurses. *Am J Crit Care*. 2018;27(4):295–302.
10. Hamric AB, Epstein EG. A health system wide moral distress consultation service: development and evaluation. *HEC Forum*. 2017;29(2):127–143.
11. Browning ED, Cruz JS. Reflective debriefing: a social work intervention addressing moral distress among ICU nurses. *J Soc Work End-of-Life Palliat Care*. 2018;14(1):44–72.
12. Savel RH, Munro CL. Moral distress, moral courage. *Am J Crit Care*. 2015;24(4):276–278.
13. American Nurses Association. A call to action: exploring moral resilience toward a culture of ethical practice. https://www.nursingworld.org/~4907b6/globalassets/docs/ana/ana-call-to-action-exploring-moral-resilience-final.pdf. Accessed September 15, 2019.
14. Wocial LD. Resilience as an incomplete strategy for coping with moral distress in critical care nurses. *Crit Care Nurse*. 2020;40(6):62–66.
15. DeGrazia M. Building moral resilience through the nurse education and support initiative. *Amer J Crit Care*. 2021;30(2):95–102.
16. Lachman VD, et al. Doing the right thing: pathways to moral courage. *Am Nurse Today*. 2012;7(5):24.
17. American Nurses Association. *Code of ethics for nurses with interpretative statements*; 2015. www.nursingworld.org/practice-policy/nursing-excellence/ethics/code-of-ethics-for-nurses/coe-view-only/.
18. Dineen KK. Addressing prescription opioid abuse concerns in context: synchronizing policy solutions to multiple complex public health problems. *Law Psychol Rev*. 2016;30(1).
19. Benjamin M. Curtis. J. *Ethics in Nursing: Cases, Principles, and Reasoning*. 4th ed. New York: Oxford; 2010.
20. Jonsen A, Siegler M, Winslade W. *Clinical Ethics: A Practical Approach to Ethical Decisions in Clinical Medicine*. 6th ed. New York: McGraw Hill; 2006.
21. Deleted in review.
22. Schneiderman LJ, Jecker NS, Jonsen AR. Medical futility: its meaning and ethical implications. *Ann Intern Med*. 1990;112(12):949.
23. Bernat JL. Medical futility: definition, determination, and disputed in critical care. *Neurocrit Care*. 2005;2(2):198.
24. Jox RJ, Schaider A, Marckmann G, Borasio GD. Medical futility at the end of life: perspectives of intensive care and palliative care clinicians. *J Med Ethics*. 2012;38(9):540–545.
25. Schwarzkopf D, Felfe J, Hartog C, Bloos F. Making it safe: speak up about futile care: a multiperspective survey on leadership, psychological safety and perceived futile care in the ICU. *Crit Care*. 2015;19(supp 1):P567.
26. Hofmann PB, Schneiderman LJ. Physicians should not always pursue a good "clinical" outcome. *Hastings Cent Rep*. 2007;37(3):inside back cover.
27. Lachman VD. Practical use of the nursing code of ethics: part I. *Medsurg Nurs*. 2009;18(1):55.
28. Winland-Brown J, Lachman VD, Swanson EO. The new code of ethics for nurses with interpretative statements (2015): practical clinical application, part 1. *Medsurg Nurs*. 2015;24(4):268.

29. Pavlish C, Brown-Saltzman K, Hersh M, Shirk M, Nudelman O. Early indicators and risk factors for ethical issues in clinical practice. *Image J Nurs Sch.* 2011;43(1):13.

30. Pavlish CL, Hellyer JH, Brown-Saltzman K, Miers AG, Squire K. Screening situations for risk of ethical conflicts: a pilot study. *Am J Crit Care.* 2015;24(3):248–256.

31. U.S. Department of Veterans Affairs. Preventive ethics. www.ethics.va.gov/integratedethics/PEC.asp. Accessed August 28, 2021.

32. Epstein EG. Preventative ethics in the intensive care unit. *AACN Adv Crit Care.* 2012;23(2):217.

33. Rushton CH. Ethical discernment and action: the art of pause. *AACN Adv Crit Care.* 2009;20(1):108.

34. Robichaux C. Developing ethical skills: from sensitivity to action. *Crit Care Nurse.* 2012;32(2):65.

35. Pavlish C, Brown-Saltzman K, Hersh M, Shirk M, Rounkle AM. Nursing priorities, actions, and regrets for ethical situations in clinical practice. *Image J Nurs Sch.* 2011;43(4):385.

36. National Council of the State Boards of Nursing (NCSBN). *NCSBN Model Act.* Chicago, IL: NCSBN; 2012, updated 2014:2.

37. American Association of Critical-Care Nurses (AACN). *AACN Scope and Standards for Progressive and Critical Care Nursing Practice.* Aliso Viejo, CA: AACN; 2019.

38. Myers LC, Heard L, Mort M. Lessons learned from medical malpractice claims involving critical care nurses. *AJCC.* 2020;29(3):174–181.

39. Painter LM, Dudjak LA, Kidwell KM, Simmons RL, Kidwell RP. The nurse's role in the causation of compensable injury. *J Nurs Care Qual.* 2011;26(4):311–319.

40. *Lattimore V Dickey*, 23 Cal. App. 4th 959, 968 (2015).

41. For example, California: *Ybarra v Spangard*, 154 P.2d 687 (1944); Colorado: *Wood v Rowland*, 592 P.2d 1332 (1978); Delaware: *Larrimore V Homeopathic Hospital Association*, 176 A.2d 362 (1962); Minnesota: *Plutshack v University of Minnesota* Hospital, 316 NW2d 1 (1982); Montana: *Hunsaker v Bozeman Deaconess Foundation*, 588 P.2d 493 (1978); Pennsylvania: *Baur v Mesta Machine Co.,* 176 A.2d 684 (1962); Texas: *Childs V Greenville Hospital Authority*, 479 S.W.2d 399 (1972); and Washington: *Stone v Sisters of Charity of the House of Providence*, 469 P.2d 229 (1970).

42. *Clough v Lively*, 387 SE2d 573 (Ga. 1989).

43. *Keyser v Garner*, 922 P.2d 409 (Idaho 1996).

44. *Long v Methodist Hospital of Indiana*, 699 NE2d 1164 (Ind. 1998).

45. *Richardson V Miller*, 44 SW3d 1 (Tenn. 2000).

46. *Ginsberg v St. Michaels Hospital*, 678 A.2d 271 (NJ, 1996).

47. *G.S. v Dep't of Human Servs., Div. of Youth & Family Servs.*, 723 A.2d 612 (NJ, 1999).

48. *The Health Insurance Portability and Accountability Act of 1996 (HIPAA), Public Law 104-191.* 1996. Enacted on August 21.

49. Restatement of Torts (2nd), American Law Institute, §§ Vol. 13, 21 (1965).

50. *Owensboro Mercy Health System v Payne*, 24 SW3d 675 (Ky. 1999).

51. Berg JW, Appelbaum PS, Grisso T. Constructing competence: formulating standards of legal competence to make medical decisions. *Rutgers L Rev.* 1996;48:345.

52. *Patient Self Determination Act, Omnibus Budget Reconciliation Act of 1990.* Pub. L; 1990:101–508.

53. *Uniform Determination of Death Act.* 1981.

54. Wijdicks EF, Varelas PN, Gronseth GS, Greer DM, American Academy of Neurology. Evidence-based guideline update: determining brain death in adults, report of the Quality Standards Subcommittee of the American Academy of Neurology. *Neurology.* 2010;74:1912.

Facilitating Care Transitions

Kimberly Sanchez, Kathrine Anne Winnie, and Natalie B. de Haas-Rowland

CARE TRANSITIONS

Care transitions have been defined as changes in the setting where care is delivered[1] or as changes to the extent of health care services provided, including the degree of monitoring, assessing, planning, intervening, and evaluating.[2] Care transitions to and from critical care are determined by the severity of illness and intensity of services, with patients transitioning into critical care for advanced monitoring and technologies and from critical care when these requirements lessen.[3] See Table 3.1 for transitional locations and levels of care.

Fragmented care transitions negatively affect patients, families, health care professionals, and health care systems.[17] General examples include a lack of patient and caregiver engagement, poor continuity of care, insufficient patient knowledge regarding symptom management, lack of coordination of services, poor communication between the care team and patient/family, mismanaged chronic health conditions, and poor communication of treatment regimens.[18] Quality care transitions require a multifaceted approach that accounts for core components and patient-specific considerations.

CORE COMPONENTS TO ANY CARE TRANSITION

Management of Complex Health Issues and Medications

Recognition of patients at risk for poor outcomes is a strategy for managing complex health issues.[18] Patients with multiple chronic conditions, cognitive deficits, history of mental health issues, and frequent hospitalizations; those unable to independently perform activities of daily living; and older adults have been identified as being at high risk for complications in care transitions.[19] Once risk has been recognized, transitional care interventions for those patients are prioritized to reduce threats to safety and improve outcomes. Patient management is initiated with the assessment of health issues and, when necessary, early treatment of chronic conditions and symptoms. Routinely reviewing the appropriateness of ordered medications and dosages can prevent errors.[18]

Medication Reconciliation

According to The Joint Commission (TJC),[20] medication reconciliation is the process by which a provider compares a patient's current medication regimen to new medications that are ordered for the patient and resolves any discrepancies. A careful medication reconciliation should address duplications, omissions, possible interactions between medications, and the need to continue current medications. Medication errors on admission are frequent[21] with the most common error being that of omission.[22]

Successful performance of a thorough medication reconciliation can be affected by several factors: interfacility/intrafacility process variation, lack of agreement or understanding of each profession's role in the reconciliation process, dependence on the patient's ability to provide accurate medication information, time, and personnel.[22] Additionally, the introduction and expansion of the use of technology in the health care setting has brought its own set of challenges, including inadequate design, poor usability, and lack of evidence for user satisfaction. In addition to the barriers listed earlier, the importance of patient and family knowledge and motivation to maintain an updated list of all medications cannot be understated.

Patient and Family Education Strategies and Evaluation

The nurse must leverage every teachable moment and take advantage of the patient's readiness and willingness to learn without providing an overload of information that will then be easily forgotten. Nurses must recognize that learning does not usually take place in one session. Patients may be able to remember only two to three pieces of information in one education session, and a method such as teach-back may be needed to verify comprehension.[23] In verifying comprehension, the patient or family is asked to teach-back the information given and receive additional education if they are unable. These steps of asking the patient or family, gauging comprehension, and providing additional education are then repeated with the intent that the patient will be able to teach-back the content. When educating patients and families, nurses need to use teaching strategies and consider individual learning styles to facilitate the transfer of information.

Health Care Team Member Accountability

Interprofessional teams are made up of individuals from different professions and occupations with varied and specialized knowledge, skills, and approaches to providing care who communicate and work together as colleagues, to provide quality, individualized care for patients.[24] The purpose of the interprofessional health care team is to enhance patient outcomes through collaboration, communication, shared decision making, and shared goal setting.[25] Interprofessional team members offer recommendations specific to their scope of practice, participate in goal setting, and provide input on safety and quality issues.[25]

Common members of the interprofessional team in critical care areas include patients, families, nurses, providers, pharmacists, respiratory care practitioners, social workers, dietitians, physical therapists, occupational therapists, speech therapists, case managers, clergy, and representatives from other professions or occupations. During care transitions extending throughout the continuity of care from inpatient to outpatient settings, a specific individual may be tasked with additional

TABLE 3.1 Transitional Locations and Levels of Care

Acute Care Description

Other critical care area	Provides specialized monitoring and/or technology, advanced cardiopulmonary life support, and stabilization or management of complex acute injury and/or illness.[4] Transferring between critical care areas may be necessary to provide specific specialty care (e.g., stroke management),[5] when patients and their families prefer a hospital closer to home, or when type of insurance dictates facility used.
Step-down area	Provides intermediate services for unstable patients who no longer require critical care services or have deteriorated in telemetry or medical-surgical areas.[5,6]
Telemetry area	Provides stable patients with continuous electrocardiographic monitoring and/or interventions of greater intensity than those provided in medical-surgical areas.[5,7]
Medical-surgical area	Provides general medical and surgical care for stable patients with a wide variety of illnesses.[8]
Long-term acute care hospital (LTAC or LTACH) or long-term care hospital (LTCH)	Provides stable patients with time and services to address more than one chronic condition before returning home, usually necessitating a hospitalization longer than 25 days.[9]

Postacute Care

Inpatient rehabilitation area	Provides nursing services along with physical, occupational, and/or speech therapy after discharge from the acute phase of hospitalization with the goal of restoring optimal function before returning home. Patients admitted to a rehabilitation area must be able to tolerate and benefit from 3 hours of therapy each day at least 5 days per week.[9,10]
Subacute care area	Provides nursing and rehabilitation services after discharge from an acute hospitalization of 3 or more days before returning home. Patients admitted to a subacute care area require fewer hours of therapy per day than an inpatient rehabilitation area and more intense skilled care than a skilled nursing facility.[10,11]
Assisted living area	Provides a combination of housing, assistance with daily activities, and supportive wellness activities, which may or may not include health care services, with the goal of maximizing independence.[12]

Additional Services Provided in Various Settings (e.g., stand-alone facilities or within facilities or home)

Skilled care	Service provided daily by licensed professionals.[11] Skilled nursing care may include wound care treatments, intravenous therapy, and injections.
Palliative care	Provides relief from the symptoms of serious illness rather than focusing on the underlying disease process.[13]
Hospice care	Provides comprehensive medical and social support services throughout the dying process. Hospice services are normally rendered when life expectancy is less than 6 months.[13,14]
Custodial care (i.e., long-term care services)	Provides assistance with activities of daily living and does not require skilled care services.[11]

Additional Locations Within a Health Care Facility

Operating room	Where surgical procedures are performed and require an aseptic field.[15]
Procedural area	Where procedures are performed without requiring an aseptic field (e.g., interventional radiology).[15]
Emergency department	Provides 24-hour unscheduled medical care for patients experiencing trauma, acute illnesses, or other emergent conditions.[16]

responsibilities varying from performing supplemental assessments and interventions,[18] providing follow-up phone calls or home visits,[26] and coordinating care.[26] In some instances, this specific individual is an advanced practice nurse, such as a clinical nurse specialist or nurse practitioner,[18,26] a registered nurse or social worker,[26] or other health care (e.g., transitions navigator) or non–health care team members (e.g., care coordinator). Interprofessional teams work together and maintain mutual accountability for meeting team goals.[25] See Chapter 1 for further discussion regarding teamwork and collaboration.

Handoff

When a transfer of care is performed, the involved caregivers participate in a handoff process in which the sender will communicate sufficient breadth and depth of information to assist the receiver in safely and effectively performing patient care responsibilities. The sender should always encourage the receiver to ask questions and clarify discussion points.[27] Transitions from the operating room to critical care are unique, in that multiple members of the health care team will be giving handoff at the same time.[28] To reduce the fragmented approach to care, the operating room nurse, critical care nurse, critical care

provider, anesthesia provider, and surgeon should participate in one comprehensive postoperative handoff that addresses all aspects of the surgical case performed and the updated plan of care.[28] Team training focusing on effective communication may be necessary if the group handoff process is new to the organization.[28] A comprehensive process for handoff is important[27] to maintain and transfer responsibility among and between health care team members.[28]

Standardizing Handoffs

Using standardized elements and available documentation while providing verbal handoff communication at the bedside is preferred[28] and has been shown to improve the handoff process by reducing omissions of relevant information.[29] Standardized elements may be compiled in checklist, template, or script format and often incorporate a mnemonic such as SBAR (situation, background, assessment, and recommendation) or I-PASS (illness severity, patient summary, action list, situation awareness and contingency plans, and synthesis by the receiver)[27,28] to prompt the sharing of important information. Although the current plan of care, treatment goals, medical and psychosocial history, and current medications should be incorporated into and reviewed during the handoff process, other content to be shared may vary based on the patient's severity of illness and the intensity of services required.[27] Each care setting, level of care, or work group may adjust their standardized tool to fit the needs of their work area.[27] A standardized handoff communication process for transitions should be followed to reduce communication failures or misunderstandings that could lead to safety events.[27]

Continuity of Care

Planning for care transitions includes a robust consideration of patient and family needs for the next phase of their care. Many times this plan of care outlines the need for ensuring comprehension and implementation of self-management strategies, ordering and delivering necessary supplies, scheduling of additional services and follow-up appointments,[21] and evaluating the risks for mortality and readmission.[5] However, this plan is dependent on where the patient is on the continuum of care. The successful implementation of a patient's plan of care is also dependent on health care team members' knowledge, ability, and willingness to execute the plan as mutually agreed on to attain a shared patient goal.

Coordination of Physical Transport

Patients are at higher risk for adverse events during transport.[30] Commonly noted patient-centric adverse events during transport included physiologic alterations such as hypotension, increased oxygen requirements or decreased oxygen saturation, temperature alterations, patient discomfort, tissue damage, and anxiety or agitation. Non–patient-specific adverse events include equipment malfunctions such as battery failure, depletion of portable oxygen supplies,[31] tangling of lines, and accidental dislodgement of catheters or drains.

Transport protocols should include pretransport communication and coordination, a list of necessary equipment, monitoring guidelines, expected documentation, required transport personnel, and training.[31] Before patient transport, an analysis should be conducted to determine whether the benefit of the transport outweighs the risk.

It is recommended that a checklist be used when the decision is made to transport a patient.[30,32] The use of a checklist ensures that all appropriate safety measures are in place, thus reducing the risk of adverse events. The use of a checklist can also assist in identifying transports that may be considered higher risk. A comprehensive checklist should include physiologic red flags, such as high ventilator support requirements, unstable cervical fractures, and new or increasing vasopressor requirements.[31] These physiologic red flags can prompt the care team to consider additional safety measures for transport, such as the addition of a physician to the transport team for patients who are at higher likelihood of deterioration during transport.

The 2004 Critical Care Medicine Guidelines for Transport[33] recommend that at least two personnel accompany all critical care patients during transport. At least one team member should be a critical care nurse. The second team member may be a respiratory therapist or technician. In many institutions, a respiratory therapist must accompany patients who are mechanically ventilated during transport. The checklist should also incorporate a list of necessary equipment for safe transport and ensure that test-specific items such as the completion of a magnetic resonance imaging (MRI) safety screening or establishing working intravenous access for contrast administration are met before patient transport.

Critical care patients must receive the same physiologic monitoring during transport as in the critical care unit. When a patient is placed on different equipment for transport, such as switching from a bedside monitor to a portable monitor, it is recommended that the patient be monitored on the new equipment for a short trial before beginning transport to ensure all equipment is in working order. Monitoring and alarm parameters must also be checked, and patient-specific alarm settings must be programmed before transport.

Consideration should also be given to the availability of monitoring at the receiving destination. At a minimum the destination should have an oxygen source, suction, accessible electrical outlets, monitors with the same monitoring capabilities as critical care unit monitors, and a code cart.[31] In addition to standard electrocardiogram, pulse oximetry, and end-tidal CO_2 monitoring, critically ill patients often have additional monitoring parameters and equipment that have specific safety considerations. See Box 3.1 for special equipment considerations when transporting patients. Box 3.2 describes issues to consider when transporting isolation patients.

QSEN | **BOX 3.1   Safety**

Special Equipment Considerations for Transport

Urinary catheter: To reduce the risk of catheter-associated urinary tract infections (CAUTI), empty the urinary catheter drainage bag before transport[34] and avoid placing urinary catheter drainage bag on the gurney or bed during transport. Maintain the collection bag below the level of the bladder.[35] Ensure that the urinary catheter is secured to the patient's thigh to minimize the risk of trauma or dislodgement during transport.

Chest tubes: Take precautions to ensure that chest tubes are not dislodged during transport. Ensure that the chest tube drainage system is kept below the level of the chest to prevent backflow if the patient's chest tube is to water seal. Do not clamp chest tubes during transport. Portable suction should be used for patients with pneumothoraxes with large air leaks, high ventilatory requirements, or high chest tube output. Patients without these complications are typically safe to transport without suction until they arrive at the receiving destination, but a brief trial on water seal is recommended before transport.[31]

Pulmonary arterial lines: Pulmonary arterial lines must be continuously monitored during transport to ensure immediate identification of migration to the right ventricle, which may cause arrhythmias, and migration to the continuous wedge position, which may cause pulmonary artery infarct or perforation.[31]

Arterial lines: Arterial lines should be continuously monitored to ensure identification of arterial catheter dislodgement, which may result in significant blood loss.[33]

External ventricular drainage device (EVD)/lumbar drain: All patients with an EVD should have intracranial pressure (ICP) monitoring during transport. Traditionally, routine clamping of EVDs and lumbar drains has been recommended during transport to avoid complications associated with the overdrainage of cerebrospinal fluid (CSF). However, more recent literature suggests that routine clamping of EVDs and lumbar drains during transport may lead to elevated ICP or CSF measurements during transport, increasing the risk for further cerebrovascular injury. It is recommended that a trial be performed before transport to assess patient tolerance of a clamped EVD or lumbar drain before the decision to clamp the drain during transport.[36]

Extracorporeal Membrane Oxygenation (ECMO): Extracorporeal life support organization (ELSO) provides guidelines for the intrahospital transport of patients undergoing ECMO. https://www.elso.org/default.aspx.

QSEN BOX 3.2 **SAFETY**

Transporting Isolation Patients[37]

Contact Precautions

- Use personal protective equipment (PPE) appropriately, including gloves and gown. Wear a gown and gloves for all interactions that may involve contact with the patient or the patient's environment. Donning PPE upon room entry and properly discarding before exiting the patient room is done to contain pathogens.
- Limit transport and movement of patients outside of the room to medically necessary purposes. When transport or movement is necessary, cover or contain the infected or colonized areas of the patient's body. Remove and dispose of contaminated PPE and perform hand hygiene before transporting patients on contact precautions. Don clean PPE to handle the patient at the transport location.

Droplet Precautions

- Limit transport and movement of patients outside of the room to medically necessary purposes. If transport or movement outside of the room is necessary, instruct patient to wear a mask and follow respiratory hygiene/cough etiquette.

Airborne Precautions

- Limit transport and movement of patients outside of the room to medically necessary purposes. If transport or movement outside an airborne infection isolation room (AIIR) is necessary, instruct patients to wear a surgical mask, if possible, and observe respiratory hygiene/cough etiquette. Health care personnel transporting patients who are on airborne precautions do not need to wear a mask or respirator during transport if the patient is wearing a mask and infectious skin lesions are covered.

The availability of basic emergency medications should be considered before every transport. In addition to emergency medications, the transport team should ensure that enough quantities of all continuously infusing medications are available while the patient is receiving care outside of the critical care unit. Ensure that other important pretransport medications are considered, including analgesics and antianxiety medications, because these medications may not be readily available at the receiving destination. Lastly, if a patient is going to be in a procedural or diagnostic area for an extended period, any antibiotic medication that is scheduled during the off-unit time should be readily available and administered per provider orders.

SPECIAL CONSIDERATIONS DURING CARE TRANSITIONS

Changes in Baseline Physical and Cognitive Function

Frailty is an age- or disease-related state in which physiologic reserves have decreased, increasing a patient's risk for morbidity and mortality

TRENDING PRIORITIES IN HEALTHCARE

Patients Experiencing Homelessness

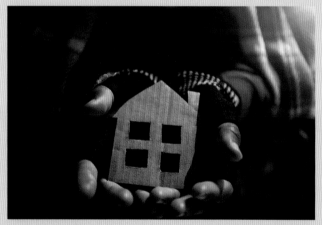

iStock.com/JubJob.

After a decade of decline from 2007–2016, homelessness has increased nationwide for the last several years beginning in 2017, with a little over 580,000 people experiencing homelessness in January 2020.[1] About 75% of the homeless population were adults over the age of 24 and most of them were in unsheltered locations such as streets or uninhabitable buildings.[1] Shelters for people experiencing homelessness are primarily emergency shelters, providing overnight beds, and transitional housing, providing up to 24 months of shelter and services.[1]

Discharge planning is needed for all patients admitted to the hospital. For patients experiencing homelessness, medical respite programs offer a short-term residence with access to medical and supportive care.[2] Patients experiencing homelessness who are ready to be discharged from the hospital but not

fully recovered to return to the streets or shelters may benefit from transitioning into a medical respite program.[2] Medical respite care is offered in a variety of settings, including stand-alone facilities, motels, or shelters,[2,3] with a varying extent of services provided, including clinical or support services.[3]

When patients experiencing homelessness are not transitioned into medical respite programs when indicated, they experience frustrations and stress from fragmented care, contributing to a transition to a suboptimal and unsafe environment for recovery.[4] There are 117 medical respite programs listed in the National Institute for Medical Respite Care directory, with 30 of those programs being operated by health centers.[3] In order to promote optimal care transitions, one must have knowledge of available resources and services for discharge planning, irrespective of the patient's housing situation.

For additional information about homelessness, check out the following website:

- National HealthCare for the Homeless Council—https://nhchc.org/.

References

1. United States Department of Housing and Urban Development. The 2020 annual homeless assessment report to congress. www.huduser.gov/portal/sites/default/files/pdf/2020-AHAR-Part-1.pdf. Accessed October 17, 2021.
2. National Institute for Medical Respite Care. Standards for medical respite/recuperative care programs. https://nimrc.org/wp-content/uploads/2021/09/Standards-for-Medical-Respite-Programs_2021_final.pdf. Accessed October 17, 2021.
3. National Institute for Medical Respite Care. State of medical respite/recuperative care programs. https://nimrc.org/wp-content/uploads/2021/08/State-of-Medical-Respite_Recup-Care-01.2021.pdf. Accessed October 17, 2021.
4. Biederman DJ, Gamble J, Manson M, Taylor D. Assessing the need for a medical respite: perceptions of service providers and homeless persons. J Community Health Nurs. 2014;31(3):145—156.

when exposed to internal or external stressors.[38] Up to 40% of frail patients experience prolonged lengths of stay in hospitals and higher readmissions from physical and cognitive complications compared with patients of the same age who are not frail.[38] When admitted to critical care areas, frail patients are at an increased risk of in-hospital deaths and reduced likelihood of survival after discharge.[38] The contributing factors of frailty should be addressed by an interprofessional team with the goal to restore optimal physical and cognitive function. Cognitive complications such as delirium are further addressed in Chapter 8.

Older Adults

As individuals age, cognitive, physiologic, and psychologic changes occur that must be considered during care transitions. Nates et al.[5] suggest decisions regarding critical care admission or discharge of adults over the age of 80 be inclusive of comorbidities, severity of illness, baseline functional status, and preferences—and not be based on age alone. See Chapter 6 for detailed information on best practices when providing care for the older adult patient.

Racial and Ethnic Disparities

Black and Hispanic individuals are at an increased risk for being admitted to the hospital compared with non-Hispanic White individuals.[39] Black patients with chronic conditions such as diabetes, hypertension, and asthma are three to five times more likely to be admitted to the hospital compared with non-Hispanic White patients.[39] Hispanic patients with the same chronic conditions are two to three times more likely to be admitted to the hospital compared with non-Hispanic White patients.[39] Once hospitalized, non-Hispanic White patients are 1.23 times more likely to receive referrals to home health care services than Hispanic patients after controlling for gender, insurance type, age, and length of stay.[40] Not having insurance was linked more to the observed disparities than was being Hispanic and should be considered when planning care transitions for this population.[40] Both Black and Hispanic patients had higher rates of preventable hospitalizations compared with non-Hispanic White individuals.[39] Asians, on the other hand, have lower rates of preventable hospitalizations compared with non-Hispanic White individuals.[39]

End of Life

Providing care at the end of life is an important and complex component of acute and critical care nursing. See Chapter 9 for detailed information on best practices in end-of-life and hospice care.

BOX 3.3 Informatics

Internet Resources: Facilitating Care Transitions
- Case Management Society of America: https://www.cmsa.org/
- Institute for Healthcare Improvement: www.ihi.org/knowledge/Pages/Tools/HowtoGuideImprovingTransitionstoReduceAvoidableRehospitalizations.aspx
- Quality Improvement Organizations: https://www.cms.gov/Medicare/Quality-Initiatives-Patient-Assessment-Instruments/QualityImprovementOrgs
- Stratis Health: http://www.stratishealth.org/index.html
- The Care Transitions Program: https://caretransitions.org/
- The National Transitions of Care Coalition: https://www.ntocc.org/
- World Health Organization: https://apps.who.int/iris/handle/10665/252272

ADDITIONAL RESOURCES

Refer to Box 3.3 for Internet resources related to facilitating care transitions.

REFERENCES

1. Coffey A, Mulcaby H, Savage E, et al. Transitional care interventions: relevance for nursing in the community. *Public Health Nurs.* 2017;34:454–460.
2. National Association of Clinical Nurse Specialists. Definitions of transitional care. 2020. https://nacns.org/professional-resources/toolkits-and-reports/transitions-of-care/definitions-of-transitional-care/.
3. Stacy K. Progressive care units: different but the same. *Crit Care Nurse.* 2011;31(3):77–83.
4. Society of Critical Care Medicine. Critical care statistics. n.d. https://www.sccm.org/Communications/Critical-Care-Statistics.
5. Nates JL, Nunnally M, Kleinpell R, et al. ICU admission, discharge, and triage guidelines: a framework to enhance clinical operations, development of institutional policies, and further research. *Crit Care Med.* 2016;44(8):1553–1602.
6. Prin M, Wunsch H. The role of stepdown beds in hospital care. *Am J Respir Crit Care Med.* 2014;190(11):1210–1216.
7. Chen EH, Hollander JE. When do patients need admission to a telemetry bed? *J Emerg Med.* 2007;33(1):53–60.
8. Academy of Medical-Surgical Nurses. *What is medical-surgical nursing?* 2020. https://www.amsn.org/practice-resources/what-medical-surgical-nursing.
9. Centers for Medicare & Medicaid Services. What are long-term care hospitals? 2019. https://www.medicare.gov/pubs/pdf/11347-Long-Term-Care-Hospitals.pdf.
10. Stefanacci RG. Admission criteria for facility-based post-acute services. *Ann Long-Term Care: Clin Care Aging.* 2015;23(11):18–20.
11. The Commission for Case Management Certification. Glossary of terms. n.d. https://ccmcertification.org/sites/default/files/docs/2019/ccmc-19-glossaryupdate.pdf.
12. National Centers for Assisted Living. What is assisted living 2020. https://www.ahcancal.org/ncal/about/assistedliving/Pages/What-is-Assisted-Living.aspx.
13. Buss MK, Rock LK, McCarthy EP. Understanding palliative care and hospice: a review for primary care providers. *Mayo Clin Proc.* 2017;92(2):280–286.
14. Bonebrake D, Culver C, Call K, Ward-Smith P. Clinically differentiating palliative care and hospice. *Clin J Oncol Nurs.* 2010;14(3):273–275.
15. Burlingame B. Facility Guidelines Institute Guidelines. Operating room requirements for 2014 and beyond. 2014. https://www.fgiguidelines.org/wp-content/uploads/2015/10/FGI_Update_ORs_140915.pdf.
16. Agency for Healthcare Research and Quality. *Emergency department performance measures and benchmarking summit: the consensus statement.* 2006. https://qualityindicators.ahrq.gov/Downloads/Resources/Publications/2006/EDPerformanceMeasures-ConsensusStatement.pdf.
17. Group Health's MacColl Institute for Healthcare Innovation. *Reducing care fragmentation: a toolkit for coordinating care.* Supported by The Commonwealth Fund; 2011. http://www.improvingchroniccare.org/index.php?p=Care_Coordination&s=326.
18. Naylor MD, Shaid EC, Carpenter D, et al. Components of comprehensive and effective transitional care. *J Am Geriatr Soc.* 2017;65:1119–1125.
19. Hirschman KB, Shaid E, McCauley K, Pauly MV, Naylor MD. Continuity of care: the transitional care model. *Online J Issues Nurs.* 2015;20(3):1.
20. The Joint Commission. *Sentinel event alert #35: using medication reconciliation to prevent errors*; 2005. https://www.jointcommission.org/-/media/tjc/documents/resources/patient-safety-topics/sentinel-event/sea_58_hand_off_comms_9_6_17_final_(1).pdf?db=web&hash=5642D63C1A5017BD214701514DA00139.
21. Rochester-Eyeguokan CD, Pincus KJ, Patel RS, Reitz SJ. The current landscape of transitions of care practice models: a scoping review. *Pharmacotherapy.* 2016;36(1):117–133.

22. Rungvivatjarus T, Kuelbs CL, Miller L, et al. Medication reconciliation improvement utilizing process redesign and clinical decision support. *Joint Comm J Qual Patient Saf*. 2020;46:27–36.

23. Agency for Healthcare Research and Quality. Use the teach-back method: tool #5. Content last reviewed February 2015. Rockville, MD; 2015. www.ahrq.gov/health-literacy/quality-resources/tools/literacy-toolkit/health-littoolkit2-tool5.html.

24. Institute of Medicine (US) Committee on the Health Professions Education Summit. Greiner AC, Knebel E. In: *Health Professions Education: A Bridge to Quality*. Washington, (DC): National Academies Press; 2003. www.ncbi.nlm.nih.gov/books/NBK221528/.

25. Franklin CM, Bernhardt JM, Lopez RP, Long-Middleton ER, Davis S. Interprofessional teamwork and collaboration between community health workers and healthcare teams: an integrative review. *Health Serv Res Manag Epidemiol*. 2015;2: 2333392815573312.

26. Enderlin CA, McLeskey N, Rooker JL, et al. Review of current conceptual models and frameworks to guide transitions of care in older adults. *Geriatr Nurs*. 2013;34(1):47–52.

27. Jewell JA, AAP Committee on Hospital Care. Standardization of inpatient handoff communication. *Pediatrics*. 2016;138(5):e20162681.

28. Rhudy L. Handoff from operating room to intensive care unit: specific pathways to decrease patient adverse events. *Nurs Clin North Am*. 2019;54:335–345.

29. Rhudy LM, Johston MR, Kreckle CA, et al. Change-of-shift nursing handoff interruptions: implications for evidence-based practice. *Worldviews Evid Based Nurs*. 2019;0:1–9.

30. Comeau OY, Armendariz-Batiste J, Woodby SA. Safety first! Using a checklist for intrafacility transport of adult intensive care patients. *Crit Care Nurse*. 2015;35(5):16–25.

31. Day D. Keeping patients safe during intrahospital transport. *Crit Care Nurse*. 2010;30(4):18–32.

32. Williams P, Karuppiah S, Greentree K, Darvall J. A checklist for intra-hospital transport of critically ill patients improves compliance with transportation safety guidelines. *Aust Crit Care*. 2020;33:20–24.

33. Warren J, Fromm RE, Orr RA, Rotello LC, Horst M, American College of Critical Care Medicine. Guidelines for the inter- and intrahospital transport of critically ill patients. *Crit Care Med*. 2004;32(1):256–262.

34. Gould CV, Umscheid C, Agarwal RK, Kuntz G, Pegues DA. The healthcare infection control practices committee. Indications for an indwelling (foley) catheter. *UroToday*. 2013.

35. Gould CV, Umscheid C, Agarwal RK, Kuntz G, Pegues DA. The Healthcare Infection Control Practices Committee. Guideline for prevention of catheter-associated urinary tract infections. Centers for Disease Control & the Department of Health & Human Services; 2009. www.cdc.gov/infectioncontrol/pdf/guidelines/cauti-guidelines-H.pdf. Updated 2019.

36. Chaikittisilpa N, Lele AV, Lyons VH, et al. Risk of routinely clamping external ventricular drains for intrahospital transport in neurocritically ill cerebrovascular patients. *Neurocritical Care*. 2017;26:196–204.

37. Centers for Disease Control and Prevention. Transmission-based precautions; 2016. www.cdc.gov/infectioncontrol/basics/Transmission-based-precautions.html.

38. Gibson JA, Crowe S. Frailty in critical care: examining implications for clinical practices. *Crit Care Nurse*. 2018;38(3):29–35.

39. Russo CA, Andrews RM, Coffey RM. Racial and ethnic disparities in potentially preventable hospitalizations, 2003. HCUP statistical brief #10. Rockville, MD: Agency for Healthcare Research and Quality; 2006. https://www.ncbi.nlm.nih.gov/books/NBK63497/.

40. Crist JD, Koerner KM, Hepworth JT, et al. Differences in transitional care provided to mexican american and non-Hispanic White older adults. *J Transcult Nurs*. 2017;28(2):159–167.

Psychosocial and Spiritual Considerations

Margaret J. Halter and Carrie J. Scotto

STRESS

The term *stress* is usually used to indicate a negative experience or internal tension. However, stress may also indicate an acute stress response that is an essential and protective reaction to a stressor, designed to mobilize the body's response to threats for the purpose of survival.

Stress is more formally defined as a nonspecific response to any demand placed on a person to adapt or change and can come from physical, emotional, social, spiritual, cultural, chemical, or environmental sources.[1]

Another term associated with the concept of stress is *stressor*. A stressor is any event or condition in the environment that brings about anxiety or stress. It is useful to note that responses to environmental events or conditions are highly individual. What one person perceives as stressful may not be anxiety producing to others. For example, some people are terribly afraid of injections, whereas others seem to be unfazed by them.

Stress Response

Stress of any type, whether positive or negative, biologic, psychologic, spiritual, or social, elicits the same physical responses. Classic stress theory describes stress as a stimulus, a response, and a transaction. Selye[2] was one of the first to describe the body's responses to stress. He identified three stages in the stress response: alarm, resistance, and exhaustion. Collectively, these stages are known as the general adaptation syndrome. In this chapter, these stages are described in terms of the body's neurohormonal response to stress. These responses begin with the initial event and may progress to the compensatory phase, progressive phase, and refractory stage.

Initial Event

An *initial event*, such as trauma, infection, or hypersensitivity, sets the stress response in motion. The stress response begins with the release of the two major neurotransmitters in the sympathetic nervous system, epinephrine and norepinephrine, which work to maintain normal cardiovascular function until the stress resolves. The *sympathetic response* is a highly integrated cardiovascular and endocrine event that produces elevations in blood pressure, respiratory rate, heart rate, and glucose production. Individuals experiencing this response may sweat profusely, exhibit tremors, and feel nauseated.

Compensatory Phase

During the *compensatory phase*, the body's resources work to counteract the effects of stress. However, people cannot sustain this level of responsiveness for long because resources become depleted. If relief is not achieved, the individual moves to the next phase of the stress response.

Progressive Phase

In the *progressive phase*, the body's resources are nearly depleted, and the individual relies on health care personnel to sustain them. Critical care treatment that includes vigilant assessment, fluids and medications, and technology is required to sustain the individual through the crisis and to restore homeostasis.

Refractory Stage

If the stressor persists or the treatment is ineffective in resolving the patient's problem, the individual moves into the refractory stage. The *refractory stage* signals the beginning of systems failure. At this point, it is not possible to recover from the illness or injury.

STRESSORS IN CRITICAL CARE

Critically ill patients experience distressing physical reactions, lack of control, fear of medical equipment, loss of meaning, and disturbed relationships during and after treatment in a critical care unit. Box 4.1 identifies stressors faced by critical care patients. See Appendix A, Patient Care Management Plan: Stress Overload.

COPING WITH STRESS AND ILLNESS

Coping Mechanisms

Coping mechanisms are conscious and unconscious processes used to adjust, adapt, and navigate life stressors. Each person's response to stress is unique and depends on a variety of internal and external variables. These variables include developmental life stages, cognitive ability, perception of the stressors, and degrees of support.

People who cope effectively tend to be comfortable with themselves and others. They are able to accurately interpret stressors, make decisions consistent with personal preferences and values, and access external resources.

BOX 4.1 Common Stressors for Patients in Critical Care Units

- Pain, discomfort, and physical restrictions
- Unfamiliar environments with excessive light, noises, alarms, and distressing events
- Loss of ability to express oneself verbally when intubated
- Unfamiliar bodily sensations resulting from bed rest, medications, surgery, or symptoms
- Threat of death
- Lack of sleep
- Loss of autonomy and control over one's body, environment, privacy, and daily activities
- Boredom broken only by brief visits, threatening stimuli, and procedural touch
- Separation from family, friends, and meaningful social roles and work
- Loss of dignity, embarrassing exposures, and a sense of vulnerability
- Worry about finances, potential job loss, and stress on loved ones
- Uncertainty about future and fear of permanent residual health deficits
- Unanswered spiritual questions and concerns about meaning of the events and life

Individual response to stressors depends on:
- Individual's perception of stressors
- Acute or chronic nature of stressors
- Cumulative effect of multiple stressors
- Effectiveness of the individual's usual coping strategies and style
- Degree of social support

Psychologic Responses

Psychologic Defense Mechanisms

Psychologic defense mechanisms are automatic coping methods that protect people from anxiety. Adaptive defense mechanisms are considered to be healthy. Maladaptive defensive mechanisms are considered unhealthy. They occur when one or more defense mechanisms are used to excess, especially immature defense mechanisms. Two common maladaptive defense mechanisms common to critical care settings are regression and denial.

Regression. Regression is an unconscious defense mechanism. It is characterized by reverting to an earlier developmental level in response to stress. Regression often occurs when patients are forced to give up former roles, autonomy, and privacy. This type of regression is natural as patients relinquish control and rely on others for the most basic needs.

In a way, regression is actually adaptive. To stay in control and resist the care that others provide could jeopardize a patient's health. However, too much regression may result in patients abandoning all control and responsibility for themselves and becoming excessively dependent on others. Behaviors such as complaining, moaning, and excessive emotion can interfere with recovery. Extreme regression may also negatively affect nurse-patient relationships.

Denial. Denial is conscious and unconscious attempts to escape unpleasant or anxiety-provoking thoughts, needs, feelings, and wishes by ignoring their existence.[1] Critically ill patients or their family members may use denial as a defense mechanism to protect against an overwhelming sense of threat brought on by illness, injury, or impending death.

Denial may be healthy and protective, allowing people to accept realities gradually. It allows the unconscious mind to absorb and process distressing information. *Unhealthy denial* is excessive. Too much denial prevents people from acting when they need to.

Family members and significant others also use denial. If they are unable to cope with a loved one's serious, possibly irreversible illness, they may only focus on recovery. Manifestations of denial include resisting realistic discussions about the patient's prognosis, insisting on resuscitation no matter how grave the condition, or investing in home remodeling to support the patient's return. Mistrust and hostility may be directed at caregivers who do not share the same hope. Family members are best supported by caregivers who recognize the protectiveness of denial. See Appendix A, Patient Care Management Plan: Impaired Family Coping.

Anxiety

Anxiety is a normal subjective human response to a perceived or actual response and can range from a vague, generalized feeling of discomfort to a state of panic and loss of control. Feelings of anxiety are common in critically ill patients but are often undetected by care providers.[3]

Anxiety and agitation in critical care patients can complicate patient recovery secondary to unplanned extubating, episodes of shortness of breath, and behavioral changes.[4] The physiologic effects of anxiety can produce negative effects in critically ill patients by activating the sympathetic nervous system, as previously discussed.

Somatic symptoms such as headache, nausea, dizziness, and insomnia may increase. Patients in severe levels of anxiety may have a pounding heart, hyperventilation, and a sense of doom.

Critical care nurses most often rely on behavioral indicators, such as agitation and restlessness, and physiologic parameters, such as increased heart rate and blood pressure, to gauge anxiety.[5] However, behavioral or vital sign changes do not provide consistently reliable indicators of anxiety and may lead to underestimation of the extent of anxiety in critical care patients.

ALTERATIONS IN SELF-CONCEPT

The stressors imposed by serious illness, trauma, and surgical procedures can cause disturbances in the patient's self-concept. *Self-concept* is a perception of one's own behavior, abilities, and unique characteristics. It develops as a result of a person's own experiences, interactions with others and the environment, and how those interactions are valued. Self-concept also includes body image, self-esteem, and self-identity.[1]

Self-concept evolves over the lifespan. Patients admitted to critical care settings may experience self-concept challenges as their self-perceptions shift according to circumstances. Patients in critical care units have little time to adjust to their altered health status, and they may be unable to clearly understand the implications of the situation. Self-concept constructs of particular relevance for critical care patients include body image, self-esteem, and personal identity.

Disturbed Body Image

The physical body is central to an individual's self-concept. *Body image* is the mental picture we have of our bodies and its physical functioning at a given time. Body image includes attitudes and feelings about one's appearance, abilities, and gender. Body image evolves over time. It is influenced by interpersonal and environmental interactions and emotional experiences and aspirations both past and present.

Bodily sensations in a state of illness are often unfamiliar and may not make sense to the patient, which creates a cascade of stress responses.[6] Patients in critical care units experience prolonged confinement to the bed, position disorientation, sensory deprivation, muscle atrophy, metabolic pattern alteration, mechanical ventilation, pain, profound weakness, nutritional alterations, and medication-induced physical symptoms.

Disturbances in body image in critical care arise when the person fails to perceive or adapt to the changes that are imposed by the situation. In some instances, the individuals may feel betrayed by a body that no longer seems under control. Body image issues often emerge and resolve over time. See Appendix A, Patient Care Management Plan: Disturbed Body Image.

Low Self-Esteem

Self-esteem refers to how well one's behavior correlates with a sense of the ideal self and is closely linked to one's sense of self-worth. Maslow[7] identified self-esteem as an important component in his hierarchy of human needs. Having a strong self-esteem helps a person deal with maturational and situational life crises more easily.

The effect of self-esteem on a patient's energy and recovery is significant. Illness robs a person of perspective, often leading to a situational low self-esteem and feelings of powerlessness, helplessness, and depression. Low self-esteem impairs one's ability to adapt. A patient may refuse to participate in self-care, exhibit self-destructive behavior, or become passive, asking no questions and permitting others to make all decisions.

A comprehensive approach to recovery includes the provision of ongoing supportive measures designed to help patients promote and maintain self-esteem. See Appendix A, Patient Care Management Plan: Situational Low Self-Esteem.

Disturbed Personal Identity

Disturbed personal identity is the inability of a person to differentiate the self as a unique and separate human being from others within a social environment. The sense of depersonalization that accompanies identity disturbance results in high levels of anxiety.

Personal identity disturbance can result from the effects of psychoactive medications; biochemical imbalances in the brain; and organic brain disorders, dementia, traumatic brain injury, amnesia, or delirium (see Chapters 4, 8, and 17).

A careful nursing assessment, including the use of psychiatric or neurologic consultation, is essential in cases of identity disturbance. Disorientation and confusion—common in patients in critical care settings—are influenced by several factors, including the severity of the physical problem, chemical imbalances, sensory overload or deprivation, and previous illness or health care experiences.

COMPROMISED DIGNITY

A sense of human dignity is the foundation for self-concept. A *sense of dignity* includes a person's positive self-regard, an ability to invest in one's own life, and feeling valued by others. When people are treated with dignity and respect, they are put in the best position to recover their health and well-being.

During a critical health care stay, patients are subjected to intense physical, psychologic, and lifestyle scrutiny.[8] They are literally and figuratively exposed at a highly vulnerable moment. Patients in acute care settings must, by necessity, give up the things that give them a sense of self: clothing, daily habits, and privacy. Their bodies are frequently uncovered to people who assess them for pathology and irregularities.

Often patients cannot communicate their preferences or give permission for assessments, tests, or interventions. Family members and other support people have restricted access to patients and are unable to speak on the patient's behalf.

The critical care environment has its own culture that influences the behaviors of the health care providers. The cultural rules of critical care environments include objectification of the person for more precise physiologic management, disempowerment, distancing the self from the experience of others, and indifference.

Supporting and maintaining dignity and privacy is a basic role of nurses. In the critical care setting, nurses practicing dignity-conserving care seek to identify sources of threats to dignity inherent in health care contexts, including the level of a person's independence and symptoms of distress.[8] Caregivers who are more aware of their own feelings and humanity are less likely to unintentionally minimize patients' emotions and experiences.[8,9]

Powerlessness

Control, a person's ability to determine the use of time, space, and resources, is compromised in the critical care unit. Basic issues such as the choice of clothing and use of other personal belongings are restricted. Patients cannot decide who enters the room, who provides personal care, or who intrudes with painful treatments.

Perception of control is dependent on a person's locus of control.[10] Individuals who have an internal locus of control perceive themselves to be responsible for the outcome of events. Individuals with an external locus of control believe that their actions have no effect on the outcome of a situation.

Patients who believe they can do nothing to change or control their circumstances are at risk for powerlessness. The degree of powerlessness a person experiences depends on a perceived sense of control, the type of loss that was experienced, and the availability of social support.

Powerlessness can be manifested by a refusal to participate in decision making, disengagement from the plan of care, expressions of self-doubt, or a seeming lack of interest in recovery. Frustration, anger, and resentment over being dependent on others often occur and are exhibited in verbal expressions regarding dissatisfaction with care.

Poor interactions with health care providers who are perceived as imposing restrictions can make the situation worse. Patients may react aggressively, may try bargaining, or may refuse to comply with diagnostic and treatment regimens. Patients may become apathetic regarding areas of life over which they still maintain some influence because so much control has been taken from them. See Appendix A, Patient Care Management Plan: Powerlessness.

SPIRITUAL RESPONSES

Many of the psychosocial issues already discussed in this chapter are rooted in the spiritual dimension of life, an area with the deepest importance for many people. The spiritual dimension encompasses the elements of life that provide meaning, purpose, hope, and connectedness to others and a higher power.[11] Providing spiritual care is an essential aspect for patient recovery in critical care units.

Spiritual Distress

Spiritual distress is a disruption in the life principle that defines a person and transcends the biologic and psychosocial nature. Physical or psychiatric illness, prolonged pain, and suffering can challenge a person's spirituality. Separation from religious or spiritual practices and rituals, coupled with pain, may bring about spiritual distress for both patients and their families.

Patients experiencing spiritual distress may question the meaning of suffering and death in relation to their personal belief system. They may wonder why the illness or injury has happened to them or may believe that a higher power has failed them in the time of greatest need.

Some people may question their existence, verbalize a wish to die, or express anger. Unresolved spiritual distress may lead to a sense of hopelessness and an unwillingness to consent to further treatment. See Appendix A, Patient Care Management: Impaired Spiritual Status.

Hopelessness

Hope is a subjective, dynamic internal process essential to life. Considered to be a spiritual process, hope arises out of a sense of being meaningfully connected to one's self, others, and powers greater than the self. With hope, a person is able to transition from a state of vulnerability to a point of being able to live as fully as possible.[12] The need for hope is stimulated by a demand to adapt or change in unexpected situations, as is the case for people who are critically ill.

Hope underlies many coping mechanisms. When people have hope and belief in their goals, they are empowered to engage in their own recovery. Although hope has a future orientation, it also has a present orientation that affects people in the here and now. Through observations of people in extreme circumstances, an element of hope must be maintained for survival[13] and is an essential component in the successful treatment of illness.

By contrast, *hopelessness* is a subjective state in which an individual sees extremely limited or no alternatives and is unable to mobilize energy. Feelings of hopelessness can greatly hinder recovery.[14] Conditions that increase a person's risk for feeling hopeless include a loss of dignity, long-term stress, loss of self-esteem, spiritual distress, and isolation, all of which can occur in a critical care experience.

PSYCHOSOCIAL SUPPORT

Providing Holistic Care

Critical care nurses possess sophisticated knowledge of anatomy and physiology, the pathophysiology of disease processes, and appropriate nursing interventions. In addition, nurses who practice holistic critical care also need the knowledge, wisdom, and skills to interpret the internal human responses to experiences of serious illness or injury.

Attention to the whole patient is the ultimate goal of nursing care and is vitally important for critical care patients, families, and nurses. Essential skills that underlie nursing interventions for psychosocial-spiritual care include using communication patterns based on compassion and care, practicing dignity-enhancing care, supporting patient coping, using a family-centered focus, and engaging spiritual resources.

Complementary and Alternative Therapies

Integrative health care practices involve a blending of allopathic medical health care methods with patient-identified complementary therapies.[15] The type of complementary or integrative therapies used depends on a patient's preferences, coping style, physical capabilities, and personality type.

Although more research is needed to support the value of complementary therapies on selected outcomes in critically ill hospitalized patients, early studies support their potential as therapeutic nursing interventions (also see Chapter 1).

Psychosocial Interventions

Although physical care is essential to preserving life, psychosocial interventions are not only life affirming but are also life sustaining. Feeling alone, marginalized, and powerless may result in losing the will to live and cause increased physical compromise and decline.

Fortunately, despite the fast-paced environment of critical care settings, the relatively small nurse-to-patient ratio may provide the time necessary for emotional and spiritual support. This type of support can even be provided while providing physical care. The following paragraphs summarize essential psychosocial interventions.

Therapeutic Communication

Therapeutic verbal and nonverbal communication are essential elements of patient care in the critical care environment. In fact, patients and family members rank their needs for communication with health care providers as one of the most important aspects of feeling cared for in the critical care setting. Facilitating communication rises to a new level when caring for patients who are unable to speak.[16–19]

Nelson et al.[20] described the top challenges to providing care in the critical areas, especially for seriously ill patients. None of the most common challenges had to do with technical issues of medical management. Instead, the top challenges include areas that relate specifically to communication. See Box 4.2, Challenges in Providing Caring Communication.

Patients also reported less stress when they perceived nurses as caring, warm, and competent, and when nurses demonstrated respect.[21] Patients interpret a nurse's expression of empathy and physical contact as evidence of caring and support.[21]

Sharing concerns with an attentive and responsive listener helps to reduce emotional or spiritual distress. Patients are comforted knowing that they are not alone when they sense that someone knows and cares about their feelings and experiences.

Although patients may share concerns with family members, they may be reluctant to burden them and may find that talking to a nurse feels emotionally safer. Most patients need to talk about their fears and prefer conversations that balance their needs for honesty with their need to maintain hope.[22]

Careful medical and nursing assessments, use of family and team conferences, and consulting a pastoral care provider lead to more effective crisis and decision-making conversations. Box 4.3 contains strategies for communicating with patients and family members in critical care settings.

Promoting Trust

Effective verbal and nonverbal communication are essential for the development of trust in a nurse-patient relationship. *Trust* manifests itself in the belief of critical care patients that the people they depend on will get them through the illness and will be able to manage complications.

BOX 4.2 Challenges to Providing Therapeutic Communication

- Impaired verbal communication due to mechanical ventilation
- Diminished quality of communication due to clinical condition (e.g., sedation, fatigue, delirium, neurologic disease)
- Inadequate communication between the family members and staff
- Insufficient knowledge or prioritization of effective communication by the staff
- Unrealistic family and provider expectations
- Family conflict regarding approaches to patient care and decision making (e.g., end-of-life care)
- Lack of advance directives
- Challenging environment for meaningful conversations

QSEN

BOX 4.3   Patient-Centered Care

Strategies for Communicating With Patients and Family Members

- Be patient. What is routine for caregivers can be stressful and new to patients and family members.
- Repeat information as many times as necessary. Stress reduces concentration, memory, and comprehension, especially in unfamiliar situations.
- Assess patient and family knowledge level and prior experience with critical care.
- Use understandable language and define medical terms without talking down.
- Ask clarifying questions to help validate understanding.
- Use a welcoming, open communication style. Critical care units can feel intimidating to people unfamiliar with the environment.
- Offer frequent updates regarding the patient's condition, even if not asked.
- Engage in conversations of meaning with patients and family members, even if brief. Often critical care conversations are reduced to conveying only technical aspects of care.
- Honor privacy and provide space for family conferences.
- Speak to patients, even if they are unconscious. This conveys caring to family, and words may comfort the patient even if there is no response.
- Use communication boards or other devices with patients who are unable to speak.
- Give patients time to respond and ask questions they can answer easily.
- Speak slowly and look at patients when communicating. Gestures, lip movements, and facial expressions convey important messages.

A patient needs to trust the nurse's competence in the physical and technical aspects of care and rely on what the nurse says. Trust and hope are decreased when inaccurate information is given or nurses do not follow through on what they say. See Appendix A, Patient Care Management Plan: Impaired Verbal Communication.

Enhancing Dignity

The practice of care that enhances a patient's dignity is anchored in authentic human presence, the giving of one's whole attention and being to another person in a given moment. When authentically present, a nurse goes beyond scientific information and is attuned to a patient's needs, experiences, and emotions in a way that facilitates healing.[23]

Dignity-enhancing perspectives include the need a person has to maintain a continuity of the self, one's roles, and legacy. Dignity-enhancing care has four components: attitude, behaviors, compassion, and dialogue. A nurse's first step in providing dignity-conserving care involves reflecting on personal attitudes and assumptions about other people and their situations.

Dignity-enhancing care is manifest in behaviors. Attending to the patient's physical appearance affirms the person's self-esteem and a healthy body image. Cleanliness and absence of body odors give patients a sense of worth. When providing physical care, provide privacy, respect social boundaries, and ask permission before touching when possible.

Validate the patient by respecting personal preferences. Simply spending time with patients as they share their life stories helps the nurse know the patient better and facilitates the development of patient-centered interventions. Calling them by their preferred names or titles helps to reinforce the patient's self-concept and identity.

Obtain the patient's permission to include others in private conversations.[21]

Communicating With Compassion

Compassion refers to the awareness of another person's suffering coupled with a sincere intention to alleviate emotional and physical distress. In compassion, caregivers are able to identify with another person and recognize a shared humanity. Showing compassion can be simple, in acts of consideration, kindness, or a simple touch.

Critical care nurses frequently touch people in the completion of procedures and caregiving activities. Keeping in mind individual and cultural differences, nurses include nonprocedural touch in their care. The use of touch intended to communicate care and comfort can be an important part of patient healing and interpersonal connection.

Compassion is also evidenced in dialogue, the fourth element of dignity-conserving care. At the most basic level, patients and family members need timely updates, explanations, repetition of unfamiliar information, and thorough information sharing. At a deeper level, patients need to feel that they are heard by their caregivers and know that their personhood is valued and respected.

Promoting Optimal Coping

A goal of expert psychosocial-spiritual care is to promote patient and family flourishing, empowering them to experience as much control and predictability as possible. As noted earlier, coping is a dynamic process involving cognitive and behavioral efforts to manage specific internal or external demands that are perceived to exceed the person's resources. The key to effective coping is to encourage the use of the best mix of strategies appropriate for a given situation.

Most adults cope by relying on their previously developed conscious and unconscious coping strategies and defense mechanisms, which are automatically triggered in a stressful situation. Teaching new coping skills to people who are experiencing acute psychologic stress may be unrealistic. However, by using active listening skills and initiating conversations with patients and family members, the nurse can identify the coping resources, skills, and preferences that may be most helpful.

Supporting Self-Control

One of the most effective ways to decrease the stress of being in a critical care environment is giving patients as much control over their care and the environment as possible. Allow patients to make decisions as they are able, such as how and when to administer personal hygiene, diet preferences, and the timing of nursing interventions. Inform patients and family members about daily activities and the purpose and effects of tests or therapies. See Appendix A, Patient Care Management Plan: Powerlessness.

Engaging Spiritual Resources

A time of crisis can also lead to a time of positive spiritual renewal and readiness for an enhanced spiritual life. Spiritual and religious beliefs and practices often give patients and family members some measure of acceptance of an illness, a sense of mastery and control, strength to endure the stressors of illness, and a source of hope and trust beyond what medical interventions can provide.

Transformative spiritual care strategies are particularly helpful in times of crisis and uncertainty. When faced with significant life challenges, people need resources to transcend their circumstances and know that no matter what happens, they will endure. Spiritual resources include faith in a higher power, support communities, a sense of hope and meaning in life, and religious practices. Patient and family spirituality affects their ability to cope with loss.[24] See Appendix A, Patient Care Management Plan: Impaired Spiritual Status.

Environmental Support

People are continuous with their environments. Alterations in the physical environment of critical care units can provide a sense of calm, enhance patient coping, and facilitate healing.[15] Nurses can make changes in care environments to give patients a greater sense of comfort and familiarity while they are in the unit.

Critical care areas are bright, loud, and busy. Close patient doors, turn off unnecessary equipment, and limit conversation at workstations. Music can promote relaxation in critical care areas when used during waking hours and with patient consent. Allow for natural sunlight if possible, and position patients so that they can see out of windows, which helps maintain orientation to time.

Familiarize patient rooms by displaying photographs, cards, drawings, and favored items. Sleep deprivation is a serious concern in critical care environments. Plan care activities to limit nighttime interruptions and collaborate with laboratory and other staff to decrease sleep interruptions.[15] The use of earplugs during sleeping hours has been shown to improve patients' subjective experience of sleep.[25]

FAMILY-CENTERED CARE

Family-centered care, an American Association of Critical-Care Nurses (AACN) practice standard for critical care, formalizes the patient and family as the unit of care. *Family-centered care* is based on the belief that patients and families should participate in decisions together and that patients need their families for love, understanding, and support while coping with critical illness.[22]

The patient determines who counts as family. Biologic or legal issues notwithstanding, it is the nature of the patient's relationships that determines the extent of interaction with others. Nurses working in critical care settings recognize the need to expand the definition of family. This expansion reflects the reality of nontraditional combinations of people including LGBTQ2S+ families, chosen families, and multigeneration families.

The elements essential to family-centered care include respect, collaboration, and support. Research demonstrates that family members of critical care patients want understandable information that is given in a timely manner. They want reassurance that their loved one is being monitored and is receiving the best care possible.

Research has demonstrated that stressors for families of patients in the critical care setting were affected by the change in family dynamics, behavior of the patient, the care setting, and communication with the health care team.[26] They also identified repeated stress during the stay and persistent negative emotional feelings.[27] Journal writing and maintaining intensive care unit (ICU) diaries by families has been offered as a method to document experiences and interactions.[28,29]

Family members also need to be allowed access to their loved ones.[22] Some family members are reassured by helping with caregiving if this is acceptable to the patient.

Family members are particularly sensitive to a nurse's words and actions, making it essential that the nurse conveys understanding and acceptance.

Critical care nurses observe the quality of the patient-family interaction and formulate interventions that will aid the family in supporting the patient.[22] Providing interventions aimed at supporting family members is an ongoing process that continues throughout the patient's stay in the unit.

Visitation Policies

Although practices vary among critical care units, a more relaxed visitation policy humanizes the environment and facilitates healing. The AACN Practice Alert, *Family Presence: Visitation in the Adult ICU*,[30] recommends giving unrestricted access of hospitalized patients to a chosen support person. Giving family members access to their loved ones enhances patient and family satisfaction and improves safety of care.

Family members have insight into the patient's behaviors and preferences, especially with patients who are unable to communicate. Interacting with family members reduces patient anxiety and enhances a sense of control.[22] Including patients and family members in critical care interdisciplinary rounds has been shown to improve perceptions of accessibility and communication.[31]

COMORBID PSYCHIATRIC DISORDERS

Patients admitted to critical care settings may have comorbid or coexisting psychiatric disorders (i.e., having more than one condition at the same time). Major depressive disorder, bipolar disorder, substance use disorders, and suicidality may be the primary precipitants of a critical care hospitalization.

The critical care team strives to continue the use of psychotropic medications for patients during the critical care stay unless medically contraindicated. In addition to disrupting the therapeutic regimen, abruptly discontinuing medication such as antidepressants and antipsychotics may result in a discontinuation syndrome. This syndrome includes extreme discomfort along with other symptoms such as nausea, vomiting, and headaches. If the patient is unable to continue oral medications, alternative routes are explored. In the absence of alternative routes of administration, switching medications may be considered.

Alcohol Withdrawal

Nurses in critical care settings are alert to the symptoms of withdrawal from chemical substances, but a full substance use assessment is often omitted in emergency admissions. Alcohol withdrawal is of particular concern, considering that the lifetime prevalence for alcohol use disorder is nearly 30%.[32] In fact, alcohol use may affect 20% to 25% of admissions in the critical care unit.[33]

Without treatment, withdrawal from alcohol typically begins 6 to 8 hours after reducing or quitting alcohol after heavy and prolonged use. The classic sign of alcohol withdrawal is tremulousness, commonly called the shakes or the jitters. Within 24 to 72 hours, vital signs—systolic and diastolic blood pressure, pulse, and body temperature—tend to increase. Sleep disturbance, nausea and vomiting, agitation, and anxiety are other symptoms.

Psychotic and perceptual changes may begin within 2 to 4 days after heavy alcohol cessation. At this point, patients are at risk for unconsciousness and delirium. Generalized tonic-clonic seizure is another serious symptom of alcohol withdrawal. Diazepam (Valium) given intravenously is a common treatment for these seizures.

Alcohol withdrawal delirium, also known as delirium tremens (DTs), is the most serious consequence of abstaining from alcohol. This medical emergency typically begins in 3 days but may take a week or more to manifest. Individuals who progress to this level are typically older and have other physical problems, particularly brain injury and liver disease. See Box 4.4 for additional alcohol withdrawal delirium symptoms.

BOX 4.4 Additional Alcohol Withdrawal Delirium Symptoms

- Disorientation, confusion, and severe anxiety
- Longer lasting hallucinations (primarily visual)
- Profuse sweating
- Seizures
- High blood pressure
- Racing and irregular heartbeat
- Severe tremors
- Low-grade fever

Commonly used medications for withdrawal symptoms include the benzodiazepines, such as chlordiazepoxide and lorazepam. Carbamazepine, an anticonvulsant, is also used for treating withdrawal symptoms and carries minimal risk of misuse.

In the event of delirium, benzodiazepines may be given intravenously. The beta-adrenergic receptor antagonists and clonidine reduce sympathetic hyperactivity. Ondansetron and promethazine may be used for nausea. As alcohol use is often accompanied by dietary deficiencies, thiamine, folic acid, and multivitamins are often added to intravenous fluids. See also Chapter 20, Alcohol Screening Questionnaire.

Nonfatal Suicide Attempt

In 2017 there were an estimated 1,400,000 nonfatal suicide attempts and more than 47,000 deaths by suicide in the United States.[34] Firearms were the most common suicide method, followed by suffocation (e.g., hanging) and poisoning (e.g., overdose). Nonfatal injuries as the result of suicide attempts may be dramatic.

Nurses in critical care settings care for patients who survived a suicide attempt. Caregivers may, understandably, resent caring for a person whose critical condition is self-inflicted, whereas other patients want to live and are fighting for their lives. It may help consider these patients' injuries to be the result of an illness (e.g., major depressive disorder or a psychotic illness), similar to patients admitted for sepsis as the result of an illness such as pneumonia.

Typically, nothing is done to address the psychiatric aspect of suicidality during critical care stays. Although suicide is rare among hospitalized medically ill patients, people who are determined to die are still at risk. These patients are monitored for suicidal thoughts. Psychiatric consultations are valuable aspects of care for this patient population.

If the patient is willing and able, critical care nurses can be helpful by supporting the patient and encouraging expression of thoughts and feelings. Sometimes nurses feel like they are prying and may be uncomfortable addressing such personal topics. Yet the suicide attempt is the elephant in the room, and both the patient and the nurse are aware of its existence. Nurses may encourage the person to explore thoughts and feelings that precipitated the suicide attempt. They may also support a future orientation by identifying goals and plans for postdischarge. In the case of individuals who have attempted to end life, follow-up care is essential and is always a part of the treatment plan.

Nurses also care for family, friends, and significant others of people who have attempted to end their lives. This is a crisis for people who are close to the patient accompanied by shame, guilt, or anger. Nurses support the expression of these feelings and other thoughts in a private setting and establish an atmosphere of interested concern for their loved one. Nurses may encourage the use of their support system or counseling services.

POST–INTENSIVE CARE SYNDROME (PICS)

Up until now in this chapter, we have focused on patients who are coping with life-threatening illnesses and injuries in the critical care environment. What happens after a life is saved and the patient returns to the community?

Advances and improvements in critical care treatment have saved countless lives. However, this survival is often followed by profound weakness, cognitive impairment, and psychiatric impairment. Collectively, these consequences are known as *post–intensive care syndrome (PICS)*.

Family members may also experience acute and chronic cognitive impairment and psychologic distress after the discharge or death of a loved one from critical care. This PICS of a family member is abbreviated *PICS-F*. Both PICS and PICS-F result in months to years of reduced quality of life and suffering.

Critical Care Unit–Acquired Weakness

The incidence of *critical care unit–acquired weakness* is found in more than 25% of critical care unit survivors.[35] Symptoms of this weakness result in poor mobility, falls, and partial loss of functioning in two or four limbs. Risk factors for developing this muscle weakness are mechanical ventilation, multisystem organ failure, sepsis, and prolonged deep sedation.

Cognitive Impairment

The incidence of *cognitive impairment* after a critical care unit stay is alarmingly high, with estimates of 75% of survivors being affected.[35] Risk factors for cognitive impairment are related to treatment, current physical problems, and prior functioning. See Box 4.5, Risk Factors for Cognitive Impairment.

Psychiatric Conditions

The incidence of psychiatric conditions following a critical care unit stay ranges from 1% to 62%.[35] These psychiatric conditions include posttraumatic stress disorder (PTSD), major depressive disorder, and anxiety disorders. In one study, over half of the respondents indicated symptoms of these disorders.[36] In addition, these conditions often co-occur.

When symptoms of one disorder are present, there is a 65% chance that one of the other two disorders will co-occur. The risk factors for the development of psychiatric conditions mirror those for cognitive impairment. Other risk factors include lower education level, being

BOX 4.5 Risk Factors for Cognitive Impairment

- Brain dysfunction (e.g., stroke or chronic alcohol use)
- Hypoxia (e.g., acute respiratory distress or cardiac arrest)
- Hypotension (e.g., sepsis or trauma)
- Glucose dysregulation
- Prolonged mechanical ventilation
- Renal replacement therapy
- Prior cognitive impairment (e.g., preexisting cognitive deficits or premorbid health conditions)

TRENDING PRIORITIES IN HEALTHCARE

Hospitalized Patients With Underlying Mental Illness

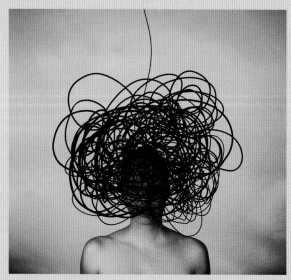

iStock.com/dragnab

According to researchers, there is an association between serious mental illness (SMI) and worse general health.[1] Those persons with SMI have more comorbidities than those without mental health issues, experience a higher mortality, and have a lower life expectancy. About half have medical comorbid conditions, and as many as 35% have undiagnosed medical comorbid conditions. Thus a very few do not have medical conditions in addition to their SMI. The leading comorbidities are urinary, digestive, neoplastic, pulmonary, and circulatory conditions.[1]

The Healthcare Cost and Utilization Project (HCUP) reported that nearly 7.7 million (21.7%) of inpatient stays consisted of mental and substance abuse secondary diagnoses in 2016.[2] Inpatient stays comprising these diagnoses were more likely to be admitted through the emergency department, and costs and length of stays were greater than those without those diagnoses. Also, in the same year, the most frequent (about one-third) secondary diagnoses were alcoholic-related conditions.[1]

Several factors must be considered when caring for critically ill patients with underlying mental health issues:

- Detailed history of both medical and mental health
- Thorough admission assessment regarding mental health issues, diagnosis(es), current treatments
- Complete appraisal of medications, including any untoward side effects, and medication interactions
- Document the patient's mental health provider(s) and supports
- Seek additional or clarifying information from the family members/significant others
- Consult in-hospital consultant as required to assist with plan of care, that is, psychologist, psychiatrist, and psychiatric nurse practitioner/clinical nurse specialist as needed
- Ensure plan of care is communicated when care is facilitated across settings
- Design discharge plan that includes importance of monitoring and addressing medical conditions as well as mental health issues when discharged
- Include family and significant others in the design and monitoring of the discharge plan

References

1. Jayatilleke N, Hayes RD, Chang CK, Stewart R. Acute general hospital admissions in people with serious mental illness. *Psychol Med.* 2018;48(16):2676–2683.
2. Owens PL, Fingar KR, McDermott KW, Muhuri PK, Heslin KC. *Inpatient Stays Involving Mental Health and Substances Disorders, 2016. HCUP Statistical Brief #249.* Rockville MD: Agency for Healthcare Quality and Research; 2019. www.hcup-us.ahrq.gov/reports/statbriefs/sb249-Mental-Substance-Use-Disorder-Hospital-Stays-2016.pdf.

---

female, preexisting psychiatric conditions, and the use of analgesia and sedation.

Stress Disorders

Serious PICS are *acute stress disorder (ASD)* and *PTSD*, which are caused by one or more traumatic events. The primary difference between ASD and PTSD is timing. ASD occurs immediately and lasts up to a month. PTSD may be a continuation of ASD or symptoms may be delayed up to 6 months. A large-scale study reported a prevalence of 22% in the 3 to 12 months after discharge from the critical care unit.[36] ASD and PTSD involve a wide range of symptoms (Box 4.6).

Family members are also at risk for developing posttraumatic stress reactions. Prolonged periods of uncertainty, anxious waiting, disrupted sleep patterns, financial concerns, witnessing emergency interventions, and confronting fears of loss and death are profoundly unsettling.

Certain populations are at greater risk for developing PTSD. These populations include patients who are young, people who have delusional memories, and individuals with preexisting psychiatric conditions.[37] There is evidence that using lighter doses of sedation—keeping patients calm but awake—may reduce the incidence of PTSD.

Critical care unit—induced PTSD is largely unidentified and untreated. Being aware of the possibility for stress overload in critical care settings is the first step to reducing PTSD. Care providers can take steps to manage or eliminate as many of those stressors as possible.

BOX 4.6 Stress Disorder Symptoms

- Recurrent intrusive recall and dreams of the distressing event
- Dissociative reactions such as flashbacks in which the individuals re-experience the traumatic event(s), depersonalization (i.e., feeling detached from the world), and derealization (i.e., experiencing the outside world as unreal or dreamlike)
- Psychologic distress and/or physiologic reactions when exposed to cues that symbolize or resemble the traumatic event(s)
- Avoidance of memories, thoughts, feelings, or reminders of the traumatic event(s)
- Negative alterations in cognitive abilities (e.g., memory of the trauma and distortions of the cause) and mood (e.g., fear, anger, guilt, detachment, and the inability to experience pleasure)
- Alterations in arousal that are evident in irritability, recklessness, hypervigilance, exaggerated startle response, poor concentration, and sleep disturbances

Data from The American Psychiatric Association. *Diagnostic and Statistical Manual of Mental Disorders.* 5th ed. Washington, DC: American Psychiatric Association; 2013.

Often patients are unaware or uncertain of what has happened to them and their bodily functions. Nurses can mediate this uncertainty by encouraging realistic discussions of the patient's experiences and explaining events carefully. Talking openly about recovery timelines and the gradual process of regaining strength, or about the process of terminal illness and final choices, will help reduce the fear of the unknown.

Prevention and Management of PICS

Two of the most important factors in preventing PICS are minimizing sedation and facilitating early mobilization during critical care stays.[35] Evaluation for signs and symptoms of PICS is an important role of critical care nurses. Even in the most ill patients, providing rehabilitation services as early as 24 to 48 hours after admission is a growing trend.[38]

Other key interventions may mitigate or prevent the development of PICS and PICS-F[39] (Table 4.1).

Early intervention can support a higher quality of life for both the patient and the patient's significant others. Education about the potential for PICS will help make potential symptoms less bewildering and increase the chances for early treatment. Critical care nurses are in a position to provide this education.

SELF-CARE FOR NURSES

Critical care nurses must be prepared to deliver urgently needed care based on sound scientific knowledge using expert clinical skills. To ensure patient safety, nurses must maintain a high level of vigilance. The environment includes involvement in persistent suffering for patients and those who love them.

Additionally, the critical care environment is disposed to events provoking moral conflict that adds to the burden of the nurse. Because of these high-stress elements, nurses need to practice self-care to maintain the ability to deliver safe and effective care.

To attain and maintain the knowledge and skills necessary for critical care, nurses need to study beyond what is required for entry-level practice. Most critical care units require a period of classroom focused on critical care and clinical precepting before solo practice. Continuing education opportunities for critical care topics are available in many formats. In addition, critical care nurses may earn critical care certification through professional accreditation (see Chapter 1).

The long hours and rapid pace of critical care call for nurses to maintain optimal health. Nurses need to give attention to balanced diet, exercise, and rest. One way to promote this is to develop a culture of health and support within the unit. Ensure that break times are used for rest and restoration. Discourage overscheduling.

Compassion Fatigue

Immersion in an environment with considerable uncertainty, suffering, and grief places nurses at risk for developing compassion fatigue, a physical, emotional, and spiritual exhaustion accompanied by emotional pain. *Compassion fatigue* refers to physical and psychologic responses that result from the type of emotional engagement necessary to provide compassionate care to relieve patients' suffering.[40]

Compassion fatigue may be thought of as losing the ability to nuture.[41] This fatigue may result in creating distance between nurses and patients or, paradoxically, nurses becoming overly involved with patients.[42,43] The critical care environment, with challenging protocols, staffing, long shifts without breaks, patient/family/colleague interactions, and workload, can negatively affect the nurse satisfaction with their jobs, leading to burnout and inability to engage effectively and express compassion.[44,45]

To avoid the extremes of either becoming overly involved in patients' suffering or detaching from them, nurses can use self-care

TABLE 4.1 Interventions to Mitigate or Prevent PICS and PICS-F.

Intervention	Rationale
Bedside report	Allows family members and patients to listen to change-of-shift reports, ask questions, and make suggestions for care
Five minutes at the bedside	At the beginning of the shift, nurses sit for 5 minutes to listen to patients and families, provide emotional support and information, and set goals
Communication board	Boards in patients' rooms can convey goals and identify tests or procedures for the day
Hourly rounding	When nurses make rounds on patients and families every hour, they can offer updates and respond to questions
Narrating care	While delivering patient care, nurses can explain and talk about what they are doing
Informal and formal education	Empowers patients and family members and increases coping strategies. Written content is helpful to reinforce learning
Patient and family diaries	Diaries document the patient's condition, treatments, and education; they reinforce real memories rather than imagined ones
Family participation in care	
Patients want to hear about life outside the critical care unit	Family members can share this information while helping with hygiene, range-of-motion, and feedings. This participation will be helpful as the patient makes the transition to home care.

PICS, Post-intensive care syndrome; *PICS-F,* post-intensive case syndrome in a family member.

activities to maintain balance. Nurses are encouraged to use *self-reflection* when feeling overwhelmed and consider the source of their feelings. There are often multiple causes for feeling overwhelmed, such as sadness about a particular patient, overwork, lateral hostility at work,[46,47] and disruptions in one's personal life.

Reflection is an important first step, because without awareness, it is difficult to identify possible solutions. Talking with friends, a spiritual care provider, or a close colleague can help the nurse recognize grief and reflect on the meaning of work.

Stress Management Techniques

Stress management techniques help restore energy and enjoyment in caring for patients. Nurses who practice self-care are more likely to experience professional and personal growth and find more meaning in their work. Maintain physical health by eating well, exercising, engaging in relaxing activities, laughing, and getting enough sleep.

Nurses can promote emotional health by participating in calming activities, such as meditation, daily gratitude reflections, deep breathing, walking, or listening to music[42] and using self-transcendence (spiritual awareness) activities, such as journal writing, sharing stories, recognizing one's own positive contributions and unique gifts, and connecting with oneself.[42]

Given the ongoing demands of critical care nursing, time at work needs to be balanced with time for recreation and relaxation. Investing time in the people and activities that nurture the spirit is crucial.

BOX 4.7   Informatics

Internet Resources: Psychosocial and Spiritual Considerations

- Critical care nurses' experiences with spiritual care: the SPIRIT study: https://aacnjournals.org/ajcconline/article-abstract/27/3/212/4199/Critical-Care-Nurses-Experiences-With-Spiritual?redirectedFrom=fulltext
- Improving the patient experience by focusing on spiritual care: http://acphospitalist.org/archives/2016/06/spiritual-care.htm
- Intensive care: a guide for patients and families: https://www.sccm.org/MyICUCare/Resources/Intensive-Care-A-Guide-for-Patients-and-Relatives#:~:text=Intensive%20Care%3A%20A%20Guide%20for%20Patients%20and%20Relatives%20is%20a,what%20recovery%20may%20be%20like
- Patient communicator app: https://www.sccm.org/MyICUCare/THRIVE/Patient-and-Family-Resources/Patient-and-Family
- Pediatric post—intensive care syndrome and the family: https://www.sccm.org/MyICUCare/Resources/Intensive-Care-A-Guide-for-Patients-and-Relatives
- Post—intensive care support group: https://www.facebook.com/groups/227842144513131/
- Spiritual support: https://intermountainhealthcare.org/services/hospice-palliative-care/services/spiritual-support/
- Ten relaxation techniques that zap stress fast: https://www.webmd.com/balance/guide/blissing-out-10-relaxation-techniques-reduce-stress-spot#1

Often, individual patient circumstances evolve, bringing about moral conflict. *Moral conflict*, also called *moral distress*, occurs when a nurse comes to a clear judgment about what course of action to take but is unable to do so because of social, institutional, or contextual constraints.[48,49] Futile care is often a source of moral distress (see Chapter 2). Unaddressed moral distress promotes negative emotional responses in nurses and can result in nurses leaving their jobs.[50,51]

When it comes to moral distress, prevention is key. Good communication among nurses, patients, and significant others goes a long way toward avoiding problematic situations. Patients and families who are aware of the patient's condition and evolving health situation will be better prepared to accept negative outcomes. Supportive professional relationships among interprofessional staff have been shown to promote discussion during stressful events.[49,50]

Box 4.7 provides Internet resources regarding psychosocial and spiritual considerations for nurses and patients in the critical care setting.

REFERENCES

1. Halter M. In: Halter M, ed. *Varcarolis' Foundations of Psychiatric-Mental Health Nursing: A Clinical Approach*. St. Louis: Elsevier; 2022.
2. Selye H. *Stress in Health and Disease*. Boston, MA: Butterworth; 1976.
3. Herman JP, McKlveen JM, Ghosal S, et al. Regulation of the hypothalamus-pituitary-adrenocortical stress response. *Compr Physiol*. 2016;6(2):603—614.
4. Perpina-Galvan J, Richart-Martinez M. Scales for evaluating self-perceived anxiety levels in patients admitted to intensive care units: a review. *Am J Crit Care*. 2009;18(6):571.
5. Jaber S, Chanques G, Altairac C, et al. A prospective study of agitation in a medical-surgical ICU: incidence, risk factors, and outcomes. *Chest*. 2005;128(4):2749.
6. Fredriksen S, Ringsberg K. Living the situation stress-experiences among intensive care patients. *Intensive Crit Care Nurs*. 2007;23:124.
7. Maslow H. *Motivation and Personality*. New York, NY: Harper & Row; 1954.
8. Husum T, Legernes E, Pederden R. "A plea for recognition": users experience of humiliation during health care. *Int J Law Psychiatry*. 2018;62:148—153. Available from: https://doi.org/10.1016/j.ijlp.11.004.
9. Malterud K, Hollnagel H. Avoiding humiliations in the clinical encounter. *Scand J Prim Health Care*. 2007;25:69.
10. Rotter JB. Generalized expectancies for internal versus external control of reinforcement. *Psychol Monogr*. 1966;80(1):1.
11. Timmins F, Kelly J. Spiritual assessment in intensive and cardiac care nursing. *Nurs Crit Care*. 2008;13(3):124—131.
12. Miller J. Hope: a construct central to nursing. *Nurs Forum*. 2007;42(1): 12—19.
13. Arnaert A, Filteau N, Sourial R. Stroke patients in the acute care phase: role of hope in self-healing. *Holist Nurs Pract*. 2006;23(3):137.
14. Wake M, Miller J. Treating hopelessness: nursing strategies from 6 countries. *Clin Nurs Res*. 1992;4910:347—365.
15. Bazuin D, Cardon K. Creating healing intensive care unit environments: physical and psychological considerations in designing critical care areas. *Crit Care Nurs Q*. 2011;24(4):259.
16. Happ MB, Garrett K, Thomas DD, et al. Nurse-patient communication interactions in the intensive care unit. *Am J Crit Care Nurs*. 2011;20(2):e28.
17. Stajduhar KI, Thorne SE, McGuinness L, Kim-Sing C. Patient perceptions of helpful communication in the context of advanced cancer. *J Clin Nurs*. 2010;19:2039.
18. Lowey S. Communication between the nurse and family caregiver in end of life care: a review of the literature. *J Hosp Palliat Nurs*. 2008;10(1):35.
19. Grossbach I. Promoting effective communication for patients receiving mechanical ventilation. *Crit Care Nurse*. 2011;31(3):46.
20. Nelson JE, Angus DC, Weissfeld LA, et al. End of life care for the critically ill: a national intensive care unit survey. *Crit Care Med*. 2006;34:2547.
21. Tulsky J. Interventions to enhance communication among patients, providers, and families. *J Palliat Med*. 2005;8(suppl 1):S95.
22. Nolan K, Waren N. Meeting the needs of family members of ICU patients. *Crit Care Nurs Q*. 2014;37(4):393—406.
23. Newman M. *Transforming Presence: The Difference that Nursing Makes*. Philadelphia, PA: FA Davis; 2008.
24. Timmins F, Naughton MT, Plakas S, Pesut B. Supporting patients' and families' religious and spiritual needs in ICU: can we do more? *Br Assoc Crit Care Nurs*. 2015;20(3):115.
25. Scotto C, et al. Earplugs improve patients' subjective experience of ICU patients during follow up sessions: A qualitative study. *Intensive Care Nurse*. 2012;40(7):2033.
26. Lebel V, Charette S. Nursing interventions to reduce stress in families of critical care patients: an integrative review. *Crit Care Nurse*. 2021;41(1):32—44.
27. Aghaie B, Anoosheh M, Foroughan M, Mohammadi E, Kazemnejad A. A whirlpool of stress in families of intensive care unit patients: a qualitative multicenter study. *Crit Care Nurse*. 2021;40(3):55—64.
28. Rogan J, Zielke M, Drrumright K, Boehm LM. Institutional challenges and solutions to evidence-based, patient-centered practice: implementing ICU diaries. *Crit Care Nurse*. 2020;40(5):47—55.
29. Nakashima H, Gallegos C. Journal writing by families of critically ill patients: an integrative review. *Crit Care Nurse*. 2020;40(5):26—37.
30. American Association of Critical-Care Nurses. Practice alert-family presence: visitation within the adult ICU. https://www.aacn.org/clinical-resources/practice-alerts/family-presence-visitation-in-the-adult-ICU. Accessed August 29, 2021.
31. Jacobowski NL, Girard TD, Mulder JA, Ely EW. Communication in critical care: family rounds in the intensive care unit. *Am J Crit Care*. 2010;19(5):421.
32. Grant BF, Goldstein RB, Saha TD, et al. Epidemiology of DSM-5 alcohol use disorder: results from the National Epidemiologic Survey on Alcohol and related conditions III. *JAMA Psychiatry*. 2015;72(8):757—766.
33. Unsaro A, Parviainen I, Tenhunen J, Ruokonen E. The proportion of intensive care unit admissions related to alcohol use: a prospective cohort study. *Acta Anaesthesiol Scand*. 2005;49:1236—1240. https://doi.org/10.1111/j.1399-6576.2005.00839.x.
34. Centers for Disease Control and Prevention. Fatal injury data. https://www.cdc.gov/injury/wisqars/fatal.html.
35. Rawal G, Yadav S, Kumar R. Post-intensive care syndrome: an overview. *J Transl Int Med*. 2017;5(2):90—92.

36. Hatch R, Young D, Barber V, Griffiths J, Harrison DA, Watkinson P. Anxiety, depression, and post traumatic stress disorder after critical illness: a UK-wide prospective cohort study. *Crit Care*. 2018;22:310. https://doi.org/10.1186/s13054-018-2223-6.

37. Battle E, James K, Bromfield T, Temblett P. Predictors of post-traumatic stress disorder following critical illness: a mixed methods study. *J Intensive Care Soc*. 2017;18(4):289—293.

38. Mayo Foundation. Improving access to rehabilitation services for ICU patients; 2019. https://www.mayoclinic.org/medical-professionals/physical-medicine-rehabilitation/news/improving-access-to-rehabilitation-services-for-icu-patients/mac-20430125#.

39. Twibell K, Petty A, Olynger A, Abebe S. Families and post-intensive care syndrome. *Am Nurse Today*. 2018;13(4). https://www.americannursetoday.com/families-post-intensive-care-syndrome/.

40. Sano R, Schiffman R, Sawin K. Negative consequences of providing nursing care in the neonatal intensive care unit. *Nurs Outlook*. 2018;66:576—585.

41. Joinson C. Coping with compassion fatigue. *Nursing*. 1992;4(116):118—120.

42. Showalter S. Compassion fatigue: what is it? Why does it matter? Recognizing the symptoms, acknowledging the impact, developing the tools to prevent compassion fatigue, and strengthen the professional already suffering from the effects. *Am J Hosp Palliat Med*. 2010;27(4):239.

43. Bush N. Compassion fatigue: are you at risk? *Oncol Nurs Forum*. 2009;26(1):24.

44. Swamy L, Mohr D, Blok A, et al. Impact of workplace climate on burnout among critical care nurses in the Veteran's Health Administration. *Am J Crit Care*. 2020;29(5):380—389.

45. Kelly LA, Johnson KL, Bay C, Todd M. Key elements of the critical care work environment associated with burnout and compassion satisfaction. *Am J Crit Care*. 2021;30(2):113—119.

46. Mealer M, Burnham EL, Goode CJ, Rothbaum B, Moss M. The prevalence and impact of post-traumatic stress disorder and burnout syndrome in nurses. *Depress Anxiety*. 2009;26:1118.

47. Alspach G. Lateral hostility between critical care nurses: a survey report. *Crit Care Nurse*. 2008;28(2):13.

48. Prentice T, Janvier A, Gillam L, Davis PG. Moral distress within neonatal and pediatric intensive care units. *Arch Dis Child*. 2016;101:701—708. https://doi.org/10.1136/archdischild-2015-309410.

49. Fumis R, Amarante G, Nascimento A, Junior J. Moral distress and its contribution to the development of burnout among critical care providers. *Ann Intensive Care*. 2017;7:71—78. https://doi.org/10.1186/s13616-017-0297-2.

50. Mealer M, Moss M. Moral distress in ICU nurses. *Intensive Care Med*. 2016;42:1615—1617. https://doi.org/10.1007/s00134-4441-1.

51. Henrich N, Dodek P, Gladstone E, et al. Consequences of moral distress in the intensive care unit. *Am J Crit Care*. 2017;26(4):48—56.

Nutritional Alterations and Management

Janine Wong Berta

NUTRIENT METABOLISM

Nutrients are chemical substances found in foods that are needed for human life, growth, maintenance, and repair of body tissues. The main nutrients in foods are carbohydrates, proteins, fats, vitamins, minerals, and water. The process by which nutrients are used at the cellular level is known as *metabolism*. The energy-yielding nutrients or macronutrients are carbohydrates, proteins, and fats. For proper metabolic functioning, adequate amounts of micronutrients, such as vitamins, minerals (including electrolytes), and trace elements must also be supplied to the human body.

PRIORITY CLINICAL ASSESSMENT OF NUTRITION STATUS

A nutrition screening should be conducted on every patient within 48 hours of admission to an acute care center.[1] A brief questionnaire to be completed by the patient or significant other, the nursing admission form, or the physician's admission note usually provide enough information to determine whether the patient is at nutrition risk (Box 5.1). Patients nutritionally at risk in critical care may need a more thorough nutrition assessment.[1]

BOX 5.1 Patients Who Are at Risk for Malnutrition

Adults Who Experience Any of the Following
- Involuntary loss or gain of a significant amount of weight (>10% of usual body weight in 6 months, >5% in 1 month), even if the weight achieved by loss or gain is appropriate for height
- Chronic disease
- Chronic use of a modified diet
- Increased metabolic requirements
- Illness or surgery that may interfere with nutrition intake
- Inadequate nutrient intake for >7 days
- Regular use of three or more medications
- Food insecurity

Anthropometric Measurements

Height and current weight are essential anthropometric measurements, and they should be measured rather than obtained through a patient or family report. The most important reason for obtaining anthropometric measurements is to be able to detect changes in the measurements over time (e.g., track response to nutrition therapy).[2]

During critical illness, changes in anthropometric measures such as weight are more likely to reflect changes in body water and its distribution. For example, edema may mask significant weight loss or underweight. Despite these limitations, weight remains an important measure of nutrition status, and any recent weight change must be evaluated.

Biochemical (Laboratory) Data

No diagnostic tests for evaluation of nutrition are perfect, and care must be taken in interpreting the results of the tests.[3] For example, albumin and prealbumin were once thought to reflect nutritional status; however, both are negative acute-phase reactants and therefore serum values are associated with inflammation rather than nutritional status.[4]

Clinical or Physical Manifestations

Clinical manifestations of nutritional alterations are listed in Box 5.2. It is especially important for the nurse to check for signs of muscle wasting, loss of subcutaneous fat, skin or hair changes, and impairment of wound healing.

Diet and Nutrition History

Information about dietary intake and significant variations in weight is a vital part of the nutrition history. Dietary intake can be evaluated in several ways, including a diet record listing food and beverage consumption usually over 3 days, a recall of food and beverage consumption over 24 hours, and a detailed interview to obtain a thorough diet history. Other information to include in a nutrition history is listed in Box 5.3.

Determining Nutrition Needs

In the inpatient setting, working with the dietitian, estimated calorie or energy needs can be measured or calculated. Various methods can be used in clinical practice to estimate caloric requirements. Indirect calorimetry, a method by which energy expenditure is calculated from oxygen consumption (VO_2) and carbon dioxide production (VCO_2), is the most accurate method for determining caloric needs.[5] Indirect calorimetry is useful in patients suspected to have a high metabolic rate or for which a validated equation does not exist. The test can be performed on spontaneously breathing patients and on patients who require mechanical ventilation. Some ventilators are constructed so that they can perform indirect calorimetry. However, for most patients, indirect calorimetry requires the use of a metabolic cart, which is not available in all institutions.

Patient calorie and protein needs are often estimated using formulas that provide allowances for increased nutrient use associated

BOX 5.2 Clinical Manifestations of Nutritional Alterations

Manifestations That May Indicate Protein-Calorie Malnutrition
- Hair loss; dull, dry, brittle hair; loss of hair pigment
- Loss of subcutaneous tissue; muscle wasting
- Poor wound healing; decubitus ulcer
- Hepatomegaly
- Edema
- Decline in functional status

Manifestations Often Present in Vitamin Deficiencies
- Conjunctival and corneal dryness (vitamin A)
- Dry, scaly skin; follicular hyperkeratosis, in which the skin appears to have gooseflesh continually (vitamin A)
- Gingivitis; poor wound healing (vitamin C)

- Petechiae; ecchymoses (vitamin C or K)
- Inflamed tongue, cracking at the corners of the mouth (riboflavin [vitamin B_2], niacin, folic acid, vitamin B_{12}, or other B vitamins)
- Edema; heart failure (thiamine [vitamin B_1])
- Confusion; confabulation (thiamine [vitamin B_1])

Manifestations Often Present in Mineral Deficiencies
- Blue sclerae; pale mucous membranes; spoon-shaped nails (iron)
- Hypogeusia, or poor sense of taste; dysgeusia, or bad taste; eczema; poor wound healing (zinc)

Manifestations Often Observed With Excessive Vitamin Intake
- Hair loss; dry skin; hepatomegaly (vitamin A)

BOX 5.3 DATA COLLECTION

Nutritional History
Inadequate Intake of Nutrients
- Alcohol abuse
- Anorexia, severe or prolonged nausea or vomiting
- Confusion, coma
- Poor dentition
- Food insecurity

Inadequate Digestion or Absorption of Nutrients
- Previous gastrointestinal operations, especially gastrectomy, jejunoileal bypass, and ileal resection
- Certain medications, especially antacids and histamine receptor antagonists (reduce upper small bowel acidity), cholestyramine (binds fat-soluble nutrients), and anticonvulsants

Increased Nutrient Losses
- Blood loss
- Severe diarrhea or vomiting
- Fistulas, draining abscesses, wounds, decubitus ulcers
- Peritoneal dialysis or hemodialysis
- Corticosteroid therapy (increased tissue catabolism)

Increased Nutrient Requirements
- Fever
- Surgery, trauma, burns, infection
- Cancer (some types)
- Physiologic demands (pregnancy, lactation, growth)

---

with injury and healing. Although indirect calorimetry is considered the most accurate method to determine energy expenditure, estimates using formulas have demonstrated reasonable accuracy.[6–8] Commonly used formulas for critically ill patients can be found in Appendix B.

Underfeeding and overfeeding must be avoided during critical illness. Overfeeding results in excessive production of carbon dioxide, which can be a burden in a patient with pulmonary compromise. Overfeeding increases fat stores, which can contribute to insulin resistance and hyperglycemia. Hyperglycemia increases the risk of postoperative infections in diabetic and nondiabetic patients.[9]

IMPLICATIONS OF UNDERNUTRITION FOR SICK OR STRESSED PATIENTS

The prevalence of malnutrition in the critical care unit ranges from 38% to 78%.[10] Iatrogenic malnutrition develops in approximately one-third of patients who were well nourished upon admission.[11] Although illness or injury is a major factor contributing to development of malnutrition, other possible contributing factors are lack of communication among the nurses, physicians, and dietitians responsible for the care of these patients; frequent diagnostic testing and procedures, which lead to interruption in feeding; medications and other therapies

that cause anorexia, nausea, or vomiting and thus interfere with food intake; insufficient monitoring of nutrient intake; and inadequate use of supplements, tube feedings, or parenteral nutrition (PN) to maintain nutrition status.

Nutrition status tends to deteriorate during hospitalization unless appropriate nutrition support is started early and continually reassessed. Malnutrition in hospitalized patients is associated with a wide variety of adverse outcomes. Wound dehiscence, pressure injuries, sepsis, infections, respiratory failure requiring ventilation, longer hospital stays, and death are more common among malnourished patients.[12–14] Decline in nutrition status during hospitalization is associated with higher incidences of complications, increased mortality rates, increased length of stay, readmission, and increased hospital costs.[10,11,15]

It is rare for a patient to exhibit a lack of only one nutrient. Nutrition deficiencies usually are combined, with the patient lacking adequate amounts of protein, calories, and possibly vitamins and minerals.

Metabolic Response to Starvation and Stress

Changes in endocrine status and metabolism together determine the onset and extent of malnutrition. Nutrition imbalance occurs when the demand for nutrients is greater than the exogenous nutrient supply. The major difference between a person who is starved and one who is starved and injured is that the latter has an increased reliance on tissue protein breakdown to provide precursors for glucose production to meet increased energy demands. Although carbohydrate and fat metabolism are also affected, the main concern is about protein metabolism and homeostasis.

During an acute, nonstressed fast, blood levels of glucose and insulin fall, and glucagon levels rise. Glucagon stimulates the liver to release glucose from its glycogen reserves, which become exhausted within a few hours. Glucagon also stimulates gluconeogenesis, and skeletal muscle provides a large amount of the substrates required for gluconeogenesis. As fasting progresses, fat becomes the primary source of fuel, and the blood ketone levels begin to increase. After the circulating ketone level rises, the brain is able to use ketones for 70% of its energy, decreasing the total body's reliance on glucose as an energy source. As gluconeogenesis from protein precursors decreases, protein breakdown and nitrogen excretion also slow. Some tissues, such as red blood cells, the renal medulla, and 30% of brain cells, are obligatory glucose users, and they continue to require a small amount of amino acids for gluconeogenesis. However, endogenous protein stores are spared from use for gluconeogenesis to a major extent, and protein homeostasis is partially restored.

Critically ill patients are at risk for a combination of starvation and the physiologic stress resulting from injury, trauma, major surgery, or sepsis. Starvation occurs because the person must have nothing by mouth (NPO) for surgical procedures, is unable to eat because of disease-related factors, or is hemodynamically too unstable to be fed. The physiologic stress causes an increased metabolic rate (hypermetabolism) that results in increased oxygen consumption and energy expenditure.

The hypermetabolic process results from increased catabolic hormone changes caused by the stressful event. The sympathetic nervous system is stimulated, causing the adrenal medulla to release catecholamines (epinephrine and norepinephrine). Other hormones released in response to stress include glucagon, adrenocorticotropic hormone, antidiuretic hormone, and glucocorticoids and mineralocorticoids (e.g., cortisol, aldosterone). Cytokines are peptide messengers secreted by macrophages as part of the inflammatory response, and they serve as hormonal regulators of the immune system. Cytokine levels increase in response to sepsis and trauma. Important cytokines include tumor necrosis factor, cachectin, interleukin-1, and interleukin-6. All these hormonal changes cause nutrient substrates, primarily amino acids, to move from peripheral tissues (e.g., skeletal muscle) to the liver for gluconeogenesis.

This mobilization of substrates occurs at the expense of body tissue and function at a time when the needs for protein synthesis (e.g., wound healing, acute-phase proteins) also are high. Hyperglycemia results from the effects of increased catecholamines, glucocorticoids, and glucagon. The body relies on its protein stores to provide substrates for gluconeogenesis because glucose becomes the major fuel source. Loss of protein results in a negative nitrogen balance and weight loss. Catabolism may be unresponsive to nutrient intake.

NUTRITION SUPPORT

Nursing Management of Nutrition Support

Nutrition support is the provision of oral, enteral, or parenteral nutrients. It is an essential adjunct in the prevention and management of malnutrition in critically ill patients.[1] The goal of nutrition support therapy is to provide enough support for body requirements, to minimize complications, and to promote rapid recovery.

Oral Supplementation

Oral supplementation may be necessary for patients who can eat and have normal digestion and absorption but cannot consume enough regular foods to meet caloric and protein needs. Patients with mild to moderate anorexia, burns, or trauma sometimes fall into this category. To improve intake and tolerance of supplements, the critical care nurse can take several steps, as follows:

1. Collaborate with the dietitian to choose appropriate products and allow the patient to participate in the selection process, if possible.
2. Offer to serve commercial supplements well chilled or on ice because this improves palatability.
3. Advise patients to sip commercial supplements slowly, consuming no more than 240 mL over 30 to 45 minutes. If formulas are consumed too quickly, rapid hydrolysis of the carbohydrate in the duodenum can contribute to dumping syndrome, characterized by abdominal cramping, weakness, tachycardia, and diarrhea.
4. Record all supplement intake separately on the intake-and-output sheet so that it can be differentiated from intake of water and other liquids.

Enteral Nutrition

Enteral nutrition or tube feedings are used for patients who have at least some digestive and absorptive capability but are unable or unwilling to consume enough by mouth. When possible, the enteral nutrition, administered within the first 24 to 48 hours of critical illness, is the preferred method of feeding over PN in critically ill patients who will be unable to meet their nutrient needs orally.[1] The proposed advantages of enteral nutrition over PN include lower cost, better maintenance of gut integrity, decreased infection, and decreased hospital length of stay.[1] A review of the literature comparing enteral nutrition and PN indicates that enteral nutrition is less expensive than PN and is associated with a lower risk of infection.[1,16]

Patients who are experiencing severe stress that greatly increases their nutrition needs (caused by major surgery, burns, or trauma) often benefit from tube feedings. Table 5.1 lists different enteral formula types and the nutrition indications for using each one. To avoid complications associated with intestinal ischemia and infarction, enteral nutrition must be initiated only after fluid resuscitation and adequate perfusion have been achieved.[1,17,18] Patients who need high doses of vasoactive medication infusions are at high risk for intestinal ischemia, and enteral feeding should be started cautiously and with a fiber-free formula.[19,20]

Enteral feeding access. Several techniques can be used to facilitate enteral access. These include surgical methods, bedside methods, fluoroscopy, endoscopy, air insufflation, and prokinetic agents.[21] Placement of feeding tubes beyond the stomach (postpyloric) eliminates some of the problems associated with gastric feeding intolerance. After the tube is placed, the correct location must be confirmed before feedings are started and regularly throughout the course of enteral feedings. After correct placement has been confirmed, marking the exit site of the tube to check for movement is helpful.

Location and type of feeding tube. Decisions regarding enteral access should be determined based on gastrointestinal (GI) anatomy, gastric emptying, and aspiration risk.[1] Nasal intubation is the simplest and most commonly used route for enteral access. This method allows access to the stomach, duodenum, or jejunum. Tube enterostomy—a gastrostomy or jejunostomy—is used primarily for long-term feedings (4–6 weeks or more) and when obstruction makes the nasoenteral route inaccessible.

Postpyloric feedings through nasoduodenal, nasojejunal, or jejunostomy tubes are commonly used when there is a high risk of

TABLE 5.1 Enteral Formulas.

Formula Type	Nutrition Uses	Clinical Examples	Examples of Commercial Products (Manufacturer)
Formulas Used When GI Tract Is Fully Functional			
Polymeric (standard): Contains whole proteins (10%–15% of calories), long-chain triglycerides (25%–40% of calories), and glucose polymers or oligosaccharides (50%–60% of calories); comes with or without fiber	Inability to ingest food Inability to consume enough to meet needs	Oral or esophageal cancer Coma, stroke Anorexia resulting from chronic illness Burns or trauma	Ensure (Abbott) Osmolite (Abbott) Jevity (Abbott) Boost (Nestlé) Nutren (Nestlé) Fibersource (Nestlé) Isosource (Nestlé)
High protein: Same as polymeric except protein provides about 25% of calories	Same as polymeric plus mild catabolism and protein deficits	Trauma or burns Sepsis	Promote (Abbott) Replete (Nestlé)
Concentrated: Same as polymeric except concentrated to 2 calories/mL	Same as polymeric but fluid restriction needed	Heart failure Neurosurgery COPD Liver disease	TwoCal HN (Abbott) Nutren 2.0 (Nestlé)
Formulas Used When GI Function Is Impaired			
Elemental or predigested: Contains hydrolyzed (partially digested) protein, peptides (short chains of amino acids) and/or amino acids, little fat (<10% of calories) or high MCT, and glucose polymers or oligosaccharides	Impaired digestion and/or absorption	Short bowel syndrome Radiation enteritis Inflammatory bowel disease	Vital (Abbott) Peptamen (Nestlé) Vivonex (Nestlé)
Diets for Specific Disease States[a]			
Kidney failure: Concentrated in calories; low sodium, potassium, magnesium, phosphorus, and vitamins A and D; low protein for renal insufficiency; higher protein formulas for dialyzed patients	Renal insufficiency Dialysis	Predialysis Hemodialysis or peritoneal dialysis	Nepro (Abbott) Suplena (Abbott) Renalcal (Nestlé) Novasource Renal (Nestlé)
Liver failure: Enriched in BCAA; low sodium	Protein intolerance	Hepatic encephalopathy	NutriHep (Nestlé)
Pulmonary dysfunction: Low carbohydrate, high fat, concentrated in calories	Respiratory insufficiency	Ventilator dependence	Pulmocare (Abbott) Nutren Pulmonary (Nestlé)
Glucose intolerance: High fat, low carbohydrate (most contain fiber and fructose)	Glucose intolerance	Individuals with diabetes mellitus whose blood sugar is poorly controlled with standard formulas	Glucerna (Abbott) Diabetisource (Nestlé) Glytrol (Nestlé)
Critical care, wound healing: High protein; most contain MCT to improve fat absorption; some have increased zinc and vitamin C for wound healing; some are high in antioxidants (vitamin E, beta-carotene); some are enriched with arginine, glutamine, or omega-3 fatty acids	Critical illness	Severe trauma or burns Sepsis Perisurgical	Pivot (Abbott) Impact (Nestlé)

[a]There is little evidence supporting the use of disease specific formulas.
BCAA, Branched chain–enriched amino acid; *COPD*, chronic obstructive pulmonary disease; *GI*, gastrointestinal; *MCT*, medium-chain triglyceride.

pulmonary aspiration, because the pyloric sphincter theoretically provides a barrier that reduces the risk of regurgitation and aspiration.[22] However, some studies have demonstrated that gastric feeding is safe and not associated with an increased risk of aspiration.[23,24] Postpyloric feedings have an advantage over intragastric feedings for patients with delayed gastric emptying, such as patients with head injury, gastroparesis, or postoperative ileus. Delivery of enteral nutrition into the small bowel is associated with improved tolerance,[25] higher calorie and protein intake,[26] and fewer GI complications.[18] Small bowel motility returns more quickly than gastric motility after surgery, and it is often possible to deliver transpyloric feedings within a few hours of injury or surgery.[22] Fig. 5.1 shows the locations of tube feeding sites.

Nursing management of enteral tube feeding complications. Nursing care of patients receiving enteral nutrition involves prevention and management of complications associated with the use of feeding tubes. Nursing management of enteral tube feeding complications is summarized in Box 5.4.

Adequacy of enteral nutrition. Critically ill patients have so many needs for care that it is easy to overlook the importance of nutrition. Many studies have shown that critically ill patients receive considerably less enteral nutrition than required.[27–30] This is a complication unique to enteral nutrition and is not observed with total parenteral nutrition (TPN). The discrepancy in nutrition intake has a variety of causes, including patient factors (e.g., high residual volumes, emesis, abdominal distention), tube-related factors (e.g., occlusion, malposition), and treatment-related factors (e.g., interruptions

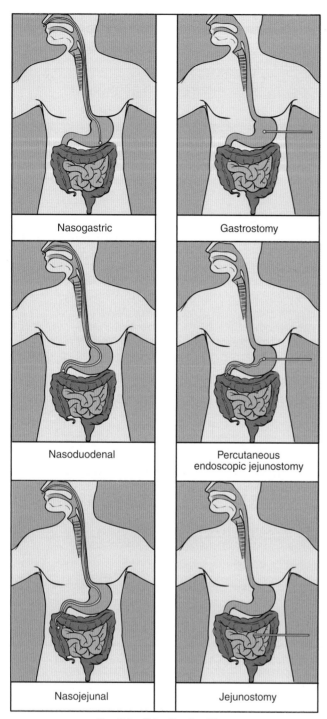

Nasogastric	Gastrostomy
Nasoduodenal	Percutaneous endoscopic jejunostomy
Nasojejunal	Jejunostomy

Fig. 5.1 Tube Feeding Sites.

caused by procedures, airway management, and medications).[28] Inadequate enteral nutrition delivery is also related to physicians' prescribing practices in the critical care unit.[30] The enteral delivery practices in the critical care unit and clinicians' concerns about aspiration may lead to inappropriate and prolonged interruptions in enteral feeding.

Parenteral Nutrition

PN refers to the delivery of all nutrients by the intravenous route. It is used when the GI tract is not functional or when nutrition needs cannot be met solely through the GI tract. Candidates for PN include patients who have severely impaired absorption (e.g., short bowel syndrome, collagen vascular diseases such as scleroderma or Ehlers-Danlos syndrome, and radiation enteritis), intestinal obstruction, peritonitis, or prolonged ileus. Some postoperative, trauma, or burn patients may need PN to supplement the nutrient intake that they are able to tolerate by the enteral route.

Types of parenteral nutrition. TPN involves administration of highly concentrated dextrose (25%—70%), providing a rich source of calories. These highly concentrated dextrose solutions are hyperosmolar, up to 1800 mOsm/L, and must be delivered through a central vein.[31] Peripheral parenteral nutrition (PPN) has a glucose concentration of 5% to 10% and may be delivered safely through a peripheral vein. PPN solution delivers nutrition support in a large volume that cannot be tolerated by patients who require fluid restriction. It provides short-term nutrition support for a few days to less than 2 weeks.

Regardless of the route of administration, PPN and TPN provide glucose, fat, protein, electrolytes, vitamins, and trace elements.

Lipid emulsion. Lipids or fat emulsions provide calories for energy and prevent essential fatty acid deficiency. There is a trend toward mixing lipid emulsions with dextrose—amino acid TPN solutions; these are called three-in-one solutions or total nutrient admixtures. Consolidating the nutrients in one container is more economical and saves nursing time, although total nutrient admixture solutions may be less stable.[31]

Nursing management of parenteral nutrition complications. Nursing care of patients receiving PN involves prevention and management of complications associated with the use of PN. Box 5.5 describes nursing management of PN complications.

Refeeding Syndrome

Refeeding syndrome is a potentially lethal condition characterized by generalized fluid and electrolyte imbalance. It occurs as a potential complication after initiation of oral, enteral, or PN in malnourished patients. During chronic starvation, several compensatory metabolic changes occur. The reintroduction of carbohydrates leads to increased insulin production. This creates an anabolic environment that increases intracellular demand for phosphorus, potassium, magnesium, vitamins, and minerals.[33] These metabolic demands result in severe shifts from the extracellular compartment. Increased insulin levels also result in fluid retention. Severe hypophosphatemia, hypokalemia, and hypomagnesemia result in altered cardiac, GI, and neurologic function. In particular, hypophosphatemia causes a decrease in 2,3-diphosphoglycerate and limits the many reactions that require adenosine triphosphate. Hypophosphatemia and other electrolyte deficiencies may lead to respiratory failure, acute heart failure, and dysrhythmias.

It is important to anticipate refeeding syndrome in patients who may be at risk. Patients with chronic malnutrition or underfeeding, chronic alcoholism, or anorexia nervosa and patients maintained NPO for several days with evidence of stress are at risk for refeeding syndrome.[34] In high-risk patients, nutrition support should be started cautiously at 25% to 50% of required calories and slowly advanced over 3 to 4 days as tolerated. Close monitoring of serum electrolytes before and during feeding is essential. Normal values do not always reflect total body stores. Correction of preexisting electrolyte imbalances is necessary before initiation of feeding. Continued monitoring and supplementation with electrolytes and vitamins are necessary throughout the first week of nutrition support.[35]

QSEN

BOX 5.4 Safety

Nursing Management of Enteral Tube Feeding Complications

Complication	Contributing Factors	Prevention or Correction
Pulmonary aspiration (signs and symptoms include tachypnea, shortness of breath, hypoxia, and infiltrate on chest radiographs)	Feeding tube positioned in esophagus or respiratory tract Regurgitation of formula	Confirm proper tube placement before administering any feeding; check tube placement at least every 4–8 hours during continuous feedings. Elevate the head to 30–45 degrees during feedings unless contraindicated. Consider giving feeding into small bowel rather than stomach in high-risk patients. Metoclopramide may improve gastric emptying and decrease risk of regurgitation. Evaluate feeding tolerance every 2 hours initially, then less frequently as condition becomes stable. Intolerance may be manifested by bloating, abdominal distention and pain, lack of stool and flatus, diminished or absent bowel sounds, tense abdomen, increased tympany, nausea and vomiting, gastric residual volume >500 mL, although a high residual volume in the absence of other abnormal findings may not be grounds for stopping feedings (measuring residual volumes is a controversial practice and is not recommended as routine practice). If intolerance is suspected, abdominal radiographs may be obtained to check for distended gastric bubble, distended loops of bowel, or air-fluid levels.
Diarrhea	Medications with GI side effects (e.g., antibiotics, digitalis, laxatives, magnesium-containing antacids, quinidine, caffeine)	Evaluate the patient's medications to determine their potential for causing diarrhea, and consult the pharmacist if necessary.
	Predisposing illness (e.g., short bowel syndrome, inflammatory bowel disease)	Use continuous feedings; consider a formula with MCT and/or soluble fiber.
	Hypertonic formula or medications (e.g., oral suspensions of antibiotics, potassium, other electrolytes), which can cause dumping syndrome	Evaluate formula administration procedures to ensure that feedings are not being given by bolus infusion; administer formula continuously or by slow intermittent infusion. Dilute enteral medications well.
	Bacterial contamination of formula	Use scrupulously clean technique in administering tube feedings; prepare formula with sterile water if there are any concerns about the safety of the water supply or if the patient is seriously immunocompromised; keep opened containers of formula refrigerated, and discard them within 24 hours; discard enteral feeding containers and administration sets every 24 hours; hang formula no more than 4–8 hours unless it comes prepackaged in sterile administration sets.
	Fecal impaction with seepage of liquid stool around impaction	Perform a digital rectal examination to rule out impaction; see guidelines for prevention of constipation below.
Constipation	Low-fiber formula, creating little fecal bulk, lack of fiber	Consider using a fiber-containing formula; ensure fluid intake is adequate; stool softeners may be beneficial.
	Medications with GI side effects (e.g., opioid pain medications)	Ensure fluid intake is adequate; stool softeners may be beneficial.
Tube occlusion	Medications administered by tube that physically plug the tube or coagulate the formula, causing it to clog the tube	If medications must be given by tube, avoid use of crushed tablets; consult with the pharmacist to determine whether medications can be dispensed as elixirs or suspensions. Dilute elixirs to prevent osmotic diarrhea. Irrigate tube with water before and after administering any medication; never add any medication to formula unless the two are known to be compatible.
	Sedimentation of formula	Irrigate tube every 4–8 hours during continuous feedings and after every intermittent feeding. If residuals are measured, flush tube thoroughly before drawing the residual and after returning formula to the stomach because gastric juices left in tube may cause precipitation of formula. Instilling pancreatic enzymes into tube can remove or prevent some occlusions.
Gastric retention	Delayed gastric emptying related to head trauma, sepsis, diabetic or uremic gastroparesis, electrolyte balance, or other illness	The cause must be corrected if possible. Consult with the physician about use of postpyloric feedings or prokinetic agents to stimulate gastric emptying. Encourage the patient to lie in the right lateral position frequently, unless contraindicated.

GI, Gastrointestinal; *MCT,* medium-chain triglyceride.

Information from *Mueller CM. American Society for Parenteral and Enteral Nutrition Adult Nutrition Support Core Curriculum.* 3rd ed. Silver Spring, MD; 2017.

BOX 5.5   Safety

Nursing Management of Parenteral Nutrition Complications

Complication	Clinical Manifestations	Prevention or Correction
Hypoglycemia	Diaphoresis, shakiness, confusion, loss of consciousness	Infuse TPN within 10% of ordered rate; monitor blood glucose until stable. If hypoglycemia is present, administer oral carbohydrate; if the patient is unconscious or oral intake is contraindicated, the physician may order an IV bolus of dextrose. Rapid cessation of TPN may lead to hypoglycemia; however, tapering the infusion over 2–4 hours is recommended.[32]
Hyperglycemia	Thirst, headache, lethargy, increased urinary output	Administer TPN within 10% of ordered rate; monitor blood glucose level at least daily until stable. The patient may require insulin added to TPN or may require a separate insulin infusion to control glucose levels if hyperglycemia is persistent; sudden appearance of hyperglycemia in a patient who was previously tolerating the same glucose load may indicate the onset of sepsis.
Hypertriglyceridemia	Serum triglyceride concentrations elevated (especially serious if >400 mg/dL); serum may appear turbid	Monitor serum triglycerides at baseline, 6 hours after lipid infusion, and at least three times weekly until stable in patients receiving lipid emulsions; reduce lipid provision in consultation with the registered dietitian.

IV, Intravenous; *TPN*, total parenteral nutrition.

NUTRITION AND CARDIOVASCULAR ALTERATIONS

Myocardial Infarction

Short-Term Interventions

In the early period after a myocardial infarction, nutrition interventions and education are designed to reduce angina, cardiac workload, and risk of dysrhythmia. Meal size, caffeine intake, and food temperatures are some dietary factors that are of concern. Small, frequent snacks are preferable to larger meals for patients with severe myocardial compromise or postprandial angina.

If caffeine is included in the diet, its effects should be monitored. Because caffeine is a stimulant, it may increase heart rate and myocardial oxygen demand. In the United States and in most industrial nations, coffee is the richest source of caffeine in the diet, with approximately 150 mg of caffeine per 180 mL (6 fluid oz) of coffee. In comparison, the caffeine content of the same volume of tea or cola is approximately 50 mg or 20 mg, respectively. Very hot or very cold foods should be avoided, because they can potentially trigger vagal or other neural input and cause cardiac dysrhythmias.

Long-Term Interventions

The focus of nutrition and lifestyle interventions for a person who has had one myocardial infarction or is at increased risk for heart disease is directed at primary and secondary prevention strategies. These strategies include lifestyle interventions, such as weight loss and decreased dietary intake of saturated fats, trans fats, and refined carbohydrates.

Heart Failure

Nutrition intervention in heart failure is designed to reduce fluid retained within the body, reducing the preload. Because fluid accompanies sodium, limitation of sodium is necessary to reduce fluid retention. Specific interventions include limiting salt intake, usually to 2 g/day or less, and limiting fluid intake as appropriate.[36] If fluid is restricted, the daily fluid allowance is usually 1.5 to 2 L/day, which includes fluids in the diet and fluids given with medications and for other purposes (see Chapter 12).

NUTRITION AND PULMONARY ALTERATIONS

Prevent or Correct Undernutrition and Underweight

The nurse and dietitian work together to encourage oral intake in undernourished or potentially undernourished patients who are capable of eating. Small, frequent feedings are especially important, because a very full stomach can interfere with diaphragmatic movement. Mouth care should be provided before meals and snacks to clear the palate of the taste of sputum and medications. Administering bronchodilators with food can help reduce the gastric irritation caused by these medications.

Many patients require enteral tube feeding because of anorexia, dyspnea, debilitation, or need for ventilatory support. It is especially important for the nurse to be alert to the risk of pulmonary aspiration in a patient with an artificial airway. To reduce the risk of pulmonary aspiration during enteral tube feeding, keep the patient's head elevated at least 30 degrees (45 degrees is preferred) during feedings unless contraindicated, keep the cuff of the artificial airway inflated during feeding if possible, monitor the patient for increasing abdominal distention, and check tube placement before each feeding (if intermittent) or at least every 4 to 8 hours if feedings are continuous.

Avoid Overfeeding

Overfeeding of total calories can impair pulmonary function. CO_2 is a metabolic byproduct of carbohydrate and lipids. VCO_2 increases when excessive calories are artificially provided. This is unlikely to be significant in a patient who is eating foods. Instead, it is an iatrogenic complication of excessive infusion of parenteral or enteral nutrition. Excessive calorie intake can increase partial pressure of carbon dioxide ($PaCO_2$) sufficiently to make it difficult to wean a patient from the ventilator. A balanced regimen with lipids and carbohydrates providing the nonprotein calories is optimal for a patient with respiratory compromise, and the patient needs to be reassessed continually to ensure that caloric intake is not excessive.[1]

Excessive lipid intake can impair capillary gas exchange in the lungs, although this is not usually sufficient to produce an increase in $PaCO_2$ or decrease in partial pressure of oxygen (PaO_2).[37] However, a patient with severe respiratory alteration may be further compromised by lipid overdose. If lipid intake is maintained at no more than 1 g/kg per day, lipid excess is rarely a problem. Serum triglyceride levels greater than 400 mg/dL may indicate inadequate lipid clearance and a need to decrease the lipid dosage.

Prevent Fluid Volume Excess

Pulmonary edema and failure of the right side of the heart, which may be precipitated by fluid volume excess, further worsen the status of a patient with respiratory compromise. Maintaining careful intake and output records allow for accurate assessment of fluid balance. Usually, the patient requires no more than 35 to 40 mL/kg per day of fluid. For a patient receiving nutrition support, fluid intake can be reduced by using concentrated TPN, by using tube feeding formulas that provide at least 1.5 to 2 calories/mL (the dietitian can recommend appropriate formulas), and by choosing oral supplements that are low in fluid. Additionally, powdered glucose polymers or powdered protein products can be used to increase caloric intake without increasing volume. The nurse plays a valuable role in continually reassessing the patient's state of hydration and alerting other team members to changes that may indicate the need for an increase or decrease in fluid intake.

NUTRITION AND NEUROLOGIC ALTERATIONS

Prevention or Correction of Nutrition Deficits
Oral Feedings

Patients with dysphagia or weakness of the swallowing musculature often experience the greatest difficulty in swallowing foods that are dry or thin liquids, such as water, that are difficult to control.

Soft, moist foods are usually easier to swallow than dry foods. An upright sitting position is preferable during meals, if possible, to allow gravity to facilitate effective swallowing. Water and other thin liquids may be especially difficult for a person with swallowing dysfunction to manage. Beverages may be thickened with commercial thickening products, with infant cereal, or with yogurt if the patient has difficulty swallowing thin fluids. Fruit nectars may be better tolerated than thinner juices.

The patient should not be rushed while eating, because this may increase the risk of pulmonary aspiration. Providing small amounts of food at frequent intervals rather than larger amounts only at mealtimes may help the patient feel less need to hurry. Suction equipment should be kept available in case aspiration occurs.

Tube Feedings

Patients who are unconscious or unable to eat because of severe dysphagia or weakness require tube feedings. Patients with neurologic alterations have an increased need for protein, calories, zinc, and vitamin C.

Prompt use of nutrition support is especially important for patients with head injuries because head injury causes marked catabolism, even in patients who receive barbiturates, which should decrease metabolic demands. Patients with head injury rapidly exhaust glycogen stores and begin to use body proteins to meet energy needs. The catabolic response is partly a result of corticosteroid therapy in patients with head injury. However, the hypermetabolism and hypercatabolism are also caused by dramatic hormonal responses to this type of injury.[38] Cortisol, epinephrine, and norepinephrine levels increase as much as seven times normal. These hormones increase the metabolic rate and caloric demands, causing mobilization of body fat and proteins to meet the increased energy needs. Patients with head injury undergo an inflammatory response and may be febrile, creating increased needs

for protein and calories. Improvement in outcome and reduction in complications have been observed in patients with head injury who receive adequate nutrition support early in the hospital course[38,39] (see Chapter 24).

Hyperglycemia is a common complication in patients receiving corticosteroids. Regular monitoring of blood glucose levels is an important part of care of such patients. They may require insulin to control hyperglycemia.

Prevention of Overweight and Obesity

Many stable patients with neurologic alterations are less active than their healthy counterparts and require fewer calories. They may become overweight or obese if given normal amounts of calories for their age and sex. Within 1 or 2 months after spinal cord injury, substantial amounts of muscle atrophy and loss of body mass begin to occur as a result of denervation and disuse. Consequently, body weight and caloric needs decline. Ideal body weights for individuals with paraplegia or quadriplegia are less than ideal body weights for healthy adults of the same height.[40] Stable, rehabilitating paraplegics need approximately 27.9 calories/kg per day, and quadriplegics need approximately 22.7 calories/kg per day.[40,41]

NUTRITION AND KIDNEY ALTERATIONS

The goal of nutrition intervention is to balance adequate calories, protein, vitamins, and minerals, while avoiding excesses of protein, fluid, electrolytes, and other nutrients with potential toxicity (see Chapter 19).

Protein

The kidney is responsible for excreting nitrogen from amino acids or proteins in the form of urea. When urinary excretion of urea is impaired in renal failure, blood urea nitrogen increases. Excessive protein intake may worsen uremia. However, patients with renal failure often have other physiologic stresses that increase protein or amino acid needs, such as losses because of dialysis, wounds, and fistulas; use of corticosteroid medications that exert a catabolic effect; increased endogenous secretion of catecholamines, corticosteroids, and glucagon, all of which can cause or aggravate catabolism; metabolic acidosis, which stimulates protein breakdown; and catabolic conditions such as trauma, surgery, and sepsis.[42] Patients with acute kidney injury need adequate amounts of protein to prevent malnutrition and other complications.[43]

Fluid

A patient with renal insufficiency usually does not require a fluid restriction until urine output begins to diminish. Patients receiving hemodialysis are limited to a fluid intake resulting in a gain of no more than 0.45 kg (1 lb) per day on the days between dialysis. This generally means a daily intake of 500 to 750 mL plus the volume lost in urine. With the use of continuous peritoneal dialysis, hemofiltration, or hemodialysis, the fluid intake can be liberalized.[44] This more liberal fluid allowance permits more adequate nutrient delivery by oral, tube, or parenteral feedings. Enteral formulas containing 1.5 to 2 calories/mL or more provide a concentrated source of calories for tube-fed patients who require fluid restriction. Intravenous lipids, particularly 20% emulsions, can be used to supply concentrated calories for the patient receiving TPN.

Energy (Calories)

Energy needs are not increased by renal failure, but adequate calories must be provided to avoid catabolism.[42,44] Catabolism reduces muscle mass and other functional body tissues, and it releases nitrogen that must be excreted by the kidney. Adults with renal insufficiency need approximately 30 to 35 calories/kg per day to prevent catabolism and ensure that all protein consumed is used for anabolism rather than to meet energy needs.[44] After renal transplantation, when the patient usually receives large doses of corticosteroids, it is especially important to ensure that caloric intake is adequate (usually 25–35 calories/kg per day) to prevent undue catabolism.

Other Nutrients

Certain nutrients such as potassium and phosphorus are restricted because they are excreted by the kidney. The patient has no specific requirement for the fat-soluble vitamins A, E, and K because they are not removed in appreciable amounts by dialysis, and restriction generally prevents development of toxicity. Patients with end-stage renal disease may have decreased clearance of vitamin A, and levels should be monitored.[45] The needs for several water-soluble vitamins and trace minerals are increased in dialysis patients because they are small enough to pass freely through the dialysis filter. Vitamins and minerals should be supplemented as necessary.[44]

NUTRITION AND GASTROINTESTINAL ALTERATIONS

Liver Failure

The liver is the most important metabolic organ. It is responsible for carbohydrate, fat, and protein metabolism; vitamin storage and activation; and detoxification of waste products. Because the diseased liver has impaired ability to deactivate hormones, levels of circulating glucagon, epinephrine, and cortisol are elevated. These hormones promote catabolism of body tissues and cause glycogen stores to be exhausted. Release of lipids from their storage depots is accelerated, but the liver has decreased ability to metabolize them for energy. Moreover, inadequate production of bile salts by the liver results in malabsorption of fat from the diet. Body proteins are used for energy sources, producing tissue wasting. The damaged liver cannot clear ammonia from the circulation adequately, and ammonia accumulates in the brain. The ammonia may contribute to the encephalopathic symptoms and to brain edema.[1,46]

Monitoring Fluid and Electrolyte Status

Ascites and edema are caused by a combination of factors. Colloid osmotic pressure in the plasma decreases because of the reduction of production of albumin and other plasma proteins by the diseased liver, increased portal pressure caused by obstruction, and renal sodium retention from secondary hyperaldosteronism. To control the fluid retention, restriction of sodium (usually 2000 mg) and fluid ($\leq$1500 mL daily) usually is necessary in conjunction with the administration of diuretics. Patients are weighed daily to evaluate the success of treatment. Physical status and laboratory data must be closely monitored for deficiencies of potassium; phosphorus; zinc; and vitamins A, D, E, and K.[1]

Provision of a Nutritious Diet and Evaluation of Response to Dietary Protein

The causes of malnutrition are complex and are usually related to decreased intake, malabsorption, maldigestion, and abnormal nutrient metabolism. A diet with adequate protein helps suppress catabolism and promote liver regeneration. Stable patients with cirrhosis usually tolerate 0.8 to 1 g of protein/kg per day. Patients with severe stress or nutrition deficits have increased needs—1.2 to 2 g of protein/kg per

day.[46] Aggressive treatment with lactulose is considered first-line therapy in the management of acute hepatic encephalopathy.

Anorexia may interfere with oral intake. Small, frequent feedings are usually better tolerated by an anorexic patient than three large meals daily. If patients are unable to meet their caloric needs, they may require oral supplements or enteral feeding. Small-bore nasoenteric feeding tubes can be used safely without increasing risk of variceal bleeding.[46] TPN should be reserved for patients who are absolutely unable to tolerate enteral feeding.[1] Diarrhea from concurrent administration of lactulose should not be confused with feeding intolerance.

A diet adequate in calories (at least 30 calories/kg daily) is provided to help prevent catabolism and to prevent the use of dietary protein for energy needs.[47] In cases of malabsorption, medium-chain triglycerides may be used to meet caloric needs. Pancreatic enzymes may also be considered for malabsorption problems.

A patient who undergoes successful liver transplantation is usually able to tolerate a regular diet with few restrictions. Intake during the postoperative period must be adequate to support nutrition repletion and healing; 1 to 1.2 g of protein/kg per day and approximately 30 calories/kg per day are usually sufficient for a well-nourished patient. Immunosuppressant therapy (corticosteroids and cyclosporine or tacrolimus) contributes to glucose intolerance. Dietary measures to control glucose intolerance include (1) obtaining approximately 30% of dietary calories from fat, (2) emphasizing complex sources of carbohydrates, and (3) eating several small meals daily. Moderate exercise often helps improve glucose tolerance.

Pancreatitis

The pancreas is an exocrine and endocrine gland required for normal digestion and metabolism of proteins, carbohydrates, and fats. Acute pancreatitis is an inflammatory process that occurs as a result of autodigestion of the pancreas by enzymes normally secreted by that organ. Food intake stimulates pancreatic secretion, increasing the damage to the pancreas and the pain associated with the disorder. Patients with the mild form of acute pancreatitis do not require nutrition support and generally resume oral feeding within 7 days. Chronic pancreatitis may develop and results in loss of exocrine and endocrine function because of the destruction of acinar and islet cells. The loss of exocrine function leads to malabsorption and steatorrhea. In chronic pancreatitis, the loss of endocrine function results in impaired glucose tolerance.[48]

Prevention of Further Damage to the Pancreas and Preventing Nutrition Deficits

The concern that feeding may stimulate the production of digestive enzymes and perpetuate tissue damage has led to the widespread use of TPN and bowel rest. Data suggest that for patients with severe pancreatitis, providing enteral nutrition support is more beneficial than prolonged bowel rest and provision of TPN.[1,49] Enteral nutrition infused into the distal jejunum bypasses the stimulatory effect of feeding on pancreatic secretion and is associated with fewer infectious and metabolic complications compared with TPN.[50,51]

The results of randomized studies comparing TPN with enteral nutrition indicate that enteral nutrition is preferable to TPN in patients with severe acute pancreatitis, reducing costs and the risk of sepsis and improving clinical outcome.[50–52] Patients unable to tolerate enteral nutrition should receive TPN, and some patients may require a combination of enteral nutrition and TPN to meet nutrition requirements.[53,54] Low-fat enteral formulas and formulas with fat provided by medium-chain triglycerides are more readily absorbed than formulas that are high in long-chain triglycerides (e.g., corn oil, sunflower oil).

When oral intake is possible, small, frequent feedings of low-fat foods are least likely to cause discomfort,[51] although the level of fat restriction should depend on the level of steatorrhea and abdominal pain the patient experiences.[49] For patients with chronic pancreatitis, pancreatic enzyme replacement therapy may be indicated.[49] Guidelines for the treatment of diabetes (discussed later) are appropriate for the care of patients with glucose intolerance or diabetes related to pancreatitis.

NUTRITION AND ENDOCRINE ALTERATIONS

Nutrition Support and Blood Glucose Control

When a patient is not expected to be able to eat for at least 5 to 7 days or inadequate intake persists for that period, initiation of nutrition support is indicated. Patients unable to tolerate oral diets or enteral feeding may require TPN to meet nutrition requirements during acute illness. No disease process benefits from starvation, and development or progression of nutrition deficits may contribute to complications such as pressure injuries, pulmonary or urinary tract infections, and sepsis, which prolong hospitalization, increase the costs of care, and may result in death.

Continuous enteral infusions are associated with improved control of blood glucose. Fiber-enriched formulas may slow the absorption of the carbohydrate, producing a more delayed and sustained glycemic response. Most standard formulas contain balanced proportions of carbohydrate, protein, and fats appropriate for diabetic patients. Specialized diabetic formulas have not shown improved outcomes compared with standard formulas.[55] Blood glucose control is especially important in the care of surgical patients. Poorly controlled diabetes reduces immune function by impairing granulocyte adherence, chemotaxis, and phagocytosis.[56,57] In surveys of critically ill patients undergoing a variety of elective operations and coronary artery surgery,[56] glucose levels of 206 to 220 mg/dL or higher during the first 24 to 36 postoperative hours were associated with higher rates of nosocomial infection than lower glucose levels.[56,58]

The following glucose goals are recommended: 140 to 180 mg/dL in critically ill patients.[59] Multiple subcutaneous insulin doses or, preferably, a continuous intravenous infusion of regular insulin may be used to maintain tight control of blood glucose in the enterally fed patient.[55] Regular insulin added to the solution is a common method of managing hyperglycemia in the patient receiving TPN.

NUTRITION AND SURGERY

Preoperative Nutrition Preparation

Patients should be allowed to consume a light meal up to 6 hours before surgery and clear liquids up to 2 hours before surgery. Administration of an oral maltodextrin beverage the evening before surgery and 2 to 3 hours before anesthesia has been demonstrated to improve postoperative insulin sensitivity, decrease protein catabolism, and maintain muscle strength. Caution should be taken when administering high-carbohydrate beverages to patients with gastroparesis.[60]

Postoperative Nutrition Interventions

Postoperative nausea and vomiting affect 50% and 30%, respectively, of all surgical patients and may result in dehydration and delayed achievement of nutritional goals. All surgical patients should be considered for prophylactic antiemetic therapy. Routine use of nasogastric decompression should be avoided. An oral diet can be initiated within 4 hours of surgery, and patients should be allowed to choose regular foods.[60,61] Allowing patients a choice in their meal selection can help optimize GI tolerance to oral intake, as patients in the postoperative period do not tend to have an appetite for high-fat or high-fiber foods and are rarely able to overconsume calories. For patients who require tube feeding, enteral nutrition can be started along the same timeline as an oral diet.

ADDITIONAL RESOURCES

See Box 5.6 for Internet resources related to nutritional alterations and management.

BOX 5.6 Informatics   QSEN

Internet Resources: Nutritional Alterations and Management

- Academy of Nutrition and Dietetics: https://www.eatright.org/
- Academy of Nutrition and Dietetics Evidence Analysis Library: https://www.andeal.org/
- American Society for Parenteral and Enteral Nutrition: http://www.nutritioncare.org/
- Dietitians on Demand: https://dietitiansondemand.com/
- Malnutrition Quality Improvement Initiative: http://malnutritionquality.org/

REFERENCES

1. McClave SA, Taylor BE, Martindale RG, et al. Guidelines for the provision and assessment of nutrition support therapy in the adult critically ill patient: Society of Critical Care Medicine (SCCM) and American Society for Parenteral and Enteral Nutrition (A.S.P.E.N.). *JPEN J Parenter Enteral Nutr.* 2016;40(2):159–211.
2. Simpson F, Doig GS, Early PN Trial Investigators Group. Physical assessment and anthropometric measures for use in critical research conducted in critically ill patient populations: an analytic observational study. *JPEN J Parenter Enteral Nutr.* 2015;39(3):313–321.
3. Mahanna E, Crimi E, White P, Mann DS, Fahy BG. Nutrition and metabolic support for critically ill patients. *Curr Opin Anesth.* 2015;28(2):131–138.
4. Soeters PB, Wolfe RR, Shenkin A. Hypoalbuminemia: pathogenesis and clinical significance. *J Parenter Enteral Nutr.* 2019;43(2):181–193.
5. Singer P, Singer J. Clinical guide for the use of metabolic carts: indirect calorimetry - no longer the orphan of energy estimation. *Nutr Clin Pract.* 2016;31:30–38.
6. Frankenfield DC, Ashcraft CM. Estimating energy needs in nutrition support patients. *J Parenter Enteral Nutr.* 2011;35:563–570.
7. Parker EA, Feinberg TM, Wappel S, Verceles AC. Consideration when using predictive equations to estimate energy needs among older, hospitalized patients: a narrative review. *Curr Nutr Rep.* 2017;6(2):102–110.
8. Dickerson RN, Patel JJ, McClain CJ. Protein and calorie requirement associated with the presence of obesity. *Nutr Clin Pract.* 2017;32(suppl 1):86S–93S.
9. Kwon S, Thompson R, Dellinger P, Yanez D, Farrohki E, Flum D. Importance of perioperative glycemic control in general surgery: a report from the Surgical Care and Outcomes Assessment Program. *Ann Surg.* 2013;257(1):8.
10. Lew CCH, Yandell R, Fraser RJL, Chua AP, Chong MFF, Miller M. Association between malnutrition and clinical outcomes in the intensive care unit: a systematic review. *J Parenter Enteral Nutr.* 2017;41(5):744–758.

11. Sharma K, Mongensen KM, Robinson MK. Pathophysiology of critical illness and role of nutrition. *Nutr Clin Pract.* 2019;34(1):12−22.

12. Philipson TJ, Snider JT, Lakdawalla DN, Stryckman B, Goldman DP. Impact of oral nutritional supplementation on hospital outcomes. *Am J Manag Care.* 2013;19(2):121−128.

13. Singer P, Anbar R, Cohen J, et al. The tight calorie control study (TICA-COS): a prospective, randomized, controlled pilot study of nutritional support in critically ill patients. *Intensive Care Med.* 2011;37(4):601−609.

14. Rubinson L, Diette GB, Song X, Brower RG, Krishnan JA. Low caloric intake is associated with nosocomial bloodstream infections in patients in the medical intensive care unit. *Crit Care Med.* 2004;32:350.

15. Mongensen KM, Malone A, Becker P, et al. Academy of Nutrition and Dietetics/American Society for Parenteral and Enteral Nutrition Consensus Malnutrition Characteristics: usability and association with outcomes. *Nutr Clin Pract.* 2019;34(5):657−665.

16. Seres DS, Valcarcel M, Guillaume A. Advantages of enteral nutrition over parenteral nutrition. *Therap Adv Gastroenterol.* 2013;6(2):157−167.

17. Yang S, Wu X, Yu W, Li J. Early enteral nutrition in critically ill patients with hemodynamic instability: an evidenced-based review and practical advice. *Nutr Clin Pract.* 2014;29(1):90−96.

18. Moore FA, Weisbrodt NW. Gut dysfunction and intolerance to enteral nutrition in critically ill patients. *Nestle Nutr Workshop Ser Clin Perform Programme.* 2003;8:149.

19. Gwon J, Lee YJ, Kyoung KH, Kim YH, Hong SK. Enteral nutrition associated non-occlusive bowel ischemia. *J Korean Surg Soc.* 2012;83:171−174.

20. Turza KC, Krenitsky J, Sawyer RG. Enteral feeding and vasoactive agents: suggested guidelines for clinicians. *Practical Gastroenterol.* 2009;78:11−22.

21. Carter M, Roberts S, Carson JA. Small-bowel feeding tube placement at bedside: electronic medical device placement and x-ray agreement. *Nutr Clin Pract.* 2018;33(2):274−280.

22. Davies AR, Morrison SS, Bailey MJ, et al. A multicenter, randomized controlled trial comparing early nasojejunal with nasogastric nutrition in critical illness. *Crit Care Med.* 2012;40(8):2342−2348.

23. Esparza J, Boivin MA, Hartshorne MF, Levy H. Equal aspiration rates in gastrically and transpylorically fed critically ill patients. *Intensive Care Med.* 2001;27:660.

24. Neumann DA, DeLegge MH. Gastric versus small-bowel tube feeding in the intensive care unit: a prospective comparison of efficacy. *Crit Care Med.* 2002;30(7):1436.

25. Davies AR, Froomes PR, French CJ, et al. Randomized comparison of nasojejunal and nasogastric feeding in critically ill patients. *Crit Care Med.* 2002;30(3):586.

26. Zhang Z, Xu X, Ding J, Ni H. Comparison of postpyloric tube feeding and gastric tube feeding in intensive care unit patients: a meta-analysis. *Nutr Clin Pract.* 2013;28(3):371−380.

27. Seron-Arbeloa C, Zamora-Elson M, Labarta-Monzon L, Mallor-Bonet T. Enteral nutrition in critical care. *J Clin Med Res.* 2013;5(1):1.

28. Engel JM, Muhling J, Junger A, Menges T, Karcher B, Hempelmann G. Enteral nutrition practice in a surgical intensive care unit: what proportion of energy expenditure is delivered enterally? *Clin Nutr.* 2003;22(2):187.

29. Krishnan JA, Muhling J, Junger A, Menges T, Karcher B, Hempelmann G. Caloric intake in medical ICU patients: consistency of care with guidelines and relationship to clinical outcomes. *Chest.* 2003;124:297.

30. Kim H, Stotts NA, Froelicher ES, Engler MM, Porter C. Why patients in critical care do not receive adequate enteral nutrition? A review of the literature. *J Crit Care.* 2012;27(6):702−713.

31. Worthington P, Gilbert KA, Wagner BA. Parenteral nutrition for the acutely ill. *AACN Clin Issues.* 2000;11(4):559.

32. Speerhas R, Wong J, Seidner D, Steiger E. Maintaining normal blood glucose concentrations with total parenteral nutrition: is it necessary to taper total parenteral nutrition? *Nutr Clin Pract.* 2003;18:414.

33. Crook MA, Hally V, Panteli JV. The importance of the refeeding syndrome. *Nutrition.* 2001;17:632.

34. Mehanna HM, Moledina J, Travis J. Refeeding syndrome: what is it, and how to prevent and treat it. *BMJ.* 2008;336:1495−1498.

35. Hearing SD. Refeeding syndrome. *BMJ.* 2004;328(7445):908.

36. Academy of Nutrition and Dietetics. Nutrition care cardiovascular disease heart failure nutrition prescription. Nutrition Care Manual. www.nutritioncaremanual.org. Accessed October 28, 2019.

37. Boisrame-Helms J, Toti F, Hasselmann M, Meziani F. Lipid emulsions for parenteral nutrition in critical illness. *Prog Lipid Res.* 2015;60:1−16.

38. Ayodele-Adesanya TM, Sullivan RC, Stawicki SPA, Evans S. Nutrition in traumatic brain injury: focus on the immune modulating supplements. In: Sadaka F, ed. *Traumatic Brain Injury [e-Book].* InTech; 2014.

39. Wang X, Dong Y, Han X, Qi XQ, Huang CG, Hou LJ. Nutritional support for patients sustaining traumatic brain injury: a systematic review and meta-analysis of prospective studies. *PLoS One.* 2013;8(3):e58838.

40. Pellicane AJ, Millis SR, Zimmerman SE, Roth EJ. Calorie and protein intake in acute rehabilitation in patients with traumatic spinal cord injury versus other diagnoses. *Top Spinal Cord Inj Rehabil.* 2013;19(3):229.

41. Aquilani R, Boschi F, Contardi A, et al. Energy expenditure and nutritional adequacy of rehabilitation paraplegics with asymptomatic bacteriuria and pressure sores. *Spinal Cord.* 2001;39:437.

42. Ikizler TA, Cano NJ, Franch H, et al. Prevention and treatment of protein energy wasting in chronic kidney disease patients: a consensus statement by the International Society of Renal Nutrition and Metabolism. *Kidney Int.* 2013;84(6):1096−1107.

43. McCarthy MS, Phipps SC. Special nutrition challenges: current approach to acute kidney injury. *Nutr Clin Pract.* 2014;29(1):56−62.

44. Cano NJM, Aparicio M, Brunori G, et al. ESPEN guidelines on parenteral nutrition: adult renal failure. *Clin Nutr.* 2009;28(4):401−414.

45. Brown RO, Compher C. The American Society for Parenteral and Enteral Nutrition (ASPEN) Board of Directors. A.S.P.E.N. clinical guideline: nutrition support in adult acute and chronic renal failure. *J Parenter Enteral Nutr.* 2010;34(4):366.

46. Patton KM, Aranda-Michel J. Nutritional aspects in liver disease and liver transplantation. *Nutr Clin Pract.* 2002;17:332.

47. Saraf N. Nutritional management of acute and chronic liver disease. *Hepat B Annu.* 2008;5(1):117−133.

48. Khokhar AS, Seidner DL. The pathophysiology of pancreatitis. *Nutr Clin Pract.* 2004;19:5.

49. Academy of Nutrition and Dietetics. Nutrition care gastrointestinal disease liver, gallbladder, and pancreas disease pancreatitis nutrition intervention. Nutrition Care Manual. www.nutritioncaremanual.org. Accessed October 28, 2019.

50. Ong JPL, Fock KM. Nutritional support in acute pancreatitis. *J Dig Dis.* 2012;13(9):445−452.

51. Russell MK. Acute pancreatitis: a review of pathophysiology and nutrition management. *Nutr Clin Pract.* 2004;19:16.

52. Al-Omran M, Albalawi ZH, Tashkandi MF, Al-Ansary LA. Enteral versus parenteral nutrition for acute pancreatitis. *Cochrane Database Syst Rev.* 2010;2010(1):CD002837.

53. Petrov MS, Pylypchuk RD, Uchugina AF. A systematic review on the timing of artificial nutrition in acute pancreatitis. *Br J Nutr.* 2009;101(6):787−793.

54. Talukdar R, Vege SS. Recent developments in acute pancreatitis. *Clin Gastroenterol Hepatol.* 2009;7(11):S3−S9.

55. Charney P, Hertzler SR. Management of blood glucose and diabetes in the critically ill patient receiving enteral feeding. *Nutr Clin Pract.* 2004;19:129.

56. Van den Berghe G, Wouters P, Weekers F, et al. Intensive insulin therapy in critically ill patients. *N Engl J Med.* 2001;345:1359.

57. Rassias AJ, Givan AL, Marrin CA, Whalen K, Pahl J, Yeager MP. Insulin increases neutrophil count and phagocytic capacity after cardiac surgery. *Anesth Analg.* 2002;94:1113.

58. Umpierrez GE, Isaacs SD, Bazargan N, You X, Thaler LM, Kitabchi AE. Hyperglycemia: an independent marker of in-hospital mortality in patients with undiagnosed diabetes. *J Clin Endocrinol Metab.* 2002;87:978.

59. American Diabetes Association. Diabetes care in the hospital: standards of medical care in diabetes - 2018. *Diabetes Care.* 2018;41(suppl 1):S144−S151.

60. Gustafsson UO, Scott MJ, Hubner M, et al. Guidelines for perioperative care in elective colorectal surgery: Enhanced Recovery after Surgery (ERAS) Society recommendations: 2018. *World J Surg.* 2019;43:659−695.

61. Warren J, Bhalla V, Cresci G. Postoperative diet advancement: surgical dogma vs evidence-based medicine. *Nutr Clin Pract.* 2011;26(2):115−125.

6

The Older Adult

Fiona Winterbottom and Misty Jenkins

CRITICAL CARE AND THE OLDER ADULT

Critical illness in the older adult can be thought of in three parts[1]:
1. predisposing factors, such as frailty;
2. precipitating factors, such as acute clinical deterioration; and
3. perpetuating factors, such as delirium and polypharmacy.

The intersection of these factors ultimately determines outcomes. Several studies have looked at very old age and outcomes, with most studies revealing that age was not an independent predictor of outcome; however, multiple preexisting comorbidities and mechanical ventilation did influence critical care outcomes.[1–3]

TRENDING PRIORITIES IN HEALTHCARE

Evidence-Based Hospital Design and the Older Adult

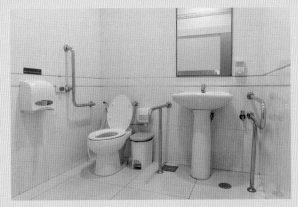

(iStock.com/pisittar.)

One of the significant issues that affect hospitalized older adults is the risk of falling. While numerous research studies have looked at potential solutions, one area getting more recognition is the design of the patient's room. Many hospitals are remodeling or constructing new buildings to meet updated regulatory standards and enhance patient centeredness.

Thus an opportunity exists to change the actual environment to enhance the safety of hospitalized older adults, notably regarding patient falls.

Various elements of the physical environment have been implicated as problematic, particularly the bathroom area. Issues with the bathroom include the bathroom's location, the toilet and sink's location, the presence and location of grab bars, and the flooring pattern.[1] In addition, manipulating an IV pole when ambulating to the bathroom and the type and swing direction of the bathroom door were other factors that further complicated the patient's environment.[1]

A recent integrative review looked at the impact of the room environment on patient falls and found limited evidence regarding the best environmental design for the bathroom to enhance fall prevention. More research is needed in this area to develop definitive guidelines.[2] However, some environmental configurations deserve further attention when redesigning a patient bathroom. Here are some items that should be considered:

- Room configurations. Use same-handed room arrangements in which all rooms within a unit are standardized such that they are all identical. With this arrangement, the door to the bathroom is always in the same place, and the bathroom configuration is always the same in every room.[2]
- Space within the bathroom area. Provide the patient sufficient room to maneuver, particularly if pushing or pulling an IV pole or using an ambulatory aid.[2]
- Space around the commode. Allow adequate space around the toilet for two health care personnel to assist the patient on and off the toilet.[3]
- Location of the toilet in relation to the sink and door. Place the toilet on the sidewall of the bathroom instead of across from the bathroom door, thus avoiding having the patient cross the room to get to the toilet.[2]
- Type, swing, and width of the bathroom door with respect to the other environmental elements in the room.[2] Consider using a barn door-type bathroom door instead of a hinged door to avoid the swing of the door.[3] Consider the width of the door frame; if it is too small, it can be challenging to get through, particularly with equipment, and if it is too wide, the door can be cumbersome.[2]
- Toilet height and manipulation. Use a toilet with a high toilet seat[3] and features that limit bending and turning to lift and close the lid and flush.[2]
- Lighting. Provide night lighting in the patient room and the bathroom to facilitate safe movement around the room at night.[3]

The configuration of a patient bathroom has a significant impact on patient safety, particularly regarding patient falls. However, more research is needed to develop consistent standards for standard bathroom configurations.

References

1. Pati D, Valipoor S, Cloutier A, et al. Physical design factors contributing to patient falls. *J Patient Saf.* 2021;17(3):e135–e142.
2. Pati D, Valipoor S, Lorusso L, et al. The impact of the built environment on patient falls in hospital rooms: an integrative review. *J Patient Saf.* 2021;17(4):273–281.
3. Lavender SA, Sommerich CM, Sanders EB, et al. Developing evidence-based design guidelines for medical/surgical hospital patient rooms that meet the needs of staff, patients, and visitors. *HERD.* 2020;13(1):145–178.

AGE-RELATED CHANGES IN THE OLDER ADULT

As adults age, reserve capacity decreases, compounded by geriatric syndromes that include delirium, sensory deficit, reduced cognition, functional decline, frailty, and multimorbidity.[1] The number of comorbidities also increases with age, which contributes to mortality and decreases physical independence.[1,4] The average number of co-morbid conditions in patients between 65 and 84 years is at least two and is more than three in those over 85 years.[4]

Neurocognitive Age-Related Changes
Physiologic Changes

The aging brain experiences physiologic changes that often present as alterations in cognition. These changes within the central nervous system (CNS) include a reduction in brain volume and weight, neurodegeneration, decrease in neurotransmitters, blood-brain barrier permeability, and cerebral blood flow.[5]

The brain decreases approximately 20% in size between 25 and 95 years of age[6] (Fig. 6.1). Reduction in brain weight may be related to the overall decrease in the number of neurons that occurs with advancing age. Portions of the cerebral cortex atrophy, predominantly the frontal and temporal cortical association areas influencing attention and executive functioning.[5]

Neurotransmitters such as acetylcholine, dopamine, serotonin, and glutamate decrease with aging. These changes have been associated with decreased cognition and motor function. Alterations in neurotransmitters are believed to play a role in delirium.[5]

Cerebral blood flow decreases with advancing age.[6] Cerebral blood flow is influenced by age-related changes in blood pressure (BP), barometric response to positional change, and severity of cerebrovascular disease (also see Chapter 16).

Cognitive Function

Cognitive function involves transforming, synthesizing, storing, and retrieving sensory input in addition to perception, attention, thinking, memory, and problem solving. A critically ill older adult is especially susceptible to acute brain dysfunction, which is commonly referred to as *delirium* (see Chapter 8). This occurs when age-related changes are coupled with the acute stress of a critical illness, resulting in an imbalance of the brain's homeostatic reserve.[5,7]

In the aging brain, a decline in hormonal and immunologic feedback mechanisms can lead to a cycle of excessive inflammatory response to an acute stress such as sepsis resulting in neurodegeneration and further inflammation.[7]

Specific risk factors for the older adult include reduced preoperative cognitive status, age greater than 75, cerebrovascular disease, and

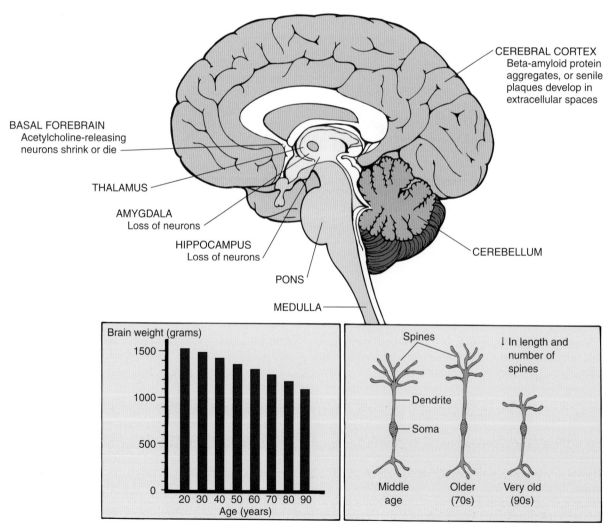

Fig. 6.1 Age-Related Changes in the Brain. (From Selkoe DJ. Aging brain, aging mind. *Sci Am.* 1992;267:134.)

frailty.[8] Baseline dementia, stress of surgery or acute illness, and hospitalization can cause cognitive decline and significantly increase risk for delirium in older adults.

Age-Related Changes of the Respiratory System and Pulmonary Disease

Significant age-related changes affect the pulmonary system, including alterations in compliance of the chest wall, strength of respiratory muscles, and static elastic recoil of the lung.[9] Additionally, arterial partial pressure of oxygen (PaO_2) and respiratory sensitivity to hypoxia and hypercarbia are reduced.[10] As a result, older adult patients have less pulmonary reserve along with increased susceptibility to infections[11,12] (Fig. 6.2).

Thoracic Wall and Respiratory Muscles

The thoracic cavity becomes progressively smaller with aging as a result of a loss of height of the intervertebral disks, leading to narrowing of the rib spaces.[12] This narrowing or kyphosis increases after 40 years of age.[12] Thoracic stiffening occurs from a decline in rib mobility secondary to contractures of intercostal muscles and calcification of costal cartilage.

Additionally, prevalence of vertebral fractures increases with age, particularly in women, as a result of osteoporosis.[9] Progressive decreases in chest wall compliance and changes in the shape of the thorax alter chest wall mechanics, leading to a deterioration in respiratory function.[9]

Strength of the diaphragm and intercostal muscles decreases with age, with a 2% annual decline in muscle function.[12] Other factors such as an increase in abdominal girth and change in posture also decrease thoracic excursion. Respiratory muscle function is affected by skeletal muscle and peripheral muscle strength.[12]

During aging, skeletal muscle progressively atrophies, and its energy metabolism decreases, which may partially explain the declining strength of the respiratory muscles.[12] Respiratory muscle strength is additionally affected by nutritional status, which is often deficient in older adults.[11]

The aging pulmonary system has a reduced ability to clear mucus from the airways. As respiratory muscle declines, the ability to generate the necessary high forced expiratory flow for an effective cough is reduced.[12] There is an increased risk of aspiration and hospital-acquired infections in older adults.[13]

Lung Parenchyma and Volumes

Diminished recoil of the lung occurs with aging, causing increased lung volume and distention of the alveolar spaces.[12] Reduced lung elasticity results from changes in the ratio of elastic to support tissue that occur with advancing age.[14]

Pulmonary Gas Exchange

Ventilation and diffusion depend on numerous factors, including lung surface area (also see Chapter 13). Capillary blood volume and surface

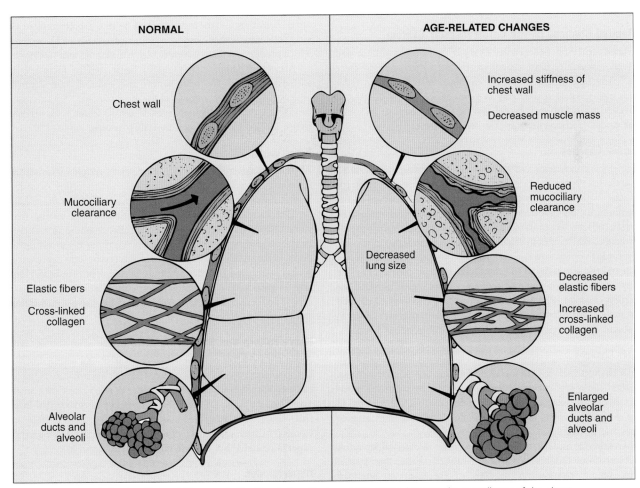

Fig. 6.2 Age-Related Changes in the Respiratory System. With advancing age, the compliance of the chest wall and lung tissue changes. There is also a reduced clearance of mucus by the cilia that line the pulmonary tree and an enlargement of the alveolar ducts and alveoli.

area have also been reported to decrease with advancing age. Changes in pulmonary circulation result in a ventilation-perfusion mismatch. Ventilation-perfusion mismatch leads to a decline in arterial partial pressure of oxygen (PaO_2) of approximately 0.3 mm Hg per year from the age of 30 years.[14]

Age-related changes in ventilation and arterial partial pressure of carbon dioxide ($PaCO_2$) occur across the adult life span. Ventilation-perfusion inequality may exist with decreased diffusion capacity of the lung for carbon monoxide and the transfer capacity of oxygen across the alveolar-capillary interface.[15]

Acute Lung Failure and Pulmonary Diseases

Critically ill older adults are at increased risk for acute lung failure. Chronic illnesses, major organ dysfunction, and decreased pulmonary reserve contribute to the incidence of acute lung failure[10] (also see Chapter 14). Chronic illnesses such as chronic obstructive pulmonary disease (COPD), pulmonary embolism, community-acquired pneumonia, and heart disease all increase with age.[10] The incidence of *COPD* is two to three times higher in people older than age 60 and is the third leading cause of death in the United States.[12]

The clinical presentation of *pneumonia* in older adults may be atypical and include a nonproductive cough, delirium, anorexia, falls, and dizziness.[16] Pneumonia has been noted to occur more frequently and with increased mortality in the older adult.[10]

The occurrence of *pulmonary embolism* is higher in older adults as a result of predisposing conditions such as malignancy, postoperative states, and immobility.

Age-Related Changes of the Cardiovascular System

Age-related structural and cellular changes in the myocardium and peripheral vasculature have a significant effect on critically ill older adults.[17] The largest risk factor for cardiovascular disease in older adults is age. Cardiac and arterial system changes result in reduced cardiovascular function and reserve, leaving an older adult at increased risk for cardiac decompensation (also see Chapter 11).

Myocardial Changes

The aging heart undergoes a modest degree of hypertrophy and thickening of the left ventricular (LV) wall without significant changes in LV cavity size.[17,18] Several other factors contribute to the changes in the myocardium, including a decrease in the number of cardiomyocytes, increase in collagen accumulation, fibrosis, increased inflammatory cells and proteins, and changes in calcium signaling of cardiomyocytes.[19]

Myocardial contraction is dependent on intracellular levels of free calcium and the sensitivity of the contractile proteins for calcium. The changes in calcium signaling lead to a prolonged duration of contraction (systole), which is caused in part by a slowed or delayed rate of myocardial relaxation.[17] In the older adult, presence of an S_4 heart sound may be evident with reduced LV compliance.[20]

Vascular Changes

Vascular changes include endothelial dysfunction and arterial stiffness. The endothelium regulates vascular homeostasis by balancing vasodilators and vasoconstrictors.[20] Endothelial dysfunction results in arterial stiffening, which reduces blood flow and promotes atherosclerosis and thrombosis.[20]

Atherosclerotic and arteriosclerotic processes in older adults cause arteries to become progressively less distensible and alter the vascular pressure-volume relationship, leading to increases in afterload and development of concentric (pressure-induced) ventricular hypertrophy.[18]

Increased arterial stiffness occurs from alterations in the arterial wall resulting in an increase in systolic BP, decrease in diastolic BP, and widening of *pulse pressure*. The effects of these changes can complicate treatment for systolic hypertension because of excessive lowering of diastolic BP and the risk for postural hypotension.[21]

Conduction and Beta-Adrenergic Changes

Heart rate modulation and adrenergic responsiveness are important changes in the aging cardiovascular system.[21] Heart rate decreases in both variability and maximal heart rate by loss of cells in the sinoatrial node, fibrosis, and hypertrophy, resulting in a slower conduction of electrical impulses throughout the heart.[22] The older adult may experience orthostatic hypotension, syncope, and cardiac decompensation from lack of cardiac reserve.[19]

Electrocardiogram Changes

Changes in the electrocardiogram (ECG) include decreased R-wave and S-wave amplitude, increased PR interval, and increased QT interval duration reflective of prolonged rate of relaxation.[17] The QRS axis shifts leftward with age, perhaps as a result of increased LV wall thickness or hypertrophy.[17]

The senescent myocardium may have a lower threshold for atrial and ventricular arrhythmias because of changes in gene expression of proteins that regulate calcium.[17] Cardiac dysrhythmias include atrial fibrillation and paroxysmal supraventricular tachycardia; the most common dysrhythmia is premature ventricular contraction.[18]

Reports show that 3% to 4% of patients over 60 years of age experience atrial fibrillation, and the incidence may be 10% in patients 80 to 89 years old.[18] Older individuals also have a high prevalence of LV hypertrophy, which predisposes them to ventricular arrhythmias and sudden death.

Atrial fibrillation is thought to be related to increased arterial stiffness, reduced LV compliance, and reduced rate control, and anticoagulation is recommended for most patients.[18,19] Age-associated cardiac conduction changes (even if asymptomatic) are predictive of future cardiac morbidity and mortality in older adults.[18,19]

Baroreceptor Changes

Abrupt changes in BP caused by changes in peripheral resistance, CO, or blood volume are sensed by *baroreceptors*, resulting in an increase in impulse frequency to the vasomotor center within the medulla.

This increase inhibits vasoconstrictor impulses arising from the vasoconstrictor region within the medulla, resulting in a decrease in heart rate and peripheral vasodilation returning BP to within normal limits.[22] Baroreflex-mediated tachycardia response to depressor agents is also attenuated in older adults. Prevalence of orthostatic hypotension is greater in older patients, especially older patients in critical care, and judicious use of antihypertensive medications is recommended.[22,23]

Heart Failure and Myocardial Infarction

Approximately 50% of heart failure cases are found within the 6% of the US population older than age 75.[17] Chronic heart failure is the leading cause of hospitalizations for adults older than 65 years, with an average 1-year mortality of 33% to 35%.[24] Incidence of myocardial infarction (MI) doubles for older men and increases more than fivefold in older women.[24] Older adults not only are more likely than young patients to experience an MI but also are more likely to die of MI.

Hypertension

Hypertension affects most individuals older than 65 years of age.[22] Pathophysiology of hypertension in older adults results from changes in arterial structure and function that decrease distensibility of large vessels, reduce forward circulation flow, increase pulse wave velocity, cause late systolic BP augmentation, and increase myocardial oxygen demand, all of which limit organ perfusion.[22]

Heart Disease Management

Treatment in older adults includes aggressive treatment of dyslipidemia with lipid-lowering medication, control of blood glucose, and lifestyle modification. Treatment with medication is recommended for older adult hypertensive patients with attention to alterations in medication distribution and disposal, changes in homeostatic cardiovascular control, and quality-of-life (QOL) factors.

Cardiac Medication Considerations in Older Adults

Treatment with medication should be considered when non-pharmacologic interventions are unsuccessful. Heart rate control can be managed with beta-blockers and calcium channel blockers. Amiodarone can be used for conversion and maintenance of sinus rhythm with atrial fibrillation[22] (Table 6.1).

Combination pharmacologic therapy in older adult patients provides opportunity for enhanced efficacy, avoidance of adverse effects, enhanced convenience, and compliance.[25] Box 6.1 lists potentially inappropriate symptom medication management for older adults.

Approximately 40% of older adults are prescribed more than five medications per day, and older adults are particularly vulnerable to adverse medication interactions.[25–27] Approximately 61% of adverse events in critical care units were linked with medications.[28] Medications most often associated with adverse events include cardiovascular medications (24%), anticoagulants (20%), anti-infective agents (13%), and hypoglycemic agents.[26]

Alterations in absorption, distribution, metabolism, and excretion are responsible for many adverse events. Alterations in gastric acid secretion, solubility of medications, and hepatic and renal function result in changes to absorption rates[29] (Table 6.2).

Age-Related Changes of the Kidney System

Aging is associated with various and complex abnormalities of hormones and systems that are important in water homeostasis and is a

TABLE 6.1 Cardiac Medication Considerations in Older Adults.

Medication	Clinical Considerations
Thiazide Diuretics	
Hydrochlorothiazide	Recommended for initial hypertensive therapy
Chlorthalidone	↓ Peripheral vascular resistance
Bendrofluazide	↓ Intravascular volume
	↓ BP
	↓ Cardiovascular, cerebrovascular, renal adverse outcomes
	Generally well tolerated in older adults
	May exacerbate arrhythmias, hyperuricemia, glucose intolerance, dyslipidemia
Nonthiazide Diuretics	
Indapamide—sulfonamide diuretic	↑ Blood glucose
	Does not increase uric acid
	May cause potassium-independent prolongation of QT interval
Furosemide—loop diuretic	↑ Blood glucose
	May cause headaches, fever, anemia
	May cause electrolyte disturbances
Mineralocorticoid Antagonists	
Spironolactone/eplerenone	Useful in hypertension when combined with other agents
	Causes potassium retention
	Not associated with adverse metabolic effects
Beta-Blockers	
Metoprolol	Indicated for older adult patients with:
	• Hypertension, CAD, heart failure
	• May cause certain dysrhythmias
	• May cause migraine headaches
	• Causes senile tremor
Calcium Antagonists	
Phenylalkylamines—verapamil	Variable effects on heart muscle, sinus node function, atrioventricular conduction, peripheral arteries, coronary circulation
Benzothiazepines—diltiazem	Effective in older adult patients with hypertension due to increasing arterial stiffness, decreased vascular angina and supraventricular arrhythmias, compliance, diastolic dysfunction
Dihydropyridines—nicardipine	Should be avoided in patients with heart failure
ACE Inhibitors (ACEIs)	
Captopril (Capoten)	Blocks conversion of angiotensin I to angiotensin II in tissue and plasma
Enalapril (Vasotec)	Lowers peripheral vascular resistance and BP without reflex stimulation of heart rate and contractility
Lisinopril (Prinivil, Zestril)	Reduces morbidity and mortality in patients with heart failure, reduced systolic function, post-MI
	Retards progression of diabetic renal disease and hypertensive nephrosclerosis

Continued

TABLE 6.1 Cardiac Medication Considerations in Older Adults.—cont'd	
Medication	**Clinical Considerations**
Angiotensin Receptor Blockers	
Losartan (Cozaar)	Selectively blocks AT1 receptor subtype to:
Valsartan (Diovan)	• Reduce BP
	• Protect kidneys
	• Reduce mortality and morbidity in heart failure patients
	Considered first line and as an alternative to ACEIs in older adult hypertensive patients with diabetes mellitus, hypertension, and heart failure who cannot tolerate ACEIs
Direct Renin Inhibitors	
Aliskiren	Effective for BP lowering without dose-related increases in adverse events in older adult patients
	May be used in combination therapy
Nonspecific Vasodilators	
Hydralazine	Fourth-line antihypertensive because of unfavorable side effects
Minoxidil	Tachycardia
	Fluid accumulation and atrial arrhythmias (minoxidil) when used as part of combination regimens
	Centrally acting agents (e.g., clonidine) are not first-line treatments in older adults because of sedation and/or bradycardia
	Abrupt discontinuation leads to increased BP and heart rate, which may aggravate ischemia and/or heart failure
Centrally Acting Agents	
Clonidine	Not first-line treatments in older adults because of sedation and/or bradycardia
	Abrupt discontinuation leads to increased BP and HR

ACE, Angiotensin-converting enzyme; *BP,* blood pressure; *CAD,* coronary artery disease; *MI,* myocardial infarction.
Adapted from Aronow WS, Fleg JL, Pepine CJ, et al. ACCF/AHA 2011 expert consensus document on hypertension in the elderly: a report of the American College of Cardiology Foundation task force on clinical expert consensus documents. *J Am Coll Cardiol.* 2011;57:2037.

risk factor for chronic kidney disease (CKD).[30] The aging kidney atrophies and has reduced function similarly to other organs.[30]

This is characterized by anatomic, morphologic, and functional change. Mitochondrial energy production is reduced, affecting active transport by kidney tubules and changes in glucose reabsorption and increase protein in the urine.[31] The number of functional nephrons decreases with age, contributing to a reduced glomerular filtration rate (GFR) and creatinine clearance ratio and decreased functional reserve.[31]

Reduction in functional nephrons impairs sodium retention, affects dilution of urine, and can predispose older adults to dehydration.[31] Causes for decreased water intake in older adults include impaired thirst perception and impaired cognition in older adults or physical impairments to enabling access to fluids.[30]

The presence of cognitive and physical disability can also limit the capacity of the older patient to ingest adequate amounts of fluid. Increased water loss from urination via diuretics and poorly controlled or undiagnosed diabetes mellitus (DM) may cause dehydration in older adults. Polypharmacy can also affect water balance in older adults.

Symptoms of dehydration in adults include thirst, confusion, dizziness, and fatigue. Delirium, dementia, and cognitive dysfunction are common causes of dehydration in older adults, leading to agitation, hallucinations, and anxiety. See Box 6.2 for a screening tool for dehydration risk with the acronym DEHYDRATIONS.[32]

Acute Kidney Injury

The therapy of choice for critically ill patients with severe acute kidney injury (AKI) is renal replacement therapy (RRT). Studies have looked at RRT initiation timing, because no clear guidelines exist. Most studies to date have found no significant benefit to initiation of early RRT. Early RRT may also increase additional risk of invasive procedures and care expense.[33]

These findings would indicate that the important decision to initiate dialysis treatment in older adults could be delayed until goals of care interventions are aligned with patients and surrogate decision makers.

Age-Related Changes of the Liver

Physiologic changes in the senescent liver include a decrease in reduced liver weight, volume, blood flow, and number of hepatocytes, as well as the loss of metabolic function. Age reduces detoxification in the liver and can have significant effect on pharmacokinetics and medication uptake in the older adult. *Ascites* can cause organ compression, and edema leads to difficulty in walking and falls in older adults.

Hepatic encephalopathy is characterized by disturbance of consciousness, which can also be hazardous to older adult patients who have increased risk of falls, aspiration, and other accidental injury. Lactulose and rifaximin may be used as a therapeutic option for treatment of hepatic encephalopathy in older adult patients.

BOX 6.1 Safety

POTENTIALLY INAPPROPRIATE SYMPTOM MEDICATION MANAGEMENT FOR OLDER ADULTS

Medication	Possible Side Effect	Medication	Possible Side Effect
NSAIDs[a]		Adjuvant Medications	
Indomethacin	CNS effects (highest of all NSAIDs)[b]	Muscle relaxants (methocarbamol, carisoprodol, chlorzoxazone, metaxalone, cyclobenzaprine, baclofen)	Anticholinergic effects,[b,c] sedation,[b] weakness,[b] cognitive impairment[b]
Ketorolac	Asymptomatic gastrointestinal conditions (ulcers[b])	Tricyclic antidepressants (amitriptyline and amitriptyline compounds)	Strong anticholinergic effects[b,c]; may lead to ataxia, impaired psychomotor function, syncope, falls; cardiac arrhythmias (QT interval changes)[b]; may produce polyuria or lead to urinary incontinence[b]; may exacerbate chronic constipation
Aspirin (>325 mg)	Asymptomatic gastrointestinal conditions (ulcers[b])	Doxepin	Cardiac dysrhythmias,[b] may produce polyuria or lead to urinary incontinence,[b] may exacerbate chronic constipation
Naproxen	Gastrointestinal bleeding,[b] renal failure,[b] high blood pressure,[b] heart failure[b]	Antihistamines (diphenhydramine, hydroxyzine, promethazine)	Potent anticholinergic properties[b,c]; may lead to confusion and sedation
Opioids		Benzodiazepines	Increased sensitivity at higher doses with prolonged sedation and increased risk for falls
Meperidine	Intense side effect profile for adverse effects, especially CNS effects (seizures) Most critical in individuals with renal compromise[b]	Short acting (lorazepam ≥3 mg, oxazepam ≥60 mg, alprazolam ≥2 mg)	May produce or exacerbate depression; smaller doses may be both effective and safer
Morphine, hydromorphone, fentanyl	Intense side effect profile at higher doses, especially CNS effects (e.g., somnolence, respiratory depression, delirium)[b]	Long acting (diazepam)	CNS effects,[b] may cause or exacerbate respiratory depression in chronic obstructive pulmonary disease,[b] may produce polyuria or lead to urinary incontinence[b]
		Selective serotonin reuptake inhibitor antidepressants (fluoxetine, citalopram, paroxetine, sertraline)	May produce CNS stimulation, sleep disturbances, and increasing agitation[b]; may exacerbate or cause syndrome of inappropriate secretion of antidiuretic hormone or hyponatremia
		Decongestants	High level of CNS stimulation, which may lead to insomnia[b]
		CNS stimulants (methylphenidate)	Altered CNS function, leading to cognitive impairment[b]; appetite-suppressing effect[b]

[a]May cause or exacerbate gastric or duodenal ulcers, prolonged clotting time and international normalized ratio, and decreased platelet function.
[b]High-severity rating.
[c]Anticholinergic effects include some of the following symptoms: blurred vision, constipation, drowsiness, sedation, dry mouth, tachycardia, urinary retention, confusion, disorientation, memory impairment, dizziness, nausea, nervousness, agitation, anxiety, facial flushing, weakness, and delirium.
CNS, Central nervous system; *NSAIDs,* nonsteroidal antiinflammatory drugs.
Based on data from Fick DM, Cooper JW, Wade WE, Waller JL, Maclean JR, Beers MH. Updating the Beers criteria for potentially inappropriate medication use in older adults: results of a U.S. consensus panel of experts. *Arch Intern Med.* 2003;163(22):2716; Laroche ML, Charmes JP, Merle L. Potentially inappropriate medications in the elderly: a French consensus panel. *Eur J Clin Pharmacol.* 2007;63(8):725.

Gastrointestinal bleeding occurs due to gastroesophageal varices, portal hypertension, gastropathy, and intestinopathy, and it increases the risk of mortality in older adults.

Hepatocellular carcinoma, bacterial infections, renal impairment, cardiopulmonary dysfunction, spontaneous bacterial peritonitis, acute and chronic kidney injury, cirrhotic cardiomyopathy, hepatorenal syndrome, and hyponatremia are all complications of liver disease.[34] See Table 6.3 for complications and management of cirrhosis in the older adult.

Age-Related Changes of the Gastrointestinal System and Nutrition

Aging physiology predisposes older adults to impaired energy regulation, metabolism derangements, and malnutrition.[35] Hospitalized, malnourished older adult patients are at increased risk of morbidity and mortality than healthy older adults.[35]

Nutritional and swallow screening are necessary in all older adult hospitalized patients to identify those at higher nutritional and aspiration risk. Protein-energy malnutrition can be responsive to

TABLE 6.2 Age-Related Changes in Pharmacokinetics.

Pharmacokinetic Parameter	Definition	Age-Related Changes
Absorption	Medication moves from site of administration to bloodstream; affected by mode of administration	Decreased absorptive surface area of small intestine and gastrointestinal motility Decreased splanchnic blood flow Increased gastric acid pH Changes in body skin/fat
Distribution	Medication is delivered from bloodstream to target tissues; affected by blood flow	Decreased lean body mass and total body water Increased total body fat Decreased serum albumin/plasma proteins Decreased red blood cells
Metabolism	Metabolic breakdown of a medication that renders it active or inactive; affected by mode of administration	Decreased liver mass Decreased medication metabolism Decreased total liver blood flow
Excretion	Removal of medication through an eliminating organ, often the kidney; some medications are excreted in bile or feces, in saliva, or through the lungs	Decreased renal blood flow/glomerular filtration rate Decreased distal renal tubular secretory function

Adapted from Rodrigues DA, Herdeiro MT, Figueiras A, Coutinho P, Roque F. Elderly and polypharmacy: physiological and cognitive changes. In: Palermo S, ed. *Frailty in the Elderly—Physical, Cognitive and Emotional Domains.* London, UK: IntechOpen; 2020.

nutritional interventions in older adults. Feeding goals should be achieved within 48 hours in older adult critical care unit patients with high nutritional risk factors, with enteral nutrition via gastric feeding as the first-line choice.

DIABETES IN OLDER ADULTS

Diabetes is underdiagnosed and can be found in at least 25% of older adults, with prevalence expected to increase over the next 20 years.[36] Diabetes results in higher mortality, reduced functional status, increased risk for institutionalization, and elevated risk for acute and chronic microvascular and cardiovascular complications.[36]

Black and Hispanic older adults have a greater rate of type 2 diabetes.[36] Type 2 diabetes is more common in older adults and has been linked to obesity. Age-related changes such as insulin resistance and diminished pancreatic islet function add to the risk for developing type 2 diabetes in older adults. Older adults, particularly adults with diabetes, are more likely to require hospitalization than younger adults.

BOX 6.2 DEHYDRATION Screening Tool for Dehydration Risk

- **D**iuretics
- **E**nd of life
- **H**igh fever
- **Y**ellow urine turns dark
- **D**izziness (orthostasis)
- **R**educed oral intake
- **A**xilla dry
- **T**achycardia
- **I**ncontinence (fear of)
- **O**ral problems (sippers)
- **N**eurologic impairment (confusion)
- Sunken eyes

Peripheral neuropathy occurs in 50% to 70% of older adults with diabetes and can cause significant pain, falls, and fractures.[36] For older adult patients who require insulin, it is important to remember that insulin therapy requires good visual and motor coordination, which may be challenging for some older adults.[36]

Age-Related Changes in the Immune System

Infections in older adults are generally more complicated, serious, and lethal than infections in younger individuals.[37] Adults older than 65 years of age are three to five times more likely to die of an infection than younger adults.[37] Older adult patients with sepsis often present with nonspecific symptoms, including altered mental status, anorexia, and generalized weakness. Approximately 60% of hospitalized patients with sepsis are over 65 years of age.[37]

Age-Related Changes in the Skin

The skin is very important in the older adult, because it protects the body through thermoregulation, fluid regulation, and sensation. The skin becomes less elastic, drier, and more fragile as the epidermis thins with age. Moisture in the stratum corneum decreases, blood vessels break easily, and risk for skin breakdown increases.

Skin disorders common in older adults include seborrheic keratosis, xerosis (dry skin), Campbell de Morgan spots, and other dermatologic disorders caused by degenerative and metabolic changes.[38]

Skin elasticity decreases as a result of collagen depletion affecting the skin's protective capability.[38] Dry aging skin is prone to separation of the dermal-epidermal junction, reduction in subcutaneous blood flow, and decreased dermal lymphatic drainage that leads to acute and chronic wounds.

Annual prevalence of chronic wounds in older adults is approximately 10% to 35%.[39] Wound healing is diminished because of decreased cytokine and growth factor production, diminished inflammatory response, and reduction of cell proliferation.[39] Diminished wound healing is particularly important in the critical care environment, where there is increased opportunity to develop pressure injuries and infections.

TABLE 6.3   Table Complications and Management of Liver Cirrhosis in Older Adults.

Complication	Management (General)	Considerations
Ascites	Sodium restrictions	Electrolyte abnormalities
	Antimineral corticoid	Changes in circulation dynamics
	Furosemide	Body weight
	Torsemide	Pulse and blood pressure
	Albumin infusion	Verification of blood biochemistry and urinalysis
Hepatic encephalopathy	Optimization of bowel movement	Diarrhea
	Laxatives	Frequent diarrhea that causes electrolyte
	Branched-chain amino acids	abnormalities
	Synthetic disaccharide lactulose	Skin troubles from frequent defecation
	Rifaximin	Dehydration
	Intravenous drip infusion of Fischer solution	Cardiac stress and fluctuation of electrolytes
Gastrointestinal bleeding/varices	Nonselective beta-blockers	Arrhythmia
	Endoscopic therapy	Fluctuation of blood pressure
		Heart failure
		Aspiration pneumonia
Sarcopenia	Risk of fall-related injury	Nutritional monitoring (serum markers including the
		albumin, cholesterol level)
		Muscle volume
		Administration of branched-chain amino acid
		preparations
Skin symptoms	Skin moisturizers	Likely to have dry skin
	Bile salts	Frequently suffer from wound infections and
	Rifampicin	persistent skin inflammation
	Antihistamines	Nalfurafine hydrochloride
Hepatocellular carcinoma	Use of phase contrast for the diagnosis	Renal function
	Surgical therapy	Cardiac function
	Transarterial chemotherapy	Bone marrow function
	Needle-guided local therapy	History of cerebral bleeding
	Molecular targeted therapies	Hypertension
		Renal function
Cirrhotic cardiomyopathy		Cardiac function
Spontaneous bacterial peritonitis		Sarcopenia
Hepatorenal syndrome		Further clinical trials and information from
Acute and chronic kidney injury		retrospective studies are necessary
Hyponatremia		

From Brennan-Cook J, Turner RL. Promoting skin care for older adults. *Home Healthc Now.* 2019;37(1):10–16.

Critical care unit patients are at high risk of pressure injury due to criticality of condition, immobility, and medications such as vasopressors (Table 6.4). Comprehensive risk assessment, appropriate support surface selection, and pressure relief to areas of risk are foundational pressure injury–prevention practices. The most common areas for pressure injury are heels, sacrum, and buttocks.

Skin tears are a significant problem for older adult critical care unit patients with friable skin. A skin tear is a wound caused by shear, friction, and/or blunt force resulting in separation of skin layers.[40]

A skin tear can be partial thickness, where there is separation of the epidermis from the dermis, or full thickness, where there is separation of both the epidermis and dermis from underlying structures.[40] Evidence suggests that skin tears may occur more frequently than pressure injuries.[40]

Age-Related Changes in the Musculoskeletal System

Falls can be particularly damaging to older adults; 25% of older Americans experience falls with injury that result in cognitive and physical dysfunction and loss of independence.[1] The critical care unit and acute care settings are particularly dangerous for older adults with cognitive impairment because they have increased risk of falling compared with older adults without cognitive impairment. See Box 6.3 for fall risk factors.

Functional decline and frailty contribute to negative health care outcomes, with up to 80% of hospitalized older adults being considered frail. *Frailty* describes a state or syndrome of decreased physical and cognitive reserve characterized by decreased mobility, weakness, reduced muscle mass, poor nutritional status, and diminished cognitive function.[41] Frailty is increasingly recognized as a risk factor for poor outcomes across many disease states and for individuals developing critical illness.

The number of frail patients admitted to the critical care unit is increasing, with a concomitant rise in mortality, resource utilization, and prolonged postacute and custodial care.[41] Use of life-sustaining critical care unit therapies continues, but outcomes of life support interventions in critically ill frail patients are unclear.[41]

TABLE 6.4 Age-Related Changes That May Affect Skin Integrity.

Body System	Age-Related Changes	Effects on Skin
Cardiac	Decreased blood flow	Delayed wound healing
	Fragile capillaries	Increased bruising
Neurologic	Decreased sensation	Increased risk of physical injury (burns)
	Decreased memory	May not sense skin breakdown
	Increased confusion	May forget to care for skin
	Decreased vision	Risk for falls and skin damage
		May not visualize skin breakdown
Musculoskeletal	Decreased mobility	Increased risk for skin breakdown and pressure injuries
		May have difficulty reaching areas for good skin care
Genitourinary	Increased incontinence	Risk for skin breakdown and increased irritation
	Increased moisture	Risk for infection
	Dehydration	Dry scaly skin
Gastrointestinal	Increased incontinence and diarrhea episodes	Risk for skin irritation and breakdown
	Decreased appetite	Delayed wound healing
	Decreased intake/malnutrition	
	Decreased chewing ability with less dentition	
Immune	Decreased immunity	Risk for skin infection
	Decreased ability to regulate temperature	Increased risk for skin cancer

Adapted from Brennan-Cook J, Turner RL. Promoting skin care for older adults. *Home Healthc Now.* 2019;37(1):10–16.

QSEN ## BOX 6.3 Safety

Factors Associated With an Increased Risk of Falling

Biologic/Intrinsic
- Impaired mobility
- Balance deficit
- Gait deficit
- Muscle weakness
- Advanced age
- Chronic illness/disability:
  - Cognitive impairment
  - Stroke
  - Parkinson disease
  - Diabetes
  - Arthritis
  - Heart disease
  - Incontinence
  - Foot disorders
  - Visual impairment
- Acute illness

Behavioral
- History of falls
- Fear of falling
- Polypharmacy
- Use of:
  - Antipsychotics
  - Sedatives/hypnotics
  - Antidepressants
- Excessive alcohol
- Risk-taking behaviors

- Lack of exercise
- Inappropriate footwear/clothing
- Inappropriate assistive devices use
- Poor nutrition or hydration
- Lack of sleep

Social and Economic
- Low income
- Lower level of education
- Illiteracy/language barriers
- Poor living conditions
- Living alone
- Lack of support networks and social interaction
- Lack of transportation
- Cultural/ethnicity

Environmental
- Poor building design and/or maintenance
- Inadequate building codes
- Stairs
- Home hazards
- Lack of:
  - Handrails
  - Curb ramps
  - Rest areas
  - Grab bars
  - Good lighting or sharp contrasts
- Slippery or uneven surfaces
- Obstacles and tripping hazards

Source: Public Health Agency of Canada. Seniors' falls in Canada, a second report. Ottawa, ON, Canada; 2014; Cheung C. Older adults, falls, and skin integrity. *Adv Skin Wound Care.* 2017;30(1):40–46.

QSEN BOX 6.4   Evidence-Based Practice

RECOMMENDATIONS FOR PERIOPERATIVE CARE OF THE OLDER ADULT

Problem	Prevention Strategy
Aspiration	Dysphagia screen
	Head of bed elevation
	Out of bed for meals
Delirium	Limit sedation
	Reduce ventilator time
	Encourage early mobility
	Promote sleep and normal circadian rhythm
	Regional pain management
Pressure injury	Select support surfaces
	Limit hypothermia
	Frequent repositioning
	Reduce friction, shear, and moisture
	Avoid alkaline and fragranced soaps
Falls	Frequent toileting
	Use assistive devices (glasses, hearing aids)
	Avoid opioids and benzodiazepines
	Reduce immobility/bed rest

Data from Mohanty S, Rosenthal RA, Russell MM, Neuman MD, Ko CY, Esnaola NF. Optimal perioperative management of the geriatric patient: best practices guideline from the ACS NSQIP/American Geriatrics Society. *J Am Coll Surg.* 2016;222(5):930–947.

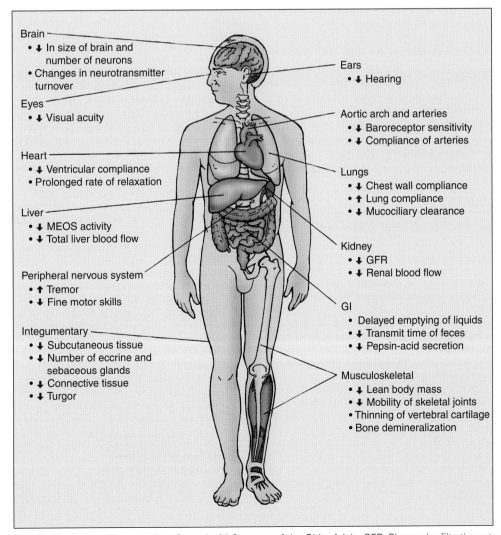

Fig. 6.3 Physiologic Changes That Occur in All Systems of the Older Adult. *GFR,* Glomerular filtration rate; *GI,* gastrointestinal; *MEOS,* microsomal enzyme oxidative system.

BOX 6.5   **Informatics**

Internet Resources: The Older Adult Patient
- Advocacy Centre for the Elderly: http://www.advocacycentreelderly.org/
- American College of Surgeons National Surgical Quality Improvement Program: https://www.facs.org/quality-programs/acs-nsqip/geriatric-periop-guideline
- American Geriatrics Society: https://www.americangeriatrics.org/
- Critical Illness, Brain Dysfunction, and Survivorship (CIBS) Center: https://www.icudelirium.org/
- Center to Advance Palliative Care: https://www.capc.org/
- Choosing Wisely: http://www.choosingwisely.org/
- Wound, Ostomy, and Continence Nursing Society: https://www.wocn.org/

COMPLICATIONS OF CRITICAL CARE FOR OLDER ADULTS

Improved acute and critical care outcomes have led to increases in the number of survivors of critical illness who have long-term complications and the need for assisted care.[42,43] Functional decline can occur within 1 day of hospitalization, leading to complications of immobility that include aspiration pneumonia, falls, deep vein thrombosis, loss of independence, pulmonary emboli, deconditioning, pressure injuries, bowel paralysis, pain, and increased length of stay. See Box 6.4 for evidence-based recommendations for perioperative care of the older adult.

Also see Fig. 6.3 for physiologic changes that occur in all systems of the older adult.

Modifiable factors to reduce critical illness impairment include prevention of immobility, recognition of delirium, reduction in sleep disruption, and family involvement in care.

Functional status before illness is a strong predictor of disability after critical illness, with studies showing that at least 50% of older adult patients who are discharged from the critical care unit require caregiving assistance or die within 12 months of hospital discharge.[43]

ADDITIONAL RESOURCES

See Box 6.5 for Internet resources related to the care of older adults.

REFERENCES

1. Ball IM, Bagshaw SM, Burns KE, et al. Outcomes of elderly critically ill medical and surgical patients: a multicentre cohort study. *Can J Anesth.* 2017;64(3):260–269.
2. Le Borgne P, Maestraggi Q, Couraud S, et al. Critically ill elderly patients (≥90 years): clinical characteristics, outcome and financial implications. *PLoS One.* 2018;13(6):e0198360.
3. Heyland D, Cook D, Bagshaw SM, et al. The very elderly admitted to ICU: a quality finish? *Crit Care Med.* 2015;43(7):1352–1360.
4. Guidet B B, Vallet H H, Boddaert J J, et al. Caring for the critically ill patients over 80: a narrative review. *Ann Intensive Care.* 2018;8(1):114. 2018.
5. McGrane TJ, Pandharipande PP, Hughes CG. Neurocognitive dysfunction and geriatric neurocritical care. In: Akhtar S, Rosenbaum S, eds. *Principles of Geriatric Critical Care.* New York: Cambridge University Press; 2018.
6. Quinn J, Kaye J. The neurology of aging. *Neurol.* 2001;7:98.
7. Brummel NE, Balas MC, Morandi A, Ferrante LE, Gill TM, Ely EW. Understanding and reducing disability in older adults following critical illness. *Crit Care Med.* 2015;43(6):1265.
8. Pandharipande PP, Girard TD, Ely EW. Long-term cognitive impairment after critical illness. *N Engl J Med.* 2013;369(14):1306.
9. Janssens JP. Aging of the respiratory system: impact on pulmonary function tests and adaptation to exertion. *Clin Chest Med.* 2005;26:469.
10. Siner J, Pisani M. Respiratory critical care in the elderly. In: Akhtar S, Rosenbaum S, eds. *Principles of Geriatric Critical Care.* New York: Cambridge University Press; 2018.
11. Mohanty S, Rosenthal RA, Russell MM, Neuman MD, Ko CY, Esnaola NF. *Optimal Perioperative Management of the Geriatric Patient: Best Practices Guideline From ACS NSQIP/American Geriatrics Society;* 2016. https://www.facs.org/quality-programs/acs-nsqip/geriatric-periop-guideline.
12. Lowery EM, Brubaker AL, Kuhlmann E, Kovacs EJ. The aging lung. *Clin Interv Aging.* 2013;8:1489.
13. Marik PE. Management of the critically ill geriatric patient. *Crit Care Med.* 2006;34(9):S176.
14. Bonomo L, Larici AR, Maggi F, Schiavon F, Berletti R. Aging and the respiratory system. *Radiol Clin North Am.* 2008;46:685.
15. Fragoso CAV, Gill TM. Respiratory impairment and the aging lung: a novel paradigm for assessing pulmonary function. *J Gerontol A Biol Sci Med Sci.* 2011;67A(3):264.
16. Tyler K, Stevenson D. Respiratory emergencies in geriatric patients. *Emerg Med Clin North Am.* 2016;34(1):39.
17. Strait JB, Lakatta EG. Aging-associated cardiovascular changes and their relationship to heart failure. *Heart Fail Clin.* 2012;8(1):143.
18. North BJ. The intersection between aging and cardiovascular disease. *Circ Res.* 2012;110(8):1097.
19. Dai X, Hummel SL, Salazar JB, Taffet GE, Zieman S, Schwartz JB. Cardiovascular physiology in the older adults. *J Geriatr Cardiol.* 2015;12(3):196.
20. Francis GS, et al. Pathophysiology of heart failure. In: Fuster V, ed. *Hurst's the Heart.* New York: McGraw-Hill; 2008.
21. Hajjar I. Postural blood pressure changes and orthostatic hypotension in elderly patients: impact of antihypertensive medications. *Drugs Aging.* 2005;22(1):55.
22. Aronow WS, Fleg JL, Pepine CJ, et al. ACCF/AHA 2011 Expert consensus document on hypertension in the elderly: a report of the American College of Cardiology Foundation task force on clinical expert consensus documents. *J Am Coll Cardiol.* 2011;57(20):2037.
23. James PA, Oparil S, Carter BL, et al. 2014 Evidence-based guideline for the management of high blood pressure in adults: report from the panel members appointed to the Eighth Joint National Committee (JNC 8). *J Am Med Assoc.* 2014;311(5):507.
24. Shih H, Lee B, Lee RJ, Boyle AJ. The aging heart and post-infarction left ventricular remodeling. *J Am Coll Cardiol.* 2010;57(1):9.
25. Cooney D, Pascuzzi K. Polypharmacy in the elderly: focus on drug interactions and adherence in hypertension. *Clin Geriatr Med.* 2009;25:221.
26. Fick DM, Cooper JW, Wade WE, Waller JL, Maclean JR, Beers MH. Updating the Beers criteria for potentially inappropriate medication use in older adults: results of a US consensus panel of experts. *Arch Intern Med.* 2003;163:2716.
27. Samuel MJ. American Geriatrics Society 2019 Updated AGS Beers Criteria® for potentially inappropriate medication use in older adults. *J Am Geriatr Soc.* 2019;67(4):674–694.
28. Rothschild JM, Landrigan CP, Cronin JW, et al. The critical care safety study: the incidence and nature of adverse events and serious errors in intensive care. *Crit Care Med.* 2005;33:1694.
29. Yuen GJ. Altered pharmacokinetics in the elderly. *Clin Geriatr Med.* 1990;6:257.
30. Koch CA, Fulop T. Clinical aspects of changes in water and sodium homeostasis in the elderly. *Rev Endocr Metab Disord.* 2017;18(1):49–66.
31. Yokota LG, Sampaio BM, Rocha EP, Balbi AL, Prado IRS, Ponce D. Acute kidney injury in elderly patients: narrative review on incidence, risk factors, and mortality. *Int J Nephrol Renovascular Dis.* 2018;11:217.
32. Morley JE. Dehydration, hypernatremia, and hyponatremia. *Clin Geriatr Med.* 2015;31(3):389–399.
33. Chaudhuri D, Herritt B, Heyland D, et al. Early renal replacement therapy versus standard care in the ICU: a systematic review, meta-analysis, and cost analysis. *J Intensive Care Med.* 2019;34(4):323–329.

34. Kamimura K, Sakamaki A, Kamimura H, et al. Considerations of elderly factors to manage the complication of liver cirrhosis in elderly patients. *World J Gastroenterol.* 2019;25(15):1817.

35. Kopp Lugli A, de Watteville A, Hollinger A, Goetz N, Heidegger C. Medical nutrition therapy in critically ill patients treated on intensive and intermediate care units: a literature review. *J Clin Med.* 2019;8(9):1395.

36. Kirkman MS, Briscoe VJ, Clark N, et al. Diabetes in older adults. *Diabetes Care.* 2012;35(12):2650.

37. Mukherjee K, Burruss SK, Brooks SE, May AK. Managing infectious disease in the critically ill elderly patient. *Curr Geriatr Rep.* 2019;8(6):1–14.

38. Smith DR, Leggat PA. Prevalence of skin disease among the elderly in different clinical environments. *Australas J Ageing.* 2005;24(2):71.

39. Chaboyer WP, Thalib L, Harbeck EL, et al. Incidence and prevalence of pressure injuries in adult intensive care patients: a systematic review and meta-analysis. *Crit Care Med.* 2018;46(11):e1074–e1081.

40. Campbell KE, Baronoski S, Gloeckner M, et al. Skin tears: prediction, prevention, assessment and management. *Nurse Prescr.* 2018;16(12):600–607.

41. Muscedere J, Waters B, Varambally A, et al. The impact of frailty on intensive care unit outcomes: a systematic review and meta-analysis. *Intensive Care Med.* 2017;43(8):1105–1122.

42. Giambattista L, Howard R, Ruhe Porto R, et al. NICHE recommended care of the critically ill older adult. *Crit Care Nurs Q.* 2015;38(3):223.

43. Desai SV, Law TJ, Needham DM. Long-term complications of critical care. *Crit Care Med.* 2011;39(2):371.

7

Pain and Pain Management

Céline Gélinas

Most patients will experience some degree of pain during their stay in the critical care unit, and the prevalence of moderate to severe pain in this population is high (>50%)[1] and disturbingly similar to that described two decades ago.[2] Acute pain is an important risk factor for the development of chronic pain, and the incidence of chronic pain after discharge from the critical care unit is also high, with prevalence ranging from 33% to 73% which can negatively affect daily functioning and quality of life.[3] Therefore management of pain is crucial and must be rethought in the context of the opioid crisis in North America.[4,5] Pain treatment should not rely on opioids solely and instead be based on a multimodal approach that includes nonopioids and nonpharmacologic interventions.[6,7] The clinical practice guideline for the Prevention and Management of Pain, Agitation/Sedation, Delirium, Immobility, and Sleep Disruption (PADIS)[6] in adult critical care patients supports this approach. This chapter discusses common challenges related to pain in critical care, provides assessment tools, and describes safe evidence-based interventions for pain management in critically ill patients.

PAIN ASSESSMENT

Appropriate pain assessment is the foundation of effective pain treatment. Because pain is recognized as a personal experience, the patient's self-report is considered the most valid measure for pain and should be obtained as often as possible.[8] In critical care, many factors, such as the administration of sedative agents, the use of mechanical ventilation, altered levels of consciousness, and delirium, alter communication with patients.[9] These obstacles make pain assessment more complex. Nevertheless, except for being unable to speak, many mechanically ventilated patients can communicate that they are in pain by head nodding, hand motions, or seeking attention with other movements.[9,10]

Self-report pain intensity scales have been used with postoperative mechanically ventilated patients who were asked to point on a scale.[1] When the patient is unable to communicate in any way, observable behavioral indicators become unique indices for pain assessment and are part of clinical guidelines and recommendations.[6,11–13] Because pain is frequently encountered in critical care, there is increased emphasis on the professional responsibility to provide effective and safe management of pain.

DEFINITION AND DESCRIPTION OF PAIN

According to the updated 2020 definition by the International Association for Study on Pain (IASP), pain is described as an unpleasant sensory and emotional experience associated with, or resembling that associated with, actual or potential tissue damage.[8] Pain has also been described as a distressing experience associated with actual or potential tissue damage with sensory, emotional, cognitive, and social/behavioral components.[14] This definition implies that pain is whatever the person experiencing it says it is, and that it exists whenever he or she says it does.[15] Therefore the patient's report of an experience as painful should be respected.[8]

However, in the critical care context, many patients are unable to self-report their pain.[16] The IASP has acknowledged that the inability to communicate verbally does not negate the possibility that an individual is experiencing pain.[8] Pain assessment must be designed to conform to the communication capabilities of the patient.

Components of Pain

The experience of pain has multiple components[17]:
- **Sensory**: Perception of pain characteristics such as intensity, location, and quality
- **Emotional**: Negative emotions such as unpleasantness, distress, anxiety, and fear associated with anticipation of pain
- **Cognitive**: Interpretation or meaning of pain by the person experiencing it
- **Behavioral**: Behaviors used to express, avoid, or control pain
- **Physiologic**: Nociception

Types of Pain

Pain can be acute or chronic, with different sensations related to the origin of the pain: nociceptive, neuropathic, or nociplastic.[8] A patient may present with different types of pain simultaneously, known as mixed pain.[18]

Acute Pain

Acute pain has a short duration, it usually corresponds to the healing process (30 days), and it should not exceed 6 months.[19] It implies tissue damage that is usually from an identifiable cause.

Chronic Pain

Chronic pain persists for more than 6 months after the healing process from the original injury, and it may or may not be associated with an illness.[19] It develops when the healing process is incomplete or when acute pain is poorly managed.

Nociceptive Pain

Nociceptive pain arises from activation of nociceptors, and can be somatic or visceral[8,20]:
- Somatic pain involves superficial tissues such as the skin, muscles, joints, and bones. The location is well defined.

- Visceral pain involves organs such as the heart, stomach, and liver. The location is diffuse, and may be referred to a different location in the body.

Not all organs are sensitive to pain, and some can be damaged extensively without the patient feeling anything. For example, many diseases of the liver, lungs, or kidneys are completely painless, and the only symptoms arise from the organ dysfunction. Relatively minor lesions in viscera such as the stomach, the bladder, or the ureters can produce excruciating pain, as these organs are abundantly innervated by sensory neurons that signal harmful events.[21]

Neuropathic Pain

Neuropathic pain arises from a lesion or disease affecting the somatosensory system.[8] The origin of neuropathic pain may be peripheral or central:

- Peripheral neuropathic pain: This involves damage of the peripheral somatosensory system such as neuralgia and neuropathy.
- Central neuropathic pain: This involves the central somatosensory cortex and can be experienced by patients after a cerebral stroke.

Neuropathic pain can be difficult to manage and frequently requires a multimodal approach (i.e., combinations of several pharmacologic or nonpharmacologic treatments).[20]

Nociplastic Pain

Nociplastic pain is in the IASP terminology of pain. This type of pain arises from an alteration of the nociceptive function, despite no clear evidence of tissue damage causing the activation of nociceptors or evidence for disease or lesion of the somatosensory system causing the pain.[8] Fibromyalgia is an example of nociplastic pain.

Physiology of Pain

Nociception

Nociception represents the neural processes of encoding and processing noxious stimuli necessary, but not sufficient, for pain.[8] Pain results from the integration of the nociceptive signal into specific cortical areas of the brain associated with higher mental processes and consciousness. In other words, pain is the conscious experience that emerges from nociception.

Four processes are involved in nociception[20]:

1. transduction
2. transmission
3. perception
4. modulation

The four processes are shown in Fig. 7.1 with pain assessment integrated with nociception.

Transduction

Transduction refers to mechanical (e.g., surgical incision), thermal (e.g., burn), or chemical (e.g., toxic substance) stimuli that damage tissues. In critical care, many nociceptive stimuli exist that stimulate the liberation of chemical substances, such as prostaglandins, bradykinin, serotonin, histamine, glutamate, and substance P. These neurotransmitters stimulate peripheral nociceptive receptors and initiate nociceptive transmission (see Fig. 7.1).

Transmission

As a result of transduction, an action potential is produced and is transmitted by nociceptive nerve fibers in the spinal cord that reach higher centers of the brain. The principal nociceptive fibers are the A-delta (Aδ) and C fibers. Large-diameter, myelinated Aδ fibers that transmit well-localized, sharp pain are involved in "first pain" sensation, which leads to reflex withdrawal. Small-diameter, unmyelinated C fibers transmit diffuse, dull, aching pain, which is referred to as "second pain." These fibers transmit the noxious sensation from the periphery through the dorsal root of the spinal cord. With the liberation of substance P, these fibers then synapse with ascending spinothalamic fibers to the central nervous system (see Fig. 7.1). These spinothalamic fibers are clustered into two specific pathways: neospinothalamic (NS) and paleospinothalamic (PS) pathways. Generally, the Aδ fibers transmit the pain sensation to the brain within the NS pathway, and the C fibers use the PS pathway.[22]

Through synapsing of nociceptive fibers with motor fibers in the spinal cord, muscle rigidity can appear because of a reflex activity.[23] Muscle rigidity is a behavioral indicator associated with pain.[24] It can contribute to immobility and decrease diaphragmatic excursion. This can lead to hypoventilation and hypoxemia. Hypoxemia can be detected by a pulse oximeter (SpO$_2$) and by monitoring of arterial partial pressure of oxygen (PaO$_2$). The interaction of a ventilated patient with the machine (e.g., activation of alarms, fighting the ventilator) also may indicate the presence of pain.[25]

Perception

The pain message is transmitted by the spinothalamic pathways to centers in the brain, where it is perceived (see Fig. 7.1). Pain sensation transmitted by the NS pathway reaches the thalamus, and the pain sensation transmitted by the PS pathway reaches the brainstem, hypothalamus, and thalamus.[22] These parts of the central nervous system influence the initial perception of pain. Projections to the limbic system and the frontal cortex allow expression of the emotional component of pain.[26] Projections to the sensory cortex located in the parietal lobe allow the patient to describe the sensory characteristics of pain, such as location, intensity, and quality.[26,27] The cognitive component of pain involves many parts of the cerebral cortex and is complex. Three components (emotional, cognitive, and sensory) represent the personal experience of pain. Parallel to this perception process, certain facial expressions and body movements are behavioral indicators of pain occurring from pain fiber projections to the motor cortex in the frontal lobe.

Modulation

Modulation is a process by which noxious stimuli traveling from the nociceptive receptors to the central nervous system are enhanced or inhibited. Pain can be modulated by ascending and descending mechanisms. A typical example of ascending pain modulation is rubbing an injury site, which activates large A-beta (Aβ) fibers in the periphery. Stimulation of these fibers activates inhibitory interneurons in the dorsal horn of the spinal cord, preventing nociceptive signal transmission from the periphery to the higher brain regions.[28]

Analgesia may also be produced at the level of the spinal cord and brainstem (spinothalamic pathway) via the release of endogenous opioids and neurotransmitters (see Fig. 7.1). Endogenous opioids are naturally occurring morphine-like pentapeptides found throughout the nervous system and exist in three general classes: beta-endorphins, enkephalins, and dynorphins. These substances block neuronal activity related to nociceptive impulses by binding to opioid mu (μ) receptor sites in the central and peripheral nervous systems.[22] The use of distraction, relaxation, and imagery techniques can facilitate the release of endogenous opioids that may reduce the overall pain experience.[29]

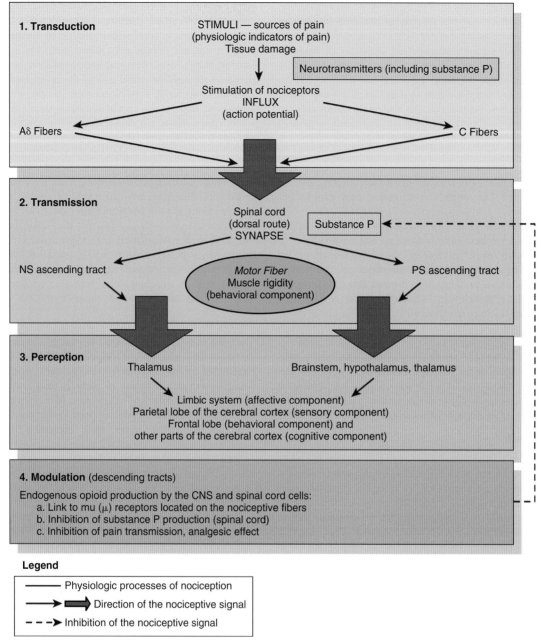

Fig. 7.1 Integration of pain assessment in the four processes of nociception. *CNS,* Central nervous system; *NS,* neospinothalamic pathway; *PS,* paleospinothalamic pathway. (Courtesy Céline Gélinas, Ingram School of Nursing, McGill University, Canada.)

PAIN ASSESSMENT

Pain assessment is an integral part of nursing care and is a prerequisite for pain control. Pain assessment has two major components: (1) reported by the patient and (2) observed by another person. In the following sections, assessment and management are addressed, and recommendations are proposed.

Pain Assessment
Patient Self-Report

Pain is known as a personal experience. This refers to the patient's self-report about his or her sensorial, emotional, and cognitive experience of pain. Because it is considered the most valid measure of pain, the patient's self-report must be obtained whenever possible.[12,30]

If sedation and cognition levels allow the patient to give more information about pain, a multidimensional assessment can be documented. Multidimensional pain assessment tools include sensorial, emotional, and cognitive components.[2,20,31,32] Or, the patient's self-report of pain can be obtained by asking questions using the mnemonic PQRSTUV[33]:

- **P:** Provocative and palliative or aggravating factors
- **Q:** Quality
- **R:** Region or location, radiation
- **S:** Severity and other symptoms

- **T:** Timing
- **U:** Understanding
- **V:** Values

Begin by asking, "Do you have pain?" The use of a simple yes or no question allows the patient to answer verbally or to indicate a response by nodding the head or by other signs. This enables mechanically ventilated patients to communicate nonverbally. Pain intensity and location also are necessary to assess for the initial assessment of pain.

Observable or Objective Component of Pain Assessment

Behavioral Indicators of Pain

When a patient's self-report is impossible to obtain, nurses can rely on the observation of behavioral indicators.[6,11–13] Pain-related behaviors have been studied in critically ill patients in the AACN Thunder Project II[34] and more recently in the *Europain* study.[1] Behaviors including facial expressions, muscle rigidity, and vocalization were associated with self-reported pain and were significant predictors of pain intensity and pain distress.

Several behavioral scales have been developed for assessing pain in critically ill adult patients unable to self-report.[35] The clinical guidelines of the Society of Critical Care Medicine (SCCM)[6] recommend both the Behavioral Pain Scale (BPS)[36] and its version for the non-intubated patient (BPS-NI)[37] and the Critical-Care Pain Observation Tool (CPOT)[38] for clinical use in critically ill adult patients unable to self-report.[6,39]

Behavioral Pain Scale

The BPS[36] and its adapted version for the nonintubated patient (BPS-NI)[37] are shown in Table 7.1, and was validated in various critical care patient groups in different countries.[35] Both versions of the tool have shown high interrater reliability with trained critical care nurses and other health professionals. The validity of the use of the BPS and BPS-NI has been supported by the association of significantly higher BPS scores during nociceptive procedures (e.g., turning, endotracheal suctioning, peripheral venous cannulation) compared with rest or non-nociceptive procedures (e.g., arterial catheter dressing change, compression stocking applications, eye care). Positive associations were also found between BPS/BPS-NI score and patients' self-report of pain intensity during nociceptive procedures. A cut-off score greater than 5 for the presence of pain was established with the BPS.[35] The BPS can be used quickly, and most clinicians were satisfied with its ease of use.[40]

Critical-Care Pain Observation Tool

The CPOT[38] shown in Table 7.2 was tested widely in various critical care patient groups in multiple countries.[35] The CPOT has good interrater reliability scores with trained critical care nurses. Validity of the CPOT use was supported with significantly higher CPOT scores during a nociceptive procedure (e.g., turning with or without other care, endotracheal suctioning) compared with rest or a non-nociceptive procedure (e.g., taking blood pressure, central catheter dressing change). Positive associations were found between the CPOT scores and the patient's self-report of pain intensity during nociceptive procedures. A cut-off score greater than 2 for the presence of pain was established with the CPOT.[35] Feasibility and clinical utility of the CPOT were positively evaluated by critical care nurses, which was sustained at 12 months after implementation of the tool.[41] Nurses agreed that the CPOT was quick enough to be used in the critical care unit, simple to understand, easy to complete, and helpful for nursing practice. An online teaching video to learn how to use the CPOT at the bedside is available (see Table 7.2).

TABLE 7.1 Behavioral Pain Scale.

Item	Description	Score
Facial expression	Relaxed	1
	Partially tightened (e.g., brow lowering)	2
	Fully tightened (e.g., eyelid closing)	3
	Grimacing	4
Upper limbs	No movement	1
	Partially bent	2
	Fully bent with finger flexion	3
	Permanently retracted	4
Compliance with ventilation	Tolerating movement	1
	Coughing but tolerating ventilation for most of the time	2
	Fighting ventilator	3
	Unable to control ventilation	4
OR		
Vocalization	No pain vocalization	1
	Moaning not frequent (<3/min) or not prolonged (<3 seconds)	2
	Moaning frequent (>3/min) or prolonged (>3 seconds)	3
	Howling or verbal complaint including "Ow! Ouch!" or breath holding	4
Total		**3–12**

Modified from Payen JF, Bru O, Bosson JL, et al. Assessing pain in critically ill sedated patients by using a behavioral pain scale. *Crit Care Med.* 2001;29(12):2258.

Use of Cut-off Scores in Behavioral Pain Scales

A cut-off score refers to the score on a specific scale associated with the best probability of correctly ruling in or ruling out a patient with a specific condition—in this case, pain. Cut-off scores are established using a criterion (i.e., a gold standard in the field).

Behavioral pain scores should be interpreted differently from the patient's self-report pain intensity scores. Although they both represent pain scores, they are measuring different dimensions of pain that are interrelated. More specifically, behavioral scores based on the nurse's observations are associated with the behavioral dimension of pain. In contrast, the patient's self-report of pain intensity relates to the sensory dimension of pain.[14]

Although self-reported pain intensity scores and behavioral pain scores move in the same direction (i.e., when one score increases, the other score increases as well), they are not equal scores.[11,12] Therefore it is important to know that BPS only allow the detection of the presence versus absence of pain. Box 7.1 provides a case example showing how a cut-off score can be used in practice.

Limitations Related to the Use of Behavioral Pain Scales

BPS have been validated for pain assessment in critically ill patients, but they have some limitations. They are impossible to monitor in patients unable to respond behaviorally to pain, such as patients with paralysis or under the effects of neuromuscular blocking agents. Also, behavioral responses may be blurred with the administration of high doses of sedative agents. Minimal behavioral responses to painful procedures were found in unconscious, mechanically ventilated, critically ill adults who were more heavily sedated compared with conscious patients.[25]

TABLE 7.2   Critical-Care Pain Observation Tool.

Indicator	SCORE		Description
Facial expression	Relaxed, neutral	0	No muscle tension observed
	Tense	1	Contraction of the upper face: brow lowering, lid tightening
	Grimacing	2	Contraction of the upper and the lower face: brow lowering, lid tightening, eyes tightly closed, nasolabial furrow, mouth opening or biting on the endotracheal tube
Body movements	Absence of movements or normal position	0	Does not move at all (does not necessarily mean absence of pain) or normal position (movements not aimed toward the pain site or not made for the purpose of protection)
	Protection	1	Slow, cautious movements, touching or rubbing the pain site, seeking attention through movements
	Restlessness/agitation	2	Pulling tube, attempting to sit up, moving limbs/thrashing, not following commands, striking at staff, trying to climb out of bed
Compliance with the ventilator (intubated patients)	Tolerating ventilator or movement	0	Alarms not activated, easy ventilation
	Coughing but tolerating	1	Coughing, alarms may be activated but stop spontaneously
	Fighting ventilator	2	Asynchrony: blocking ventilation, alarms frequently activated
	To be aligned with Vocalization	0	Talking in normal tone or no sound
OR			
Vocalization (nonintubated patients)	Sighing, moaning	1	Sighing, moaning
	Crying out, sobbing	2	Crying out, sobbing
Muscle tension	Relaxed	0	No resistance to passive movements
	Tense, rigid	1	Resistance to passive movements
	Very tense or rigid	2	Strong resistance to passive movements, incapacity to complete them
Total		/8	

1. The patient must be observed at rest for 1 minute to obtain a baseline value of the CPOT.
   1.1 Observation of patient at rest (baseline).
   The nurse looks at the patient's face and body to note any visible reactions for an observation period of 1 minute. The nurse gives a score for all items except for muscle tension. At the end of the 1-minute period, the nurse holds the patient's arm in both hands. The nurse places one hand at the elbow and uses the other one to hold the patient's hand. Then the nurse performs a passive flexion and extension of the upper limb and feels any resistance the patient may exhibit. If the movements are performed easily, the patient is found to be relaxed with no resistance (score 0). If the movements can still be performed but with more strength, then it is concluded that the patient is showing resistance to movements (score 1). If the nurse cannot complete the movements, strong resistance is felt (score 2). This can be observed when the patient clenches his or her fists.
2. Then the patient should be observed during nociceptive procedures (e.g., turning, wound care) to detect any changes in the patient's behaviors.
   2.1 Observation of patient during a nociceptive procedure.
   While performing a nociceptive procedure known to be painful, the nurse looks at the patient's face to note any reactions such as brow lowering or grimacing. These reactions may be brief or can last longer. The nurse also looks out for body movements. For instance, he or she looks for protective movements such as the patient trying to reach or touching the pain site (e.g., surgical incision, injury site). In the mechanically ventilated patient, the nurse pays attention to alarms and if they stop spontaneously or require that he or she intervenes (e.g., reassurance, administering medication). It is important that the nurse auscultates the patient to check for the position of the endotracheal tube and the presence of secretions, because these factors may influence this item without being indicative of pain. According to muscle tension, the nurse can feel if the patient is resisting against the movement. When turning the patient in bed, a score of 2 is given when the patient is resisting against the movement and attempts to get on his or her back.

TABLE 7.2 Critical-Care Pain Observation Tool.—cont'd

Indicator	SCORE	Description

3. The patient should be evaluated before and at the peak effect of an analgesic agent to assess whether the treatment was effective in relieving pain.
4. The patient should be attributed the highest score observed during the observation period.
5. The patient should be attributed a score for each behavior included in the CPOT. Muscle tension should be evaluated last because it may lead to behavioral reactions not necessarily related to pain but more to the actual stimulation. According to compliance with the ventilator, the nurse must check that the endotracheal tube is well positioned and for the presence of secretions, which could lead to higher scores for this item.

An online teaching video funded and created by Kaiser Permanente Northern California Nursing Research (KPNCNR) to learn how to use the CPOT at the bedside is available on the ICU Liberation website at https://www.sccm.org/ICULiberation/Resources/Critical-Care-Pain-Observation-Tool-How-to-Use-it.
Modified from Gélinas C, Fillion L, Puntillo KA, Viens C, Fortier M. Validation of the Critical-Care Pain Observation Tool (CPOT) in adult patients. *Am J Crit Care.* 2006;15:420. Figure of facial expressions courtesy Céline Gélinas, Ingram School of Nursing, McGill University, Canada.

In addition, BPS developed for nonverbal critically ill patients may have to be adapted for patients with a brain injury and an altered level of consciousness, because they were found to exhibit different behavioral responses to pain.[42,43] Instead of grimacing, brain-injured patients with altered levels of consciousness seemed to react mostly by lowering their eyebrows, showing face flushing, tearing, and exhibiting limb flexion when exposed to pain. Conscious brain-injured patients were more likely to exhibit grimacing and touching the pain site in response to pain.[42] The content of existing BPS may need to be adjusted for use in this specific vulnerable group. The CPOT was recently adapted for critically ill patients with a brain injury and this version of the tool is called CPOT-Neuro.[44]

When selecting a scale, nurses should make sure that it has been tested in the patient population and context in which they plan to use it. A scale can be shown to be valid only with a specific group of people and in a given context.[44] Nurses should also consult family members to better understand the patient's pain behaviors and their specific reactions at rest and during activity.[11–13]

Physiologic Indicators

When patients cannot react behaviorally to pain, the only possible clues left for the detection of pain are physiologic indicators.

Vital signs. Vital signs (i.e., blood pressure, heart rate, respiratory rate) have received some attention; however, their validity in the pain assessment process is not supported. Although vital sign values generally increase during nociceptive procedures, they have also been found to decrease or to remain stable. Moreover, vital signs are not consistently related to the patient's self-report of pain, and they are not predictive of pain.[9]

In the American Society for Pain Management Nursing (ASPMN) recommendations[12] and the SCCM guidelines,[6] it is stated that vital signs should not be considered as primary indicators of pain because they can be attributed to other distress conditions, homeostatic changes, and medications. Instead, changes in vital signs should be considered a cue to begin further assessment of pain with appropriate tools.[6,11,12]

Pupil dilation index. Besides vital signs, the pupil dilation reflex (PDR) has been studied in relation to the assessment of pain in critical care patients. The increase in PDR was found to be associated with nociceptive procedures[45] or pain scores[46–48] in surgical critical care patients. However, a recent study showed poor performance of video pupillometry in the prediction of nociception in brain-injured critical care patients.[49] PDR may be influenced by factors other than pain, such as the administration of high doses of opioids and brain injury.

Nociception indices. Other innovative technology may have some potential. The Analgesia Nociception Index (which is based on heart rate variability) and the Nociception Level Index (which is based on multiple parameters related to heart rate, heart rate variability, galvanic skin response, and peripheral temperature) have been shown to be useful in detecting nociceptive procedures and was associated with pain scores in critically ill adults,[50–52] but more research is needed.

Patient-Related Challenges to Pain Assessment and Management

Communication

The most obvious patient barrier to the assessment of pain in critical care patients is an alteration in the ability to communicate. With patients unable to self-report, the nurse relies on validated BPS such as the BPS/BPS-NI[36,37] and the CPOT[38] to assess the presence of pain.[6,11,12,53–55]

The patient's family can contribute to the assessment of pain.[53–55] A family member's impression of a patient's pain should be considered in the pain assessment process of a critically ill patient.[6,11,12,53–55]

Altered Level of Consciousness and Unconsciousness

A patient who either is unconscious or has an altered level of consciousness presents a dilemma for all clinicians. Experts recommend

BOX 7.1 Case Example of Using a Cut-Off Score With the Critical-Care Pain Observation Tool (CPOT)

A patient is admitted to the critical care unit after cardiac surgery. He is mechanically ventilated and too drowsy to communicate effectively with the nurse using signs (e.g., head nodding or pointing on a communication board). However, he seems to be uncomfortable, as he becomes agitated each time he is touched. The nurse in charge is puzzled about the need to administer an analgesic or a sedative—both prescribed on the postoperative care protocol. She first assesses for the presence of pain and gets a score of 4 out of 8 on the CPOT as the patient grimaces and attempts to sit in the bed. Considering that a CPOT score higher than 2 strongly suggests the presence of pain, the nurse gives a dose of subcutaneous analgesic. The patient has a relaxed face and is cautiously moving his hand from time to time toward the surgical wound on his chest 30 minutes after the administration of the analgesic. The CPOT score is now 1 out of 8, indicating pain relief, as it dropped from 4 to 1 (i.e., more than 2 points).

assuming that patients who are unconscious or with an altered level of consciousness have pain and that they be treated the same way as conscious patients are treated when they are exposed to sources of pain.[12] Interviews with 100 patients who recalled their experiences from a time when they were unconscious revealed that 25% could hear, understand, and respond emotionally to what was being said.[56]

Moreover, it has been shown that some cortical activation related to pain perception is still present in unconscious patients in a neurovegetative state.[57] Knowing this, the critical care nurse can initiate a discussion with the other members of the health care team to formulate a plan of care for the patient's comfort.

Older Adult Patients

Many older adult patients do not complain much about pain. Misconceptions such as believing that pain is a normal consequence of aging or being afraid to disturb the health care team are barriers to pain expression for older adults.[20]

Cognitive impairment. Cognitive deficits present additional pain assessment barriers. Many older adult patients with mild to moderate cognitive impairments and even some with severe impairment are able to use pain intensity scales.[58-60] Vertical pain intensity scales are more easily understood by older adults and are recommended (Fig. 7.2).[59] Older patients with cognitive deficits should receive repeated instructions and be given sufficient time to respond.

When the self-report of pain is impossible to obtain, direct observation of pain-related behaviors is recommended.[12,58] More than 20 behavioral tools have been developed for older patients with cognitive deficits.[60-63]

Delirium

Delirium is a form of transient cognitive impairment that is highly prevalent in critically ill patients.[6] Not much evidence is available on pain assessment tools that are valid for use in delirium. The BPS-NI

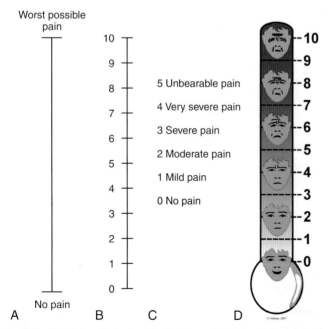

Fig. 7.2 Pain Intensity Scales (Vertical Format). (A) Visual Analog Scale (VAS). (B) Numeric Rating Scale (NRS). (C) Descriptive Rating Scale (DRS). (D) Faces Pain Thermometer. (Courtesy Céline Gélinas, Ingram School of Nursing, McGill University, Canada.)

was initially tested in 30 critically ill patients with 84% being positive for delirium.[37] Higher BPS-NI scores were found during turning compared with rest and catheter dressing change, a non-nociceptive procedure, supporting its ability to discriminate between nociceptive and non-nociceptive conditions. Findings with the CPOT in 40 delirious critically ill patients were similar. Higher CPOT scores were found during nociceptive procedures (e.g., repositioning, endotracheal suctioning, and dressing change of a wound) compared with a non-nociceptive procedure (e.g., taking blood pressure).[64]

Language Differences

Another barrier to accurate pain assessment is cultural influences on pain and pain reporting.[65] To facilitate communication, the use of a pain intensity scale in the patient's language is vital. The 0-to-10 numeric pain scales have been translated into many different languages.[20]

Cultural Influences

When assessing a patient from a cultural group different from your own, it should not be assumed the patient will have a specific response to pain or exhibit a particular behavior because of his or her culture. Patients have individual responses to pain. The health care practitioner may wrongfully assign or expect behaviors that a patient will not exhibit. The complexities and intricacies of cultural beliefs require more extensive discussion than is possible here. It is important for the nurse to support, whenever possible, the special beliefs and needs of the patient and his or her family to provide the most therapeutic environment for healing to occur.

Opioid Use Considerations

Opioid-Related Iatrogenic Withdrawal Syndrome

Physical dependence and tolerance to opioids may develop if opioids are administered over a long period. Physical dependence is manifested by withdrawal symptoms when opioids are abruptly stopped. This is known as *iatrogenic withdrawal syndrome* (IWS). Patients at higher risk of IWS are current opioid users and those who are opioid-naïve (i.e., never used or have not used in the previous 6 months) and who received opioids during a prolonged critical care unit hospitalization. Signs and symptoms of IWS are multisystemic, including central nervous system irritability (e.g., restlessness, insomnia), sympathetic nervous system activation (e.g., diaphoresis, lacrimation, piloerection, yawning), and gastrointestinal system (e.g., diarrhea, nausea, and vomiting).[66-68] These signs and symptoms are not specific to IWS and can occur in many other clinical conditions.

Criteria in the *Diagnostic and Statistical Manual of Mental Disorders* 5th edition (DSM-5) established to identify IWS include the following:
- Reduction or discontinuation of opioids after high or prolonged use
- Development of three or more manifestations of IWS
- Determination that manifestations are not related to other clinical conditions[67]

Withdrawal may be avoided by a planned slow wean from the opioid to allow the brain to reestablish neurochemical balance without opioid influence.[20] Preventive strategies may be used to minimize the use of opioids. Practice guidelines promote the use of non-pharmacologic interventions (e.g., massage, music therapy, relaxation techniques) and of nonopioids.[6]

Opioid Use Disorder and Opioid Misuse

In a national report analyzing data from 2009 to 2015 in the United States, critical care admissions for opioid overdoses increased over the study period by 34%, from 44 per 10,000 to 59 per 10,000 admissions.[5] The mortality rate of critical care admissions related to opioid overdoses increased and reached 10% in 2015.[5]

Opioid use disorder. Opioid use disorder (previously known as opioid addiction) is defined as a problematic pattern of opioid use that leads to serious impairment or distress.[67,69]

Opioid misuse. Opioid misuse can be described as the use of opioids in a manner other than as directed by a physician, such as use in higher doses, more frequent doses, or longer than indicated or using someone else's medication. Guidelines recommend a reduction of opioid prescription for chronic pain,[70] and this is also in alignment with the PADIS guidelines recommending the use of a multimodal analgesia approach with low doses of opioids when appropriate.[6]

Assessment of opioid disorder and misuse. Tools are available to assist the patient's level of risk of opioid use disorder and opioid misuse. Some include the Screener and Opioid Assessment for Patients with Pain (SOAPP-R),[71] the Opioid Risk Tool for Opioid Use Disorder (ORT-OUD),[72] and the Opioid Compliance Checklist (OCC).[73] Medication use and opioid risk assessment should be performed by the critical care team at admission and before discharge to ensure that appropriate and safe follow-up is provided.[74]

PAIN MANAGEMENT

The management of pain in a critically ill patient is as multidimensional as its assessment and is a multidisciplinary team effort.[75] A multimodal analgesic approach based on pharmacologic and nonpharmacologic interventions should be adopted to achieve optimal pain management while using the lowest effective doses of opioids when appropriate.[6] Pain management decisions should be based on pain assessment findings, and reassessment of pain at the peak effect of analgesics determines the effectiveness of analgesia.

Pain Management Algorithm

The pain management algorithm using the 0-to-10 NRS and CPOT is provided in Fig. 7.3. The algorithm includes regular pain assessments at rest and during standard care procedures.

Low Pain Score

When a low pain score is obtained (i.e., NRS = 1–3, CPOT = 1–2), a nonopioid analgesic and/or nonpharmacologic interventions may be used.

Higher Pain Score

When a significant pain score is detected (i.e., NRS >3, CPOT >2), the administration of a nonopioid and/or low dose of opioid may be considered, and subsequent reassessment of pain (ideally at the peak effect of the opioid or within 1 hour after administration) is necessary to determine the effectiveness of analgesia.

Effectiveness of analgesia is considered if a reduction in greater than three points on the NRS[76] or greater than two on the CPOT[77] or a score of 0 on either scale is achieved.

Pharmacologic Control of Pain

Pharmacologic management of pain has infinite variety in the critical care unit. Although this chapter is not an in-depth discussion of pharmacology, some commonly administered agents are discussed. Pain pharmacology is divided into two categories of action: opioid agonists and nonopioids. Elements of the PADIS guidelines[6] for the treatment of pain in critically ill adults are presented in Box 7.2. How pain is approached and managed is a progression or combination of the available agents, the type of pain, and the patient response to treatment.

Opioid Analgesics

The opioids recommended as first-line analgesics are the agonists. These opioids bind to mu receptors (transmission process), which

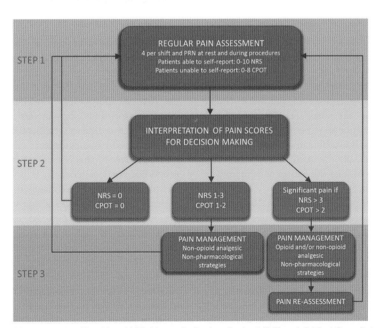

Fig. 7.3 Pain Management Algorithm With Numeric Rating Scale *(NRS)* and Critical-Care Pain Observation Tool *(CPOT)*. (From Gélinas C. Pain assessment in the critically ill adult: recent evidence and new trends. *Intensive Crit Care Nurs.* 2016;34:4.)

BOX 7.2 Summary of Pain Management Guidelines[6]

- Patients in critical care routinely experience pain at rest and during procedures, including regular activities (e.g., endotracheal suctioning, turning) and discrete procedures (e.g., tube or drain removal, arterial catheter insertion).
  1. Perform routine pain assessment in all patients.
  2. In patients who are able to self-report their level of pain, use a 0-to-10 numerical rating scale, either verbally or visually.
  3. The BPS/BPS-NI (scale 3–12) and CPOT (scale 0–8) are the most valid and reliable behavioral pain scales. A BPS/BPS-NI >5 or a CPOT >2 indicates that the patient has significant pain.
  4. When the patient is unable to self-report, the family can be involved in their loved one's pain assessment process if they feel comfortable doing so.
  5. Vital signs should be used only as a cue for further pain assessment using appropriate and validated methods such as the patient's self-report (whenever possible) or a behavioral scale (i.e., BPS/BPS-NI, CPOT).
- An assessment-driven, protocol-based, stepwise approach for pain and sedation management in critically ill adults is recommended.
- A multimodal analgesic approach to pain management is encouraged.
- Adjuvants to opioid therapy include acetaminophen, ketamine (in postsurgical critical care patients), and neuropathic pain medication (e.g., gabapentin, carbamazepine, pregabalin) for neuropathic pain management or after cardiovascular surgery.
- The lowest effective dose of an opioid may be used for procedural pain management, and NSAIDs may be used for discrete and infrequent procedures (e.g., chest tube removal).
- Massage, music, relaxation techniques, and ice therapy are effective and feasible nonpharmacologic interventions for procedural and/or nonprocedural pain management.

appear to be responsible for pain relief. Additional pharmacologic information is presented in Table 7.3.

Morphine. Because of its water solubility, morphine has a slower onset of action and a longer duration compared with the lipid-soluble opioids (e.g., fentanyl). Morphine has two main metabolites: morphine-3-glucuronide (M3G, inactive) and morphine-6-glucuronide (M6G, active). M6G is responsible for the analgesic effect but may accumulate and cause excessive sedation in patients with renal failure or hepatic dysfunction.[78] Morphine is available in a variety of delivery methods. It is the standard by which all other opioids are measured. It is also the agent that most closely mimics the endogenous opioids in the human pain modulation system.

Morphine is indicated for severe pain. It has additional actions that are helpful for managing other symptoms. Morphine dilates peripheral veins and arteries, making it useful in reducing myocardial workload. Morphine is also viewed as an antianxiety agent because of the calming effect it produces.

Many side effects have been reported with the use of morphine (see Table 7.3). The hypotensive effect can be particularly problematic in a patient who is hypovolemic. The vasodilation effect is potentiated in volume-depleted patients, and the hemodynamic status must be carefully monitored. Volume resuscitation restores blood pressure in the event of a prolonged hypotensive response.

Fentanyl. Fentanyl is a synthetic opioid preferred for critically ill patients with hemodynamic instability or morphine allergy. It is a lipid-soluble agent that has a more rapid onset than morphine and a shorter duration. The metabolites of fentanyl are largely inactive and nontoxic, which makes it an effective and safe opioid. Fentanyl and hydromorphone are preferred in hemodynamically unstable patients and in patients with impaired kidney function.[79] It is available in intravenous (IV), intraspinal, and transdermal forms. The transdermal form is commonly referred to as the "Duragesic patch" or the "72-hour patch."

When fentanyl is given by rapid administration and at higher doses, it has been associated with the additional hazard of bradycardia and rigidity in the chest wall muscles.[80] The use of transdermal fentanyl is rarely indicated in critically ill patients. The customary use of the "fentanyl patch" is for patients experiencing chronic pain or cancer pain; in critical care, it is used for patients who require extended pain control. Transdermal delivery requires 12 to 16 hours for onset of action, and the patch has a duration of action of 72 hours.[20] If this delivery method is used, the patient will require other opioid management until the transdermal fentanyl takes effect.

Hydromorphone. Hydromorphone is a semisynthetic opioid; the onset of action and duration are similar to morphine.[20] It is an effective opioid with multiple routes of delivery. It is more potent than morphine. Hydromorphone produces an inactive metabolite (i.e., hydromorphone-3-glucuronide), making it the opioid of choice for use in patients with end-stage renal disease.[80]

Meperidine. Meperidine (Demerol) is a less potent opioid with agonist effects similar to those of morphine. It is considered the weakest of the opioids, and it must be administered in large doses to be equivalent in action to morphine. Because the duration of action is short, dosing is frequent. A major concern with this medication is the metabolite *normeperidine*, which is neurotoxic. At high doses in patients with kidney failure or liver dysfunction or in older adults, this metabolite may induce neurotoxicity, including irritability, muscle spasticity, tremors, agitation, and seizures.[20] Although meperidine is useful in short-term specific conditions (e.g., treating postoperative shivering),[81] it should not be used routinely for analgesia in the critical care unit.[79–81]

Codeine. Codeine has limited use in the management of severe pain. It is rarely used in the critical care unit. It provides analgesia for mild to moderate pain, and it is usually compounded with a nonopioid (e.g., acetaminophen). To be active, codeine must be metabolized in the liver to morphine.[20] Codeine is available only through oral, intramuscular, and subcutaneous routes, and its absorption can be reduced in a critical care patient by altered gastrointestinal motility and decreased tissue perfusion.

Methadone. Methadone is a synthetic opioid with morphine-like properties but less sedation. It is longer acting than morphine and has a long half-life; this makes it difficult to titrate in critical care patients. Methadone lacks active metabolites, and routes other than the kidney eliminate 60% of the medication. This means that methadone does not accumulate in patients with kidney failure. Methadone can be used to treat chronic pain syndromes when patients experience tolerance with other opioids and may help facilitate the down-titration of opioid infusions in critical care patients.[80] However, prolongation of the QT interval, which can lead to torsades de pointes, has been reported with its use.[78]

More potent opioids: remifentanil and sufentanil. Remifentanil and sufentanil are opioid agonists. The use of these potent medications has been studied in critically ill patients.

Remifentanil is 250 times more potent than morphine, and it has a rapid onset and predictable offset of action. For this reason, it allows a

TABLE 7.3 Pharmacologic Management Pain.

Medication	Dosage	Onset (min)	Duration (h)	Available Routes	Properties	Side Effects and Comments
Morphine	1—4 mg IV bolus	5—10	3—4	PO, SL, R, IV, IM, SC, EA, IA	Analgesia, antianxiety	Standard for comparison Side effects: sedation, respiratory depression, euphoria or dysphoria, hypotension, nausea, vomiting, pruritus, constipation, urinary retention 1—10 mg/h IV infusion M6G can accumulate in patients with renal failure or hepatic dysfunction
Fentanyl	25—100 mcg IV bolus 25—200 mcg/h IV infusion	1—5	0.5—4	OTFC, IV, IM, TD, EA, IA	Analgesia, antianxiety	Same side effects as morphine Rigidity with high doses
Hydromorphone (Dilaudid)	0.2—1 mg IV bolus 0.2—2 mg/h IV infusion	5	3—4	PO, R, IV, IM, SC, EA, IA	Analgesia, antianxiety	Same side effects as morphine
Codeine	15—30 mg IM, SC	10—20	3—4	PO, IM, SC	Analgesia (mild to moderate pain)	Lacks potency (unpredictable absorption; not all patients convert it to active form to achieve analgesia) Most common side effects: light-headedness, dizziness, shortness of breath, sedation, nausea, vomiting
Acetaminophen	325—1000 mg maximum of 4 g/day	20—30	4—6	PO, R	Analgesia, antipyretic	Rare side effects Hepatotoxicity
Ketorolac (Toradol)	15—30 mg IV	<10	6—8	PO, IM, IV	Analgesia, minimum antiinflammatory effect	Short-term use (<5 days) Side effects: gastric ulceration, bleeding, exacerbation of renal insufficiency Use with care in older adult and renal failure patients

EA, Epidural analgesia; *IA,* intrathecal analgesia; *IM,* intramuscular; *IV,* intravenous; *M6G,* morphine-6-glucuronide; *OTFC,* oral transmucosal fentanyl citrate; *PO,* oral; *R,* rectal; *SC,* subcutaneous; *SL,* sublingual; *TD,* transdermal.

rapid emergence from sedation, facilitating the evaluation of the neurologic state of the patient after stopping the infusion.[82,83] As opposed to fentanyl, the use of remifentanil was associated with a lower incidence of postoperative delirium.[84]

Sufentanil is 7 to 13 times more potent than fentanyl and 500 to 1000 times more potent than morphine. It has more pronounced sedation properties than fentanyl and other opioids. Patients given sufentanil require minimal sedative agent doses to achieve an adequate sedation level. It has a rapid distribution and a high clearance rate, preventing accumulation when given for a long period.[85] Sufentanil has a longer emergence from sedation compared with remifentanil, but it has a longer analgesic effect after its administration is stopped.[83]

Preventing and Treating Opioid-Induced Respiratory Depression

Respiratory depression is the most life-threatening opioid side effect. Although no universal definition of respiratory depression exists, it is usually described in terms of decreased respiratory rate (fewer than 8 or 10 breaths/min), decreased SpO_2 levels, or elevated end-tidal carbon dioxide ($ETCO_2$) levels.[20] A change in the patient's level of consciousness or an increase in sedation normally precedes respiratory depression.

Many risk factors for opioid-induced respiratory depression have been identified. Patients at risk include those with advanced age; obesity; sleep apnea; impaired kidney, pulmonary, liver, or cardiac function; patients in whom pain is controlled after a period of poor control; opioid-naïve patients (i.e., receiving opioids for less than a week); patients with concurrent use of other central nervous system depressants; and those at postoperative day 1.[86] The risk of respiratory depression increases when other medications with sedative effects (e.g., benzodiazepines, antiemetics, neuroleptics, antihistamines) are concomitantly administered.

Monitoring. Guidelines on monitoring for patients receiving opioid analgesia were revised by ASPMN.[86] In addition to assessing pain intensity as a targeted outcome of analgesia, regular sedation and respiratory assessments are necessary. Respirations should be evaluated over

1 minute and qualified according to rate, rhythm, and depth of chest excursion. Technology-supported monitoring (e.g., continuous pulse oximetry and capnography) can be useful in high-risk patients.

Opioid reversal. Critical respiratory depression can be readily reversed with administration of the opioid antagonist naloxone.[20] The usual dose is 0.4 mg, which is mixed with 10 mL of normal saline (for a concentration of 0.04 mg/mL). Naloxone is normally given intravenously very slowly (0.5 mL over 2 minutes) while the patient is carefully monitored. Naloxone administration can be discontinued as soon as the patient is responsive to physical stimulation and able to take deep breaths. However, the medication should be kept nearby. Because the duration of naloxone is shorter than most opioids, another dose may be needed 30 minutes after the first dose. The benefits of reversing respiratory depression with naloxone must be carefully weighed against the risk of a sudden onset of pain and the difficulty achieving pain relief. To prevent this from occurring, it is important to provide a nonopioid medication for pain control. Moreover, the use of naloxone is not recommended after prolonged analgesia because it can induce withdrawal and may cause nausea and cardiovascular dysrhythmias.

Sedative With Analgesic Properties: Dexmedetomidine

Dexmedetomidine (Precedex) is a short-acting alpha-2 agonist that is indicated for short-term sedation of mechanically ventilated patients in the critical care unit. Its mechanism of action is unique and differs from the mechanism of action of other commonly used sedatives in critical care. Compared with midazolam (Versed) or lorazepam (Ativan), whose hypnotic effects act mainly on the limbic system, the cortex, or both, the effect of dexmedetomidine is located in the locus caeruleus section of the brainstem. As a result, patients receiving dexmedetomidine IV infusions are calm and sleepy, yet remain easily arousable.[87] For this reason, dexmedetomidine is ideal for mild to moderate sedation, often referred to as conscious sedation. Refer to Chapter 8 for details on dosage and administration.

Dexmedetomidine also possesses an analgesic property. The analgesic effects of dexmedetomidine are principally due to spinal antinociception via binding to non-noradrenergic receptors (heteroreceptors) located on the dorsal horn neurons of the spinal cord.[87] Dexmedetomidine has been reported to decrease postoperative opioid requirements in adults.[88] Although dexmedetomidine use is increasing in critical care, it is not without risk. Inhibition of noradrenergic receptors in the brainstem and the spinal cord can cause hypotension and bradycardia.[87]

Nonopioid Analgesics

In the PADIS guidelines, the use of nonopioids or adjuvants in combination with an opioid is recommended to reduce opioid requirements and opioid-related side effects.[6] This strategy provides greater analgesic effect through action at the peripheral and central levels. Pharmacologic information is presented in Table 7.3.

Acetaminophen. Acetaminophen is an analgesic used to treat mild to moderate pain and is a suggested adjunct to an opioid for pain management in critically ill adults.[6] It inhibits the synthesis of neurotransmitter prostaglandins in the central nervous system, and has no antiinflammatory properties.[20] Acetaminophen is metabolized by two pathways: major (nontoxic metabolite) and minor (toxic metabolite that is rapidly converted into a nontoxic form by glutathione). In an acetaminophen overdose, a larger amount is processed by the minor pathway, which results in a larger quantity of toxic metabolites and may cause damage to the liver. Side effects are rare at therapeutic doses (total daily dose should not exceed 4 g in 24 hours).

When calculating the total daily dose of acetaminophen all products containing acetaminophen are included. Special care must be taken for patients with liver dysfunction, malnutrition, or a history of excess alcohol consumption; total dose of acetaminophen in these patients should not exceed 2 g/day.[20]

Nonsteroidal antiinflammatory drugs. The use of nonsteroidal antiinflammatory drugs (NSAIDs) are indicated in combination with opioids in patients with acute musculoskeletal and soft tissue inflammation.[20] The use of an NSAID is suggested as an alternative for pain management during discrete and infrequent procedures in critically ill adults.[6] The mechanism of action of NSAIDs is to block the action of cyclooxygenase (COX), the enzyme that converts arachidonic acid to prostaglandins. The production of prostaglandins (transduction process) is inhibited by blocking the action of COX (Fig. 7.4).

Ketorolac is the most appropriate NSAID for use in the critical care setting. Not all critically ill patients are candidates for ketorolac therapy because of its side effects. Caution is advised for older adults or patients with kidney dysfunction because of slower clearance rates. Because ketorolac is an NSAID, monitoring for clumping of platelets is of primary importance. Laboratory data should be evaluated for an increase in bleeding time, with monitoring for signs of abnormal bleeding. Prolonged use of ketorolac for more than 5 days is associated with an increase in kidney failure and bleeding.[89]

Ketamine. Low-dose ketamine is suggested as an adjunct to opioid therapy in postsurgical critical care adult patients.[6] Ketamine is a dissociative anesthetic agent that has analgesic properties. It was traditionally used intravenously for procedural pain in burn patients. It is also available in enteral routes. Compared with opioids, ketamine has the benefit of sparing the respiratory drive, but it has many side effects related to the release of catecholamines and the emergence of delirium. For this reason, ketamine is not recommended for routine therapy in critically ill patients. Before ketamine is administered, the dissociative state should be explained to the patient. A *dissociative state* refers to the feelings of separateness from the environment, loss of control, hallucinations, and vivid dreams. The use of benzodiazepines (e.g., midazolam) can reduce the incidence of this unpleasant effect.[20]

Lidocaine. Lidocaine is another anesthetic that can be used for procedural and acute pain or for some patients with chronic neuropathic pain.[20] When used locally, anesthetics act through the transduction process (see Fig. 7.4). The routine use of IV lidocaine is not suggested for pain management in critically ill adults.[6]

Anticonvulsants. Anticonvulsants (e.g., carbamazepine, gabapentin, pregabalin) are first-line analgesics for lancing neuropathic pain. Their use in combination with opioids is recommended for neuropathic pain management in critically ill adults and is suggested for use in adults after cardiovascular surgery.[6] Even if the specific mechanism for pain relief is unknown, analgesia probably results from the suppression of sodium ion (Na+) discharges, reducing the neuronal hyperexcitability (action potential) in the transduction process (see Fig. 7.4).[20]

Antidepressants. Antidepressants are also considered as analgesics in various chronic pain syndromes such as headache, fibromyalgia, low back pain, neuropathy, central pain, and cancer pain. The analgesic dose is often lower than the dose required to treat depression. Antidepressant adjuvant analgesics are usually divided into two main groups: tricyclic antidepressants (e.g., amitriptyline, imipramine, desipramine) and biogenic amine reuptake inhibitors (e.g., venlafaxine, paroxetine, sertraline). The mechanism of analgesia most widely accepted is the ability

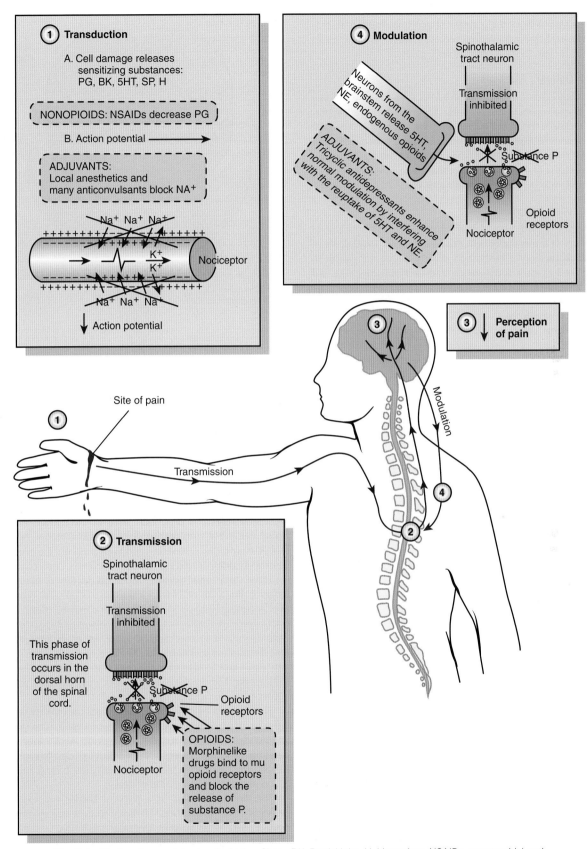

Fig. 7.4 Nociception and Analgesic Action Sites. *BK,* Bradykinin; *H,* histamine; *NSAIDs,* nonsteroidal anti-inflammatory drugs; *PG,* prostaglandins; *SP,* substance P; *5HT,* serotonin. (From McCaffery M, Pasero C. *Pain: Clinical Manual for Nursing Practice.* 2nd ed. St. Louis: Mosby; 1999.)

of antidepressants to block the reuptake of neurotransmitters serotonin and norepinephrine in the central nervous system.[20] This increases the activity of the modulation process (see Fig. 7.4).

Medication Delivery Methods

The most common route for medication administration is the IV route by means of continuous infusion, bolus administration, or patient-controlled analgesia (PCA). Traditionally, the choice has been IV bolus administration. The benefits of this method are the rapid onset of action and the ease of titration. The major disadvantage is the increase and decrease of the serum level of the opioid, leading to periods of pain control with periods of breakthrough pain.

Patient-Controlled Analgesia

PCA is a method of medication delivery that uses the IV route and an infusion pump. It allows the patient to self-administer small doses of analgesics. This method of medication delivery allows the patient to control the level of pain and sedation and to avoid the peaks and valleys of intermittent dosing by the health care professional. The patient can self-administer a bolus of medication the moment the pain begins, acting preemptively.

Certain patients are not candidates for PCA. Patients with alterations in the level of consciousness or mentation are unable to understand the use of the equipment. Very elderly patients and patients with kidney or liver dysfunction may require careful screening for PCA.

Allowing the patient to self-administer opioid doses does not diminish the role of the critical care nurse in pain management. The nurse advises about necessary changes to the prescription and continues to monitor the effects of the medication and doses. The patient is closely monitored during the first 2 hours of therapy and after every change in the prescription. If the patient's pain does not respond within the first 2 hours of therapy, a total reassessment of the pain state is essential. The nurse monitors the number of boluses the patient delivers. If the patient is pressing the button to bolus medication more often than the prescription, the dose may be insufficient to maintain pain control.

Naloxone must be readily available to reverse opioid-induced respiratory depression. Ideally, a patient undergoing an elective procedure requiring opioid analgesia postoperatively is instructed in the use of PCA during preoperative teaching.

Intraspinal Pain Control

Intraspinal anesthesia uses the concept that the spinal cord is the primary link in nociceptive transmission. The goal is to mimic the body's endogenous opioid pain modification system by interfering with the transmission of pain and providing an opioid receptor binding agent directly into the spinal cord. The hemodynamic status of the patient changes very little.

Intraspinal anesthesia is particularly appropriate for pain in the thorax, upper abdomen, and lower extremities. The two intraspinal routes are intrathecal and epidural (Fig. 7.5). Regardless of the route, the effects of the opioid agonist used are similar, and assessment parameters are the same as those used for other routes.

Intrathecal Analgesia

Intrathecal (subarachnoid) opioids are placed directly into the cerebrospinal fluid and attach to spinal cord receptor sites. Opioids introduced at this site act quickly at the dorsal horn. The dural sheath is punctured, eliminating the barrier for pathogens between the

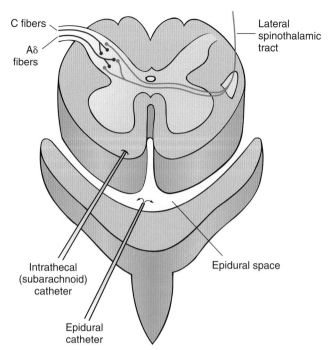

Fig. 7.5 Intraspinal catheter placement in a spinal cord cross-section.

environment and the cerebrospinal fluid. This creates the risk of serious infections. The intrathecal route is usually reserved for intraoperative use. Single-bolus dosing provides short-term relief for short-lived pain (the pain of labor and delivery is well managed using this regimen). Side effects of intrathecal pain control include postdural puncture headache and infection.

Epidural Analgesia

Epidural analgesia is commonly used in the critical care unit after major abdominal surgery, nephrectomy, thoracotomy, and major orthopedic procedures. Certain conditions preclude the use of this pain control method, including systemic infection, anticoagulation, and increased intracranial pressure. Epidural delivery of opioids provides longer lasting pain relief with less dosing of opioids. When delivered into the epidural space, 5 mg of morphine may be effective for 6 to 24 hours compared with 3 to 4 hours when delivered intravenously. Opioids infused in the epidural space are more unpredictable than opioids administered intrathecally. The epidural space is filled with fatty tissue and is external to the dura mater. The fatty tissue interferes with uptake, and the dura mater acts as a barrier to diffusion, making diffusion rate difficult to predict.

The type of medication used determines the rapidity of medication diffusion. Hydrophilic medications (e.g., morphine) are water soluble and penetrate the dura mater slowly, giving them a longer onset and duration of action. Lipophilic medications (e.g., fentanyl) are lipid soluble; they penetrate the dura rapidly and have a rapid onset of action and a shorter duration of action.

The dura mater acts as a physical barrier and causes delay in diffusion of the medication. Medications delivered epidurally may be administered by bolus or by continuous infusion.

Respiratory depression may occur early in the therapy or within 24 hours after initiation. The epidural catheter also puts the patient at risk for infection. The efficiency of this pain control method and the increased mobility of the patient do not diminish the nurse's responsibility to monitor and evaluate the outcomes of the pain management protocol in use.

Equianalgesia

When a modification of opioid is considered, the nurse must be aware of equianalgesic dosages. In doing any conversion, the goal is to provide equal analgesic effects with the new agents. This concept is referred to as *equianalgesia*. Morphine is the standard for the conversion of opioids. Prescribed dosages must consider the patient's age and health status.[20] The critical care nurse must have access to a chart on the unit for easy referral to administer the correct dosages of opioids to critically ill patients. Because of the variety of agents and routes, the professional pain organizations have developed equianalgesia charts for use by health care professionals. All critical care units need to have an equianalgesic chart posted for easy reference. Box 7.3 presents a guide to using these charts. Table 7.4 provides the equianalgesic dose for different medications used in clinical practice. Table 7.5 presents an equianalgesic chart with oral nonopioid and opioid doses for mild to moderate pain.

NONPHARMACOLOGIC PAIN MANAGEMENT

Although numerous methods of pain management other than medications are mentioned in the critical care literature,[90] only few studies have been done to provide evidence of their effectiveness in the critical care setting.[91] Many nonpharmacologic interventions, including massage, ice therapy, music, and relaxation techniques, are suggested in the PADIS guidelines for procedural and/or nonprocedural pain management and are part of the "ICU Liberation Bundle" because they are simple and safe to use.[6,7] It is crucial that nurses be provided with the appropriate training and equipment required to apply nonpharmacologic interventions for pain management in critically ill patients. There must also be some commitment to the treatment from the patient. The family and significant others may be involved also.[92]

Physical Techniques

Stimulating other non-pain sensory fibers (Aβ) in the periphery modifies pain transmission. These fibers are stimulated by thermal changes, as in simple massage and ice therapy.

Massage

The effect of massage on pain relief was mainly tested in postoperative critical care patients following cardiac surgery. A systematic review and meta-analysis of 12 randomized controlled trials (RCTs) revealed that massage was effective in reducing postoperative pain in critical care cardiac surgery patients compared with usual care or sham massage (e.g., hand holding).[93] Duration of massage (10–30 minutes), frequency (single or repeated administration), and body area (back, feet and hands, or only hands) varied across RCTs. Massage can be administered by nurses following minimal training (3–6 hours).

Ice Therapy

Ice therapy applied for 10 to 20 minutes was found to be helpful to reduce procedural pain (e.g., chest tube removal) when used in combination with an analgesia in critically ill patients.[6]

BOX 7.3   Guide to Using Equianalgesic Charts

- Equianalgesic means approximately the same pain relief.
- The equianalgesic chart is a guideline. Doses and intervals between doses are titrated according to the individual's response.
- The equianalgesic chart is helpful when switching from one medication to another or when switching from one route of administration to another.
- Dosages in the equianalgesic chart for moderate to severe pain are not necessarily starting doses. The doses suggest a ratio for comparing the analgesia of one medication with another.
- For older patients, initially reduce the recommended adult opioid dose for moderate to severe pain by 25%–50%.
- The longer the patient has been receiving opioids, the more conservative the starting dose of a *new* opioid should be.

Cognitive-Behavioral Techniques

Using the cortical interpretation of pain as the foundation, several interventions can reduce the patient's pain report, including cognitive techniques such as relaxation and music.

Relaxation and Deep Breathing

Breathing techniques were found to reduce procedural pain (chest tube removal) when timed with an opioid in cardiac surgery critical care patients.[6] Relaxation decreases oxygen consumption and muscle tone, and can decrease heart rate and blood pressure. Deep-breathing exercises can be as simple as teaching the patient to inhale slowly through the nose and to exhale through pursed lips.[94]

Music

Music is a commonly used intervention for relaxation. In a systematic review and meta-analysis of 18 RCTs, the administration of 20 to 30 minutes of music has been found to be effective in reducing pain in critically ill adults.[95] The music should be supplied by a small set of headphones or earbuds. It is important to educate the patient and family and to provide music of the patient's choice.[95] The family of a patient unable to self-report may suggest music based on the patient's preferences.[92]

Bundle Interventions

Combining interventions is also effective at reducing pain. Two RCTs tested a combination of three interventions as a bundle and reduced pain scores on a 0-to-10 NRS for cardiac surgery critical care patients,[96] and on both the 0-to-10 NRS and the CPOT in a heterogeneous patient sample.[97]

Bundled interventions follow the same schedule and require the same resources as those of single interventions.

ADDITIONAL RESOURCES

See Box 7.4 for Internet resources related to pain and pain management.

TABLE 7.4 Equianalgesic Chart Approximate Equivalent Doses of Opioids for Moderate to Severe Pain.

Analgesic	Parenteral (IM, SC, IV) Route (mg)[a,b]	PO Route (mg)[a]	Comments
Mu Opioid Agonists			
Morphine	10	30	Standard for comparison; multiple routes of administration; available in immediate-release and controlled-release formulations; active metabolite M6G can accumulate with repeated dosing in renal failure
Codeine	130	200 NR	IM has unpredictable absorption and high side effect profile; use PO for mild to moderate pain; usually compounded with nonopioid (e.g., Tylenol No. 3)
Fentanyl	100 mcg/h parenterally and transdermally ≅ 4 mg/h morphine parenterally; 1 mcg/h transdermally ≅ 2 mg/24 h morphine PO	—	Short half-life, but at steady state, slow elimination from tissues can lead to prolonged half-life (up to 12 h); start opioid-naïve patients on no more than 25 mcg/h transdermally; transdermal fentanyl NR for acute pain management; available by oral transmucosal route
Hydromorphone (Dilaudid)	1.5	7.5	Useful alternative to morphine; no evidence that metabolites are clinically relevant; shorter duration than morphine; available in high-potency parenteral formulation (10 mg/mL) useful for SC infusion; 3 mg rectal ≅ 650 mg aspirin PO; with repeated dosing (e.g., PCA), it is more likely than 2–3 mg parenteral hydromorphone = 10 mg parenteral morphine
Levorphanol (Levo-Dromoran)	2	4	Longer acting than morphine when given repeatedly; long half-life can lead to accumulation within 2–3 days of repeated dosing
Meperidine	75	300 NR	No longer preferred as first-line opioid for management of acute or chronic pain because of potential toxicity from accumulation of metabolite, normeperidine; normeperidine has 15–20 h half-life and is not reversed by naloxone; NR in elderly patients or patients with impaired renal function; NR by continuous IV infusion
Oxycodone	—	20	Used for moderate pain when combined with nonopioid (e.g., Percocet, Tylox); available as single entity in immediate-release and controlled-release formulations (e.g., OxyContin); can be used similar to PO morphine for severe pain
Oxymorphone (Numorphan)	1	10 rectal	Used for moderate to severe pain; no PO formulation
Agonist-Antagonist Opioids[c]			
Buprenorphine (Buprenex)	0.4	—	Not readily reversed by naloxone; NR for laboring patients
Butorphanol (Stadol)	2	—	Available in nasal spray
Dezocine (Dalgan)	10	—	
Nalbuphine (Nubain)	10	—	
Pentazocine (Talwin)	30	50	

[a]Duration of analgesia is dose dependent; the higher the dose, usually the longer the duration.

[b]IV boluses may be used to produce analgesia that lasts approximately as long as IM or SC doses. However, of all routes of administration, IV produces the highest peak concentration of the medication, and the peak concentration is associated with the highest level of toxicity (e.g., sedation). To decrease the peak effect and reduce the level of toxicity, IV boluses may be administered more slowly (e.g., 10 mg of morphine over a 15-minute period), or smaller doses may be administered more often (e.g., 5 mg of morphine every 1–1.5 hours).

[c]Not recommended for severe, escalating pain. If used in combination with mu agonists, may reverse analgesia and precipitate withdrawal in opioid-dependent patients.

FDA, US Food and Drug Administration; IM, intramuscular; IV, intravenous; M6G, morphine-6-glucuronide; NR, not recommended; PCA, patient-controlled analgesia; PO, per os (by mouth); PRN, pro re nata (as needed); SC, subcutaneous.

From Pasero C, McCaffery M. Pain Assessment and Pharmacologic Management. St. Louis: Elsevier; 2011.

TABLE 7.5 Equianalgesic Chart Approximate Equivalent Doses of PO Nonopioids and Opioids for Mild to Moderate Pain.

Analgesic	PO Dosage (mg)
Nonopioids	
Acetaminophen	650
Aspirin (ASA)	650
Opioids[a]	
Codeine	32–60
Hydrocodone[b]	5
Meperidine (Demerol)	50
Oxycodone[c]	3–5
Propoxyphene (Darvon)	65–100

[a]Often combined with acetaminophen; avoid exceeding maximum total daily dose of acetaminophen (4000 mg/day).

[b]Combined with acetaminophen (e.g., Vicodin, Lortab).

[c]Combined with acetaminophen (e.g., Percocet, Tylox); also available alone as controlled-release OxyContin and immediate-release formulations.

ASA, Acetylsalicylic acid; *PO,* per os (oral).

Selected references for more information: McCaffery M, Pasero C. Acetaminophen and NSAIDS: adult dosing information. In: Pasero C, McCaffery M, eds. *Pain Assessment and Pharmacologic Management.* St. Louis: Mosby; 2011: 211; American Pain Society (APS). *Principles of Analgesic Use in the Treatment of Acute Pain and Cancer Pain.* 3rd ed. Glenview, IL: APS; 1992; Sunshine A, Olson NZ, Colon A, et al. Analgesic efficacy of controlled-release (CR) oxycodone and CR morphine. *Clin Pharmacol Ther.* 1996;59:130.

Modified from Pasero C, McCaffery M. *Pain Assessment and Pharmacologic Management.* St. Louis: Elsevier; 2011.

QSEN

BOX 7.4 Informatics

Internet Resources: Pain and Pain Management

- American Society for Pain Management Nursing (ASPMN): http://www.aspmn.org/
- Canadian Pain Society (CPS): https://www.canadianpainsociety.ca/
- International Association for the Study on Pain (IASP): https://www.iasp-pain.org/
- Joint Commission: https://www.jointcommission.org/
- Society of Critical Care Medicine (SCCM): https://www.sccm.org/
- PADIS Guidelines: https://www.sccm.org/ICULiberation/Guidelines

---

REFERENCES

1. Puntillo KA, Max A, Timsit JF, et al. Determinants of procedural pain intensity in the intensive care unit: the Europain study. *Am J Respir Crit Care Med.* 2014;189(1):39–47.
2. Puntillo KA, White C, Morris AB, et al. Patients' perceptions and responses to procedural pain: results from Thunder Project II. *Am J Crit Care.* 2001;10(4):238–251.
3. Stamenkovic DM, Laycock H, Karanikolas M, Ladjevic NG, Neskovic V, Bantel C. Chronic pain and chronic opioid use after intensive care discharge—is it time to change practice? *Front Pharmacol.* 2019;10:23.
4. Belzak L, Halverson J. The opioid crisis in Canada: a national perspective. *Health Promot Chronic Dis Prev Can.* 2018;38(6):224–233.
5. Stevens JP, Wall MJ, Novack L, Marshall J, Hsu DJ, Howell MD. The critical care crisis of opioid overdoses in the United States. 2017;1(12):1803–1809.

6. Devlin JW, Skrobik Y, Gélinas C, et al. Clinical practice guidelines for the prevention and management of pain, agitation/sedation, delirium, immobility, and sleep disruption in adult patients in the ICU. *Crit Care Med.* 2018;46(9):e825–e873.
7. Holden DN, Retelski J. *The ICU liberation bundle: an emphasis on non-pharmacologic intervention*; 2020. https://www.sccm.org/Communications/Critical-Connections/Archives/2019/The-ICU-Liberation-Bundle-An-Emphasis-on-Nonpharm.
8. International Association for the Study of Pain. IASP terminology. https://www.iasp-pain.org/Education/Content.aspx?ItemNumber=1698. Accessed November 11, 2021.
9. Gélinas C. Pain assessment in the critically ill adult: recent evidence and new trends. *Intensive Crit Care Nurs.* 2016;34:1–11.
10. Khalaila R, Zbidat W, Anwar K, Bayya A, Linton DM, Sviri S. Communication difficulties and psychoemotional distress in patients receiving mechanical ventilation. *Am J Crit Care.* 2011;20(6):470–479.
11. Assessing pain in critically ill adults. *Crit Care Nurse.* 2018;38(6):e13–e16.
12. Herr K, Coyne PJ, Ely E, Gélinas C, Manworren RCB. Pain assessment in the patient unable to self-report: clinical practice recommendations in support of the ASPMN 2019 position statement. *Pain Manag Nurs.* 2019;20(5):404–417.
13. Herr K, Coyne PJ, Ely E, Gélinas C, Manworren RCB. ASPMN 2019 position statement: pain assessment in the patient unable to self-report. *Pain Manag Nurs.* 2019;20(5):402–403.
14. Williams AC, Craig KD. Updating the definition of pain. *Pain.* 2016;157(11):2420–2423.
15. McCaffery M. *Nursing Management of the Patient with Pain.* 2nd ed. Philadelphia: Lippincott; 1979.
16. Anand KJ, Craig KD. New perspectives on the definition of pain. *Pain.* 1996;67(1):3–6.
17. McGuire DB. Comprehensive and multidimensional assessment and measurement of pain. *J Pain Symptom Manage.* 1992;7(5):312–319.
18. Freynhagen R, Parada HA, Calderon-Ospina CA, et al. Current understanding of the mixed pain concept: a brief narrative review. *Curr Med Res Opin.* 2019;35(6):1011–1018.
19. Lynch ME, Craig KD, Peng PWH. *Clinical Pain Management: A Practical Guide.* Chichester, West Sussex, UK: Blackwell Pub; 2011.
20. Pasero C, McCaffery M. *Pain Assessment and Pharmacologic Management.* St. Louis: Elsevier/Mosby; 2011.
21. Cervero F, Laird JM. Visceral pain. *Lancet.* 1999;353(9170):2145–2148.
22. Melzack R, Wall PD. *The challenge of Pain.* Updated. 2nd ed. London, England: Penguin Books; 1996.
23. Carr DB, Goudas LC. Acute pain. *Lancet.* 1999;353(9169):2051–2058.
24. Gélinas C, Puntillo KA, Levin P, Azoulay E. The behavior pain assessment tool for critically ill adults: a validation study in 28 countries. *Pain.* 2017;158(5):811–821.
25. Gélinas C, Arbour C. Behavioral and physiologic indicators during a nociceptive procedure in conscious and unconscious mechanically ventilated adults: similar or different? *J Crit Care.* 2009;24(4):628.e627, 617.
26. Rainville P. Brain mechanisms of pain affect and pain modulation. *Curr Opin Neurobiol.* 2002;12(2):195–204.
27. Derbyshire SW, Osborn J. Modeling pain circuits: how imaging may modify perception. *Neuroimaging Clin N Am.* 2007;17(4):485–493.
28. Melzack R, Wall PD. Pain mechanisms: a new theory. *Science.* 1965;150(3699):971–979.
29. Lorenz J, Minoshima S, Casey KL. Keeping pain out of mind: the role of the dorsolateral prefrontal cortex in pain modulation. *Brain.* 2003;126(Pt 5):1079–1091.
30. Puntillo KA, Pasero C, Li D, et al. Evaluation of pain in ICU patients. *Chest.* 2009;135(4):1069–1074.
31. Daut RL, Cleeland CS. The prevalence and severity of pain in cancer. *Cancer.* 1982;50(9):1913–1918.
32. Melzack R. The short-form McGill pain questionnaire. *Pain.* 1987;30(2):191–197.
33. Jarvis C. *Physical Examination & Health Assessment.* 7th ed. St. Louis: Elsevier; 2016.

34. Puntillo KA, Morris AB, Thompson CL, Stanik-Hutt J, White CA, Wild LR. Pain behaviors observed during six common procedures: results from Thunder Project II. *Crit Care Med.* 2004;32(2):421–427.

35. Gélinas C, Joffe AM, Szumita PM, et al. A psychometric analysis update of behavioral pain assessment tools in noncommunicative, critically ill adults. *AACN Adv Crit Care.* 2019;30(4):365–387.

36. Payen JF, Bru O, Bosson JL, et al. Assessing pain in critically ill sedated patients by using a behavioral pain scale. *Crit Care Med.* 2001;29(12):2258–2263.

37. Chanques G, Payen JF, Mercier G, et al. Assessing pain in non-intubated critically ill patients unable to self report: an adaptation of the Behavioral Pain Scale. *Intensive Care Med.* 2009;35(12):2060–2067.

38. Gélinas C, Fillion L, Puntillo KA, Viens C, Fortier M. Validation of the critical-care pain observation tool in adult patients. *Am J Crit Care.* 2006;15(4):420–427.

39. Georgiou E, Hadjibalassi M, Lambrinou E, Andreou P, Papathanassoglou ED. The impact of pain assessment on critically ill patients' outcomes: a systematic review. *BioMed Res Int.* 2015;2015:503830.

40. Chanques G, Pohlman A, Kress JP, et al. Psychometric comparison of three behavioural scales for the assessment of pain in critically ill patients unable to self-report. *Crit Care.* 2014;18(5):R160.

41. Gélinas C, Ross M, Boitor M, Desjardins S, Vaillant F, Michaud C. Nurses' evaluations of the CPOT use at 12-month post-implementation in the intensive care unit. *Nurs Crit Care.* 2014;19(6):272–280.

42. Gélinas C, Boitor M, Puntillo KA, et al. Behaviors indicative of pain in brain-injured adult patients with different levels of consciousness in the intensive care unit. *J Pain Symptom Manage.* 2019;57(4):761–773.

43. Roulin MJ, Ramelet AS. Behavioral changes in brain-injured critical care adults with different levels of consciousness during nociceptive stimulation: an observational study. *Intensive Care Med.* 2014;40:1115–1123.

44. Gélinas C, Bérubé M, Puntillo KA, et al. Validation of the Critical-Care Pain Observation Tool-Neuro for the assessment of pain in brain-injured adults in the intensive care unit: a prospective cohort study. *BMC Crit Care.* 2021;25:142.

45. Li D, Miaskowski C, Burkhardt D, Puntillo K. Evaluations of physiologic reactivity and reflexive behaviors during noxious procedures in sedated critically ill patients. *J Crit Care.* 2009;24(3):472.e479, 472.e413.

46. Lukaszewicz AC, Dereu D, Gayat E, Payen D. The relevance of pupillometry for evaluation of analgesia before noxious procedures in the intensive care unit. *Anesth Analg.* 2015;120(6):1297–1300.

47. Paulus J, Roquilly A, Beloeil H, Theraud J, Asehnoune K, Lejus C. Pupillary reflex measurement predicts insufficient analgesia before endotracheal suctioning in critically ill patients. *Crit Care.* 2013;17(4):R161.

48. Aissou M, Snauwaert A, Dupuis C, Atchabahian A, Aubrun F, Beaussier M. Objective assessment of the immediate postoperative analgesia using pupillary reflex measurement: a prospective and observational study. *Anesthesiology.* 2012;116(5):1006–1012.

49. Bernard C, Delmas V, Duflos C, et al. Assessing pain in critically ill brain-injured patients: a psychometric comparison of 3 pain scales and video-pupillometry. *Pain.* 2019;160(11):2535–2543.

50. Chanques G, Tarri T, Ride A, et al. Analgesia nociception index for the assessment of pain in critically ill patients: a diagnostic accuracy study. *Br J Anaesth.* 2017;119(4):812–820.

51. Gélinas C, Shahiri TS, Richard-Lalonde M, et al. Exploration of a Multi-Parameter Technology for Pain Assessment in Postoperative Patients After Cardiac Surgery in the Intensive Care Unit: The Nociception Level Index (NOL)TM. *J Pain Res.* 2021;14:3723–3731.

52. Shahiri S, Richard-Lalonde M, Richebé P, Gélinas C. Exploration of the Nociception Level (NOL™) Index for pain assessment during endotracheal suctioning in mechanically ventilated patients in the intensive care unit: an observational and feasibility study. *Pain Manag Nurs.* 2020;21(5):428–434.

53. Vanderbyl B, Gélinas C. Family perspectives of traumatically brain injured patient pain behaviors in the intensive care unit. *Pain Manag Nurs.* 2017;18(4):202–213.

54. Richard-Lalonde M, Boitor M, Mohand-Said S, Gélinas C. Family members' perceptions of pain behaviors and pain management of adult patients unable to self-report in the intensive care unit: a qualitative descriptive study. *Can J Pain.* 2018;2(1):315e323.

55. Mohand-Saïd S, Richard-Lalonde M, Boitor M, Gélinas C. Family members' experiences with observing pain behaviors using the Critical-Care Pain Observation Tool. *Pain Manag Nurs.* 2019;20(5):455–461.

56. Lawrence M. The unconscious experience. *Am J Crit Care.* 1995;4:227–232.

57. Laureys S, Faymonville ME, Peigneux P, et al. Cortical processing of noxious somatosensory stimuli in the persistent vegetative state. *Neuroimage.* 2002;17:732–741.

58. Hadjistavropoulos T, Herr K, Prkachin KM, et al. Pain assessment in elderly adults with dementia. *Lancet Neurol.* 2014;13:1216–1227.

59. Herr K. Pain assessment strategies in older adults. *J Pain.* 2011;3(suppl 1):S3–S13.

60. Zwakhalen SM, Hamers JP, Abu-Saad HH, Berger MP. Pain in elderly people with severe dementia: a systematic review of behavioral pain assessment tools. *BMC Geriatr.* 2006;6:1.

61. Fuchs-Labelle S, Hadjistavropoulos T. Development and preliminary validation of the pain assessment checklist for seniors with limited ability to communicate (PACSLAC). *Pain Manag Nurs.* 2004;5:37–49.

62. Warden V, Hurley AC, Volicer L. Development and psychometric evaluation of the Pain Assessment in Advanced Dementia (PAINAD) scale. *J Am Med Dir Assoc.* 2003;4:9–15.

63. Herr K, Bursch H, Ersek M, et al. Use of pain-behavioral assessment tools in the nursing home: expert consensus recommendations for practice. *J Gerontol Nurs.* 2010;36:18–29.

64. Kanji S, MacPhee H, Singh A, et al. Validation of the critical care pain observation tool in critically ill patients with delirium: a prospective cohort study. *Crit Care Med.* 2016;44(5):943–947.

65. Davidhizar R, Giger JN. A review of the literature on care of clients in pain who are culturally diverse. *Int Nurs Rev.* 2004;51:47–55.

66. Cammarano WB, Pittet JF, Weitz S, Schlobohm RM, Marks JD. Acute withdrawal syndrome related to the administration of analgesic and sedative medications in adult intensive care unit patients. *Crit Care Med.* 1998;26(4):676–684.

67. American Psychiatric Association. *Diagnostic and Statistical Manual of Mental Disorders (DSM-5®).* 5th ed. Washington, DC: American Psychiatric Publishing; 2013.

68. Arroyo-Novoa M, Figueroa-Ramos MI, Puntillo KA. Opioid and benzodiazepine iatrogenic withdrawal syndrome in patients in the intensive care unit. *AACN Adv Crit Care.* 2019;30(4):353–364.

69. Centers for Disease Control and Prevention. Opioid overdose: commonly used terms. https://www.cdc.gov/drugoverdose/opioids/terms.html. Accessed July 9, 2021.

70. Dowell D, Haegerich TM, Chou R. CDC guidelines for prescribing opioids for chronic pain – United States. *MMWR Recomm Rep (Morb Mortal Wkly Rep).* 2016;65(No. RR-1):1–49.

71. Butler SF, Budman SH, Fernandez K, Jamison RN. Validation of a screener and opioid assessment measure for patients with chronic pain. *Pain.* 2004;112:65–75.

72. Cheatle MD, Compton PA, Dhingra L, Wasser TE, O'Brien CP. Development of the revised opioid risk tool to predict opioid use disorder in patients with chronic non-malignant pain. *J Pain.* 2019;20(7):842–851.

73. Jamison RN, Martel MO, Huang CC, Jurcik D, Edwards RR. Efficacy of the opioid compliance checklist to monitor chronic pain patients receiving opioid therapy in primary care. *J Pain.* 2016;17(4):414–423.

74. Marie B. Assessing patients' risk for opioid use disorder. *AACN Adv Crit Care.* 2019;30(4):343–352.

75. Rose L. Interprofessional collaboration in the ICU: how to define? *Nurs Crit Care.* 2011;16:5–10.

76. Cepeda MS, Africano JM, Polo R, Alcala R, Carr DB. What decline in pain intensity is meaningful to patients with acute pain? *Pain.* 2003;105(1–2):151–157.

77. Gélinas C, Arbour C, Michaud C, Vaillant F, Desjardins S. Implementation of the Critical-Care Pain Observation Tool on pain assessment/management nursing practices in an intensive care unit with nonverbal critically ill adults: a before and after study. *Int J Nurs Stud.* 2011;48(12):1495–1504.

78. Devlin JW, Mallow-Corbett S, Riker RR. Adverse drug events associated with the use of analgesics, sedatives, and antipsychotics in the intensive care unit. *Crit Care Med.* 2010;38(suppl 6):S231–S243.

79. Brush DR, Kress JP. Sedation and analgesia for the mechanically ventilated patient. *Clin Chest Med.* 2009;30:131—141.

80. Devlin JW, Roberts RJ. Pharmacology of commonly used analgesics and sedatives in the ICU: benzodiazepines, propofol, and opioids. *Crit Care Clin.* 2009;25:431.

81. Ashley E, Given J. Pain management in the critically ill. *Br J Perioper Nurs.* 2008;18:504.

82. Cavaliere F, Antonelli M, Arcangeli A, et al. A low-dose remifentanyl infusion is well tolerated for sedation in mechanically ventilated, critically ill patients. *Can J Anaesth.* 2002;49:1088—1094.

83. Soltész S, Biedler A, Silomon M, Schöpflin I, Molter GP. Recovery after remifentanyl and sufentanyl for analgesia and sedation of mechanically ventilated patients after trauma or major surgery. *Br J Anaesth.* 2001;86:763—768.

84. Radtke FM, Franck M, Lorenz M, et al. Remifentanyl reduces the incidence of post-operative delirium. *J Int Med Res.* 2010;38:1225.

85. Ethuin F, Boudaoud S, Leblanc I, et al. Pharmacokinetics of long-term sufentanyl infusion for sedation in ICU patients. *Intensive Care Med.* 2003;29:1916—1920.

86. Jungquist CR, Quinlan-Colwell A, Vallerand A, et al. American Society for Pain Management nursing guidelines on monitoring for opioid-induced advancing sedation and respiratory depression: revisions. *Pain Manag Nurs.* 2020;21(1):7—25.

87. Gertler R, Brown HC, Mitchell DH, Silvius EN. Dexmedetomidine: a novel sedative-analgesic agent. *SAVE Proc.* 2001;14:13—21.

88. Ohtani N, Yasui Y, Watanabe D, Kitamura M, Shoji K, Masaki E. Perioperative infusion of dexmedetomidine at a high dose reduces postoperative analgesic requirements: a randomized control trial. *J Anesth.* 2011;25:872—878.

89. Macario A, Lipman AG. Ketorolac in the era of cyclo-oxygenase-2 selective nonsteroidal anti-inflammatory drugs: a systematic review of efficacy, side effects, and regulatory issues. *Pain Med.* 2001;2(4):336—351.

90. Faigeles B, Howie-Esquivel J, Miaskowski C, et al. Predictors and use of nonpharmacologic interventions for procedural pain associated with turning among hospitalized adults. *Pain Manag Nurs.* 2013;14(2):85—93.

91. Martorella G. Characteristics of nonpharmacological interventions for pain management in the ICU: a scoping review. *AACN Adv Crit Care.* 2019;30(4):388—397.

92. Gosselin E, Richard-Lalonde M. Role of family members in pain management in adult critical care. *AACN Adv Crit Care.* 2019;30(4):398—410.

93. Boitor M, Gélinas C, Richard-Lalonde M, Thombs BD. The effect of massage on acute postoperative pain in critically and acutely ill adults post-thoracic surgery: systematic review and meta-analysis of randomized controlled trials. *Heart Lung.* 2017;46:339—346.

94. Friesner SA, Curry DM, Moddeman GR. Comparison of two pain management strategies during chest tube removal: relaxation exercise with opioids and opioids alone. *Heart Lung.* 2006;35:269—276.

95. Richard-Lalonde M, Gélinas C, Boitor M, et al. The effect of music on pain in the adult intensive care unit: a systematic review of randomized controlled trials. *J Pain Symptom Manage.* 2020;59(6):1304—1309.e6.

96. Kshettry VR, Carole LF, Henly SJ, Sendelbach S, Kummer B. Complementary alternative medical therapies for heart surgery patients: feasibility, safety, and impact. *Ann Thorac Surg.* 2006;81(1):201—205.

97. Papathanassoglou EDE, Hadjibalassi M, Miltiadous P, et al. Effects of an integrative nursing intervention on pain in critically ill patients: a pilot clinical trial. *Am J Crit Care.* 2018;27(3):172—185.

8

Sedation and Delirium Management

Mary E. Lough

One of the challenges facing clinicians is how to provide a therapeutic healing environment for patients in the alarm-filled, emergency-focused critical care unit. Many critical care patients demonstrate agitation and discomfort caused by painful procedures, invasive tubes, sleep deprivation, fear, anxiety, and physiologic stress. Clinical practice guidelines have been developed by the Society of Critical Care Medicine (SCCM) to improve management of pain, agitation/sedation, delirium, immobility, and sleep disruption (PADIS) in critically ill adult patients.[1]

SEDATION

Sedation and Agitation Assessment Scales

The use of a validated scale is recommended to standardize assessments of agitation and sedation in a critically ill adult.[1-3] The Richmond Agitation-Sedation Scale (RASS)[4,5] and the Sedation-Agitation Scale (SAS)[6] are recommended in the guidelines (Table 8.1).[1] Because individuals do not metabolize sedative medications at the same rate, the use of a standardized scale ensures that continuous infusions of sedatives such as propofol or dexmedetomidine are titrated to a specific measurable outcome. Collaboratively, the critical care team is required to assign the sedation level goal that is most appropriate for each individual patient and reassess as needed. The current guidelines recommend light sedation for critically ill patients receiving mechanical ventilation.[1]

Pain Assessment Scales

The first step in assessing an agitated patient is to rule out any sensations of pain (see Chapter 7).[1] Preemptive analgesia should be provided before painful procedures.[1] The SCCM guidelines recommend that all critically ill, intubated, mechanically ventilated patients have stated goals for analgesia and sedation.[1] The next step is to determine the minimum level of sedation required for an individual patient.[1]

Levels of Sedation

In the clinical setting, depth of sedation may also be described using the general descriptive terms defined by the American Association of Anesthesiologists (Box 8.1)[7]:
- *Light sedation* (minimal sedation) refers to pharmacologic relief of anxiety (anxiolysis) so that the patient is alert and can respond to verbal commands (approximates RASS −1 to +1 and SAS 4 to 7).[1]
- *Moderate sedation* describes pharmacologic depression of patient consciousness. This is also known as *procedural sedation*, as this

is often the target level when tubes or lines are to be inserted (approximates RASS −3 and SAS 3).
- *Deep sedation* describes pharmacologic depression of patient consciousness to where the patient cannot maintain an open airway (approximates RASS −4 and SAS 2).
- *General anesthesia* describes pharmacologic depression of patient consciousness using multiple medications, administered by a physician anesthesiologist or a nurse anesthetist (approximates RASS −5 and SAS 1).

When the patient has a depressed level of consciousness because of sedative medications (moderate, deep, or general anesthesia), vigilant monitoring of cardiac and respiratory function and vital signs is required. To ensure patient safety, in addition to the clinician performing the procedure, qualified clinicians who are able to monitor and recover the patient must be present. The clinician administering the sedative medication must be qualified to manage the patient appropriate to their area of practice, licensure, and training.

Pharmacologic Management of Sedation

Achievement of the lightest possible sedation to provide comfort for an alert patient is now considered the standard in critical care.[7] To achieve this goal, it is necessary for all members of the clinical team to be familiar with the pharmacokinetics of frequently used categories of sedatives. Additionally, if the patient is experiencing pain, analgesia must be administered in addition to sedative agents (see Chapter 7).[1] Sedative medications include benzodiazepines, sedative-hypnotic agents such as propofol, and the central alpha agonist dexmedetomidine (Table 8.2). Dexmedetomidine-based and propofol-based sedative regimens are the current recommendations for sedation of mechanically ventilated adult patients.[1]

All sedatives are to be administered to a specific target level identified by a RASS or SAS level appropriate to the patient's clinical condition. A target level is specified every day and reevaluated whenever there is a change in sedation dosage or patient condition. One likely sedation goal is that the patient is awake and calm, specified as a target sedation level of RASS 0 or SAS 4. This describes a patient who follows simple verbal commands without agitation and who can sustain eye contact for at least 10 seconds, as described in Table 8.1. When the intent is to provide deep sedation for a critical illness, the target sedation level is specified as RASS −4 to −5 or SAS 1 to 2. These target values describe a mechanically ventilated patient who is not responsive to a spoken voice and who does not respond purposefully to physical stimulation. If this is not the clinically intended level of consciousness, sedative infusions should be turned down or turned off. If deep sedation or neuromuscular blockade is prescribed, a frontal electrocochleogram monitor is recommended to evaluate deeper

TABLE 8.1 Sedation Scales.

Score	Description	Definition
Richmond Agitation-Sedation Scale (RASS)[a,b]		
+4	Combative	Overtly combative, violent, immediate danger to staff
+3	Very agitated	Pulls or removes tube(s) or catheter(s); aggressive
+2	Agitated	Frequent nonpurposeful movement; fights ventilator
+1	Restless	Anxious but movements not aggressive or vigorous
0	Alert and calm	
−1	Drowsy	Not fully alert, but has sustained awakening (eye opening/eye contact) to voice (>10 seconds)
−2	Light sedation	Briefly awakens with eye contact to voice (<10 seconds)
−3	Moderate sedation	Movement or eye opening to voice (but no eye contact)
−4	Deep sedation	No response to voice, but movement or eye opening to physical stimulation
−5	Unresponsive	No response to voice or physical stimulation
Sedation-Agitation Scale (SAS)[c]		
7	Dangerously agitated	Pulls at ETT, tries to remove catheters, climbs over bed rail, strikes at staff, thrashes side to side
6	Very agitated	Does not calm despite frequent verbal reminding of limits, requires physical restraints, bites ETT
5	Agitated	Anxious or mildly agitated, attempts to sit up, calms down to verbal instructions
4	Calm and cooperative	Calm, awakens easily, follows commands
3	Sedated	Difficult to arouse, awakens to verbal stimuli or gentle shaking but drifts off again; follows simple commands
2	Very sedated	Arouses to physical stimuli but does not communicate or follow commands; may move spontaneously
1	Unarousable	Minimal or no response to noxious stimuli; does not communicate or follow commands

[a]Sessler CN, Gosnell MS, Grap MJ, et al. The Richmond Agitation-Sedation Scale: validity and reliability in adult intensive care unit patients. *Am J Respir Crit Care Med.* 2002;166:1338–1344.

[b]Ely EW, Truman B, Shintani A, et al. Monitoring sedation status over time in ICU patients: reliability and validity of the Richmond Agitation-Sedation Scale (RASS). *JAMA.* 2003;289:2983–2991.

[c]Riker RR, Picard JT, Fraser GL. Prospective evaluation of the Sedation-Agitation Scale for adult critically ill patients. *Crit Care Med.* 1999;27:1325–1329.

ETT, Endotracheal tube.

sedation levels because of the absence of patient responsiveness at RASS −5 or SAS 1.[1]

Benzodiazepines

Benzodiazepines have powerful amnesic properties that inhibit reception of new sensory information. Benzodiazepines do not confer analgesia. The most commonly used benzodiazepines are diazepam (Valium), midazolam (Versed), and lorazepam (Ativan). Previously a mainstay of sedation, benzodiazepines are no longer recommended for sedation of mechanically ventilated critically ill adults. Benzodiazepine-based sedative regimens are associated with longer duration of mechanical ventilation and delirium.[1,8]

The major unwanted side effects associated with benzodiazepines are delirium and dose-related respiratory depression and hypotension.

QSEN

BOX 8.1 Evidence-Based Practice

Levels of Sedation

Light Sedation (Minimal Sedation, Anxiolysis)

Medication-induced state during which patients respond normally to verbal commands. Although cognitive function and coordination may be impaired, ventilatory and cardiovascular functions are unaffected.

Moderate Sedation With Analgesia (Conscious Sedation, Procedural Sedation)

Medication-induced depression of consciousness during which patients respond purposefully to verbal commands, alone or accompanied by light tactile stimulation. No interventions are required to maintain a patent airway, and spontaneous ventilation is adequate. Cardiovascular function is usually maintained.

Deep Sedation and Analgesia

Medication-induced depression of consciousness during which patients cannot be easily aroused but respond purposefully after repeated or painful stimulation. The ability to maintain ventilatory function independently is impaired. Patients require assistance in maintaining a patent airway, and spontaneous ventilation may be inadequate. Cardiovascular function is usually maintained.

General Anesthesia

Medication-induced loss of consciousness during which patients are not arousable, even by painful stimulation. The ability to maintain ventilatory function independently is impaired, and assistance to maintain a patent airway is required. Positive-pressure ventilation may be required because of depressed spontaneous ventilation or medication-induced depression of neuromuscular function. Cardiovascular function may be impaired.

Data from the American Association of Anesthesiologists. Continuum of Depth of Sedation: Definition of General Anesthesia and Levels of Sedation/Analgesia. 1999; revised 2014. Practice Guidelines for Moderate Procedural Sedation and Analgesia 2018. <https://www.asahq.org/standards-and-guidelines?q=moderate%20sedation>. Accessed May 11, 2021.

TABLE 8.2   Pharmacologic Management: Sedation.

Medication	Dosage	Action	Special Considerations
Benzodiazepines			

Diazepam	Loading dose IV: 5—10 mg/kg slowly
	Intermittent maintenance dose IV:
	    0.03—0.1 mg/kg every 30 minutes to 6
	    hours as needed
		Anxiolysis
		Amnesia
		Sedation
			Onset: 2—5 minutes after IV administration
			Side effects: hypotension, respiratory depression
			Half-life: long (20—120 hours); active metabolites also contribute to prolonged sedative effect.
			Tolerance: physical tolerance develops with prolonged use, and higher doses of medication are required to achieve same effect over time; slow wean required from diazepam after continuous prolonged use; no active metabolites.
			Phlebitis occurs with peripheral IV administration.

Lorazepam	Loading dose IV: 0.02—0.04 mg/kg
	    ($\leq$2 mg) slowly
	Intermittent maintenance IV every 2—6 hours:
	    0.02—0.6 mg/kg slowly
	Continuous IV maintenance infusion:
	    0.01—0.1 mg/kg/h ($\leq$10 mg/h)
		Anxiolysis
		Amnesia
		Sedation
			Onset: 15—20 minutes after IV administration
			Side effects: hypotension, respiratory depression, propylene glycol—related acidosis, nephrotoxicity
			Half-life: relatively long (8—15 hours)
			Tolerance: physical tolerance develops with use, and higher medication dosage is required to achieve same effect over time; slow wean required from lorazepam after continuous prolonged use.
			Solvent-related acidosis and kidney failure occur at high doses.

Midazolam	Loading dose IV: 0.01—0.05 mg/kg slowly
	    over several minutes
	Continuous IV maintenance infusion:
	    0.02—0.1 mg/kg/h
		Anxiolysis
		Amnesia
		Sedation
			Onset: 2—5 minutes after IV administration
			Side effects: hypotension, respiratory depression
			Half-life: 3—11 hours; sedative effect is prolonged when midazolam infusion has continued for many days, owing to presence of active sedative metabolites; sedative effect is also prolonged in kidney failure.
			Tolerance: physical tolerance develops with prolonged use, and higher medication dosages are required to achieve same effect over time; slow wean required from midazolam after prolonged use.

Sedative-Hypnotics			

Propofol	Loading dose IV: 5 mcg/kg/min over
	    5 minutes
	Continuous IV maintenance infusion:
	    5—50 mcg/kg/min
		Anxiolysis
		Amnesia
		Sedation
			Onset: very rapid onset (1—2 minutes) after IV administration
			Side effects: hypotension, respiratory depression (patient must be intubated and mechanically ventilated to eliminate this complication), pain at injection site if administered via peripheral IV line; pancreatitis; hypertriglyceridemia, propofol-related infusion syndrome, allergic reactions
			Half-life: 1—2 minutes when used as short-term agent; with prolonged continuous IV infusion, half-life extends to 50 $\pm$ 18.6 hours.
			Effective short-term anesthetic agent, useful for rapid "wake-up" of patients for assessment; if continuous infusion is used for many days, emergence from sedation can take hours or days; sedative effect depends on dose administered, depth of sedation, and length of time sedated.
			Change IV infusion tubing every 6—12 hours.
			Requires dedicated IV catheter and tubing (do not mix with other medications).
			Monitor serum triglyceride levels.

Central Alpha-Adrenergic Receptor Agonists			
Dexmedetomidine	Loading dose IV: 1 mcg/kg over 10 minutes Continuous IV maintenance infusion: 0.2—0.7 mcg/kg/h	Anxiolysis Analgesia Sedation	Onset: 5—10 minutes Side effects: Bradycardia, hypotension, loss of airway reflexes Half-life: 1.8—3.1 hours No active metabolites Intermittent bolus dosing is not recommended. Maintenance infusion is adjusted to achieve desired level of sedation.

IV, Intravenous.

Data from Barr J, Fraser GL, Puntillo K, et al. Clinical practice guidelines for the management of pain, agitation, and delirium in adult patients in the intensive care unit. *Crit Care Med.* 2013;41:263—306.

If needed, flumazenil (Romazicon) is the antidote used to reverse benzodiazepine overdose in symptomatic patients. Flumazenil should be used with caution in patients with benzodiazepine dependence because rapid withdrawal can induce seizures and other adverse side effects.[9]

Sedative-Hypnotic Agents

Propofol is a powerful sedative and respiratory depressant used for sedation in mechanically ventilated patients in critical care.[10] It is immediately identifiable by its white milky appearance, and it is always dispensed in a glass container. At high doses (greater than 100–200 mcg/kg per minute), propofol is intended to produce a state of general anesthesia in the operating room. In the critical care unit, propofol is prescribed as a continuous infusion at lower doses (5–50 mcg/kg per minute) to induce sedation in critically ill patients. Because propofol is lipid soluble, it quickly crosses cell membranes, including the cells that compose the blood-brain barrier. This allows rapid onset of sedation (30–60 seconds) with subsequent loss of consciousness.[10,11] In addition to a rapid onset of action, propofol has a very short half-life with initial use (2–4 minutes), is rapidly eliminated from the body (30–60 minutes), and does not have active metabolites.[11] The short half-life makes propofol an ideal sedative when a patient will need to be quickly awakened for a spontaneous awakening trial (SAT) and spontaneous breathing trial or to assess neurologic status. Propofol is clinically effective because it can be titrated, or turned off, when a patient is mechanically ventilated and may decrease time to extubation.

Propofol is not an analgesic. Therefore it is important to add an opiate to ensure adequate pain control. Nor is propofol a reliable amnesic, and patients sedated with only propofol can have vivid rec-ollections of their experiences. If amnesia is required during a procedure, a short-acting opiate such as fentanyl can be administered.

The risk of complications increases with prolonged administration of propofol at doses greater than 5 mg/kg/h for longer than 48 hours.[10] The term *propofol-related infusion syndrome* describes metabolic acidosis, muscular weakness, rhabdomyolysis, myoglobinuria, acute kidney injury, and cardiovascular dysrhythmias. This condition has a mortality of 50% (48% in adults, 52% in children) based on published case reports.[12]

A rare benign effect of propofol infusion is green urine.[10] Urine discoloration occurs when the patient's liver cannot metabolize all of the propofol, and the remainder is excreted via the kidney. Propofol is not nephrotoxic, and the urine returns to a normal color when the medication is stopped. Secondary side effects related to the fat-emulsion carrier include hyperlipidemia, hypertriglyceridemia, and acute pancreatitis. Serum triglycerides should be measured on all patients who receive propofol for longer than 48 hours. Propofol should not be administered to patients with known allergies to soy or eggs, because the intralipid carrier contains soybean oil, glycerol, and egg-lecitin.[10]

Propofol is a lipid-based emulsion, a medium highly conducive to bacterial growth.[13] For this reason, the manufacturer and the Centers for Disease Control and Prevention (CDC) recommend that the tubing be changed every 12 hours to prevent catheter-related infections.[14] Use of aseptic technique is mandatory to prevent infection.[13] Nursing vigilance is required to monitor sedation levels and to be alert for the rare but significant risk of propofol-related complications. Table 8.2 provides additional information.

Central Alpha Agonists

Two central alpha-adrenergic agonists with sedative properties are available. Clonidine (Catapres) is prescribed as a patch, and dexmedetomidine (Precedex) is prescribed as a continuous infusion. Clonidine may be prescribed for patients experiencing alcohol withdrawal syndrome (AWS; see later discussion in this chapter).

Dexmedetomidine is an alpha-2 agonist that is approved by the US Food and Drug Administration for use as a short-term sedative (less than 24 hours) in mechanically ventilated patients. Sedation occurs when the medication activates postsynaptic alpha-2 receptors in the central nervous system in the brain. This activation inhibits norepinephrine release and blocks sympathetic nervous system fight-or-flight functions, leading to sedation. Sympathetic nervous system inhibition may cause hypotension and bradycardia. Analgesic effects occur because dexmedetomidine binds to alpha-2 receptors in the spinal cord. These unique mechanisms of action allow patients to be lightly sedated and also interactive, factors that are associated with a shorter time to extubation compared with traditional sedative regimens.[15–17] Dexmedetomidine may shorten the duration of delirium compared with other sedative agents.[16,17]

Dexmedetomidine is administered with a loading dose of 1 mcg/kg over 10 minutes, followed by a continuous infusion of 0.4 mcg/kg (range 0.2–0.7 mcg/kg per hour).[2] Dexmedetomidine has a short half-life (6 minutes) and is eliminated from the body in approximately 2 hours. Elimination from the body is dramatically slowed if the patient has liver failure (see Table 8.2).

Many patients have other sedatives or opiates infusing in addition to dexmedetomidine, and the combination may potentiate the overall sedative effect. Monitoring of sedation level, blood pressure, heart rate, respiratory rate, and pulse oximetry is required. Dexmedetomidine confers sedation and analgesic effects without respiratory depression. Consequently, patients can be extubated while still on a dexmedetomidine infusion. This can be helpful for patients who are anxious during ventilator weaning.

Daily Sedation Interruption

One strategy to avoid the pitfalls of sedative dependence and withdrawal is to turn off the sedative infusions once each day. This intervention has been given several names, including *sedation vacation* and *spontaneous awakening trial (SAT)*.[1] At a scheduled time, all continuously infusing sedatives are stopped. Sometimes analgesics are also stopped, depending on the hospital's protocol. The patient is allowed to regain consciousness for clinical assessment using a standardized instrument such as RASS or SAS (see Table 8.1).[1] The patient is carefully monitored, and when awareness is attained, an assessment of level of consciousness and neurologic function is performed. It is essential that a protocol be in place for the nurse to restart the sedatives if the patient experiences either a deleterious change in vital signs (high/low blood pressure or heart rate) or becomes highly agitated, pulling at lines or tubes and endangering his or her safety. In many protocols, when the sedative medications are restarted, a lower dose is used to avoid dependence.

A typical protocol is to schedule the daily sedative interruption in the morning, conduct a clinical assessment and spontaneous breathing trial, then restart the sedative and opiate infusions at 50% of the previous morning dose and adjust upward until the desired sedation goal is achieved.[18]

Other protocols forgo infusions and use intermittent intravenous push for "as-needed" sedatives and analgesics to manage pain and sedation. Another approach is to maintain the patient at a lighter level of sedation all the time rather than specifying specific times to stop the sedatives.[19]

An important nursing responsibility is to prevent the patient from coming to harm during sedative or analgesic medication withdrawal

TABLE 8.3 Signs and Symptoms of Sedative or Analgesic Medication Withdrawal[a]

System	Opiate Withdrawal	Benzodiazepine Withdrawal[b]
Neurologic	Delirium, tremors, seizures	Agitation, anxiety, delirium, tremors, myoclonus, headache, seizures, fatigue, paresthesias, sleep disturbances
Sensory	Dilation of pupils, teary eyes, irritability, increased sensitivity to pain, sweating, yawning	Increased sensitivity to light/sound, sweating
Musculoskeletal	Cramps, muscle aches	Muscle cramps
Gastrointestinal	Vomiting, diarrhea	Nausea, diarrhea
Respiratory	Tachypnea	Tachypnea

[a]Data on propofol are limited, but withdrawal symptoms after prolonged use are similar to withdrawal symptoms of benzodiazepines.
[b]Not all symptoms are seen in all patients.

(Table 8.3). If the patient is seriously agitated, it is vital to consult with the physician and pharmacist to establish an effective treatment plan that allows safe weaning from sedative medications (see Table 8.1).

AGITATION

Agitation describes hyperactive patient movements that range in intensity from slight restless hand and body movements to pulling out lines and tubes or physical aggression and self-harm. Some common causes of agitation include pain, anxiety, delirium, hypoxia, ventilator dyssynchrony, neurologic injury, uncomfortable position, full bladder, sleep deprivation, alcohol withdrawal, sepsis, medication reaction, and organ failure. In the past, when a patient showed physical signs of agitation, a benzodiazepine sedative (lorazepam or midazolam) was quickly administered to reduce the patient's mental awareness and hyperactivity (see Table 8.2). However, because benzodiazepines have been shown to induce delirium, these medications are no longer recommended.[1]

Agitation is assessed using a validated scale such as SAS or RASS (see Table 8.1). Standardized assessment scales allow clinicians to identify agitation in its milder forms and to potentially ameliorate the patient's symptoms. The goal is to treat the cause of the agitation rather than to overmedicate. When patients are dangerously agitated (SAS +7), are combative (RASS +4), or could endanger themselves or others, immediate sedation is warranted. In these extreme situations, a benzodiazepine may be administered.[2]

DELIRIUM

Delirium is a global impairment of cognitive processes, usually of sudden onset, coupled with disorientation, impaired short-term memory, altered sensory perceptions (i.e., hallucinations), abnormal thought processes, and inappropriate behavior. Routine monitoring for delirium is recommended.[1] Delirium is more prevalent than generally recognized; it is difficult to diagnose in a critically ill patient and represents acute brain dysfunction caused by sepsis, critical illness, or dysfunction of other vital organs. Greater than 50% of mechanically ventilated patients experience delirium. Delirium increases hospital stay and mortality rates for patients who are mechanically ventilated.

When patients are agitated, restless, and pulling at tubes and lines, they are often identified as being delirious. In this scenario, delirium may be described as *ICU psychosis* or *sundowner syndrome*. However, a delirious patient is not always agitated, and it is much more difficult to detect delirium when a patient is physically calm.

Specific scoring instruments are available to assess delirium, and two have been validated for use with mechanically ventilated critical care patients[1–3]: the Confusion Assessment Method for the Intensive Care Unit (CAM-ICU) (Figs. 8.1 and 8.2)[20,21] and the Intensive Care Delirium Screening Checklist (ICDSC) (Fig. 8.3).[19,22] Both of these delirium tools are used in tandem with the RASS to exclude patients in coma. Coma is a known risk factor for development of delirium. Both CAM-ICU and ICDSC provide a structured format to evaluate delirium for verbal patients and for nonverbal and mechanically ventilated patients.[1]

Pharmacologic Management of Delirium

Pharmacologic treatment of delirium is challenging.[1] The neuroleptic medication haloperidol (Haldol) has traditionally been administered to treat hyperactive delirium. More recent studies have shown that haloperidol or other atypical antipsychotics do not reduce the incidence or the duration of delirium.[1,23] An additional challenge with haloperidol is that it prolongs the Q-Tc interval, increasing the patient's risk of the ventricular dysrhythmia *torsades de pointes*.[2]

No medication has been identified that prevents delirium. Novel antipsychotic medications have not been shown to be helpful.[23] Dexmedetomidine may reduce delirium duration.[24]

Interventions to Prevent Delirium

In mechanically ventilated patients, the interventions used to decrease delirium include using light sedation, scheduling a daily sedative interruption, scheduling a spontaneous breathing trial, daily delirium monitoring, and early mobility.[1] Early mobility may prevent the muscle weakness that accompanies long periods of bed rest during critical illness and may reduce the cognitive complications associated with prolonged illness that many patients experience.[1]

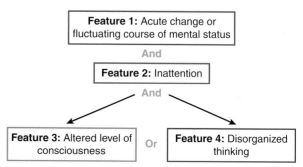

Fig. 8.1 Confusion Assessment Method for the Intensive Care Unit (CAM-ICU). Delirium is defined as positive in Feature 1 *and* Feature 2 and *either* Feature 3 *or* Feature 4. (Copyright 2002, E. Wesley Ely, MD, MPH, and Vanderbilt University. All rights reserved.)

RICHMOND AGITATION-SEDATION SCALE (RASS)

Step

1 Sedation Assessment

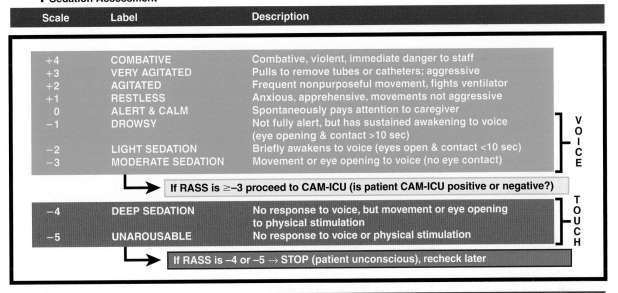

Scale	Label	Description
+4	COMBATIVE	Combative, violent, immediate danger to staff
+3	VERY AGITATED	Pulls to remove tubes or catheters; aggressive
+2	AGITATED	Frequent nonpurposeful movement, fights ventilator
+1	RESTLESS	Anxious, apprehensive, movements not aggressive
0	ALERT & CALM	Spontaneously pays attention to caregiver
−1	DROWSY	Not fully alert, but has sustained awakening to voice (eye opening & contact >10 sec)
−2	LIGHT SEDATION	Briefly awakens to voice (eyes open & contact <10 sec)
−3	MODERATE SEDATION	Movement or eye opening to voice (no eye contact)

If RASS is ≥−3 proceed to CAM-ICU (is patient CAM-ICU positive or negative?)

| −4 | DEEP SEDATION | No response to voice, but movement or eye opening to physical stimulation |
| −5 | UNAROUSABLE | No response to voice or physical stimulation |

If RASS is −4 or −5 → STOP (patient unconscious), recheck later

Confusion Assessment Method for the ICU (CAM-ICU)

Step

2 Delirium Assessment

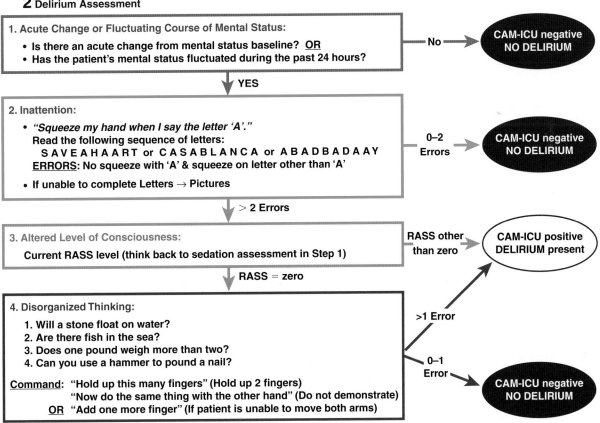

1. Acute Change or Fluctuating Course of Mental Status:
- Is there an acute change from mental status baseline? **OR**
- Has the patient's mental status fluctuated during the past 24 hours?

→ **No** → CAM-ICU negative NO DELIRIUM

↓ **YES**

2. Inattention:
- *"Squeeze my hand when I say the letter 'A'."*
  Read the following sequence of letters:
  S A V E A H A A R T or **C A S A B L A N C A** or **A B A D B A D A A Y**
  ERRORS: No squeeze with 'A' & squeeze on letter other than 'A'
- If unable to complete Letters → Pictures

→ **0–2 Errors** → CAM-ICU negative NO DELIRIUM

↓ **> 2 Errors**

3. Altered Level of Consciousness:
Current RASS level (think back to sedation assessment in Step 1)

→ **RASS other than zero** → CAM-ICU positive DELIRIUM present

↓ **RASS = zero**

4. Disorganized Thinking:
1. Will a stone float on water?
2. Are there fish in the sea?
3. Does one pound weigh more than two?
4. Can you use a hammer to pound a nail?

Command: "Hold up this many fingers" (Hold up 2 fingers)
"Now do the same thing with the other hand" (Do not demonstrate)
OR "Add one more finger" (If patient is unable to move both arms)

→ **>1 Error** → CAM-ICU positive DELIRIUM present

→ **0–1 Error** → CAM-ICU negative NO DELIRIUM

Fig. 8.2 Confusion Assessment Method for the Intensive Care Unit *(CAM-ICU)* Delirium Assessment. Step 1: Sedation Assessment; Step 2: Delirium Assessment. *RASS,* Richmond Agitation-Sedation Scale. (Copyright 2002, E. Wesley Ely, MD, MPH, and Vanderbilt University. All rights reserved.)

The Intensive Care Delirium Screening Checklist (ICDSC)

1. Altered level of consciousness

(A) No response or (B) the need for vigorous stimulation in order to obtain any response signified a severe alteration in the level of consciousness precluding evaluation. If there is coma (A) or stupor (B) most of the time period, then a dash (—) is entered and there is no further evaluation for that period.

(C) Drowsiness or response to a mild to moderate stimulation implies an altered level of consciousness and scores 1 point.

(D) Wakefulness or sleeping state that could easily be aroused is considered normal and scores zero points.

(E) Hypervigilance is rated as an abnormal level of consciousness and scores 1 point.

2. Inattention

Difficulty in following a conversation or instruction, easily distracted by external stimuli, or difficulty in shifting focus scores 1 point.

3. Disorientation

Any obvious mistake in time, place, or person scores 1 point.

4. Hallucination, delusion, or psychosis

The unequivocal clinical manifestation of hallucination or of behavior probably due to hallucination (eg, trying to catch a nonexistent object) or delusion or gross impairment in reality testing scores 1 point.

5. Psychomotor agitation or retardation

Hyperactivity requiring the use of additional sedative drugs or restraints in order to control potential danger (eg, pulling out IV lines, hitting staff), hypoactivity, or clinically noticeable psychomotor slowing scores 1 point.

6. Inappropriate speech or mood

Inappropriate, disorganized, or incoherent speech or inappropriate mood related to events or situation scores 1 point.

7. Sleep/wake cycle disturbance

Sleeping less than four hours, waking frequently at night (do not consider wakefulness initiated by medical staff or loud environment), or sleeping during most of the day scores 1 point.

8. Symptom fluctuation

Fluctuation of the manifestation of any item or symptom over 24 hours (eg, from one shift to another) scores 1 point.

How to Calculate a Score for the ICDSC*

Patient Evaluation	Day 1	Day 2	Day 3	Day 4	Day 5
Altered level of consciousness (A–E)*					
Inattention					
Disorientation					
Hallucination, delusion, psychosis					
Psychomotor agitation or retardation					
Inappropriate speech or mood					
Sleep-wake cycle disturbance					
Symptom fluctuation					
Total Score (0–8)					

*Level of Consciousness	Score
A: no response	–
B: response to intense and repeated stimulation (loud voice and pain)	–
C: response to mild or moderate stimulation	1
D: normal wakefulness	0
E: exaggerated response to normal stimulation	1
If **A** or **B**, do not complete patient evaluation for the period.	

Scoring System

The scale is completed based on information collected from each 8-hour shift or from the previous 24 hours. Obvious manifestation of an item = 1 point. No manifestation of an item or no assessment possible = 0 points. The score of each item is entered in the corresponding space and is 0 or 1. A total score of ≥4 on any given day has a 99% sensitivity for correlation with a psychiatric diagnosis of delirium.

*The ICDSC is also used in tandem with the RASS (see Table 8.1) to assess sedation-agitation in addition to delirium.

Fig. 8.3 Intensive Care Delirium Screening Checklist *(ICDSC)*. (From Bergeron N, Dubois MJ, Dumont M, Dial S, Skrobik Y. Intensive Care Delirium Screening Checklist: evaluation of a new screening tool.) *Intensive Care Med.* 2001;27:859.

Sleep protocols are used in many critical care units to increase the opportunity for patients to sleep at night. The protocols include dimming lights at night, ensuring there are periods of time when tubes are not manipulated, providing earplugs or eye masks, and clustering nursing care interventions to provide uninterrupted rest periods.

Physical restraints are often used in critical care units to avoid patient self-removal of lines or tubes. However, to prevent unpleasant patient memories of being restrained, avoidance of physical restraint is recommended in current delirium management guidelines.[1]

Critical care patient diaries are written in everyday language and will be used to answer questions such as, "What happened when I was attached to the breathing machine?" The diary is typically created by family members and staff writing about events during the period of critical illness. Although there is no evidence that creating a patient diary reduces delirium, it can provide a way to later describe the many events the patient may not remember.[25,26] This is important because many patients experience depression and other cognitive changes after a critical illness, now named *post–intensive care syndrome* (PICS).

ALCOHOL WITHDRAWAL SYNDROME AND DELIRIUM TREMENS

Critically ill patients who are alcohol dependent and were drinking before hospital admission are at risk of severe AWS.[27,28] AWS is associated with an increased risk of delirium, hallucinations, seizures, need for mechanical ventilation, and death. When hyperactive agitated delirium is caused by alcohol withdrawal, it is termed *delirium tremens* (DTs).[28] After hospital admission, approximately 50% of alcohol-dependent patients experience AWS-related symptoms with decreasing blood alcohol concentration.[28] Fewer than 5% experience severe complications such as delirium or a seizure.[28] Screening tools to identify alcohol dependence, such as the Alcohol Use Disorders Identification Test (AUDIT) discussed in the chapter on Trauma (see Chapter 24), are very helpful.[28] Management of alcohol withdrawal involves close monitoring of AWS-related agitation and administration of intravenous benzodiazepines, generally diazepam or lorazepam. Diazepam has the advantage of a longer half-life and high lipid solubility. Lipid-soluble medications quickly cross the blood-brain barrier and enter the central nervous system to produce a sedative effect. Benzodiazepines should be administered in response to increased signs of agitation associated with DTs, with dosage guided by a clinical protocol. This is known as an *AWS symptom-triggered* approach.[28,29] Additionally, a variety of nonbenzodiazepine adjunctive medications may be added to protocols, including dexmedetomidine, clonidine, propofol, ketamine, barbiturates, and haloperidol.[30]

The severity of alcohol withdrawal can be assessed with a scale such as the Clinical Institute Withdrawal Assessment of Alcohol Scale (revised).[31] Multivitamins, including thiamine (vitamin B_1), are administered prophylactically to prevent additional neurologic sequelae.[27] Delirium related to alcohol withdrawal is pharmacologically managed very differently from delirium from other causes. Long-acting benzodiazepines are the medications of choice in AWS.[27,30] In contrast, benzodiazepines are contraindicated for treatment of delirium from nonalcohol-related causes.

COLLABORATIVE MANAGEMENT

Collaborative management of anxiety, agitation, sedation, and delirium is a responsibility shared by all members of the health care

---

BOX 8.2 Evidence-Based Practice QSEN

Summary of Guidelines for Assessment and Treatment of Agitation and Delirium

- Agitation in critically ill patients may result from inadequately treated pain, anxiety, delirium, or ventilator dyssynchrony.
- Detection and treatment of pain, agitation, and delirium should be reassessed often.
- Patients should be awake and able to purposely follow commands to participate in their care unless a clinical indication for deeper sedation exists.

Agitation

- Depth and quality of sedation should be routinely assessed in all critical care patients.
- RASS and SAS are the most valid and reliable scales for assessing quality and depth of sedation in critically ill patients.
- Target lightest possible level of sedation and/or use daily sedative interruption.
- Use sedation protocols and checklists to facilitate sedation management.
- Suggest using analgesia-first sedation for intubated and mechanically ventilated critically ill patients.
- Suggest using nonbenzodiazepines for sedation (either propofol or dexmedetomidine) rather than benzodiazepines (either midazolam or lorazepam) in mechanically ventilated adult patients.

Delirium

- Delirium assessment should be routinely performed in all critically ill patients.
- CAM-ICU and ICDSC delirium monitoring tools are the most valid and reliable scales to assess delirium in mechanically ventilated patients.
- Mobilize critical care patients as early as possible to reduce incidence and duration of delirium and to improve functional outcomes.
- Promote sleep in critically ill patients by controlling light and noise, clustering patient care activities, and decreasing stimuli at night.
- Avoid use of antipsychotics in patients who are at risk for torsades de pointes.
- Suggest not using benzodiazepines in critically ill patients with delirium unrelated to alcohol/benzodiazepine withdrawal.

CSM-ICU, Confusion Assessment Method for the Intensive Care Unit; *ICDSC*, Intensive Care Delirium Screening Checklist; *RASS*, Richmond Agitation-Sedation Scale; *SAS*, Sedation-Agitation Scale.
From Barr J, Fraser GL, Puntillo K, et al. Clinical practice guidelines for the management of pain, agitation, and delirium in adult patients in the intensive care unit. *Crit Care Med.* 2013;41:263; Devlin JW, Skrobik Y, Gélinas C, et al. Clinical practice guidelines for the prevention and management of pain, agitation/sedation, delirium, immobility, and sleep disruption in adult patients in the ICU. *Crit Care Med.* 2018;46(9):e825–e873.

---

team, as indicated by the clinical practice guidelines summarized in Box 8.2. Recognition of the problem is the first step toward a solution to establish a more effective standard of patient care in management of sedation, analgesia, and delirium.

ADDITIONAL RESOURCES

See Box 8.3 for Internet resources related to sedation, agitation, and delirium management.

BOX 8.3 **Informatics**

Internet Resources: Sedation, Agitation, and Delirium Management
- Delirium/Sedation: https://www.icudelirium.org/
- Pain Agitation/Delirium Guidelines: https://www.sccm.org/Research/Guidelines
- The Joint Commission: https://www.jointcommission.org/en/resources/for-consumers/speak-up-campaigns/anesthesia-and-sedation

REFERENCES

1. Devlin JW, Skrobik Y, Gélinas C, et al. Clinical practice guidelines for the prevention and management of pain, agitation/sedation, delirium, immobility, and sleep disruption in adult patients in the ICU. *Crit Care Med.* 2018;46(9):e825–e873.
2. Barr J, Fraser GL, Puntillo K, et al. Clinical practice guidelines for the management of pain, agitation, and delirium in adult patients in the intensive care unit. *Crit Care Med.* 2013;41(1):263–306.
3. Gelinas C, Berube M, Chevrier A, et al. Delirium assessment tools for use in critically ill adults: a psychometric analysis and systematic review. *Crit Care Nurse.* 2018;38(1):38–49.
4. Sessler CN, Gosnell MS, Grap MJ, et al. The Richmond Agitation-Sedation Scale: validity and reliability in adult intensive care unit patients. *Am J Respir Crit Care Med.* 2002;166(10):1338–1344.
5. Ely EW, Truman B, Shintani A, et al. Monitoring sedation status over time in ICU patients: reliability and validity of the Richmond Agitation-Sedation Scale (RASS). *J Am Med Assoc.* 2003;289(22):2983–2991.
6. Riker RR, Picard JT, Fraser GL. Prospective evaluation of the sedation-agitation scale for adult critically ill patients. *Crit Care Med.* 1999;27(7):1325–1329.
7. American Association of Anesthesiologists (ASA). Continuum of depth of sedation: definition of general anesthesia and levels of sedation/analgesia. https://www.asahq.org/standards-and-guidelines?q=moderate%20sedation. Accessed October 5, 2019.
8. Pandharipande PP, Girard TD, Jackson JC, et al. Long-term cognitive impairment after critical illness. *N Engl J Med.* 2013;369(14):1306–1316.
9. Penninga EI, Graudal N, Ladekarl MB, Jurgens G. Adverse events associated with flumazenil treatment for the management of suspected benzodiazepine intoxication-a systematic review with meta-analyses of randomised trials. *Basic Clin Pharmacol Toxicol.* 2016;118(1):37–44.
10. Sahinovic MM, Struys M, Absalom AR. Clinical pharmacokinetics and pharmacodynamics of propofol. *Clin Pharmacokinet.* 2018;57(12):1539–1558.
11. Dinis-Oliveira RJ. Metabolic profiles of propofol and fospropofol: clinical and forensic interpretative aspects. *BioMed Res Int.* 2018;2018:6852857.
12. Hemphill S, McMenamin L, Bellamy MC, Hopkins PM. Propofol infusion syndrome: a structured literature review and analysis of published case reports. *Br J Anaesth.* 2019;122(4):448–459.

13. Zorrilla-Vaca A, Arevalo JJ, Escandon-Vargas K, Soltanifar D, Mirski MA. Infectious disease risk associated with contaminated propofol anesthesia, 1989-2014(1). *Emerg Infect Dis.* 2016;22(6):981–992.
14. Adler AC. Propofol: review of potential risks during administration. *AANA J (Am Assoc Nurse Anesth).* 2017;85(2):104–107.
15. Keating GM. Dexmedetomidine: a review of its use for sedation in the intensive care setting. *Drugs.* 2015;75(10):1119–1130.
16. Flükiger J, Hollinger A, Speich B, et al. Dexmedetomidine in prevention and treatment of postoperative and intensive care unit delirium: a systematic review and meta-analysis. *Ann Intensive Care.* 2018;8(1):92.
17. Duan X, Coburn M, Rossaint R, Sanders RD, Waesberghe JV, Kowark A. Efficacy of perioperative dexmedetomidine on postoperative delirium: systematic review and meta-analysis with trial sequential analysis of randomised controlled trials. *Br J Anaesth.* 2018;121(2):384–397.
18. Girard TD, Kress JP, Fuchs BD, et al. Efficacy and safety of a paired sedation and ventilator weaning protocol for mechanically ventilated patients in intensive care (Awakening and Breathing Controlled trial): a randomised controlled trial. *Lancet.* 2008;371(9607):126–134.
19. Bergeron N, Dubois MJ, Dumont M, Dial S, Skrobik Y. Intensive care delirium screening checklist: evaluation of a new screening tool. *Intensive Care Med.* 2001;27(5):859–864.
20. Ely EW, Margolin R, Francis J, et al. Evaluation of delirium in critically ill patients: validation of the Confusion Assessment Method for the Intensive Care Unit (CAM-ICU). *Crit Care Med.* 2001;29(7):1370–1379.
21. Ely EW, Inouye SK, Bernard GR, et al. Delirium in mechanically ventilated patients: validity and reliability of the confusion assessment method for the intensive care unit (CAM-ICU). *J Am Med Assoc.* 2001;286(21):2703–2710.
22. Ouimet S, Riker R, Bergeron N, Cossette M, Kavanagh B, Skrobik Y. Subsyndromal delirium in the ICU: evidence for a disease spectrum. *Intensive Care Med.* 2007;33(6):1007–1013.
23. Girard TD, Exline MC, Carson SS, et al. Haloperidol and ziprasidone for treatment of delirium in critical illness. *N Engl J Med.* 2018;379(26):2506–2516.
24. Ungarian J, Rankin JA, Then KL. Delirium in the intensive care unit: is dexmedetomidine effective? *Crit Care Nurse.* 2019;39(4):e8–e21.
25. Halm MA. Intensive Care Unit Diaries, Part 1: constructing illness narratives to promote recovery after critical illness. *Am J Crit Care.* 2019;28(4):319–323.
26. Levine SA, Reilly KM, Nedder MM, Avery KR. The patient's perspective of the intensive care unit diary in the cardiac intensive care unit. *Crit Care Nurse.* 2018;38(4):28–36.
27. Dixit D, Endicott J, Burry L, et al. Management of acute alcohol withdrawal syndrome in critically ill patients. *Pharmacotherapy.* 2016;36(7):797–822.
28. Schuckit MA. Recognition and management of withdrawal delirium (delirium tremens). *N Engl J Med.* 2014;371(22):2109–2113.
29. Holleck JL, Merchant N, Gunderson CG. Symptom-triggered therapy for alcohol withdrawal syndrome: a systematic review and meta-analysis of randomized controlled trials. *J Gen Intern Med.* 2019;34(6):1018–1024.
30. Foertsch MJ, Winter JB, Rhoades AG, Martin LT, Droege CA, Ernst NE. Recognition, assessment, and pharmacotherapeutic treatment of alcohol withdrawal syndrome in the intensive care unit. *Crit Care Nurs Q.* 2019;42(1):12–29.
31. Sen S, Grgurich P, Tulolo A, et al. A symptom-triggered benzodiazepine protocol utilizing SAS and CIWA-Ar scoring for the treatment of alcohol withdrawal syndrome in the critically ill. *Ann Pharmacother.* 2017;51(2):101–110.

9

Palliative and End-of-Life Care

Caroline Etland

PALLIATIVE CARE

An important shift in care of terminally ill patients in the critical care unit has occurred with the growth of palliative care programs in the United States. The rapid expansion of this new specialty has decreased the mortality rate in critical care units for patients followed by palliative care services through transfer to lower acuity units and has decreased the costs associated with higher acuity critical care beds, pharmacy, laboratory, and diagnostic costs.

Patients who are identified as being near the end of life require aggressive care for symptom management provided by a team of health professionals. Palliative care guidelines have been released by a consortium of organizations concerned with palliative care and end-of-life care, and they may provide guidance when the usual first-line treatments do not promote comfort for critically ill patients who are near death.[1] Strategies that are based on research evidence and expert opinion for specific conditions such as delirium, opioid dose escalation, and dyspnea at the end of life are outlined on the Palliative Care Network of Wisconsin website, which provides access to evidence-based and expert-based Fast Facts that address a wide variety of clinical, ethical, and psychosocial problems that arise with the care of seriously ill and dying patients.[2]

Symptom Management

It has long been in question whether critical care patients can accurately report their symptoms because of the effects of sedating medications, severe illness, and organ dysfunction. Kalowes[3] studied critical care unit patients with a diagnosis other than cancer during a daily wake-up and compared their report of symptoms with reports of their family members. Almost all patients had more than 10 symptoms, and there was 85.5% congruence between patient and family report of physiologic and psychological symptoms. Overall, patients experienced significant symptom burden near the end of life but received limited treatment to alleviate suffering.

Pain

Many critical care patients are unconscious, so assessment of pain and other symptoms becomes more difficult (see Chapter 7).[4] Because opioids provide sedation, anxiolysis, and analgesia, they are particularly beneficial in ventilated patients. Morphine is the medication of choice, and there is no upper limit in dosing. However, in higher doses, morphine metabolites can cause myoclonus, hyperalgesia, and allodynia. In a paralyzed patient, this may not be detectable, but it can be uncomfortable on some level for the patient, perhaps evident in vital signs or response to ventilator settings. Careful assessment of patients' vital signs may reveal suspected discomfort that necessitates an opioid switch to hydromorphone or fentanyl. In nonventilated patients, sedation may cause respiratory depression, and nonopioids or specific anesthetic agents may be more appropriate. Antiinflammatory medications or neuroleptic agents often provide significant comfort for inflammatory conditions or neurologic pain. Titration of intravenous infusions to achieve maximum effect with minimum sedation is an inexact science. Critical care nurses should assume that pain is present in an immobile patient and administer routine analgesics to prevent suffering.

Dyspnea

A systematic review and meta-analysis of cancer-related dyspnea interventions critically examined the common interventions used by many practitioners.[5] Dyspnea is best managed with close evaluation of the patient and the use of opioids, sedatives, and nonpharmacologic interventions (oxygen, positioning, and increased ambient air flow). Morphine reduces anxiety and muscle tension and increases pulmonary vasodilation but is ineffective when inhaled. Benzodiazepines, particularly midazolam, may be used in patients who are unable to take opioids or for whom the respiratory effects are minimal. Midazolam has been shown to be at least equally effective as morphine and, in some studies, superior to morphine.[6] Benzodiazepines and opioids should be titrated to effect. Oxygen did not prove to be superior in the studies reviewed, but ambient air movement of some sort often provides relief. Treatment efforts should be aimed at the patient's expression of dyspnea rather than at respiratory rates or oxygen levels.

Nausea and Vomiting

Nausea and vomiting are common and should be treated with antiemetics. The cause of nausea and vomiting may be intestinal obstruction or increased intracranial pressure. Treatment for decompression may be uncomfortable in dying patients, and its use should be weighed using a benefit-to-burden ratio. In certain circumstances, an intervention to provide percutaneous drainage for decompression may be used in a patient who is not imminently dying.

Fever and Infection

Fever and infection necessitate evaluation of the benefits of continuing antibiotics so as not to prolong the dying process. Management of fever with antipyretics may be appropriate for the patient's comfort, but other methods such as ice or hypothermia blankets should be balanced against the amount of distress the patient may experience.

Edema

Edema may cause discomfort, and diuretics may be effective if kidney function is intact. Dialysis is not warranted at the end of life. The use of intravenous fluids may contribute to the edema when kidney function is impaired, and the body is slowing its functions.

Anxiety

Anxiety should be assessed verbally, if possible, or by changes in vital signs or restlessness. Benzodiazepines, especially midazolam with its rapid onset and short half-life, are commonly used. Minimizing noxious sounds and playing a patient's favorite music or aromatherapy may help soothe anxiety.

Delirium

Delirium is commonly observed in critically ill and dying patients (see Chapter 8). Haloperidol and benzodiazepines (e.g., midazolam, lorazepam) have traditionally been used to manage delirium but have side effects that can be problematic. To ensure accurate trending of delirium, a standardized assessment tool such as the Confusion Assessment Method for the ICU is recommended to adequately assess delirium.[7] Evidence-based strategies to minimize and shorten the duration of delirium should be used.

END-OF-LIFE CARE

Attention to end of life of hospitalized patients has increased since the publication of the Study to Understand Prognoses and Preferences for Outcomes and Risks of Treatment (SUPPORT).[8] In this major report, more than 9000 seriously ill patients in five medical centers were studied. Despite an intervention to improve communication regarding preferences for life-sustaining treatments, shortcomings were found; aggressive treatment was common, only half of the physicians knew their patients' preferences to avoid cardiopulmonary resuscitation (CPR), more than one-third of patients who died spent at least 10 days in a critical care unit, and family members of half of conscious patients reported moderate to severe pain at least half of the time.

Soon after the publication of the SUPPORT study, the Institute of Medicine (IOM) released a report, *Approaching Death: Improving Care at the End of Life*,[9] followed by an updated report in 2014.[10] Based on the growth of palliative care programs and developing research on end-of-life care, the recommendations changed to highlight new priorities. Recommendations from the IOM reports are summarized in Table 9.1, which reflects advances in the science of palliative and end-of-life care.

Advance Directives

Although advance directives (ADs), also known as a *living will* or a *health care power of attorney*, were intended to ensure that patients received the care they desired at the end of life, the enactment of structures and processes to support completion of ADs has been suboptimal. Traditionally, AD completion rates in adults range from 16% to 36% overall, with less than one-half of seriously or terminally ill patients having documented their wishes.[11] A 2014 study revealed that AD completion has increased to 72% with a decrease of in-hospital deaths from 45% to 35% in the older-adult study sample.[11] Another study demonstrated that patients with limited English proficiency (LEP) had a lower percentage of completed ADs, suggesting a disparity in care because their wishes for life-sustaining treatment were not known.[12] Most patients have expressed a desire to avoid "general life support" if dying or permanently unconscious, but few have specified preferences regarding specific life-sustaining treatments. A large study of veterans found that veterans who had living wills or who had appointed a surrogate decision maker were much less likely to experience aggressive care at the end of life.[13] Even when ADs are present, the question arises about whether they are applicable for current care decisions; in other words, is this a terminal illness? To address this problem, the state of California has enacted legislation that requires physicians, nurse practitioners, and physician assistants to inform patients when a terminal illness is diagnosed and that they have a right to comprehensive information and counseling regarding end-of-life care.[14] This type of regulation supports discussion of wanted versus unwanted care at the time of diagnosis. However, many providers remain reluctant to document this information in the medical record.

Physician Orders for Life-Sustaining Treatment

The Physician Orders for Life-Sustaining Treatment (POLST)[15] is different from an AD. POLST forms are medical orders that are honored across all treatment settings and are especially important to emergency responders in the community. Also, they are completed by the patient and provider in the presence of a serious chronic illness and should be incorporated into medical orders on admission to the hospital or skilled nursing facility. POLST forms are more easily read than an AD in that they are formatted as checkboxes with specific directions. States that have approved use of POLST-type forms through legislation or specific regulations have witnessed a shift in proactive discussions of patients' wishes for life-sustaining treatment.[16-18]

TABLE 9.1 Comparison of Death in America Reports.

Approaching Death Report (1997)	Dying in America Report (2014)
• Patients with fatal illnesses and their family should receive reliable, skillful, and supportive care.	• Coordinate person-centered, family oriented end-of-life care
• Health professionals should improve care for dying patients.	• Improve clinician-patient communication, including robust advance care planning processes.
• Policymakers and consumers should work with health professionals to improve quality and financing of care.	• Improve access to palliative care training for physicians and nurses.
• Health profession education should include end-of-life content.	• Implement models of care to provide services that patients and families need that are not covered by existing insurance plans.
• Palliative care should be developed, possibly as a medical specialty.	• Implement culturally appropriate public education and public engagement strategies.
• Research on end of life should be funded.	
• The public should communicate more about the experience of dying and options available.	

Adapted from Field MJ, Cassell CK, eds. *Approaching Death: Improving Care at the End of Life.* Washington, DC: National Academy Press; 1997; Dying in America and Committee on Approaching Death, Addressing Key End of Life Issues, Institute of Medicine. *Dying in America: Improving Quality and Honoring Individual Preferences Near the End of Life.* Washington, DC: National Academies Press; 2015.

Advance Care Planning

Although cultural influences in the United States discourage discussion of death, societal trends are shifting awareness regarding quality-of-life decision making and unintended consequences of aggressive medical treatment. Planning for decisions to be made at a later date if one is unable to speak for oneself is a difficult process, but this knowledge helps family members to make the treatment decisions if a patient cannot communicate. Advance care planning (ACP) for patients with chronic illness is advantageous for all involved. A systematic review of the effects of ACP on end-of-life care revealed that ACP decreases life-sustaining treatment, increases use of hospice and palliative care, and prevents hospitalization.[19] When surrogates hear the patient's wishes for end-of-life care, they can be more knowledgeable and less conflicted when asked to make decisions that may result in a loved one's death during a serious illness (Box 9.1).

Communication of the patient's wishes among family members, primary care providers, and intensivists is critical. If patients have stated desires, they should be communicated when patients are entering or are transferred out of the critical care unit. If the patient has not specified his or her preferences, that information also is important and should be communicated to new health care providers; the level of care patients desire should be offered as appropriate. Families and care providers should be informed if patients decline aggressive care so that families will not be left with difficult decisions in emergency situations. Emotional support for the patient and the family is important as they discuss ACP in the critical care setting.

COMFORT CARE

The decision to withdraw life-sustaining treatments and transition to comfort care at the end of life should be made with as much involvement of the patient as possible, including physical presence of the patient in decision making or procuring paper documents if the patient is unable to participate; the patient's wishes as understood from prior discussions with the patient should guide the decision about whether to withdraw treatment. Withholding and withdrawing treatment are considered to be morally and legally equivalent.[20] However, because families experience more stress in withdrawing treatments than in withholding them,[21] treatments should not be started that the patient would not want or that would not be of benefit. Prigerson et al.[22] are currently studying surrogate decision-makers of critical care unit patients in a randomized controlled trial to determine

whether an intervention can reduce the stress associated with decision making and anticipatory grief and prevent the severity of postdeath surrogate health outcomes and psychologic stress. A standardized approach to supporting surrogate decision-makers throughout the critical care unit stay is aligned with transparency in clinician-family communication and ethical principles.

The goal of withdrawal of life-sustaining treatments is to remove treatments that are not beneficial and may be uncomfortable. Any treatment in this circumstance may be withheld or withdrawn. After the goal of comfort has been chosen, each procedure and medication should be evaluated to determine whether it is necessary or causes discomfort. Treatments that cause discomfort do not need to be continued. Another defining question is whether treatments are prolonging the dying process. When disagreements arise, ethics consultations have been found to be helpful in resolving conflicts regarding inappropriately prolonged, nonbeneficial, or unwanted treatments in the critical care unit, shifting the focus to more appropriate comfort care.[23]

Forgoing life-sustaining treatments is not the same as active euthanasia or self-initiated consumption of lethal medications. Direct actions to cause another's death are fundamentally different from allowing a person to die by withholding or withdrawing life-sustaining treatment or avoiding any intervention that interferes with a natural death after illness or trauma.[24]

Effect of Do Not Resuscitate Orders

As a patient clinically declines and death approaches, the decision to initiate a do not resuscitate (DNR) order is influenced by many factors, including goals of care, comorbidities, pace of clinical decline, availability of surrogate decision-makers, and provider practice patterns. Critical care nurses often initiate discussion of DNR status and play a key role in collaborating with physicians to identify which therapies remain useful to the patient.

"DNR" and "withdrawal of life-sustaining treatment" are not synonymous. Nurses should demonstrate to families that loved ones are receiving aggressive comfort interventions and any treatments that remain part of the plan of care. Once a decision is made to withdraw life-sustaining treatment, comfort orders should be implemented before withdrawal of treatment. A best practice for minimizing pain and suffering of both the patient and family is to use standardized order sets for consistency in practice.

Prognostication and Prognostic Tools

Most patients in the critical care unit have one or more chronic illnesses that greatly affect long-term recovery from major health events such as respiratory failure, myocardial infarction, or sepsis. Because humans and their course of illness can be unpredictable, physicians' ability to prognosticate the length of time before death is limited,[25] and the time to death usually is overestimated to patients and families and in the medical record.

Severity scoring systems belong to one of five classes: prognostic, disease-specific, single-organ failure, trauma scores, and organ dysfunction.[26] Two common tools for estimating critical care unit mortality are the Acute Physiology and Chronic Health Evaluation (APACHE) and multiple-organ dysfunction score.[27,28] In addition to use of prognostic tools specific to the critical care unit, it makes sense to incorporate prognostic tools for chronic illnesses into overall decision making and the communication process with patients and families. Scoring diagnoses with a traditionally poor prognosis or a consistent trajectory of functional decline can be helpful in comparing current health status with the health status at the time of diagnosis.

QSEN | BOX 9.1 **Patient-Centered Care**

Principles of a Good Death

- Anticipate and be able to prepare for a good death.
- Retain some control.
- Be afforded dignity and privacy.
- Have symptom control, including pain relief.
- Choose place of death when possible.
- Have access to information and expertise when necessary.
- Have emotional and spiritual support.
- Have access to hospice care.
- Have control over who is present at death.
- Respect the wishes of the dying patient through advance directives.
- Have time to say good-bye.
- Be able to die rather than pointlessly prolonging life.

Adapted from Smith R. A good death. An important aim for health services and for us all. *BMJ*. 2000;320:129–130.

TABLE 9.2　Selected Prognostic Scales.

Prognostic Scale	Disease/Clinical Condition	Prognostic Scale	Disease/Clinical Condition
Palliative Prognostic Scale (PPS)	Any hospice population; palliative care patients	Lung Cancer Prognostic Model (LCPM)	Terminal lung cancer patients
Palliative Prognostic Index (PPI)	Terminal cancer patients	Dementia Prognostic Model (DPM)	Demographic, diagnosis, laboratory, and functional data on dementia residents
Palliative Prognostic Score (PaP)	Terminal cancer patients	Prognostic Index for One-Year Mortality in Older Adults (PIMOA)	Adults older than 70 years with previous stay in hospital
Seattle Heart Failure Model; Heart Failure Risk Scoring System (HFRSS)	Acute heart failure	Cancer Prognostic Scale (CPS)	Terminal cancer patients in progressive care unit
BODE Scale	Chronic obstructive pulmonary disease	Mortality Risk Index Score (MRIS)	New admission to nursing home

Adapted from Lau F, Cloutier-Fisher D, Kuziemsky C, et al. A systematic review of prognostic tools for estimating survival time in palliative care. *J Palliat Care.* 2007;23(2):93–112.

Loved ones of critically ill patients have witnessed the functional decline and may have hoped for improvement despite advancement of disease. Use of prognostic scales can add meaningful information to help patients and families make informed decisions. Some more commonly used prognostic scales are listed in Table 9.2.

Despite this information and these tools, uncertainty remains a major issue in decision making for physicians, patients, and families. Because of uncertainty and because some patients who were never thought likely to survive actually return to a critical care unit, professionals are not always confident about issues of survivability. Moreover, many families cling to small hopes of survival and recovery.

DECISION MAKING

Communication and Decision Making

Communication with the patient and family is critical. Regardless of the health literacy of the patient or family, explanations of life-sustaining treatments such as CPR, ventilation, and tube feedings in simple language are necessary for effective communication. Many patients and families experience a "data dump" during communication with health care providers, who focus on reporting vital statistics and odds of success. Several organizations have made available education handouts that explain life-sustaining treatments in realistic terms.[29,30] These materials are excellent visual tools during a discussion with a health care provider. Handouts are written at a low reading level and are available in several languages. Focusing on improving critical care unit communication when patients are dying increases family satisfaction, decreases family stress, and decreases days of nonbeneficial treatment.[31]

Most physicians and nurses have not been taught how to conduct this type of dialogue effectively during training. There are many options to gain the training and experience necessary to shift the decision making from a purely clinical perspective to a more humanistic view. Programs such as Education in Palliative and End-of-Life Care,[32] End-of-Life Nursing Education Consortium (ELNEC),[33] and Center to Advance Palliative Care Palliative Care Leadership Center[34] training are cost-effective methods to educate and support clinicians to communicate more effectively with patients and families at the end of life. Additional information on ethical and legal issues is provided in Chapter 2.

Patients

Patients' capacity for decision making is limited by illness severity and cognitive deficits accentuated by medications and the environment. When decision making is required, the patient is the first person to be approached if able to speak for himself or herself. When the patient is unable to safely make health care decisions because of disease progression or the therapy used for treatment, written documents such as a living will or a health care power of attorney should be obtained when possible. Additional information on power of attorney for health care can be found in the previous section on ACP. Without those documents, wishes of the patient should be ascertained from individuals closest to the patient. Some patients have neither capacity nor surrogates to assist in decision making; this was the case in 27% of deaths in one study.[35] In the absence of a surrogate decision maker, care decisions for unrepresented patients may be delayed, and discharge to another care setting can prove difficult. Only five states have empowered existing institutional committees to make decisions for unrepresented patients, illustrating the need for transparent and fair processes to be developed.[36]

Families

Family members continue to report dissatisfaction with communication and decision making.[37] Increasing the frequency of communication and sharing concerns early in the hospitalization make subsequent discussions easier for the patient, family, and health professional. Families have commonly complained about infrequent physician communication,[38] unmet communication needs in the shift from aggressive to end-of-life care, and lacking or inadequate communication.[39] Sometimes families are not ready to receive the prognosis and engage in decision making. Communication seems to be the most common source of complaints in families.

Family Meetings

Family meetings in the presence of the critical care team is another method used to arrive at a common understanding of the patient's prognosis and goals for future care. A research analysis of the amount of time families were able to speak in these meetings revealed that when families had greater opportunity to talk, their satisfaction with physician communication increased, and their ratings of conflict with the physician decreased.[40,41]

Curtis et al.[42] studied the process of family meetings and how to improve them to promote better end-of-life care for patients in the critical care unit and their families. They found that the missed opportunities that occur during these meetings were occasions to listen to family; to acknowledge and address emotions; and to pursue key tenets of palliative care such as patient preferences, surrogate decision making, and nonabandonment. As families make decisions, they appreciate support for those decisions because the support can reduce the burden they experience. The health care team can reinforce the legitimacy of the family expressing feelings of disappointment, sadness, and loss. It is important that the family is made aware that the patient was more than a clinical disease and that he or she was recognized as an individual while in the critical care unit.

Cultural and Spiritual Influences on Communication

Cultural and spiritual influences on attitudes and beliefs about death and dying differ dramatically. The cultures of the predominant religions in the surrounding community should be familiar to the local health care team. Globalization patterns have altered the cultural and religious diversity of communities in the United States, necessitating that nurses partner more closely with spiritual care resources and community liaisons to better understand family structures and decision making. These differences may affect how the health care team is viewed, how decisions are made, whether aggressive treatment is preferred, how death is met, and how grieving will occur.[43,44] Patients who do not follow a particular religion should be assessed for their individual spiritual beliefs or lack thereof. The plan of care should also include evaluation of spiritual and religious support of the patient's family. A literature review revealed that religious or spiritual practices of families were highly important to many, yet only 4% of physicians requested a chaplain visit to critical care unit patients.[45] Identifying sources of spiritual comfort strengthens the bond between caregivers, patients, or family. Satisfaction with critical care unit care has been associated with the extent to which the family is satisfied with their spiritual care, especially when the patient is near death.[46] Staff members' own attitudes about the specific practices of a culture should be carefully monitored[44] and tempered with respect and humility. Interpreters are necessary when the patient or the family members do not speak English. A cultural and religious assessment is warranted in all situations, because cultural or religious affiliation does not imply that patients or families follow all of the tenets of that group.

Hospice Information

Although hospice care has been available for many years, patients and families often consider this method of care only in the last weeks or months of an end-stage illness, and they commonly view hospice care as "giving up," or outright abandonment. Health professionals can assist patients and families by providing information about the benefits of hospice, particularly regarding aggressive symptom management and family support. Some hospices are offering to partner with critical care units in the provision of end-of-life care and in the process of withdrawal of ventilatory support. Hospice care is an option that should be considered, especially in end-stage illness, and the benefit to surviving family members should be emphasized. In some circumstances, alert patients may express a wish to die at home even while still ventilated. Hospice-to-home programs have demonstrated that granting this wish may be feasible with coordinated effort.

WITHDRAWAL OR WITHHOLDING OF TREATMENT

Discussions about the potential for impending death are never held early enough. The first discussion about prognosis often occurs in conjunction with the topic of the discontinuation of life support. Some family members dread such conversations but are grateful to discuss the uncertainty of their loved one's future. Physicians should give families time to adjust to this information and make preparations by providing early discussions about prognosis, goals of therapy, and the patient's wishes.[47]

Proactive Approach

When patients are admitted to the critical care unit with serious illnesses and are likely to die, a proactive approach to palliative care has been found to shorten critical care unit stays without a significant difference in mortality rates or discharge disposition.[48,49] The use of nonbeneficial resources decreases, and prolonged dying is avoided. Rapid response team daily rounds on noncritical care units have proven to be anecdotally effective in early identification of patients showing early signs of clinical deterioration. Communication with the provider at this time can avert an admission to a critical care unit, possibly even averting a Code Blue event.

Patients with assistive cardiac devices present a different challenge in discussion of withdrawal of life support. These patients often are cognitively intact and must consent to removal of technology that is keeping them alive. To reduce confusion and distress among clinicians, protocols for discontinuation of organ-assistance devices are recommended as a standard of care.

Futility and Nonbeneficial Care Discussions

Nurses and physicians frequently disagree about the futility of interventions. Sometimes nurses consider withdrawal before physicians and patients do, and they then feel the care they are giving is unnecessary and possibly harmful. Nurses in one study were found to be more pessimistic but more often correct than physicians about the prognoses of dying patients, but nurses have also proposed treatment withdrawal for some very sick patients who survived.[50] Nurses described acknowledging futility and acting on the patient's distress, being ideally placed to advocate with specialists. At the same time, nurses describe the tension that can result in recommending palliative care or hospice to the medical staff.[51]

Steps Toward Comfort Care

Once a decision has been made to withdraw life-sustaining therapies, each intervention should be evaluated to determine whether it still provides any benefit.[52] In a patient who has received life support for a prolonged time, a staged withdrawal of interventions such as removal of ventilator support via terminal weaning allows for better symptom control. For families, seeing a loved one look peaceful as life support is withdrawn ultimately helps with grief resolution in the future. Usually, routine interventions (e.g., laboratory tests, imaging, cardiac monitoring) are removed first, followed by respiratory support devices. Withdrawal of specific treatments may produce effects necessitating symptom management. Withdrawal of dialysis may cause dyspnea from volume overload, which may require the use of opioids or benzodiazepines. Efforts to discontinue artificial feeding may be met with concern from the family, because offering food has great social significance. It is essential to share information with family and providers regarding the potential benefits of withholding nutrition and fluids in the days immediately before death to prevent unnecessary suffering.[53] Critical care patients who survive withdrawal of life support measures may continue to remain in critical care for a period of time before dying or being transferred to a less acute setting. During this time, various symptoms may occur that can be distressing for patients, families, and nursing staff.

Withdrawal of Mechanical Ventilation

A dramatic geographic variation exists in practices surrounding withdrawal of life-sustaining therapies. Some evidence suggests that this variation may be driven more by physicians' attitudes and biases than by factors such as patients' preferences or cultural differences. This inconsistency in care further complicates a difficult process. From clinical, ethical, and legal perspectives, standardized withdrawal from life-support order sets is recommended to direct and support nursing judgment in this complex and emotional clinical situation.

At the heart of the difficulty of conversations about withdrawal of life support is the pattern and selection of language to address the decision. Recommendations for creating a supportive atmosphere during withdrawal discussions included taking a moment at the beginning of the conversation to inquire about the family's emotional state, acknowledging verbal and nonverbal expressions of emotion and using that to support families, and acknowledging that most family members face a significant emotional burden when a loved one is critically ill or dying.

During the family meeting in which a decision to withdraw life support is made, a time to initiate withdrawal is usually established. For example, a distant family member may need to arrive, and then the procedure will occur. It is helpful if other staff members are alerted to the fact that a withdrawal is occurring. A neutral sign hung on the door or use of a special room may caution staff to avoid loud conversations and laughter, which is quite upsetting to grieving families. Nurses can support the family by suggesting specific measures to modify the environment and minimize symptoms that the family might perceive as suffering of their loved one.

After the decision to remove ventilatory support is made and the family is gathered, the family should be told what the impending death will be like. When the patient is dependent on ventilatory support or vasopressors and that support is removed, death typically follows in minutes. The patient appears as if sleeping, and the usual signs of color and skin temperature changes will not be seen before death. The opposite is true if the patient is not ventilator dependent. When the patient is to be extubated at the beginning of the withdrawal process, the family should be prepared for respiratory noises and gasping respirations. These signs are less likely when the endotracheal tube is removed near the end of the withdrawal process, as is more commonly done. When assessing how prepared family members felt for what would happen during withdrawal of life support, Kirchhoff et al.[54] found that families who did not receive preparatory information before the withdrawal of life support requested this information during interviews 2 to 4 weeks after the patient's death. Family members who received this recommended information reported they felt significantly more prepared. Providing information to families for the experience of withdrawal alerts them to what the patient may exhibit as death approaches, reducing the distress families may feel during the withdrawal process.

Pacemakers or implantable cardioverter defibrillators should be turned off to prevent patient discomfort or distress from the shocks firing[55] and to avoid interfering with the pronouncement of death. Neuromuscular blocking agents should be discontinued before removal of ventilator support, because paralysis precludes the assessment of the patient's discomfort and the means of the patient to communicate with loved ones.[56]

The removal of monitors is usually recommended. However, physicians and nurses may use the monitor to assess the distress of the patient during the withdrawal process and to adjust the amount of medication needed for symptom management. Families may glance at the monitor to verify that electrical activity has ceased, because the appearance of death may be too subtle to detect. If not needed, monitors should be removed to make the room appear as normal as possible.

Sedation During Withdrawal of Life Support

Opioids and benzodiazepines are the most commonly administered medications, because dyspnea and anxiety are the usual symptoms related to ventilator withdrawal. von Gunten and Weissman[57] recommend sedating all patients, even patients who are comatose. Recommended dosing is a bolus intravenous dose of morphine (2–10 mg) and a continuous morphine infusion at 50% of the bolus dose per hour. An intravenous dose of midazolam (1–2 mg) is administered, followed by an infusion at 1 mg/h. The intent is to provide good symptom control, so doses accelerate until the patient's comfort is achieved. Additional medication should be available at the bedside for immediate administration if discomfort is observed in the patient. In one study, the use of opioids or benzodiazepines to treat discomfort after the withdrawal of life support did not hasten death in critically ill patients.[58] A standardized withdrawal order set with titration parameters minimizes variation and subjectivity among the physician's orders and the nurse's implementation of the orders.

Ventilator Settings

After the patient's comfort is achieved, ventilator settings are reduced. An experienced physician, a respiratory therapist, and a nurse should be present during this time. Ventilator alarms should be turned off. The method of withdrawal adopted is usually determined by the clinician's preference. The choice of terminal wean as opposed to extubation is based on considerations of access for suctioning, appearance of the patient for the family, how long the patient is likely to survive off the ventilator, and whether the patient has the ability to communicate with loved ones at the bedside.

If terminal wean is used, positive end-expiratory pressure is reduced to normal, and then the mode is set to patient control. Next, the fraction of inspired oxygen is reduced to 0.21 (21%). All these steps are taken slowly while observing the patient for distress or anxiety. If extubation is performed immediately rather than at the end of the terminal wean, the family should be prepared for airway compromise and the appearance of the patient. The terminal wean offers the most control over secretions, respiratory noises, and gasping.

Terminal extubation of alert patients can be difficult, because there is uncertainty about the amount and type of medications to provide. Billings outlined the issues surrounding the terminal extubation procedure.[59] Patients indicating the desire to remove life support retain the need for comfort medications to control dyspnea and secretions until death. Some health care providers may believe this is a moral "gray area" and relate the process to assisted suicide. However, patients with decisional capacity may elect to discontinue life support, which has been supported by court decisions and bioethical opinion.

PROFESSIONAL ISSUES

Health Care Settings

Professional issues surround the provision of end-of-life and palliative care within traditional acute and clinical settings. In critical care units, care may be managed by an intensivist or by a committee of specialists but seldom by the family physician who knows the patient. The use of consultants may be limited. Palliative care specialists may be available at certain times, but they are often considered "outsiders," although the trend to use this specialty service is increasing with the availability of programs in US hospitals. How the consultation is arranged may vary by institution. Turf issues should not compromise patient care. Having a clear plan for withdrawal and better preparation of the family may assist the professionals involved in feeling more comfortable with the care provided.[60] Expert nurses should advocate for vulnerable patients by communicating the patient's wishes and presenting a realistic picture to family members.[61]

Some interventions have been found to be helpful for health professionals in improving patient care. Although it did not improve nurses' assessment of patients' dying experience, a standardized order form for withdrawal was found to increase the amount of medications nurses administered for sedation.[62]

Emotional Support for the Nurse

Nurses who care for dying patients need to have their work valued as highly as other high-tech functions in the critical care unit. Critical care units usually have several nurses who are looked to by other staff to provide end-of-life care or to assist with withdrawal of life support. When several deaths occur close together, those nurses may be called on frequently. Some consideration in assignment should be given when a nurse has more than one death in a shift or a week. Taking a new admission is also difficult immediately after a death, and it can occur before the family has left the unit. Nurse administrators can provide some additional resources, debriefing, or time off when the burden has been high. Hearing supportive words from colleagues has been reported by critical care nurses as helpful in coping with the death of a patient.[63] Often, critical care nurses experience moral distress because of the severity of patients' illnesses and the requirement of technology to maintain vital organ function. Collaborative strategies for minimizing moral distress rely on the bedside nurse and critical care leadership to implement individual and organizational changes.[64]

FAMILY CARE

In this chapter, the term *family* means whatever the patient states is the family. An integral part of the patient-family dyad, families expect a cure for any condition the patient may have; they do not expect to receive bad news. They look for the good news in any message received from caregivers and are surprised when told that death is the only outcome possible.[54] Families need assistance in forming their expectations about outcomes. Ongoing communication about the patient's progress is preferable to waiting until the patient is near death and then communicating with the family. Most studies of families at this time are descriptive, and interventions need to be developed to help them.[65]

One intervention used with families at the end of life is a grieving or comfort cart. In one critical care unit, the cart has a top drawer with multiple language versions of the Bible, Koran, and Book of Mormon, and pamphlets about grief and bereavement.[66] The lower portion of the cart holds paper cups, napkins, and condiments. Fresh coffee and tea are brewed on the unit and served with muffins and cookies from the cafeteria. Family responses have been positive, because they do not want to leave the bedside despite their hunger. Another strategy is to provide nursing units with supplies including religious items and music to support the emotional and spiritual needs of families at the end of life.[67,68]

Waiting for Good News

Patients and families do not come to the critical care unit with the expectation of death. Even patients who have had previous admissions

expect to be "saved." Having this in mind while talking to families may assist professionals in interpreting families' responses. Preparing families for changes in the patient as the health condition deteriorates helps them make plans. They need to know whether other family members should be called, whether someone should spend the night, or whether financial arrangements should be changed before an impending death (e.g., to enable the surviving spouse to have access to funds). Anticipated changes can be described to prepare families. Emotional support and grieving can be facilitated through discussion of the dying patient and their unique qualities and families' memories.

Families may refuse to forgo life-supporting treatments and want "everything done" for a variety of reasons. Effective communication throughout the hospitalization and information provided throughout the stay predispose the family to better acceptance of news as the patient deteriorates. Family satisfaction is increased when they feel supported during their decision making or hear more empathic statements from physicians.[69,70]

Families in Crisis

Families may experience a sense of crisis as emergencies occur or as the patient deteriorates and dies. Responses to the news of the death vary. Family members may show anger or be quiet, exhibit emotions or stoicism. Culture or religious beliefs may affect their response to news. It is helpful to ask whether family members would like to see a chaplain or a social worker. Quiet and calm, some privacy, and support are always appreciated.

After Death

After the death, the family may wish to spend time at the bedside. Family members' time with the body should be unhurried and private. They need adequate room to sit and spend time. They can be asked if they need assistance or resources and whether they wish to be alone or have someone nearby. Frequently, the bed is needed for another patient, and coordination is required to ensure that the family has sufficient time even as another patient needs to be admitted. Supporting families after a death involves immediate bereavement support, information on what to do about the death, bereavement support for the future, contact with the family after death, and assessment of the quality of care the patient experienced.[71] Having material already prepared with the necessary after-death information is quite helpful at this time. Most hospices offer bereavement support groups that are available to any member of the community free of charge, regardless of whether a loved one was enrolled in hospice. Nurses need to be aware of their own judgment on what is an appropriate response, because individuals respond differently to the same news, even within the same family.

COLLABORATIVE CARE

The ability to provide collaborative, compassionate end-of-life care is the responsibility of all clinicians who work with critically ill patients. Interdisciplinary collaborative efforts are associated with improvement in care.[72] In 2008 the Society of Critical Care Medicine (SCCM) published a revised guideline, "Recommendations for End-of-Life Care in the Intensive Care Unit," to provide guidance for end-of-life care for the team.[52] The evidence-based practice feature on end-of-life care provides a summary of the topics included (Box 9.2). Critical care unit staff can assess the quality of their care by assessing perceptions of families and staff, auditing documentation, or making observations of care.[73] The same attention should be directed toward improving end-of-life care that is directed toward skills of electrocardiogram interpretation or hemodynamic monitoring.

QSEN | **BOX 9.2 Evidence-Based Practice**

Guidelines for End-of-Life Care in the Critical Care Unit

Key topics of the guidelines for end-of-life care in the critical care unit, based on research and expert panel review, are categorized.

Patient-Centered and Family-Centered Care and Decision Making: Comprehensive Ideal for End-of-Life Care
- Use legal standards for decision making.
- Resolve conflict.
- Communicate with families.

Ethical Principles Related to Withdrawal of Life-Sustaining Treatment
- Withholding versus withdrawing
- Killing versus allowing to die
- Intended versus merely foreseen consequences

Practical Aspects of Withdrawing Life-Sustaining Treatments in Critical Care Unit
- Procedure

- Specific issues
- Use of paralytics

Symptom Management in End-of-Life Care
- Pain and dyspnea
- Delirium
- Medications used

Considerations at Time of Death
- Notification of death
- Brain death
- Organ donation
- Bereavement and support
- Needs of interdisciplinary team

Research, Quality Improvement, and Education
- Develop interventions likely to improve quality of care.
- Develop education programs.

Data from Truog RD, Campbell ML, Curtis JR, et al. Recommendations for end-of-life care in the intensive care unit: a consensus statement by the American Academy of Critical Care Medicine. *Crit Care Med.* 2008;36(3):953—963.

QSEN | **BOX 9.3 Informatics**

Internet Resources: Palliative and End-of-Life Care
- American Academy of Hospice and Palliative Care Medicine (AAHPM): www.aahpm.org
- End-of-Life Nursing Education Consortium (ELNEC): www.aacnnursing.org/ELNEC
- Center to Advance Palliative Care (CAPC): www.capc.org/
- Hospice and Palliative Care Nurses Association (HPNA): advancingexpertcare.org
- NIH: National Institute on Aging: www.nia.nih.gov/health/end-of-life
- Palliative Care Network of Wisconsin: www.mypcnow.org

ADDITIONAL RESOURCES

See Box 9.3 for Internet resources pertaining to palliative and end-of-life care.

REFERENCES

1. Abbasi J. New guidelines aim to expand palliative care beyond specialists. *JAMA.* 2019;322(3):193—195. https://doi.org/10.1001/jama.2019.5939.
2. Palliative Care Network of Wisconsin. Fast facts and concepts. https://www.mypcnow.org/fast-facts/ Accessed January 9, 2021.
3. Kalowes P. *Doctoral Dissertation. Symptom Burden at the End of Life in Patients with Terminal and Life Threatening Illness in Intensive Care Units.* San Diego, CA: University of San Diego; 2007.
4. Barr J, Fraser GL, Puntillo K, et al. Clinical practice guidelines for the management of pain, agitation, and delirium in adult patients in the intensive care unit. *Crit Care Med.* 2013;41(1):263—306. https://doi.org/10.1097/CCM.0b013e3182783b72.
5. Ben-Aharon I, Gafter-Gvili A, Leibovici L, Stemmer SM. Interventions for alleviating cancer-related dyspnea: a systematic review and meta-analysis. *Acta Oncol.* 2012;51(8):996—1008. https://doi.org/10.3109/0284186X.2012.709638.
6. Del Fabbro E, Dalal S, Bruera E. Symptom control in palliative care, part III: dyspnea and delirium. *J Palliat Med.* 2006;9(2):422—436.
7. Vanderbilt University Medical Center. *Confusion assessment method for the ICU (CAM-ICU): the complete training manual*; 2016. www.icudelirium.org/medical-professionals/delirium/monitoring-delirium-in-the-icu.
8. SUPPORT Investigators. A controlled trial to improve care for seriously ill hospitalized patients. The Study to Understand Prognoses and Preferences for Outcomes and Risks of Treatments (SUPPORT). *JAMA.* 1995;274(20):1591—1598.
9. Field MJ, Cassell CK, eds. *Approaching Death: Improving Care at the End of Life.* Washington, DC: National Academy Press; 1997.
10. Committee on Approaching Death. *Addressing key end of life issues, Institute of medicine. Dying in America: Improving Quality and Honoring Individual Preferences Near the End of Life.* Washington DC: National Academies Press; 2015.
11. Department of Health and Human Services. *Advance Directives and Advance Care Planning: Report to Congress*; 2008. https://aspe.hhs.gov/reports/advance-directives-advance-care-planning-report-congress-0.
12. Barwise A, Jaramillo C, Novotny P, et al. Differences in code status and end of life decision making in patients with limited English proficiency in the intensive care unit. *Mayo Clin Proc.* 2018;93(9):1271—1281. https://doi.org/10.1016/j.mayocp.2018.04.021.
13. Silveria MJ, Kim SY, Langa KM. Advance directives and outcomes of surrogate decision making before death. *N Engl J Med.* 2015;362(13):1211—1218. https://doi.org/10.1056/NEJMsa0907901.
14. California Legislative Information. *AB-2139, Eggman. End of Life Care: Patient Notification.* California Legislative Information; 2014. https://leginfo.legislature.ca.gov/faces/billNavClient.xhtml?bill_id=201320140AB2139.
15. Center for ethics in health care. Oregon POLST program. Center for Ethics in Health Care. https://www.ohsu.edu/center-for-ethics/oregon-polst-program. Accessed January 9, 2021.
16. Hickman SE, Nelson CA, Moss AH, Tolle SW, Perrin NA, Hammes BJ. The consistency between treatments provided to nursing facility residents and orders on the Physician Orders for Life Sustaining Treatment form. *J Am Geriatr Soc.* 2011;59(11):2091—2099. https://doi.org/10.1111/j.1532-5415.2011.03656.x.
17. Hickman SE, Nelson CA, Perrin NA, Moss AH, Hammes BJ, Tolle SW. A comparison of methods to communicate treatment preferences in nursing facilities: traditional practices versus the Physician Orders for Life

Sustaining Treatment program. *J Am Geriatr Soc.* 2010;58(7):1241−1248. https://doi.org/10.1111/j.1532-5415.2010.02955.x.

18. Briggs LA, Kirchhoff KT, Hammes BJ, Song MK, Colvin ER. Patient-centered advance care planning in special patient populations: a pilot study. *J Prof Nurs.* 2004;20(1):47−58.

19. Brinkman-Stoppelenburg A, Rietjens J, van der Heide A. The effects of advance care planning on end of life care: a systematic review. *Palliat Med.* 2014;228(8):1000−1025. https://doi.org/10.1177/0269216314526272.

20. Rubenfeld GD. Principles and practice of withdrawing life sustaining treatments. *Crit Care Clin.* 2004;20(3):435−451.

21. Tilden V, Tolle SW, Nelson CA, Fields J. Family decision-making to withdraw life-sustaining treatments from hospitalized patients. *Nurs Res.* 2001;50(2):105−115.

22. Prigerson HG, Viola M, Brewin CR, et al. Enhancing and mobilizing the potential for wellness and emotional resilience (EMPOWER) among surrogate decision makers of ICU patients: study protocol for a randomized controlled trial. *Trials.* 2019;20(408):1−13. https://doi.org/10.1186/s13063-019-3515-0.

23. Voigt LP, Rajendram P, Shuman AG, et al. Characteristics and outcomes of ethics consultations in an oncologic intensive care unit. *J Intensive Care Med.* 2014;1:436−442. https://doi.org/10.1177/0885066614538389.

24. Campbell ML. *Forgoing Life-Sustaining Therapy: How to Care for the Patient Who Is Near Death.* Aliso Viejo, CA: American Association of Critical-Care Nurses; 1998.

25. Christakis NA, Lamont EB. Extent and determinants of error in doctors' prognoses in terminally ill patients: prospective cohort study. *BMJ.* 2000;320(7233):469−472.

26. Lau F, Cloutier-Fisher D, Kuziemsky C, et al. A systematic review of prognostic tools for estimating survival time in palliative care. *J Palliat Care.* 2007;23(2):93−112.

27. Strand K, Flaatten H. Severity scoring in the ICU: a review. *Acta Anaesthesiol Scand.* 2008;52(4):467−478. https://doi.org/10.1111/j.1399-6576.2008.01586.x.

28. Marshall JC, Cook DJ, Christou NV, Bernard GR, Sprung CL, Sibbald WJ. Multiple organ dysfunction score: a reliable descriptor of a complex clinical outcome. *Crit Care Med.* 1995;23(10):1638−1652.

29. Coalition for Compassionate Care of California. *Decision Aids for Healthcare Providers*; 2019. https://coalitionccc.org/CCCC/Resources/Decision-Aids-for-Healthcare-Providers/CCCC/Resources/Decision-Aids-for-Healthcare-Providers.aspx?hkey=e1004f2b-3e6f-4569-93f4-b9e92ef7ed43.

30. Family Caregiver Alliance. *Fact and Tip Sheets*; 2019. www.caregiver.org/fact-sheets.

31. Treece PD. Communication in the intensive care unit about the end of life. *AACN Adv Crit Care.* 2007;18(4):406−414.

32. Northwestern Medicine Feinberg School of Medicine. EPEC: education in palliative and end-of-life care. www.bioethics.northwestern.edu/programs/epec/. Accessed January 9, 2021.

33. American Association of Colleges of Nursing. End-of-life Nursing Education Consortium (ELNEC). www.aacnnursing.org/ELNEC. Accessed January 9, 2021.

34. Palliative Care Leadership Centers. Overview. https://www.capc.org/palliative-care-leadership-centers/. Accessed January 9, 2021.

35. White DB, Curtis JR, Lo B, Luce JM. Decisions to limit life-sustaining treatment for critically ill patients who lack both decision-making capacity and surrogate decision-makers. *Crit Care Med.* 2006;4(8):2053−2059.

36. Pope TM. Making medical decisions for patients without surrogates. *N Engl J Med.* 2013;269(21):1976−1978. https://doi.org/10.1056/NEJMp1308197.

37. Sharma RK, Dy SM. Cross-cultural communication and use of the family meeting in palliative care. *Am J Hosp Palliat Med.* 2011;28(6):437−444. https://doi.org/10.1177/1049909110394158.

38. Baker R, Wu AW, Teno JM, et al. Family satisfaction with end-of-life care in seriously ill hospitalized adults. *J Am Geriatr Soc.* 2000;48(suppl 5):S61−S69.

39. Curtis JR. Communicating about end-of-life care with patients and families in the intensive care unit. *Crit Care Clin.* 2004;20(3):363−380.

40. Curtis JR, Patrick DL, Shannon SE, Treece PD, Engelberg RA, Rubenfeld GD. The family conference as a focus to improve communication about end-of-life care in the intensive care unit: opportunities for improvement. *Crit Care Med.* 2001;29(suppl 2):N26−N33.

41. Abbott KH, Sago JG, Breen CM, Abernethy AP, Tulsky JA. Families looking back: one year after discussion of withdrawal or withholding of life-sustaining support. *Crit Care Med.* 2001;29(1):197−201.

42. Curtis JR, Engelberg RA, Wenrich MD, Shannon SE, Treece PD, Rubenfeld GD. Missed opportunities during family conferences about end-of-life care in the intensive care unit. *Am J Respir Crit Care Med.* 2005;171(8):844−849.

43. Degenholtz HB, Thomas SB, Miller MJ. Race and the intensive care unit: disparities and preferences for end-of-life care. *Crit Care Med.* 2003; 31(suppl 5):S373−S378.

44. Lipson JG, Dibble SL, Minarik PA. *Culture and Nursing Care: A Pocket Guide.* San Francisco CA: University of California San Francisco Nursing Press; 1996.

45. Gordon B, Keogh M, Davidson Z, et al. Addressing spirituality during critical illness: a review of current literature. *J Crit Care.* 2018;45:76−81. https://doi.org/10.1016/j.jcrc.2018.01.015.

46. Wall RJ, Engelberg RA, Gries CJ, Glavan B, Curtis JR. Spiritual care of families in the intensive care unit. *Crit Care Med.* 2007;35(4):1084−1090.

47. Scheunemann LP, Ernecoff NC, Buddadhumaruk P, et al. Clinician-family communication about patient values and preferences in intensive care units. *JAMA.* 2019;179(5):676−684. https://doi.org/10.1001/jamainternmed.2019.0027.

48. Campbell ML, Guzman JA. Impact of a proactive approach to improve end-of-life care in a medical ICU. *Chest.* 2003;123(1):266−271.

49. Norton SA, Hogan LA, Holloway RG, Temkin-Greener H, Buckley MJ, Quill TE. Proactive palliative care in the medical intensive care unit: effects on length of stay for selected high-risk patients. *Crit Care Med.* 2007;35(6):1530−1535.

50. Frick S, Uehlinger DE, Zuercher Zenklusen RM. Medical futility: predicting outcome of intensive care unit patients by nurses and doctors—a prospective comparative study. *Crit Care Med.* 2003;31(2):456−461.

51. Broom A, Kirby E, Good P, Wootton J, Yates P, Hardy J. Negotiating futility, managing emotions: nursing the transition to palliative care. *Qual Health Res.* 2015;25(3):299−309. https://doi.org/10.1177/1049732314553123.

52. Truog RD, Campbell ML, Curtis JR, et al. Recommendations for end of life care in the intensive care unit: a consensus statement by the American College of Critical Care Medicine. *Crit Care Med.* 2008;36(30):953−963.

53. Hospice and Palliative Nurses Association. Artificial nutrition and hydration in end-of-life care. HPNA position paper. *Home Healthc Nurse.* 2004;22(5):341−345.

54. Kirchhoff KT, Palzkill J, Kowalkowski J, Mork A, Gretarsdottir E. Preparing families of intensive care patients for withdrawal of life support: a pilot study. *Am J Crit Care.* 2008;17(2):113−121.

55. Goldstein NE, Lambert R, Bradley E, Lynn J, Krumholz HM. Management of implantable cardioverter defibrillators in end-of-life care. *Ann Intern Med.* 2004;141(11):835−838.

56. Campbell ML. How to withdraw mechanical ventilation: a systematic review of the literature. *AACN Adv Crit Care.* 2007;18(4):397−403.

57. von Gunten CF, Weissman DE. *Fast facts and concepts #34. Symptom control for ventilator withdrawal in the dying patient*; 2015. https://www.mypcnow.org/fast-fact/symptom-control-for-ventilator-withdrawal-in-the-dying-patient/.

58. Chan JD, Treece PD, Engelberg RA, et al. Narcotic and benzodiazepine use after withdrawal of life support: association with time to death? *Chest.* 2004;126(1):286−293.

59. Billings A. Terminal extubation of the alert patient. *J Palliat Care.* 2011;14(7):800−801. https://doi.org/10.1089/jpm.2011.9676.

60. Rocker GM, Cook DJ, O'Callaghan CJ, et al. Canadian nurses' and respiratory therapists' perspectives on withdrawal of life support in the intensive care unit. *J Crit Care.* 2005;20(1):59−65.

61. Robichaux CM, Clark AP. Practice of expert critical care nurses in situations of prognostic conflict at the end of life. *Am J Crit Care.* 2006;15(5):480−489.

62. Treece PD, Engelberg RA, Crowley L, et al. Evaluation of a standardized order form for the withdrawal of life support in the intensive care unit. *Crit Care Med.* 2004;32(5):1141−1148.

63. Kisorio LC, Langley GC. Intensive care nurses' experiences of end-of-life care. *Intensive Crit Care Nurs.* 2016;33:30−38. https://doi.org/10.1016/j.iccn.2015.11.002.

64. American Association of Critical-Care Nurses. Resources for moral distress. https://www.aacn.org/clinical-resources/moral-distress. Accessed January 9, 2021.

65. Wiegand D. Families and withdrawal of life-sustaining therapy: state of the science. *J Fam Nurs.* 2006;12(2):165–184.

66. Whitmer M, Hurst S, Stadler K, Ide R. Caring in the curing environment. *J Hosp Palliat Nurs.* 2007;9(6):329–333. https://doi.org/10.1097/01.NJH. 0000299318.30009.f7.

67. Davidson J. Family-centered care: meeting the needs of patients' families and helping families adapt to critical illness. *Crit Care Nurse.* 2009;29(3): 28–34. https://doi.org/10.4037/ccn2009611.

68. Davidson JE, Boyer ML, Casey D, Matzel SC, Walden CD. Gap analysis of cultural and religious needs of hospitalized patients. *Crit Care Nurs Q.* 2008;31(2):119–126. https://doi.org/10.1097/01.CNQ.0000314472.33883.d4.

69. Gries CJ, Curtis JR, Wall RJ, Engelberg RA. Family member satisfaction with end-of-life decision making in the ICU. *Chest.* 2008;133(3):704–712. https://doi.org/10.1378/chest.07-1773.

70. Stapleton RD, Engelberg RA, Wenrich MD, Goss CH, Curtis JR. Clinician statements and family satisfaction with family conferences in the intensive care unit. *Crit Care Med.* 2006;34(6):1679–1685.

71. Shannon S. Helping families cope with death in the ICU. In: Curtis JR, Rubenfeld GD, eds. *Managing Death in the Intensive Care Unit: The Transition from Cure to Comfort.* Oxford: Oxford University Press; 2001.

72. Baggs JG, Norton SA, Schmitt MH, Sellers CR. The dying patient in the ICU: role of the interdisciplinary team. *Crit Care Clin.* 2004;20(3):525–540.

73. Kirchhoff KT, Anumandla PR, Foth KT, Lues SN, Gilbertson-White SH. Documentation on withdrawal of life support in adult patients in the intensive care unit. *Am J Crit Care.* 2004;13(4):328–334.

10

Cardiovascular Clinical Assessment and Diagnostic Procedures

Mary E. Lough, Sarah J. Berger, Amy Larsen, and Cass Piper Sandoval

The different procedures used in the diagnosis and management of critically ill patients are discussed under the major headings of Cardiovascular Clinical Assessment, Hemodynamic Monitoring, Electrocardiography, Laboratory Tests, and Diagnostic Procedures.

CARDIOVASCULAR CLINICAL ASSESSMENT

Physical assessment of a patient with cardiovascular disease is a vital clinical skill to master. The process is both detailed and systematic.

History

Data collected from a thorough, thoughtful history taking contribute to both nursing and medical decisions about therapeutic interventions. For a patient in acute distress, the history taking is shortened to just a few questions about the patient's chief complaint, precipitating events, and current medications (Box 10.1—Data Collection). For a patient who is not in obvious distress, the history focuses on the following four areas:

1. Review of the patient's present illness
2. Overview of the patient's general cardiovascular status, including previous cardiac diagnostic studies, interventional procedures, cardiac surgeries, and current medications (i.e., cardiac, noncardiac, and over-the-counter medications)
3. Review of the patient's general health status, including family history of coronary artery disease (CAD), hypertension, diabetes, peripheral arterial disease, or stroke
4. Survey of the patient's lifestyle, including risk factors for CAD

One unique challenge in cardiovascular assessment is identifying when "chest pain" is of cardiac origin and when it is not.[1] Almost eight million patients come to hospital emergency departments with a chief complaint of chest pain.[2] Only approximately 10% of these patients are experiencing an acute cardiac event. In most cases, the chest pain is from another cause such as gastroesophageal reflux disease. For this reason, identifying those patients who are experiencing an acute coronary syndrome (ACS) is crucial.[2]

The following safety information should always be considered:

- If any evidence of CAD or risk of heart disease exists, assume that the chest pain is caused by myocardial ischemia until proven otherwise.
- Questions to elicit the nature of the chest pain cover five basic areas: (1) quality of the pain, (2) location of the pain, (3) duration of the pain, (4) factors that provoke the pain, and (5) factors that relieve the pain.
- Little correlation may exist between the severity of chest discomfort and the gravity of its cause. This is a result of the subjective nature of pain and the unique presentation of ischemic disease in women, older patients, and patients with diabetes.
- Subjective descriptors vary greatly among individuals. Not all patients use the word "pain"; some may describe their problem as "pressure," "heaviness," "discomfort," or "indigestion."
- Other nonpainful symptoms that may signal cardiac dysfunction are dyspnea, palpitations, cough, fatigue, edema, ischemic leg pain, nocturia, cyanosis, and a history of syncope.
- In the evaluation of acute chest pain, a 12-lead electrocardiogram (ECG) to diagnose ST segment changes must be obtained within 10 minutes of arrival at an emergency department.[3,4]

Physical Examination

A comprehensive physical assessment is fundamental to arriving at an accurate diagnosis. A nurse who has developed the skills of *inspection, palpation,* and *auscultation* can be confident when assessing patients with cardiovascular disease. *Percussion,* another physical assessment skill, is not used when assessing the cardiovascular system.

Inspection

Assessing general appearance. The face is observed for skin color (i.e., cyanotic, pale, or jaundiced) and for an apprehensive or painful expression. The patient's skin, lips, tongue, and mucous membranes are inspected for pallor or cyanosis. *Central cyanosis* is a bluish discoloration of the tongue and sublingual area. Central cyanosis is a medical emergency indicating hypoxemia. Pulse oximetry, arterial blood gas analysis, and treatment with 100% oxygen must be instituted immediately.

BOX 10.1   DATA COLLECTION

Cardiovascular History

Common Cardiovascular Symptoms

- Chest pains
- Palpitations
- Dyspnea
- Cough, hemoptysis
- Nausea
- Nocturia
- Edema
- Dizziness, syncope, visual changes
- Leg claudication (pain) or paresthesias
- Fatigue

Patient Lifestyle

- Baseline cognitive functioning
- Health habits
- Use of tea and coffee, over-the-counter medication use, smoking, exercise, sleep, dietary habits
- Use of illegal drugs (e.g., cocaine)
- Use of alcohol (daily quantity)
- Lifestyle pattern and responsibilities
- Working, relaxing, coping, cultural habits
- Social support systems
- Recent life changes within past 12 months
- Emotional state
- Evidence of psychologic stress, anger, anxiety, depression
- Perception of illness and its meaning for the future

Cardiovascular Risk Factors

- Sex
- Age
- Cultural identity
- Family history of premature CAD (age 65 years or younger)
- Smoking history
- Hypertension
- Hyperlipidemia
- Sedentary lifestyle
- Diabetes mellitus
- Obesity
- Kidney failure

Medical History

Child

- Murmurs, cyanosis, streptococcal infections, rheumatic fever

Adult

- Diseases and abnormalities
- Heart failure (right- or left-sided), CAD, heart valve disease, mitral valve prolapse, myocardial infarction, peripheral vascular disease (arterial or venous), diabetes mellitus, hypertension, hyperlipidemia, dysrhythmias, murmurs, endocarditis, visual defects, recent weight changes, psychiatric illnesses, thrombophlebitis, deep vein thrombosis, systemic or pulmonary emboli
- Surgical history

- *Cardiovascular:* Coronary artery bypass grafting, valvular placement, peripheral vascular bypasses or repairs, pacemaker, defibrillator implant (ICD)
- *Other body systems:* Neurologic, gastrointestinal, musculoskeletal, pulmonary, renal, immunologic, hematologic
- Allergies, especially to emergency medications (lidocaine, morphine), radiographic contrast agents, or iodine (shellfish)
- Recent dental work or infection

Family History

- CAD at age 65 years or younger
- Myocardial infarction
- Early death of unknown origin
- Hypertension
- Stroke
- Diabetes mellitus
- Lipid disorders
- Collagen vascular disease

Current Medication Use

- Angiotensin-converting enzyme (ACE) inhibitors
- Anticoagulants
- Antidysrhythmics
- Antihypertensives
- Antiplatelet agents
- Angiotensin-receptor blockers
- Beta-blockers
- Calcium channel blockers
- Cholesterol-lowering agents
- Digitalis
- Diuretics
- Nitrates
- Hormone replacement therapy
- Oral contraceptives
- Potassium, calcium
- Nonprescription medications or herbal remedies

Cardiac Studies or Interventions Completed in the Past

- Cardiac catheterization
- Electrophysiology study
- Cardiac ultrasound (echocardiogram)
- 12-lead electroencephalogram
- Exercise ECG (stress test)
- Myocardial imaging with radiographic isotopes (e.g., thallium, dipyridamole, dobutamine)
- Fibrinolytic therapy
- Percutaneous transluminal coronary angioplasty
- Atherectomy
- Stent placement
- Valvuloplasty

CAD, Coronary artery disease; *ECG,* electrocardiogram; *ICD,* implantable cardioverter defibrillator.

The anterior thorax and posterior thorax are inspected for skeletal deformities that may displace the heart and cause cardiac compromise. The skin on the chest wall and abdomen is inspected for scars, wounds, and bulges associated with pacemaker or defibrillator implants.

Body posture can provide information about the amount of effort it takes to breathe. For example, sitting upright to breathe may be necessary for a patient with acute heart failure. Leaning forward may be the least painful position for a patient with pericarditis.

Body weight in proportion to height is assessed to determine whether the patient is obese, a risk factor for cardiovascular disease,[5] or severely underweight (cachectic).[6] Respiratory rate, pattern, and effort are also observed and recorded.

The abdomen is assessed for signs of distention or ascites, which may be associated with right-sided heart failure. Abdominal adiposity is a known risk factor for CAD.

Examining the extremities. The nail beds are inspected for signs of discoloration or cyanosis. *Clubbing* in the nail bed is a sign associated with long-standing central cyanotic heart disease or pulmonary disease with hypoxemia. Clubbing of the nail refers to a nail that has lost the normal angle between the finger and the nail root; the nail becomes wide and convex. The terminal phalanx of the finger also becomes bulbous and swollen. Clubbing is rare and is a sign of severe central cyanosis (Fig. 10.1). *Peripheral cyanosis*, a bluish discoloration of the nail bed, is a more common sign. Peripheral cyanosis results from a reduction in the quantity of oxygen in the peripheral extremities from arterial disease or decreased cardiac output (CO). Clubbing never occurs because of peripheral cyanosis.

Lower extremities. Legs are inspected for both signs of peripheral arterial disease and venous disease. The visible signs of peripheral arterial vascular disease include pale, shiny legs with sparse hair growth.[7] Research suggests that women can have peripheral atherosclerosis with less obvious signs of peripheral arterial disease.[8] If untreated, peripheral arterial disease can lead to critical limb ischemia, decreased quality of life, and premature death.[9]

Venous disease is caused by failure of the valves in the veins leading to bleeding into the surrounding tissues. Increasing pressure in the tissues causes edema, brown skin discoloration from red blood cell (RBC) destruction, dependent rubor, and frequently nonhealing leg ulcers.[10]

A comparison of typical assessment findings in peripheral arterial and venous diseases is presented in Table 10.1.

Estimating jugular vein distention and central venous pressure. The jugular veins of the neck are inspected for a noninvasive estimate of intravascular volume and pressure.[11] The internal jugular (IJ) veins are observed for signs of jugular vein distention (JVD), as shown in Fig. 10.2 and Box 10.2, caused by an elevation in jugular venous pressure (JVP). Elevated JVP can be observed as a sign without measurement. JVP is best observed in the right jugular vein.[11] The most common causes of JVP elevation are fluid volume overload and right ventricular failure.

The right IJ vein can be palpated to permit noninvasive measurement of elevated central venous pressure (CVP) in centimeters (Fig. 10.3 and Box 10.3).[12] Any elevation greater than 8 cm is considered high.[11] Bedside ultrasound can also be used to evaluate JVD and to estimate CVP.[13] The combination of peripheral edema and JVD identifies a potential for poor clinical outcomes.[14,15]

Thoracic reference points. The thoracic cage is divided with imaginary vertical lines (sternal, midclavicular, axillary, vertebral, and scapular), and the intercostal spaces are numbered below each rib. The second rib is the easiest to locate because it is attached to the sternum at the angle of Louis. This angle (also called the *sternal angle*) is the

Clubbing of Nail Beds

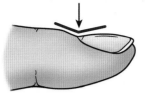

Normal nail shows a slight angle between root of nail bed and finger.

Normal Finger and Nail Bed

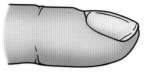

Early clubbing shows loss of angle at root of nail bed. Fingertip is of normal size.

Early Clubbing

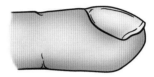

Moderate clubbing shows bulging of angle at root of nail bed. Distal finger/toe is enlarged.

Moderate Clubbing

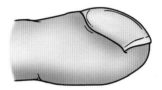

Advanced clubbing shows bulging and widening of nail bed. Distal finger/toe is bulbous.

Advanced Clubbing

Fig. 10.1 Clubbing of Nail Beds.

bony ridge on the sternum that lies approximately 2 inches below the sternal notch. After the second rib has been located, it can be used as a reference point to count off the other ribs and intercostal spaces.

Observing the apical impulse. The anterior thorax is inspected for the apical impulse, sometimes referred to as the *point of maximal impulse*. The apical impulse occurs as the left ventricle contracts during systole and rotates forward, causing the left ventricular apex of the heart to hit the chest wall. The apical impulse is a quick, localized, outward movement normally located just lateral to the left midclavicular line at the fifth intercostal space in an adult patient (Fig. 10.4).[11] The apical impulse is the only normal pulsation visualized on the chest wall. In a patient without cardiac disease, point of maximal impulse may not be noticeable (see Fig. 10.4).

Palpation

Palpation is a technique that uses the sense of touch in the tips of the fingers and the palm of the hand.

Assessing arterial pulses. Seven pairs of bilateral arterial pulses are normally palpated. The examination incorporates bilateral assessment of the carotid, brachial, radial, ulnar, popliteal, posterior tibial, and dorsalis pedis arterial pulses. The pulses are palpated separately and

TABLE 10.1 Comparison of Peripheral Arterial and Venous Disease Signs and Symptoms in Legs.

Signs and Symptoms	Peripheral Arterial Disease	Peripheral Venous Disease
Skin	Shiny dry appearance	Brown patches on skin at ankles and lower leg
	Pallor with elevation	Mottled rubor (brown/red) appearance, especially when dependent
		Skin texture may be hard and fibrotic
		Flaking skin, dermatitis
Hair on leg	Decreased hair growth	Decreased hair growth
Ulcers on leg or foot	Foot or toe wounds (ulcers) that do not heal	Venous ulcers at ankle or lower leg
	Gangrene on toes	Moist with copious drainage
Nails	Slow nail growth	Normal
	Thick, opaque nails	
Varicose veins	No	Present
Temperature	Cold compared with rest of the body	Warm
Capillary refill	Slow ($\geq$3 seconds)	Normal (<3 seconds)
Edema	None	Legs and feet are swollen and edematous
Pulses	Weak or absent	Normal
Pain	Burning sensation in feet	Legs can feel heavy, aching, tired, with burning or itching from swelling
	Leg cramps when walking: intermittent claudication	
	Leg cramps at rest: ischemic claudication	
	Numbness	
Associated conditions	Diabetes	Diabetes
	Atherosclerotic disease	Varicose veins

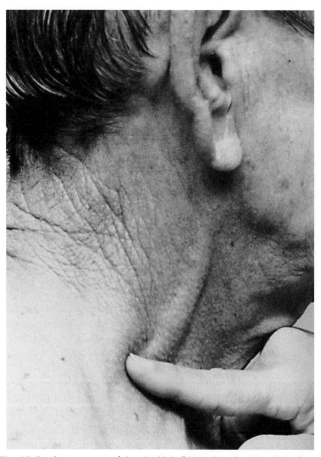

Fig. 10.2 Assessment of Jugular Vein Distention. Applying light finger pressure over the sternocleidomastoid muscle, parallel to the clavicle, helps identify the external jugular vein by occluding flow and distending it. The finger pressure is released, and the patient is observed for true distention. If the patient's trunk is elevated to 30 degrees or more, jugular vein distention should not be present.

BOX 10.2 Procedure for Assessing Jugular Vein Distention

1. The patient reclines at 30- to 45-degree angle.
2. The examiner stands on the patient's right side and turns the patient's head slightly toward the left.
3. If the jugular vein is not visible, light finger pressure is applied across the sternocleidomastoid muscle just above and parallel to the clavicle. This pressure fills the external jugular vein by obstructing flow (see Fig. 10.2).
4. After the location of the vein has been identified, the pressure is released, and the presence of jugular vein distention (JVD) is assessed.
5. Because inhalation decreases venous pressure, JVD should be assessed at end-exhalation.
6. Any fullness in the vein extending more than 3 cm above the sternal angle is evidence of increased venous pressure. Generally, the higher the sitting angle of the patient when JVD is visualized, the higher is the central venous pressure.
7. *Documentation:* JVD is reported by including the angle of the head of the bed at the time JVD was evaluated (e.g., "Presence of JVD with head of bed elevated to 45 degrees").

compared bilaterally to check for consistency. Pulse volume is graded on a scale of 0 to 3+ with specific descriptors:

- 0 Not palpable
- 1+ Faintly palpable, weak and thready
- 2+ Palpable, normal pulse
- 3+ Bounding hyperdynamic pulse

Evaluating capillary refill. Capillary refill assessment is an assessment technique that uses the patient's nail beds to evaluate arterial circulation to the extremity and determine overall perfusion. The nail bed is compressed to produce blanching, after which release of the pressure should result in the return of blood flow and baseline nail color in less than 2 seconds. Capillary refill time of greater than 5 seconds has been associated with more severe organ failure[16] and increased mortality.[10] Capillary refill is a standard component of the cardiovascular physical examination.

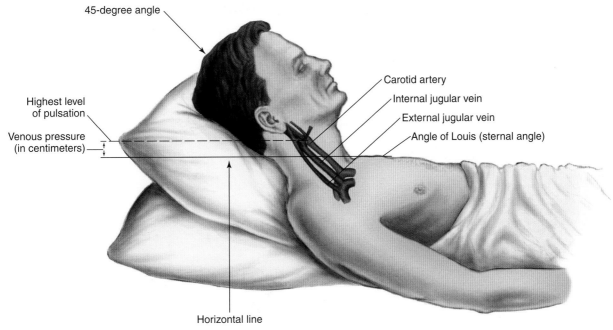

Fig. 10.3 Position of Internal and External Jugular Veins. Pulsation in the internal jugular vein can be used to estimate central venous pressure. (Modified from Thompson JM, McFarland GK, Hirsch JE, et al. *Mosby's Clinical Nursing.* 5th ed. St. Louis: Mosby; 2002.)

BOX 10.3 Procedure for Assessing Central Venous Pressure

1. The patient reclines in the bed. The highest point of pulsation in the internal jugular vein is observed during exhalation.
2. The vertical distance between this pulsation (top of the fluid level) and the sternal angle is estimated or measured in centimeters.
3. This number is added to 5 cm for an estimation of central venous pressure (CVP); 5 cm is the approximate distance of the sternal angle above the level of the right atrium (see Fig. 10.3).
4. *Documentation:* The degree of elevation of the patient is included in the report (e.g., "CVP estimated at 13 cm, using internal jugular vein pulsation, with head of bed elevated 45 degrees").

Estimating edema. Edema is fluid accumulation in the extravascular spaces of the body. The dependent tissues within the legs and sacrum are particularly susceptible. Edema may be dependent, unilateral, or bilateral, and pitting or nonpitting. The amount of edema is quantified by measuring the circumference of the limb or by pressing the skin of the feet, ankles, and shins against underlying bone. Edema is a symptom associated with several diseases, and further diagnostic evaluation is required to determine the cause. Although no universal scale for pitting edema exists, typical scales use a system ranging from 0 to 4+ (Table 10.2).

Auscultation

Measuring blood pressure. Blood pressure (BP) measurement is an essential component of every complete physical examination. A normal BP is below 120/80 mm Hg. In patients with chronic kidney disease or diabetes, the goal is a BP less than 140/90 mm Hg.[17]

Detecting orthostatic hypotension. Postural (orthostatic) hypotension occurs when the systolic BP (SBP) falls 20 mm Hg or the diastolic BP falls 10 mm Hg with a change in position to standing (Box 10.4).[18] Orthostatic hypotension is accompanied by dizziness, lightheadedness, or syncope. The most common causes of orthostatic vital sign changes (i.e., decrease in BP and increase in heart rate [HR]) seen in the critical care unit are:

- Intravascular volume depletion or fluid loss caused by bleeding, diuresis, or fever
- Inadequate vascular vasoconstrictor mechanisms to constrict the arterial bed, which can occur after prolonged immobility or because of a spinal cord injury
- Autonomic insufficiency caused by administration of pharmacologic agents such as beta-blockers, angiotensin-converting enzyme inhibitors, and calcium channel blockers

Evaluating pulse pressure. Pulse pressure describes the difference between systolic and diastolic values. The normal pulse pressure is 40 mm Hg and represents the difference between an SBP of 120 mm Hg and a diastolic BP of 80 mm Hg. In a critically ill patient, a low BP is frequently associated with a narrow pulse pressure. For example, a patient with a BP of 90/72 mm Hg has a pulse pressure of 18 mm Hg. The narrowed pulse pressure is a temporary compensatory mechanism caused by arterial vasoconstriction resulting from volume depletion or heart failure. The narrow pulse pressure ensures that the mean arterial pressure (MAP, 78 mm Hg in this example) remains in a therapeutic range to provide adequate organ perfusion.

In contrast, a hypotensive patient with sepsis who exhibits vasodilation may have a wide pulse pressure. If the BP is 90/36 mm Hg, the pulse pressure is 54 mm Hg, and the MAP is an inadequate 54 mm Hg. In both examples, the SBP is the same (90 mm Hg); the difference in pulse pressure is caused by differences in intravascular volume and vascular tone.

Detecting pulsus paradoxus. In normal physiology, the strength of the pulse fluctuates throughout the respiratory cycle. When the "pulse" is measured using the SBP, the pressure is observed to decrease slightly

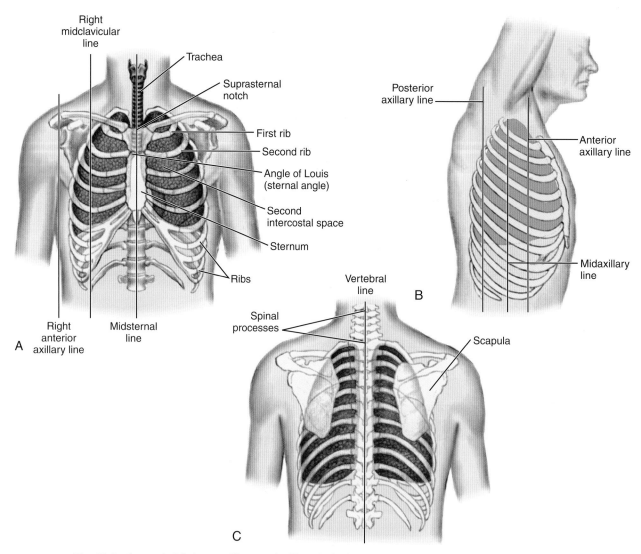

Fig. 10.4 Anatomical Reference Lines on the Thoracic Surface. (A) The anterior view has a midsternal line, and two midclavicular lines (right is shown). (B) The lateral view has three lines, anterior axillary, mid-axillary and posterior axillary. C The posterior view has a vertebral line aligned with the spine.

TABLE 10.2   Pitting Edema Scale.

| Scale | Edema | INDENTATION DEPTH | | Time to Baseline |
		English Units	Metric Units	
0	None	0	0	
1+	Trace	0–0.25 inch	<6.5 mm	Rapid
2+	Mild	0.25–0.5 inch	6.5–12.5 mm	10–15 seconds
3+	Moderate	0.5–1 inch	12.5 mm–2.5 cm	1–2 minutes
4+	Severe	>1 inch	>2.5 cm	2–5 minutes

during inspiration and to increase slightly during respiratory exhalation. The normal difference is 2 to 4 mm Hg. In some clinical conditions such as cardiac tamponade, the BP decline is abnormally large during inspiration. In general, an inspiratory decline of SBP greater than 10 mm Hg is considered diagnostic of pulsus paradoxus.[19] The techniques for measuring pulsus paradoxus using a sphygmomanometer, BP cuff, and pulse oximetry waveform are described in Box 10.5. If the patient is hypotensive, pulsus paradoxus is more accurately assessed in the critical

care unit by monitoring a pulse oximetry waveform or an indwelling arterial catheter waveform.

Assessing heart sounds. Auscultation of the heart with a stethoscope is considered the most challenging part of the cardiac physical examination. Handheld ultrasound devices increasingly are used at the bedside to augment cardiac auscultation findings.[20] A summary of the advice given by most experts to effectively acquire the skills of cardiac auscultation is:

BOX 10.4   Measurement of Postural (Orthostatic) Vital Signs

Guidelines
1. Record BP and HR in each position.
2. Do not remove cuff between measurements.
3. Record all associated signs and symptoms.
4. Clearly document patient position.

Lying	Sitting	Standing
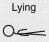		

Technique
1. Keep the patient as flat as possible for 10 minutes before the initial assessment.
2. Patient supine: Obtain initial BP and HR measurements.
3. Patient sitting with legs hanging: Measure immediately and after 2 minutes.
4. Patient standing: Measure immediately and after 2 minutes. If BP and HR are stable but orthostasis is suspected, BP and HR can be repeated every 2 minutes. This is rarely practical for a critically ill patient.

Results
Normal Changes
1. HR increases by 5 to 20 beats/min (transiently).
2. Systolic BP decreases by 10 mm Hg.
3. Diastolic BP decreases by 5 mm Hg.

Positive Orthostasis
1. Decrease in systolic BP by more than 20 mm Hg.
2. Decrease in diastolic BP by more than 10 mm Hg within 3 minutes.

BP, Blood pressure; *HR,* heart rate.

BOX 10.5   Procedure for Measuring Pulsus Paradoxus

Measurement With Sphygmomanometer
1. The patient should be lying supine in a comfortable position.
2. The breathing pattern should be of normal depth and rate to avoid excessive respiratory interference.
3. The sphygmomanometer cuff is inflated to a pressure greater than systolic blood pressure (BP), and Korotkoff sounds are auscultated over the brachial artery while the cuff is deflated at a rate of approximately 2 to 3 mm Hg per heartbeat.
4. The peak systolic BP during expiration (i.e., pressure at which Korotkoff sounds are heard only during expiration) should be identified and then reconfirmed.
5. The cuff is deflated slowly to establish systolic BP at which Korotkoff sounds become audible during both inspiration and expiration.
6. If the auscultated difference between these two systolic BP values exceeds 10 mm Hg during quiet respiration, a paradoxical pulse is present.

Measurement by Waveform Analysis
1. A pulse oximetry sensor with a visible pulse waveform can be used as an additional measurement device.
2. In the critical care unit, an arterial waveform from an indwelling arterial catheter (if present) can be used to measure the difference in systolic BP between expiration and inspiration.

BOX 10.6   Characteristics of First and Second Heart Sounds

First Heart Sound (S₁)	Second Heart Sound (S₂)
High pitched	High pitched
Loudest in mitral area (apex)	Loudest in aortic area (base)
Split S₁	Split S₂
Normal split less than 20 ms	Normal split less than 30 ms
Split heard best in tricuspid area	Split heard best in pulmonic area
Important to differentiate between split S₁ and S₄	↑ Split with inhalation
Occurs immediately before carotid upstroke	↓ Split with exhalation

↑, Increased; ↓, decreased; *ms,* milliseconds.

1. Auscultate systematically across the precordium.
2. Visualize the cardiac anatomy under each point of auscultation, expecting to hear the physiologically associated sounds.
3. Memorize the cardiac cycle to enhance the ability to hear abnormal sounds.
4. Practice, practice, practice.

First and second heart sounds. Normal heart sounds are referred to as the *first heart sound* (S₁) and the *second heart sound* (S₂). S₁ is the sound associated with mitral and tricuspid valve closure and is heard most clearly in the mitral and tricuspid areas. S₂ (aortic and pulmonic closure) can be heard best at the second intercostal space to the right and left of the sternum (see Fig. 10.4). Both S₁ and S₂ are high pitched sounds that are heard best with the diaphragm of the stethoscope (Box 10.6). Each sound is loudest in an auscultation area located downstream from the actual valvular component of the sound, as shown in Fig. 10.5.

Abnormal heart sounds. **Third and fourth heart sounds.** Abnormal heart sounds are known as the *third heart sound* (S₃) and the *fourth heart sound* (S₄); they are referred to as *gallops* when auscultated during an episode of tachycardia (Fig. 10.6). These low-pitched sounds occur during diastole and are best heard with the bell of the stethoscope positioned lightly over the apical impulse. The characteristics of S₃ and S₄ are described in detail in Box 10.7. The presence of S₃ may be normal in children, young adults, and pregnant women because of rapid filling of the ventricle in a young, healthy heart. However, S₃ in

the presence of cardiac symptoms is an indicator of heart failure in a noncompliant ventricle with fluid overload.[21]

Auscultation of S₄ also leads the examiner to suspect heart failure and decreased ventricular compliance. Also referred to as an *atrial gallop*, S₄ occurs at the end of diastole (just before S₁), when the ventricle is full. It is associated with atrial contraction, also called *atrial kick*.

Heart murmurs. Heart valve murmurs are prolonged extra sounds that occur during systole or diastole and are typically a sign of either ventricular dysfunction or valvular heart disease.[22,23] Mortality is increased with multivalve disease.[24]

Murmurs are produced by turbulent blood flow through the chambers of the heart, from forward flow through narrowed or irregular valve openings, or backward regurgitant flow through an incompetent valve. Murmurs occur in both systole and diastole (Table 10.3). Most murmurs are caused by structural valvular changes

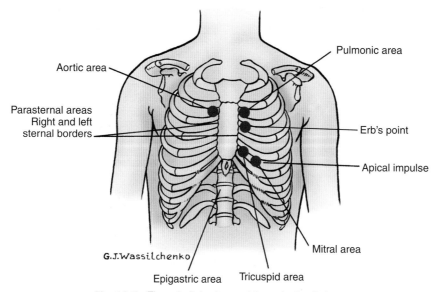

Fig. 10.5 Thoracic Palpation and Auscultation Points.

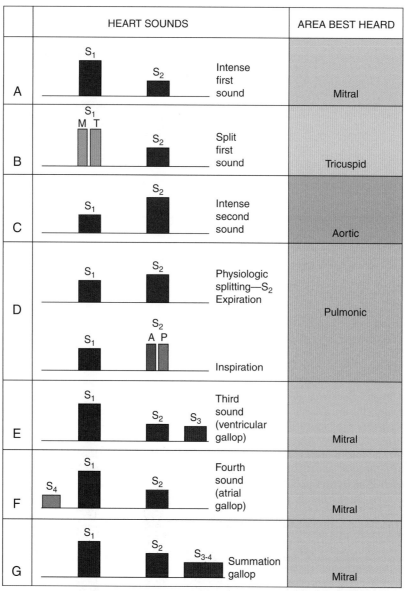

Fig. 10.6 Characteristics of Normal and Abnormal Heart Sounds, Heart Murmurs, and Associated Auscultatory Areas: Where Each Is Best Heard With a Stethoscope.

BOX 10.7 Characteristics of Third and Fourth Heart Sounds

Third Heart Sound (S₃)	Fourth Heart Sound (S₄)
Physiologic Causes	**Physiologic Causes**
Related to diastolic motion and rapid filling of ventricles in early diastole	Related to diastolic motion and ventricular dilation with atrial contraction in late diastole
	May occur with or without cardiac decompensation
Can be normal in children and young adults (<40 years old)	Ventricular hypertrophy with decrease in ventricular compliance (CAD, systemic hypertension, cardiomyopathy, aortic or pulmonary stenosis, increase in intensity with acute MI or angina)
Physiologic Causes	
Ventricular dysfunction with increase in end-systolic volume (MI, heart failure, valvular disease, systemic or pulmonary hypertension)	Hyperkinetic states (anemia, thyrotoxicosis, arteriovenous fistula)
Hyperdynamic states (anemia, thyrotoxicosis, mitral or tricuspid regurgitation)	Acute valvular regurgitation
Rhythmic Word Association	
"Kentucky": S_1, S_2, S_3	"Tennessee": S_4, S_1, S_2
Synonyms	
Ventricular gallop	Atrial gallop
Protodiastolic gallop	Presystolic gallop

CAD, Coronary artery disease; *MI,* myocardial infarction.

TABLE 10.3 Characteristics of Heart Murmurs.

Defects	Timing in Cardiac Cycle	Pitch; Intensity; Quality	Location; Radiation
Systolic Murmurs			
Mitral regurgitation	S_1 — S_2	High; harsh; blowing	Mitral area; may radiate to axilla
Tricuspid regurgitation	S_1 — S_2	High; often faint, but varies; blowing	Tricuspid RLSB, apex, LLSB, epigastric areas; little radiation
Ventricular septal defect	S_1 — S_2	High; loud; blowing	Left sternal border
Aortic stenosis	S_1 ◇ S_2	"Chhhh hh;" medium; rough, harsh	Aortic area to suprasternal notch, right side of neck, apex
Pulmonary stenosis	S_1 ◇ S_2	Low to medium; loud; harsh, grinding	Pulmonic area; no radiation
Diastolic Murmurs			
Mitral stenosis	Atrial kick S_2 — S_1	Low; quiet to loud with thrill; rough rumble	Mitral area; usually no radiation
Tricuspid stenosis	Atrial kick S_2 — S_1	Medium; quiet; louder with inspiration; rumble	Tricuspid area or epigastrium; little radiation
Aortic regurgitation	S_2 — S_1	High; faint to medium; blowing	Aortic area to LLSB and aorta; Erb's point
Pulmonic regurgitation	S_2 — S_1	Medium; faint; blowing	Pulmonic area; no radiation

LLSB, Left lower sternal border; *RLSB,* right lower sternal border.

BOX 10.8 Technique of Auscultation of Heart Sounds and Murmurs

1. **Stethoscope**
   - Diaphragm
   - Larger surface area
   - Brings out higher frequency and filters out lower frequency
   - Use for listening to S_1/S_2 (split S_1/S_2), loud murmurs, pericardial friction rubs
   - Bell
   - Smaller surface area
   - Filters out high-frequency sounds and accentuates low-frequency sounds
   - Rest lightly on area (or else it becomes a diaphragm)
2. **Location: Heart sounds auscultated at APTM**
   - *A:* Aortic area (second right ICS along sternal border)
   - *P:* Pulmonic area (second left ICS along sternal border)
   - *T:* Tricuspid area (fourth left ICS along sternal border)
   - *M:* Mitral area (fifth ICS at MCL)
3. **"Know your bases"**
   - Base of the heart refers to the right and left second ICS beside the sternum S_2 where the aortic or pulmonic sounds are auscultated
   - Apex or left ventricular area refers to the fifth ICS along the MCL
   - Most commonly referred to as PMI
   - Also referred to as mitral area
   - S_1 and mitral sounds are loudest here
   - Erb's point: Second aortic area (third left ICS along sternal border); pericardial friction rubs are heard best here
4. **Palpation**
   - Location
   - Palpate carotid pulse (or watch ECG to identify S_1 and S_2)
5. **Be quiet and patient**
   - Listen for S_1 and S_2 first, ignoring all other sounds
   - Inching technique
   - After you are sure which is S_1 or S_2, try to determine when the other sound comes in
   - Is it systolic or diastolic?
   - S_3 and S_4 are best heard with patient in left lateral decubitus position; note the location (suggests origin of sound)
   - Note the timing (S_4 comes just before S_1, and S_3 comes just after S_2)
6. **Interpret the sounds based on the clinical condition**

ECG, Electrocardiogram; *ICS,* intercostal space; *MCL,* midclavicular line; *PMI,* point of maximal impulse.

BOX 10.9 Grading of Cardiac Murmurs

Grade	Description
1	Very faint; may be heard only in quiet environment
2	Quiet but clearly audible
3	Moderately loud
4	Loud; may be associated with palpable thrill
5	Very loud; thrill easily palpable
6	Very loud; may be heard with stethoscope off the chest; thrill palpable and visible

systolic and diastolic, corresponding with cardiac motion within the pericardial sac. It is often associated with chest pain, which can be aggravated by deep inspiration, coughing, swallowing, and changing position. It is important to differentiate pericarditis from acute myocardial ischemia, and the detection of a pericardial friction rub through auscultation can assist in this differentiation, leading to effective diagnosis and treatment.[25]

HEMODYNAMIC MONITORING

Hemodynamic monitoring is described across a spectrum of very invasive, moderately invasive, minimally invasive, and noninvasive methods (Fig. 10.7). Every method has advantages and disadvantages, and all require an understanding of the physiologic principles that guide diagnostic assessment and management. In clinical practice, there is tremendous variation in the technologies used depending on the setting and patient acuity. In general, cardiovascular surgical units use more-invasive hemodynamic monitoring, whereas nonsurgical critical care areas begin with less-invasive monitoring, adding invasive technologies based on the patient's physiologic requirements. Hemodynamic technologies are discussed in this chapter following a more-invasive to less-invasive trajectory.

Hemodynamic Monitoring Equipment

A traditional invasive hemodynamic monitoring system has four component parts (Fig. 10.8):
- An invasive catheter and high-pressure tubing connect the patient to the transducer.
- The transducer receives the physiologic signal from the catheter and tubing and converts it into electrical energy.
- The flush system maintains patency of the fluid-filled system and catheter.
- The bedside monitor contains the amplifier with recorder, which increases the volume of the electrical signal and displays it on an oscilloscope and on a digital scale in millimeters of mercury (mm Hg).

Although many different types of invasive catheters can be inserted to monitor hemodynamic pressures, all such catheters are connected to similar equipment (see Fig. 10.8). However, there is variation in the way different hospitals configure their hemodynamic systems. The basic setup consists of the following:
- A bag of 0.9% sodium chloride (also known as *normal saline*) is used as a flush solution, delivered at approximately 3 mL/h. In some hospitals, heparin is added as an anticoagulant. A pressure infusion cuff covers the bag of flush solution, and the cuff is inflated to 300 mm Hg.

(see Fig. 10.5 and Fig. 10.6). The steps to auscultate effectively and accurately for cardiac murmurs are listed in Box 10.8. Murmurs are characterized by specific criteria:
- *Timing:* Place in the cardiac cycle (systole/diastole)
- *Location:* Where the sound is auscultated on the chest wall (mitral or aortic area)
- *Radiation:* How far the sound spreads across the chest wall
- *Quality:* Whether the murmur is blowing, grating, or harsh
- *Pitch:* Whether the tone is high or low
- *Intensity:* Loudness is graded on a scale of 1 to 6; a higher number denotes a louder murmur (Box 10.9; see Table 10.3).

Pericardial friction rub. A pericardial friction rub is a sound that can occur 2 to 7 days after a myocardial infarction (MI). The friction rub results from pericardial inflammation (pericarditis).[25] A pericardial friction rub can be auscultated in many cases. Classically, a pericardial friction rub is a grating or scratching sound that is both

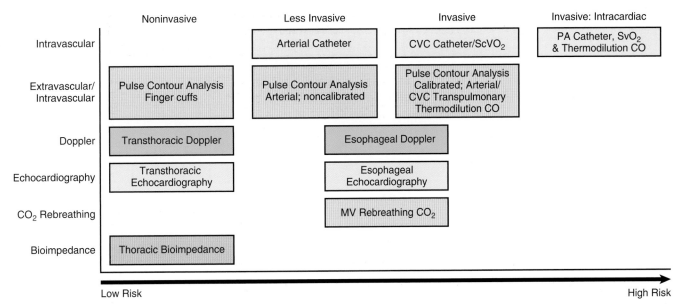

Fig. 10.7 Overview of options for hemodynamic monitoring in critical care from noninvasive to highly invasive, from low risk to high risk, and listing the different monitoring options that are available. *CO*, Cardiac output; *CO₂*, carbon dioxide; *CVC*, central venous catheter; *MV*, mechanical ventilation; *ScVO₂*, mixed venous oxygen saturation.

- The system contains intravenous (IV) tubing, three-way stopcocks, and an in-line flow device attached for continuous fluid infusion and manual flush. High-pressure tubing must be used to connect the invasive catheter to the transducer to prevent damping (flattening) of the waveform.
- A pressure transducer is used. Transducers are disposable and use a silicon chip.

Heparin

The use of the anticoagulant heparin added to the normal saline flush setup to maintain catheter patency is controversial.[26,27] Although many units do add heparin to flush solutions, other critical care units avoid heparin because of concern about development of heparin-induced antibodies that can trigger an autoimmune condition known as heparin-induced thrombocytopenia (HIT).[28] HIT is associated with a decrease in platelet count of more than 50% accompanied by thrombus formation.[28] If heparin is used in the flush infusion, ongoing monitoring of the platelet count is recommended.

Flush solutions, lines, stopcocks, and disposable transducers are changed every 96 hours per current US Centers for Disease Control and Prevention guidelines.[29,30] However, there is variation in practice among hospitals; some change the flush solutions every 24 hours. For this reason, it is essential to be familiar with the specific written procedures that concern hemodynamic monitoring equipment in each critical care unit. Dextrose solutions are not recommended as flush solutions in monitoring catheters.[29,30]

Calibration of Hemodynamic Monitoring Equipment

To ensure accuracy of hemodynamic pressure readings, two baseline measurements are necessary:
- Calibration of the system to atmospheric pressure, also known as *zeroing the transducer*
- Determination of the midaxillary axis for transducer height placement, necessary to accurately *level the transducer*[31]

Zeroing the transducer. To calibrate the equipment to atmospheric pressure, referred to as *zeroing the transducer*, the three-way stopcock nearest to the transducer is turned simultaneously to open the transducer to air (atmospheric pressure) and to close it to the patient and the flush system. The monitor is adjusted so that "0" is displayed, which equals local atmospheric pressure. Atmospheric pressure is not zero; it is 760 mm Hg at sea level. Using zero to represent current atmospheric pressure provides a convenient baseline for hemodynamic measurement purposes.

Some monitors also require calibration of the upper scale limit while the system remains open to air. At the end of the calibration procedure, the stopcock is returned to the closed position, and a closed cap is placed over the open port. At this point, the patient's waveform and hemodynamic pressures are displayed.

Disposable transducers are very accurate, and after they are calibrated to atmospheric pressure, drift from the zero baseline is minimal. Although in theory this means that repeated calibration is unnecessary, clinical protocols in most units require the nurse to calibrate the transducer at the beginning of each shift for quality assurance.

Midaxillary line (phlebostatic axis). The *midaxillary line*, also known as the *phlebostatic axis*, describes a reference point on the side of the chest that is used for consistent transducer height placement. To locate the axis, a theoretical line is drawn from the fourth sternal intercostal space, where it joins the sternum, to a theoretical line on the side of the chest that is one-half of the depth of the lateral chest wall.[31] This theoretical line approximates the level of the atria, as shown in Fig. 10.8. It is used as the reference mark for CVP and pulmonary artery (PA) catheter transducers. The transducer "air reference stopcock" approximates the position of the tip of an invasive hemodynamic monitoring catheter within the chest.

Leveling the transducer. Leveling the transducer is different from zeroing. This process aligns the transducer with the level of the left atrium. The purpose is to line up the air-fluid interface with the left

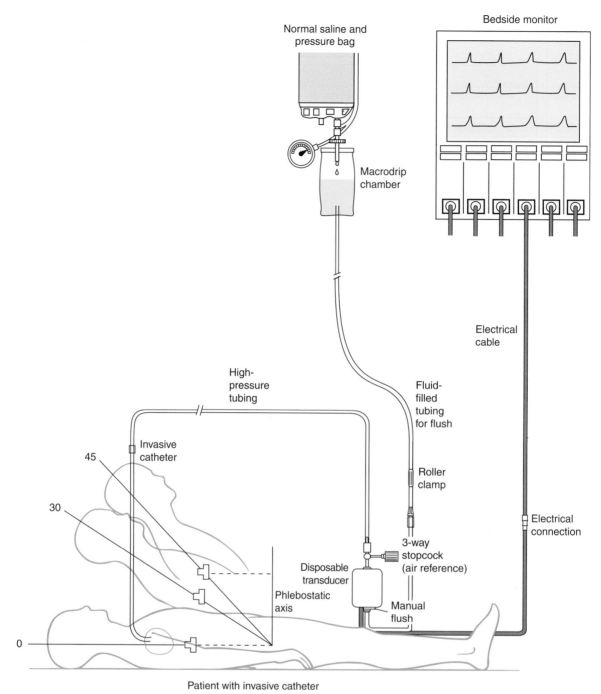

Fig. 10.8 The four parts of a hemodynamic monitoring system include an invasive catheter attached to high-pressure tubing to connect to the transducer; a transducer; a flush system, including a manual flush; and a bedside monitor.

atrium to correct for changes in hydrostatic pressure in blood vessels above and below the level of the heart.[31]

A carpenter's level or laser-light level can be used to ensure that the transducer is parallel with the midaxillary line (phlebostatic axis). Research has shown that estimating the position of the transducer relative to the midaxillary line can lead to inaccurate placement.[32] Errors in measurement can occur if the transducer is placed below the midaxillary line, because the fluid in the system weighs on the transducer, creating additional hydrostatic pressure, and produces a falsely high reading. For every inch the transducer is below the tip of the catheter, the fluid pressure in the system increases the measurement by 1.87 mm Hg. For example, if the transducer is positioned 6 inches below the tip of the catheter, this falsely elevates the displayed pressure by 11 mm Hg.

If the transducer is placed above this atrial level, gravity and lack of fluid pressure give an erroneously low reading. For every inch the transducer is positioned above the catheter tip, the measurement is 1.87 mm Hg less than the true value. If several clinicians are taking measurements, the reference point can be marked on the side of the patient's chest to ensure accurate measurements. When there is a change in the patient's position, the transducer must be leveled again to ensure that accurate hemodynamic pressure measurements are recorded.[31]

Patient Position During Hemodynamic Monitoring

The position of the patient during hemodynamic monitoring would not be an issue if critical care patients remained supine. The emphasis on raising the head of the bed above 30 degrees to prevent aspiration, and position changes to prevent sacral skin pressure injury, requires a re-evaluation of transducer level with each position change.

Head-of-bed backrest position. Nurse researchers have determined that the CVP, pulmonary artery pressure (PAP), and pulmonary artery occlusion pressure (PAOP), also known as *pulmonary artery wedge pressure*, can be reliably measured at head-of-bed backrest positions from 0 (flat) to 60 degrees if the patient is lying on his or her back (supine).[31] If the patient is normovolemic and hemodynamically stable, raising the head of the bed usually does not affect hemodynamic pressure measurements. If the patient is so hemodynamically unstable or hypovolemic that raising the head of the bed negatively affects intravascular volume distribution, the first priority is to correct the hemodynamic instability and leave the patient in a lower backrest position. Most patients do not need the head of the bed to be lowered to 0 degrees to obtain accurate CVP, PAP, or PAOP readings, as long as the midaxillary line is used as the reference point.[31]

Lateral position. The landmarks for leveling the transducer are different if the patient is turned to the side. Researchers have evaluated hemodynamic pressure measurement readings with patients in the 30-degree and 90-degree lateral positions with the head of the bed flat, and they found the measurements to be reliable.[31] In the 30-degree angle position, the landmark to use for leveling the transducer is one-half of the distance from the surface of the bed to the left sternal border.[31] In the 90-degree right-lateral position, the transducer fluid-air interface was positioned at the fourth intercostal space at the midsternum. In the 90-degree left lateral position, the transducer was positioned at the left parasternal border (beside the sternum).[31] It is important to know that measurements can be recorded in nonsupine positions, because critically ill patients must be turned to prevent development of pressure injury and other complications of immobility.

Intraarterial Blood Pressure Monitoring

Indications

Intraarterial BP monitoring is considered minimally invasive compared with catheters placed into a central vein. Arterial BP monitoring is indicated for any major medical or surgical condition that has the potential to alter BP or CO, tissue perfusion, or fluid volume status. The system is designed for continuous measurement of three BP parameters: systole, diastole, and MAP. The direct arterial access is helpful in the management of patients with acute lung failure who require frequent arterial blood gas measurements.[27]

Insertion of an Arterial Catheter

The size of the catheter is proportionate to the diameter of the cannulated artery.

Catheter-over-needle insertion technique. Arterial catheters are often inserted in the smaller arteries, using a "catheter-over-needle" unit in which the needle is used as a temporary guide for catheter placement. With this method, after the unit has been inserted into the artery, the needle is withdrawn, leaving the supple plastic catheter in place. This method is used for catheter insertion and monitoring from the radial artery.

Seldinger insertion technique. To insert a catheter into a larger artery, the Seldinger technique is typically used, which involves the following steps:

- Entry into the artery using a needle
- Passage of a supple guidewire through the needle into the artery
- Removal of the needle
- Passage of the catheter over the guidewire
- Removal of the guidewire, leaving the catheter in the artery

The femoral artery is a large vessel that is cannulated using the Seldinger technique.

Other smaller arteries such as the dorsalis pedis, axillary, or brachial arteries are generally used only when other arterial access is unavailable.[27]

Insertion and Allen test. Several major peripheral arteries are suitable for receiving a catheter and for long-term hemodynamic monitoring. The most frequently used site for arterial pressure monitoring is the radial artery. Before insertion of an arterial catheter in the radial artery, the integrity of the arterial blood supply to the hand is assessed by a procedure known as the modified Allen test as described in Box 10.10.

The major advantage of the radial artery is the supply of collateral circulation to the hand provided by the ulnar artery through the

---

BOX 10.10 Procedure for Assessment of Arterial Blood Supply to the Hand: Allen Test (Modified)

Before a radial artery is punctured or cannulated, the Allen test is performed to assess blood flow to the hand and to ensure that it is adequate.

Allen Test by Visual Inspection

1. If the patient is alert and cooperative, he or she is asked to repeatedly make a tight fist to squeeze the blood out of the hand.
2. The radial artery is compressed with firm thumb pressure by the examiner.
3. The patient is requested to open the hand palm side up while the radial artery is still occluded.
4. Pressure is released, and the time it takes for color to return to the hand is noted.

If the ulnar artery is patent, color will return within 3 seconds. The patient may describe a tingling in the palm as blood flow returns. Delayed color return (a "failed" Allen test) implies that the ulnar artery is inadequate. This means the radial artery is the only reliable source of arterial blood flow to the hand, and therefore it must not be punctured or cannulated.

Allen Test With Pulse Oximetry

1. If the patient is unable to cooperate to make a fist, an alternative approach is to use a pulse oximeter that displays a pulse waveform.
2. Place the pulse oximeter on the patient's middle finger, and establish an adequate pulse amplitude display on the monitor.
3. Simultaneously compress the radial and ulnar arteries until the waveform clearly decreases or vanishes.
4. Release pressure off the ulnar artery only. If the ulnar artery is patent, the pulse amplitude recovers its normal appearance.
5. Repeat the procedure with the radial artery.
6. Arterial catheterization of the radial artery can be accomplished safely only if blood supply to the hand is adequate.

palmar arch in most people. Before radial artery cannulation, collateral circulation must be assessed by using Doppler flow or by the modified Allen test according to institutional protocol. In the Allen test, the radial and ulnar arteries are compressed simultaneously. The patient is asked to clench and unclench the hand until it blanches. One of the arteries is then released, and the hand should immediately flush from that side. The same procedure is repeated for the remaining artery.[27]

Nursing Management

Intraarterial BP monitoring is designed for continuous assessment of arterial perfusion to the major organ systems of the body. MAP is the clinical parameter most often used to assess perfusion, because MAP represents perfusion pressure throughout the cardiac cycle. Because one-third of the cardiac cycle is spent in systole and two-thirds is spent in diastole, the MAP calculation must reflect the greater amount of time spent in diastole. This MAP formula can be calculated by hand or with a calculator, where diastole times 2 plus systole is divided by 3, as shown in the following formula:

$$\frac{(\text{Diastole} \times 2) + (\text{Systole} \times 1)}{3} = \text{MAP}$$

A BP of 120/60 mm Hg produces a MAP of 80 mm Hg. However, the bedside hemodynamic monitor may show a slightly different digital number, because bedside monitoring computers calculate the area under the curve of the arterial line tracing.

Preventing infection in arterial catheters. Infection was once believed to be rare in arterial catheters because of the rapid arterial blood flow. New evidence suggests that an arterial catheters is associated with the same risk of bloodstream infections as a central venous catheter (CVC).[28] Therefore infection prevention measures must be just as meticulous for arterial catheters as for central catheters.[28]

Assessing arterial perfusion pressure. A MAP greater than 60 mm Hg is necessary to perfuse the coronary arteries. A higher MAP may be required to perfuse the brain and the kidneys. A MAP between 70 and 90 mm Hg is preferable for a patient with heart disease to decrease LV workload. After carotid endarterectomy or neurosurgery, a higher MAP of 90 to 110 mm Hg may be more appropriate to increase cerebral perfusion pressure. Systolic and diastolic pressures are monitored in conjunction with the MAP. If CO decreases, the body compensates by constricting peripheral vessels to maintain a stable perfusion pressure. However, the pulse pressure (difference between systolic and diastolic pressures) narrows. The following examples explain this point:

Mr. A: BP 90/70 mm Hg; MAP 76 mm Hg
Mr. B: BP 150/40 mm Hg; MAP 76 mm Hg

Both patients have a mean perfusion pressure of 76 mm Hg, but they are clinically very different. Mr. A is peripherally vasoconstricted, as is demonstrated by the narrow pulse pressure (90/70 mm Hg). His skin is cool to touch, and he has weak peripheral pulses. Mr. B has a wide pulse pressure (150/40 mm Hg), warm skin, and normally palpable peripheral pulses. Nursing assessment includes comparison of clinical findings with arterial line readings.

Interpreting the arterial pressure waveform. As the aortic valve opens, blood is ejected from the left ventricle and is recorded as an increase of pressure in the arterial system producing a characteristic waveform (Fig. 10.9).

- *Systole:* The highest point recorded
- *Dicrotic notch:* A notch visible on the downstroke of the arterial waveform signifies closure of the aortic valve and the start of blood flowing into the arterial vasculature
- *Diastole:* The lowest point recorded

Troubleshooting arterial pressure monitoring problems. Major complications associated with arterial pressure monitoring are rare. The most life-threatening risk is exsanguination if the Luer-Lock connections are not tight or if an in-line stopcock is inadvertently opened to air. Pressure alarm limits must always be active with clinical alarm limits (high and low) set at a safe audible warning range for each patient. See Box 10.11 for Quality and Safety Education for Nurses (QSEN) about Clinical Alarm Systems.

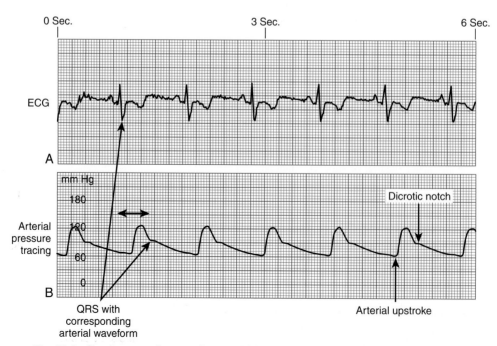

Fig. 10.9 Simultaneous electrocardiogram *(ECG)* (A) and normal arterial pressure (B) tracings.

QSEN

BOX 10.11 Safety

Clinical Alarm Systems
Clinical Alarm System Effectiveness
1. Implement regular preventive maintenance and testing of alarm systems.
2. Ensure that alarms are activated with appropriate settings and are sufficiently audible with respect to distances and competing noise within the unit. (See Alarm Fatigue in Chapter 1.)

Clinical Alarm Safety
Alarm Identification
1. Audible and visual indication should be present for any condition that poses a risk to the patient. Indicators should be visible from at least 10 ft (3 m).
2. Cause of the alarm must be easily identifiable by the health care practitioner.
3. Life-threatening conditions should be clearly differentiated from noncritical alarm situations.
4. High-priority alarms should override low-priority alarms.
5. Alarm must be sufficiently loud or distinctive to be heard over the environmental noise of a busy critical care unit.
6. It should never be possible to turn the volume control to "off."

Disabling and Silencing Alarms
1. Alarm silence must have visual indicator to clearly show it is disabled.
2. Critical alarms should not be permanently overridden (turned "off").
3. New, life-threatening alarm conditions should override a silenced alarm.

Power
Battery units should initiate an alarm before a unit stops working effectively.

Alarm Limits
1. Alarm limits can be adjusted to meet the clinical needs of a patient. The system should default to standard settings between patients.
2. Alarm limits should preferably be displayed on the monitor.

When the digital monitor displays a low BP digital reading, it is a nursing responsibility to determine whether this is a true patient problem or a problem with the monitoring equipment. A damped waveform occurs when communication from the artery to the transducer is interrupted and produces falsely lower values on the monitor and oscilloscope (Table 10.4).

An underdamped arterial waveform produces inaccurate high values due to increased dynamic response or increased oscillations within the system. Other issues that require assessment and troubleshooting are described in Table 10.4.

Fast-flush square waveform test. The dynamic response of the monitoring system can be verified for accuracy at the bedside by the fast-flush square waveform test, also called the *dynamic frequency response test*.[31] The nurse performs this test to ensure that the patient pressures and waveform shown on the bedside monitor are accurate.[31] The test makes use of the manual flush system on the transducer. Normally, the flush device allows only 3 mL of fluid per hour. With the normal waveform displayed, the manual fast-flush procedure is used to generate a rapid increase in pressure, which is displayed on the monitor oscilloscope. As shown in Fig. 10.10, the normal dynamic response waveform shows a square pattern with one or two oscillations before the return of the arterial waveform. If the system is overdamped, a sloped (rather than square) pattern is seen. If the system is underdamped, additional oscillations, or vibrations, are seen

on the fast-flush square wave test. This test can be performed with any hemodynamic monitoring system. If air bubbles, clots, or kinks are in the system, the waveform becomes damped, or flattened, and this is reflected in the square waveform result.

This is an easy test to perform, and it should be incorporated into nursing care procedures at the bedside when the hemodynamic system is first set up, at least once per shift, after opening the system for any reason, and when there is concern about the accuracy of the waveform.[31] If the pressure waveform is distorted or the digital display is inaccurate, the troubleshooting methods described in Table 10.4 can be implemented. The nurse caring for a patient with an arterial line must be able to assess whether a low MAP or narrowed perfusion pressure represents decreased arterial perfusion or equipment malfunction. Assessment of the arterial waveform on the oscilloscope, in combination with clinical assessment, and use of the square waveform test will yield the answer.

Hemodynamic Monitoring Alarm Safety

All critically ill patients must have the hemodynamic monitoring alarms on and adjusted to sound an audible alarm if the patient should experience a change in BP, HR, respiratory rate, or other significant monitored variable. A National Patient Safety Goal mandates reducing harm associated with clinical alarms. Alarm limits must be customized to the patient's physiologic baseline to reduce false-positive alarms. The key issues concerning clinical monitor alarms are presented in Box 10.10.

Invasive Hemodynamic Monitoring

Invasive hemodynamic monitoring refers to monitoring situations where catheters are placed into central veins, or pass through the right-heart chambers (see Fig. 10.7). This predominantly describes CVCs, pulmonary artery catheters, and thermodilution CO. Some of the newer monitoring methods that combine arterial and central venous monitoring systems, also are considered invasive (see Fig. 10.7).

Central Venous Pressure Monitoring
Indications

When a major IV line is required for volume replacement, a CVC is used, because large volumes of fluid can be delivered easily. Because of the risks associated with central lines during insertion and maintenance, this is considered an invasive form of hemodynamic monitoring. The CVC can also be attached to a pressure monitoring system and to monitor the central venous waveform.

Central Venous Catheters

The range of available CVC options includes single-lumen, double-lumen, triple-lumen, and quad-lumen infusion catheters, depending on the specific needs of the patient. CVCs are made from a variety of materials ranging from polyurethane to silicone; most are soft and flexible. Antimicrobial-impregnated or heparin-coated catheters have a lower rate of bloodstream infections.[32]

Insertion Sites

The large veins of the upper thorax, the subclavian (SC) and IJ, are most commonly used for percutaneous CVC line insertion.[29,30] The femoral vein in the groin is used when the thoracic veins are not accessible. All three major sites have different advantages and disadvantages.

Internal jugular vein. The IJ vein is the most frequently used access site for CVC insertion. Compared with the other thoracic veins, it is

TABLE 10.4   Nursing Measures to Ensure Patient Safety and to Troubleshoot Problems With Hemodynamic Monitoring Equipment.

Problem	Prevention	Rationale	Troubleshooting
Overdamping of waveform	Provide continuous infusion of solution containing heparin through an in-line flush device (1 unit of heparin for each 1 mL of flush solution).	Ensure that recorded pressures and waveform are accurate, because a damped waveform gives inaccurate readings.	Before insertion, completely flush the line and/or catheter. In a line attached to a patient, back flush through the system to clear bubbles from tubing or transducer.
Underdamping ("overshoot" or "fling")	Use short lengths of noncompliant tubing. Use fast-flush square wave test to demonstrate optimal system damping. Verify arterial waveform accuracy with the cuff blood pressure.	If the monitoring system is underdamped, the systolic and diastolic values will be overestimated by the waveform and the digital values. False high systolic values may lead to clinical decisions based on erroneous data.	Perform the fast-flush square wave test to verify optimal damping of the monitoring system.
Clot formation at end of the catheter	Provide continuous infusion of solution containing heparin through an in-line flush device (1 unit of heparin for each 1 mL of flush solution).	Any foreign object placed in the body can cause local activation of the patient's coagulation system as a normal defense mechanism. The clots that are formed may be dangerous if they break off and travel to other parts of the body.	If a clot in the catheter is suspected because of a damped waveform or resistance to forward flush of the system, gently aspirate the line using a small syringe inserted into the proximal stopcock. Flush the line again after the clot is removed, and inspect the waveform. It should return to a normal pattern.
Hemorrhage	Use Luer-Lock (screw) connections in-line setup. Close and cap stopcocks when not in use.	A loose connection or open stopcock creates a low-pressure sump effect, causing blood to back into the line and into the open air. If a catheter is accidently removed, the vessel can bleed profusely, especially with an arterial line or if the patient has abnormal coagulation factors (resulting from heparin in the line) or has hypertension.	After a blood leak is recognized, tighten all connections, flush the line, and estimate blood loss.
	Ensure that the catheter is sutured or securely taped in position.		If the catheter has been inadvertently removed, put pressure on the cannulation site. When bleeding has stopped, apply a sterile dressing, estimate blood loss, and inform the physician. If the patient is restless, an armboard may protect lines inserted in the arm.
Air emboli	Ensure that all air bubbles are purged from a new line setup before attachment to an indwelling catheter.	Air can be introduced at several times, including when CVP tubing comes apart, when a new line setup is attached, or when a new CVP or PA line is inserted. During insertion of a CVP or PA line, the patient may be asked to hold his or her breath at specific times to prevent drawing air into the chest during inhalation.	Because it is impossible to get the air back after it has been introduced into the bloodstream, prevention is the best cure.
	Ensure that the drip chamber from the bag of flush solution is more than one-half full before using the in-line, fast-flush system.	In-line, fast-flush devices are designed to permit clearing of blood from the line after withdrawal of blood samples.	If air bubbles occur, they must be vented through the in-line stopcocks, and the drip chamber must be filled.
	Some sources recommend removing all air from the bag of flush solution before assembling the system.	If the chamber of the intravenous tubing is too low or empty, the rapid flow of fluid will create turbulence and cause flushing of air bubbles into the system and into the bloodstream.	The LAP line setup is the only system that includes an air filter specifically to prevent air emboli.

TABLE 10.4 Nursing Measures to Ensure Patient Safety and to Troubleshoot Problems With Hemodynamic Monitoring Equipment.—cont'd

Problem	Prevention	Rationale	Troubleshooting
Normal waveform with *low* digital pressure	Ensure that the system is calibrated to atmospheric pressure.	This will provide a 0 baseline relative to atmospheric pressure.	Recalibrate the equipment if transducer drift has occurred.
	Ensure that the transducer is placed at the level of the phlebostatic axis.	If the transducer has been placed *higher* than the phlebostatic level, gravity and the lack of hydrostatic pressure will produce a false *low* reading.	Reposition the transducer at the level of the phlebostatic axis. Misplacement can occur if the patient moves from the bed to the chair or if the bed is placed in a Trendelenburg position.
Normal waveform with *high* digital pressure	Ensure that the system is calibrated to atmospheric pressure.	This will provide a 0 baseline relative to atmospheric pressure.	Recalibrate the equipment if transducer drift has occurred.
	Ensure that the transducer is placed at the level of the phlebostatic axis.	If the transducer has been placed *lower* than the phlebostatic level, the weight of hydrostatic pressure on the transducer will produce a false *high* reading.	Reposition the transducer at the level of the phlebostatic axis.
			This situation can occur if the head of the bed was raised and the transducer was not repositioned. Some centers require attachment of the transducer to the patient's chest to avoid this problem.
Loss of waveform	Always have the hemodynamic waveform monitored so that changes or loss can be quickly noted.	The catheter may be kinked, or a stopcock may be turned off.	Check the line setup to ensure that all stopcocks are turned in the correct position and that the tubing is not kinked. Sometimes the catheter migrates against a vessel wall, and having the patient change position restores the waveform.

CVP, Central venous pressure; *LAP*, left atrial pressure; *PA*, pulmonary artery.

the easiest to canalize. If the IJ vein is unavailable, the external jugular vein may be accessed, although blood flow is significantly higher in the IJ vein, making it the preferred site. Another advantage of the IJ vein is that the risk of creating an iatrogenic pneumothorax is small. Disadvantages to the IJ vein are patient discomfort from the indwelling catheter when moving the head or neck and contamination of the IJ vein site from oral or tracheal secretions, especially if the patient is intubated or has a tracheostomy.

Subclavian vein. The SC site produces the least patient discomfort from the catheter. The disadvantages are that the SC vein is more difficult to access and carries a higher risk of iatrogenic pneumothorax or hemothorax, although the risk varies greatly depending on the experience and skill of the physician inserting the catheter.

Femoral vein. The femoral vein is considered the easiest cannulation site, because there are no curves in the insertion route. Because there is a higher rate of nosocomial infection with femoral catheters, this site is not recommended.[29,30] If a femoral venous access has been used, the CVC should be changed to either the SC or IJ location as soon as the patient is hemodynamically stable.[29,30]

Insertion

During insertion of a catheter in the SC or IJ vein, the patient may be placed in a Trendelenburg position. Placing the head in a dependent position causes the IJ veins in the neck to become more prominent, facilitating line placement. To minimize the risk of air embolus during the procedure, the patient may be asked to "take a deep breath and hold it" any time the needle or catheter is open to air. The tip of the catheter is designed to remain in the vena cava and should not migrate into the right atrium. Because many patients are awake and alert when a CVC is inserted, a brief explanation about the procedure can minimize patient anxiety and result in cooperation during the insertion. This cooperation is important, because CVC insertion is a sterile procedure and because the supine or Trendelenburg position may be uncomfortable for many patients. The ECG should be monitored during CVC insertion because of the associated risk of dysrhythmias.

All CVCs are designed for placement by percutaneous injection after skin preparation and administration of a local anesthetic. Visualization of the vessel using bedside ultrasound before insertion is recommended to reduce CVC placement attempts.[29,30] A prepackaged CVC kit contains sterile towels, chlorhexidine and alcohol for skin preparation, a needle introducer, a syringe, a guidewire, and a catheter. The Seldinger technique, in which the vein is located by using a "seeking" needle and syringe, is the preferred method of placement. A guidewire is passed through the needle, the needle is removed, and the catheter is passed over the guidewire. After the tip of the catheter is correctly placed in the vena cava, the guidewire is removed. Sterile IV tubing with solution is attached, and the catheter is sutured in place. A

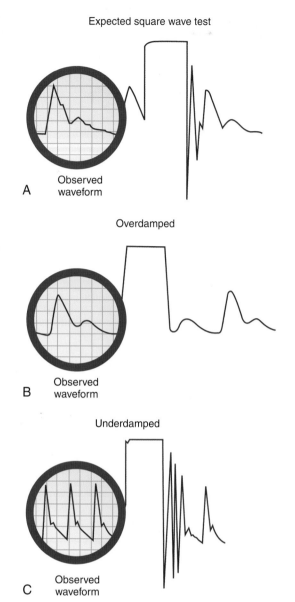

Expected square wave test

A Observed waveform

Overdamped

B Observed waveform

Underdamped

C Observed waveform

Fig. 10.10 Square Wave Test. (A) Expected square wave test result. (B) Overdamped. (C) Underdamped. (From Darovic GO. *Hemodynamic Monitoring: Invasive and Noninvasive Clinical Application.* 3rd ed. Philadelphia: Saunders; 2002.)

chest radiograph is obtained after upper thoracic CVC placement to verify placement and the absence of an iatrogenic hemothorax or pneumothorax, especially if the SC vein was accessed.

Nursing Management

Nursing priorities for the patient with a CVC and CVP monitoring focus on (1) preventing CVC-associated complications, (2) assessing fluid volume status, (3) accommodating changes in patient position, (4) accurately interpreting CVP waveforms, and (5) safely removing CVCs.

Preventing central venous catheter complications. The CVC is an essential tool in the care of a critically ill patient, but it is associated with some risks, and it is the responsibility of all clinicians to be informed about these hazards and to follow hospital procedures to avoid iatrogenic complications. CVC complications include air embolus, catheter-associated thrombus formation, and infection.

Air embolus. The risk of air embolus, although uncommon, is always present for a patient with a central venous line in place. Air can enter during insertion through a disconnected or broken catheter by means of an open stopcock, or air can enter along the path of a removed CVC. This is more likely if the patient is in an upright position because air can be pulled into the venous system with the increase in negative intrathoracic pressure during inhalation. If a large volume of air is inadvertently infused rapidly, it can become trapped in the right ventricular outflow tract, stopping blood flow from the right side of the heart to the lungs. Based on animal studies, this volume is approximately 4 mL/kg, and in humans an air volume of 300 to 500 mL would likely be fatal.[33,34] If the air embolus is large, the patient will experience respiratory distress and cardiovascular collapse. An auscultatory clinical sign specifically associated with a large venous air embolism is the *mill wheel murmur.*[34] A mill wheel murmur is a loud, churning sound heard over the middle chest, caused by a large obstruction to right ventricular outflow. Treatment involves immediately occluding the external site where air is entering, administering 100% oxygen, and placing the patient on the left side with the head downward (left lateral Trendelenburg position).[34] This position displaces the air from the right ventricular outflow tract to the apex of the heart, where the air may be aspirated by catheter intervention or gradually absorbed by the bloodstream as the patient remains in the left lateral Trendelenburg position. Precautions to prevent an air embolism in a central line include using only screw (Luer-Lock) connections and using only closed-top screw caps on all three-way stopcocks.

Thrombus formation. Clot formation (thrombus) at the CVC site is common. Thrombus formation is not uniform; it may involve development of a *fibrin sleeve* around the catheter, or the thrombus may be attached directly to the vessel wall.[35] Other factors that promote clot formation include rupture of vascular endothelium, interruption of laminar blood flow, and physical presence of the catheter, all of which activate the coagulation cascade. Gradual thrombus formation may lead to "sudden" CVC occlusion. Usually, it becomes more difficult to withdraw blood from the CVC, or the CVP waveform becomes intermittently damped over a period of hours or even 1 to 2 days and is reported as "needing frequent flushes" to remain patent. This may be caused by the continued lengthening of a fibrin sleeve that extends along the catheter length from the insertion site past the catheter tip. CVC complications can be additive; for example, the risk of catheter-related infection is increased in the presence of thrombi, where the thrombus likely serves as a culture medium for bacterial growth. Because of concerns over the development of HIT, many hospitals use a saline-only flush to maintain CVC patency.

Central line–associated bloodstream infection. Infection related to the use of CVCs is a major problem, commonly known as *central line–associated bloodstream infection (CLABSI).* The infection incidence strongly correlates with the length of time the CVC has been inserted, with longer insertion times associated with higher infection rates.[29,30] CVC-related infection is identified at the catheter insertion site or as a bloodstream infection (septicemia). Systemic manifestations of infection can be present without inflammation at the catheter site. No decrease in bloodstream infections was found when catheters were routinely changed, and this practice is no longer recommended.[29,30] When a CVC is infected, it must be removed, and a new catheter must be inserted in a different site. If a catheter infection is suspected, the CVC should not be changed over a guidewire because of the risk of transferring the infection.[29,30]

Most infections are transmitted from the skin, and infection prevention begins before insertion of the CVC. Insertion guidelines state that the physician must use effective handwashing procedures, clean the insertion site with 2% chlorhexidine gluconate in 70% isopropyl, use sterile technique during catheter insertion, and maintain maximal sterile barrier precautions.[29,30] In most hospitals, the nurse is authorized to stop the insertion procedure if these insertion infection control guidelines are not followed. A daily review to determine whether the central line is still required is recommended to ensure that CVCs are removed promptly when no longer needed (Box 10.12—**QSEN** Safety Box: Prevention of CLABSI).[29] All clinicians must use good handwashing technique and follow aseptic procedures during site care and any time the CVC system is entered to withdraw blood, administer medications, or change tubing.[29,30] Site dressings impregnated with chlorhexidine are recommended to reduce CVC infection rates.[29,30] To decrease the infection risk, most hospitals routinely audit use of CVCs to reduce the CVC duration to the absolute minimum, as fewer insertion days means fewer CLABSIs.[36]

Assessing fluid volume status. Use of the CVP value to assess volume status is considered inaccurate.[37] A landmark systematic review of the literature revealed a weak relationship between the CVP measurement and blood volume.[37] Furthermore, a low CVP value is not always reliable in predicting which patients will respond to a fluid challenge.[37] Among patients with a CVP between 0 and 5 mm Hg, up to 25% do not respond to a fluid challenge as expected.[38] Only approximately

half of critically ill patients respond as expected to a fluid challenge.[37] In this situation, the clinician must look at other indices of poor tissue perfusion such as an elevated lactate level, low base deficit, or decreased urine output.[38]

Passive leg raise. Another method to assess fluid responsiveness is to passively raise and support the patient's legs to allow the venous blood from the lower extremities to flow rapidly into the vena cava and return to the right heart. This method has the advantage of not infusing any IV fluid.[39] If this maneuver significantly increases the CVP, this may suggest that the patient would have a positive response to an IV fluid bolus.[40] However, a change in the CVP value is not considered as reliable as using real-time monitoring of CO using a pulse wave analysis method, as described later.[39]

Accommodating changes in patient position. To achieve accurate CVP measurements, the midaxillary line (phlebostatic axis) is used as a reference point on the body, and the transducer or water manometer zero must be level with this point. If the midaxillary line is used and the transducer is correctly aligned, any head-of-bed position up to 60 degrees may be used for accurate CVP readings for most patients who are hemodynamically stable. Elevating the head of the bed is especially helpful for a patient with cardiopulmonary illness who cannot tolerate a flat position.

Interpreting central venous pressure waveforms. The normal right atrial (CVP) waveform has three positive deflections—a, c, and v waves—that correspond to specific atrial events in the cardiac cycle (Fig. 10.11). The *a*

QSEN | BOX 10.12 **Safety**

Prevention of Central Line–Associated Bloodstream Infections (CLABSI)

1. **Education, Training, and Staffing**
   a. Nurses and other health care providers should receive education about indications for central venous catheter (CVC) use, maintenance, and infection prevention.
   b. Only trained personnel should insert and maintain CVCs.
   c. Adequate staffing levels in critical care units are associated with fewer catheter-related bloodstream infections (CRBSIs).
2. **Selection of Catheters and Sites**
   a. Use subclavian site rather than jugular or femoral insertion sites to minimize infection risk.
   b. Use ultrasound guidance to place CVCs.
   c. Remove any catheter that is no longer essential.
   d. If a CVC was placed in a medical emergency when aseptic technique was not assured, replace CVC within 48 hours.
3. **Hand Hygiene and Aseptic Technique**
   a. Perform hand hygiene procedures by washing hands with soap and water or alcohol-based hand rub (ABHR) before and after palpating the CVC site, dressing the site, or any other intervention.
   b. New sterile gloves must be worn by the professional inserting the CVC.
   c. New sterile gloves must be donned before touching a new catheter for CVC exchange over a guidewire.
   d. Wear clean or sterile gloves when changing the catheter dressing.
4. **Maximal Sterile Barrier Precautions**
   a. For insertion, use maximal sterile barrier precautions including cap, mask, sterile gown, sterile gloves, and full-body drape.
5. **Skin Preparation**
   a. Prepare clean skin with greater than 0.5% chlorhexidine preparation with alcohol before CVC insertion.

   b. Antiseptics should be allowed to dry according to the manufacturer's recommendation before CVC insertion.
6. **Catheter Site Dressing Regimens**
   a. Transparent, semipermeable polyurethane dressings permit continuous visualization of the CVC insertion site.
   b. Replace transparent dressings on CVC sites at least every 7 days.
   c. Monitor the site when changing the dressing or by palpation through an intact dressing.
   d. Replace catheter site dressing whenever the dressing becomes damp, loose, or soiled.
   e. Do not use topical antibiotic ointment or creams on insertion sites (except for dialysis catheters) because of increased fungal infection risk.
   f. Use a chlorhexidine-impregnated sponge dressing at CVC site if CRBSI rate is not decreasing by other means (no recommendation for other types of chlorhexidine dressings).
7. **Cleansing of the Insertion Site**
   a. Use 2% chlorhexidine wash for daily skin cleaning to reduce CRBSIs.
8. **Catheter Securement Device**
   a. Use a sutureless catheter securement device to reduce catheter movement, which may reduce infection risk.
9. **Antimicrobial Strategies**
   a. Use an antimicrobial-impregnated CVC when catheters are expected to remain in place for longer than 5 days.
   b. Do not administer systemic antimicrobial prophylaxis to prevent CRBSIs.
   c. Do not routinely use anticoagulant therapy to prevent CRBSIs.
10. **No Routine CVC Replacement**
   a. Do not routinely replace CVCs.
   b. Do not replace CVCs on the basis of fever alone.

From O'Grady NP, Alexander M, Burns LA, et al. Guidelines for the prevention of intravascular catheter-related infections. *Am J Infect Control.* 2011;39(4):S1–S34.

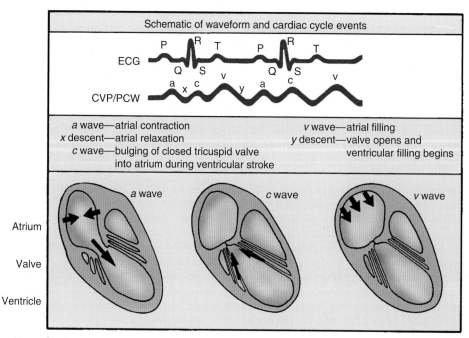

Fig. 10.11 Cardiac Events That Produce Central Venous Pressure Waveform With *a, c,* and *v* Waves. The *a* wave represents atrial contraction. The *x* descent represents atrial relaxation. The *c* wave represents the bulging of the closed tricuspid valve into the right atrium during ventricular systole. The *v* wave represents atrial filling. The *y* descent represents opening of the tricuspid valve and filling of the ventricle. *CVP,* Central venous pressure; *ECG,* electrocardiogram; *PCW,* pulmonary capillary wedge pressure.

wave reflects atrial contraction and follows the P wave seen on the ECG. The downslope of this wave is called the *x descent* and represents atrial relaxation. The *c wave* reflects the bulging of the closed tricuspid valve into the right atrium during ventricular contraction; this wave is small and not always visible but corresponds to the QRS-T interval on the ECG. The *v wave* represents atrial filling and increased pressure against the closed tricuspid valve in early diastole. The downslope of the v wave is named the *y descent* and represents the fall in pressure as the tricuspid valve opens and blood flows from the right atrium to the right ventricle.

Cannon waves. Dysrhythmias can change the pattern of the CVP waveform. In a junctional rhythm or following a premature ventricular contraction (PVC), the atria are depolarized after the ventricles when retrograde conduction to the atria occurs. This may be seen as a retrograde P wave on the ECG and as a large combined *ac* or *cannon wave* on the CVP waveform (Fig. 10.12). These cannon waves are observed as large pulses in the jugular veins. Other pathologic conditions, such as advanced right ventricular failure or tricuspid valve insufficiency, allow regurgitant backflow of blood from the right ventricle to the right atrium during ventricular contraction, producing large v waves on the right atrial waveform. In atrial fibrillation, the CVP waveform has no recognizable pattern because of the disorganization of the atrial rhythm.

Safely removing central venous catheters. Removal of the CVC usually is a nursing responsibility. Complications are uncommon, and the ones to anticipate are bleeding and air embolus. Recommended techniques to avoid air embolus during CVC removal include removing the catheter when the patient is supine in bed (not in a chair) and placing the patient flat if tolerated. Patients with heart failure, pulmonary disease, and neurologic conditions with raised intracranial pressure should not be placed flat. If the patient is alert and able to cooperate, he or she is asked to take a deep breath to raise intrathoracic pressure during removal. After removal, to decrease the risk of air entering by a "track" or bleeding, firm pressure is applied, and the site is covered by an occlusive dressing.

Pulmonary Artery Pressure Monitoring

The pulmonary artery catheter (PA-Catheter) is the most invasive of the critical care monitoring catheters (see Fig. 10.7). It is also known as a *right-heart catheter* or *Swan-Ganz catheter* (named after the catheter's inventors).[41] PA-Catheters are predominantly inserted during open-heart surgery,[42] in management of acute heart failure,[43,44] and in management of acute pulmonary hypertension. The PA-Catheter is invasive. It previously seemed intuitive that the diagnostic information provided would confer a survival advantage over less-invasive methods, but research has shown this is not the case.[45] Consequently routine use of PA-Catheters has decreased dramatically.[45]

In noncardiac critical care units, the PA-Catheter has been replaced by less-invasive technologies, discussed later in this chapter.

Indications

The thermodilution PA-Catheter is reserved for the most hemodynamically unstable patients for the diagnosis and evaluation of cardiogenic shock, pulmonary hypertension, and management during and after heart surgery.[45] The PA-Catheter can provide information about PAP (systolic, diastolic, mean), PAOP (wedge pressure), and CO.

The traditional PA-Catheter, invented by Swan and Ganz, has four lumens that obtain different measurements from different locations: Right atrial pressure (similar to CVP), PAP, PAOP, and CO (Fig. 10.13A). Multifunction PA-Catheters may have additional lumens, which can be used for IV infusion and to measure continuous mixed venous oxygen, right ventricular volume, and continuous CO

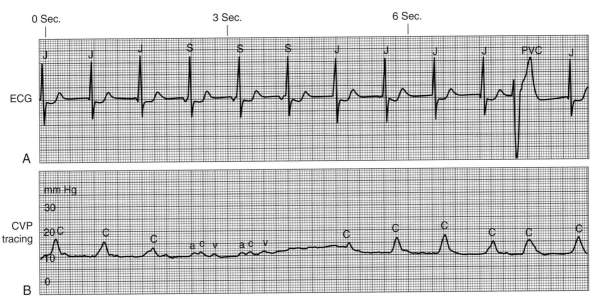

Fig. 10.12 Simultaneous electrocardiogram *(ECG)* (A) and central venous pressure *(CVP)* (B) tracings. The CVP waveform shows large cannon waves corresponding to the junctional beats or premature ventricular contractions *(bottom strip)*. When there are retrograde p waves present, the CVP waveform has a normal configuration. *ac,* Normal right atrial pressure tracing; *C,* cannon waves on CVP tracing; *J,* junctional rhythm followed by cannon waves on CVP waveform; *PVC,* premature ventricular contraction followed by cannon wave on CVP; *S,* retrograde p waves, produce an atrial contraction as evidenced by the normal CVP tracing with a, c, and v waves.

(Fig. 10.13C). Other PA-Catheters include transvenous pacing electrodes to pace the heart if needed.

The PA-Catheter is typically a 110 cm in length. The usual size for adults is 7.5 or 8.0 Fr, although 5.0 and 7.0 Fr sizes are available. Each of the four lumens exits into the heart or pulmonary artery at a different point, graduated along the catheter length.

Right atrial lumen. The proximal lumen is situated in the right atrium and is used for IV infusion, CVP measurement, withdrawal of venous blood samples, and injection of fluid for CO determinations. This port is often described as the *right atrial port.*

Pulmonary artery lumen. The distal PA lumen is located at the tip of the PA-Catheter and is situated in the pulmonary artery. It is used to record pressures within the pulmonary artery.

Balloon lumen. The third lumen opens into a balloon at the end of the catheter that can be inflated with 0.8 mL (7 Fr) to 1.5 mL (7.5 Fr) of air. The balloon is inflated during catheter insertion after the catheter reaches the right atrium to assist in forward flow of the catheter and to minimize right ventricular ectopy from the catheter tip. The balloon is also inflated to obtain the PAOP measurements when the PA-Catheter is correctly positioned in the pulmonary artery.

Thermistor lumen. The fourth lumen is a thermistor (temperature sensor) used to measure changes in blood temperature. It is located 4 cm from the catheter tip and is used to measure thermodilution CO.

Insertion. If a PA-Catheter is to be inserted into a patient who is awake, some brief explanations about the procedure are helpful to ensure that the patient understands what is going to happen. The initial insertion techniques used for placement of a PA-Catheter are similar to those described for CVC insertion. Because the PA-Catheter passes within the right-heart chambers and pulmonary artery, the catheter insertion is monitored using fluoroscopy or waveform analysis on the bedside monitor (Fig. 10.14). In most insertions, the PA-Catheter floats into the right pulmonary artery.

Before inserting the catheter into the vein, the physician—using sterile technique—tests the balloon for inflation and flushes the catheter with physiologic saline to remove any air. The PA-Catheter is then attached to the bedside hemodynamic line setup and monitor so that the waveforms can be visualized as the catheter is advanced through the right side of the heart (see Fig. 10.14). A larger introducer sheath (8.5 Fr), which has the tip positioned in the vena cava and has an additional IV side-port lumen, is often used to cannulate the vein first. This introducer sheath is known by several different names in clinical practice, including *sheath, cordis, introducer,* or *side port.* This introducer sheath remains in place, and the supple PA-Catheter is threaded through it into the vena cava and into the right side of the heart.

Nursing Management

Nursing priorities for the patient with a PA-Catheter focus on (1) accurately interpreting pulmonary artery waveforms, (2) verifying PA-Catheter position, (3) accommodating changes in patient position, (4) recognizing respiratory changes on waveforms, (5) preventing PA-Catheter associated complications, (6) monitoring cardiac output, (7) evaluating hemodynamic performance, and (8) safely removing the PA-Catheter.

Accurately interpreting pulmonary artery waveforms. Each chamber of the heart has a distinctive waveform with recognizable characteristics. It is the responsibility of the critical care nurse to recognize each waveform displayed on the bedside monitor when the catheter enters the corresponding chamber during insertion and during routine monitoring. The waveforms are monitored in sequence during the PA-Catheter insertion procedure.

Right atrial waveform. As the PA-Catheter is advanced into the right atrium during insertion, a right atrial waveform must be visible on the monitor, with recognizable a, c, and v waves (see Fig. 10.14). Normal mean pressure in the right atrium is 2 to 5 mm Hg. Before

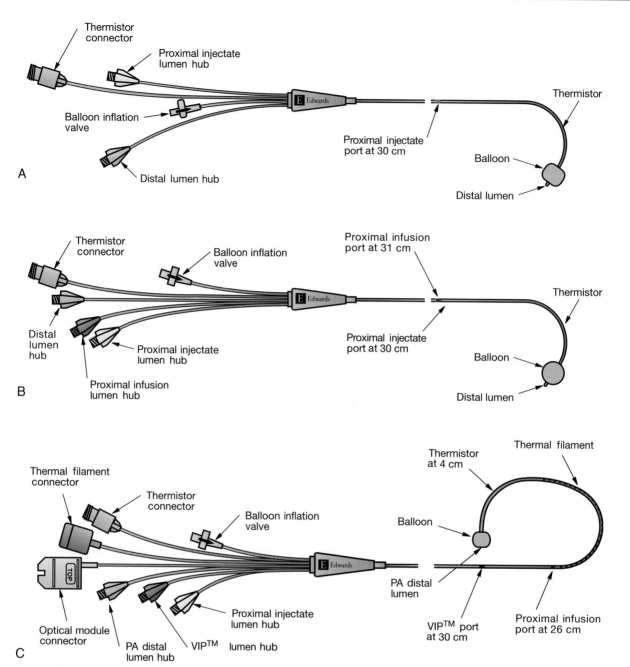

Fig. 10.13 Types of Pulmonary Artery Catheters. (A) Four-lumen catheter. (B) Five-lumen catheter that includes additional venous infusion port *(VIP)* into the right atrium. (C) Seven-lumen catheter that includes a VIP port and two additional lumens, as well as a thermal filament for continuous cardiac output (CCO) and internal fiberoptic strands for continuous mixed venous oxygen saturation (Svo$_2$) monitoring (i.e., optical module connector). An additional option is to combine the use of the CCO filament and the thermistor response time to calculate continuous right ventricular end-diastolic volume and right ventricular ejection fraction. *PA*, Pulmonary artery. (Copyright 2001 Edwards Lifesciences LLC. All rights reserved. Reprinted with permission of Edwards Lifesciences, Swan-Ganz is a trademark of Edwards Lifesciences Corporation, registered in the US Patent and Trademark Office.)

passage through the tricuspid valve, the balloon at the tip of the catheter is inflated for two reasons. First, it cushions the pointed tip of the PA-Catheter so that if the tip touches the right ventricular wall, it will cause less myocardial irritability and consequently fewer ventricular dysrhythmias. Second, inflation of the balloon assists the catheter to float with the flow of blood from the right ventricle into the pulmonary artery. Because of these features and the balloon, PA-Catheters are also described as *flow-directional catheters.*

Right ventricular waveform. The right ventricular waveform is distinctly pulsatile, with distinct systolic and diastolic pressures. Normal right ventricular pressures are 20 to 30 mm Hg systolic and 0 to 5 mm Hg diastolic. Even with the balloon inflated, it is common

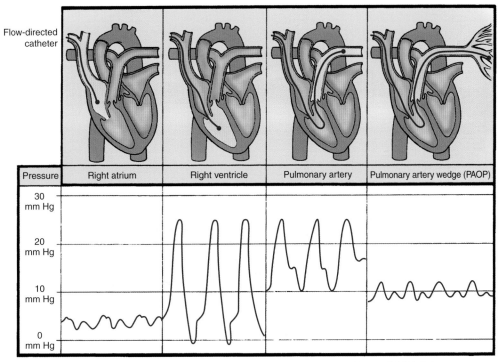

Fig. 10.14 Pulmonary Artery Catheter Insertion With Corresponding Waveforms. *PAOP,* Pulmonary artery occlusion pressure.

for ventricular ectopy to occur during passage through the right ventricle. All patients who have a PA-Catheter inserted must have simultaneous ECG monitoring, with defibrillator and emergency resuscitation equipment nearby.

Pulmonary artery waveform. As the catheter enters the pulmonary artery, the waveform again changes. The diastolic pressure rises. Normal pressures in the pulmonary artery range from 20 to 30 mm Hg systolic over 10 mm Hg diastolic. A dicrotic notch, visible on the downslope of the waveform, represents closure of the pulmonic valve.

Pulmonary artery occlusion waveform (wedge). While the balloon remains inflated, the catheter is advanced into the wedge position. This maneuver produces the PAOP. The waveform decreases in size and is nonpulsatile, reflecting a normal left atrial tracing with a and v wave deflections. This is known as a *wedge tracing* because the balloon is "wedged" into a small pulmonary vessel, but it is technically described as the PAOP (see Fig. 10.14). The balloon occludes the pulmonary vessel so that the PA-Catheter tip and lumen are exposed only to left atrial pressure and are protected from the pulsatile influence of the right ventricle and pulmonary artery. When the balloon is deflated, the catheter should spontaneously float back into the pulmonary artery. When the balloon is reinflated, the catheter should move forward into a small artery and the wedge tracing should be visible on the monitor. Normal PAOP ranges from 5 to 12 mm Hg.

Verifying pulmonary artery catheter position. After insertion, the introducer is sutured to the skin, and the catheter, which lies within the introducer, is secured with a catheter securement device. If the tip of the PA-Catheter is advanced too far into the pulmonary microvasculature, the patient is at risk for pulmonary infarction. If the PA-Catheter is not advanced sufficiently into the pulmonary artery, it will not be useful for PAOP readings.

PAD-PADP relationship. In many critical care units, if the patient's pulmonary artery diastolic pressure (PADP) and PAOP values are approximate (within 0–3 mm Hg), the PADP is reliably used to

follow the trend of LV filling pressure (preload). This practice prevents possible trauma from frequent balloon inflation; in such a situation, the PA-Catheter is consciously pulled back into a safe position within the pulmonary artery so that wedging cannot occur.

PA-Catheter position. After insertion of the catheter, the chest radiograph or fluoroscopy is used to verify the PA-Catheter position to ensure that it is not looped or knotted in the right ventricle and to rule out pneumothorax or hemorrhagic complications. A thin plastic sleeve is placed on the outside of the catheter when it is inserted to maintain sterility of the part of the PA-Catheter that exits from the patient. If the PA-Catheter is not in the desired position or if it migrates out of position, it can be repositioned. Use of this external sleeve on PA-Catheters has been associated with lower rates of bloodstream infection.[32]

Accommodating changes in patient position with a PA-Catheter. The patient does not need to be flat for accurate pressure readings to be obtained. In the supine position, when the transducer is placed at the level of the midaxillary line (phlebostatic axis), a head-of-bed position from flat up to 60 degrees is appropriate for most patients.[31] PADP and PAOP measurements in the lateral position may be significantly different from measurements taken when the patient is lying supine. If there is concern about the validity of pressure readings in a particular patient, it is more reliable to take measurements with the patient on his or her back, with the head of bed elevated from flat to 60 degrees as tolerated. After a patient changes position, a stabilization period of 5 to 15 minutes is recommended before taking pressure readings.[31]

Recognizing respiratory variation in pulmonary artery waveforms. All PADP and PAOP (wedge) tracings are subject to respiratory interference, especially when the patient is on a positive-pressure, volume-cycled ventilator. During the positive-pressure inhalation phase, the increase in intrathoracic pressure may "push up" the PA-Catheter tracing, producing an artificially high reading (Fig. 10.15A). During

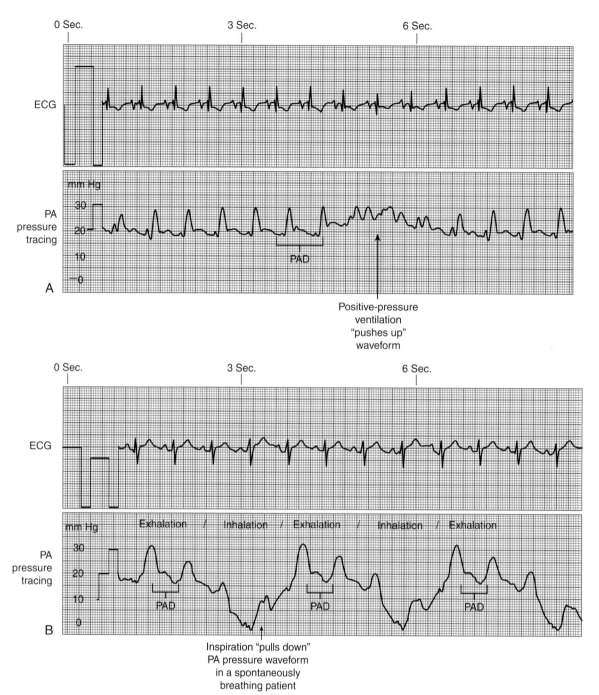

Fig. 10.15 Pulmonary Artery *(PA)* Waveforms That Demonstrate the Effect of Mechanical Ventilation on PA Pressures. For accuracy, PA pressures are read at the end of exhalation. (A) In positive-pressure ventilation, the increase in intrathoracic pressure during inhalation "pushes up" the PA waveform, creating a falsely high reading. (B) In spontaneous breathing, the decrease in intrathoracic pressure during normal inhalation "pulls down" the PA waveform, creating a falsely low reading. *ECG,* Electrocardiogram; *PADP,* pulmonary artery diastolic pressure.

inhalation with spontaneous breaths, negative intrathoracic pressure "pulls down" the waveform, producing an erroneously low measurement (Fig. 10.15B). To minimize the effect of respiratory variation, the PADP is read at end-expiration, which is the most stable point in the respiratory cycle when intrapleural pressures are close to zero. If the digital number fluctuates with respiration, a printed readout on paper can be obtained to verify true PADP. In

some clinical settings, ECG signals or airway pressure and flow are recorded simultaneously with the PADP/PAOP tracing to identify end-expiration.[31] Respiratory variation on the PA-Catheter waveform is particularly noticeable with larger tidal volumes.

Positive end-expiratory pressure. Some clinical diagnoses, such as acute respiratory distress syndrome (ARDS), require the use of high levels of positive end-expiratory pressure (PEEP) set with the ventilator to treat refractory hypoxemia. If a PEEP of greater than 10 cm H_2O is used, PAOP (wedge) and PAPs will be artificially elevated, and CO may be negatively affected. However, it is important *not* to disconnect a patient from the ventilator just to record PAP measurements, because this will close alveoli, will decrease the patient's oxygenation level, and may result in persistent hypoxemia.

Because patients remain on PEEP for treatment, they remain on it during measurement of PAP. In this situation, the trend of PA-Catheter readings is more important than one individual measurement. The trend of the measurements is used as a basis for clinical interventions to support and improve cardiopulmonary function in the critically ill patient.

Preventing pulmonary artery catheter complications. Potential cardiac complications include ventricular dysrhythmias, endocarditis, valvular damage, cardiac rupture, and cardiac tamponade. Serious pulmonary complications include rupture of a PA-Catheter balloon, thrombosis, embolism or hemorrhage of the pulmonary artery, and infarction of a segment of lung. The PA-Catheter tracing is continuously monitored to ensure that the catheter does not migrate forward into a spontaneous wedge or PAOP position. A segment of lung can infarct if the wedged catheter occludes a segment of the lung vasculature for a prolonged period. If the catheter is spontaneously wedged, the catheter must be gently pulled back out of the wedge position to prevent pulmonary infarction.

Infection is always a risk with a PA-Catheter, as it is considered a central line (see Box 10.12).

Measuring cardiac output with a pulmonary artery catheter. The PA-Catheter is used to measure CO using an intermittent bolus method, or by a continuous readout from thermistors incorporated into the catheter.

Thermodilution cardiac output bolus measurement. The bolus thermodilution method is performed at the bedside and results in CO calculated in liters per minute. Three CO values that are within a 10% mean range are obtained at one time and are averaged to calculate CO. The thermodilution CO is very accurate when several injectate values are averaged.[46] A known amount, usually 10 mL, of room temperature physiologic saline solution is injected into the proximal lumen of the PA-Catheter. The injectate exits into the right atrium and travels with the flow of blood past the thermistor (temperature sensor) located at the distal end of the PA-Catheter. The injectate is delivered by hand injection from a closed in-line system attached to a 500-mL bag of 0.9% saline to deliver the individual injections (bolus method).

Cardiac output curve. The thermodilution CO method uses the indicator-dilution method, in which a known temperature is the indicator. It is based on the principle that the change in temperature over time is inversely proportional to blood flow. Blood flow can be diagrammatically represented as a CO curve on which temperature is plotted against time (Fig. 10.16). Most hemodynamic monitors display this CO curve, which must then be interpreted to determine whether the CO injection is valid. The normal curve has a smooth upstroke, with a rounded peak and a gradually tapering downslope. If the curve has an uneven pattern, it may indicate faulty injection technique, and the CO measurement must be repeated. Patient movement or coughing also alters the CO measurement.

Injectate temperature. If the CO is within the normal range, it is equally accurate whether iced or room temperature injectate is used. However, if the CO values are extremely high or very low, iced injectate may be more accurate. To ensure accurate readings, the difference between injectate temperature and body temperature must be at least 10°C, and the injectate must be delivered within 4 seconds, with minimal handling of the syringe to prevent warming of the

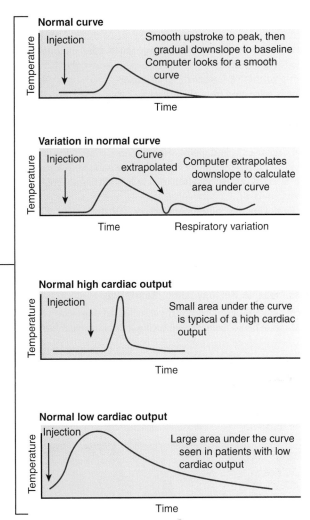

Fig. 10.16 A Cardiac Thermodilution Bolus Output Curve.

solution. This is particularly important if iced injectate is used. With all delivery systems, the injectate is delivered at the same point in the respiratory cycle, usually end-exhalation.

Patient position and cardiac output. In a stable patient with a normal volume status, reliable CO measurements can be obtained in a supine position (patient lying on his or her back) with the head of the bed elevated up to 60 degrees. If the patient is hypovolemic or unstable, leaving the head of the bed in a flat position or only slightly elevated is the most clinically appropriate choice. CO measurements performed when the patient is turned to the side are not considered as accurate as measurements performed with the patient in the supine position.

Clinical conditions that alter cardiac output. Two clinical conditions produce errors in the thermodilution CO measurement: tricuspid valve regurgitation and ventricular septal rupture. If the patient has tricuspid valve regurgitation, the expected flow of blood from the right atrium to the pulmonary artery is disrupted by backflow from the right ventricle to the right atrium. This creates a lower CO measurement than the patient's actual output. If the person has an intracardiac left-to-right shunt, as occurs after ventricular septal rupture, the thermodilution CO measures the large right-to-left shunt volume and records a higher CO than the patient's true systemic output.

Continuous invasive cardiac output measurement. The bolus thermodilution method is reliable but performed intermittently.

Continuous CO monitoring using a PA-Catheter is also frequently used in clinical practice. One method uses a thermal filament on the PA-Catheter to emit small energy signals (the indicator) into the bloodstream. These signals are then detected by the thermistor near the tip of the PA-Catheter. An indicator curve is created, and a CO value is calculated from these data.

Calculated hemodynamic profiles using a pulmonary artery catheter. For a patient with a thermodilution PA-Catheter in place, additional hemodynamic information can be calculated using routine vital signs, CO, and body surface area. These measurements are calculated using specific formulas that are indexed to a patient's body size. Selected calculated values used in hemodynamic profiles are listed in Appendix B.

Removing the pulmonary artery catheter safely. PA-Catheters can be safely removed from the patient by critical care nurses competent in this procedure.[31] Removal is not usually associated with major complications. Rarely, PVCs occur as the catheter is pulled through the right ventricle.[31]

Less-Invasive Hemodynamic Monitoring

Tremendous progress has been made in the development of less-invasive methods of hemodynamic monitoring. The newer monitoring methods range from completely noninvasive to methods that, although less invasive than a PA-Catheter, involve insertion of intravascular catheters or esophageal probes to gather monitoring information (Table 10.5). All newer monitoring methods that estimate CO have been compared with the PA-Catheter thermodilution CO method.

The latest innovation is to provide a suite of hemodynamic monitoring options using similar technologies with different ranges of invasiveness, as diagrammed in Fig. 10.7. This range of hemodynamic options allows the critical care team to tailor the invasiveness and diagnostic capabilities of the monitoring system to the clinical needs of the patient.

Arterial Waveform—Based Hemodynamic Monitoring and Cardiac Output Methods

Arterial pressure—based systems are revolutionizing hemodynamic monitoring as proprietary technologies from different companies showcase new technologies with options ranging from noninvasive to invasive (see Fig. 10.7 and Table 10.5).

Finger cuff hemodynamic monitoring systems. Finger cuff systems are noninvasive and trend continuous BP, stroke volume (SV), stroke volume variation (SVV), and CO. These systems are designed for short-term use to monitor hemodynamic variables without inserting

---

TABLE 10.5 Cardiac Output Measurement: Noninvasive and Minimally Invasive Methods.

Device Name	Probe Placement	Method	Cardiac Output Calculation	Clinical Issues
Noninvasive Methods				
Bioimpedance	External electrodes placed on the neck and chest	Thoracic electrical bioimpedance	A small alternating current is applied across the chest by skin electrodes.	Noninvasive
Pressure and Pulse Contour (ClearSight, Edwards Lifesciences, CA)	Fingers	External finger cuffs	Pulsatile changes in thoracic blood volume result in changes in electrical impedance. The rate of change of impedance during systole is measured and used to calculate CO. Pulsatile changes on finger arteries are used to calculate BP, CO, SVV.	Less accurate with low body temperature. One cuff used up to 8 hours on a finger. With two cuffs, change fingers each hour.
Minimally Invasive Methods				
Pulse Contour Waveform Methods				
LiDCO (LiDCO Ltd., Cambridge, United Kingdom)	Requires a venous access catheter (central or peripheral) and an arterial catheter with a lithium-monitoring sensor attached (calibrated)	Pulse contour waveform analysis method (calibrated)	Independent calibration with a lithium dilution technique is initially required. A small, subtherapeutic dose of isotonic lithium chloride is injected through the venous catheter. The lithium is detected at the arterial sensor (femoral artery), where a fixed flow pump ensures constant flow. A concentration-time curve is produced for lithium before recirculation. CO is calculated based on lithium dose given and the measurement of the area under the curve. A noncalibrated system is also available.	Easy to set up; uses conventional venous and arterial catheters. Can measure extravascular lung water for patients with pulmonary edema. CO measurement affected by artifact on arterial waveform and by irregular and damped arterial waveforms. Can be used in conscious and in unresponsive patients. Requires calibration at least every 8 hours to maintain accuracy; cannot be used in patients on lithium therapy because this interferes with calibration

TABLE 10.5 Cardiac Output Measurement: Noninvasive and Minimally Invasive Methods.—cont'd

Device Name	Probe Placement	Method	Cardiac Output Calculation	Clinical Issues
PiCCO (Pulsion Medical Systems, Munich, Germany)	Requires a central venous access catheter and uses a specialized arterial thermistor-tipped catheter in the femoral artery	Pulse contour waveform analysis method that uses transpulmonary thermodilution	A set volume of cold saline is injected through the central venous catheter. The arterial thermistor-tipped catheter detects the blood temperature change. Continuous CO measurements are achieved by analyzing the systolic component of the arterial waveform. A noncalibrated system is also available.	CO measurement affected by artifact on arterial waveform and irregular arterial waveforms. Three calibrations required initially; frequent recalibration required to maintain accuracy
FloTrac, Vigileo (Edward Lifesciences, Irvine, CA)	Requires a functional arterial catheter	Pulse contour waveform analysis method (does not require calibration)	Calculates CO by use of arterial pressure waveform analysis in conjunction with patient data (age, sex, height, weight). Uses an internal proprietary algorithm based on the principle that pulse pressure (difference between systolic and diastolic pressure) is proportional to SV and inversely proportional to aortic compliance. Aortic pressure is sampled at 100 Hz and is updated every 20 seconds.	Does not require external calibration, but requires zeroing of the transducer. Lack of calibration procedures controversial

Esophageal Probe Methods

Device Name	Probe Placement	Method	Cardiac Output Calculation	Clinical Issues
Esophageal Doppler	Ultrasound probe placed in the lower esophagus	SV calculated by measurement of the aortic blood velocity in the descending thoracic aorta (by continuous wave Doppler) plus calculation of the cross-sectional area of the aorta; CO calculated based on these values	The aorta cross-sectional area, measured using M-mode ultrasound, is multiplied by blood velocity to calculate flow or CO. The value of total CO is derived from a nomogram using aortic blood velocity, height, weight, and age.	Useful in the operating room or with deeply sedated patients. Stiff probe; placement not well tolerated by conscious patients
TEE	Ultrasound probe placed in esophagus	Probe placement allows imaging of LV outflow tract; SV measured by Doppler	The LV outflow tract area is measured; this value is squared and multiplied by the velocity time interval of blood flow and HR. LV SV can be measured, as can HR to use the SV × HR = CO formula.	Useful in the operating room or with deeply sedated patients. Stiff probe; placement not well tolerated by conscious patients. Requires skill to accurately position probe to visualize LV outflow tract

Partial CO_2 Rebreathing Method

Device Name	Probe Placement	Method	Cardiac Output Calculation	Clinical Issues
NICO$_2$ (Philips, Respironics) Amsterdam, Netherlands	Addition of partial CO_2 rebreathing circuit to ventilator	Partial CO_2 rebreathing method	CO measurement is based on changes in respiratory CO_2 concentration obtained from a short period of rebreathing. CO_2 elimination is calculated by sensors that measure flow, airway pressure, and CO_2 concentration. These variables are used in the Fick partial rebreathing formula to calculate CO.	Can be used only in intubated and ventilated patients. Specialized additional tubing setup on ventilator. Cannot be used in patients who cannot tolerate hypercapnia (elevated CO_2). CO measurement altered by intrapulmonary shunt

BP, Blood pressure; *CO,* cardiac output; *CO_2,* carbon dioxide; *HR,* heart rate; *LV,* left ventricular; *SV,* stroke volume; *SVV,* stroke volume variation; *TEE,* transesophageal echocardiography.

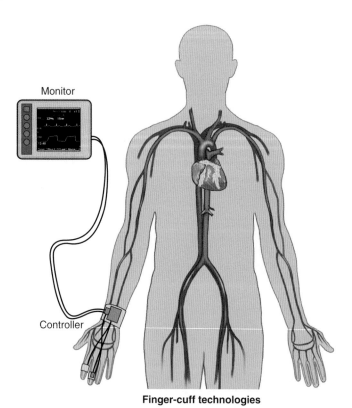

Finger-cuff technologies

Fig. 10.17 Finger Cuff Arterial Pressure—Based Monitoring. Noninvasive systems that can measure blood pressure and heart rate and calculate stroke volume variation and cardiac output. (From Lough ME. *Hemodynamic Monitoring: Evolving Technologies and Clinical Practice.* Philadelphia: Elsevier; 2016.)

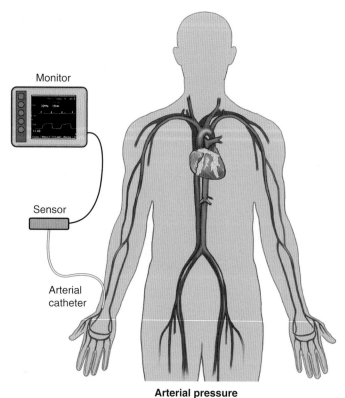

Arterial pressure

Fig. 10.18 Arterial Waveform and Pressure-Based Monitoring. Less-invasive systems that use a specialized transducer and arterial catheter sensor to calculate stroke volume, stroke volume variation, cardiac output, and cardiac index. Both calibrated and noncalibrated hemodynamic systems are available. (From Lough ME. *Hemodynamic Monitoring: Evolving Technologies and Clinical Practice.* Philadelphia: Elsevier; 2016.)

any invasive lines. They are the first step in a suite of devices that use arterial waveform analysis (Fig. 10.17).[47] Finger cuff devices may be particularly helpful during initial hemodynamic assessment or when invasive monitoring is not readily available.

Arterial pulse analysis hemodynamic monitoring systems. Arterial waveform—based systems require insertion of an arterial catheter fitted with specialized sensors that use the arterial pressure and pulse waveform to provide real-time data. The systems use proprietary thermistors, software, and bedside computer systems (Fig. 10.18). The different technologies and the systems may be described as *pulse contour analysis, pulse wave analysis,* or *pulse power analysis.* Arterial pressure—based systems trend continuous BP, SV, SVV, pulse pressure variation, and CO. A significant advantage is that the patient does not have to be intubated or sedated to tolerate the monitoring system. Another advantage is that the CO values are recorded in real time and change with breathing pattern and fluid volume interventions. The continuous SVV and CO values are sometimes referred to as *functional hemodynamics.* These values can be used in the assessment of *fluid volume responsiveness* using the *passive leg raise maneuver* (Fig. 10.19).[40] Real-time hemodynamic monitoring systems are especially well suited to this bedside examination. The increase in central blood volume as the legs are raised should increase SV and decrease SVV if a patient is fluid responsive (Fig. 10.20).

These systems are generally noncalibrated and considered minimally invasive.[48,49] In general, noncalibrated systems are reported to have lower levels of CO accuracy compared with bolus thermodilution methods.[48,49] However, the tradeoff is that noncalibrated systems offer

a less invasive method of trending CO. Pulse waveform—based methods are less accurate with dysrhythmias because of the irregularity in the shape of the arterial waveform.[48,49]

The nursing management of an arterial catheter described in the earlier section on arterial pressure monitoring also applies here. If the arterial waveform is not pristine, the hemodynamic data will be compromised. The position of the transducer is also important. If the transducer level is misaligned by more than 4 inches (10 cm), inaccurate measurements can result.[50]

Transpulmonary thermodilution monitoring systems. Transpulmonary thermodilution monitoring systems are calibrated and more invasive, as they require both arterial and central venous access (see Fig. 10.7). As explained earlier, the system may be described by specific pulse analysis terms depending on the manufacturer. Transpulmonary thermodilution systems are used when more exact (calibrated) information is required. The calibration methods vary from cold saline to lithium depending on the system used. Systems should be calibrated at least every 8 hours.

To obtain a CO using the transpulmonary thermodilution technique, a bolus of cold saline is injected into the CVC and measured at a femoral arterial thermistor-tipped catheter. Injectate temperature and transit time are used to generate a thermodilution temperature curve to calculate CO (Fig. 10.21).

The transpulmonary thermodilution method uses a CVC and an arterial catheter but avoids placing a catheter into the right-heart

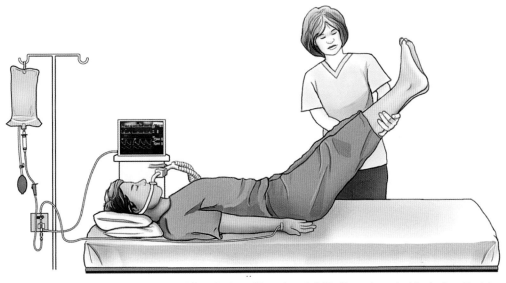

Fig. 10.19 Passive Leg Raise in Intubated Patient. (From Lough ME. *Hemodynamic Monitoring: Evolving Technologies and Clinical Practice.* Philadelphia: Elsevier; 2016.)

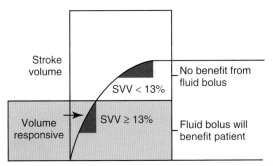

Fig. 10.20 Stroke Volume Variation *(SVV)* in Response to a Volume Challenge. (From Lough ME. *Hemodynamic Monitoring: Evolving Technologies and Clinical Practice.* Philadelphia: Elsevier; 2016.)

chambers, which is considered a benefit because it is less invasive. Transpulmonary thermodilution systems also provide different data from the traditional PA-Catheter. The *extravascular lung water index* measures the volume and percentage of water in lung tissue; a higher index value is a marker of pulmonary edema. Lung water content increases in conditions such as heart failure and ARDS. Higher lung water content is associated with higher mortality. Knowledge of extravascular lung water may influence whether to administer diuretics or administer volume.

Pulse contour analysis enables the use of SVV to assess volume status. SVV measures the difference between the highest and lowest SV over the previous 30 seconds. The caveat is that for this to be considered truly accurate, the patient must be mechanically ventilated and not overbreathing the ventilator. This requirement restricts accurate SVV monitoring to patients during anesthesia, deep sedation, or pharmacologic paralysis.

Visual Hemodynamic Monitoring Methods

Transesophageal echocardiography. Traditionally, echocardiography would not have been described as a primary hemodynamic monitoring modality, although this perspective has changed in many settings. This is because transesophageal echocardiography (TEE) monitoring during cardiac surgery has increased, with more patients returning to the cardiac critical care unit with an esophageal probe in place.[51] Generally, surgical patients monitored with TEE are mechanically ventilated and anesthetized after surgery. Because of the close anatomic relationship between the heart and the esophagus, TEE produces images of very high quality of the heart chambers, heart valves, and thoracic aorta without the interference of the chest wall, bone, or air-filled lung (Fig. 10.22). TEE has the advantage of displaying a real-time image of the heart in motion. This allows real-time assessment of LV cardiac contractility. Additional information specific to noninvasive transthoracic echocardiography (TTE) is provided later in this chapter.

Ultrasound-based hemodynamic monitoring. Handheld ultrasound has become an essential noninvasive component of beside hemodynamic assessment in many critical care units.[52] Critical care societies now recommend that all medical trainees learn the basic skills of ultrasonography.[52] One of the most useful ultrasound skills is the assessment of fluid volume status by examination of the inferior vena cava (IVC) during the respiratory cycle.

In a mechanically ventilated patient, intrathoracic pressure is highest during inspiration and lowest at end-expiration. At the point of lowest pressure, preload volume is rapidly drawn into the right atrium, causing the IVC to "collapse." This IVC collapse or narrowing is more obvious in a patient with hypovolemia. In a patient with normal volume status or hypervolemia, the IVC walls have less movement with breathing (Fig. 10.23).[52]

In a spontaneously breathing patient, the respiratory mechanics are different. The lowest pressure occurs during inspiration; with hypovolemia, the IVC walls may be seen to narrow or "collapse".[52] This measurement is considered less reliable in a spontaneously breathing patient.[53]

Ultrasound is a frequency greater than 20,000 Hz, which is above the range of human hearing. Ultrasound is reflected visibly at interfaces between tissues that have different densities. Many ultrasound protocols have been developed to guide clinical management and are increasingly used in the initial assessment of hemodynamic instability. Protocols are used to ensure that all practitioners use ultrasound-guided diagnosis in a consistent manner. One of the earliest uses of ultrasound was in trauma. The noninvasive Focused

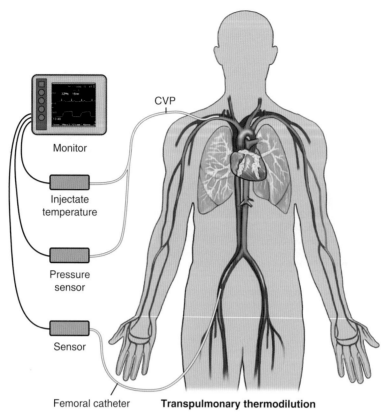

Fig. 10.21 Transpulmonary Thermodilution Arterial Waveform Pressure–Based Monitoring. More-invasive calibrated systems that use an arterial catheter and central venous catheter *(CVC)* to obtain a transpulmonary thermodilution (TPTD) cardiac output (CVC through pulmonary vascular system to arterial catheter with sensor). (From Lough ME. *Hemodynamic Monitoring: Evolving Technologies and Clinical Practice.* Philadelphia: Elsevier; 2016.)

Assessment by Sonography for Trauma (FAST) protocol is used in trauma to evaluate intraabdominal blood as described for trauma in Chapter 24.

Doppler-Based Hemodynamic Monitoring Methods

Doppler offers another method to trend CO. This modality can be noninvasive or invasive. The esophagus is used as the monitoring site for patients who are deeply sedated or are under general anesthesia in the operating room. The esophageal Doppler probe (Fig. 10.24) is generally described as minimally invasive compared with a PA-Catheter (see Figs. 10.13–10.15).[54] Insertion of the esophageal Doppler probe is similar to insertion of a gastric tube, although the probe is relatively inflexible and stiff.[54] The probe is inserted 35 to 40 cm from the teeth. The tip of the probe rests near T5-T6 on the vertebral column, where the esophagus typically is parallel with the descending aorta. When the probe is correctly placed, this method has a high degree of accuracy for CO measurement. Accurate CO values depend on correct placement and on the skill of the operator.[54]

Intermittent SV and CO information can also be obtained using a noninvasive transthoracic Doppler. This technique is more frequently used in pediatric and non–critical care settings.

ELECTROCARDIOGRAPHY

Nursing priorities for the patient with bedside ECG monitoring focus on accurate (1) selection of the ECG lead, (2) interpretation of the

ECG rhythm, and (3) initiation of emergency measures to treat dysrhythmias when required.

Selecting Electrocardiogram Leads

All electrocardiographs use a system of one or more leads.

3-Lead ECG System

The basic 3-lead ECG system consists of three bipolar electrodes that are applied to the chest wall as shown in Fig. 10.25A. The 3-lead system is rarely used today except in transport monitors.

5-Lead ECG System

The five ECG system electrodes are typically color-coded to avoid errors when placed on the chest. The electrode locations are right arm (RA); left arm (LA); left leg (LL) that is placed on the left abdomen below the diaphragm preferably lower than the umbilicus; right leg (RL), placed on the right abdomen below the diaphragm; and a chest electrode often placed in the V1 position at the fourth intercostal space right sternal border, as shown in Fig. 10.25B.

Electrode Care

Electrodes do not transmit any electricity to the patient; rather, they sense and record intrinsic cardiac electrical activity from the body's surface. Lead wires can be disposable or reusable.[55] There is no difference in infection rates provided the nondisposable ECG lead wires

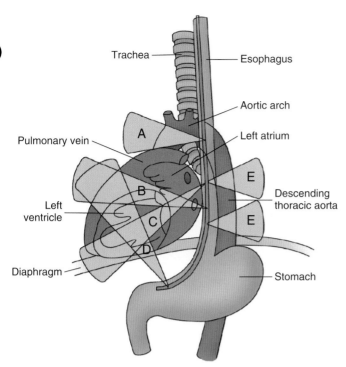

Fig. 10.22 Diagram of Common Scan Planes During a Transesophageal Echocardiogram With a Two-Dimensional View. *A,* Horizontal scan plane of the aortic arch and distal portion of aorta. *B,* Basal short-axis (transverse), long-axis (sagittal), and short-axis views of both atria. *C,* Four-chamber and left atrioventricular long-axis views. A sagittal scan plane can image a cross section of the left ventricle. *D,* Transgastric, short-axis view of the left and right ventricles. *E,* Transverse and sagittal scan sections of the descending aorta.

and connectors are thoroughly cleaned between each patient use.[56] The ECG skin electrode patch that touches the patient's skin is always disposable. Disposable leads or electrodes should be changed or replaced per manufacturer's guidelines. It is important to properly prepare the patient's skin before placing the electrodes, because this

will improve signal quality, thereby decreasing erroneous alarms. Proper preparation includes washing the electrode area with soap and water and wiping with a washcloth or gauze. Do not use alcohol for skin preparation, because it dries out the skin. Excessive hair at the electrode site should be clipped.

Alarm fatigue is a serious patient safety issue that has direct effects on nursing practice and care. See **QSEN** Box 10.13 for more information on alarm management.

Electrocardiogram Paper

ECG paper records the speed and magnitude of electrical impulses on a grid composed of small and large boxes. At a standard paper speed of 25 mm/s, looking at the ECG paper from left to right, one small box (1-mm wide) is equivalent to 0.04 second, and one large box (5-mm wide) represents 0.20 second. These ECG boxes represent the time it takes for the electrical impulse to travel through a particular part of the heart and are stated in seconds rather than in millimeters or number of boxes. The vertical scale represents the magnitude, or amplitude, of the electrical signal. The vertical scale is standardized to a specific calibration. Standard calibration is 10mm/mV.

Interpreting Electrocardiograph Waveforms

The analysis of waveforms and intervals provides the basis for ECG interpretation (Fig. 10.26).

Waveform Recognition

P wave. The P wave represents atrial depolarization.

QRS complex. The QRS complex represents ventricular depolarization, corresponding to phase 0 of the ventricular action potential. It is referred to as a *complex* because it consists of several different waves. The letter *Q* is used to describe an initial negative deflection; the first deflection from the baseline is labeled a Q wave only if it is negative. The letter *R* applies to any positive deflection from baseline. If there are two positive deflections in one QRS complex, the second is labeled *R'* ("R prime") and is commonly seen in lead V_1 in patients with right bundle branch block (RBBB). The letter *S* refers to any subsequent negative deflections. Any combination of these deflections can occur

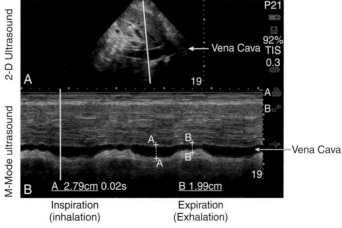

Fig. 10.23 Respiratory Changes in Intrathoracic Pressure on Inferior Vena Cava (IVC) Diameter Viewed by Ultrasound. (A) The upper image shows a two-dimensional ultrasound of the IVC from the subxiphoid view in a spontaneously breathing patient. A *yellow line* passes through the vena cava, and the open appearance of the vena cava indicates it is filled with blood, suggesting the patient has taken a deep breath. (B) The lower image shows M-mode ultrasound indicating changes in the IVC diameter with breathing. The *yellow line* passing through the vena cava is in the same position as in the upper image. *Position A* at 2.79 cm diameter indicates inspiration (inhalation). *Position B* at 1.99 cm diameter indicates expiration (exhalation). (From Lough ME. *Hemodynamic Monitoring: Evolving Technologies and Clinical Practice.* Philadelphia: Elsevier; 2016.)

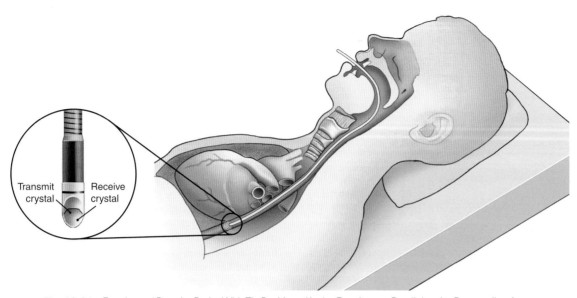

Fig. 10.24 Esophageal Doppler Probe With Tip Positioned in the Esophagus, Parallel to the Descending Aorta.

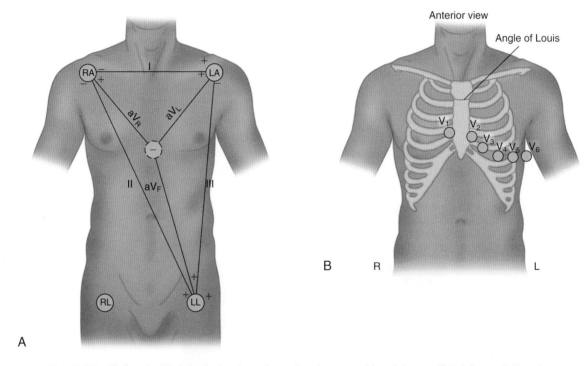

Fig. 10.25 (A) Standard limb leads. Leads are located on the extremities: right arm *(RA)*, left arm *(LA)*, and left leg *(LL)*. The right leg *(RL)* electrode serves as a ground. Leads I, II, and III are bipolar, with each using a positive electrode and a negative electrode. Leads aVR, aVL, and aVF are augmented unipolar leads that use the calculated center of the heart as their negative electrode. (B) Precordial leads. V_1 to V_6 are the six standard precordial leads and are placed as follows: V_1, fourth intercostal space, right sternal border; V_2, fourth intercostal space, left sternal border; V_3, equidistant between V_2 and V_4; V_4, fifth intercostal space, left midclavicular line; V_5, anterior axillary line, same horizontal level as V_4; V_6, midaxillary line, same horizontal level as V_4. Color-coded cable attachments allow quick identification and accurate electrode placement.

and is collectively called the *QRS complex* (Fig. 10.27). The QRS complex duration is normally less than 0.11 second (2.5 small boxes).

T wave. The T wave represents ventricular repolarization, corresponding to phase 3 of the ventricular action potential. The onset of the QRS complex to approximately the midpoint or peak of the T wave represents an absolute refractory period, during which the heart muscle cannot respond to another stimulus no matter how strong that stimulus may be (Fig. 10.28). From the midpoint to the end of the T wave, the heart muscle is in the relative refractory period. The heart muscle has not yet fully recovered, but it can be depolarized again if a strong enough stimulus is received. This can be a particularly dangerous time for ventricular ectopy to occur, especially if any portion of the

BOX 10.13 Safety

Alarm Fatigue and Alarm Management

Alarm fatigue is a significant patient safety risk. Adverse patient events, including death, have occurred as the result of improper alarm management in the acute care setting. Recent studies have demonstrated that over 85% (and possibly even up to 99%) of alarms are clinically nonactionable, resulting in desensitization to alarms. The concern over alarm fatigue needs to be balanced with the need to continuously monitor patients that are critically ill. Evidence-based strategies to reduce alarm fatigue include:

- Following proper skin preparation steps when applying ECG monitoring leads. Replace leads on a routine basis as outlined by institutional guidelines.
- Personalizing alarm parameters for individual patients based on patient condition and institutional guidelines.
- Diligent use of continuous monitoring. Once no longer clinically indicated, continuous monitoring should be discontinued.

American Association of Critical-Care Nurses (AACN). Managing alarms in acute care across the lifespan: electrocardiography and pulse oximetry: AACN Practice Alert. *Crit Care Nurse.* 2018;38(2):e16–e20.

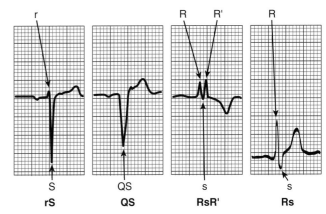

Fig. 10.27 Examples of QRS Complexes. Small deflections (less than 5 mm) are labeled with lowercase letters, and uppercase letters are used for larger deflections (greater than 5mm). A second upward deflection is labeled R'.

myocardium is ischemic, because the ischemic muscle takes even longer to fully repolarize. An impulse arriving during this period is known as *R on T* and may cause disorganized, self-perpetuating depolarizations of various sections of the myocardium and lead to ventricular tachycardia (VT) or ventricular fibrillation (VF).

Intervals between waveforms. The intervals between waveforms are evaluated to determine the time it takes for cardiac activation (see Fig. 10.26).

PR interval. The PR interval is measured from the beginning of the P wave to the beginning of the QRS complex. The PR interval is normally 0.12 to 0.20 seconds long and represents the time it takes for the electrical impulse to travel from the sinoatrial (SA) node to the atrioventricular (AV) node. Because this period includes any delay of the impulse within the AV node to initiate ventricular depolarization, the PR interval is an indicator of AV node function.

QRS. As mentioned previously, the QRS complex duration is normally less than 0.11 second (2.5 small boxes). The QRS duration is widened in bundle branch block (BBB; right or left) or ventricular preexcitation, as would be present in Wolff-Parkinson-White syndrome. Ventricular paced rhythms also cause a wide QRS complex.

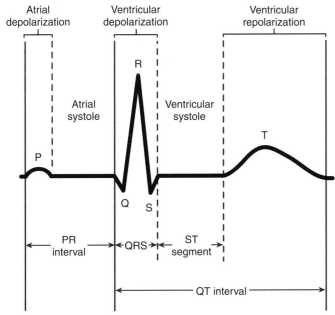

Fig. 10.26 Normal Electrocardiogram (ECG) Waveforms, Intervals, and Correlation With Events of Cardiac Cycle. The *P wave* represents atrial depolarization, followed immediately by atrial systole. The *QRS complex* represents ventricular depolarization, followed immediately by ventricular systole. The *ST segment* corresponds to phase 2 of the action potential, during which time the heart muscle is completely depolarized and contraction normally occurs. The *T wave* represents ventricular repolarization. The *PR interval*, measured from the beginning of the P wave to the beginning of the QRS complex, corresponds to atrial depolarization and impulse delay in the atrioventricular node. The *QT interval*, measured from the beginning of the QRS complex to the end of the T wave, represents the time from initial depolarization of the ventricles to the end of ventricular repolarization.

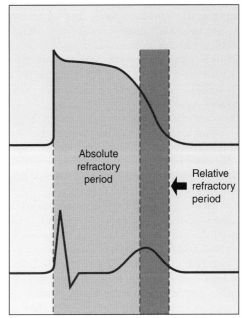

Fig. 10.28 Absolute and relative refractory periods are correlated with the cardiac muscle action potential and with an electrocardiogram tracing.

ST segment. The ST segment is the portion of the ECG waveform that extends from the end of the QRS complex to the beginning of the T wave. Its duration is not measured. Instead, its shape and amplitude are evaluated. The ST segment is normally flat and at the same level as the isoelectric baseline measured at the PR segment or the TP segment. Any change (i.e., elevation or depression) from baseline is expressed in millimeters and may indicate myocardial ischemia (one small box equals 1 mm). ST segment elevation of 1 to 2 mm is associated with acute myocardial injury, acute MI, and pericarditis. ST segment depression (decrease from baseline more than 1–2 mm) is associated with myocardial ischemia.[57] The ST segment must be monitored carefully in high-risk patients (described later).

QT interval. *Measuring the QT interval.* The QT interval is measured from the beginning of the QRS complex to the end of the T wave and indicates the total time from the onset of ventricular depolarization to the completion of ventricular repolarization. While there is no established bedside monitoring lead recommended for measuring the QT interval, the lead with the longest T wave should be selected. Avoid leads with a U wave following the QT, because it can be difficult to determine the end of the QT interval.[58] An important point is that each clinician must measure the QT interval using the same ECG lead.[58] The length of a QT interval depends on the HR and must be adjusted according to the HR to be evaluated in a clinically meaningful way.

Corrected QT interval. Because the QT interval shortens at faster HRs and lengthens with slower HRs, it is often written as a "corrected" value (QTc), meaning the QT value was mathematically corrected to a HR of 60 beats/min. This allows comparison of the QTc interval across a range of HRs. The QTc interval is most commonly calculated by Bazett's formula, which divides the measured QT interval (in seconds) by the square root of the R-R cycle length.[58] A QTc interval of greater than 0.47 second (470 ms) in women and greater than 0.45 second (450 ms) in men is considered prolonged.[58] In clinical practice a QTc time interval of 500 ms is often used. A prolonged QTc interval is significant because it can predispose the patient to the development of polymorphic VT, known also as *torsades de pointes.*

QT interval and medications. Many antidysrhythmic medications can prolong the QT interval, notably class Ia antidysrhythmics (quinidine, procainamide, disopyramide) and class III antidysrhythmics (amiodarone, dronedarone, ibutilide, dofetilide, sotalol). Not all QT-prolonging medications are antidysrhythmics. Other classes of medications known to cause QT prolongation include anesthetics, antibiotics, antidepressants, antiemetics, antipsychotics, opioids, and sedatives.

When medications associated with a high risk of QT prolongation are started, it is important to record the premedication baseline QTc interval and to regularly monitor and record the QTc interval during treatment. The risk of torsades de pointes is increased with prolongation of the QTc interval beyond 0.5 second (500 ms) or an increase of 60 ms compared with the baseline QTc interval.[59]

QT and torsades de pointes. The risk of torsades de pointe increases with electrolyte abnormalities, including hypokalemia, hypomagnesemia, and hypocalcemia.[60] Risk increases in the presence of bradycardia, heart block with pauses, and premature ventricular beats with short-long-short cycles.[60] Another risk factor may be genetics; 10% to 15% of patients with acquired long QT syndrome (medication induced) carry a genetic predisposition for the syndrome.[60]

Acute therapy is directed at increasing the HR, which shortens the QT interval, stopping culprit medications, and correcting electrolyte abnormalities. It may also include placement of a temporary pacemaker and administering IV magnesium, especially if serum levels of magnesium are low.

Dysrhythmia Interpretation

In clinical practice, the terms *dysrhythmia* and *arrhythmia* often are used interchangeably. Which term is more accurate is a matter of debate. Both are considered clinically correct, and either may be used in practice. In this textbook, dysrhythmia is the more commonly used term. A dysrhythmia is any disturbance in the normal cardiac conduction pathway. Dysrhythmias can be detected on a 12-lead ECG, but they often occur only sporadically. For this reason, patients in a critical care unit are monitored continuously using a single-lead or dual-lead system, and rhythm strips are routinely recorded per organization standards. Dysrhythmias occur frequently in cardiac and noncardiac critically ill patients. A systematic approach to assess a rhythm disturbance is an indispensable skill. Steps to accurately interpret a rhythm strip are introduced first, followed by specific criteria to evaluate common dysrhythmias encountered in clinical practice.

Heart Rate Determination

The first thing to assess when evaluating a rhythm strip is the ventricular rate. Regardless of the dysrhythmia involved, the ventricular rate and BP are key to whether the patient can tolerate the dysrhythmia (i.e., maintain CO and mentation). Once the patient can no longer tolerate the dysrhythmia, often a ventricular rate greater than 200 or less than 30, emergency measures must be started to correct the condition. A detailed analysis of the underlying rhythm disturbance can occur later, once the patient's clinical condition has stabilized.

The three methods for calculating rate (Fig. 10.29A) are as follows:

1. Number of R-R intervals in 6 seconds multiplied by 10. ECG paper is usually marked at the top in 3-second increments, making a 6-second interval easy to identify.
2. Number of large boxes between QRS complexes divided into 300. This can also be counted out between two QRS complexes. Begin with the first QRS complex to occur on a line and count the large boxes in sequence as 300, 150, 100, 75, 60, 50, 43, 37 bpm, or until the following QRS.
3. Number of small boxes between QRS complexes divided into 1500.

In a healthy heart, the atrial rate and the ventricular rate are the same. However, in many dysrhythmias, the atrial and ventricular rates are different, and both must be calculated. To find the atrial rate, the P-P interval, instead of the R-R interval, is used in one of the three methods listed for determining rate.

The choice of method for calculating the HR depends on the regularity of the rhythm. If the rhythm is irregular, it may be helpful to count for 30 seconds; or the first method (R-R intervals in 6 seconds multiplied by 10) can be used (Fig. 10.29B). If the rhythm is regular, any of the methods can be used.

Rhythm Determination

The term *rhythm* refers to the regularity with which the P waves or R waves occur. Calipers assist in determining rhythm. One point of the calipers is placed on the beginning of one R wave, and the other point is placed on the next R wave. Leaving the calipers "set" at this interval, each succeeding R-R interval is checked to be sure it is the same width as the first one measured.

In describing the rhythm, three terms are used:

- *Regular rhythm.* R-R intervals are the same, within 10%.
- *Regularly irregular.* R-R intervals are not the same, but a pattern is involved, which could be grouping, rhythmic speeding up and slowing down, or another consistent pattern.

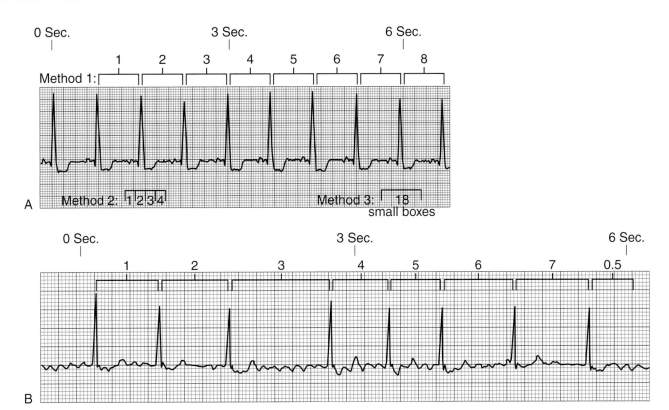

Fig. 10.29 (A) Calculation of heart rate if the rhythm is regular. *Method 1*: Number of R-R intervals in 6 seconds multiplied by 10 (e.g., 8 × 10 = 80/min). *Method 2*: Number of large boxes between QRS complexes divided into 300 (e.g., 300 ÷ 4 = 75/min). A variation on this method is to count large boxes between QRS complexes starting with the first QRS complex to occur on a vertical line. Two QRS complexes that are one box apart is a rate of 300; two boxes apart is a rate of 150; three boxes apart is a rate of 100 bpm. The full sequence is 300, 150, 100, 75, 60, 50, 43, 37 bpm, between QRS complexes. *Method 3*: Number of small boxes between QRS complexes divided into 1500 (e.g., 1500 ÷ 18 = 84/min). (B) Rate calculation if the rhythm is irregular. Only method 1 can be used (e.g., 7.5 intervals × 10 = 75/min).

- *Irregularly irregular.* R-R intervals are not the same, and no pattern can be found.

P wave evaluation. The P wave is analyzed by considering whether the P wave is present or absent. If present, is each P wave associated with a QRS complex? It is expected that one P wave will be in front of every QRS. Sometimes, two, three, or four P waves may be in front of every QRS complex. If this pattern is consistent, the P waves and QRS are still associated, although not on a 1:1 basis.

PR interval evaluation. The duration of the PR interval, which normally is 0.12 to 0.20 second (120–200 ms), is measured first. This is measured from the start of a visible P wave to the beginning of the next QRS complex (see Fig. 10.26). All PR intervals on the strip are verified to be sure they have the same duration as the original interval.

QRS complex evaluation. The entire ECG strip must be evaluated to ascertain that the QRS complexes are consistently the same shape and width. The normal QRS complex duration is 0.06 to 0.10 second (60–110 ms). Any QRS longer than 0.10 second is considered abnormal. If more than one QRS shape is visible on the strip, each QRS complex must be measured. The QRS complex is measured from where it leaves the baseline to where it returns to the baseline (see Fig. 10.26).

QT interval evaluation. The length of the QT interval varies with the HR. The QT interval is shorter when the HR is faster. A QT interval corrected for HR (QTc interval) that is longer than 0.50 second (500 ms) is of concern, as discussed in the section on QT interval.

Sinus Rhythms

The cardiac cycle begins when an impulse originates in the sinus node. The wave of depolarization spreading through the atria results in a P wave on the ECG. The impulse is delayed briefly in the AV node, which corresponds to the PR interval on the ECG. After leaving the AV node, the wave of depolarization spreads rapidly through the bundle of His and the bundle branches and causes ventricular depolarization, which is recorded as a QRS complex by the ECG. Contraction immediately follows depolarization. Contraction is terminated by repolarization, which is demonstrated as a T wave on the ECG.

Normal Sinus Rhythm

If all the events described for sinus rhythms occur in their normal sequence with normal rates and intervals, the patient is in normal sinus rhythm. The criteria for normal sinus rhythm are as follows:

Rate: Intrinsic rate of the sinus node is 60 to 100 beats/min. External factors such as medications, fever, or exercise can affect the intrinsic rate.

Rhythm: Rhythm is regular, within 10%.

P wave: P waves are present, and only one precedes each QRS complex.

PR interval: The PR interval represents the expected delay in the AV node. In normal sinus rhythm, the PR interval is 0.12 to 0.20 second.

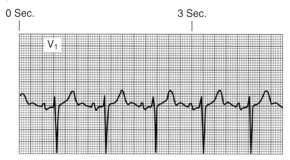

Fig. 10.30 Normal Sinus Rhythm. The rate is 70, and the rhythm is regular. One P wave is present before each QRS complex. The PR interval is 0.18 seconds and does not vary throughout the strip. The QRS complex duration is 0.08 seconds. All evaluation criteria are within normal limits.

QRS complex: All QRS complexes must look alike. If conduction through the ventricles is normal, the QRS complex duration is 0.06 to 0.10 second. Fig. 10.30 is an example of normal sinus rhythm in V_1.

Sinus Bradycardia

Sinus bradycardia meets all the criteria for normal sinus rhythm except that the rate is less than 60 beats/min (Table 10.6):
Rate: Intrinsic rate of the sinus node is less than 60 beats/min.
Rhythm: Rhythm is regular, within 10%.
P wave: P waves are present, and only one precedes every QRS complex.
PR interval: PR interval is 0.12 to 0.20 second.
QRS complex: All QRS complexes look alike, QRS complex duration is 0.06 to 0.10 second.

Clinical significance. Sinus bradycardia may occur with vagal stimulation, increased intracranial pressure, medication therapy with digoxin or beta-blockers, and ischemia of the sinus node. Sinus bradycardia is not treated unless the patient displays symptoms of hypoperfusion, such as hypotension, dizziness, chest pain, or changes in level of consciousness.

Sinus bradycardia occurs in healthy trained athletes at rest, and this does not require treatment. However, this is not the typical case in critical care.

Sinus Tachycardia

Sinus tachycardia meets all the criteria for normal sinus rhythm except that the rate is greater than 100 beats/min (see Table 10.6):
Rate: Intrinsic sinus node rate is greater than 100 beats/min.
Rhythm: Rhythm is regular, within 10%.
P wave: P waves are present, and only one precedes each QRS complex.
PR interval: PR interval is 0.12 to 0.20 second.
QRS complex: All QRS complexes look alike, QRS complex duration is 0.06 to 0.10 second.

Clinical significance. Sinus tachycardia may occur with pain, fever, hemorrhage, shock, heart failure, and thyrotoxicosis.[61] Tachycardia is detrimental to anyone with ischemic heart disease because it decreases the time for ventricular filling, decreases SV, and compromises CO. Tachycardia increases heart work and myocardial oxygen demand, while decreasing oxygen supply by decreasing coronary artery filling time, especially in a person with structural heart disease.

Sinus Dysrhythmia

Sinus dysrhythmia, commonly called *sinus arrhythmia* in clinical practice, meets all the criteria for normal sinus rhythm except that the rhythm is irregular (see Table 10.6). This irregularity coincides with the respiratory pattern; HR increases with inhalation and decreases with exhalation (Fig. 10.31). Sinus dysrhythmia often occurs in children and young adults, and the incidence decreases with age. No treatment is required. To avoid being misled by other rhythm disturbances, look at all P waves closely to verify that they are the same shape and that the PR intervals are consistent.

TABLE 10.6	Sinus Rhythms.			
Parameter	**Normal Sinus Rhythm**	**Sinus Bradycardia**	**Sinus Tachycardia**	**Sinus Dysrhythmia**
Rate	60–100 beats/min	<60 beats/min	>100 beats/min	Variable
Rhythm	Regular	Regular	Regular	Irregular; respiratory variation
P wave	Present, with 1 per QRS complex	Present, with 1 per QRS complex	Present, with 1 per QRS complex	Present, with 1 per QRS complex
P-R interval	0.12–0.20 second and constant	0.12–0.20 second and constant	0.12–0.20 second and constant	0.12–0.20 second and constant
QRS complex	0.06–0.10 second	0.06–0.10 second	0.06–0.10 second	0.06–0.10 second

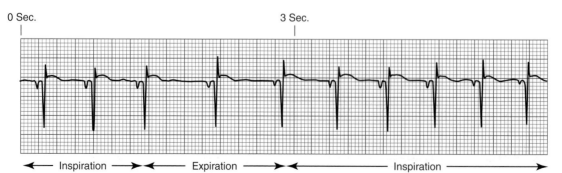

Fig. 10.31 Sinus Dysrhythmia. The heart rate is increased during inspiration and decreased during expiration. This pattern is also known as *sinus arrhythmia* in clinical practice. The p wave in lead V1 can be positive, negative (shown here) or biphasic.

Atrial Dysrhythmias

Atrial dysrhythmias originate from an ectopic focus in the atria somewhere other than the sinus node. The ectopic impulse occurs prematurely, before the normal sinus impulse occurs. The premature atrial depolarization may initiate a normal QRS complex, an abnormal or aberrant pattern, or a supraventricular tachycardia (SVT). Huge advances have been made in the understanding of the pathogenesis and management of atrial dysrhythmias.

Premature Atrial Contractions

Premature atrial contractions (PACs) are isolated early beats from an ectopic focus in the atria. The underlying rhythm is usually sinus. The regular sinus rhythm is interrupted by an early, abnormally shaped atrial P wave. The early atrial wave usually looks different from the sinus P wave and may be inverted. The PR interval may be longer, shorter, or the same as the PR interval of a sinus impulse. The QRS complex that follows the ectopic atrial P wave can vary in shape depending on the degree of refractoriness of the AV node:

- *PAC with a narrow QRS complex:* If the atrial impulse arrives in the AV node after the AV node is fully repolarized, the impulse is conducted to the ventricles as a normal QRS complex. If the ventricles are also fully repolarized, conduction through the bundle branches is expected, and a normal QRS complex is recorded on the ECG (Fig. 10.32A).
- *PAC with a wide QRS complex:* Occasionally, the early ectopic P wave can be conducted through the AV node, but part of the conduction pathway through the ventricular bundle branches is blocked. This produces a wide QRS (Fig. 10.32B). Conduction through the ventricles that is different from normal is referred to as *aberrant*. Consequently, these early, abnormally conducted PACs are often described as *aberrantly conducted PACs*.
- *PAC non-conducted:* The ectopic P wave sometimes arrives so early that the AV node is still in its absolute refractory period. In this case the wave of depolarization does not move past the AV node, and no QRS complex follows. All that is seen on the ECG is an early, abnormal P wave followed by a pause until the next sinus P wave occurs (Fig. 10.32C). This is called a *nonconducted PAC.* Usually, these P waves are so early that they are superimposed on the T wave of the previous beat, making them difficult to find. The pause that follows is still clearly seen. Whenever an unexpected pause occurs in a rhythm, the T wave preceding the pause must be examined very carefully and compared with other T waves on the same strip to locate distortions that may reveal a hidden early P wave.

Occasional PACs can occur in individuals with normal hearts. PACs may be exacerbated by emotional upheaval, nicotine, caffeine, and some medications. Heart failure can cause PACs because of increased pressure within the atria. As atrial pressure begins to rise, the atrial walls are stretched, causing irritability of atrial cells and the occurrence of PACs.

Supraventricular Tachycardia

SVT describes a varied group of dysrhythmias that originate above the AV node. SVT is not a specific term; it includes sinus tachycardia, atrial tachycardia, multifocal atrial tachycardia, atrial flutter, atrial fibrillation, and junctional tachycardia. Initially, the SVT may be described as a narrow complex tachycardia.

Narrow complex tachycardia. An SVT narrow complex tachycardia has a rate greater than 100 and a QRS complex less than 0.12 second (120 ms).[61] Women are affected by episodic SVT at approximately twice the rate of men.[61]

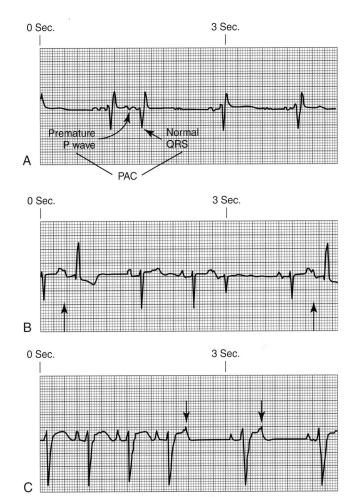

Fig. 10.32 Premature Atrial Contractions *(PACs).* (A) Normally conducted PAC. The early P wave is indicated by the *arrow,* and the QRS complex that follows has a normal shape and duration. (B) Aberrantly conducted PAC. Early PACs that are abnormally conducted, identified by *arrows,* are described as *aberrantly conducted PACs.* (C) Nonconducted PACs. The early P waves arrive at the AV node too early to be conducted and distort the T waves, making them appear peaked compared with the normal T waves. These are known as *nonconducted* or *blocked PACs* and are indicated by *arrows.*

SVT is not always benign. Approximately 14% of people with SVT report that they have experienced syncope (lost consciousness) while driving, and 50% have experienced symptoms of near-syncope.[61] Medications are used to limit the SVT rate and prevent "blackouts" or syncope. SVT that is persistent for weeks or months may lead to a tachycardia-mediated cardiomyopathy. A baseline 12-lead ECG is helpful, and a 12-lead ECG obtained during the palpitations is diagnostically helpful.[61]

Supraventricular tachycardia with aberrant conduction. If the QRS complex in SVT is wider than 0.12 second, it is important to differentiate between SVT with aberrant conduction and VT (discussed later). SVT with aberrant conduction includes SVT with a BBB and SVT that uses an anomalous congenital additional fiber (accessory pathway), such as Wolff-Parkinson-White syndrome. Patients with SVT with aberrant conduction are frequently misdiagnosed, and evaluation by a specialist is highly recommended.[61]

Paroxysmal supraventricular tachycardia. *Paroxysmal* means starting and stopping abruptly. *Paroxysmal supraventricular tachycardia*

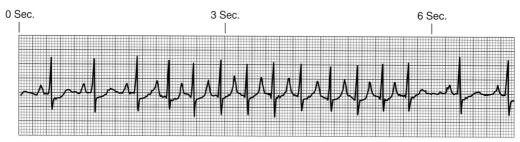

Fig. 10.33 Paroxysmal Supraventricular Tachycardia. The atrial rate during tachycardia is 158 beats/min. The run starts and stops abruptly.

(PSVT) refers to the sudden interruption of sinus rhythm by an atrial ectopic focus that fires repetitively at a rate of 150 to 250 beats/min and eventually stops as suddenly as it began (Fig. 10.33). The rhythm of PSVT is perfectly regular because the reentry loop has a specific length; each circuit through the loop requires exactly the same amount of time to complete. Reentry within the atria itself or involving the AV node is responsible for most SVTs, including PSVT.

PSVT usually responds rapidly to medical management, which initially includes the use of vagal maneuvers.[61] Vagal maneuvers used in critical care include the following:

- *Valsalva maneuver:* The patient is asked to "bear down," as if going to the bathroom.
- *Modified Valsalva maneuver:* A newer method of Valsalva maneuver has shown increased efficacy for converting PSVT to normal sinus rhythm. This method involves performing the standard Valsalva by asking the patient to bear down; then, immediately after, the patient is positioned flat and a passive leg raise of 45 degrees for 15 seconds is performed.[62]
- *Carotid sinus massage:* This maneuver is performed on only one side of the neck over the carotid artery by a physician, on a patient with a monitored ECG. It is not used on older patients who may have atherosclerotic disease of the carotid arteries.

Adenosine for PSVT diagnosis. If vagal maneuvers are unsuccessful at terminating the PSVT, the next step usually is the use of IV medications if the patient is hemodynamically stable. The IV medication of choice to briefly block conduction through the AV node is adenosine.[61] In PSVT, adenosine alone is often sufficient to restore normal sinus rhythm, but if not, it will unmask the ectopic P waves and confirm or provide strong clues to diagnose the SVT. The usual dose is 6 mg given intravenously by rapid push, followed by a normal saline flush. If the 6 mg adenosine does not create a temporary AV block or restore sinus rhythm, a 12-mg IV dose is administered. Continuous cardiac monitoring is essential when administering adenosine. Potential dysrhythmic side effects of adenosine include a 1% to 15% chance of initiating atrial fibrillation. Adenosine should be used with caution for patients with severe asthma or chronic obstructive pulmonary disease (COPD).

Medications for PSVT rate control. Other IV medications that may be used to slow the rate in PSVT include amiodarone, a class III antidysrhythmic with a rapid onset and a short half-life. Beta-blockers, such as metoprolol, are also commonly used to slow conduction. Alternatively, diltiazem, a class IV calcium channel blocker in the nondihydropyridine group, can be administered. However, extreme caution should be taken when administering calcium channel blockers if any beta-blockade has already been administered, and vice versa. The action of these medications is to slow conduction through the AV node. If IV medications do not convert the PSVT or sustained SVT, or

if the patient becomes hemodynamically unstable, the next step is electrical cardioversion.[61]

Atrial Flutter

Atrial flutter is recognized on the ECG by the *sawtooth* atrial pattern. These sawtooth-shaped atrial wavelets are not P waves; they are more appropriately called F waves (atrial flutter waves), as shown in Fig. 10.34. The AV node does not allow conduction of all flutter waves to the ventricles:

Atrial rate: 250 to 300 atrial flutter waves per minute.

Ventricular rate: Ventricular rate varies based on conduction through the AV node.

Rhythm: Rhythm varies based on conduction through the AV node (may have a pattern).

P wave: P waves are replaced by flutter waves that arise from an ectopic atrial site best seen in leads II, III, AVF.

PR interval: No longer applies, instead calculate the ratio of flutter waves to QRS complexes (2:1; 3:1; 4:1…).

QRS complex: QRS complex is typically narrow.

Clinical significance. Atrial flutter can be started by any isolated atrial impulse, but to be maintained, the atrial flutter requires a reentry circular pathway around macroscopic structures in the atria. Typically,

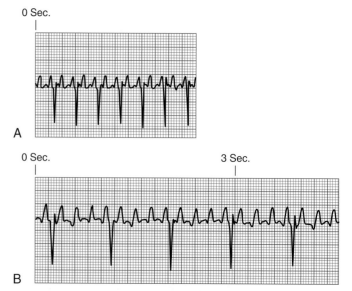

Fig. 10.34 (A) The initial strip shows atrial flutter with 2:1 conduction through the atrioventricular (AV) node. (B) During carotid sinus massage, the AV conduction rate is decreased, revealing the flutter waves more clearly.

TABLE 10.7 **Atrial Dysrhythmias.**				
Parameter	**Paroxysmal Supraventricular Tachycardia**	**Multifocal Atrial Tachycardia**	**Atrial Flutter**	**Atrial Fibrillation**
Rate				
Atrial	150–250 beats/min	100–160 beats/min	250–350 beats/min	>350 beats/min (unable to count it)
Ventricular	Same or less	Same	250–350 beats/min, one-half or less	100–180 beats/min (uncontrolled); <100 beats/min (controlled)
Rhythm	Regular	Irregular	Atrial, regular; ventricular, may or may not be regular	Irregularly irregular
P wave	Present; abnormally shaped	Present; three or more different shapes	F waves	Fibrillatory baseline
PR interval	May be normal or prolonged	Variable	Conduction ratio: flutter waves per QRS complex	Absent
QRS complex	0.06–0.10 second	0.06–0.10 second	0.06–0.10 second	0.06–0.10 second

these structures are in the right atrium and in 75% of cases involve the vena cava and the tricuspid valve in an area known as the *cavotricuspid isthmus*.[61] Clinical presentation will vary based on the presence or absence of underlying heart disease and the ventricular rate.

Evaluating atrial and ventricular rates in atrial flutter. **Conduction ratio in atrial flutter.** When describing atrial flutter, the term *PR interval* no longer applies; instead, a conduction ratio, such as 3:1 or 4:1 (ratio of atrial waves to QRS complexes) is used. The number of flutter waves that arrive at the AV node before one is conducted to the ventricles is a measure of AV node conduction or refractoriness (Table 10.7). Sometimes the conduction is regular, or in a pattern, sometimes it is irregular. Atrial flutter and atrial fibrillation can coexist in the same patient.[61]

Ventricular rate in atrial flutter. The major factor underlying atrial flutter symptoms is the ventricular response rate. If the atrial rate is 300 beats/min and the AV conduction ratio is 4:1, the ventricular response rate is 75 beats/min and should be well tolerated. However, if the atrial rate is 300 beats/min but the AV conduction ratio is 2:1, the corresponding ventricular rate of 150 beats/min may cause angina, acute heart failure, or other signs of cardiac decompensation. An atrial rate of 250 beats/min with a 1:1 AV conduction ratio yields a ventricular response rate of 250 beats/min; the patient is extremely symptomatic, and emergency measures are needed to decrease the ventricular rate.

Sometimes it is difficult to identify the flutter waves, especially if the conduction ratio is 2:1 (see Fig. 10.34A). Vagal maneuvers or adenosine can be useful diagnostic tools to allow better visualization of the flutter waves. Vagal maneuvers or IV adenosine cannot terminate atrial flutter but do create a temporary AV block to permit visualization of the atrial waveform and thereby facilitate accurate diagnosis, as seen in Fig. 10.34B.

Atrial flutter management. Antidysrhythmic medications are prescribed in two ways to treat atrial flutter: to convert the rhythm to sinus rhythm (rhythm control) and to slow conduction through the AV node (rate control):

- *Atrial flutter rhythm control:* The most effective medications for rhythm control are amiodarone, dofetilide, and sotalol; flecainide or propafenone can be used in the absence of structural heart disease.
- *Atrial flutter rate control:* Medications that slow conduction through the AV node are used to control the ventricular rate, including calcium channel blockers and beta-blockers.[61] Amiodarone shares both properties. It can slow conduction through the AV node and convert the atrial dysrhythmia. Amiodarone is preferred when the atrial flutter creates hemodynamic instability.[61]

Table 12.14 in Chapter 12 contains additional information about antidysrhythmic medications.

- *Atrial flutter cardioversion:* If at any time a patient with atrial flutter becomes hemodynamically unstable, electrical cardioversion is the recommended emergency intervention.[61]
- *Atrial flutter thrombosis risk:* If atrial flutter has been present for more than 48 hours, one-third of patients will have thrombi in the atria, and anticoagulation is mandated before pharmacologic or electrical cardioversion.[61]
- *Atrial flutter radiofrequency ablation:* For atrial flutter unrelated to an acute disease process, permanent termination of the atrial flutter circuit can be achieved by radiofrequency catheter ablation. Catheter ablation is used to create a line of conduction block across one or more sections of the reentry pathway.

Atrial Fibrillation

The ECG tracing in atrial fibrillation has an uneven atrial baseline that lacks clearly defined P waves and instead shows rapid oscillations or fibrillation wavelets that vary in size, shape, and frequency (Fig. 10.35). The atrial fibrillation wavelets are particularly visible in the inferior ECG leads II, III, and AVF.

Atrial Fibrillation Criteria

Atrial rate: 240 to 400 atrial wavelets per minute; irregular

Ventricular rate (controlled): 60 to 100 per minute; irregular R-R intervals

Ventricular rate (uncontrolled): >100 per minute; irregular R-R intervals

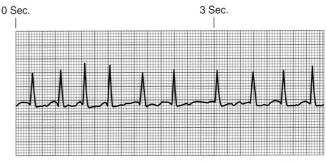

0 Sec.   3 Sec.

Fig. 10.35 Atrial Fibrillation. A fibrillating atrial baseline with an irregular ventricular rate and narrow QRS complex.

Rhythm: Irregularly irregular ventricular rhythm (no pattern)
P wave: Replaced by a fibrillating atrial baseline
PR interval: No longer applies
QRS complex: QRS complex is typically narrow

Clinical significance. Atrial fibrillation is either associated with underlying structural heart disease such as a mitral valve stenosis or described as *nonvalvular atrial fibrillation.*[63] Atrial fibrillation may also be classified under the broad category of SVT, when the HR is rapid and associated with symptoms of hypotension and breathlessness, especially during paroxysmal atrial fibrillation uncontrolled by medication (see Table 10.7).

Pathogenesis of atrial fibrillation. The pathogenesis of atrial fibrillation has traditionally been ascribed to random electrical foci firing in the atria. Research using high-density atrial mapping, high-speed video recordings, and ECG analysis has uncovered distinct spatial organization within the atria.[63] Atrial fibrillation involves several reentry circuits within the atria, and in some cases, they originate at specific anatomic sites. The four pulmonary veins that drain into the left atrium are a trigger site for early atrial foci to initiate and propagate reentry circuits to maintain atrial fibrillation.[63] The earliest atrial ectopic foci have been electrically mapped 2 to 4 cm within the pulmonary veins. The affected pulmonary veins contain thin myocardial sleeves that project into the pulmonary veins from the left atrium. This ectopic tissue resembles discontinuous finger-like projections approximately 5 mm thick that extend 4.5 cm into one or more pulmonary veins. The tissue ultimately becomes part of the venous wall. The spread of atrial fibrillation to the rest of the atria is thought to occur through multiple reentry wavelets that are maintained in perpetual motion by a dominant reentry circuit, which functions at a higher frequency and perpetuates the atrial fibrillation.

When a single focus can be identified, it is possible to encircle that area and isolate that site using radiofrequency catheter ablation. Several different catheter ablation designs are used to isolate foci that originate in the four pulmonary veins, encircling all four veins together or isolating individual or pairs of pulmonary veins.[63]

The atria demonstrate other pathologic changes in atrial fibrillation, typically atrial fibrosis and loss of atrial muscle mass.[63] Any change in atrial architecture increases the risk of atrial fibrillation.[63] An enlarged atrium is an independent risk factor for atrial fibrillation. Conversely, ongoing atrial fibrillation can contribute to pathologic atrial enlargement.

Atrial fibrillation risk factors. Atrial fibrillation is most common in older adults. Less than 1% of adults younger than 60 years have atrial fibrillation. In contrast, almost one-third of adults older than 80 years have atrial fibrillation.[63] Atrial fibrillation is the most common cardiac dysrhythmia in the United States and is responsible for most dysrhythmia-related hospital admissions. There are known risk factors that increase the risk of developing atrial fibrillation, notably structural heart disease, including hypertension, ischemic heart disease, hyperlipidemia, and heart failure. Other disease states associated with higher risk include diabetes mellitus, chronic kidney disease, anemia, arthritis, and COPD.[63]

Atrial fibrillation management. Debate continues about the most effective treatment approach for atrial fibrillation. In the past, the gold standard goal has been to convert the patient out of atrial fibrillation back to sinus rhythm. However, for many older adults, remaining out of atrial fibrillation is an unattainable goal. The major therapeutic decision is whether it is possible to achieve *rhythm* control or ventricular *rate* control. The risk of stroke increases fivefold with atrial fibrillation.[63] Therefore all patients with atrial fibrillation require anticoagulation to prevent development of atrial thrombi, thrombotic embolism, and stroke.[63]

Atrial fibrillation rhythm control. For a hospitalized patient with new-onset atrial fibrillation with unstable hemodynamic values, the primary focus is generally on rhythm control (conversion to sinus rhythm) using antidysrhythmic medications or electrical cardioversion. Emergency medications used to convert atrial fibrillation to sinus rhythm, also known as a *chemical cardioversion*, include amiodarone and ibutilide. Antidysrhythmic medications used long-term to maintain sinus rhythm include amiodarone, dronedarone, disopyramide, flecainide, propafenone, quinidine, sotalol, and dofetilide. Selection of the optimal medication depends on whether the patient has underlying structural heart disease.[63] Even with medication therapy, recurrence of atrial fibrillation is likely. Electrical cardioversion may be successful in converting the atria to sinus rhythm if attempted within a few days or weeks of the onset of atrial fibrillation. Success is less likely if atrial fibrillation has existed for a long time.[63]

Atrial fibrillation rate control. Medications used to control the ventricular rate in atrial fibrillation include calcium channel blockers, beta-blockers, and digoxin. These medications work to slow conduction through the AV node. They have no effect on the fibrillating atria. In the past, it was assumed that rate control was an inferior strategy, because the patient stayed in atrial fibrillation, lost "atrial kick," and was presumed to have an increased risk of embolic stroke. Two multicenter trials have altered that perception: the *Atrial Fibrillation Follow-up: Investigation of Rhythm Management* (AFFIRM) and the *RAte Control versus Electrical Cardioversion for Persistent Atrial Fibrillation* (RACE). These two trials found similar morbidity, mortality, and quality of life in patients treated with rhythm conversion or rate control. For long-term management of permanent atrial fibrillation, rate control is the recommended approach, and therapeutic anticoagulation to prevent embolic stroke is mandatory.[64] Antidysrhythmic and antithrombotic medications used to manage atrial fibrillation are listed in Table 12.17 in Chapter 12.

Stroke risk assessment and antithrombotic therapy in atrial fibrillation. Atrial fibrillation, because of the development of thrombi in the atria, greatly increases the risk of embolic stroke. Electrical and chemical (medication induced) forms of cardioversion entail the threat of precipitating emboli into the systemic circulation. During atrial fibrillation, the atria do not contract effectively, and blood may pool and promote clots that attach to the atrial walls (mural thrombi). If cardioversion is successful and normal sinus rhythm is restored, the atria again contract forcibly and, if thrombus formation has occurred, may send clots traveling through the pulmonary or systemic circulation.

To prevent embolic stroke, it is important to pay attention to the 48-hour rule. Patients who have been in atrial fibrillation for greater than 48 hours, or an unknown timeframe, must be adequately anticoagulated with an oral vitamin K antagonist (warfarin) to a goal international normalized ratio (INR) of 2.0 to 3.0, or administered a factor Xa inhibitor, or a direct thrombin inhibitor for at least 3 weeks before elective cardioversion.[65] After successful cardioversion, patients should be anticoagulated for an additional 4 weeks.[64]

TEE is helpful in identifying the presence or absence of thrombi in fibrillating atria and is recommended as a screening tool before elective cardioversion.[64] It is especially helpful for patients in atrial fibrillation for less than 48 hours who, in the absence of atrial thrombi, may undergo cardioversion without anticoagulation.[64] TEE is described in more detail later in this chapter.

Patients who experience episodes of rapid atrial fibrillation for only a few hours or days at a time and then convert back to sinus rhythm spontaneously (paroxysmal atrial fibrillation) are also at risk for embolic stroke. Several scoring mechanisms have been developed to help predict which patients with atrial fibrillation require prophylactic anticoagulation. The CHADS2 and CHA2DS2-VASc are discussed in the following sections. The atrial fibrillation antithrombotic recommendations apply equally to patients with atrial flutter.[64,65]

CHADS2. The acronym *CHADS2* is an easy-to-remember risk assessment tool used to predict stroke risk in atrial fibrillation and to guide antithrombotic therapy (Box 10.14). The letters stand for *cardiac failure, hypertension, age, diabetes, stroke* (double points).[64] The score ranges from 0 to 6.

CHA2DS2-VASc. The CHA2DS2-VASc has an expanded risk factor profile that includes acute heart failure, hypertension, age 75 years or older (double points), diabetes, stroke (double points), vascular disease, age 65 to 74 years, and sex (female) (see Box 10.14).[65] Anticoagulant therapy is based on risk stratification score and patient-specific comorbidities.

Atrial fibrillation catheter ablation procedures. Many factors must be considered before choosing radiofrequency catheter ablation. Type of atrial fibrillation, degree of symptoms, presence of structural heart disease, candidacy for alternative options, candidacy for anticoagulation, and patient preference must all be assessed. The goal of radiofrequency catheter ablation is to reduce clinical symptoms associated with atrial fibrillation. Based on the results of published studies, 57% of patients have reduced symptoms after ablation even without antidysrhythmic medications.[66] When multiple ablation procedures are performed, the success rate increases to 71% without antidysrhythmic medications and to 77% with antidysrhythmics.[66]

Junctional Dysrhythmias

Only certain areas of the AV node have the property of automaticity. The entire area around the AV node is collectively called the *junction*. After an ectopic electrical impulse arises in the junction, it spreads in two directions at once, both retrograde and antegrade:

BOX 10.14 CHADS2 and CHA2DS2-VASc Score

CHADS2		
Letter	Risk Factor	Score
C	Chronic heart failure	1
H	Hypertension	1
A	Age >75 years	1
D	Diabetes mellitus	1
S	Stroke or TIA	2

CHA2DS2-VASC		
Letter	Risk Factor	Score
C	Chronic heart failure	1
H	Hypertension	1
A	Age >75 years	2
D	Diabetes mellitus	1
S	Stroke or TIA	2
V	Vascular disease	1
A	Age 65–74	1
Sc	Sex category (female)	1

TIA, Transient ischemic attack.

- *Retrograde (backward) conduction*: One wave of depolarization spreads upward to depolarize the atria causing the recording of a P wave on the ECG and the P wave is inverted when viewed in lead II.
- *Antegrade (forward) conduction*: At the same time, another wave of depolarization spreads downward into the ventricles through the normal conduction pathway, producing a normal QRS complex.

In a junctional rhythm, depending on the location, the P wave may vary:
- P wave before the QRS complex, with a short PR interval of less than 0.12 second
- P wave hidden entirely by the QRS complex
- P wave seen after the QRS complex

Premature Junctional Contraction

If only a single ectopic impulse originates in the junction, it is simply called a *premature junctional contraction*. On the ECG, the rhythm is regular from the sinus node except for one early QRS complex of normal shape and duration. The P wave can be entirely absent. If a P wave can be found, it very closely precedes or follows the QRS complex. In lead II, the P wave appears inverted (having a negative deflection) because the atria are being depolarized from the AV node upward, which is the opposite direction from the wave of depolarization that occurs when triggered by the sinus node. If the P wave appears before the QRS complex, the PR interval is less than 0.12 second.

Junctional Escape Rhythm

Sometimes the junction becomes the dominant pacemaker of the heart (Table 10.8). The intrinsic rate of the junction normally is 40 to 60 beats/min.

Junctional escape rhythm criteria.

Rate: Intrinsic rate of junction is 40 to 60 beats per minute if it is the dominant pacemaker of the heart.

Rhythm: Regular.

P wave: May be seen before the QRS, obscured by the QRS, or follow the QRS.

PR interval: Absent or very short if present.

QRS complex: QRS complex is typically narrow, 0.16 to 0.10 second.

Clinical significance. A junctional escape rhythm is a protective mechanism that occurs when the sinus node fails. Generally, a junctional escape rhythm (Fig. 10.36) is well tolerated hemodynamically, although efforts must be directed toward restoring sinus rhythm.

Junctional Tachycardia and Accelerated Junctional Rhythm

A junctional rhythm can also occur at a faster rate (see Table 10.8). The term *tachycardia* is reserved for rates greater than 100 beats/min. *Junctional tachycardia* is a narrow complex rhythm that arises from the AV junction nearer to the bundle of His area. The rate is rapid (120–220 beats/min).[64] Junctional tachycardia may cause hemodynamic compromise, depending on the rate and the patient's underlying cardiac reserve.

When the junctional rate is greater than 60 beats/min and less than 100 beats/min, it is described as an *accelerated junctional rhythm*. The BP is usually maintained in an accelerated junctional rhythm, because the HR is within the normal range to allow adequate diastolic filling time.

Ventricular Dysrhythmias

Ventricular dysrhythmias result from an ectopic focus in any portion of the ventricular myocardium. The usual conduction pathway

TABLE 10.8 Junctional Rhythms.

Parameter	Junctional Escape Rhythm	Accelerated Junctional Rhythm	Junctional Tachycardia
Rate	40–60 beats/min	60–100 beats/min	>100 beats/min
Rhythm	Regular	Regular	Regular
P waves	May be present or absent; inverted in lead II	May be present or absent; inverted in lead II	May be present or absent; inverted in lead II
P-R interval	<0.12 second	<0.12 second	<0.12 second
QRS complex	0.06–0.10 second	0.06–0.10 second	0.06–0.10 second

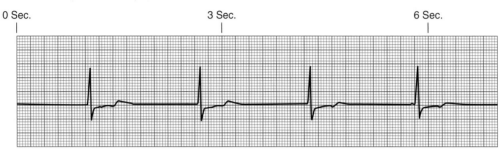

Fig. 10.36 Junctional Escape Rhythm. The ventricular rate is 38 beats/min. P waves are absent, and the QRS complex is narrow with a normal width.

through the ventricles is not used, and the wave of depolarization must spread from cell to cell. As a result, the QRS complex is prolonged and is always greater than 0.12 second. The width of the QRS complex, not the height, is important in the diagnosis of ventricular ectopy. In general, ventricular dysrhythmias have more serious implications than atrial or junctional dysrhythmias and occur only rarely in healthy individuals.

Premature Ventricular Contractions

A PVC is a single ectopic impulse originating in the ventricles. Some PVCs are very small in height but are wider than 0.12 second. If there is doubt, a different lead is evaluated. The shape of the QRS complex depends on the location of the ectopic focus:

- Unifocal PVCs: If all the ventricular ectopic beats look the same in a particular lead, they are called *unifocal*, which means that all result from the same irritable focus (Fig. 10.37A).
- Multifocal PVCs: When the ventricular ectopic beats have various shapes in the same lead, they are called *multifocal* (Fig. 10.37B). Multifocal ventricular ectopic beats are more serious than unifocal ventricular ectopic beats, because they indicate a greater area of irritable myocardial tissue and are more likely to deteriorate into VT or VF. There are many ways that ventricular ectopy may be identified in clincal practice, as described in the following examples.

PVC with compensatory pause. When the impulse from the sinus node meets depolarized myocardium from a PVC, a compensatory pause will occur. A full compensatory pause is shown and described in Fig. 10.38A.

Interpolated PVC. The conduction of the SA node is not disturbed and the R-R intervals before and after the PVC are unchanged. The normal sinus P wave that occurs immediately after the PVC finds the ventricles depolarized and responsive to another impulse, a normal QRS complex results, and the PVC is "sandwiched" between two normal beats without disturbing the underlying sinus rhythm (Fig. 10.38B). This PVC is referred to as *interpolated* (meaning "between"). Interpolated PVCs occur when the normal sinus rate is relatively slow as in sinus bradycardia.

Ventricular bigeminy. When a PVC follows each normally conducted beat, ventricular bigeminy is present (Fig. 10.39).

Ventricular trigeminy. If a PVC follows every two normal beats, it is called *ventricular trigeminy.*

Consecutive PVCs. Two consecutive PVCs are described as a *couplet*, and three consecutive PVCs are called a *triplet* or a *three-beat run of VT.*

R-on-T PVC. The *relative refractory period*, represented on the ECG by the last half of the T wave, is a vulnerable time for ectopy to occur, because repolarization is incomplete (see Fig. 10.28). This is called the *R-on-T phenomenon.*

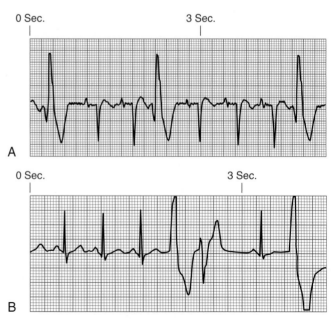

Fig. 10.37 (A) Unifocal premature ventricular contractions (PVCs). (B) Multifocal PVCs.

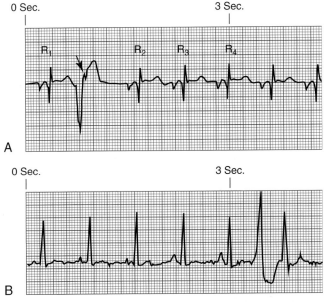

A

B

Fig. 10.38 (A) Premature ventricular contraction (PVC) with fully compensatory pause. The interval between the two sinus beats that surround the PVC (R_1 and R_2) is exactly two times the normal interval between sinus beats (R_3 and R_4). The fully compensatory pause occurs because the sinus node continues to pace despite the PVC. The sinus P wave *(arrow)* is hidden in the ST segment of the PVC. This P wave did not conduct through to the ventricles because they had just been depolarized and were still in the absolute refractory period. (B) Interpolated PVC. The PVC falls between two normally conducted QRS complexes without disturbing the sinus rhythm. The RR interval between sinus beats remains the same.

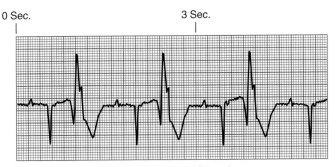

Fig. 10.39 Ventricular Bigeminy.

Causes of premature ventricular contractions. PVCs can result from many causes. They can occur in healthy individuals with no evidence of heart disease. The critical care nurse has an important role in identifying factors that may be causing or contributing to PVCs.

PVCs and myocardial ischemia. Acute ischemia is the most dangerous cause of ventricular ectopy. Ischemia alters cell membrane permeability, giving rise to early depolarization and the initiation of ectopic impulses. Ventricular ectopy that occurs during an acute ischemic event may require treatment with IV amiodarone or other antidysrhythmic medications.

PVCs and electrolyte imbalance. Metabolic abnormalities are common causes of PVCs. Hypokalemia, hypoxemia, and acidosis predispose the cell membrane to instability and may cause ventricular ectopy. Treatment is directed toward identifying the metabolic disturbance and correcting it. The ability of oxygen and potassium values to change very rapidly in a critically ill patient cannot be underestimated.

Invasive procedures, such as insertion of a PA-Catheter or cardiac catheterization, can cause PVCs by mechanically irritating the ventricular muscle. In these situations, the ectopy usually resolves with removal or advancement of the catheter.

PVCs and medications. Certain medications can cause ventricular ectopy. Digitalis toxicity may precipitate PVCs, which are resistant to conventional antidysrhythmic therapy. Some class I antidysrhythmic medications can cause more serious dysrhythmias than the dysrhythmias they were intended to treat. This is called a *prodysrhythmic effect* (also described as a *proarrhythmic effect*), and it can sometimes be fatal. Class 1a medications prolong the QT interval by lengthening the ventricular refractory period. This is a therapeutic effect, but when the QT interval prolongation becomes excessive, a characteristic form of polymorphic VT called *torsades de pointes* develops (Fig. 10.40). In this dysrhythmia, VT is very rapid, and QRS complexes appear to twist in a spiral pattern around the baseline. Torsades de pointes results in hemodynamic instability because of the extremely rapid rate. If torsades de pointes is not terminated, death ensues. Sometimes torsades de pointes stops spontaneously, although the patient may experience a syncopal episode or seizure at the time of the dysrhythmia. Risk factors for development of torsades de pointes are listed in Box 10.15.

Idioventricular rhythms. Sometimes an ectopic focus in the ventricle can become the dominant pacemaker of the heart (Table 10.9). If the sinus node and the AV junction fail, the ventricles depolarize at their own intrinsic rate of 20 to 40 times per minute. This is called an *idioventricular rhythm* and is a naturally protective mechanism.

Criteria for Idioventricular Rhythms.

Rhythm: Regular

P wave: Not associated with the QRS

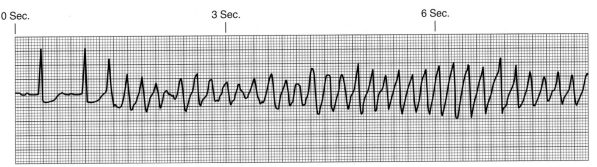

Fig. 10.40 Torsades de Pointes.

BOX 10.15 Risk Factors for Torsades de Pointes

Prolonged QTc Interval
- QTc interval $\geq$ 500 ms

Medications
- Use of QT interval–prolonging medications
- Rapid intravenous infusion of QT interval–prolonging medications
- Diuretics

Structural Heart Conditions
- Heart failure
- Myocardial infarction

Metabolic Conditions
- Hypokalemia
- Hypomagnesemia
- Hypocalcemia
- Liver failure with decreased medication metabolism
- Bradycardia
- Sinus bradycardia
- Complete heart block
- Incomplete heart block with pauses
- Premature complexes leading to short-long-short cycles

Genetic Predisposition
- Occult (latent) congenital long-QT syndrome
- Genetic polymorphisms (reduced repolarization reserve)

Age and Sex
- Advanced age
- Female sex

Torsades de pointes risk increases with a higher number of risk factors, some of which may be clinically silent and difficult to detect.

From Drew BJ, Ackerman MJ, Funk M, et al. Prevention of torsade de pointes in hospital settings: a scientific statement from the American Heart Association and the American College of Cardiology Foundation. *Circulation.* 2010;121(8):1047.

PR interval: Absent

QRS duration: Greater than 0.12 second, complexes are wide because the impulses originate in the ventricles

Clinical significance. Rather than trying to abolish the ventricular beats, the aim of treatment is to increase the effective HR and reestablish dominance of a higher pacing site such as the sinus node or the AV junction. Usually, a temporary pacemaker is used to increase the HR until the underlying problems that caused failure of the other pacing sites can be resolved.

Accelerated idioventricular rhythm. An accelerated idioventricular rhythm (AIVR) occurs when a ventricular focus assumes control of the heart at a rate greater than its intrinsic rate of 40 beats/min but less than 100 beats/min (Fig. 10.41). The patient with AIVR must be closely observed for changes in rate and/or hemodynamic deterioration. IV lidocaine must never be administered to a patient with an idioventricular rhythm, because lidocaine suppresses the ventricular pacemaker and converts the rhythm to asystole.

Ventricular tachycardia. VT is caused by a ventricular pacing site firing at a rate of 100 times or more per minute, usually maintained by a reentry mechanism within the ventricular tissue (Fig. 10.42). The complexes are wide, and the rhythm may be slightly irregular, often accelerating as the tachycardia continues (see Table 10.9).

Ventricular tachycardia criteria.

Rate: Greater than 100 bpm

Rhythm: Mostly regular, may have some irregular beats

P wave: Not related to the QRS. Sinus node may continue to function normally.

PR interval: Absent

QRS duration: Greater than 0.12 second

Clinical significance. The clinical significance of VT depends on many factors as described in more detail below. VT poses a higher risk when it is sustained and associated with ischemia or structural heart disease, versus nonsustained or from a reversible cause.

Nonsustained VT: A brief episode with a duration of less than 30 seconds is described as nonsustained VT.

Sustained VT: A life-threatening VT lasting longer than 30 seconds that must be terminated quickly, or the VT is likely to degenerate into VF and death.

Fusion beats: If the sinus impulse and the ventricular ectopic impulse meet in the middle of the ventricles, a fusion beat may occur. Fusion beats are narrower than ventricular beats and the shape is a combination of the patient's sinus QRS complex and the ventricular ectopic QRS complex. When present, P waves and fusion beats are helpful in verifying the diagnosis of VT as opposed to SVT.

Emergency treatment for VT: Clinical management of VT depends on whether the patient is stable or unstable and whether a pulse and adequate BP are present. Pulseless VT is a life-threatening condition. The patient loses consciousness and needs immediate cardiopulmonary resuscitation and defibrillation as described in the American Heart Association (AHA) protocols for advanced cardiac life support (ACLS).

After the acute episode is over, patients who have already experienced sustained VT or cardiac arrest continue to be at risk for sudden cardiac death. An extensive clinical evaluation is warranted, including cardiac catheterization and electrophysiologic testing with programmed ventricular stimulation. Therapy is aimed at preventing a recurrence of sustained VT or VF. It may include treating the underlying cause, administering antidysrhythmic medications, performing ablation of the reentrant pathway within the ventricle, or inserting an implantable cardioverter defibrillator (ICD). Chapter 12 provides more information on ICDs (see Fig. 12.5).

TABLE 10.9 Ventricular Rhythms.

Parameter	Idioventricular Rhythm	Accelerated Idioventricular Rhythm	Ventricular Tachycardia	Ventricular Fibrillation
Rate	20–40 beats/min	40–100 beats/min	>100 beats/min	None
Rhythm	Usually regular	Usually regular	Usually regular	Irregular
P waves	Absent or retrograde	Absent or retrograde	Absent or retrograde	None
PR interval	None	None	None	None
QRS complex	>0.12 second	>0.12 second	>0.12 second	Fibrillatory waves

Page RL, Joglar JA, Caldwell MA, et al. 2015 ACC/AHA/HRS Guideline for the Management of Adult Patients With Supraventricular Tachycardia: A Report of the American College of Cardiology/American Heart Association Task Force on Clinical Practice Guidelines and the Heart Rhythm Society. *J Am Coll Cardiol.* 2016;67(13):e27-e115.

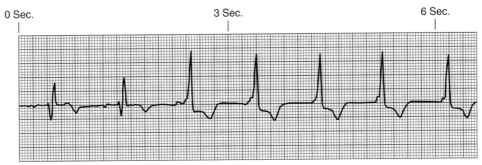

Fig. 10.41 Accelerated Idioventricular Rhythm. The QRS complex duration is 0.14 second, and the ventricular rate is 65 beats/min.

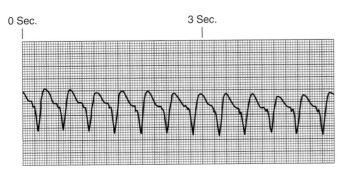

Fig. 10.42 Ventricular Tachycardia.

Fig. 10.43 Ventricular Fibrillation.

Ventricular fibrillation. VF is the result of chaotic electrical activity in the ventricles that causes the ventricles to quiver and no forward flow of blood occurs. On the ECG, VF appears as a continuous, undulating pattern without clear P wave, QRS complex, or T wave (Fig. 10.43).

Criteria for ventricular fibrillation.

Rate: Indeterminate
Rhythm: Irregular wavy baseline without recognizable QRS complexes
P wave: Absent, cannot be distinguished from fibrillating baseline
PR interval: Absent
QRS duration: Absent, no QRS complexes are present
QRS complex: Wavy baseline, no QRS complexes are present

Clinical significance. When VF occurs in the setting of an acute ischemic event and is accompanied by a significant amount of myocardial damage, the survival rate is poor. Resuscitation is often unsuccessful; recurrence rates are high for patients who are resuscitated. VF appears on the ECG as large, erratic undulations of the baseline (coarse VF) or as a mild tremor (fine VF). In VF, the patient does not have a pulse, no blood is being pumped forward, and defibrillation is the only definitive therapy. Defibrillation is more likely to be successful with coarse VF. The AHA-ACLS protocol should be followed. As with any cardiac arrest situation, supportive measures such as cardiopulmonary resuscitation, intubation, and correction of metabolic abnormalities are performed concurrently with definitive therapy.

Atrioventricular Blocks

On the ECG, the ability of the AV node to conduct is evaluated by measuring the PR interval and the relationship of P waves to QRS complexes (Table 10.10). The normal PR interval, measured from the beginning of the P wave to the beginning of the QRS complex, ranges from 0.12 to 0.20 second. When the normal conduction of the AV node is impaired, the PR interval will be greater than 0.2 second, resulting in a heart block.

First-Degree Atrioventricular Block

When all atrial impulses are conducted to the ventricles and the PR interval is greater than 0.20 second, a condition known as *first-degree AV block* exists (Fig. 10.44).

Criteria for first-degree AV block.

Rate: Depends on the underlying rhythm, usually sinus rhythm
Rhythm: Regular if sinus rhythm
P wave: Present, normal shape
PR interval: Greater than 0.20 second
QRS duration: 0.06 to 0.10 second
QRS complex: Normal appearance generally

Clinical significance. First-degree AV block represents slowed conduction through the AV node. If the HR is adequate this may not be a problem. However, if the associated QRS complex is widened, it is likely that there is also damage to the bundle branches from sclerosis, ischemia, or infarction.

Second-Degree Atrioventricular Block

Second-degree AV block can be broadly defined as a condition in which some atrial impulses are conducted to the ventricles, but others are "blocked" at the AV node. This description of intermittent AV conduction covers two patterns with markedly different clinical significance: Second-degree AV block is divided into Mobitz type I (also known as *Wenckebach block*) and Mobitz type II.

Mobitz type I. In Mobitz type I block, the AV conduction times progressively lengthen until a P wave is not conducted. This typically occurs in a pattern of *grouped beats* and is observed on the ECG by a gradually lengthening PR interval, until ultimately the final P wave in the group fails to conduct. In Mobitz type I, the QRS complex is generally of normal width and appearance. Several criteria must be present for Mobitz I (Wenckebach) to be diagnosed, as follows:

TABLE 10.10   Atrioventricular Block.

Parameter	First-Degree	Second-Degree Mobitz I (Wenckebach)	Second-Degree Mobitz II	Third-Degree (Complete)
PR interval	>0.20 second and constant	Increases with each consecutively conducted P wave	Constant	Varies randomly
P waves	One P wave for each QRS complex	Intermittently not conducted, yielding more P waves than QRS complexes	Intermittently not conducted, yielding more P waves than QRS complexes	P waves independent and not related to QRS complexes
QRS complex	0.06—0.10 second	0.06—0.10 second	May be normal, but usually coexists with BBB (>0.12 second)	0.06—0.10 second if junctional escape pacemaker activates ventricles >0.12 second if ventricular escape pacemaker activates ventricles

BBB, Bundle branch block.

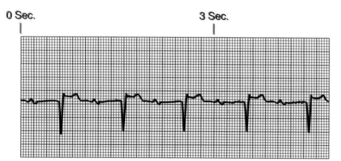

0 Sec.   3 Sec.

Fig. 10.44   First-Degree Atrioventricular Block. The PR interval is prolonged to 0.44 second.

Criteria for second-degree AV block—Mobitz I (Wenckebach).
Rate: Grouped beats with a P wave: QRS pattern of 3:2, 4:3, or 5:4.
Rhythm: Beats have a grouped pattern followed by a pause due to a nonconducted P wave.
P wave: More P waves than QRS complexes. P-to-P interval is normal.
PR interval: The PR interval progressively lengthens until there is a nonconducted P wave often described as a pause. The first P-R interval is the shortest in the group; the last PR interval is the longest in the group.
QRS duration: 0.06 to 0.10 second.
QRS complex: Normal shape and width.
   Clinical significance. Mobitz I indicates that there is injury to the AV node. If the HR is maintained above 60 bpm the patient may not experience symptoms. However, this rhythm should not be ignored as the degree of AV block may progress.

Mobitz I block has a specific, repeating pattern that catches the eye. The expected groups are 3:2, 4:3, or 5:4. For example, if four P waves are conducted to the ventricles and the fifth one is not, a 5:4 conduction ratio is present (five P waves to four QRS complexes). The nonconducted P wave ends a group. After the pause, the cycle repeats itself (Fig. 10.45).
   Mobitz type II. Mobitz type II block is always anatomically located below the AV node in the bundle of His, in the bundle branches, or in the Purkinje fibers. This results in an all-or-nothing situation with respect to AV conduction. When conduction does occur, all PR intervals are the same. Because of the anatomic location of the block, the PR interval is constant and the QRS complexes are wide on the ECG (Fig. 10.46).
   Criteria for second-degree AV block—Mobitz II.
Rate: Varies depending on the conduction rate from atria to ventricles
Rhythm: May have a pattern if the AV node consistently conducts every second or third P wave. Irregular if P waves are conducted inconsistently.
P wave: Present, normal shape.
PR interval: Normal interval for P waves that are conducted (0.12—0.20 second).
QRS duration: 0.06 to 0.10 second or wider. The QRS may be wider depending on the location of the block.
QRS complex: May be normal or widened. Shape may vary depending on the location of the block.
   Clinical significance. Mobitz II block is more ominous clinically than Mobitz I and may progress to complete AV block. For this reason, it is important to prepare for transcutaneous cardiac pacing (TCP), via pad electrodes applied to the chest. Also, consider the possibility that a temporary transvenous pacemaker may be placed, or a permanent pacemaker may be required before hospital discharge.

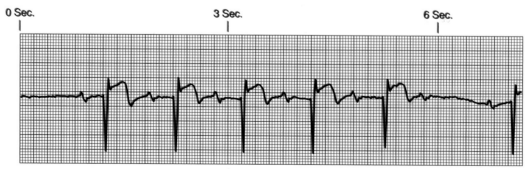

0 Sec.   3 Sec.   6 Sec.

Fig. 10.45   Mobitz type I (Wenckebach) Second-Degree Atrioventricular Block. The PR intervals gradually increase from 0.36 to 0.46 second until a P wave is not conducted to the ventricles.

0 Sec.　　　　　　　　　　3 Sec.

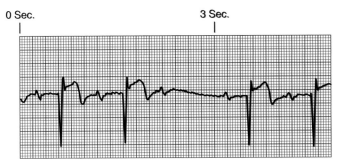

Fig. 10.46 Mobitz Type II Second-Degree Atrioventricular Block. The PR intervals remain constant.

Third-Degree Atrioventricular Block

Third-degree, or complete, AV block is a condition in which no atrial impulses can conduct from the atria to the ventricles. This condition is also described by the terms *complete heart block* or *AV dissociation* to indicate that different cardiac pacemakers control the atrial rate and the ventricular rate. The block can be located at the level of the AV node or below the node within the bundle of His or the bundle branches.

Criteria for Third-degree AV block.
Rate: Depends on underlying ventricular rate
Rhythm: Regular at intrinsic ventricular rate of 20 to 40 beats/min
P wave: Present, normal shape, unrelated to QRS complexes
PR interval: Absent
QRS duration: QRS wide, greater than 0.10 second
QRS complex: Usually wider than the normal QRS is the pacing focus is from the ventricles.

Clinical significance. When a ventricular focus is pacing the heart, the QRS complex is wide and unrelated to the P waves (Fig. 10.47). Pacemaker support is often necessary to maintain an adequate CO.

LABORATORY TESTS

Laboratory assessment of cardiovascular status is obtained through studies of blood serum. Accurate interpretation of these laboratory studies, along with the clinical picture, enables the critical care team to diagnose, treat, and assess the response to therapeutic interventions.

Laboratory studies of blood serum are performed to assess the following:

1. Electrolyte levels that can alter cardiac muscle contraction
2. Cardiac biomarkers that reflect myocardial cellular integrity or infarction
3. Hematologic status to evaluate risk of anemia and infection
4. Coagulation times
5. Serum lipid levels
6. Status of other organ systems that can secondarily affect cardiac function

Interpreting Serum Electrolyte Values
Potassium

During depolarization and repolarization of nerve and muscle fiber, potassium and sodium exchange occurs intracellularly and extracellularly. The potassium gradient across the cell membrane determines conduction velocity and helps confine pacing activity to the sinus node. Excess or deficiency of potassium can alter myocardial muscle function. Normal serum potassium (K^+) levels are generally 3.5 to 4.5 mEq/L, although definitions may vary slightly between institutions. Table 10.11 lists electrolyte values that affect cardiac contractility.

Hyperkalemia. Elevated serum potassium (higher than 4.5 mEq/L), called *hyperkalemia*, can be caused by various conditions, including excess potassium administration, extensive skeletal muscle destruction (rhabdomyolysis), tumor lysis syndrome, and kidney failure. Some medications may induce hyperkalemia, including potassium-sparing diuretics, angiotensin-converting enzyme inhibitors, and angiotensin-receptor blockers.[67]

ECG changes in hyperkalemia. Hyperkalemia can elicit significant changes in the ECG because it decreases AV conduction velocity, slows ventricular depolarization, and accelerates repolarization. As the serum levels of potassium rise, tall, narrow peaked T waves may be seen and are followed by prolongation of the PR interval, loss of the P wave, widening of the QRS complex, heart block, and eventually asystole (Fig. 10.48A). Severely elevated serum potassium (greater than 8 mEq/L) causes a wide QRS complex tachycardia, as shown in the 12-lead ECG in Fig. 10.48B. If not corrected, severe hyperkalemia can lead to VF or cardiac standstill. Evidence of hyperkalemia is not always visible on the ECG, and ECG waveform changes are not always a sensitive indicator of elevated potassium levels.

Emergency treatment of hyperkalemia. Extreme hyperkalemia can be acutely managed with IV insulin to drive the potassium inside the cell and temporarily out of the plasma. Glucose must be administered at the same time to avoid hypoglycemia as a secondary complication. Potassium is permanently removed from the bloodstream by cation-exchange resin products, such as sodium polystyrene sulfonate (Kayexalate), placed into the gastrointestinal tract or by

0 Sec.　　　　　　　　　　3 Sec.

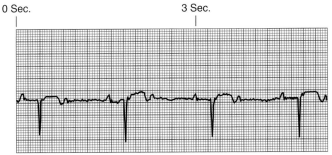

Fig. 10.47 Third-Degree (Complete) Heart Block. The atrial rate (P waves) and ventricular rate (QRSs) are consistent but are not in synchrony.

TABLE 10.11 Chemistry Values That Affect Cardiac Contractility and Conduction.			
	NORMAL RANGES[a]		
Electrolyte	**mEq/L**	**mg/dL**	**mmol/L**
Potassium (K^+)	3.5–4.5		3.50–4.50
Ionized calcium (Ca)		4.0–5.0	1.00–1.30
Total calcium (Ca^{2+})		8.5–10.5	2.00–2.60
Magnesium (Mg^{2+})	1.5–2.0	1.8–2.4	0.70–1.10

[a]Laboratory values may be reported as mEq/L, mg/dL, or mmol/L. Each measurement parameter used produces a different value. Some electrolytes are reported with more than one reference value. Different clinical laboratories use different reference values, and the cited reference values may vary slightly between clinical laboratories.

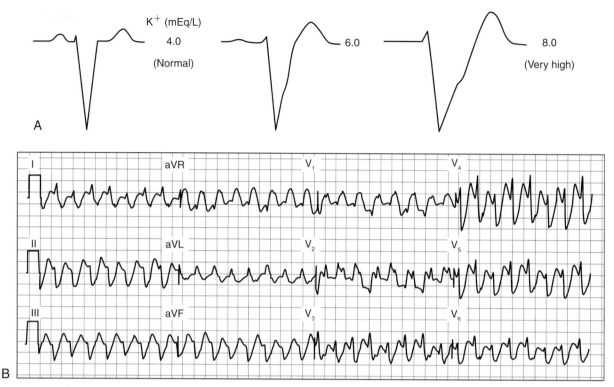

Fig. 10.48 Effects of Hyperkalemia on an Electrocardiogram (ECG). (A) Stages in hyperkalemia from normal potassium levels to plasma levels of 8 mEq/L. At approximately 6 mEq/L, the P wave flattens, the QRS complex broadens, and the ST segment disappears, with the S wave flowing into the tall, tented T wave. (B) A 12-lead ECG of a patient with a serum potassium level of 9.1 mEq/L.

hemodialysis.[68] Coexisting low serum sodium, calcium, or pH levels potentiate the cardiac effects of hyperkalemia.

Hypokalemia. A low serum potassium level, called *hypokalemia* (less than 3.5 mEq/L), is commonly caused by diuretic therapy with insufficient replacement, gastrointestinal losses, and some medications.[68]

ECG changes in hypokalemia. The earliest ECG change is often the appearance of PVCs, which can deteriorate into VT or VF without appropriate potassium replacement. Hypokalemia impairs myocardial conduction and prolongs ventricular repolarization; this can be seen by a prominent U wave, which is a positive deflection after the T wave on the ECG (Fig. 10.49). The U wave is not unique to hypokalemia, but its presence is a signal for the clinician to check the serum potassium level. Serum potassium levels must be closely monitored, and replacement administered as needed. Great care must be taken with administration of concentrated electrolytes to prevent complications. Potassium is a high-alert medication, and additional safety procedures are recommended for replacement of this electrolyte (Box 10.16— **QSEN** Safety: Medication Administration).

Calcium

Calcium (Ca^{2+}) is an important cation in the body. Calcium metabolism is controlled by many factors, including normal parathyroid hormone function, calcitonin, and vitamin D acting on target organs such as the kidney, bone, and gastrointestinal tract. Calcium is an important mediator of many cardiovascular functions because of its effect on vascular tone, myocardial contractility, and cardiac excitability.

Serum calcium values can be recorded in three ways, depending on the hospital laboratory: milliequivalents per liter (mEq/L), milligrams

per deciliter (mg/dL), or millimoles per liter (mmol/L). In the bloodstream, approximately 50% of calcium is biologically active, known as *ionized calcium*.[69] The remaining calcium is bound to protein (primarily albumin) and inorganic ions such as sulfate and phosphate. Calcium is not biologically active in its bound state.[69] The normal values for total and ionized serum calcium levels are listed in Table 10.11. The normal serum concentration of ionized calcium is maintained within very narrow limits; changes in ionized calcium level are responsible for the clinical effects of hypercalcemia and hypocalcemia. The only accurate way to determine the level of ionized calcium, described as *physiologically active, unbound,* or *free,* is to measure the ionized serum value with a laboratory assay.[69] The mathematically calculated values that extrapolate from total calcium and serum albumin levels have been shown to be inaccurate and should not be used with critically ill patients.[70]

Hypercalcemia. Hypercalcemia is defined as increased amounts of ionized calcium (greater than 4.8 mg/dL or 1.30 mmol/L) or increased amounts of total serum calcium (greater than 10.5 mg/dL or 2.60 mmol/L). Serum calcium levels are increased by bone tumors; primary hyperparathyroidism caused by elevated parathyroid hormone levels; excessive intake of supplemental calcium and vitamin D, usually in oral antacids; hypomagnesemia; and as a complication of kidney failure from decreased excretion of calcium. Hypercalcemia affects many organs; causes smooth muscle relaxation; and can lead to neurologic changes such as lethargy, confusion, and even coma.

ECG changes in hypercalcemia. Cardiovascular effects of elevated serum calcium include strengthening contractility and shortening ventricular repolarization, demonstrated on the ECG by a shortened QTc interval. Rhythm disturbances may include bradycardia;

Hypokalemia

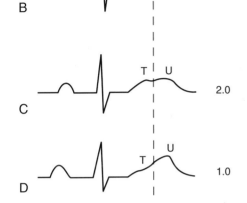

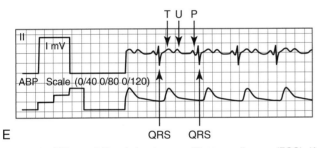

Fig. 10.49 Effects of Hypokalemia on an Electrocardiogram (ECG). (A) At a normal serum concentration of 3.5 to 4.5 mEq/L, the amplitude of the T wave is appreciably greater than that of the U wave. (B) By the time the serum potassium level has decreased to 3 mEq/L, the amplitudes of the T and U waves are approaching each other. (C and D) With a further decrease in the level of potassium, the U wave begins to tower over and fuse with the T wave. (E) ECG tracing from a patient with a serum potassium of 2.6 mEq/L shows a prominent U wave.

first-degree, second-degree, and third-degree heart block; and BBB. Hypercalcemia can potentiate the effects of digitalis and cause hypertension.[71]

Management of symptomatic hypercalcemia involves promotion of calcium excretion by diuretics and infusion of a large volume of normal saline if tolerated by the heart, lungs, and kidneys. Patients who cannot tolerate this clinical regimen may receive hemodialysis using a low-calcium dialysate.

Hypocalcemia. Hypocalcemia is defined as an ionized calcium level below normal (less than 1.05 mmol/L) or a low total serum calcium level. Hypocalcemia (measured by ionized calcium) is a common finding and was found in 55% of critically ill patients on admission to the critical care unit in one study.[70] The more severe the patient's

illness, the greater the risk of developing hypocalcemia.[70] Transfusions of blood from the blood bank lower serum calcium levels, because the citrate used as an anticoagulant in banked blood binds to the calcium.[71] This is called *citrate chelation*. If citrate is used during hemodialysis or plasmapheresis, it has the same calcium-binding (chelating) effect. Phosphate also binds to calcium and can lower the serum calcium level. Metabolic alkalosis often coexists with hypocalcemia. The cardiovascular effects of hypocalcemia include decreased myocardial contractility, decreased CO, and hypotension.

ECG changes in hypocalcemia. Rhythm disturbances with severe hypocalcemia are variable, ranging from bradycardia to VT and asystole. When ionized calcium is low, the ECG may show a prolonged QTc interval. A prolonged QTc predisposes a patient to torsades de pointes (see Fig. 10.40).

Emergency treatment of hypocalcemia. Management of hypocalcemia, especially when ionized calcium is low, involves infusion of IV calcium chloride or IV calcium gluconate[71]:

- Calcium chloride provides 27 mg of elemental calcium/mL (272 mg in 10 mL).
- Calcium gluconate provides 9 mg of elemental calcium/mL (90 mg in 10 mL).

Magnesium

Magnesium (Mg^{2+}) is essential for many enzyme, protein, lipid, and carbohydrate functions in the body and is critical for the production and use of energy.[72] The body stores most magnesium in bone (50%–60%), muscle, and soft tissues, with less than 1% present in blood.[72] As with other electrolytes, the ionized portion of serum magnesium is the biologically active component that is available for biochemical processes. Due to limited availability, only 2% of clinical laboratories in the United States measure ionized magnesium[72]; routine blood tests measure total serum magnesium.[72] Serum magnesium can be reported in units of mEq/L, mg/dL, or mmol/L, depending on the laboratory running the analysis. The normal serum range is 1.5 to 2 mEq/L, 1.8 to 2.4 mg/dL, or 0.7 to 1.1 mmol/L. Normal reference values vary between hospital laboratories.

Hypermagnesemia. Hypermagnesemia is rare in critical care patients. It results from kidney failure, tumor lysis syndrome, or iatrogenic overtreatment.

Hypomagnesemia. Hypomagnesemia is defined as a total serum magnesium concentration less than 1.5 mEq/L. It is commonly associated with other electrolyte imbalances, most notably alterations in potassium, calcium, and phosphorus. Low serum magnesium levels can result from many causes. Aggressive diuresis with loop diuretics can lower serum levels.[72] Diarrhea can be a significant cause of magnesium loss, because lower gastrointestinal fluids contain up to 15 mEq/L of magnesium; vomiting or gastric suction causes less depletion, because upper gastrointestinal fluids contain approximately 1 mEq/L. Another cause of magnesium depletion is rapid administration of citrated blood products, which results in citrate chelation. Insufficient dietary magnesium intake and chronic alcohol abuse are also risk factors. Hypomagnesemia can also occur in patients who take proton-pump inhibitor medications to reduce production of gastric acid. This condition improves when the proton-pump inhibitors are stopped. In chronic hypomagnesemia, serum levels are replenished from the bone stores.[72]

ECG changes in hypomagnesemia. In hypomagnesemia, the ECG changes are similar to changes seen with hypokalemia and hypocalcemia: prolonged PR and QTc intervals, presence of U waves, T wave flattening, and widened QRS complex. Cardiac dysrhythmias may be

QSEN BOX 10.16 **Safety**

Medication Administration

1. **Accurate Patient Identification**
   - Use at least two patient identifiers (not the patient's room number) when taking blood samples or administering medications or blood products. Examples include the patient's name or date of birth. In many hospitals in addition to verbal confirmation, a bar-code scanner or QR code reader that is linked to the documentation system is used to verify the patient's armband at the point of care.

2. **Effective Communication Among Caregivers**
   - An organizational method to decrease the number of medication errors is the use of *computerized physician order entry.*
   - Hospitals should have a process for taking verbal or telephone orders that requires a verification "read back" of the complete order by the person receiving the order.
   - The Institute of Safe Medication Practices (ISMP) maintains a list of medications with similar-sounding names, as name confusion can lead to medication errors. The list is available on the ISMP website at www. ismp.org/tools/confuseddrugnames.pdf. Medication errors can be reported to the Medication Errors Reporting Program.
   - Standardize the abbreviations, acronyms, and symbols used throughout the organization, including a list of abbreviations, acronyms, and symbols not to use.
   - Examples of problematic abbreviations include "U" for units and "μg" for micrograms. When handwritten, a capital U can be mistaken for a zero (0); in numerous case reports, an insulin dosage written in U was interpreted as 0. Using the abbreviation "μg" instead of "mcg" for micrograms is also problematic; when handwritten, the Greek letter μ can look like an "m." The error-prone abbreviations list is available on the ISMP website at www.ismp.org/tools/errorproneabbreviations.pdf.
   - Use of trailing zeros (e.g., 2.0 vs. 2) and use of a leading decimal point without a leading zero (e.g., .2 instead of 0.2) are dangerous prescription-writing practices. Misinterpretation has caused 10-fold dosing errors.

3. **High-Alert Medication Safety**
   - Remove concentrated electrolytes (including, but not limited to, potassium chloride [KCl], potassium phosphate, and hypertonic sodium chloride) from patient care units.

   - Standardize and limit the number of medication concentrations available in the organization.
   - In the first 2 years after enacting a *sentinel event reporting mechanism*, the most common category was medication errors, and the most frequently implicated medication was KCl. The Joint Commission reviewed 10 incidents of patient death resulting from misadministration of KCl. Eight deaths were the result of direct infusion of concentrated KCl. In six of the eight cases, KCl was mistaken for another medication, primarily because of similarities in packaging and labeling. Most often, KCl was mistaken for sodium chloride, heparin, or furosemide (Lasix).
   - The Joint Commission suggests that health care organizations *not* make concentrated KCl available outside the pharmacy unless appropriate, specific safeguards are in place.
   - A list of high-alert medications is available on the ISMP website www.ismp.org.

3. **Infusion Pump Safety**
   - Ensure free-flow protection on all general-use and patient-controlled analgesia intravenous (IV) infusion pumps used in the organization.
   - Infusion pumps that do not provide protection from the free flow of IV fluid or medication into the patient are hazardous.
   - *Free flow* occurs when IV solution flows freely under the force of gravity without being controlled by the infusion pump. Free flow typically occurs after the administration set is temporarily removed from the pump to transfer a patient to another area, change a patient's gown, or place a patient on a radiography table. Clinicians can greatly reduce this risk by using administration sets with set-based anti—free-flow mechanisms that prevent gravity free flow by closing off the IV tubing to **prohibit flow when the administration set is removed from the pump.**

4. **Hospital Safety**
   - The Joint Commission develops Hospital National Patient Safety Goals (see Chapter 1) each year that incorporate medication safety requirements.

---

supraventricular or ventricular and include the polymorphic ventricular rhythm torsades de pointes (see Fig. 10.40).

Emergency treatment of hypomagnesemia. Routine use of magnesium in cardiac arrest is not recommended. However, in cardiac arrest with torsades de pointes, administration of magnesium may be considered.[73] It is important to evaluate kidney function and to monitor magnesium blood levels.

Cardiac Biomarker Studies

Cardiac Biomarkers in Acute Coronary Syndrome

Cardiac biomarkers are proteins that are released from damaged myocardial cells.[74] When myocardial cells are damaged, they release detectable proteins into the bloodstream, so an increase in biomarkers can be correlated with heart muscle injury. The biomarkers that are routinely measured include cardiac troponin I and cardiac troponin T. Table 10.12 summarizes the cardiac biomarkers related to myocardial injury and MI.

Troponin T and troponin I. The troponins are biomarkers for myocardial damage. The elevation of troponin I and troponin T occurs 3 to 6 hours after acute myocardial damage.[74] Troponin levels are measured at symptom onset in the hospital or when the patient

comes to the emergency department. Serial troponin values are measured at specific time intervals per institutional protocol until values peak.

Because troponin I is found only in cardiac muscle, it is a highly specific biomarker for myocardial damage. The advantage to using a

TABLE 10.12 Serum Biomarkers After Acute Myocardial Infarction.

Serum Biomarker	Time to Initial Elevation (hours[a])	Peak Elevation[b] (hours[a])	Return to Baseline (days[a])
Cardiac troponin I	3—12	24	5—10
Cardiac troponin T	3—12	12—48	5—14
CK-MB[c]	3—12	24	2—3

[a]Time periods represent average reported values.
[b]Does not include patients who have had reperfusion therapy.
[c]The creatine kinase (CK) enzyme consists of two subunits, the brain type (B) and the muscle type (M).

more sensitive biomarker test is that more patients with ACS will be identified, although this will not eliminate the requirement for astute clinical assessment because of the many other conditions associated with elevated troponin levels. A negative high-sensitivity troponin result eliminates acute MI as a diagnosis in most cases.

Natriuretic Peptide Biomarkers in Heart Failure: BNP and NT-proBNP

Natriuretic peptides are biomarkers that provide additional information for accurate evaluation of a patient with acute shortness of breath.[75] It can be difficult to identify whether a patient with shortness of breath has a primary pulmonary problem or has symptoms of acute heart failure with pulmonary edema. In decompensated heart failure, ventricular distention from volume overload, or pressure overload, causes myocytes in the ventricle to release B-type natriuretic peptide (BNP). Several laboratory assays are commercially available to measure BNP, including a point-of-care test, a central laboratory test for BNP, and a laboratory test to measure the N-terminal fragment of proBNP (NT-proBNP).[75] BNP has a half-life of approximately 20 minutes, whereas NT-proBNP has a longer half-life of 1 to 2 hours.

With greater ventricular wall stress, more natriuretic peptide is released from the myocardium, reflected as an elevated BNP/NT-proBNP blood level. This value is combined with the physical examination, 12-lead ECG, and chest radiograph to increase the accuracy of heart failure diagnosis. The choice of test generally depends on what is available in the hospital clinical laboratory.

There are some caveats to the use of natriuretic peptides as biomarkers principally because they are not unique to the heart. Natriuretic peptides are also released from the endothelium and from the kidney, and this can alter the measured BNP levels. Filtration by the kidney is one of the mechanisms by which BNP is cleared from the bloodstream. BNP levels are higher in patients with kidney failure, especially if the glomerular filtration rate is less than 60 mL/min/1.7 m^2.

B-type natriuretic peptide. A symptomatic patient with a BNP level less than 100 pg/mL is unlikely to be in heart failure. Conversely, a patient with a BNP level greater than 400 pg/dL is almost definitely in heart failure. BNP is an excellent test to rule out acute heart failure. The challenge lies in interpreting the results of patients with a BNP level of 100 to 400 pg/mL, sometimes described as the *gray zone*. This intermediate gray zone highlights the importance of using a spectrum of clinical and diagnostic tests. As the symptoms of heart failure are successfully treated, the BNP level usually decreases toward the normal range.

N-terminal fragment of pro-B-type natriuretic peptide. A symptomatic patient with a NT-proBNP below 300 pg/mL is unlikely to be in heart failure. Notably, NT-proBNP is often stratified by age, and threshold values may vary by clinical laboratory. For example, in a patient younger than 50 years, a NT-proBNP level of 450 pg/mL suggests heart failure. In a patient older than 50 years, the threshold for heart failure rises to 900 pg/mL. In a patient older than 75 years the NT-proBNP threshold as an indicator of heart failure rises to 1800 pg/mL.

Hematologic Studies

Hematologic laboratory studies that are routinely ordered for the management of patients with altered cardiovascular status are RBC or erythrocyte level, hemoglobin level, hematocrit level, and white blood cell (WBC) or leukocyte level.

Red Blood Cells

The normal number of RBCs in a person varies with age, sex, environmental temperature, altitude, and exercise. Men produce 4.5 to 6

million RBCs/mm^3, whereas the normal level for women is 4 to 5.5 million RBCs/mm^3. Anemia is the clinical condition that occurs when insufficient RBCs are available to carry oxygen to the tissues. Polycythemia is the condition that occurs when excess RBCs are produced.

Hemoglobin. Hemoglobin is a measure of the oxygen carrying capacity of the RBCs. Hemoglobin levels normally range from 14 to 18 g/dL in men and from 12 to 16 g/dL in women.

Hematocrit. The hematocrit is the volume percentage of RBCs in whole blood. The value is 40% to 54% for men and 38% to 48% for women.

White Blood Cells

Most inflammatory processes that produce necrotic tissue within the heart muscle, such as rheumatic fever, endocarditis, and MI, increase the WBC, or leukocyte, level. The WBC level also increases in response to infection. The normal WBC level for men and women is 5000 to 10,000 cells/mm^3.

Platelets

The normal platelet count is 150,000 to 400,000 cells/mm^3. Less commonly, the normal platelet count range is written as 150 to 400 × 10^9/L. There is no routine test available that can evaluate platelet functionality. The reported laboratory value is simply a total count of platelets. Platelets are important because they are the first cells to be activated when the coagulation system is stimulated. Many medications inhibit platelet function and make the platelets "slippery" so that they do not clump together to activate the clotting process. The antiplatelet action of a medication sometimes is its intended role, such as with aspirin used to prevent ACS, or it can be an unintended side effect. A low platelet count is called *thrombocytopenia.*

Blood Coagulation Studies

Coagulation studies are ordered to determine blood-clotting effectiveness. Anticoagulants, most notably heparin, direct thrombin inhibitors, warfarin, and platelet inhibitory agents, are administered daily in critical care units for many clinical reasons. It is essential to understand the laboratory tests that are used to monitor the effectiveness of therapeutic anticoagulation.

Prothrombin time. Most coagulation study results are reported as the length of time in seconds it takes for blood to form a clot in the laboratory test tube. The prothrombin time is not directly used to determine the therapeutic dosage of warfarin (Coumadin) necessary to achieve anticoagulation. Because the prothrombin time is not standardized between laboratories, the result of this test is reported as a standardized INR.[76]

International normalized ratio. The INR was developed by the World Health Organization (WHO) in 1982 to standardize PT results among clinical laboratories worldwide. Table 10.13 shows target INR ranges for therapeutic anticoagulation with warfarin.[77,78]

When a patient first begins warfarin therapy, it can take 72 hours or more to achieve a therapeutic level of anticoagulation. This is because the half-life of prothrombin is 36 to 42 hours. This delay in anticoagulation effectiveness also occurs if a patient is being converted from heparin-based anticoagulation, monitored by activated partial thromboplastin time, to warfarin-based anticoagulation (monitored by INR). To ensure a safe transition, a period of 48 to 72 hours is required to obtain a therapeutic INR value before the heparin is discontinued.

Activated partial thromboplastin time. The activated partial thromboplastin time is used to measure the effectiveness of IV or subcutaneous unfractionated heparin therapy.[76] Coagulation monitoring is required with unfractionated heparin, although not with subcutaneous

TABLE 10.13 Normal and Therapeutic Coagulation Values.

Test	Normal Value	Therapeutic Anticoagulant Target Value
INR	<1.0	2.0–3.0
aPTT	28–38 seconds	1.5–2.5 × normal
PTT	60–90 seconds	1.5–2.0 × normal
ACT[a]	0–120 seconds	150–300 seconds
Anti-Factor Xa	0	0.35–0.7 IU/mL for unfractionated heparin
		0.5–1.0 IU/mL for low–molecular-weight heparin

[a]ACT is normal, but therapeutic values may vary with type of activator used.

ACT, Activated coagulation time; *aPPT,* activated partial thromboplastin time; *INR,* international normalized ratio; *PTT,* partial thromboplastin time.

low–molecular-weight heparin because of lower levels of plasma protein binding. In cases of over-anticoagulation with heparin, the antidote is protamine sulfate

Activated clotting time. The activated clotting time (ACT) is a point-of-care test that is performed outside of the laboratory setting in areas such as the cardiac catheterization laboratory, operating room, or critical care unit. Normal and therapeutic values for ACT coagulation studies are shown in Table 10.13.

Anti-Factor Xa assay. Another method of measuring anticoagulant effectiveness is anti-Factor Xa serum level. For patients in whom aPTT may not be accurate due to physiologic factors (clotting factor deficiencies, liver disease, renal impairment, obesity, and lupus, among others), anti-Factor Xa monitoring may provide more accurate assessment of anticoagulation status. Anti-Factor Xa measures plasma heparin levels and may be used to monitor unfractionated and low–molecular-weight heparin. Therapeutic ranges for anti-Factor Xa for unfractionated heparin are 0.35 to 0.7 IU/mL and for low–molecular-weight heparin are 0.5 to 1.0 IU/mL.[79]

Serum Lipid Studies

Four primary blood lipid levels are important in evaluating an individual's risk of developing or having progression of CAD: total cholesterol, low-density lipoprotein cholesterol (LDL-C), triglycerides, and high-density lipoprotein cholesterol (HDL-C). When levels of cholesterol LDLs and triglycerides are elevated or the level of HDLs is low, the patient is considered at risk for developing or having progression of CAD and is offered intensive interventions involving diet therapy, exercise prescription, and medication therapy.[80] The following lipid biomarkers are commonly ordered together as a "lipid panel."

Total Cholesterol

Cholesterol is a type of lipid (sterol) that is present in cell membranes, is produced by the liver, and is a precursor of bile acids and steroid hormones. The cholesterol level in the blood is determined partly by genetics and partly by acquired factors such as diet, calorie balance, and level of physical activity. Cholesterol in excess amounts (greater than 200 mg/dL) in the serum accelerates the progression of atherosclerosis (atherogenesis).

Low-Density Lipoproteins

Approximately 60% to 70% of the total serum cholesterol is carried in the bloodstream, complexed as LDL-C. The LDL-C and total serum cholesterol levels are directly correlated with risk for CAD, and high levels of each are significant predictors of future acute MI in individuals with established coronary artery atherosclerosis. LDL-C is the major atherogenic lipoprotein and is the primary target for cholesterol-lowering efforts.[80] Guidelines recommend maintaining an LDL-C level below 130 mg/dL for a patient with no history of atherosclerotic disease. A patient with known CAD but who is not high risk should aim for an LDL-C level below 100 mg/dL. The recommended target LDL-C level for high-risk patients with CAD or diabetes is 70 mg/dL.[80]

Very-Low-Density Lipoproteins and Triglycerides

Very-low-density lipoproteins contain 10% to 15% of the total serum cholesterol along with most of the triglycerides in fasting serum.

High-Density Lipoproteins

HDLs are particles that carry 20% to 30% of the total serum cholesterol. Although higher levels of HDL seem to carry a relation to reduced atherosclerotic risk, the evidence is not currently conclusive.[81]

Triglycerides

Triglycerides are another form of lipid in the bloodstream that is normally included in the lipid assessment panel. Current guidelines recommend beginning medical management for triglyceride levels greater than 150 mg/dL.[80] Elevated triglyceride levels are associated with diabetes mellitus and an increased risk of atherosclerotic disease.

DIAGNOSTIC PROCEDURES

Cardiac Catheterization and Coronary Arteriography

Cardiac catheterization and coronary arteriography are routine diagnostic procedures for patients with known or suspected heart disease. Clinical indications for cardiac catheterization include ACS, positive findings on noninvasive cardiac stress testing or imaging, after cardiac arrest with unclear etiology, pulmonary hypertension, pericardial disease, heart failure with a history suggestive of CAD, cardiomyopathy or valvular heart disease, and congenital heart disease. Cardiac catheterization is also common as part of the perioperative evaluation before cardiac and noncardiac surgery. Cardiac catheterization is used to describe anatomic and hemodynamic findings and to provide a baseline for medical or surgical therapy.[82–84]

Left-Heart Catheterization

During catheterization of the left side of the heart, hemodynamic pressure measurements are taken in the aortic root, the left ventricle, and the left atrium.[85] Access is obtained via the radial, brachial, or femoral artery. Radiopaque contrast dye is used to visualize the left ventricle (ventriculogram). This information is also used to calculate the LV ejection fraction. The coronary arteries are visualized, and contrast dye is injected directly into each arterial system. The general term for vessel imaging is *angiogram* (veins and arteries), but a more specific term used to describe visualization of arteries is *arteriogram*.

Right-Heart Catheterization

Catheterization of the right side of the heart is performed using a thermodilution PA-Catheter. Access is obtained via the brachial, IJ, or femoral vein. Information obtained includes hemodynamic pressure measurements in the right atrium, the right ventricle, the pulmonary artery, in the PA-Catheter occlusion wedge position, and measurement of CO, calculated hemodynamic values, and oxygen saturations. An angiogram of the right-heart chambers using radiopaque contrast dye may also be performed.

Electrophysiology Study

An electrophysiology study (EPS) is an invasive diagnostic procedure used to record intracardiac electrical activity within the heart chambers. An EPS may be indicated after a syncopal episode (loss of consciousness); rapid wide complex tachycardia; or other cardiac electrical problems not diagnosed by noninvasive studies such as the 12-lead ECG, treadmill stress test, or remote continuous ECG monitoring.

An EPS is performed in a specially equipped cardiac catheterization or electrophysiology laboratory.[86] The EPS catheters are similar to pacing catheters, placed at specific anatomic sites within the heart to record the earliest electrical activity. Catheter placements are illustrated in Fig. 10.50, with catheter tip positions shown at the following locations:

1. High right atrium near the SA node
2. AV node
3. Coronary sinus behind the left atrial/ventricular border
4. Bundle of His near the tricuspid valve
5. Right ventricle near the apex

During an EPS, programmed electrical stimulation is used to trigger the dysrhythmia. This technique delivers pulses of early paced beats via a specific catheter to the selected area of myocardium. The electrophysiologist simultaneously looks for a site of early electrical activation that stimulates the myocardium before the SA node. The goal of an EPS is to discover the origin of dysrhythmias that cannot be evaluated from the surface ECG alone.

When a follow-up EPS is required for a patient with an ICD, the device can substitute for the electrophysiology catheters. The ICD has

sensing leads, pace termination, backup bradycardia pacing, and cardioversion and defibrillation capabilities. The EPS can be performed by the external ICD programmer in the electrophysiology laboratory. The ICD generator and leads perform programmed electrical stimulation in a manner similar to a full EPS. Chapter 12 provides more information on the therapeutic uses of ICDs.

Ambulatory Electrocardiography

Before coming to the critical care unit, a patient might have had other ECG tests to determine the degree of cardiovascular disease. Ambulatory electrocardiography is a technique that records the ECG of patients while they perform their usual activities. It is designed to document abnormal cardiac rhythms that occur randomly or that are induced by specific circumstances such as emotional stress or physical activity. Clinical indications include palpitations, dizziness, syncope, and pacemaker evaluation. Two types of recording systems are available: continuous and intermittent.

Continuous Electrocardiogram Recording Systems

Patch monitors represent a newer generation of noninvasive ECG monitor that a patient wears on the chest continuously for up to 14 days to record their ECG during normal daily activity. Continuous recording systems capture every heartbeat, do not require active participation of the patient, and do not miss asymptomatic ECG changes that may be accompanied by a loss of consciousness. The patient can also press a button to time-mark symptoms and complete a patient symptom log.

Echocardiography

Echocardiography uses waves of ultrasound to obtain and display images of cardiac structures. Normal human hearing occurs at a sound frequency of 20 to 20,000 cycles per second (Hz). Ultrasound uses sound frequencies above 20,000 Hz. Ultrasound is reflected best at interfaces between tissues that have different densities. In the heart, these are the blood, cardiac valves, myocardium, and pericardium. Because all these structures differ in density, their borders can be seen on the echocardiogram. Echocardiography is used to detect structural heart abnormalities such as mitral valve stenosis and regurgitation, prolapse of mitral valve leaflets, aortic stenosis and insufficiency, hypertrophic cardiomyopathy, atrial septal defect, thoracic aortic dissection, cardiac tamponade, and pericardial effusion. There are several methods for obtaining images of cardiac structures with echocardiography, including transthoracic (TTE), transesophageal (TEE), intravascular (IVUS), and intracardiac (ICE). There are also several basic modes of echocardiography used to image the heart: two-dimensional, three-dimensional, motion-mode (M-mode), and Doppler. Echocardiography can also be performed during stress testing to noninvasively evaluate patients for ischemic heart disease. The protocols used for echocardiographic exercise stress testing are very similar to the protocols used in the ECG stress test setting and are described in Table 10.14.

Transthoracic Echocardiography

When TTE is performed, the patient is in a supine, left lateral, or semirecumbent position. The position used depends on the patient's clinical condition and on which structures are to be examined. A transducer is placed on the skin, with lubricant between the transducer and the skin to improve contact and reduce artifact. The active element in the transducer is a piezoelectric crystal. *Piezoelectric* refers to the ability to transform electrical energy into mechanical energy (in this case, sound energy). The transducer emits ultrasound waves and

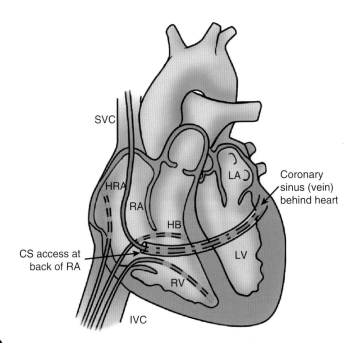

Fig. 10.50 Catheter Placement Within the Heart During an Electrophysiology Study. *CS,* Coronary sinus; *HB,* His bundle; *HRA,* high right atrium; *IVC,* inferior vena cava; *LA,* left atrium; *LV,* left ventricle; *RA,* right atrium; *RV,* right ventricle; *SVC,* superior vena cava.

TABLE 10.14	Stress Testing Methods.		
Test Parameters	**Stress Electrocardiography**	**Stress Echocardiography**	**Stress Radionuclide Imaging**
Exercise stress test	3-, 5-, or 12-lead ECG leads are attached to the chest and limbs to monitor the ECG *during* exercise protocol.	Patient exercises according to protocol. Echocardiogram is recorded immediately *after* exercise.	Radiopharmaceutical (thallium-201 or technetium-99m) is injected before exercise. Patient exercises according to the protocol. Heart is scanned *after* exercise to view uptake of radiotracer.
Pharmacologic stress test	Patient is at rest. IV medications stimulate HR and contractility: Dosage starts with dobutamine at 5 mcg/kg/min and is increased as needed to increase HR. ECG pattern is monitored during the medication infusions. Other medications include adenosine, regadenoson, and dipyridamole.	Patient is at rest. IV medications stimulate HR and contractility: Dosage starts with dobutamine at 5 mcg/kg/min and is increased as needed to increase HR. Echocardiogram is recorded during and after the medication infusions. Other medications include adenosine, regadenoson, and dipyridamole.	Patient is at rest. IV medications simulate exercise: Dosage starts with dobutamine 5 mcg/kg/min and is increased as needed to increase HR. Radionuclide image is scanned during and after pharmacologic stress. Other medications include adenosine, regadenoson, and dipyridamole.
Clinical indications	Used to rule out CAD. Not as helpful if patient has a distorted ECG pattern at baseline owing to LBBB, RBBB, or internal ventricular pacemaker because ST segment changes are obscured.	Useful for patients with LBBB, RBBB, and implanted pacemaker because the wall motion is visualized directly.	Helpful for patients with LBBB, RBBB, and implanted pacemaker. It is useful before CABG to determine whether bypass graft will supply blood to an ischemic area. There is no benefit in grafting an artery to an infarcted area.
Clinical outcome of a positive test result	Chest pain develops. ST segment ECG pattern changes.	Chest pain develops. Wall-motion abnormalities are visualized.	Areas of the heart that do not take up radiotracer are called *cold spots*. A cold spot is ischemic or infarcted tissue. A follow-up scan later the same day (or the next day with some radiotracers) shows whether the cold spot has filled in; if yes, the area is ischemic; if it remains cold, the area is infarcted.

CABG, Coronary artery bypass graft; *CAD,* coronary artery disease; *ECG,* electrocardiogram; *HR,* heart rate; *IV,* intravenous; *LBBB,* left bundle branch block; *RBBB,* right bundle branch block.

receives a signal from the reflected sound waves. Periods of sound transmission alternate with periods of sound reception.

Ultrasonic waves do not travel through air very well, and they cannot penetrate very dense structures such as bone. In adults, the transducer is usually placed in the third or fourth intercostal space to the left of the sternum, because at that point the pericardium is in direct contact with the chest wall, and the ultrasonic waves are not obstructed by air or bone. Other positions are sometimes used if the standard location does not provide adequate visualization of the cardiac structures. In the critical care unit, the echocardiograph machine is usually brought to the bedside. The lighting in the room can be dimmed to improve the visual clarity of the images displayed on the screen.

Nursing care consists of monitoring the patient during the procedure, which is usually performed by an echocardiography technician. TTE is completely noninvasive; the nurse explains this and the purpose of the test to the patient and family. The procedure is not uncomfortable, but it may be tiring for certain patients because of the length of the procedure, which is usually 30 to 60 minutes.

Transesophageal Echocardiography

TEE is a technique in which the transducer (single-plane, biplane, or multiplane device) is mounted on a flexible shaft similar to an endoscope and advanced into the esophagus, from where cardiac structures

can be more clearly visualized. The multiplane transducer has a single array of crystals that can be rotated in a 180-degree arc, requiring less manipulation of the probe within the esophagus. Because of the close anatomic relationship between the heart and the esophagus, TEE produces high-quality images of intracardiac structures and the thoracic aorta without the interference of the chest wall, bone, or air-filled lung.

A soft bite block is inserted between the teeth to prevent damage to the echoscope or the patient's mouth. As the echoscope is inserted, the patient is asked to swallow. The echoscope is advanced to 25 cm from the mouth, and imaging is begun. The location is similar to the Doppler probe shown in Fig. 10.22. TEE is also used intraoperatively during cardiac surgery for monitoring valve repair and replacement.

During TEE, vital signs are closely monitored with ECG, BP, and clinical observation. Emergency resuscitation equipment must be present in case of a severe vasovagal episode, typically bradycardia and hypotension. Suction equipment must be at the bedside in the event of emesis, excessive oral secretions, or for emergency support.

Intravascular Ultrasound

Intravascular ultrasound (IVUS) is used as an adjunct diagnostic technique during coronary angiography or during a percutaneous coronary procedure. A miniature, flexible ultrasound catheter that incorporates a high-frequency transducer (20–40 MHz) provides high-resolution images of the coronary arterial wall. This technology is not an alternative to angiography but is used as a complementary diagnostic technique. IVUS permits an anatomic view of the interior of the coronary artery. The cardiologist can visualize the exact location of atherosclerotic plaque or see whether a coronary stent has deployed (expanded) correctly against the vessel wall.

Intracardiac Ultrasound

The use of intracardiac ultrasound, also known as intracardiac echocardiography (ICE), is increasing. Flexible ultrasound catheters can be directed into the atria and ventricles. Diagnostic uses include direct visualization of intracardiac structures, replacement for TEE during interventional or selected surgical procedures, and views of the atrial or ventricular septum during a repair procedure.

Two-Dimensional and Three-Dimensional Echocardiograms

The two-dimensional echocardiogram uses crystals in the transducer to create a cross-sectional imaging plane. Sections of the heart are then viewed from numerous different angles. The picture is displayed on an oscilloscope, and digital photographs are taken to serve as a permanent record. The two-dimensional echocardiogram images a whole "slice" of the heart at once and is used for direct measurement of LV volumes and wall mass. The two-dimensional slice also permits visualization of the cardiac structures in relation to each other and readily identifies valvular dysfunction and wall-motion abnormalities after MI. A more recent innovation is a real-time three-dimensional echocardiogram. It produces more realistic images, especially when imaging cardiac valves or congenital anomalies.

Two-Dimensional Motion-Mode Echocardiography

M-mode two-dimensional echocardiography is noninvasive and allows visualization of specific cardiac structures over time. A handheld crystal transducer is placed against the chest wall to direct a thin beam of ultrasound through the heart. As the ultrasound beam encounters different interfaces, it is reflected back (echo) as a dot and recorded as the heart beats. Fig. 10.51A shows the labeled structures and Fig. 10.51B shows the ultrasound visualization via the line of the transducer. In M-mode, each echo-dot becomes a line on an oscilloscope recording motion and measurement of the mitral valve, the intraventricular septum, and other structures the ultrasound beam encounters over time (Fig. 10.51C). M-mode echocardiograms are particularly useful in detecting small pericardial effusions and cardiac tamponade.

Phonocardiogram

Phonocardiography is combined with echocardiography to evaluate valvular dysfunction. A phonocardiogram (*phono* [sound], *cardio* [heart], and *gram* [recording]) provides a graphic display of the sounds that occur in the heart and great vessels. The transducer is placed on the chest wall to record heart sounds that correspond to auscultation with a traditional stethoscope.

Color-Flow Doppler Echocardiography

Doppler echocardiography provides a special kind of echocardiogram that assesses blood flow. It uses a pulsed or continuous wave of ultrasound that records frequency shifts of reflected sound waves, showing velocity and direction of blood flow relative to the transducer. Doppler signals are usually displayed in color. Known as *color-flow mapping* or *imaging*, this technique analyzes Doppler signals from multiple intracardiac sites simultaneously. The Doppler tracing for each site is displayed in a color-coded format superimposed on a real-time two-dimensional echocardiographic image. Flow toward the transducer is displayed in one color, whereas flow away from the transducer is displayed in a contrasting color. The brightness of the color varies to signify different flow velocities.

Doppler echocardiography is especially useful in individuals with valvular heart disease. The blood flow associated with regurgitation and stenosis can be detected, and estimates can be made of the severity of the disease. Doppler can accurately estimate right ventricular systolic pressure. When several valves are involved, the Doppler technique can clarify the extent of damage to the individual valves. Other uses for Doppler echocardiography include evaluation of congenital shunts, measurement of volume flow and CO, and assessment of new structural abnormalities after acute MI. By measuring flow velocity in the right ventricular outflow tract, mean PAP can be estimated.

Magnetic Resonance Imaging

Magnetic resonance imaging (MRI) is a noninvasive imaging technique that can obtain specific biochemical information from body tissue without the use of ionizing radiation. The procedure does not present any known hazard to living cells. Often the image is superior to radiography and ultrasonography because bone does not interfere with MRI.

Metal Objects and Patient Safety

MRI is a safe procedure. The main hazard is related to the presence of metal substances in the environment. Because the magnetism used is approximately 40,000 times stronger than the magnetic field of the earth, metal objects such as IV line poles, infusion pumps, or oxygen tanks can become projectiles if they come close enough to the magnet's pull. No metal objects are permitted in the area of the MRI scanner including any metallic implants or other metal (residual bullet or shrapnel) that may be moved by the magnetic force during the scan. Aneurysm clips are composed of ferromagnetic materials and can experience significant torque when exposed to the magnetic field. Most contemporary cardiac electronic devices that are implanted are MRI safe, but older pacemakers or ICDs may malfunction during exposure to the strong magnetic field.

Cardiovascular Magnetic Resonance

Cardiac MRI, also known as *cardiovascular magnetic resonance (CMR)*, is useful in diagnosing complications of MI such as pericarditis or pericardial effusion, valvular dysfunction, ventricular septal rupture, aneurysm, and intracardiac thrombus. Blood that is actively flowing does not emit a magnetic resonance signal; it provides a natural dark contrast material in the lumen of proximal coronary arteries. As a result, abnormalities of lumen size such as narrowing, which may provide evidence of obstruction, can be visualized. Pharmacologic stress imaging can also be done during CMR using an inotrope such as dobutamine or alternate vasodilating agents.

Cardiac Computed Tomography

Cardiac computed tomography (CT) is a widely available noninvasive examination that is usually used to evaluate patients for CAD but can also be used to assess ventricular function, morphology, and myocardial perfusion. When used to assess the coronary arteries, it is also known as *coronary CT angiography (CCTA)*. Before the CCTA procedure, sublingual nitroglycerin is used to dilate the coronary arteries, and beta-blockers to reduce the HR may be administered to allow for better visualization. During the study, IV contrast dye is

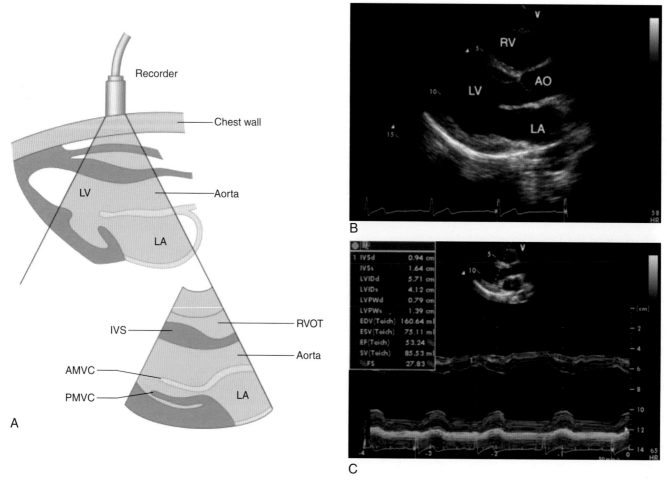

Fig. 10.51 Two-Dimensional Echocardiography and M-Mode Echocardiography. (A) Schematic of long-axis view of normal cardiac structures traversed by a two-dimensional ultrasound beam, as the heart beats. The transducer is repositioned on the chest to allow visualization of different structures. (B) Two-dimensional echocardiography recording of a normal heart. (C) M-mode echocardiograph recording of a normal heart. The transducer ultrasound beam traverses the left ventricle slightly below the mitral valve. *AMVC,* Anterior mitral valve cusp; *AO,* aorta; *IVS,* interventricular septum; *LA,* left atrium; *LV,* left ventricle; *LV(d),* left ventricular end-diastolic dimensions; *LV(s),* left ventricular end-systolic dimensions; *MV,* mitral valve; *PM,* papillary muscle; *PMVC,* posterior mitral valve cusp; *PVW,* posterior ventricular wall; *RA,* right atrium; *RV,* right ventricle; *RVOT,* right ventricular outflow tract. (From Kumar P, Clark M, eds. *Kumar and Clarke's Clinical Medicine.* 9th ed. St. Louis: Elsevier; 2017.)

injected to help delineate the presence of plaques or stenosis, as well as the extent of disease. Patients must be able to lie still and hold their breath periodically. Contraindications include kidney disease due to the administration of contrast dye, and tachyarrhythmias.

Coronary artery calcium score. Cardiac CT is also used to calculate the coronary artery calcium score (CACS).[87] The quantity of calcium in atherosclerotic plaque is measured using multidetector CT, then the CACS is calculated. A score less than 100 is considered low risk, whereas a score greater than 300 indicates high risk of a future coronary event. Clinically, the CACS is considered along with other risk factor information to evaluate individual risk from atherosclerotic coronary disease.

Cardiac Radionuclide Imaging Studies

Several types of radionuclide imaging tests are available. As with diagnostic ECG and echocardiography, many of the radionuclide tests can be performed both at rest and during exercise.

Purpose of Radionuclide Scans

The purpose of a radionuclide scan, also known as *nuclear myocardial perfusion imaging,* is to determine whether there is a perfusion defect in cardiac muscle (Fig. 10.52). A scan is indicated for a symptomatic patient with known or suspected CAD. The radionuclide scan is especially helpful for a patient who has a coexisting LBBB or a permanent pacemaker where the QRS complex shape is distorted. Both situations make interpretation of acute angina or equivalent symptoms challenging to interpret accurately on the 12-lead ECG or during ECG stress testing. This has opened a window of opportunity for radionuclide imaging, in which the myocardial ability to receive blood flow is visualized directly.

Blockage of an artery can lead to a discrete myocardial perfusion defect, meaning that the blood supply to this area is decreased (ischemic) or absent (infarcted). Although coronary arteriography defines the anatomy of the coronary arteries, it does not show how effectively the arteries perfuse the portion of cardiac muscle they

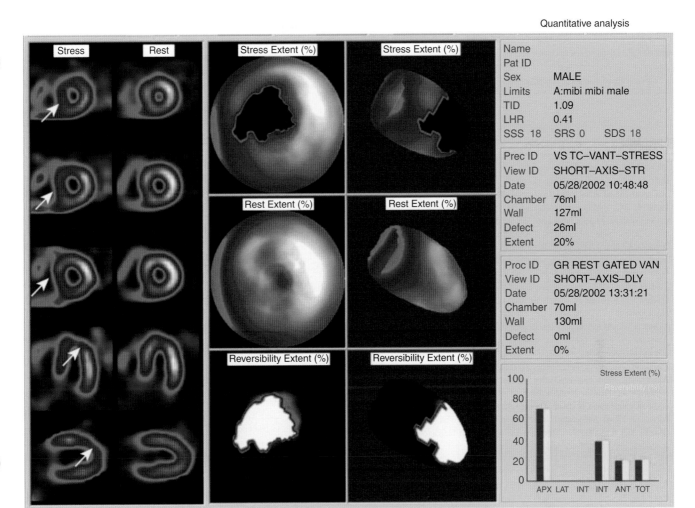

Fig. 10.52 Radionuclide Isotope and Myocardial Perfusion Viability. *Left panel*: From top to bottom, three short-axis views and two vertical-axis views of the heart after stress. The *white arrow* shows areas of poor myocardial perfusion. The matching scans are taken after rest and reinjection of the tracer. The images at rest show normal perfusion and tracer uptake. *Bright orange* indicates normal myocardial uptake, while *blue-purple* indicates ischemic tissue with poor tracer uptake. *Middle panel*: From top to bottom, polar maps of the entire myocardium localize the ischemic area normally supplied by the left anterior descending (LAD) artery. *Right panel*: Quantitative analysis of myocardial viability. (From Kumar P, Clark M, eds. *Kumar and Clarke's Clinical Medicine*. 9th ed. St. Louis: Elsevier; 2017.)

supply. Radionuclide imaging can help determine whether there are ischemic areas of the heart that are still viable and amenable to revascularization.

Radionuclide Isotopes

The radioisotopes used in cardiac diagnostic imaging are very different from the radioisotopes used in oncology for tumor ablation. Diagnostic isotopes have a short half-life (minutes to hours) and are used in very small amounts to minimize radioactivity risk. Patients do not need to be isolated, and no specific precautions are required for blood, urine, stool, or other body fluids.

Thallium-201. Thallium-201 (^{201}Tl) is a low-energy radioactive isotope. It is an analog of potassium and acts like potassium when injected into the bloodstream. Because thallium is similar to potassium, it is absorbed from the bloodstream by cardiac muscle cells as part of the sodium-potassium adenosine triphosphatase (ATPase) pump. Thallium uptake depends on two factors: the patency of the coronary arteries and the amount of healthy myocardium with a

functional sodium-potassium ATPase pump. Areas of infarcted myocardium (dead tissue) do not take up thallium. After thallium has been injected, a specialized scintillation camera and associated computer system are used to scan the myocardium.

Technetium-99m. Technetium-99m (^{99m}Tc) is also used frequently. It is often attached to other trace substances for diagnostic imaging (^{99m}Tc-sestamibi or ^{99m}Tc-tetrofosmin). These substances may be described as *radiopharmaceuticals*. ^{99m}Tc tracers are highly suited to imaging myocardium during ACS, because the tracers do not redistribute over time (they remain in myocardium), allowing a second scan to be performed many hours later if needed (see Fig. 10.52). The protocols used for stress testing are similar and are described in Table 10.14.

ADDITIONAL RESOURCES

See Box 10.17 for Internet resources related to cardiovascular diagnostic procedures.

BOX 10.17 **Informatics**

Internet Resources: Cardiovascular Diagnostic Procedures
- American Association of Critical-Care Nurses (AACN): https://www.aacn.org
- American Heart Association (AHA): https://www.heart.org/en/professional

REFERENCES

1. Wertli MM, Dangma TD, Müller SE, et al. Non-cardiac chest pain patients in the emergency department: do physicians have a plan how to diagnose and treat them? A retrospective study. *PLoS One.* 2019;14(2):e0211615.
2. Fanaroff AC, Rymer JA, Goldstein SA, Simel DL, Newby LK. Does this patient with chest pain have acute coronary syndrome? The rational clinical examination systematic review. *J Am Med Assoc.* 2015;314(18):1955–1965.
3. Amsterdam EA, Wenger NK, Brindis RG, et al. AHA/ACC guideline for the management of patients with non-ST-elevation acute coronary syndromes: a report of the American College of Cardiology/American Heart Association Task Force on practice guidelines. *J Am Coll Cardiol.* 2014;64(24):e139–e228.
4. O'Gara PT, Kushner FG, Ascheim DD, et al. ACCF/AHA guideline for the management of ST-elevation myocardial infarction: executive summary: a report of the American College of Cardiology Foundation/American Heart Association Task Force on practice guidelines. *J Am Coll Cardiol.* 2013;61(4):485–510.
5. Rao G, Powell-Wiley TM, Ancheta I, et al, and on behalf of American Heart Association Obesity Committee of the Council on Lifestyle and Cardiometabolic Health. Identification of obesity and cardiovascular risk in ethnically and racially diverse populations: a scientific statement from the American Heart Association. *Circulation.* 2015;132(5):457–472.
6. Okoshi MP, Capalbo RV, Romeiro FG, Okoshi K. Cardiac cachexia: perspectives for prevention and treatment. *Arq Bras Cardiol.* 2017;108(1):74–80.
7. Gogalniceanu P, Lancaster RT, Patel VI. Clinical assessment of peripheral arterial disease of the lower limbs. *N Engl J Med.* 2018;378(18):e24.
8. Coke LA, Dennison-Himmelfarb C. Peripheral arterial disease prevention in women: awareness and action. *J Cardiovasc Nurs.* 2019;34(6):427–429.
9. Duff S, Mafilios MS, Bhounsule P, Hasegawa JT. The burden of critical limb ischemia: a review of recent literature. *Vasc Health Risk Manag.* 2019;15:187–208.
10. Mrgan M, Rytter D, Brabrand M. Capillary refill time is a predictor of short-term mortality for adult patients admitted to a medical department: an observational cohort study. *Emerg Med J.* 2014;31(12):954–958.
11. Higgins J. Physical examination of the cardiovascular system. *Int J Clin Cardiol.* 2015;2(1):1–7.
12. Thibodeau JT, Drazner MH. The role of the clinical examination in patients with heart failure. *JACC Heart Fail.* 2018;6(7):543–551.
13. Saugel B, Scheeren TWL, Teboul JL. Ultrasound-guided central venous catheter placement: a structured review and recommendations for clinical practice. *Crit Care.* 2017;21(1):225.
14. Fudim M, Parikh KS, Dunning A, et al. Relation of volume overload to clinical outcomes in acute heart failure (from ASCEND-HF). *Am J Cardiol.* 2018;122(9):1506–1512.
15. Chernomordik F, Berkovitch A, Schwammenthal E, et al. Short- and long-term prognostic implications of jugular venous distension in patients hospitalized with acute heart failure. *Am J Cardiol.* 2016;118(2):226–231.
16. Lima A, Bakker J. Clinical assessment of peripheral circulation. *Curr Opin Crit Care.* 2015;21(3):226–231.
17. Whelton PK, Carey RM, Aronow WS, et al. 2017 ACC/AHA/AAPA/ABC/ACPM/AGS/APhA/ASH/ASPC/NMA/PCNA guideline for the prevention, detection, evaluation, and management of high blood pressure in adults: a report of the American College of Cardiology/American heart association task force on clinical practice guidelines. *J Am Coll Cardiol.* 2018;71(19):e127–e248.
18. Freeman R, Abuzinadah AR, Gibbons C, Jones P, Miglis MG, Sinn DI. Orthostatic hypotension: JACC state-of-the-art review. *J Am Coll Cardiol.* 2018;72(11):1294–1309.
19. Hamzaoui O, Monnet X, Teboul JL. Pulsus paradoxus. *Eur Respir J.* 2013;42(6):1696–1705.
20. Price S, Platz E, Cullen L, et al. Acute heart failure study group of the European Society of Cardiology Acute Cardiovascular Care A. Expert consensus document: echocardiography and lung ultrasonography for the assessment and management of acute heart failure. *Nat Rev Cardiol.* 2017;14(7):427–440.
21. Minami Y, Kajimoto K, Sato N, et al. Third heart sound in hospitalised patients with acute heart failure: insights from the ATTEND study. *Int J Clin Pract.* 2015;69(8):820–828.
22. Nishimura RA, Otto CM, Bonow RO, et al. AHA/ACC guideline for the management of patients with valvular heart disease: a report of the American College of Cardiology/American heart association Task force on practice guidelines. *Circulation.* 2014;129(23):e521–643.
23. Nishimura RA, Otto CM, Bonow RO, et al. AHA/ACC focused update of the 2014 AHA/ACC guideline for the management of patients with valvular heart disease: a report of the American College of Cardiology/American Heart Association Task Force on Clinical Practice Guidelines. *Circulation.* 2017;135(25):e1159–e1195.
24. Unger P, Clavel MA, Lindman BR, Mathieu P, Pibarot P. Pathophysiology and management of multivalvular disease. *Nat Rev Cardiol.* 2016;13(7):429–440.
25. Montrief T, Davis WT, Koyfman A, Long B. Mechanical, inflammatory, and embolic complications of myocardial infarction: an emergency medicine review. *Am J Emerg Med.* 2019;37(6):1175–1183.
26. Robertson-Malt S, Malt GN, Farquhar V, Greer W. Heparin versus normal saline for patency of arterial lines. *Cochrane Database Syst Rev.* 2014;(5):CD007364.
27. Lough ME. Arterial pressure monitoring. In: *Hemodynamic Monitoring: Evolving Technologies and Clinical Practice.* 1st ed. Philadelphia: Elsevier; 2016:55–88.
28. East JM, Cserti-Gazdewich CM, Granton JT. Heparin-induced thrombocytopenia in the critically ill patient. *Chest.* 2018;154(3):678–690.
29. O'Grady NP, Alexander M, Burns LA, et al. Guidelines for the prevention of intravascular catheter-related infections. *Am J Infect Control.* 2011;39(4 suppl 1):S1–S34.
30. Centers for Disease Control and Prevention. Guidelines for the Prevention of Intravascular Catheter-Related Infections (2011); Summary of Recommendations (Edit 2017). https://www.cdc.gov/infectioncontrol/guidelines/bsi/recommendations.html; Accessed June 28, 2022.
31. Barros L, Bridges E, Cockerham M, Greco S, Herrera FNS. Pulmonary artery/central venous pressure monitoring in adults. *AACN Practice Alerts.* https://www.aacn.org/~/media/aacn-website/clincial-resources/practice-alerts/pap2017practicealert.pdf. Accessed March 15, 2022.
32. Sjodin C, Sondergaard S, Johansson L. Variability in alignment of central venous pressure transducer to physiologic reference point in the intensive care unit—a descriptive and correlational study. *Aust Crit Care.* 2019;32(3):213–217.
33. Wang AZ, Zhou M, Jiang W, Zhang WX. The differences between venous air embolism and fat embolism in routine intraoperative monitoring methods, transesophageal echocardiography, and fatal volume in pigs. *J Trauma.* 2008;65(2):416–423.
34. Brull SJ, Prielipp RC. Vascular air embolism: a silent hazard to patient safety. *J Crit Care.* 2017;42:255–263.
35. Sinno MC, Alam M. Echocardiographically detected fibrinous sheaths associated with central venous catheters. *Echocardiography.* 2012;29(3):E56–E59.
36. Xiong Z, Chen H. Interventions to reduce unnecessary central venous catheter use to prevent central-line-associated bloodstream infections in adults: a systematic review. *Infect Control Hosp Epidemiol.* 2018;39(12):1442–1448.
37. Marik PE, Baram M, Vahid B. Does central venous pressure predict fluid responsiveness? A systematic review of the literature and the tale of seven mares. *Chest.* 2008;134(1):172–178.
38. Kupchik N, Bridges E. Critical analysis, critical care: central venous pressure monitoring: what's the evidence? *Am J Nurs.* 2012;112(1):58–61.
39. Monnet X, Teboul JL. Passive leg raising: five rules, not a drop of fluid. *Crit Care.* 2015;19:18.
40. Pickett JD, Bridges E, Kritek PA, Whitney JD. Passive leg-raising and prediction of fluid responsiveness: systematic review. *Crit Care Nurse.* 2017;37(2):32–47.

41. Kubiak GM, Ciarka A, Biniecka M, Ceranowicz P. Right heart catheterization-background, physiological basics, and clinical implications. *J Clin Med.* 2019;8(9):1331.

42. Marik PE. Obituary: pulmonary artery catheter 1970 to 2013. *Ann Intensive Care.* 2013;3(1):38.

43. Sotomi Y, Sato N, Kajimoto K, et al. Impact of pulmonary artery catheter on outcome in patients with acute heart failure syndromes with hypotension or receiving inotropes: from the ATTEND Registry. *Int J Cardiol.* 2014;172(1):165–172.

44. Ikuta K, Wang Y, Robinson A, Ahmad T, Krumholz HM, Desai NR. National trends in use and outcomes of pulmonary artery catheters among Medicare beneficiaries, 1999-2013. *JAMA Cardiol.* 2017;2(8):908–913.

45. De Backer D, Vincent JL. The pulmonary artery catheter: is it still alive? *Curr Opin Crit Care.* 2018;24(3):204–208.

46. Giraud R, Siegenthaler N, Merlani P, Bendjelid K. Reproducibility of transpulmonary thermodilution cardiac output measurements in clinical practice: a systematic review. *J Clin Monit Comput.* 2017;31(1):43–51.

47. Headley JM. Arterial waveform and pressure-based technologies. In: Lough ME, ed. *Hemodynamic Monitoring: Evolving Technologies and Clinical Practice.* Philadelphia: Elsevier; 2016:341–369.

48. Peeters Y, Bernards J, Mekeirele M, Hoffmann B, De Raes M, Malbrain ML. Hemodynamic monitoring: to calibrate or not to calibrate? Part 1—Calibrated techniques. *Anaesthesiol Intensive Ther.* 2015;47(5):487–500.

49. Bernards J, Mekeirele M, Hoffmann B, Peeters Y, De Raes M, Malbrain ML. Hemodynamic monitoring: to calibrate or not to calibrate? Part 2—Noncalibrated techniques. *Anaesthesiol Intensive Ther.* 2015;47(5):501–516.

50. He HW, Liu DW, Long Y, Wang XT, Zhao ML, Lai XL. The effect of variable arterial transducer level on the accuracy of pulse contour waveform-derived measurements in critically ill patients. *J Clin Monit Comput.* 2016;30(5):569–575.

51. Sidebotham DA, Allen SJ, Gerber IL, Fayers T. Intraoperative transesophageal echocardiography for surgical repair of mitral regurgitation. *J Am Soc Echocardiogr.* 2014;27(4):345–366.

52. Turner EE, Tarabichi YNP. Ultrasonography-based, hemodynamic monitoring. In: Lough ME, ed. *Hemodynamic Monitoring: Evolving Technologies and Clinical Practice.* Philadelphia: Elsevier; 2016:307–340.

53. Airapetian N, Maizel J, Alyamani O, et al. Does inferior vena cava respiratory variability predict fluid responsiveness in spontaneously breathing patients? *Crit Care.* 2015;19:400.

54. Philips R. Doppler based hemodynamic monitoring. In: Lough ME, ed. *Hemodynamic Monitoring: Evolving Technologies and Clinical Practice.* Philadelphia: Elsevier; 2016:281–306.

55. Albert NM, Murray T, Bena JF, et al. Differences in alarm events between disposable and reusable electrocardiography lead wires. *Am J Crit Care.* 2015;24(1):67–73, quiz 74.

56. Albert NM, Slifcak E, Roach JD, et al. Infection rates in intensive care units by electrocardiographic lead wire type: disposable vs reusable. *Am J Crit Care.* 2014;23(6):460–468.

57. American Association of Critical-Care Nurses (AACN). Ensuring accurate ST-segment monitoring: AACN Practice Alert. http://www.aacn.org/wd/practice/docs/practicealerts/st-segment-monitoring.pdf?menu=aboutus. Accessed June 28, 2022.

58. Sandau KE, Funk M, Auerbach A, et al. Update to practice standards for electrocardiographic monitoring in hospital settings: a scientific statement from the American Heart Association. *Circulation.* 2017;136(19):e273–e344.

59. Sommargren CE, Drew BJ. Preventing torsades de pointes by careful cardiac monitoring in hospital settings. *AACN Adv Crit Care.* 2007;18(3):285–293.

60. Drew BJ, Ackerman MJ, Funk M, et al. Prevention of torsade de pointes in hospital settings: a scientific statement from the American Heart Association and the American College of Cardiology Foundation. *Circulation.* 2010;121(8):1047–1060.

61. Page RL, Joglar JA, Caldwell MA, et al. 2015 ACC/AHA/HRS guideline for the management of adult patients with supraventricular tachycardia: a report of the American College of Cardiology/American Heart Association Task Force on Clinical Practice Guidelines and the Heart Rhythm Society. *Circulation.* 2016;133(14):e506–e574.

62. Appelboam A, Reuben A, Mann C, et al. Postural modification to the standard Valsalva manoeuvre for emergency treatment of supraventricular tachycardias (REVERT): a randomised controlled trial. *Lancet.* 2015;386(10005):1747–1753.

63. January CT, Wann LS, Alpert JS, et al. 2014 AHA/ACC/HRS guideline for the management of patients with atrial fibrillation: a report of the American College of Cardiology/American Heart Association Task Force on practice guidelines and the Heart Rhythm Society. *Circulation.* 2014;130(23):e199–e267.

64. You JJ, Singer DE, Howard PA, et al. Antithrombotic therapy for atrial fibrillation: antithrombotic therapy and prevention of thrombosis, 9th ed: American College of Chest Physicians Evidence-Based Clinical Practice Guidelines. *Chest.* 2012;141(suppl 2):e531S–e575S.

65. Camm AJ, Lip GY, De Caterina R, et al, Guidelines ESCCfP. 2012 focused update of the ESC Guidelines for the management of atrial fibrillation: an update of the 2010 ESC Guidelines for the management of atrial fibrillation. developed with the special contribution of the European Heart Rhythm Association. *Eur Heart J.* 2012;33(21):2719–2747.

66. Calkins H. Catheter ablation to maintain sinus rhythm. *Circulation.* 2012;125(11):1439–1445.

67. Raebel MA. Hyperkalemia associated with use of angiotensin-converting enzyme inhibitors and angiotensin receptor blockers. *Cardiovasc Ther.* 2012;30(3):e156–e166.

68. Kovesdy CP. Management of hyperkalemia: an update for the internist. *Am J Med.* 2015;128(12):1281–1287.

69. Baird GS. Ionized calcium. *Clin Chim Acta.* 2011;412(9–10):696–701.

70. Steele T, Kolamunnage-Dona R, Downey C, Toh CH, Welters I. Assessment and clinical course of hypocalcemia in critical illness. *Crit Care.* 2013;17(3):R106.

71. Kelly A, Levine MA. Hypocalcemia in the critically ill patient. *J Intensive Care Med.* 2013;28(3):166–177.

72. de Baaij JH, Hoenderop JG, Bindels RJ. Magnesium in man: implications for health and disease. *Physiol Rev.* 2015;95(1):1–46.

73. Panchal AR, Berg KM, Kudenchuk PJ. American heart association focused update on advanced cardiovascular life support use of antiarrhythmic drugs during and immediately after cardiac arrest: an update to the american heart association guidelines for cardiopulmonary resuscitation and emergency cardiovascular care. *Circulation.* 2018;138(23):e740–e749.

74. Amundson BE, Apple FS. Cardiac troponin assays: a review of quantitative point-of-care devices and their efficacy in the diagnosis of myocardial infarction. *Clin Chem Lab Med.* 2015;53(5):665–676.

75. Maisel A, Xue Y, Greene SJ, et al. The potential role of natriuretic peptide-guided management for patients hospitalized for heart failure. *J Card Fail.* 2015;21(3):233–239.

76. Tripodi A, Lippi G, Plebani M. How to report results of prothrombin and activated partial thromboplastin times. *Clin Chem Lab Med.* 2016;54(2):215–222.

77. Holbrook A, Schulman S, Witt DM, et al. Evidence-based management of anticoagulant therapy: antithrombotic therapy and prevention of thrombosis, 9th ed: American College of chest physicians evidence-based clinical practice guidelines. *Chest.* 2012;141(suppl 2):e152S–e184S.

78. Whitlock RP, Sun JC, Fremes SE, Rubens FD, Teoh KH. Antithrombotic and thrombolytic therapy for valvular disease: antithrombotic therapy and prevention of thrombosis, 9th ed: American College of chest physicians evidence-based clinical practice guidelines. *Chest.* 2012;141(suppl 2):e576S–e600S.

79. Linkins LA, Dans AL, Moores LK, et al. Treatment and prevention of heparin-induced thrombocytopenia: antithrombotic therapy and prevention of thrombosis, 9th ed: American College of chest physicians evidence-based clinical practice guidelines. *Chest.* 2012;141(suppl 2):e495S–e530S.

80. Grundy SM, Stone NJ, Bailey AL, et al. 2018 AHA/ACC/AACVPR/AAPA/ABC/ACPM/ADA/AGS/APhA/ASPC/NLA/PCNA guideline on the management of blood cholesterol: a report of the American College of Cardiology/American heart association Task force on clinical practice guidelines. *J Am Coll Cardiol.* 2019;73(24):e285–e350.

81. Rosenson RS. The high-density lipoprotein puzzle: why classic epidemiology, genetic epidemiology, and clinical trials conflict? *Arterioscler Thromb Vasc Biol.* 2016;36(5):777–782.

82. Fihn SD, Blankenship JC, Alexander KP, et al. 2014 ACC/AHA/AATS/PCNA/SCAI/STS focused update of the guideline for the diagnosis and management of patients with stable ischemic heart disease: a report of the American College of Cardiology/American Heart Association Task Force on practice guidelines, and the American association for thoracic surgery, preventive cardiovascular nurses association, society for cardiovascular angiography and interventions, and society of thoracic Surgeons. *J Thorac Cardiovasc Surg*. 2015;149(3):e5–e23.

83. Patel MR, Bailey SR, Bonow RO, et al. ACCF/SCAI/AATS/AHA/ASE/ASNC/HFSA/HRS/SCCM/SCCT/SCMR/STS 2012 appropriate use criteria for diagnostic catheterization: a report of the American College of Cardiology Foundation appropriate Use criteria Task force, society for cardiovascular angiography and interventions, American Association for Thoracic Surgery, American Heart Association, American Society of Echocardiography, American Society of Nuclear Cardiology, Heart Failure Society of America, heart rhythm society, society of critical care medicine, society of cardiovascular computed tomography, society for cardiovascular magnetic resonance, and society of thoracic surgeons. *J Am Coll Cardiol*. 2012;59(22):1995–2027.

84. Sanborn TA, Tcheng JE, Anderson HV, et al. ACC/AHA/SCAI 2014 health policy statement on structured reporting for the cardiac catheterization laboratory: a report of the American College of Cardiology Clinical Quality Committee. *Circulation*. 2014;129(24):2578–2609.

85. Nishimura RA, Carabello BA. Hemodynamics in the cardiac catheterization laboratory of the 21st century. *Circulation*. 2012;125(17):2138–2150.

86. Haines DE, Beheiry S, Akar JG, et al. Heart Rhythm Society expert consensus statement on electrophysiology laboratory standards: process, protocols, equipment, personnel, and safety. *Heart Rhythm*. 2014;11(8):e9–e51.

87. Grayburn PA. Interpreting the coronary-artery calcium score. *N Engl J Med*. 2012;366(4):294–296.

11

Cardiovascular Disorders

Annette Haynes and Patricia Henry

PREVENTING CARDIOVASCULAR DISEASE

Cardiovascular disease (CVD) remains the leading cause of death in the United States. From 2006 to 2016, the overall rate of CVD mortality in the United States declined by 31.8%.[1] Globally, 17.6 million deaths occur secondary to CVD occur each year, which is a 14.5% increase worldwide.[1]

The American Heart Association (AHA) has evolved from focusing only on prevention of disease to an emphasis on cardiovascular health and achievement of a healthy lifestyle, maintaining health factors, and population-level health promotion:

- *Healthy lifestyle*: healthy diet, weight, physical activity, and not smoking.
- *Health factor goals*: optimal cholesterol levels, blood pressure (BP), and glucose control.
- *Population health*: improving cardiovascular health of the public.

The seven metrics of a healthy lifestyle and health factors are the basis of the AHA's 2020 Impact Goals to improve cardiovascular health for all Americans by 20% and decrease deaths from CVD and stroke by 20% by 2020.[2]

ATHEROSCLEROTIC CARDIOVASCULAR DISEASE

The prevalence of atherosclerotic cardiovascular disease (ASCVD), which includes coronary heart disease (CHD), heart failure (HF), stroke, and hypertension in adults (>20 years old), was 48% (121.5 million) in 2016. Hypertension demonstrated the greatest effect on ASCVD, with 24.3 million.[1] Treatments have evolved with age-specific and sex-specific guidelines and campaigns including Go Red for Women. The World Health Organization's global action plan targets preventable risk factors (tobacco and alcohol use, salt intake, obesity, elevated BP, and glucose) to reduce premature mortality by 25% by 2025, also known as the 25 by 25 campaign.[3]

CORONARY ARTERY DISEASE

Description and Etiology

The biggest contributor to cardiovascular system—related morbidity and mortality is *coronary artery disease* (CAD). *Atherosclerosis* is a progressive disease that affects arteries throughout the body. In the heart, atherosclerotic changes are clinically known as *CAD*. This disease process is also known by the term *CHD*, because other heart structures ultimately become involved as the disease progresses.

Risk Factors

The atherosclerotic vascular changes that lead to CAD may begin in childhood. Research and epidemiologic data collected during the past 50 years have demonstrated a strong association between preventable (*modifiable*) risk factors and nonpreventable (*nonmodifiable*) risk factors and the development of CAD[1,4] (Box 11.1):

- *Nonmodifiable risk factors*: Age, family history, race, and sex.
- *Modifiable risk factors*: Diabetes (Table 11.1), hyperlipidemia (Table 11.2), hypertension (Table 11.3), cigarette smoking, obesity, and physical inactivity (see Box 11.1).[1–16] Other risk factors include two CAD disease risk equivalents: chronic kidney disease and diabetes.

Women and Heart Disease

Substantial progress has been made in the awareness, treatment, and prevention of CVD in women.[17] CVD still causes approximately more than one-third of female deaths in the United States.[1] After age 65 years, a higher percentage of women than men have hypertension. Average body weight continues to increase. Nearly two out of every three women in the United States older than age 20 years are overweight or obese.[17] The average age for first acute myocardial infarction (MI) in men is 65 years; in women, it is 71.8 years.[1]

The Nurses' Health Study identified that early menarche (monthly period onset) younger than 10 years old increased CVD risk by up to 20%. Early menopause (less than 40 years old) increased CVD risk by 32%.[18] The incidence of CVD is 2 to 3 times higher among postmenopausal women than among women who are premenopausal.[1] In the past, it seemed logical to prescribe *hormone replacement therapy* (HRT) to treat the symptoms of menopause.[18] Current guidelines do not recommend the use of HRT for primary or secondary prevention of CVD.[18] Diabetes, smoking, and hyperlipidemia all increase the cardiovascular risk for women.[19] Data from the Framingham Heart Study indicate the lifetime risk for CVD is more than one in two for women.[19,20] Optimum prevention strategies for women following the AHAs Life's Simple 7 model are often delayed or inadequate.[20] Women lag 10 years behind men for total CHD risk and more than 20 years for MI and sudden death.

In the 2011 update of *Effectiveness Based Guidelines for the Prevention of CVD in Women*,[17] a new algorithm for risk classification in women was adopted that stratified women's risk into the following three categories:

- *Women at high risk*: Documented CHD, CVD, peripheral artery disease (PAD), abdominal aortic aneurysm, diabetes mellitus,

BOX 11.1 Coronary Artery Disease Risk Factors[1–16]

Age
- Coronary artery disease (CAD) disease generally first manifests after age 45 years.
- Men tend to develop CAD symptoms 5–10 years earlier than women.
- Rate of cardiovascular disease (CVD) in women increases after age 75 years.
- CAD rate is 2–3 times greater in postmenopausal women compared with premenopausal women.

Family History
- Positive family history is defined as a close blood relative who has a myocardial infarction (MI) or stroke before age 60 years.
- Family history suggests genetic or lifestyle predisposition for development of CAD.
- Patients with CAD family history have a 50% greater risk of having an MI.

Diabetes Mellitus
- Elevated blood glucose is a known risk factor for development of vascular inflammation associated with atherosclerosis.
- The American Diabetes Association recommends use of the hemoglobin A_{1c} test with a threshold of 6.5% or greater, fasting blood glucose 126 mg/dL or greater, or 2-hour plasma glucose 200 mg/dL during an oral glucose tolerance test to diagnose diabetes.
- Diabetics have increased risk of developing CAD and worse clinical outcomes after acute coronary syndrome (ACS) events.
- See Table 11.1 for fasting blood glucose levels and risk for CAD.

Physical Activity
- A sedentary lifestyle has negative effects regardless of age, sex, body mass index (BMI), and smoking status.
- Regular vigorous physical activity using large muscle groups promotes adaptation to aerobic exercise, which can prevent development of CAD and reduce symptoms in patients with established CVD.
- Exercise, decreased low-density lipoprotein (LDL) and triglyceride levels, and increased high-density lipoprotein (HDL) cholesterol reduce insulin resistance at the cellular level, lowering the risk for developing type 2 diabetes.
- Lifelong physical activity is necessary to prevent atherosclerotic CAD and stroke.

Obesity
- Two-thirds of US adults are overweight.
- BMI greater than 30 kg/m^2 is considered obese.
- Obesity is associated with a sedentary lifestyle, calories consumed, and portion size.
- Normal BMI is 18.5–25 kg/m^2 (weight/height^2)

Fat Pattern Distribution
- Higher weight carried in the abdominal area has greater risk of CAD.
- Large waist (apple body shape)—excess abdominal adiposity—indicates added fat around the abdominal organs.
- Smaller waist and larger hips (pear body shape) is associated with lower risk of CAD.
- Goal waist measurements are less than 40 inches for men and less than 35 inches for women.

High-Fat Diet
- A diet rich in saturated fats leads to elevated cholesterol levels.
- A low-fat, high-fiber diet and increased physical activity are the first line of treatment.
- If these are ineffective, lipid-lowering medications are indicated.
- Less than 50% of patients prescribed reduction therapy take their medications.
- Only one-third of treated patients reach their LDL target value.

Hyperlipidemia
- Hyperlipidemia causes severe atherosclerosis and development of CAD.
- Total cholesterol is the sum of HDL, LDL, and VLDL cholesterol (goal <200 mg/dL).

HDL (Goal >40 mg/dL for Men; >50 mg/dL for Women)
- HDL is known as *good cholesterol*; a higher serum level protects against atherosclerotic events.
- HDL promotes efflux of cholesterol from cells.
- HDL has antiinflammatory and antioxidant effects on the arterial wall.

LDL (Goal <100 mg/dL)
- LDL is known as *bad cholesterol* because high serum levels are associated with increased risk of ACS, stroke, and peripheral artery disease.
- LDL initiates atherosclerosis by infiltrating the vessel wall and inflammatory vessel effects.
- Initial efforts to decrease LDL are based on weight loss, smoking cessation, low-fat diet, physical exercise, and maintaining normal body size.
- If lifestyle changes are not effective in decreasing LDL, the medication category of choice is statins.
- See Table 11.2 for lipid guidelines and risk for CAD.

Triglycerides (Ideal Goal <100 mg/dL)
- Triglyceride level greater than 150 mg/dL increases risk for heart disease and stroke.
- Mean triglyceride level in men older than 20 years is 108.8 mg/dL.

Lipoprotein(a) (Goal <30 mg/dL)
- Lp(a) is one of the lipid particles that makes up total LDL value.
- Lp(a) is described verbally as "LP little a."
- It is manufactured in the liver and circulates bound to a large glycoprotein called *apolipoprotein A*.
- It is elevated in the presence of inflammation.
- Lp(a) stimulates atheroma and clot formation in inflamed arteries.
- Elevated Lp(a) is the most frequently encountered genetic lipid disorder in families with premature CAD.
- Medication treatment is high doses (1500–2000 mg/day) of extended-release nicotinic acid (niacin).

Metabolic Syndrome
- *Metabolic syndrome* refers to clustering of risk factors associated with CVD and type 2 diabetes.
- Approximately one-third of people in the United States have metabolic syndrome.
- Risk factors include:
  - Fasting plasma glucose greater than 100 mg/dL or taking medications to lower elevated blood glucose
  - HDL cholesterol less than 40 mg/dL in men and less than 50 mg/dL in women
  - Triglycerides greater than 150 mg/dL or taking medications to lower elevated triglycerides
  - Waist circumference greater than 40 inches (102 cm) in men or greater than 35 inches (88 cm) in women
  - Blood pressure (BP) greater than 130 mm Hg systolic or greater than 85 mm Hg diastolic or taking antihypertensive medications

Cigarette Smoking
- Smoking unfavorably alters lipid profile by decreasing HDL and increasing LDL and triglyceride levels.
- The greater number of cigarettes smoked per day, the greater risk of developing CAD, acute MI, and stroke.
- Smoking fewer than five cigarettes per day increases risk.

BOX 11.1 Coronary Artery Disease Risk Factors—cont'd

- Smokers are 2–4 times more likely to develop CAD compared with nonsmokers.
- Passive secondhand smoke exposure also increases CVD risk for nonsmoking adults with up to 30% increased risk of coronary heart disease.
- Of US adults, 20% are current smokers.
- Within 1 year of giving up cigarettes, an ex-smoker's risk of developing CAD decreases significantly.
- Nicotine is addictive, and giving up smoking is difficult.
- People need tremendous support to be able to "kick the habit."

Hypertension

- Hypertension is defined as systolic BP greater than 120 mm Hg and/or diastolic BP greater than 90 mm Hg.
- Increased systolic pressure damages endothelium, leading to vascular inflammation and plaque development.
- Hypertension is known as the silent killer because 28% of patients without CAD and 51% of patients with CVD are unaware of having hypertension.

- Initial treatments aim at lifestyle changes including physical activity, low sodium diet, limiting alcohol intake, and achieving normal body weight.
- Most patients are started on a diuretic; if this is insufficient, an angiotensin-converting enzyme inhibitor, angiotensin receptor blocker, beta-blocker, or calcium channel blocker may be added.
- Most patients require at least two medications from different classifications to normalize their BP.
- See Table 11.3 for BP guidelines and CAD risk.

Risk Equivalents for CAD

- Medical conditions in which patients have as much risk of experiencing a coronary event as if they already had CAD include:
  - Chronic kidney disease—risk for death from acute MI rises as serum creatinine level increases
  - Diabetes mellitus
  - Peripheral artery disease
  - Cerebrovascular disease

TABLE 11.1 Diabetes: Fasting Blood Glucose and Risk for Coronary Artery Disease.

Blood Glucose Level	Fasting Plasma Glucose Level[a] (mg/dL)	Risk of CAD
Normal	70–100	Low
Prediabetes	101–125	Intermediate
Diabetes	126 or greater	High

[a]Values greater than normal increase the risk for coronary artery disease and kidney failure.
CAD, Coronary artery disease.

end-stage or chronic kidney disease, or 10-year predicted risk for CHD greater than 10%

- *Women at risk:* Cigarette smoking; systolic BP 120 mm Hg or greater, diastolic BP 80 mm Hg or greater, or treated hypertension; total cholesterol 200 mg/dL or greater, high-density lipoprotein (HDL) C less than 50 mg/dL, or treated for dyslipidemia; obesity, particularly central adiposity; poor diet; physical inactivity; family history of premature CVD occurring in first-degree relatives in men younger than 55 years old or women younger than 65 years old; metabolic syndrome; evidence of advanced subclinical atherosclerosis (e.g., coronary calcification, carotid plaque, or thickened

TABLE 11.2 Hyperlipidemia: Treatment of Blood Cholesterol to Decrease Atherosclerotic Cardiovascular Risk Disease.[6–14]

Patient Characteristics	Intensity of Statins Needed
Age 75 years or less and no safety concerns	High-intensity statin
Age more than 75 years or safety concerns	Moderate-intensity statin
Primary Prevention for LDL-C >190 mg/dL	
Age >21 years	High-intensity statins to achieve 50% decrease in LDL-C; consider nonstatin therapy
Diabetes; age 40–75 years; LDL-C 70–189 mg/dL	Moderate-intensity statins; high-intensity statins when 10-year ASCVD risk is greater than 7.5%
No diabetes; age 40–75 years; LDL-C 70–189 mg/dL	Moderate-intensity statins; if 10-year ASCVD risk is more than 7.5%, moderate- to high-intensity statins; if 10-year ASCVD risk is 0.5%–7.5%, moderate-intensity steroids
Other Factors to Consider	
LDL-C ≥160 mg/dL	Family history; premature ASCVD; hs-CRP 2 or greater; CAC Agatston score >300; ABI <0.9; or lifetime ASCVD risk
LDL-C <190 mg/dL	Age less than 40 years or greater than 75 years; or <5% 10-year ASCVD risk
Clinical ASCVD Risk Factors	
ACS	
History of MI	
Stable or unstable angina	
Coronary or other arterial revascularization	
Stroke	
TIA	
PAD	

ABI, Ankle-brachial index; *ACS,* acute coronary syndrome; *ASCVD,* atherosclerotic cardiovascular disease; *CAC,* coronary artery calcium; *hs-CRP,* high-sensitivity C-reactive protein; *LDL-C,* low-density lipoprotein cholesterol; *MI,* myocardial infarction; *PAD,* peripheral artery disease; *TIA,* transient ischemic attack.

TABLE 11.3 Hypertension Management Guidelines.[15]			
GENERAL POPULATION (NO DIABETES OR CKD) LOW RISK OF CAD		**DIABETES OR CKD PRESENT HIGH RISK OF CAD**	
Age ≥60 Years	**Age <60 Years**	**All Ages; Diabetes Present; No CVD**	**All Ages; CKD Present With or Without Diabetes**
BP goal[a]: SBP <150 DBP <90	BP goal: SBP <140 DBP <90	BP goal: SBP <140 DBP <90	BP goal: SBP <140 DBP <90

[a]BP values greater than normal increase the risk for coronary artery disease and heart failure. All BP values are reported in mm Hg.
BP, Blood pressure; *CKD,* chronic kidney disease; *CVD,* cardiovascular disease; *DBP,* diastolic blood pressure; *SBP,* systolic blood pressure. Information from James PA. Evidence-based guidelines for the management of high blood pressure in adults. Report from the panel members appointed to the Eighth Joint National Committee (JNC8). *JAMA.* 2014; 311(5): 507-520.

intimal mean thickness); systemic autoimmune collagen vascular disease (e.g., lupus or rheumatoid arthritis); history of pre-eclampsia, gestational diabetes, or pregnancy-induced hypertension; or poor exercise tolerance with treadmill testing

- *Women's ideal cardiovascular health:* Framingham risk score less than 10%, absence of major CVD risk factors, and engagement in a healthy lifestyle[1,17]

In 2011, these guidelines added several 10-year risk equations for the prediction of 10-year global CVD risk, such as the updated Framingham CVD risk profile and the Reynolds Risk Score for women.[17,19]

The AHA defined a new concept of ideal cardiovascular health in women as follows:

- Absence of clinical CVD and presence of all ideal levels of total cholesterol (less than 200 mg/dL)
- BP less than 120/80 mm Hg
- Fasting blood glucose less than 100 mg/dL
- Adherence to healthy behaviors
- Lean body mass index less than 25 kg/m^2
- Participation in physical activity at recommended levels
- Cessation of smoking
- Pursuit of eating pattern as suggested by *Dietary Approaches to Stop Hypertension* (DASH) diet[20]

Almost 400,000 women die of CVD annually in the United States. Mortality rates for women after an acute MI are higher than for men: 26% compared with 14.9%.[21] The risk factors hypertension, diabetes mellitus, alcohol intake, and physical inactivity are more strongly associated with acute MI in women than in men.[17,20] Many reasons contribute to the higher mortality from acute MI in women, including waiting longer to seek medical care, having smaller coronary arteries, being older when symptoms occur, and experiencing very different symptoms from those of men of similar age.[19,20]

Vascular Inflammation and C-Reactive Protein

The link between vascular inflammation and atherosclerotic disease is well established.[22] The inflammatory marker most frequently cited is C-reactive protein (CRP). It is measured as high-sensitivity CRP (hs-CRP).[22] CRP is associated with an increased risk for development of other cardiovascular risk factors, including diabetes, hypertension, and weight gain. The higher the hs-CRP value, the greater the risk of a coronary event, especially if all other potential causes of systemic inflammation, such as infection, can be ruled out. If other systemic inflammatory conditions such as bronchitis or urinary tract infection are present, the hs-CRP test loses all predictive value. CRP and other inflammatory markers are used to estimate the probability of future acute coronary events.[22–25] During acute coronary syndrome (ACS) events, there is widespread activation of neutrophils in the cardiac circulation (measured from the coronary sinus), which suggests that inflammation is not limited to one unstable plaque.[22]

Coronary Artery Disease Risk Equivalents

Certain medical conditions are risk equivalents of CAD. A *risk equivalent* means the person has the same risk of having an acute MI as if he or she already had CHD. Two noncardiac medical conditions considered risk equivalents for CAD are diabetes mellitus and chronic kidney disease.[26] PAD and cerebrovascular disease are atherosclerotic conditions that are also considered CAD risk equivalents.[26]

Multifactorial Risk

CAD has multifactorial causation, the greater the number of risk factors, the greater the risk of developing CAD. The best time for an individual to make lifestyle changes is *before* the symptoms of CAD occur. Patients with two or more risk factors or with one or more CAD risk-equivalent diseases have the greatest potential to benefit from risk factor reduction and lifestyle change.[26] The major risk factors for developing CAD have been extensively documented in large epidemiologic studies and include smoking, family history, adverse lipid profile, and elevated BP.

Primary Versus Secondary Prevention of Coronary Artery Disease

If a person has symptoms of CAD or has previously had an ACS event, the goal of any lifestyle change or medication is called *secondary prevention*, or preventing another heart attack.[11] If an individual matches the risk profile described previously but does *not* have symptoms of CAD or has *not* had an acute MI, the treatment plan is described as *primary prevention*. The constellation of cardiac risk factors is well established and can predict development of CAD for most populations in the developed world.

Pathophysiology of Coronary Artery Disease

CAD is a progressive atherosclerotic disorder of the coronary arteries that results in narrowing or complete occlusion. *Atherosclerosis* affects the medium-sized arteries that perfuse the heart and other major organs. Normal arterial walls are composed of three layers: (1) the *intima* (inner lining), (2) the *media* (middle muscular layer), and (3) the *adventitia* (outer coat).

Development of Atherosclerosis

Atherosclerosis is a chronic inflammatory disorder that is characterized by an accumulation of macrophages and T lymphocytes in the arterial intimal wall. One of the triggers of vascular inflammation is a high low-density lipoprotein (LDL) cholesterol concentration. The inflammation injures the wall, allowing the LDL cholesterol to move into the vessel wall below the endothelial surface. Blood monocytes adhere to endothelial cells and migrate into the vessel wall. Within the artery wall, some monocytes differentiate into macrophages that unite with and then internalize LDL cholesterol. The *foam cells* that result are the marker cells of atherosclerosis.

TRENDING PRIORITIES IN HEALTHCARE

Health Equity

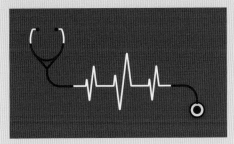

iStock.com/filo

Health equity covers many areas of life in the United States. Health disparities were exposed to a greater degree during the COVID-19 pandemic because this issue was in the forefront of the national consciousness every day. Health equity is relevant to critical care because many patients who contracted COVID-19 required mechanical ventilation.[1,3–5]

Access to critical care beds: In an examination of intensive care unit (ICU) bed availability across the United States (US), researchers found that only half (51%) of low-income communities have hospitals with ICU beds close by. In contrast, in higher-income communities, almost all (97%) have hospitals with ICU beds nearby.[1] This disparity was more acute in rural areas compared with cities and urban areas.[1]

Digital health equity: Unequal access to computers, and lack of digital literacy and skills limits patients' access to vital health care information.[2] Up to a quarter of the population in the United States does not have broadband Internet service, a gap that is associated with a lower household income.[2] Hospitals increasingly use digital portals and electronic messaging to remind patients to take medications, prepare for appointments, and pay bills. Increasingly, patients who do not have access to this technology will be at a disadvantage in managing their healthcare.

Race, ethnicity, and critical care outcomes in COVID-19: There is strong evidence that Hispanic and Black populations had higher rates of COVID-19 positivity.[3] However, what is not known is the impact of race and ethnicity on critical care outcomes. This question is actively being investigated following the COVID-19 pandemic.[4–6]

In general, these early published accounts describe the outcomes of individual hospital critical care units with a wide variation in outcomes.[3–5] In one study of a large cohort of patients who tested positive for COVID-19 in the early days of the pandemic, being black, male, and older than 60 years increased the likelihood of hospital admission, but only poverty was associated with ICU admission.[3] Another study found no statistical difference in the in-hospital mortality between White patients and others following ICU admission for COVID-19.[4] In contrast, a different hospital reported a much higher mortality in Black and Hispanic patients than in White patients following mechanical ventilation for complications of COVID-19.[5] The reasons for these differing outcomes are not known. One reason may be that not all hospitals have access to the same level of critical care resources. Critically ill Black and Hispanic patients are predominantly cared for in minority-serving hospitals, which have shown less improvement over the last decade compared to non-minority hospitals.[7] Many factors contribute to disparities in critical care outcomes and the reasons are important to investigate and correct.

A positive outcome from the COVID-19 pandemic is that it exposed the issue of health inequity, in terms of access to hospitals.[1] Whether treatment varies based on race or ethnicity once a patient is admitted to a critical care unit is unknown. Henceforth, reporting of race and ethnicity will be a standard feature of any patient research report and this question will be answered.

Race and cardiovascular disease outcomes: The American Heart Association (AHA) scientific statement on the cardiovascular (CV) health of African Americans emphasizes the higher risk profile for CV disease in this population including hypertension, diabetes mellitus, and obesity.[8] These risk factors contribute to an increased atherosclerotic risk profile and earlier onset of CV disease, including stroke, heart failure, and peripheral artery disease.[8] Disease management is less effective and mortality is higher in the African American population.[8]

References

1. Kanter GP, Segal AG, Groeneveld PW. Income disparities in access to critical care services. *Health Aff (Millwood)*. 2020;39(8):1362–1367.
2. Sieck CJ, Sheon A, Ancker JS, Castek J, Callahan B, Siefer A. Digital inclusion as a social determinant of health. *NPJ Digit Med*. 2021;4(1):52.
3. Magesh S, John D, Li WT, et al. Disparities in COVID-19 outcomes by race, ethnicity, and socioeconomic status: a systematic-review and meta-analysis. *JAMA Network Open*. 2021;4(11):e2134147.
4. Muñoz-Price LS, Nattinger AB, Rivera F, et al. Racial disparities in incidence and outcomes among patients with COVID-19. *JAMA Network Open*. 2020;3(9):e2021892.
5. Lazar MH, Fadel R, Gardner-Gray J, et al. Racial differences in a Detroit, MI, ICU population of coronavirus disease 2019 patients. *Crit Care Med*. 2021;49(3):482–489.
6. Olanipekun T, Abe T, Sobukonla T, et al. Association between race and risk of ICU mortality in mechanically ventilated COVID-19 patients at a safety net hospital. *J Natl Med Assoc*. 2022;114(1):18–25.
7. Danziger J, Ángel Armengol de la Hoz M, Li W, et al. Temporal trends in critical care outcomes in U.S. minority-serving hospitals. *Am J Respir Crit Care Med*. 2020;201(6):681–687.
8. Carnethon MR, Pu J, Howard G, et al. Cardiovascular health in African Americans: a scientific statement from the American Heart Association. *Circulation*. 2017;136(21):e393–e423.

Elevated LDL cholesterol levels promote low-level endothelial inflammation, which allows lipoproteins to infiltrate the intimal vessel wall. After it has infiltrated under the endothelium, LDL cholesterol tends to stay within the vessel wall rather than return to the circulation. This contrasts with the actions of HDL cholesterol, which enters the vessel wall, helps efflux cholesterol from cells, and then returns to the circulation.[7] The actions of HDL cholesterol may help minimize the number of foam cells in the artery wall.[7]

Atherosclerotic Plaque Rupture

When a mature atherosclerotic plaque develops, it is not uniform in composition. It has a lipid liquid center filled with procoagulant factors. A connective tissue *fibrous cap* covers the top of the fluid lipid center.[27] The abrupt rupture of this cap allows procoagulant lipids to flood into the vessel lumen and rapidly form a coronary thrombosis, as shown in Table 11.4. As the enlarging clot blocks blood flow through the coronary artery, an MI will occur unless adequate collateral circulation from other coronary vessels occurs. Symptoms and suggested cardiac interventions at appropriate stages in development of CAD are also listed in Table 11.4.

Plaques that are likely to rupture are saturated with macrophages and other inflammatory cells. These *vulnerable plaques* are usually not obstructive and are situated at bends or branch points in the arterial tree.[26] It is unknown what factors increase erosion or rupture of the

TABLE 11.4   Coronary Artery Disease: Pathogenesis, Symptoms, Diagnosis, and Management Timeline.

	Pathology of CAD	Symptoms of CAD	Diagnosis of CAD	Management of CAD
	Normal coronary artery seen in young healthy children	No symptoms	None	• Healthy lifestyle • Obesity prevention
	Fatty streaks on intima of aorta and coronary arteries in many young adults	No symptoms	None	Preventive measures with a focus on a healthy lifestyle
	Atherosclerotic plaque increases in size but does not occlude blood flow	• No symptoms • Most adults are unaware they have CAD	None	Cardiac risk factor management
	Atherosclerotic plaque occludes more than 70% of coronary artery lumen. Stable cap on lipid plaque interior.	Stable angina • Chest pain or pressure with exertion or exercise	ECG stress test Elective coronary arteriogram	• Aggressive risk factor management • Sublingual nitroglycerin for angina • Elective PCI with stent
	Atherosclerotic plaque becomes fibrous and calcified. Plaque has a large procoagulant lipid core. Cap has thinned with cracks, allowing platelets and fibrin to aggregate.	Unstable angina/ACS • Change in chest pain/pressure symptoms • Chest pain/pressure at rest • Symptoms not relieved by NTG	• 12-lead ECG • Coronary arteriogram • Biomarkers	• Emergency PCI with stent • Aggressive risk factor management • Aggressive risk factor management
	Atherosclerotic cap ruptures and the procoagulant lipid core is released forming a thrombosis that blocks blood flow.	STEMI or NSTEMI • Abrupt onset of chest pain or pressure or symptoms at rest • Angina not relieved by NTG • Sudden shortness of breath, cold sweat	• Emergency 12-lead ECG • Emergency coronary arteriogram • Biomarkers	• Emergency PCI with stent • Aggressive risk factor management

ACS, Acute coronary syndrome; *CAD,* coronary artery disease; *ECG*, electrocardiogram; *NSTEMI*, non–ST segment elevation myocardial infarction; *NTG*, nitroglycerin; *PCI*, percutaneous coronary intervention; *STEMI*, ST segment elevation myocardial infarction.

fibrous cap. As deep fissures in the cap expose the procoagulant factors to the blood plasma, an unstoppable cycle is put into motion. When platelets in the bloodstream are exposed to collagen, necrotic debris, von Willebrand factor, and thromboxane, a clot is formed and can occlude the coronary artery. Highly fibrotic plaques do not rupture. The type of atherosclerotic plaque that is prone to rupture has a weak fibrous cap and holds a large amount of liquid cholesterol within the plaque (see Table 11.4).

Plaque Regression

A reduction in blood cholesterol decreases atherosclerotic plaque size by decreasing the amount of liquid cholesterol within the plaque core.[6] Lowering cholesterol levels does not change the dimensions of the fibrous or calcified portions of the plaque. However, lower cholesterol levels reduce vascular inflammation and make vulnerable plaque less likely to rupture.

Acute Coronary Syndrome

The term *acute coronary syndrome* (ACS) is used to describe the array of clinical presentations of CAD that range from unstable angina to acute MI.[1,26] An acute MI is generally described by patients as a "heart attack." This section discusses stable manifestations of CAD (stable angina) and acute manifestations described as an ACS (unstable angina and acute MI). Fig. 11.1 provides a summary of priority diagnostic assessment and priority nursing interventions in ACS.

Angina

Angina pectoris, or chest pain, caused by myocardial ischemia is not a separate disease but rather a symptom of CAD. It is caused by a blockage or spasm of a coronary artery, leading to diminished myocardial blood supply. The lack of oxygen causes myocardial ischemia, which is felt as chest discomfort, pressure, or pain. Angina may occur anywhere in the chest, neck, arms, or back, but the most commonly described location is pain or pressure behind the sternum. The pain often radiates to the left arm but can also radiate down both arms and to the back, shoulder, jaw, or neck (Fig. 11.2). Angina

symptoms are not the same for all individuals. Many patients may describe pressure or discomfort rather than pain, and presenting symptoms can be highly individualized, as described in Box 11.2. Patients and families must be taught that angina does not always present in the dramatic heart attack scenario as often portrayed on television and in movies, in which the person clutches the throat or chest and exhibits extreme distress.[26,28]

Angina symptom equivalents. Men and women should be informed of angina symptom equivalents, such as unexpected shortness of breath; breaking out in a cold sweat; or sudden fatigue, nausea, or lightheadedness.[28]

Women and angina. Many women experience a variety of symptoms before an acute MI and during the acute event, as shown in Box 11.3.[19,20] The recognition and publicity about the fact that many women have atypical symptoms but do not experience "crushing chest pain" is important to understand to avoid a woman's symptoms being trivialized by health care clinicians.[19] It is vital that women are made aware of the *angina symptom equivalents* of unexplained shortness of breath; breaking out in a cold sweat; or sudden fatigue, nausea, or lightheadedness.[26,28] More women die of ACS every year in the United States compared with men, a fact that is largely unknown by health care providers.[19,20]

Stable angina. *Stable angina* is predictable and caused by similar precipitating factors each time; typically, it is exercise induced. Patients become used to the pattern of this type of angina and may describe it as "my usual chest pain." Pain control should be achieved within 5 minutes of rest and by taking sublingual nitroglycerin. Ischemia and chest pain occur when myocardial demand from exertion exceeds the fixed blood oxygen supply.

Unstable angina. *Unstable angina* is defined as a change in a previously established stable pattern of angina. It is part of the continuum of ACS. Unstable angina usually is more intense than stable angina, may awaken the person from sleep, or may necessitate more than nitrates for pain relief. A change in the level or frequency of symptoms requires immediate medical evaluation. Severe angina that persists for more than 5 minutes, worsens in intensity, and is not relieved by one nitroglycerin tablet is a medical emergency, and the patient or a family

---

Acute Coronary Syndrome

Priority Diagnostic assessment	STEMI	Priority nursing interventions

• Vital signs
• 12 lead ECG
• Troponins x 3
• IV access
• Clinical assessment
• History and risk factors
  ○ Diabetes mellitus
  ○ Kidney disease
  ○ Previous MI or HF
• Additional cardiac tests:
  ○ Cardiac echocardiogram
  ○ Cardiac catheterization
	• ST segment elevation
	• Q waves not always present
	• Troponins elevated
	• Ongoing ischemic chest pain
	
	Non-STEMI
	• ST segment normal
	• Q waves not always present
	• Troponins elevated
	• Ongoing ischemic chest pain
		• Continuous ECG monitoring of atrial and ventricular dysrhythmias
		• Maintain SpO2 >90% with supplemental oxygen as needed
		• NTG sublingual to dilate coronary arteries
		• Morphine for pain
		• Monitor electrolytes: K+, Mg++
		• Plan for immediate medical intervention to open coronary artery
		• Patient and family education

Fig. 11.1 Acute Coronary Syndrome: Priority Diagnostic Assessments and Priority Nursing Interventions. *CVC,* Central venous catheter; *ECG,* electrocardiogram; *HF,* heart failure; *IV,* intravenous; *MI,* myocardial Infarction; *NTG,* nitroglycerin; *non-STEMI,* non–ST segment elevation myocardial infarction; *SPO₂,* saturation of hemoglobin with oxygen measured by pulse oximetry; *STEMI,* ST segment elevation myocardial infarction.

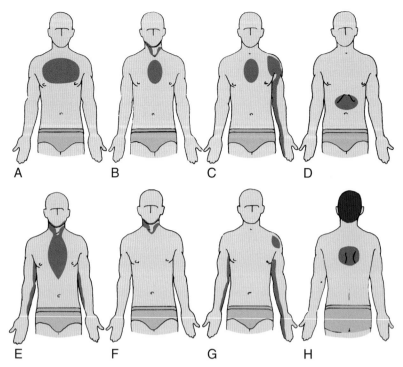

Fig. 11.2 Common Sites for Anginal Pain. (A) Upper part of chest. (B) Beneath sternum, radiating to neck and jaw. (C) Beneath sternum, radiating down left arm. (D) Epigastric. (E) Epigastric, radiating to neck, jaw, and arms. (F) Neck and jaw. (G) Left shoulder. (H) Intrascapular.

member must call 911 immediately.[27] The 911 (Emergency Medical Services [EMS]) system is available to 98% of the population of the United States.[28] Family and friends are discouraged from driving a person experiencing unstable angina to the hospital and instead are urged to call 911. Patients should be instructed never to drive themselves but to contact the EMS by calling 911. Delay in reperfusion,

cardiac arrest in a personal car, and mortality are all increased when EMS is not called.[28]

Unstable angina is an indication of atherosclerotic plaque instability. It can signal atherosclerotic plaque rupture and thrombus formation that can lead to MI. A patient who comes to the emergency department with recent-onset unstable angina but who has nonspecific or

---

BOX 11.2   Characteristics of Angina Pectoris (Chest Pain)

Location
- Beneath sternum, radiating to neck and jaw
- Upper chest
- Beneath sternum, radiating down left arm
- Epigastric
- Epigastric, radiating to neck, jaw, and arms
- Neck and jaw
- Left shoulder, inner aspect of both arms
- Intrascapular

Duration
- Less than 5 minutes (stable)
- Longer than 5 minutes or worsening symptoms without relief from rest or sublingual nitroglycerin indicates preinfarction symptoms (unstable)

Quality
- Sensation of pressure or heavy weight on the chest
- Feeling of tightness like a vise
- Visceral quality (deep, heavy, squeezing, aching)
- Burning sensation
- Shortness of breath, with feeling of suffocation
- Most severe pain ever experienced

Radiation
- Medial aspect of left arm
- Jaw
- Left shoulder
- Right arm

Precipitating Factors
- Exertion or exercise
- Cold weather
- Exercising after large, heavy meal
- Walking against the wind
- Emotional upset
- Fright, anger
- Coitus

Medication Relief
- Usually within 45 seconds to 5 minutes after sublingual nitroglycerin administration

BOX 11.3 Cardiovascular Symptoms Experienced by Women Before Acute Myocardial Infarction

Generalized Symptoms Before Acute Myocardial Infarction	Discomfort/Pain Symptoms During Acute Myocardial Infarction
Unusual fatigue	Centered high in chest
Dizzy or faint	Under left breast
Hot, flushed	Back/between shoulder blades
Indigestion	Neck/throat
Heart racing	Generalized chest
Numbness in hands/fingers	Leg(s)
Vomiting	Both arms
Loss of appetite	Top of shoulders
New vision problems	Right arm or shoulder
Headache	Jaw/teeth
Coughing	
Choking sensation	

From McSweeney JC. Preventing and experiencing ischemic heart disease as a woman: state of the science. A scientific statement from the American Heart Association. *Circulation.* 2016;133:1302.

nonelevated ST segment changes on a 12-lead electrocardiogram (ECG) may be admitted to the critical care unit to rule out MI. If the symptoms are typical of MI, it is important to treat the patient according to the latest published guidelines, because not all patients who experience MI have ST segment elevation on the 12-lead ECG.[17,27]

Variant angina. Variant angina, or Prinzmetal angina, is caused by a dynamic obstruction from intense vasoconstriction of a coronary artery.[29] Spasm can occur with or without atherosclerotic lesions. Variant angina commonly occurs when the individual is at rest, and it is often cyclic, occurring at the same time every day. Smoking, alcohol use, and illegal stimulant drug (cocaine, methamphetamine) use may precipitate spasm. A definitive diagnosis of variant angina is made during a cardiac catheterization study. Signs of spasm include ST segment elevation and chest pain. Coronary artery spasm can occur with or without CAD. The prognosis is excellent when no significant coronary artery stenosis exists. Coronary artery spasm is treated with nitroglycerin or calcium channel blockers to vasodilate the coronary arteries.

Silent ischemia. Silent ischemia describes a situation in which objective evidence of ischemia is observed on an ECG monitor, but the person does not complain of anginal symptoms. One-third of patients who are having an MI do not report chest pain as a symptom.[26] Patients with diabetes are at particular risk for silent ischemia. Many patients who had type 2 diabetes for more than 10 years have developed *autonomic neuropathy*, which decreases their ability to experience chest pain. Patients with diabetes may misinterpret angina symptom equivalents such as nausea, vomiting, and diaphoresis as signaling a disruption in glucose control rather than a sign of myocardial ischemia.

Medical Management

Accurate assessment of chest pain symptoms is essential if unstable angina is to be recognized and treated effectively. An important reason to ask questions about the chest pain is to differentiate between stable and unstable angina. The change from stable to unstable angina is potentially life threatening for the patient. If the ST segments are elevated or a newly documented left bundle branch block (LBBB) is seen on the 12-lead ECG, the patient should be treated for acute MI.[28] However, if these classic ECG signs are missing and the chest pain continues, the current pharmacologic treatment of choice is aspirin (if the patient cannot tolerate aspirin, a thienopyridine such as clopidogrel can be given).

Patients with definite unstable angina or non–ST segment elevation myocardial infarction (NSTEMI) should receive dual antiplatelet therapy on admission if an invasive strategy is imminent. A glycoprotein (GP) IIb/IIIa inhibitor or direct thrombin inhibitor such as bivalirudin is administered; a loading dose of clopidogrel is given at least 6 hours before the procedure. Patients undergoing noninvasive treatment should receive aspirin and a thienopyridine (clopidogrel, prasugrel, or ticagrelor) for 1 month and ideally up to 1 year. If symptoms persist, diagnostic angiography is performed. A stress test should be performed on patients who are not undergoing invasive therapy for unstable angina or NSTEMI; if the stress test is negative, the GP IIb/IIIa inhibitor can be discontinued, and unfractionated heparin (UFH) administered for 48 hours.

Nursing Management

Care management for a patient with CAD and angina incorporates a variety of patient care diagnoses (Box 11.4). Nursing priorities focus on early identification of myocardial ischemia, control of chest pain, recognition of complications, maintenance of a calm environment, and patient and family education. See Appendix A for patient care management plans specific to patients with CAD.

Recognizing Myocardial Ischemia

Complaints of chest discomfort (angina) must be evaluated quickly, because angina is an indicator of myocardial ischemia. The patient is asked to rate the intensity of the chest discomfort on a scale of 0 to 10. Pain levels must be assessed with sensitivity to differences in cultural manifestations of pain. The term *chest pain* is not to be used exclusively, because some patients describe their angina as "pressure" or "heaviness."

It is important to document the characteristics of the pain and the patient's heart rate and rhythm, BP, respirations, temperature, skin color, peripheral pulses, urine output, mentation, and overall tissue perfusion. A 12-lead ECG is used to identify the area of ischemic myocardium. The major concern is that the chest pain may represent preinfarction angina, and early identification is essential so that the patient can be immediately treated. Treatment may include transfer to the cardiac catheterization laboratory for a coronary arteriogram and opening of a blocked artery. If the hospital does not have a cardiac catheterization laboratory, GP IIb/IIIa receptor blockers may be infused to prevent the evolution of the acute MI before transfer.[27,28]

Relieving Chest Pain

In the critical care unit, control of angina is achieved by a combination of supplemental oxygen, nitrates, analgesia, and surveillance of angina and of the effects of pharmacologic therapy.

- *Oxygen:* All patients with acute ischemic pain are administered supplemental oxygen to increase myocardial oxygenation. Pulse oximetry is used to guide therapy and maintain oxygen saturation above 90% unless the patient has a history of chronic obstructive pulmonary disease and is a carbon dioxide retainer.

QSEN   BOX 11.4   **Evidence-Based Practice**

Coronary Artery Disease and Stable Angina

Strong evidence exists that the following lifestyle interventions help prevent coronary artery disease (CAD).

- Diet:
  - Diet low in salt and high in fiber, fruit, vegetables, and grains
  - All dietary fat less than 30% of total calories; saturated fat less than 7%
  - Limit glucose in diet (simple sugars)
  - Limit calories if overweight
  - Omega-3 fatty acids included in diet
- Exercise:
  - Start by walking more often and increase physical exercise from there.
  - Refer to cardiac rehabilitation program.
- Obesity:
  - Achieve healthy body weight.
- Addiction:
  - Stop cigarette smoking.
  - Avoid exposure to environmental (secondhand) tobacco smoke at home and at work.
  - Limit alcohol intake.

Strong evidence exists that the following diagnostic procedures help the patient with angina.

- When a patient presents with chest pain, quickly obtaining a detailed history of symptoms, focused physical examination, and risk factor assessment can help determine whether the probability of CAD is low, intermediate, or high.
- Initial laboratory tests include hemoglobin, fasting blood glucose, lipid panel, and cardiac enzymes.
- Obtain a baseline 12-lead electrocardiogram (ECG) at rest, even if chest pain is not present.
- Obtain a 12-lead ECG during an episode of chest pain.
- Obtain a chest radiograph if symptoms of heart failure are present.
- Obtain an exercise 12-lead ECG if the patient's condition is stable and symptoms suggest CAD or if the patient's condition is stable with complete left bundle branch block or right bundle branch block that makes the ECG difficult to interpret for ischemia.
- Obtain cardiac echocardiography for a patient with a systolic murmur suggestive of aortic stenosis.
- Use cardiac echocardiography to determine the extent of left ventricular (LV) hypertrophy or dysfunction.
- Stress cardiac echocardiography is recommended for patients with greater than 1 mm of ST segment depression at rest (stress may be induced by physical exercise or by pharmacologic stimulation).
- Coronary angiography (typically as part of a cardiac catheterization procedure) is recommended for patients at high risk for adverse coronary events.

Initial Pharmacologic and Lifestyle Treatment Recommendations

- The goal of treatment is to eliminate chest pain.
- The 10 most important elements of CAD and stable angina management can be remembered using the following A–E mnemonic:

  A—Aspirin and antianginal medications: Prescribe daily low-dose (75–325 mg) aspirin, oral nitrates, and sublingual nitroglycerin for episodes of angina.

  B—Beta-blockers and blood pressure: Use angiotensin-converting enzyme inhibitors and beta-blockers to decrease blood pressure to less than 140/90 mm Hg if no other CAD risk factors are present and to less than 130/80 mm Hg if diabetes or kidney disease is present.

  C—Cholesterol and cigarettes: Obtain a fasting lipid profile. Recommend diet or lipid reduction medication therapy (statin) to lower low-density lipoprotein cholesterol (LDL-C) to less than 100 mg/dL (<70 mg/dL if achievable), increase high-density lipoprotein cholesterol to more than 40 mg/dL for men or more than 50 mg/dL for women, and reduce triglycerides to less than 150 mg/dL. Recommend adding plant stanols or sterols (2 g/day) or viscous fiber (>10 g/day), or both, to diet to further lower LDL-C; add dietary omega-3 fatty acids in the form of fish or capsule (1 g/day). Always ask about tobacco use, and strongly recommend smoking cessation; encourage nicotine replacement therapy (nicotine patches or gum) as needed.

  D—Diet and diabetes: Prescribe a low-fat, calorie-appropriate diet and provide nutritional consultation as needed to achieve a fasting blood glucose level of 70–100 mg/dL and hemoglobin A_{1c} of less than 6.5%.

  E—Education and exercise: Provide education about risk factor modification and the CAD disease process; recommend daily exercise for 30–60 minutes (ideal) or at least seven times each week (minimum of 5 days per week). A body mass index between 18.5 kg/m² and 24.9 kg/m² and waist circumference less than 40 inches for men or less than 35 inches for women should be recommended. Treat depression, if present. Hormone replacement therapy is not recommended as a treatment for symptoms of coronary heart disease. Influenza vaccination is recommended.

Interventional and Surgical Recommendations for Stable High-Risk Patients

Patients are risk stratified according to their symptoms and the results of cardiac diagnostic tests.

- Percutaneous catheter intervention (PCI):
  - PCI is more frequently performed than open-heart surgery for relief of anginal symptoms.
- Coronary artery bypass graft surgery:
  - For patients with left main occlusion or multivessel disease.
  - For patients with two-vessel disease who have significant proximal left anterior descending coronary artery stenosis and an LV ejection fraction less than 50%.

References

Amsterdam EA, Wenger NK, Brindis RG, et al. 2014 AHA/ACC guideline for the management of patients with non-ST elevation acute coronary syndromes. A report of the American College of Cardiology/American Heart Association task force on practice guidelines. *Circulation*. 2014;130:e344–e426.

Fihn SD, Gardin JM, Abrams J, et al. 2012 ACCF/AHA/ACP/AATS/PCNA/SCAI/STS guideline for the diagnosis and management of patients with stable ischemic heart disease: a report of the American College of Cardiology Foundation/American Heart Association task force on practice guidelines, and the American College of Physicians, American Association for Thoracic Surgery, Preventive Cardiovascular Nurses Association, Society for Cardiovascular Angiography and Interventions, and Society of Thoracic Surgeons. *Circulation*. 2012;126(25):e354.

O'Gara PT, Kushner FG, Ascheim DD, et al. 2013 ACCF/AHA guideline for the management of ST-elevation myocardial infarction: a report of the American College of Cardiology Foundation/American Heart Association task force on practice guidelines. *Circulation*. 2013;127(4):e362.

- *Nitrates:* A combination of intravenous and sublingual nitroglycerin is used to vasodilate the coronary arteries and decrease pain. After nitrate administration, the critical care nurse closely observes the patient for relief of chest pain, for return of the ST segment to baseline, and for the potential development of unwanted side effects such as hypotension and headache. Administration of a nitrate is avoided if the systolic BP is less than 90 mm Hg. Medication interactions with nitrates are another potential cause for concern. The phosphodiesterase inhibitor medication *sildenafil* is prescribed for several conditions including pulmonary hypertension (PH) (Revatio) and erectile dysfunction (Viagra). Sildenafil and nitrates in combination may contribute to a precipitous fall in BP.[3]
- *Analgesia:* Morphine (2–4 mg given intravenously) is the analgesic opiate of choice for preinfarction angina. It relieves pain and decreases fear and anxiety. After administration, the critical care nurse assesses the patient for pain relief and the development of unwanted side effects such as hypotension and respiratory depression.[26]
- *Aspirin:* Chewing an oral non–enteric-coated aspirin (162–325 mg) at the beginning of chest pain has been shown to reduce mortality. The nonenteric formulation is preferred because it increases absorption in the mouth when chewed, not swallowed.[26,28]

Maintaining a Calm Environment

Patients admitted to a critical care unit with unstable angina experience extreme anxiety and fear of death. The critical care nurse is faced with the challenge of ensuring that the elements of a calm environment to alleviate the patient's fear and anxiety are maintained, while being ready at all times to respond to an acute emergency such as a cardiac arrest or to assist with emergency intubation or insertion of hemodynamic monitoring catheters.

Educate the Patient and Family

In the critical care unit, the patient's ability to retain educational information is severely affected by stress and pain. Education topics that should be discussed when the clinical condition has stabilized are listed in Box 11.5. It is essential to teach avoidance of the Valsalva maneuver, which is defined as forced expiration against a closed glottis. This can be explained to the patient as "bearing down" during defecation or breath holding when repositioning in bed. The Valsalva maneuver causes an increase in intrathoracic pressure, which decreases venous return to the right side of the heart and can be associated with low BP and symptomatic bradycardia.

After the anginal pain is controlled, longer-term education of the patient and the family can begin. Points to cover include (1) risk factor modification, (2) signs and symptoms of angina, (3) when to call the physician, (4) medications, and (5) dealing with emotions and stress. However, because the acute hospital length of stay for uncomplicated angina is usually less than 3 days, referral to a cardiac rehabilitation program for a controlled exercise program and risk factor modification after discharge may be the most helpful teaching intervention a critical care nurse can provide.

Evidence-Based Practice for CAD and Stable Angina

Evidence-based practice management for CAD and stable angina is described in Box 11.6.

◎ BOX 11.5 PRIORITY PATIENT CARE MANAGEMENT

Coronary Artery Disease and Angina
- Acute Pain due to transmission and perception of cutaneous, visceral, muscular, or ischemic impulses
- Ineffective Tissue Perfusion due to decreased myocardial blood flow
- Activity Intolerance due to cardiopulmonary dysfunction
- Powerlessness due to lack of control over current situation or disease progression
- Anxiety due to threat to biologic, psychologic, or social integrity
- Lack of Knowledge of Treatment Regime due to lack of previous exposure to information (see Box 11.6, Patient and Family Education Plan: Coronary Artery Disease and Angina)

Patient Care Management plans are located in Appendix A.

MYOCARDIAL INFARCTION

Description and Etiology

Myocardial infarction is the term used to describe irreversible myocardial necrosis (cell death) that results from an abrupt decrease

---

✳ BOX 11.6 PRIORITY PATIENT AND FAMILY EDUCATION

Coronary Artery Disease and Angina
Before discharge, the patient should be able to teach back the following topics:
- Angina: Describe signs and symptoms such as pain, pressure, and heaviness in chest, arms, or jaw.
- Preinfarction or unstable angina: Any chest pain that is not relieved by a sublingual nitroglycerin (NTG) tablet taken 5 minutes apart times three doses provides a reason to call 911 (emergency services).
- Use of the 0–10 pain scale: Notify critical care nurse or emergency personnel of any changes in pain intensity.
- Use of sublingual NTG for angina: Pain intensity should decrease on pain scale after NTG administration. At home, NTG must be kept in a dark, airtight container, or it loses its potency. To ensure potency, the NTG supply must be replaced approximately every 6 months. Active NTG has a slight burning sensation when placed under the tongue.
- Avoid Valsalva maneuver.
- Risk factor modification tailored to the patient's individual risk factor profile:
  - Decrease fat intake to 30% of total calories a day.
  - Stop smoking.
  - Reduce salt intake.
  - Control hypertension.
  - Treat diabetes and control blood glucose levels (if patient has diabetes).
  - Increase physical activity; achieve ideal body weight.
- Intention to attend a cardiac rehabilitation program
- Medication teaching about indications and side effects
- Follow-up care after discharge
- Symptoms to report to a health care professional
- Discussion of how to handle emotional stress and anger

or total cessation of coronary blood flow to a specific area of the myocardium. In the hospital, this is often referred to as an *acute MI*, indicating the sudden onset and the life-threatening nature of the event. Increasingly, an acute MI is described in relation to whether ST segment elevation is seen on a diagnostic 12-lead ECG. It may be labeled an *acute NSTEMI*[27] or an *acute STEMI* (ST segment elevation MI).[28]

Three mechanisms can block the coronary artery and are responsible for the acute reduction in oxygen delivery to the myocardium: (1) plaque rupture, (2) new coronary artery thrombosis, and (3) coronary artery spasm close to the ruptured plaque.

Myocardial tissue can best be salvaged within the first 2 hours after the onset of anginal symptoms, as illustrated in Fig. 11.3.[30] The earlier the myocardium is revascularized, the better the chances of survival. However, many people do not seek treatment until the acute phase has passed or delay seeking treatment because of denial or lack of understanding of their symptoms.

Pathophysiology

Ischemia

The outer region of the infarcted myocardial area is the *zone of ischemia*, or penumbra, as illustrated in Fig. 11.4. It is composed of viable cells. Priority interventions are targeted to save this viable muscle. Repolarization in this zone is temporarily impaired but eventually is restored to normal. Repolarization of the cells in this area manifests as T-wave inversion on the ECG (Fig. 11.5B).

Injury

The infarcted zone is surrounded by injured but still potentially viable tissue in an area known as the *zone of injury* (see Fig. 11.4). Cells in this area do not fully repolarize because of the deficient blood supply. This is recorded on the ECG as elevation of the ST segment (Fig. 11.5C).

Infarction

The area of dead muscle (necrosis) in the myocardium is known as the *zone of infarction* (see Fig. 11.4). On the ECG, evidence of this zone is seen as new pathologic Q waves, which reflect a lack of depolarization from the cardiac surface involved in the MI (Fig. 11.5D). As healing takes place, the cells in this area are replaced by scar tissue.

Q Wave Myocardial Infarction

MIs are classified according to the location on the myocardial surface and the muscle layers affected. Not all infarctions cause necrosis in all layers, as shown in Fig. 11.6. A transmural MI involves all three cardiac layers: *endocardium, myocardium,* and *epicardium*. A transmural or full wall-thickness, MI usually provokes significant ECG changes (see Fig. 11.5). This is also described as a *Q wave MI*. Not every acute MI produces a recognizable series of Q waves on the 12-lead ECG. Some patients who had a demonstrated Q wave on a 12-lead ECG as a result of an acute MI lose the Q wave months or years later. The reasons for this are unknown, but it may represent the development of collateral circulation.

Twelve-Lead Electrocardiogram Changes

The ECG changes produced by an MI demonstrate alteration in myocardial depolarization (QRS complex) and repolarization (ST segment). The changes in repolarization are seen by the presence of new Q waves. These new, pathologic Q waves are deeper and wider than the tiny Q waves found on a normal 12-lead ECG.[26,27]

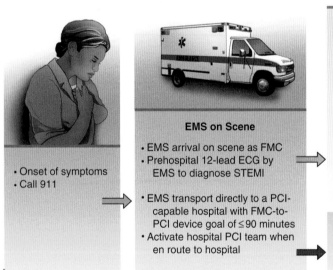
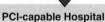
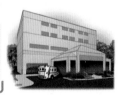
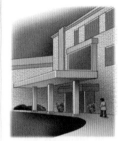

Non-PCI Capable Hospital
- Immediate interhospital transport to a PCI-capable hospital for patients with STEMI
- Goal is FMC-to-PCI device time of ≤120 minutes.
- When unavoidable time delays will make the FMC-to-PCI device time longer than 120 minutes, fibrinolysis should be selected as the method of reperfusion for patients without contraindications.
- IV fibrinolysis should start within 30 minutes of arrival.

EMS on Scene
- EMS arrival on scene as FMC
- Prehospital 12-lead ECG by EMS to diagnose STEMI

- EMS transport directly to a PCI-capable hospital with FMC-to-PCI device goal of ≤90 minutes
- Activate hospital PCI team when en route to hospital

- Onset of symptoms
- Call 911

PCI-capable Hospital
- When a patient is initially seen at a PCI-capable hospital, the goal is a door-to-PCI device time of under 90 minutes.

Goal Is Total Ischemic Time ≤ 120 Minutes

Fig. 11.3 Evaluation of Prehospital Chest Pain and Acute Coronary Syndrome and Treatment Options. The first step is to call 911 *(green arrow)*. Transport to a PCI-capable hospital is always the optimal first choice when available *(red arrows)*. Transport to a non–PCI-capable hospital is considered when other options are unavailable *(yellow arrow* and *yellow box)*. *ECG,* Electrocardiogram; *EMS,* emergency medical services; *FMC,* first medical contact; *PCI,* percutaneous coronary intervention; *STEMI,* ST segment elevation myocardial infarction.

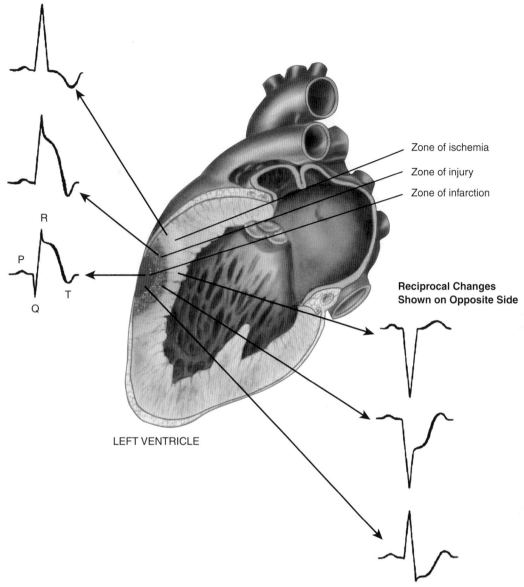

Fig. 11.4 Zone of ischemia, zone of injury, and zone of infarction are shown through electrocardiogram waveforms and reciprocal waveforms corresponding to each zone.

Myocardial Infarction Location

The location of infarction is determined by correlating the ECG leads with Q waves and the ST segment and T-wave abnormalities (Table 11.5). The ECG manifestations that are used to diagnose MI and pinpoint the area of damaged ventricle include inverted T waves, ST segment elevation, and pathologic Q waves in specific lead groupings, as described subsequently.

Anterior wall infarction. Anterior wall infarction results from occlusion of the proximal left anterior descending artery (see Table 11.5). ST segment elevation is expected in leads V_1 through V_4 on the 12-lead ECG, as shown in Fig. 11.7. If the left main coronary artery is occluded, the ECG manifestations will involve almost all precordial leads V_1 through V_6 and leads I and aVL (see Table 11.5). These specific groups of ECG changes that help locate the part of the heart that is experiencing infarction are called *indicative changes.* A large

anterior wall MI may be associated with left ventricular pump failure, cardiogenic shock, or death.

Left lateral wall infarction. Left lateral wall infarction occurs as a result of occlusion of the circumflex coronary artery. On a 12-lead ECG, new Q waves and ST segment T-wave changes are seen in leads I, aVL, V_5, and V_6 (Fig. 11.8). In reality, few patients present with only lateral wall ECG changes, and some anterior wall leads (V_3 and V_4) may show evidence of injury or infarction.

Inferior wall infarction. Inferior wall infarction occurs with occlusion of the right coronary artery. This infarction manifests by ECG changes in leads II, III, and aV_F (Fig. 11.9). Conduction disturbances are expected with an inferior wall MI and are related to the anatomy of the coronary arterial supply. Because the right coronary artery perfuses the sinoatrial node in slightly more than half of the population and supplies the proximal bundle of His and the atrioventricular (AV) node in more

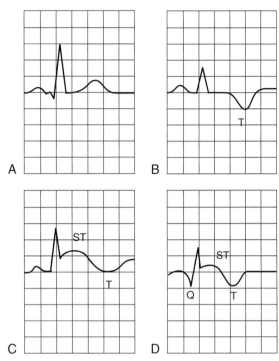

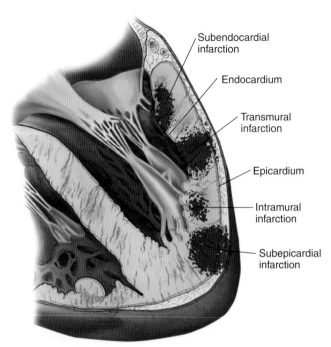

Fig. 11.6 Location of Infarctions in Myocardium.

Fig. 11.5 Electrocardiogram (ECG) Changes Indicative of Ischemia, Injury, and Infarction (Necrosis) of the Myocardium. (A) Normal ECG. (B) Ischemia indicated by inversion of the T wave. (C) Ischemia and current of injury indicated by T-wave inversion and ST segment elevation. The ST segment may be elevated above or depressed below the baseline, depending on whether the tracing is from a lead facing toward or away from the infarcted area and depending on whether epicardial or endocardial injury occurs. Epicardial injury causes ST segment elevation in leads facing the epicardium. (D) Ischemia, injury, and myocardial necrosis. The Q wave indicates necrosis of the myocardium.

than 90% of individuals, heart block and other conduction disturbances should be anticipated.

Non—ST Segment Elevation Myocardial Infarction

The 12-lead ECG is a highly useful diagnostic tool. For many years, it was considered the gold standard when diagnosing acute MI. However, the ST segment is not elevated in every acute MI. One reason for the lack of ST segment elevation may be that the infarction and subsequent necrosis are not full-thickness lesions. Because some of the muscle in the area can still be depolarized, ST segment elevation may not occur. This type of MI is also less likely to develop Q waves on a subsequent 12-lead ECG after the acute phase has passed. This situation is diagnostically known as an *NSTEMI*.[27] This condition has previously been described by several names including nontransmural MI, non—Q wave MI, and subendocardial MI. Because patients who sustain an NSTEMI do have CAD, it is important that they be treated aggressively to minimize the size of the infarcted area. Without the visual clue of ST segment elevation on the 12-lead ECG, the patients cannot receive immediate intravenous fibrinolytic agents, but they can be appropriately managed in an interventional catheterization laboratory and receive GP IIb/IIIa inhibitor therapy, as illustrated in the timeline in Fig. 11.3. The 12-lead ECG plays a vital role in identifying the treatment plan for a patient with ACS. Visualizing ST segment elevation when present is helpful. Patients without ST segment elevation may still be at risk for becoming unstable and are also

TABLE 11.5	**Correlations Among Ventricular Surfaces, Electrocardiogram Leads, and Coronary Arteries.**	
Surface of Left Ventricle	**ECG Leads**	**Usually Involved**
Inferior	II, III, aVF	Right coronary artery
Lateral	V$_5$ and V$_6$, I, aVL	Left circumflex artery
Anterior	V$_2$, V$_3$, V$_4$	Left anterior descending artery
Anterior lateral	V$_1$ through V$_6$, I, aVL	Left main coronary artery
Septal	V$_1$ and V$_2$	Left anterior descending artery
Posterior	V$_1$ and V$_2$	Left circumflex or right coronary artery (reciprocal changes)
	V$_7$, V$_8$, V$_9$ (direct)	

I lateral	aVR	V$_1$ septal	V$_4$ anterior
II inferior	aVL lateral	V$_2$ septal	V$_5$ lateral
III inferior	aVF inferior	V$_3$ anterior	V$_6$ lateral

ECG, Electrocardiogram.

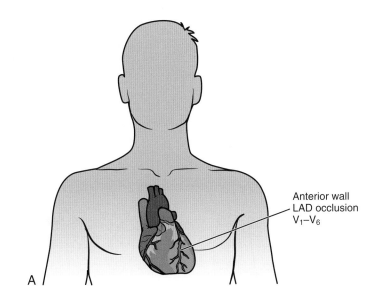

A

LIMB LEADS		PRECORDIAL LEADS	
Lead I	AV_R	V_1	V_4
Lead II	AV_L	V_2	V_5
Lead III	AV_F	V_3	V_6

B

Example of an Acute Anterior Wall MI

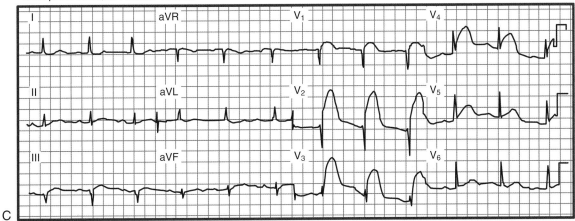

C

Fig. 11.7   Changes Seen on 12-Lead Electrocardiogram (ECG) With Anterior Wall Myocardial Infarction (MI).
(A) Infarction location on the cardiac wall. (B) ECG leads with expected ST segment elevation. (C) A 12-lead
ECG from a patient experiencing left anterior wall MI. *LAD,* Left anterior descending artery.

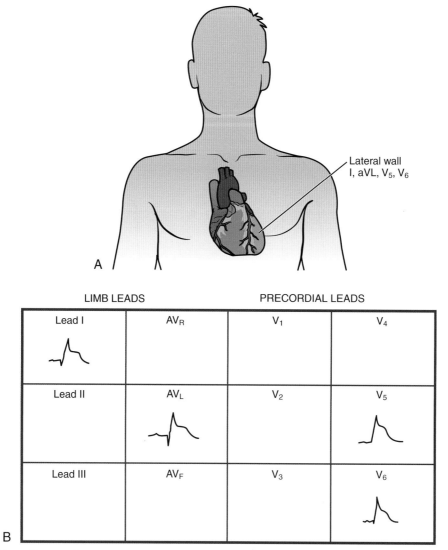

Fig. 11.8 Changes Seen on 12-Lead Electrocardiogram (ECG) With Lateral Wall ST Segment Elevation Myocardial Infarction. (A) Infarction location on the cardiac wall. (B) ECG leads with expected ST segment elevation.

monitored (Fig. 11.10). In this case, the definitive diagnosis may be made in the cardiac catheterization laboratory or by elevation of specific cardiac biomarkers.

Cardiac Biomarkers During Myocardial Infarction

Cardiac biomarkers are released in the presence of damage and necrosis of the myocardium. These biomarkers are also called *cardiac enzymes*. To confirm the diagnosis of acute MI, the serum biomarkers troponin I or troponin T are measured by a blood test. Troponins begin to rise within 3 to 4 hours of STEMI. Elevated troponins are detectable for 7 to 10 days. Creatine kinase—muscle/brain (CK-MB) is an older cardiac biomarker that is less frequently measured.

If the coronary artery is opened by fibrinolytic therapy or a percutaneous catheter intervention (PCI), the biomarkers exhibit a more rapid increase and dramatic decrease (Fig. 11.11).

Complications of Acute Myocardial Infarction

Many patients experience complications occurring early or late in the post-MI course. These complications may result from electrical dysfunction or from a cardiac contractility problem. Electrical dysfunctions include bradycardia, bundle branch blocks, and various degrees of heart block. Pumping complications can cause heart failure, pulmonary edema, and cardiogenic shock. The presence of a new murmur in a patient with an acute MI warrants special attention, as it may indicate rupture of the papillary muscle. The murmur can be indicative of severe damage and impending complications such as heart failure and pulmonary edema.

Sinus bradycardia. Sinus bradycardia (heart rate less than 60 beats/min) occurs frequently in patients who sustain an acute MI. It is more prevalent with an inferior wall infarction in the first hour after STEMI. Symptomatic bradycardia with hypotension and low cardiac output is treated with atropine (0.5—1.0 mg by intravenous push), repeated every 3 to 5 minutes to a maximum dose of 0.03 mg/kg (e.g., 2 mg for a person who weighs 70 kg) per advanced cardiac life support guidelines.

Sinus tachycardia. Sinus tachycardia (heart rate greater than 100 beats/min) most often occurs with an anterior wall MI. Anterior infarction impairs left ventricular pumping ability, reducing the

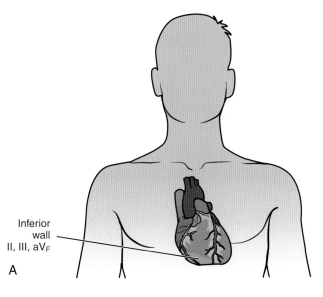

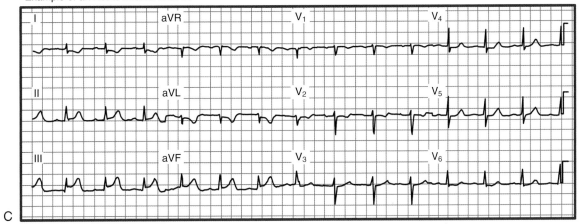

Fig. 11.9 Changes Seen on 12-Lead Electrocardiogram (ECG) With Inferior Wall Myocardial Infarction (MI). (A) Infarction location on the cardiac wall. (B) ECG leads with expected ST segment elevation. (C) A 12-lead ECG from a patient experiencing inferior wall MI.

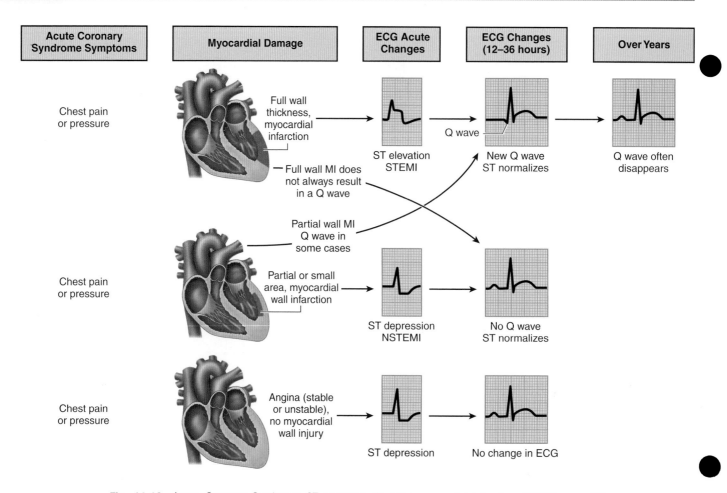

Acute Coronary Syndrome Symptoms	Myocardial Damage	ECG Acute Changes	ECG Changes (12–36 hours)	Over Years

Chest pain or pressure — Full wall thickness, myocardial infarction — Full wall MI does not always result in a Q wave — ST elevation STEMI — New Q wave ST normalizes — Q wave often disappears

Q wave

Partial wall MI Q wave in some cases

Chest pain or pressure — Partial or small area, myocardial wall infarction — ST depression NSTEMI — No Q wave ST normalizes

Chest pain or pressure — Angina (stable or unstable), no myocardial wall injury — ST depression — No change in ECG

Fig. 11.10 Acute Coronary Syndrome: ST segment elevation myocardial infarction (STEMI), non–ST segment elevation myocardial infarction (NSTEMI), Unstable Angina, Electrocardiography Changes Over Time. *ECG,* Electrocardiogram.

ejection fraction and the stroke volume. In an attempt to maintain cardiac output, the heart rate increases. Sinus tachycardia is corrected by treating the underlying cause, as it greatly increases myocardial oxygen consumption, leading to further ischemia.

Atrial dysrhythmias. Premature atrial contractions occur frequently in patients who sustain an acute MI. Atrial fibrillation is also common and may occur spontaneously or may be preceded by premature atrial contractions. With the onset of atrial fibrillation, the loss of organized atrial contraction decreases cardiac output by up to 20%. Patients with new-onset or preexisting atrial fibrillation have higher morbidity rates than patients in sinus rhythm during an ACS event. Patients with ACS and new-onset atrial fibrillation experience a greater number of in-hospital adverse events, such as reinfarction, shock, pulmonary edema, bleeding, and stroke. Management of atrial fibrillation includes rate control and rhythm control.[31]

Ventricular dysrhythmias. Premature ventricular contractions are seen in almost all patients within the first few hours after MI. They are initially controlled through administration of oxygen to reduce myocardial hypoxia and by correcting acid–base or electrolyte imbalances. In the setting of an acute MI, premature ventricular contractions are pharmacologically treated if they have the following characteristics: frequent (more than 6 per minute), closely coupled (R-on-T phenomenon), multiform shapes, and occurrence in bursts of three or more, increasing the risk of sustained ventricular tachycardia (VT). Ventricular fibrillation (VF) is a life-threatening dysrhythmia associated with high mortality in acute MI. Beta-blockers are prescribed after acute MI to decrease mortality from ventricular dysrhythmias.

Atrioventricular heart block during myocardial infarction. Heart block can occur in 6% to 14% of patients with STEMI, and these patients have increased mortality rates. In STEMI, AV block most often occurs after an inferior wall MI. Because the right coronary artery supplies the AV node in 90% of the population, right coronary artery occlusion leads to ischemia and infarction of the AV node cells. The development of sudden heart block has become much less common, because most patients receive fibrinolysis or undergo PCI to open the occluded vessel. In most cases, transcutaneous pacing is the primary intervention; transvenous pacemakers are used less frequently.

Ventricular aneurysm after myocardial infarction. A ventricular aneurysm (Fig. 11.12) is a noncontractile, thinned left ventricular wall that results from an acute transmural infarction. It is a rare event that occurs in the setting of an acute left anterior descending artery occlusion with a wide area of infarcted myocardium. The most effective prevention is early reperfusion of the myocardium, accomplished by opening the thrombosed coronary artery. The most common complications of a ventricular aneurysm are acute heart failure, systemic emboli, angina, and VT. Treatment is directed toward management of these complications and surgical repair by left ventricular aneurysmectomy. The affected area may be described as *hypokinetic* (contracts poorly), *akinetic* (noncontractile scar tissue), or *dyskinetic* (scar tissue that moves in

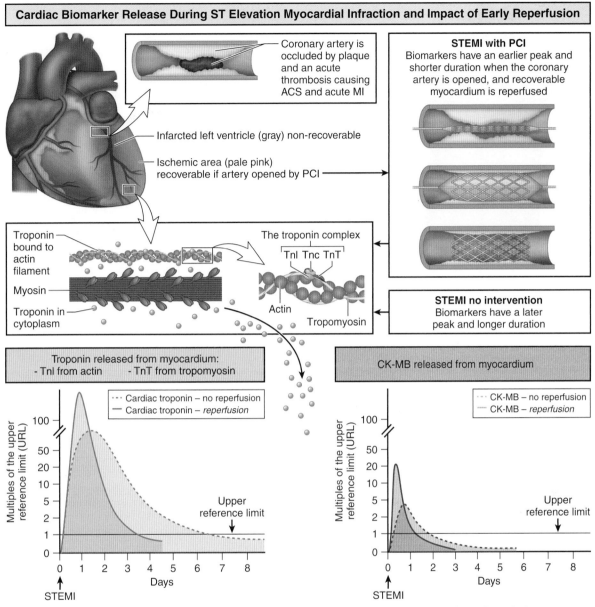

Cardiac Biomarker Release During ST Elevation Myocardial Infraction and Impact of Early Reperfusion

- Coronary artery is occluded by plaque and an acute thrombosis causing ACS and acute MI

- Infarcted left ventricle (gray) non-recoverable

- Ischemic area (pale pink) recoverable if artery opened by PCI

STEMI with PCI
Biomarkers have an earlier peak and shorter duration when the coronary artery is opened, and recoverable myocardium is reperfused

Troponin bound to actin filament

Myosin

Troponin in cytoplasm

The troponin complex

TnI Tnc TnT

Actin

Tropomyosin

STEMI no intervention
Biomarkers have a later peak and longer duration

Troponin released from myocardium:
- TnI from actin   - TnT from tropomyosin

CK-MB released from myocardium

··· Cardiac troponin – no reperfusion
— Cardiac troponin – *reperfusion*

··· CK-MB – no reperfusion
— CK-MB – *reperfusion*

Fig. 11.11 Cardiac Biomarkers During ST Elevation Myocardial Infarction and the Effect of Early Reperfusion. *ACS*, Acute coronary syndrome; *CK-MB*, creatinine–kinase: muscle/brain; *MI*, myocardial infarction; *PCI*, percutaneous coronary intervention; *STEMI*, ST segment elevation myocardial infarction; *TnC*, troponin C; *TnI*, troponin I; *TnT*, troponin T.

the opposite direction to the normal contractile myocardium). The prognosis depends on the size of the aneurysm, the level of overall left ventricular dysfunction, and the severity of coexisting CAD.

Ventricular septal rupture after myocardial infarction. Rupture of the ventricular septal wall after MI is a rare but potentially lethal complication of an acute anterior wall MI (Fig. 11.13). *Ventricular septal rupture*, also known as *acquired ventricular septal defect*, is an abnormal communication between the right and left ventricle. Studies report this complication occurs in less than 0.2% to 3.9% of all MIs, and the incidence has declined because most patients with STEMI have the blocked coronary artery opened through PCI or fibrinolysis within a short timeframe after diagnosis.[32] Nevertheless, rupture of the ventricular septum carries an extremely high mortality rate.

Mortality rates between 35% and 73% are typical.[32] Most patients with septal rupture also have signs and symptoms of cardiogenic shock. Ventricular septal rupture manifests as severe chest pain, syncope, hypotension, and sudden hemodynamic deterioration caused by shunting of blood from the high-pressure left ventricle into the low-pressure right ventricle through the new septal opening. A holosystolic murmur (often accompanied by a thrill) can be auscultated and is best heard along the left sternal border. Rupture of the septum is a medical and surgical emergency. The patient's condition is stabilized with vasodilators and an intra-aortic balloon pump (IABP) to decrease afterload. The goal of afterload reduction in this patient population is to decrease the amount of blood being shunted to the right side of the heart and consequently to increase

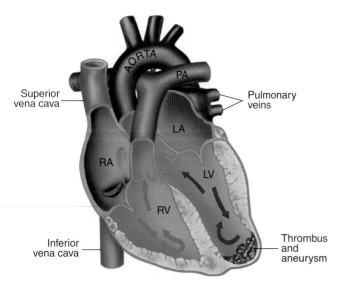

Fig. 11.12 Ventricular Aneurysm After Acute Myocardial Infarction. *LA*, Left atrium; *LV*, left ventricle; *PA*, pulmonary artery; *RA*, right atrium; *RV*, right ventricle.

the flow of blood to the systemic circulation. Survival improves if the septal rupture is very small, and the patient's condition is sufficiently stable to wait for scar tissue to form before surgical repair. When the septal opening is large, the massive left-to-right shunt across the septum makes the chances of survival dismal with or without surgery.[32]

Papillary muscle rupture after myocardial infarction. Papillary muscle rupture can occur when the infarct involves the area around one of the papillary muscles that support the mitral valve. Infarction of the papillary muscles results in ineffective mitral valve closure, and blood is forced back into the low-pressure left atrium during ventricular systole. The rupture may be partial or complete. Complete rupture

is catastrophic and precipitates severe acute mitral regurgitation, cardiogenic shock, and high risk of death.

Partial rupture (Fig. 11.14) also results in mitral regurgitation, but the condition can be stabilized with aggressive medical management using an IABP and vasodilators. Urgent surgical intervention is required to replace the mitral valve.[33]

Cardiac wall rupture after myocardial infarction. The incidence of cardiac wall rupture has two peak times. The first occurs within the first 24 hours, and the second occurs between 3 and 5 days after infarction, when leukocyte scavenger cells are removing necrotic debris, thinning the myocardial wall. The onset is sudden and usually catastrophic. Bleeding into the pericardial sac results in cardiac tamponade, cardiogenic shock, pulseless electrical activity, and death. Survival is rare. If rupture occurs in the hospital, emergency pericardiocentesis is required to relieve the tamponade until a surgical repair can be attempted. The best prevention is early reperfusion of the myocardium.

Pericarditis after myocardial infarction. Pericarditis is inflammation of the pericardial sac. It can occur during or after acute MI. The damaged epicardium becomes rough and inflamed and irritates the pericardium lying adjacent to it, precipitating pericarditis. Pain is the most common symptom of pericarditis, and a pericardial friction rub is the most common initial sign. The friction rub is best auscultated with a stethoscope at the sternal border and is described as a grating, scraping, or leathery scratching. Pericarditis frequently produces a pericardial effusion.[34] After the effusion occurs, the friction rub may disappear. On a 12-lead ECG, pericarditis may manifest as elevation of the ST segment in all the typically upright leads.[35] Pericarditis is treated with nonsteroidal anti-inflammatory drugs, aspirin, and rest. Pericarditis that occurs as a late complication of acute MI is known as *Dressler syndrome*.

Heart failure and acute myocardial infarction. Many patients with acute STEMI also have acute heart failure on admission to the hospital. These patients have often waited longer to come to the hospital and are older and more likely to be female. Compared with patients with acute MI but not heart failure, these patients have a higher risk of adverse in-hospital events and have longer lengths of stay and higher in-hospital mortality rates. More detailed information about heart failure is presented later in this chapter.

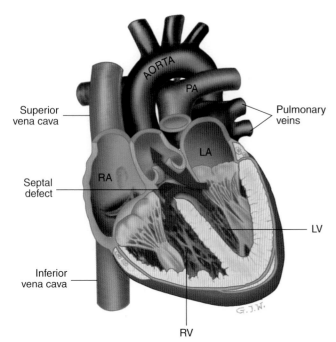

Fig. 11.13 Ventricular Septal Rupture After Acute Myocardial Infarction. *LA*, Left atrium; *LV*, left ventricle; *PA*, pulmonary artery; *RA*, right atrium; *RV*, right ventricle.

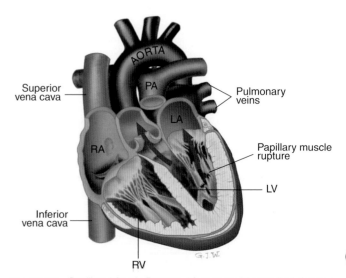

Fig. 11.14 Papillary Muscle Rupture After Acute Myocardial Infarction. *LA*, Left atrium; *LV*, left ventricle; *PA*, pulmonary artery; *RA*, right atrium; *RV*, right ventricle.

Medical Management

Quality outcomes research shows that compliance with the guidelines developed by the American College of Cardiology (ACC) and the AHA decreases in-hospital mortality after acute MI.[36] When the AHA/ACC guidelines for treatment of STEMI or NSTEMI are followed, patients admitted to hospitals have an 8.3% in-hospital mortality rate compared with a 15.3% mortality rate in patients treated at hospitals where the most recent guidelines are not fully used.[36] The guidelines are research based and are designed to improve the outcome of patients admitted to the hospital with acute MI. Clinical guidelines address the issues of interventions to open the coronary artery, anticoagulation, prevention of dysrhythmias, intensive glucose control, and prevention of ventricular remodeling after STEMI. To facilitate rapid coronary artery revascularization in STEMI, local hospitals are encouraged to develop a coordinated patient transfer strategy between PCI-capable and non–PCI-capable hospitals, as illustrated in Fig. 11.3.[28]

Recanalization of Coronary Artery

The essential immediate interventions for a patient with an acute STEMI are fibrinolytic therapy or PCI to open the occluded artery.[28] All clinical guidelines emphasize the need for patients with symptoms of ACS to be rapidly triaged and treated.[28]

Anticoagulation

In the acute phase after STEMI, heparin is administered in combination with fibrinolytic therapy to recanalize (open) the coronary artery.[28] For patients who will receive fibrinolytic therapy, an initial heparin bolus of 60 units/kg (maximum 4000 units) is given intravenously, followed by a continuous heparin drip at 12 units/kg per hour (maximum 1000 units/hour) to maintain an activated partial thromboplastin time (aPTT) between 50 and 70 seconds (1.5–2.0 times control) for 48 hours or until revascularization.[28]

It is also prudent to administer intravenous UFH or subcutaneous low–molecular-weight heparin (LMWH) if the patient is at risk for thrombus development. For patients with known heparin-induced thrombocytopenia, as an alternative to LMWH or UFH, a third class of antithrombotic medications is available: direct antithrombotic agents (e.g., bivalirudin, argatroban). Patients at risk for thrombotic emboli include patients with an anterior wall infarction, atrial fibrillation, previous embolus, cardiomyopathy, or cardiogenic shock.

Dysrhythmia Prevention

The antidysrhythmic with the best safety record after STEMI is amiodarone. Beta-blockers are another class of antidysrhythmics that are recommended for all patients after STEMI. Beta-blockers prevent ventricular dysrhythmias, lower BP, and prevent reinfarction, especially in patients with left ventricular dysfunction.[28]

Prevention of Ventricular Remodeling

Many patients are at risk for development of ventricular remodeling after STEMI. Vasodilating medications (angiotensin-converting enzyme inhibitors [ACEIs] or angiotensin II receptor blockers [ARBs]) can stop or limit the ventricular remodeling that leads to heart failure. *Ventricular remodeling* refers to progressive changes in the size, architecture, and shape of the myocardium and occurs because of an injury such as MI. Ventricular remodeling is modulated by catecholamines and activation of neurohormonal compensatory mechanisms. The heart chamber walls ultimately become dilated, thinned, and poorly contractile. An ACEI or, if it is not tolerated, an ARB is indicated for all patients after STEMI.[28]

◎ BOX 11.7   PRIORITY PATIENT CARE MANAGEMENT

Myocardial Infarction

- Acute Pain due to transmission and perception of cutaneous, visceral, muscular, or ischemic impulses
- Impaired Cardiac Output due to alterations in preload
- Impaired Cardiac Output due to alterations in afterload
- Impaired Cardiac Output due to alterations in contractility
- Impaired Cardiac Output due to alterations in heart rate or rhythm
- Impaired Cardiac Output due to sympathetic blockade
- Ineffective Tissue Perfusion due to decreased myocardial blood flow
- Activity Intolerance due to cardiopulmonary dysfunction
- Impaired Sleep due to fragmented sleep
- Anxiety due to threat to biologic, psychologic, or social integrity
- Lack of Knowledge of Treatment Regime due to lack of previous exposure to information (see Box 11.8, Patient and Family Education Plan: Myocardial Infarction)

Patient Care Management plans are located in Appendix A.

Information about the clinical effects of heart failure is provided later in this chapter.

Evidence-Based Practice for Myocardial Infarction

A summary of evidence-based practice for management of MI is in Box 11.7.

Nursing Management

Care management for a patient with an acute MI incorporates a variety of patient diagnoses (Box 11.8). Nursing priorities focus on achieving a balance between myocardial oxygen supply and demand, preventing complications, and providing patient and family education. See Appendix A for patient care management plans specific to patients with acute MI.

Balancing Myocardial Oxygen Supply and Demand

In the acute period, if severe heart muscle damage has occurred, myocardial oxygen supply is increased by the administration of supplemental oxygen to prevent tissue hypoxia. Cardiac medications play an increasingly important role in balancing supply and demand, and the critical care nurse administers and monitors the effectiveness of these agents. For a patient with a low cardiac output, positive inotropic medications such as dobutamine, dopamine, or both may be administered. Milrinone, a phosphodiesterase inhibitor that increases contractility by improving sarcolemma calcium uptake and causes positive inotropic effects in the myocardium, may be prescribed.

In contrast to dobutamine and dopamine, milrinone does not compete for receptor sites in patients taking beta-blockers. These inotropic agents are used to increase cardiac contractility in the healthy areas of the heart (increasing oxygen supply) while avoiding damage to the recently infarcted areas. Myocardial oxygen supply can be further enhanced with coronary artery vasodilators. Nitroglycerin is often administered for the first 48 hours to increase vasodilation and prevent myocardial ischemia. Research evidence supports the administration of early beta-blockade therapy to decrease myocardial workload and to prevent dysrhythmias. However, if the patient is in cardiogenic shock, beta-blockers are withheld until the cardiac output has improved.[28] Other interventions to decrease cardiac work and

---

✳ **BOX 11.8   PRIORITY PATIENT AND FAMILY EDUCATION**

Myocardial Infarction

Before discharge, the patient should be able to teach back the following topics:

- Pathophysiology of coronary artery disease, angina, and acute myocardial infarction
- Angina: Describe signs and symptoms such as pain, pressure, or heaviness in chest, arms, or jaw.
- Use of 0–10 pain scale: Notify critical care nurse or emergency personnel of any changes in chest pain intensity.
- Avoid Valsalva maneuver.
- Risk factor modification tailored to the patient's individual risk factor profile:
  - Decrease daily fat intake to less than 30% of total calories.
  - Reduce total serum cholesterol to less than 200 mg/dL.

- Reduce low-density lipoprotein cholesterol to less than 70 mg/dL.
- Stop smoking.
- Reduce salt intake.
- Control hypertension.
- Control diabetes (if patient has diabetes).
- Increase physical activity.
- Achieve ideal body weight, if overweight.
- Referral to cardiac rehabilitation program
- Medication teaching about indications and side effects
- Follow-up care after discharge
- Symptoms to report to a health care professional
- Discussion of how to handle emotional stress and anger

---

myocardial oxygen consumption include bed rest with bedside commode privileges when the patient is clinically stable.

Preventing Complications

A thorough grasp of the range of potential complications that can occur after STEMI is essential. Cardiac monitoring for early detection of ventricular dysrhythmias is ongoing. Assessment for signs of continued ischemic pain is important, because angina is a warning sign of myocardium being at risk. In response to angina, a 12-lead ECG is obtained to determine whether an extension of the infarct exists, nitroglycerin is administered, and the physician is notified immediately so that interventions may be initiated to limit the size of the MI. Heart failure is a serious complication after STEMI. When the patient's BP is stable, treatment with ACEIs is initiated. These vasodilators are used to prevent left ventricular remodeling and dilation that occurs in many patients after acute MI. Hypotension is a potential complication of ACEIs, especially with the first dose. It is an important nursing responsibility to monitor BP and patient symptoms after taking an ACEI. Surveillance to detect obvious and subtle signs of bleeding is also a priority, because so many patients with acute MI receive antiplatelet, anticoagulant, and fibrinolytic medications.[26,28]

In the first 24 hours after an MI, diet is progressed as tolerated. Preventing hospital-acquired pneumonia and deep vein thrombosis (DVT) is facilitated by early mobilization and raising the head of the bed 30 degrees or more. An upright position facilitates decrease in venous return, lowering of preload, and decrease in the workload of the myocardium. The patient is taught to avoid increasing intra-abdominal pressure (Valsalva maneuver). Stool softeners may be given to the patient to lessen the risk of constipation from analgesics and bed rest and to decrease the risk of straining. Providing a calming and quiet environment that focuses on the well-being of the patient assists in the recovery phase.

Depression After Myocardial Infarction

Depression is a condition that occurs across a wide spectrum of human experiences. Depression is a risk factor for development of CAD and impedes recovery after acute MI.[37] Key symptoms that are mentioned frequently include fatigue, change in appetite, and sleep disturbance.

Educate the Patient and Family

After the acute phase of an MI, patient and family education becomes a priority. Education focuses on the following key elements: (1) risk factor reduction, (2) manifestations of angina, (3) when to call a physician or emergency services, (4) medications, and (5) resumption of physical and sexual activities (Box 11.9). It is recommended that a referral be made to a cardiac rehabilitation program to reinforce education that was initiated during hospitalization.[38]

CARDIAC ARREST AND SUDDEN CARDIAC DEATH

Description

Of the patients who die suddenly each year of CHD, 50% of men and 64% of women have no previous symptoms of the disease. Of sudden cardiac deaths (SCDs), 70% to 89% occur in men, and the annual incidence is 3 to 4 times higher in men than in women; however, this disparity decreases with advancing age. People who have had an MI with symptoms that last less than 1 hour or occur in a hospital emergency department have an SCD rate 4 to 6 times higher than that of the general population. SCD represents approximately 50% of all cardiovascular deaths each year, and 25% of these are first symptomatic cardiac event.[39]

When the onset of symptoms is rapid, the most likely mechanism of SCD is VT, which degenerates into VF. Despite aggressive cardiopulmonary resuscitation (CPR) initiated outside the hospital, few individuals who sustain an out-of-hospital cardiac arrest survive to hospital discharge. Strategies that have been shown to improve resuscitation survival involve huge community-wide programs to teach laypersons CPR and how to use an automated external defibrillator. These programs assist with survival to hospital discharge.[40]

Etiology

Most SCD incidents occur in patients with preexisting ventricular dysfunction resulting from heart disease. Specific SCD risk factors include extensive coronary atherosclerosis with or without a history of acute MI; dilated or hypertrophic cardiomyopathy (HCM); valvular heart disease; autonomic nervous system abnormalities; electrical system abnormalities such as AV block, Wolff-Parkinson-White syndrome, long QT syndrome, or Brugada syndrome; and taking medications that prolong the QT interval.[40–42] An ejection fraction less than 30% and a history of ventricular dysrhythmias are powerful predictors of SCD. Other risk factors are listed in Box 11.10. Many individuals are unaware of their risk for SCD.

QSEN **BOX 11.9** **Evidence-Based Practice**

Acute Coronary Syndrome and Acute Myocardial Infarction (Non-STEMI and STEMI)

Prevention of Acute Coronary Syndrome

The term *acute coronary syndrome* (ACS) is used to define the life-threatening consequences of coronary artery disease (CAD), notably unstable angina, non—ST segment elevation myocardial infarction (non-STEMI), and ST segment elevation myocardial infarction (STEMI):

- *Unstable angina* is a term that denotes chest pain that is not relieved by sublingual nitroglycerin or rest within 5 minutes.
- Non-STEMI is an acute myocardial infarction (MI) *without* ST segment elevation on the 12-lead electrocardiogram (ECG).
- STEMI is an acute MI *with* ST segment elevation on the 12-lead ECG.

All recommendations are class I, meaning that there is strong research evidence to support these recommendations.

Recommendations That Decrease Risk of Developing Non-STEMI and STEMI

- Primary care providers should evaluate CAD risk factors for all patients every 3—5 years using a validated risk assessment scoring tool.
- The 10-year risk of ACS and acute MI should be assessed for all patients who have more than two major risk factors through the use of evidence-based risk assessment tools.
- An intensive risk factor modification program is recommended for patients with established CAD or high-risk equivalents such as diabetes or chronic kidney disease.

Recommendations About Emergency ACS Symptoms

- A patient who has previously diagnosed CAD should take one sublingual nitroglycerin dose, and the patient (if alone) or a friend or relative should call 911 if chest pain or discomfort is unrelieved or worsening in 5 minutes.
- The same recommendation applies to a patient without known CAD. If pain is unrelieved with rest or worsening at 5 minutes, the patient (if alone) or a friend or relative should call 911.
- Patients with chest discomfort should be transported to the hospital by ambulance rather than be driven by a friend or relative.
- Family members should be advised to take a cardiopulmonary resuscitation (CPR) course before an ACS emergency occurs. This course teaches CPR skills, demonstrates use of an automated external defibrillator (AED), and educates participants about the "chain of survival" concept.

Recommendations for Prehospital EMS Paramedic First Responders

- First responders such as emergency medical services (EMS) paramedics can provide early defibrillation and advanced cardiac life support (ACLS) for patients in cardiac arrest.
- EMS personnel should administer 162—325 mg of nonenteric aspirin (chewed, not swallowed) to patients with chest pain and suspected STEMI.
- A prehospital fibrinolysis protocol is reasonable for patients with STEMI if there are physicians in the ambulance or if there is a well-organized EMS service with full-time paramedics plus 12-lead ECG transmission capability and online medical direction.
- Patients older than 75 years and patients with cardiogenic shock should be transported to a hospital with the capability to provide fibrinolytics, emergency percutaneous coronary intervention (PCI), or emergency coronary artery bypass graft (CABG) surgery.
- Patients with STEMI who have a contraindication to fibrinolytic therapy should be brought to a hospital with the capability to provide emergency PCI or CABG surgery. At the scene, the door-to-departure time should be *less than 30 minutes*. PCI should be initiated *within 90 minutes* after initial medical contact.

Recommendations for Initial Emergency Clinical Management

- Hospitals should establish multidisciplinary teams to facilitate rapid triage of patients who present to the emergency department (ED) with chest pain.
- Use of written protocols is recommended to standardize care. An immediate cardiology consultation is advised if the patient's symptoms fall outside the written protocol.

STEMI

- *Fibrinolytics for STEMI:* Time from coming into contact with the health care system (paramedics or ED) to receiving fibrinolytics should be *less than 30 minutes*. A brief, focused neurologic examination to determine prior stroke or presence of cognitive defects is necessary before administration of fibrinolytics.
- *PCI for STEMI:* Time from coming into contact with the health care system (paramedics or ED) to balloon inflation PCI should be *less than 90 minutes*.

Non-STEMI

- If the level of risk for a patient with non-STEMI is not immediately apparent, a "chest pain unit" within the ED permits close surveillance by competent clinicians without immediate hospital admission.
- Glycoprotein IIb/IIIa inhibitors for non-STEMI, in addition to aspirin and heparin, are indicated if cardiac catheterization or PCI is planned.
- PCI may be indicated for non-STEMI.

Recommendations for Initial Emergency Physical Assessment
Vital Signs

- Heart rate, blood pressure, respiratory rate, temperature, oxygen saturation with pulse oximetry (SpO_2), and ECG monitoring to detect presence of dysrhythmias are obtained.

Physical Assessment

- Assess for warm or cool skin, color, capillary refill, and peripheral pulses.
- Auscultate heart for cardiac murmur or new S_3 or S_4.
- Auscultate lungs for air entry plus crackles and wheezes.
- Observe for breathlessness and frothy pink sputum (pulmonary edema).
- Ask patient, family, or significant others for relevant history.

Recommendations for Emergency Diagnostics
12-Lead ECG

- For all patients with chest discomfort or angina-equivalent symptoms, a 12-lead ECG should be obtained and shown to the ED physician within 10 minutes after the patient's arrival in the ED.
- If the first ECG is normal, but the patient continues to have symptoms of chest pain or discomfort, the 12-lead ECG should be repeated at 5—10-minute intervals, *or* continuous 12-lead ECG monitoring can be used.
- In patients with inferior wall infarction, right ventricular infarction must be suspected and right-sided ECG leads recorded. V_4R is the diagnostic lead of choice to diagnose ST segment elevation in the right ventricle.

Laboratory Studies

- Laboratory tests should be performed as part of the general management of STEMI but should not delay the administration of reperfusion therapy.

Cardiac Biomarkers

- Measurement of cardiac-specific troponins is recommended for patients with coexistent skeletal muscle injury. Clinicians are advised not to wait for results of the biomarker assay before initiating reperfusion therapy. Point-of-care (handheld) biomarker assay results can be used for rapid determination

Continued

QSEN | BOX 11.9 Evidence-Based Practice—cont'd

of treatment, but subsequent biomarker assays should be done by quantitative laboratory analysis.

Imaging Studies

- *Portable chest radiograph:* Obtaining a chest radiograph must not delay reperfusion therapy unless a major complication such as aortic dissection is suspected.
- *Portable echocardiography (transthoracic echocardiogram or transesophageal echocardiogram) or magnetic resonance imaging:* A scan should be obtained to distinguish aortic dissection from STEMI for patients in whom the symptoms are unclear.

Recommendations for Care
Prevent Hypoxia

- Supplemental oxygen is administered to maintain oxygen saturation greater than 90%.

Coronary Vasodilation

- Sublingual nitroglycerin (0.04 mg every 5 minutes × 3 doses) is administered. If chest pain or discomfort is ongoing, start a peripheral intravenous (IV) line. Administer IV nitroglycerin for relief of chest pain, control of hypertension, or relief of pulmonary congestion.

Pain Control

- Intravenous morphine sulfate (2–4 mg) is administered; dosage can be increased by 2–8-mg IV increments at 5–15-minute intervals for STEMI pain control.

NSAIDs

- Discontinue nonsteroidal antiinflammatory drugs (NSAIDs; except for aspirin), both nonselective and cyclooxygenase 2 selective agents, at time of presentation with STEMI because of increased risk of mortality, reinfarction, hypertension, heart failure, and myocardial rupture associated with NSAID use.

Aspirin

- Aspirin 162 mg is chewed by patient for rapid buccal absorption.

Beta-Blockers

- Oral beta-blocker therapy is administered to patients with STEMI who do not have contraindications to beta blockade, regardless of fibrinolytic or primary PCI reperfusion.
- Contraindications for beta blockade with STEMI include signs of heart failure, low cardiac output, cardiogenic shock risk, heart block or prolonged P-R interval (>0.24 seconds), and active asthma or reactive airways disease.
- While considering the options for reperfusion, beta-blockers are given if the patient has tachycardia or hypertension; otherwise, they are started as soon as possible after STEMI.

Angiotensin-Converting Enzyme Inhibitors

- Oral angiotensin-converting enzyme inhibitors (ACEIs) are indicated within the first 24 hours after STEMI unless contraindicated.

Recommendations for Emergency Interventions for STEMI
Fibrinolytic Medications

- Fibrinolytic medications are administered to patients with STEMI (if PCI is unavailable) with ST segment elevation greater than 0.1 mV (1 mm or one small box) in two contiguous precordial (chest) leads *or* two adjacent limb leads, new left bundle branch block (LBBB) or presumed new LBBB, and onset of symptoms less than 12 hours earlier.
- Before administration of fibrinolytic therapy, rule out neurologic contraindications.

- Rule out facial trauma, uncontrolled hypertension, or ischemic stroke within the past 3 months.
- If contraindications to fibrinolysis are present, PCI is the preferred method of reperfusion.

PCI

- Emergency diagnostic coronary angiography should be performed to identify blocked coronary artery before PCI.
- Emergency PCI is recommended over fibrinolytic therapy if symptom onset was longer than 3 hours ago.
- Emergency PCI can be performed within 12 hours after symptom onset for patients with new LBBB or presumed new LBBB.
- Emergency PCI balloon inflation should be done within 90 minutes after arrival at the hospital.

Cardiac Surgery

Emergency CABG surgery is undertaken for specific indications in STEMI:
- Failed PCI with persistent pain or hemodynamic instability
- Recurrent ischemia refractory to medical therapy in patients with suitable anatomy who are not candidates for PCI
- Post-MI ventricular septal rupture or papillary muscle rupture, both of which frequently lead to cardiogenic shock
- Cardiogenic shock less than 36 hours after MI, in patients younger than 75 years with ST segment elevation, or in patients with new LBBB who have multivessel or left main disease
- Recurrent ventricular dysrhythmias in patients with 50% or greater left main coronary artery lesion or triple-vessel disease or both

Recommendations for Secondary Prevention of Complications
Medications

- ACEIs to prevent ventricular remodeling
- Beta-blockers to prevent ventricular dysrhythmias
- Diuretics if heart failure has developed
- Antihyperlipidemics if total cholesterol, low-density lipoprotein cholesterol, or triglycerides are elevated

Recommendations for Management of Complications After STEMI
Cardiogenic Shock

- Intra-aortic balloon pump for patients with hypotension (blood pressure of 90 mm Hg or systolic blood pressure of 30 mm Hg below baseline).

Ventricular Arrhythmias

- Ventricular fibrillation (VF) or pulseless ventricular tachycardia (VT) is managed by standard ACLS criteria.
- Patients with hemodynamically significant VT more than 2 days after STEMI who have ongoing ventricular dysrhythmias are considered for implantation of an implantable cardioverter defibrillator (ICD).
- Patients with an ejection fraction (EF) between 30% and 40% at 1 month after STEMI should undergo an electrophysiology study; if they are inducible to VT/VF, an ICD is recommended to reduce risk of sudden cardiac death (SCD).
- Patients with an EF of less than 30% at 1 month after STEMI are at high risk for SCD.

AV Block

- Transvenous pacemaker (emergency) or permanent pacemaker (later elective) is inserted for symptomatic second-degree or third-degree atrioventricular block.
- All patients who require permanent pacing after STEMI should also be evaluated for ICD indications.

BOX 11.9 Evidence-Based Practice—cont'd

Provide Relevant Education
Medications
- Provide written and verbal instructions about medication dosages, administration, and side effects.

Emergency Information
- Give the patient and family information about calling 911 if pain/angina-equivalent symptoms persist or worsen after 5 minutes.
- Family members of high-risk patients are advised to take a CPR class and learn about AEDs.

Risk Factors
- Provide education to reduce risk factors including education on smoking cessation, hypertension control, weight control, normal blood glucose, low-fat diet, and normal lipid panel.

- Patients are advised to increase physical activity.
- Women are advised to avoid new hormone replacement therapy.

Cardiac Rehabilitation
- Participation in a cardiac rehabilitation program will help the patient continue the process of risk factor and lifestyle modification.

References
Amsterdam EA, Wenger NK, Brindis RG, et al. 2014 AHA/ACC guideline for the management of patients with non-ST elevation acute coronary syndromes. A report of the American College of Cardiology/American Heart Association task force on practice guidelines. *Circulation*. 2014;130:e344—e426.

O'Gara PT, Kushner FG, Ascheim DD, et al. 2013 ACCF/AHA guideline for the management of ST-elevation myocardial infarction: a report of the American College of Cardiology foundation/American Heart Association task force on practice guidelines. *Circulation*. 2013;127(4):e362.

BOX 11.10 Causes of Sudden Cardiac Death

Acquired SCD Risk
Most patients with sudden cardiac death (SCD) are older adults and have a history of coronary artery disease (CAD), myocardial infarction (MI), and subsequent heart failure.
- Heart failure:
  - Ejection fraction less than 30%
  - Heart structure is abnormal (systolic or diastolic ventricular dysfunction).
  - CAD and a history of MI that has produced scar tissue is the most common cause of ventricular tachycardia (VT)/ventricular fibrillation (VF) leading to SCD.
- Cardiomyopathy (dilated or ischemic):
  - Patients who are inducible for VT/VF in electrophysiology study (EPS) are at highest risk.
  - Risk is decreased by implantation of an implantable cardioverter defibrillator (ICD) and antidysrhythmic medication therapy.

Genetic SCD Risk
Genetic cardiovascular disease accounts for 40% of SCD in young adults.
- Brugada syndrome:
  - Electrocardiogram (ECG) signs: Coved-type ST segment elevation (>2 mm) in right precordial leads, although ECG variations also occur.
  - Heart structure appears normal.
  - High risk of VT or VF in otherwise young healthy adults.
  - VT/VF often occurs at night or at rest.
  - Represents 4% of all SCD; average age is 41 years.
  - Represents up to 20% of genetic SCD patients.

- Hereditary: Autosomal-dominant genetic transmission.
- Five times more common in men.
- Patients who are inducible in EPS are at increased risk.
- Risk reduced by implantation of an ICD.
- Wolff-Parkinson-White (WPW) syndrome:
  - Congenital accessory conduction pathway connects atria and ventricles.
  - Accessory pathway is *in addition* to the normal conduction system.
  - Accessory pathway allows very rapid transmission of impulses leading to "pre-excitation" of the ventricle that can degenerate into VT/VF, especially if atrial dysrhythmias are present.
  - WPW syndrome is usually identified when the patient is a teenager or young adult.
  - WPW syndrome is often recognized during exercise by palpitations or breathlessness.
  - Cure is possible in many cases by radiofrequency ablation of the accessory pathway.
- Hypertrophic cardiomyopathy (HCM):
  - Risk of VT/VF with exercise exists.
  - The obstructive form of HCM can be cured in many cases by alcohol ablation of the enlarged ventricular septum.
  - For other patients with HCM, the risk is reduced by implantation of an ICD.
- Long QT syndrome:
  - Risk of VT/VF with exercise exists.
  - Risk is reduced by implantation of an ICD.

Medical Management

Depending on the length of time the patient was unconscious after the cardiac arrest, cognitive defects may be present because of the lack of cerebral blood flow and resultant hypoxia. The cardiac arrest may also have damaged the myocardium and other tissues. Therapy is tailored to the needs of the patient.[43,44] For comatose patients at high risk for hypoxic brain injury after cardiac arrest, therapeutic hypothermia is initiated to preserve brain function. In the Framingham study, women experienced SCD at half the rate of men and were on average 6 to 10 years older than men when they experienced the event.[39] Prevention focuses on identification and treatment of high-risk cardiac patients

(see sections Implantable Cardioverter Defibrillator and Antidysrhythmic Medications in Chapter 12).

HEART FAILURE

Description and Etiology

The number of patients with heart failure is increasing in the United States. More than 6 million adults (older than age 20 years) in the United States have heart failure. It is estimated that by 2030, an additional 3 million more people will be diagnosed with this condition.[1]

TABLE 11.6 New York Heart Association Functional Classification of Heart Failure.

Class	Definition
I	Normal daily activity does not initiate symptoms
II	Normal daily activities initiate onset of symptoms, but symptoms subside with rest
III	Minimal activity initiates symptoms; patients are usually symptom-free at rest
IV	Any type of activity initiates symptoms, and symptoms are present at rest

Pathophysiology

Heart failure is a response to cardiac dysfunction, a condition in which the heart cannot pump blood at a volume required to meet the body's needs. Any condition that impairs the ability of the ventricles to fill or eject blood can cause heart failure. CAD with resultant necrotic damage to the left ventricle is the underlying cause in most patients. Other major conditions that lead to heart failure include valvular dysfunction, infection (myocarditis or endocarditis), cardiomyopathy, and uncontrolled hypertension.[45] Hypertension is the precursor of heart failure in both men and women.[1]

Assessment and Diagnosis

Heart failure is typically classified by the New York Heart Association (NYHA) criteria (Table 11.6). Patients are assigned into four groups, I through IV, according to the severity of symptoms and degree of patient activity eliciting symptoms. Research-based clinical guidelines add a second level of classification that emphasizes the progressive nature of heart failure through stages identified as A, B, C, D with increasing distress and intensified clinical interventions (Table 11.7).[45]

Heart failure can manifest in many ways, depending on how far ventricular remodeling and dysfunction have advanced. This diagnosis may be discovered because of a known clinical syndrome such as acute MI or because of decreased exercise tolerance, fluid retention, or admission to a critical care unit for an unrelated condition.[45]

The first step in the diagnosis is to determine the underlying structural abnormality creating the ventricular dysfunction and symptoms. Various imaging tests are available to visualize cardiac anatomy, and laboratory tests are used to evaluate the effect of hormonal or electrolyte imbalance. The results of these tests permit the cardiology team to design a treatment plan to control symptoms and possibly correct the underlying cause, as not all HEART FAILURE has the same etiology.

Left Ventricular Failure

Failure of the left ventricle is defined as a disturbance of the contractile function of the left ventricle, resulting in a low cardiac output state. This leads to vasoconstriction of the arterial bed that increases systemic vascular resistance (SVR), a condition also described as "high afterload," and creates congestion and edema in the pulmonary circulation and alveoli. Patients presenting with left ventricular failure have one of the following: (1) decreased exercise tolerance, (2) fluid retention, or (3) discovery made during examination of noncardiac problems.[45] Clinical manifestations of left ventricular failure include decreased peripheral perfusion with weak or diminished pulses; cool, pale extremities; and, in later stages, peripheral

TABLE 11.7 Progression of Heart Failure.

Stage	Structural Heart Disorder	Symptoms	Management
A	No, but at risk because of hypertension, CAD, diabetes mellitus	None	Preventive treatment of known risk factors: • Hypertension • Lipid disorders • Cigarette smoking • Diabetes mellitus • Discourage alcohol and illicit drug use
B	Yes, but without symptoms; previous MI, family history of CM; asymptomatic valvular disease or CM	None	Treat all risk factors; if indicated, use the following: • ACEIs • Beta-blockers
C	Yes, with prior or current symptoms	Shortness of breath, fatigue, reduced exercise tolerance	Treat all risk factors and heart failure symptoms: • Diuretics • ACEIs • Beta-blockers • Digitalis • Dietary salt restriction
D	Yes, with refractory heart failure symptoms despite maximal specialized interventions (pharmacologic, medical, nursing); recurrent hospitalization for heart failure symptoms	Marked symptoms at rest despite maximal medical therapy	Refractory heart failure requires interventions from previous stages (A—C), plus the following: • Continuous IV inotropic support • Mechanical assist devices • Heart transplantation • Hospice care

ACEI, Angiotensin-converting enzyme inhibitor; *CAD,* coronary artery disease; *CM,* cardiomyopathy; *IV,* intravenous; *MI,* myocardial infarction.
Modified from Hunt SA, Abraham WT, Chin MH, et al. ACC/AHA 2005 guideline update for the diagnosis and management of chronic heart failure in the adult: a report of the American College of Cardiology/American Heart Association Task Force on Practice Guidelines. *Circulation.* 2005;112(12):e154.

TABLE 11.8 Clinical Manifestations of Right-Sided and Left-Sided Heart Failure.

LEFT VENTRICULAR FAILURE		RIGHT VENTRICULAR FAILURE	
Signs	**Symptoms**	**Signs**	**Symptoms**
Tachypnea	Fatigue	Peripheral edema	Weakness
Tachycardia	Dyspnea	Hepatomegaly	Anorexia
Cough	Orthopnea	Splenomegaly	Indigestion
Bibasilar crackles	Paroxysmal nocturnal dyspnea	Hepatojugular reflux	Weight gain
Gallop rhythms (S_3 and S_4)	Nocturia	Ascites	Mental changes
Increased pulmonary artery pressures		Jugular venous distention	
Hemoptysis		Increased central venous pressure	
Cyanosis		Pulmonary hypertension	
Pulmonary edema			

cyanosis (Table 11.8). *Hemodynamics of left ventricular failure.* Over time, with progression of the disease state, the fluid accumulation behind the dysfunctional left ventricle elevates pulmonary pressures, contributes to pulmonary congestion and edema, and produces dysfunction of the right ventricle, resulting in failure of the right side of the heart.

Right Ventricular Failure

Failure of the right side of the heart is defined as ineffective right ventricular contractile function. Pure failure of the right ventricle may result from an acute condition such as a pulmonary embolus or a right ventricular infarction, but it most commonly occurs secondary to failure of the left side of the heart. The physical signs of right ventricular failure are jugular venous distention, elevated central venous pressure, weakness, peripheral or sacral edema, hepatomegaly (enlarged liver), jaundice, and liver tenderness. Gastrointestinal symptoms include poor appetite, anorexia, nausea, and an uncomfortable feeling of fullness (see Table 11.8).[45,46]

Systolic Heart Failure

The term *systolic dysfunction* describes an abnormality of the heart muscle that markedly decreases contractility during systole (ejection) and lessens the quantity of blood that can be pumped out of the heart.

Heart failure with reduced ejection fraction. Patients with a diagnosis of systolic heart failure (SHF), also known as *heart failure with reduced ejection fraction (HFrEF)*, have signs and symptoms of heart failure combined with a below-normal ejection fraction (Fig. 11.15). It is still debated how low the ejection fraction must be to qualify as SHF, but the value usually is less than 50%; some clinicians use values below 35% or 40%.[45] Symptoms of HFrEF include dyspnea, exercise intolerance, and fluid volume overload.

CAD and its sequelae represent the underlying cause in two-thirds of patients with HFrEF.[45] The remaining patients with systolic dysfunction have *nonischemic cardiomyopathy*. This may be described as a *dilated cardiomyopathy* (DCM),[45] that results from an identifiable cause, such as hypertension, thyroid disease, cardiac valvular disease, alcohol use, or myocarditis.[45] If the cause is unknown, systolic

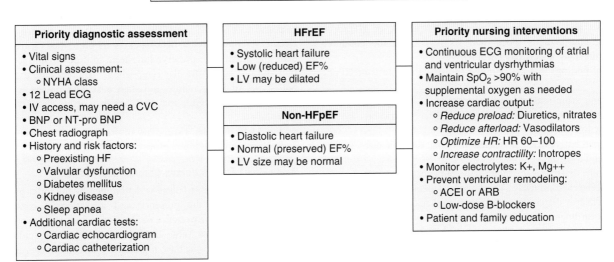

Fig. 11.15 Acute Heart Failure: Priority Diagnostic Assessment and Priority Nursing Interventions. *ARB*, Angiotensin receptor blocker; *ACEI*, angiotensin-converting enzyme inhibitors; *BNP*, B-type natriuretic peptide; *ECG*, electrocardiogram; *EF%*, ejection fraction percentage; *HF*, heart failure; *HR*, heart rate; *HFpEF*, heart failure with preserved ejection fraction; *HFrEF*, heart failure with reduced ejection fraction; *LV*, left ventricle; *NT-pro BNP*, B-type natriuretic peptide; *NYHA*, New York Heart Association; *SpO2*, pulse oximetry oxygen saturation.

dysfunction is described as *idiopathic dilated cardiomyopathy*. SHF incidence increases with age.

Clinical findings that are required to make a diagnosis of HFrEF include:

- Signs and symptoms of heart failure
- Left ventricular systolic dysfunction with an ejection fraction below normal

In HFrEF, the ventricular chambers change their shape, a detrimental development termed *ventricular remodeling*. The negative effect on the cardiac cells is different from the dysfunction and loss of myocytes from myocardial ischemia and infarction.

Hemodynamics of systolic heart failure. Significant hemodynamic changes occur as systolic dysfunction progresses. In SHF, the left ventricular end-diastolic volume is high, which increases the left ventricular end-diastolic pressure compared with a normal heart. The increase in intracardiac volume and pressure causes an increase in left atrial and pulmonary venous pressures. This means that all blood flowing into the heart through the pulmonary vascular bed is exposed to increased hydrostatic pressure, which is necessary to fill the congested heart. The increase in pulmonary vascular pressure causes transudation of fluid from the pulmonary capillaries into the alveolar interstitium, and this fluid is ultimately forced through the walls of the alveoli, causing pulmonary edema. The pulmonary complications of heart failure are described in greater detail later. The elevated left heart pressures eventually raise pressures in the right side of the heart and lead to secondary right heart failure.

Diastolic Heart Failure

The term *diastolic dysfunction* describes an abnormality of the heart muscle that makes it unable to relax, stretch, or fill during diastole.

Heart failure with preserved ejection fraction. Diastolic heart failure (DHF), also known as *heart failure with preserved ejection fraction (HFpEF)*, is caused by left ventricular dysfunction.[45] HFpEF is treated differently from HFrEF (see Fig. 11.15). Studies have shown that patients with HFpEF have a preserved ejection fraction between 40% and 55%.[45] Principal causes are similar to HFrEF (described earlier): CAD, myocardial ischemia, atrial fibrillation, advanced age (older than 75 years), obesity, hypertension, and diabetes mellitus.[45] Some conditions that are known to markedly alter diastolic function include HCM, restrictive cardiomyopathy (RCM), and infiltrative diseases such as amyloidosis and neoplastic infiltrate. The incidence of HFpEF is highest among patients older than 75 years, and the condition disproportionately affects older women.[45]

Clinical findings that are required to make a diagnosis of HFpEF include[45]:

- Signs and symptoms of heart failure
- Normal or only mildly abnormal left ventricular systolic dysfunction
- Abnormal left ventricular relaxation, filling, diastolic distensibility, or diastolic stiffness

Normally, diastole is the filling stage of the cardiac cycle when the ventricle relaxes completely. The abnormal hemodynamics of DHF can be elicited by diagnostic tests such as cardiac catheterization and a stress echocardiogram (see Stress Echocardiography and Table 10.14). An ejection fraction above the range of 40% to 50% is considered normal for this population.

Hemodynamics of diastolic heart failure. In HFpEF, the left ventricular end-diastolic pressure is high, whereas the left ventricular end-diastolic volume is paradoxically low compared with normal hearts.[45] Another diagnostic clue is that many patients with DHF have normal intracardiac pressures at rest, but during exercise, the left ventricular end-diastolic pressure and pulmonary vascular pressure rise rapidly. This occurs because the noncompliant, stiff ventricle cannot increase stroke volume during exercise; cardiac output remains low, even though physical demand is high. Patients with HFpEF often experience a sudden increase in BP and sinus tachycardia during exercise; they are exercise intolerant and experience fatigue, dyspnea, pulmonary venous congestion, and pulmonary edema.[45]

Systolic Heart Failure Versus Diastolic Heart Failure

It is impossible to accurately determine whether a patient has SHF(HFrEF) or DHF(HFpEF) from clinical assessment alone.[45] Both types of heart failure produce similar signs and symptoms. The level of symptoms and quality of life vary among individuals and between men and women, even when the ejection fraction and presumed cardiac dysfunction are the same. This variation may occur because most symptoms come from the neurohormonal compensatory mechanisms (described later) rather than the cardiac output. An elevated B-type natriuretic peptide (BNP) or NT-proBNP level is very useful to diagnose and assess severity of heart failure in patients with fluid overload and shortness of breath.[45,47] The natriuretic peptide value tends to be higher in patients with a diagnosis of HFrEF compared with patients with HFpEF, although the difference is not reliable enough to be used to differentiate the two types in clinical practice.[45,47] Briefly, the more severe the heart failure, the higher the value of BNP or NT-proBNP.

The definitive diagnosis of the type of heart failure is often made using Doppler echocardiography. A two-dimensional echocardiogram coupled with Doppler flow studies to determine whether abnormalities of the myocardium, heart valves, or pericardium are present and which chambers are involved is the single most powerful diagnostic test in the evaluation of patients with heart failure. Calculation of the ejection fraction can be determined using Doppler echocardiography or during a cardiac catheterization. These diagnostic tests also show that some patients exhibit combined HFrEF and HFpEF.[45]

It is impossible to distinguish whether a patient has SHF or DHF simply by looking at the medications they are prescribed. The same medications are used to treat the two types of heart failure, although the underlying rationales may be different.[48] For example, beta-blockers are used in DHF to slow the heart rate, to prolong diastole to give more time for ventricular filling, and to modify the ventricular response to exercise, especially for patients who have a preserved ejection fraction.[48] When beta-blockers are prescribed for treatment of SHF, the intent is to preserve long-term inotropic (contractile) function and prevent ventricular remodeling.[48] Diuretics are used to treat both types of heart failure, although a smaller dosage is generally needed in DHF.[48] ACEIs and ARBs are also used to treat both types of heart failure.

Fig. 11.15 provides a summary of priority diagnostic interventions and priority nursing interventions in acute heart failure.

Acute Heart Failure Versus Chronic Heart Failure

Acute or chronic heart failure is determined by the rapid progression of the syndrome, the presence and activation of compensatory mechanisms, and the presence or absence of fluid accumulation in the interstitial space (see Table 11.8). In clinical practice guidelines, the terms *acute* and *chronic* have replaced the older term *congestive heart failure*. However, the words congestive heart failure are still commonly used in clinical practice.

Acute heart failure has a sudden onset with no compensatory mechanisms. The patient may experience acute pulmonary edema, low cardiac output, or cardiogenic shock. Patients with chronic heart failure are hypervolemic, have sodium and water retention, and have structural heart chamber changes such as dilation or hypertrophy.[49]

Chronic heart failure is an ongoing process, with symptoms that may be made tolerable by medication, diet, and a reduced activity level. The deterioration into acute heart failure can be precipitated by the onset of dysrhythmias, acute ischemia, sudden illness, or cessation of medications. This may necessitate admission to a critical care unit. Hypertension is the primary precursor of heart failure in women, whereas CHD, specifically MI, is the primary cause of heart failure in men.[49]

Neurohormonal Compensatory Mechanisms in Heart Failure

When the heart begins to fail and the cardiac output is no longer sufficient to meet the metabolic needs of tissues, the body activates several major compensatory mechanisms: the sympathetic nervous system, the renin-angiotensin-aldosterone system (RAAS), and, if hypertension is present, the development of ventricular hypertrophy (see Table 11.8). This process ultimately reshapes the ventricle in a process described as *ventricular remodeling*. These pathophysiologic processes and the pharmacologic measures taken to limit ventricular remodeling are described in this section.[50]

Sympathetic nervous system activation. The sympathetic nervous system compensates for low cardiac output by increasing heart rate and BP. As a result, levels of circulating catecholamines are increased, leading to peripheral vasoconstriction. In addition to increasing BP and heart rate, catecholamines cause shunting of blood from nonvital organs such as the skin to vital organs such as the heart and brain. This mechanism, although initially helpful, may become a negative factor if elevation of heart rate increases myocardial oxygen demand while shortening the amount of time for diastolic filling and coronary artery perfusion.

Renin-angiotensin-aldosterone system activation. In acute and chronic heart failure, activation of the RAAS promotes fluid retention.[50] The RAAS is activated by low cardiac output that causes the hormone renin to be secreted by the kidneys. A physiologic chain of events is then set in motion that leads to volume overload. The renin acts on angiotensinogen in the bloodstream and converts it to angiotensin I; when angiotensin passes through the lung tissues, it is activated by angiotensin-converting enzyme, an enzyme that converts angiotensin I to angiotensin II, a powerful vasoconstrictor that increases SVR, BP, and the workload of the left ventricle; the increased SVR further decreases cardiac output. The mineralocorticoid hormone aldosterone is released from the adrenal glands and stimulates sodium retention via the distal tubules of the kidney. In response to the low cardiac output, the renal arterioles constrict, decrease glomerular filtration, and increase reabsorption of sodium from the proximal and distal tubules. To break the RAAS cycle of fluid retention in heart failure, two types of medications are prescribed to interrupt the steps. To inhibit the conversion of angiotensin I to angiotensin II, an ACEI is prescribed (see Table 12.21 in Chapter 12). These agents prevent arterial vasoconstriction, decrease BP and SVR, and decrease the amount of ventricular remodeling that often occurs with heart failure. A medication that inhibits angiotensin II directly may be prescribed instead. The medications in this category are ARBs.[48] Spironolactone (Aldactone) is a medication from a different category that is also prescribed to break the RAAS cycle. Spironolactone is a mineralocorticoid receptor antagonist that inhibits (blocks) the retention of sodium from the distal tubules of the kidney.[48] Fig. 11.16 depicts the mechanism of action by which these medications act on the RAAS.

Ventricular hypertrophy in heart failure. The final compensatory mechanism is ventricular hypertrophy. It is also strongly associated

with preexisting hypertension. Because myocardial hypertrophy increases the force of contraction, hypertrophy helps the ventricle overcome an increase in afterload. When this mechanism is no longer efficient for the ventricle, it will remodel by dilation.

Ventricular remodeling in heart failure. In ventricular remodeling the shape of the ventricle is changed, or remodeled, to resemble a round bowl. A dilated ventricle has poor contractility and is enlarged without hypertrophy. Research trial evidence indicates that synergistic use of medications from different categories—ACEI or ARB, spironolactone, and beta-blockers—can halt or reduce the progression of ventricular remodeling.[45,47,48]

Pulmonary Complications of Heart Failure

The clinical manifestations of acute heart failure result from tissue hypoperfusion and organ congestion and are progressive. The severity of clinical manifestations increases as heart failure worsens. Initially, manifestations appear only with exertion, but eventually, they also occur at rest.[45,47,49]

Shortness of Breath in Heart Failure

The patient experiences the feeling of shortness of breath first with exertion, but as heart failure worsens, symptoms are also present at rest. A diagnostic blood test is available to assist clinicians in differentiating whether a patient's shortness of breath is caused by heart failure or by a non-cardiac pulmonary complication. BNP, a cardiac neurohormone released by the ventricles in response to volume expansion and pressure overload, is elevated in DHF and SHF.[51] Heart failure increases left ventricular wall tension because of the excess preload in the ventricles. When the BNP blood level is greater than 100 pg/mL, the dyspnea is most likely related to heart failure rather than pulmonary failure.[45,51] The more severe the heart failure, the higher the BNP value.[51] If the patient has concomitant kidney disease, the BNP will be also elevated because of the kidney failure. A BNP value greater than 200 pg/mL is required to diagnose heart failure.[51]

Breathlessness in heart failure is described by these terms:

- *Dyspnea:* sensation of shortness of breath from pulmonary vascular congestion and decreased lung compliance
- *Orthopnea:* difficulty breathing when lying flat because of an increase in venous return that occurs in the supine position
- *Paroxysmal nocturnal dyspnea:* severe form of orthopnea in which the patient awakens from sleep gasping for air
- *Cardiac asthma:* dyspnea with wheezing, a nonproductive cough, and pulmonary crackles that progress to the gurgling sounds of pulmonary edema

Pulmonary Edema in Heart Failure

Pulmonary edema, or protein-laden fluid in the alveoli, inhibits gas exchange by impairing the diffusion pathway between the alveolus and the capillary (Fig. 11.17A). It is caused by increased left atrial and ventricular pressures and results in an excessive accumulation of serous or serosanguineous fluid in the interstitial spaces and alveoli of the lungs. The formation of pulmonary edema has two stages.

The first stage is not as severe and is characterized by interstitial edema, engorgement of the perivascular and peribronchial spaces, and increased lymphatic flow (Fig. 11.17B). The later stage is characterized by alveolar edema resulting from fluid moving into the alveoli from the interstitium (Fig. 11.17C). Eventually, blood plasma moves into the alveoli faster than the lymphatic system can clear it, interfering with diffusion of oxygen, depressing the arterial partial pressure of oxygen (PaO_2), and leading to tissue hypoxia (Fig. 11.17D).

Organs involved	Pathophysiology	Medication actions

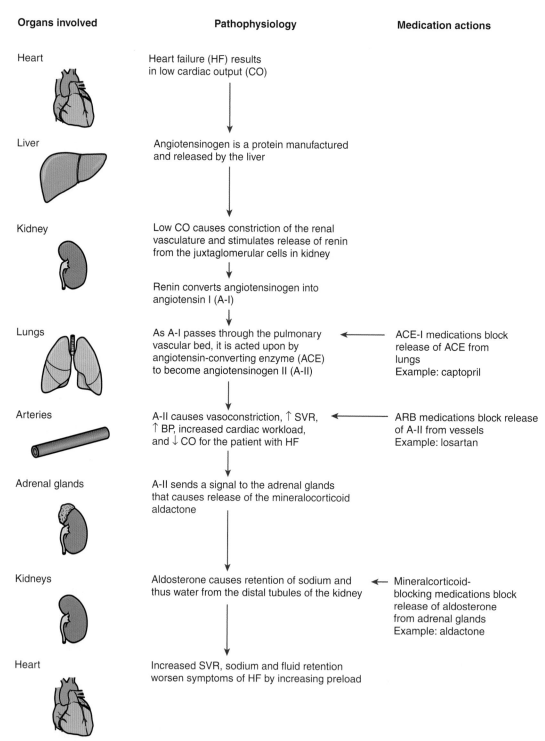

Heart — Heart failure (HF) results in low cardiac output (CO)

Liver — Angiotensinogen is a protein manufactured and released by the liver

Kidney — Low CO causes constriction of the renal vasculature and stimulates release of renin from the juxtaglomerular cells in kidney

Renin converts angiotensinogen into angiotensin I (A-I)

Lungs — As A-I passes through the pulmonary vascular bed, it is acted upon by angiotensin-converting enzyme (ACE) to become angiotensinogen II (A-II) ← ACE-I medications block release of ACE from lungs
Example: captopril

Arteries — A-II causes vasoconstriction, ↑ SVR, ↑ BP, increased cardiac workload, and ↓ CO for the patient with HF ← ARB medications block release of A-II from vessels
Example: losartan

Adrenal glands — A-II sends a signal to the adrenal glands that causes release of the mineralocorticoid aldactone

Kidneys — Aldosterone causes retention of sodium and thus water from the distal tubules of the kidney ← Mineralcorticoid-blocking medications block release of aldosterone from adrenal glands
Example: aldactone

Heart — Increased SVR, sodium and fluid retention worsen symptoms of HF by increasing preload

Fig. 11.16 Renin-Angiotensin-Aldosterone System: Role in Heart Failure and Medication Actions. *ARB*, Angiotensin receptor blocker; *BP*, blood pressure; *CO*, cardiac output; *SVR*, systemic vascular resistance.

Patients experiencing heart failure and acute pulmonary edema are extremely breathless and anxious and have a sensation of suffocation. This is a life-threatening emergency. In acute pulmonary edema, pink, frothy sputum is coughed and expectorated, and patients may be very agitated, sitting upright and gasping for breath. The respiratory rate is elevated, and accessory muscles of ventilation are used, with nasal flaring and bulging neck muscles. Respirations are characterized by loud inspiratory and expiratory gurgling sounds. Diaphoresis is profuse, and the skin is cold, ashen, and sometimes cyanotic. This reflects low cardiac output, increased sympathetic stimulation, peripheral vasoconstriction, and desaturation of arterial blood.

Arterial blood gases in pulmonary edema. Arterial blood gas values are variable. In the early stage of pulmonary edema, respiratory alkalosis may be present because of hyperventilation, which eliminates carbon

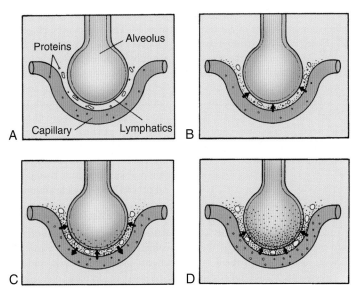

Fig. 11.17 As Pulmonary Edema Progresses, It Inhibits Oxygen and Carbon Dioxide Exchange at the Alveolar Capillary Interface. (A) Normal relationship. (B) Increased pulmonary capillary hydrostatic pressure causes fluid to move from the vascular space into the pulmonary interstitial space. (C) Lymphatic flow increases in an attempt to pull fluid back into the vascular or lymphatic space. (D) Failure of lymphatic flow and worsening of left-sided heart failure results in further movement of fluid into the interstitial space and the alveoli.

dioxide. As the pulmonary edema progresses and gas exchange becomes impaired, acidosis (pH less than 7.35) and hypoxemia ensue. A chest radiograph usually confirms an enlarged cardiac silhouette, pulmonary venous congestion, and interstitial edema.

Dysrhythmias and Heart Failure

A ventricular ejection fraction less than 30% and the presence of NYHA class III or IV heart failure are strongly associated with ventricular dysrhythmias and an increased risk for death.[52] Because sustained VT or VF initiates SCD, high-risk patients with severe heart failure are prescribed antidysrhythmic medications and have an implantable cardioverter defibrillator (ICD) inserted.[52]

Many patients with heart failure also have atrial fibrillation. Digoxin is frequently prescribed for atrial fibrillation to control ventricular heart rate. Digoxin does not prolong life, but it makes patients feel less symptomatic. Digoxin may also work synergistically with specific beta-blockers (e.g., carvedilol) and make the symptoms more tolerable for patients with severe heart failure.[48]

Medical Management

The goals of the medical management of heart failure are to relieve symptoms, enhance cardiac performance, and correct known precipitating causes.

Relief of Symptoms and Enhancement of Cardiac Performance

Control of symptoms involves management of fluid overload and improvement of cardiac output by decreasing SVR and increasing contractility. Medications are an essential tool to improve heart function. Diuretics are administered to decrease preload and to eliminate excess fluid from the body.[48] If pulmonary edema develops, additional diuretics are used. Morphine is given to facilitate peripheral dilation and decrease anxiety. Afterload is decreased by vasodilators such as sodium nitroprusside (Nipride) and nitroglycerin. Sodium nitroprusside is a balanced vasodilator medication that relaxes arterial resistance and venous capacitance vessels. By reducing both preload and afterload, it can relieve congestion and improve cardiac output, particularly in patients with increased SVR. It is useful in favorably redistributing total left ventricular stroke volume in patients with either mitral or aortic insufficiency such that regurgitant flow is reduced while forward flow is increased.[48] Nitrates are used to decrease preload and vasodilate the coronary arteries if CAD is an underlying cause of the acute heart failure.

For some patients, an IABP is temporarily required.[47] Contractility is initially increased by continuous infusion of positive inotropic medications (dopamine) or by combination inodilators such as dobutamine or milrinone, which have both inotropic and vasodilatory effects.

After the acute exacerbation is resolved, the patient is transitioned to oral agents and weaned off the intravenous medications. Before transitioning out of the critical care unit, the patient with heart failure receives ACEIs to inhibit left ventricular chamber remodeling and slow left ventricular dilation. If the patient does not tolerate ACEIs, ARBs may be substituted.[47,48] Low-dose beta-blockers such as carvedilol may also be prescribed, although strict surveillance is required to anticipate and avoid untoward negative inotropic effects.[48] Digoxin may be added to the regimen, especially if the patient has concomitant atrial fibrillation.[48]

Nonpharmacologic interventions that are increasingly used include *cardiac resynchronization therapy* (CRT).[52–55] CRT is biventricular pacing, where the right and left ventricles each have a pacing lead in contact with the myocardium. CRT has a beneficial effect on clinical symptoms, exercise capacity, and systolic left ventricular performance.[52–55]

Correction of Precipitating Causes

After symptoms of heart failure are controlled, diagnostic studies such as cardiac catheterization, echocardiography, and myocardial perfusion imaging tests, are undertaken to uncover the cause of the heart failure. The results are used to tailor long-term management to treat the cause. Some structural problems such as valvular disease may be amenable to surgical or interventional correction.

Palliative Care for End-Stage Heart Failure

A consensus statement on palliative and supportive care in advanced heart failure was published in 2004.[56] Heart failure is a progressive disease, and patients do not recover.[56,57] At a point in the disease trajectory, many patients with NYHA class IV heart failure become candidates for palliative care.[56] The primary aim of palliative care is symptom management and relief of suffering. Fundamental to all symptom management strategies for heart failure is the optimization of medications according to current guidelines.[47,48] The most common symptoms of advanced heart failure are dyspnea, pain, and fatigue.[45,47] See Chapter 9 for in-depth information on palliative care.

Nursing Management

Care management for a patient with heart failure incorporates a variety of patient diagnoses (Box 11.11). Nursing priorities are designed to achieve optimal cardiopulmonary function, promote comfort and emotional support, monitor the effectiveness of pharmacologic therapy, ensure nutrition intake is sufficient, and provide patient and family education. See Appendix A for patient care management plans specific to patients with CAD.

Optimizing Cardiopulmonary Function

The patient's ECG is evaluated for dysrhythmias that may be present as a result of medication toxicity or electrolyte imbalance. Breath sounds are auscultated frequently to determine the adequacy of respiratory effort and to assess for onset or worsening of pulmonary congestion. Oxygen is administered through a nasal cannula to relieve dyspnea. Diuretics or vasodilators are used to decrease excessive preload and afterload.[48] If the patient is not hypotensive, morphine may be administered to decrease hyperventilation and anxiety. If the patient's ventilatory status worsens, the nurse must be prepared for endotracheal intubation and mechanical ventilation. Obtaining daily weights is important until the weight stabilizes at a "dry" weight. Generally, the daily weight is used in fluid management, and a weekly weight is optimally used for tracking body weight (e.g., muscle, fat).

Promoting Comfort and Emotional Support

Activity must be restricted during periods of breathlessness. Bed rest usually is prescribed for the patient, who is positioned with the head of the bed elevated to allow for maximal lung expansion. The arms can be supported on pillows so that no undue stress is placed on the shoulder muscles. The legs may be placed in a dependent position to encourage venous pooling, decreasing venous return. Rest periods must be carefully planned and adhered to, and independence within the patient's activity prescription must be fostered. Vital signs are recorded before an activity is begun and after it is completed. Signs of activity intolerance such as dyspnea, fatigue, sustained increase in pulse, and onset of dysrhythmias are documented and reported to the physician. Activity is gradually increased according to the patient's tolerance. Skin breakdown is a risk because of the combination of bed rest, inadequate nutrition, peripheral edema, and decreased perfusion to the skin and subcutaneous tissue. Frequent position changes and mobilization can help provide comfort and prevent this complication.

Monitoring Effects of Pharmacologic Therapy

Patients experiencing acute heart failure require aggressive pharmacologic therapy.[48] The critical care nurse must know the action, side effects, therapeutic levels, and toxic effects of diuretics and venodilators used to decrease preload, positive inotropic agents used to increase ventricular contractility, vasodilators used to decrease afterload, and any antidysrhythmics used to control heart rate and prevent dysrhythmias. The patient's hemodynamic response to these agents is closely monitored. Fluid intake and output balances are tabulated daily or hourly in the critical care unit.

Nutritional Intake

Patients experiencing acute heart failure often have decreased appetite and nausea, and small, frequent meals may be more appropriate than the standard three large meals. Food must be as tasty as possible. Favorite foods and foods from home may be incorporated into the diet as long as the foods are compatible with nutritional restrictions such as low levels of sodium to decrease the risk of fluid retention. Each patient must be assessed for nutritional imbalance individually. Not all patients with heart failure have the same nutritional needs. See Chapter 7 for an in-depth discussion of nutrition in heart disease.

Educate the Patient and Family

The nurse assesses the patient's and family's understanding of the pathophysiology and individual risk factor profile for heart failure. Primary topics of education include (1) the importance of a daily weight, (2) fluid restrictions, (3) written information about the multiple medications used to control the symptoms of heart failure, (4) physical activity, and (5) when to call a health care provider (Box 11.12).[58,59] Many patients with a diagnosis of heart failure also require education about lifestyle changes such as smoking cessation, weight loss, energy conservation, and how to incorporate exercise and sodium restriction into their daily lives.[58,59] Achieving optimal outcomes for a patient with heart failure requires contributions from a team of educated health care clinicians.

Evidence-Based Practice for Heart Failure

Evidence-based practice management of heart failure is described in Box 11.13.[60]

CARDIOMYOPATHY

Description and Etiology

Cardiomyopathy is a disease of the heart muscle (*cardio-* [heart], *-myo-* [muscle], and *-pathy* [pathology]). Cardiomyopathies are classified by structural abnormalities and genotype if known. Cardiomyopathies are

---

> ## ◎ BOX 11.11 PRIORITY PATIENT CARE MANAGEMENT
>
> **Acute Heart Failure**
> - Impaired Gas Exchange due to ventilation/perfusion mismatching or intrapulmonary shunting
> - Impaired Cardiac Output due to alterations in preload
> - Impaired Cardiac Output due to alterations in contractility
> - Impaired Cardiac Output due to alterations in afterload (pulmonary circulation)
> - Impaired Cardiac Output due to alterations in heart rate or rhythm
> - Activity Intolerance due to cardiopulmonary dysfunction
> - Anxiety due to threat to biologic, psychologic, or social integrity
> - Ineffective Tissue Perfusion due to decreased myocardial blood flow
> - Lack of Knowledge of Treatment Regime due to lack of previous exposure to information (see Box 11.12, Patient and Family Education Plan: Acute Heart Failure)
>
> Patient Care Management plans are located in Appendix A.

✴ BOX 11.12 PRIORITY PATIENT AND FAMILY EDUCATION

Acute Heart Failure

The patient should be able to teach back the following topics:

- Heart failure: pathophysiology of heart failure
- Fluid balance: low-salt diet to reduce fluid retention; intake and output measurement; signs of fluid overload such as peripheral edema
- Daily weight: Increase or loss of 1–2 lb in a few days is a sign of fluid gain or loss, not true weight gain or loss.
- Breathlessness: Increasing shortness of breath, wheezing, and sleeping upright on pillows or in a recliner are symptoms that must be monitored and reported to a health care professional.
- Activity: activity conservation with rest periods as heart failure progresses
- Medications: As medications are complex, information must be given in writing and orally:
  - Preload: purpose of diuretics, increased urine output, and control of fluid volume

- Afterload: purpose of vasodilators or angiotensin-converting enzyme inhibitors in decreasing workload of the heart
- Heart rate: The purpose of digoxin is to control atrial fibrillation, a frequent dysrhythmia in heart failure.
- Contractility: With the exception of digoxin, no oral contractility medications are approved by the US Food and Drug Administration.
- Anticoagulation: Patients with distended atria and enlarged ventricles or with atrial fibrillation may be prescribed an anticoagulant such as warfarin (Coumadin); risks of bleeding, importance of correct dosages, prothrombin times, international normalized ratio, and nutritional-pharmacologic interactions are emphasized.
- Follow-up care
- Symptoms to report to a health care professional

QSEN | BOX 11.13 Evidence-Based Practice

Heart Failure

A collaborative heart failure management team provides an integrated approach to care to achieve clinical stability for the patient.

1. Ensure systematic assessment and management:
   - To achieve an absence of "congestion" and to stabilize patient's condition at the best "stage" possible when in the hospital (see Tables 11.7 and 11.8)
   - To maintain same stability once discharged home and to avoid hospital readmission
2. Counsel and educate patient and family after discharge from hospital. Patients and families should understand:
   - Heart failure disease process
   - Heart failure medications, dosages, medication schedule, medication side effects
   - Fluid balance related to salt-restriction diet (2 g/day of sodium), daily weight, diuretic regimen
   - When to call health care provider

- Risk of additional complications: sudden cardiac death; progressive heart failure; need for other cardiac procedures (pacemaker, implantable cardioverter defibrillator, percutaneous coronary intervention) or cardiac surgery (coronary artery bypass graft, valve replacement); mechanical assist device or heart transplantation, as needed by some patients
- Purpose of advance directive for health care decisions
3. Promote patient compliance with treatment regimen:
   - Patient needs support from concerned companions and health care professionals.
   - Patient should remain physically active and involved with life.
4. Facilitate hospital discharge; implement outpatient models of health care delivery:
   - Close communication between inpatient and outpatient health care providers is essential.

Reference

Yancy CW, Jessup M, Bozkurt B, et al. 2013 ACCF/AHA guideline for management of heart failure. *J Am Coll Cardiol*. 2013;62(16):e147.

---

also categorized as *extrinsic*, caused by external factors such as hypertension, ischemia, inflammation, or valvular dysfunction, or as *intrinsic*, corresponding to myocardial diseases without identifiable external causes.[61–63] Cardiomyopathy categories are hypertrophic (HCM), restrictive, and dilated (DCM), as illustrated in Fig. 11.18. The two main forms of primary cardiomyopathies are HCM and DCM. Most cases of HCM and 20% to 50% of cases of DCM are familial, showing a genetic disposition.[62]

Hypertrophic Obstructive Cardiomyopathy

HCM is a genetically inherited disease that affects the myocardial sarcomere.[62] As HCM progresses, the left ventricle becomes stiff, noncompliant, and hypertrophied, sometimes in an asymmetric fashion.[62] HCM occurs in two forms. A well-known but less frequent manifestation is a stiff, noncompliant myocardial muscle with left ventricular hypertrophy and hypertrophy of the upper ventricular septum. This left ventricular septal hypertrophy obstructs outflow

through the aortic valve, especially during exercise (see Fig. 11.18A). It also pulls the papillary muscle out of alignment, causing mitral regurgitation. Other patients with HCM have generalized left ventricular hypertrophy, but the septum is not more enlarged than the rest of the myocardium.[62] HCM causes significant diastolic dysfunction because the muscle-bound, stiff, noncompliant heart muscle does not allow adequate filling during diastole.

Two advances in diagnostic medicine have propelled understanding of the differences between these two forms of HCM. *Two-dimensional transthoracic echocardiography* (TTE) is often useful as the first diagnostic test to identify HCM.[62,63] TTE enables visualization of septal anatomy, septal movement, and ventricular wall thickness and motion. The second advance is *diagnostic genetics*. Genetic testing for HCM usually is performed at a center with expertise in this area.[63] HCM is inherited as an autosomal dominant trait, and the clinical expression is caused by mutations in any one of 12 genes.[62,63] Each gene encodes different protein components of the myocardial

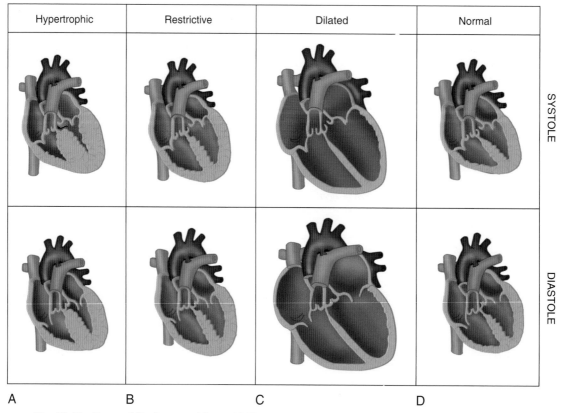

Hypertrophic	Restrictive	Dilated	Normal	
				SYSTOLE
				DIASTOLE
A	B	C	D	

Fig. 11.18 Types of Cardiomyopathies and Differences in Ventricular Diameter During Systole and Diastole Compared With a Normal Heart. (A) Hypertrophic. (B) Restrictive. (C) Dilated. (D) Normal.

sarcomere.[63] Genetic analysis is an area of ongoing research that will undoubtedly help clarify other aspects of HCM within the next decade.

In HCM, symptoms are similar to those seen with heart failure, with the addition of myocardial ischemia, supraventricular tachycardia, VT, syncope, and stroke.[62] Symptoms usually are more intense with physical exercise, especially in the obstructive form of HCM, in which the aortic outflow tract is obstructed by the enlarged left ventricular septum. Because a known association exists between HCM and SCD, limitation of physical activity may be recommended. Causes of SCD are thought to stem from ventricular dysrhythmias and atrial fibrillation.[63] The atrial dysrhythmias are related to increased age and atrial enlargement. Pharmacologic management includes beta-blockers to decrease left ventricular workload, medications to control and prevent atrial and ventricular dysrhythmias, anticoagulation if atrial fibrillation or left ventricular thrombi are present, and medications to manage heart failure. Interventional procedures include insertion of an ICD to decrease the risk of SCD and percutaneous alcohol ablation of the intraventricular septum to decrease the size of the septal wall.[62]

Dilated Cardiomyopathy

DCM is characterized by gross dilation of both ventricles without muscle hypertrophy (see Fig. 11.18C). Several distinct causes of DCM exist. DCM has both primary and secondary causes and is the most common cause of heart failure. DCM results from valvular, ischemic, toxic, metabolic, infectious, and systemic causes.[61,62,64]

Ischemic dilated cardiomyopathy. Ischemic DCM results from repeated myocardial injury or infarction resulting in reduction of ejection fraction. It is the most common cause of DCM in the United States. The patient has signs and symptoms of SHF and a low ejection fraction.[62,64] Treatment consists of the use of ACEIs in symptomatic and asymptomatic patients and beta-blockers and digoxin in symptomatic patients.

Idiopathic dilated cardiomyopathy. When the cause of DCM is unknown, it is called *idiopathic DCM*. In some cases, the occurrence is linked to genetic inheritance. Scientific advances in molecular genetics permit detailed studies of families with a high incidence of DCM. It is thought that 10% to 50% of *familial idiopathic DCM* cases reflect genetic transmission. In affected families, various genetic mutations occur in the gene that codes for the sarcomere contractile protein in the heart. The heritable trait can be expressed as an autosomal dominant or recessive inheritance pattern. Preliminary research indicates that the genetic picture is highly individual for different family groups, even if the clinical picture appears similar.

Other causes of dilated cardiomyopathy. Many other nonischemic, nongenetic causes of DCM exist. Injury can be caused by valvular heart dysfunction that has placed extreme pressure or volume on the chambers, and viral or bacterial infections such as myocarditis can lead to inflammatory changes that permanently remodel the heart.[62,64] Other noncardiac causes include infiltration by systemic collagens as in amyloidosis or sarcoidosis.[64]

In DCM, the myocardial muscle fibers contract poorly, resulting in global left ventricular dysfunction, low cardiac output, atrial and ventricular dysrhythmias, blood pooling that leads to ventricular thrombi and embolic episodes, refractory heart failure, and premature death. The goals of medical management of DCM are similar to the goals for SHF: improvement of pump function, removal of excess fluid, control of heart failure symptoms, anticipation and management of complications, and prevention of SCD.

Restrictive Cardiomyopathy

RCM is the least commonly encountered cardiomyopathy in developed countries (see Fig. 11.18B). As with the other cardiomyopathies, RCM can be idiopathic or can have a known cause. RCMs involve abnormalities of diastolic function with preserved systolic function. DHF, low cardiac output, dyspnea, orthopnea, and liver engorgement are the most common clinical manifestations of RCM. An elevated jugular venous pressure, S_4, and late S_3 may be present. Both ventricles are typically small with decreased volumes and large atria. The atrial septum and cardiac valves may be thickened, and pericardial effusion may be present. Medical management is aimed at improving symptoms and preventing tachycardia. Diuretics and nitrates reduce pulmonary pressure and fluid volume, thus relieving dyspnea. Patients are advised to reduce sodium intake, weigh daily, and restrict water intake. ACEIs and ARBs improve stroke volume and reduce myocardial oxygen demand.[61]

Nursing Management

Care management for a patient with cardiomyopathy incorporates a variety of patient diagnoses related to symptoms of heart failure as listed in (see Box 11.11). Nursing priorities are individualized according to the type of cardiomyopathy and are focused on achievement of a stable fluid balance, monitoring the effects of pharmacologic therapy, safely increasing mobility, and providing patient and family education. Cardiomyopathy produces symptoms of heart failure, and a collaborative team of compassionate, knowledgeable professionals is required to provide effective care and education for patients (Boxes 11.12 and 11.13).[60] See Appendix A for patient care management plans specific to patients with cardiomyopathy and heart failure.

ENDOCARDITIS

Description and Etiology

Endocarditis is an inflammation on the endothelial surface of the heart, specifically thrombotic-fibrin vegetation on the cardiac valves. This irritation can be related to infectious or noninfectious sources.[65,66] The older term *bacterial endocarditis* has been replaced by the term *infectious endocarditis* (IE) because nonbacterial organisms can be the infective source of the endothelial inflammation. The incidence of IE has not declined over the past 30 years, with 10,000 to 20,000 cases reported each year and a mortality rate of 20% to 40%.[67] IE is the fourth most common cause of life-threatening infectious syndromes (after urosepsis, pneumonia, and intraabdominal sepsis). The risk of acquiring IE is higher among patients with congenital heart disease, valvular heart disease, and prosthetic heart valves. Approximately 75% of patients have a preexisting structural abnormality of the involved cardiac valve. Increasing incidence of invasive health care interventions such as implantable pacemakers and ICDs, body piercings, intravenous drug abuse (IVDA), and an increase in the number of older patients with degenerative valve disease increases the numbers at risk for IE. Additional risk factors include men over 60 years of age, poor dentition, and type 2 diabetes mellitus.[67] Involvement of right heart valves is highly suspicious for IVDA.[68] Among IVDAs, the incidence of IE is 60 times that of age-matched controls.[69]

Development of IE depends on these events[67]:
- Presence of a nonbacterial thrombotic lesion on a cardiac valve or endothelium
- Bacteremia (bacteria in bloodstream)
- Bacteria attaching to the nonbacterial thrombotic lesion
- Proliferation of bacteria on and within the lesion that may develop into a *vegetation*

Research suggests the source of the organism is less likely to be related to a specific invasive procedure such as a urogenital procedure or dental work. Rather, IE results from the confluence of multiple daily bacteremic events in the presence of a susceptible cardiac lesion.[68]

Clinical manifestations of IE that may be identified on physical examination include fever, splenomegaly, and hematuria. The skin may show petechiae and splinter hemorrhages in the nail beds, or small raised, tender areas in the pads of fingers and toes. In the eyes, round or oval spots consisting of coagulated fibrin may be seen in the retina and lead to hemorrhage. A heart murmur can be auscultated. The patient may describe being tired, especially with exertion. These findings are verified with additional tests such as a cardiac echocardiogram and blood cultures.

Pathophysiology

IE results from a bacterial or fungal organism in the bloodstream that successfully colonizes the cardiac endothelium. IE is fatal if not treated. Bacterial organisms, typically streptococci, staphylococci, and enterococci, are the most common pathogens. An increase in multidrug-resistant organisms has led to increased numbers of patients, more serious complications, and higher mortality rates.[68] Sites where endocarditis vegetations occur often correlate with aberrant intracardiac flow caused by valvular damage or septal defects. After the vegetations have colonized, organisms multiply at a rapid rate inside a protective platelet-fibrin casing that sequesters the infection.[69]

Assessment and Diagnosis

Diagnosis must be made as soon as possible to initiate treatment and identify patients at high risk for complications. Diagnosis is guided by classic manifestations of bacteremia or fungemia, evidence of active valvulitis, peripheral emboli, and immunologic vascular phenomena.

Modified Duke Criteria

The 2015 AHA scientific statement on IE supports use of the modified Duke criteria for diagnosis, early identification, and treatment of IE (Table 11.9). This system stratifies patients with suspected IE into three categories: (1) definite cases, (2) possible cases, and (3) rejected cases. A definite diagnosis of IE requires two major criteria, one major and three minor criteria, or five minor criteria. A possible diagnosis of IE requires one major and one minor criteria, or three minor criteria.[65–69]

Blood Cultures

Initial symptoms include fever sometimes accompanied by rigor (shivering), fatigue, and malaise; up to 50% of patients report myalgias and joint pain.[66] Blood cultures are drawn during periods of elevated temperature to detect the infective organism. At least 10 mL of venous blood should be placed in each of the blood culture containers to ensure that the organism will be detected.[68] Culture-negative endocarditis occurs in up to one-third of cases and usually is related to prior antibiotic use or infection by a "fastidious" organism, which does not proliferate under conventional laboratory culture conditions.[67] White blood cell counts are typically elevated, and the symptoms are identified in the Duke criteria (see Table 11.9).

Chest Radiograph

Cough and pleuritic chest pain are present in 40% to 60% of cases. The first noninvasive test is often a chest radiograph to detect nodular infiltrates, cardiomegaly, and enlarged pulmonary vessels.

TABLE 11.9 Modified Duke Criteria.

Major Criteria	Minor Criteria
Blood Culture Positive for IE • Micro-organism consistent with IE from two separate blood cultures: • *Viridans streptococci* • *Streptococcus bovis* • HACEK group (*Haemophilus* species, *Aggregatibacter* species, *Cardiobacterium hominis*, *Eikenella corrodens*, and *Kingella* species) • *Staphylococcus aureus* • Community-acquired enterococci without a known primary focus **OR** • Micro-organisms consistent with IE from persistently positive blood cultures: • At least two positive cultures from blood samples drawn at least 12 hours apart • Four separate blood cultures (with first and last sample drawn at least 1 hour apart) • One positive blood culture for *Coxiella burnetii* or antiphase-I immunoglobulin G (IgG) antibody titer >1:800 **Echocardiogram Positive for IE** • TEE/TTE to visualize heart valves • TEE recommended for prosthetic valves • Oscillating intracardiac mass on valve • Intracardiac abscess • New partial dehiscence of prosthetic valve • New valvular regurgitation	**Predisposition:** Heart condition or an injectable drug user **Fever:** Temperature >38°C **Vascular phenomena:** Major arterial emboli, septic pulmonary infarcts, mycotic aneurysm, intracranial hemorrhage, conjunctival hemorrhages, and Janeway lesions **Immunologic phenomena:** Glomerulonephritis, Osler nodes, Roth spots, rheumatoid factor **Microbial evidence:** Positive blood culture that does not meet any major criterion (as described) or serologic evidence of active infection with an organism consistent with IE **Possible Rejection Criteria for IE** • Firm alternative diagnosis for IE • Resolution of IE symptoms with antibiotics ≤4 days • No pathologic evidence of IE at surgery or autopsy with antibiotics for ≤4 days.

IE, Infective endocarditis; *TEE*, transesophageal echocardiography; *TTE*, transthoracic echocardiography.

Echocardiogram

The other essential noninvasive test is an echocardiogram of the heart valves to visualize vegetations. TTE may be performed initially, but transesophageal echocardiography is more valuable because of the clarity of the heart valve images. Transesophageal echocardiography is more sensitive in detection of vegetations and abscesses.[67,68] Color-flow mapping is especially useful to visualize the severity of valvular regurgitation.

Complications

Heart failure is the most frequent complication of IE and the most frequent cause of death. Embolic complications are the second most common complication, occurring in 22% to 50% of IE cases; 65% of the emboli occur in the central nervous system (CNS) and can cause a stroke. Pulmonary embolism (PE) occurs in 66% to 75% of IVDA cases that involve vegetations on the tricuspid valve. Other organs affected by emboli include liver, spleen, kidney, abdominal mesenteric artery, and peripheral vessels. Septic emboli may be visible on the fingers and toes. The rate of emboli formation rapidly declines with appropriate intravenous antimicrobial administration.[68] Risk of death increases with the development of emboli and decreased arterial perfusion to vital organs. Even with appropriate treatment, mortality risk is almost 40% at 1 year.[67]

Medical Management

Treatment requires prolonged intravenous therapy with adequate doses of antimicrobial agents tailored to the specific IE microbe and patient circumstances. The antibiotic management of native valve endocarditis is frequently different from treatment of prosthetic valve endocarditis or IVDA endocarditis. Antibiotic treatment, administered in high doses intravenously, is prolonged and may involve combination therapy.[66-70] Best outcomes are achieved if therapy is initiated before hemodynamic compromise.

In many cases, antimicrobial medications are insufficient to cure the IE. Cardiac surgery to excise the damaged native or prosthetic valve is required for persistent vegetation, valve dysfunction, perivalvular extension, and aggressive fungal or antibiotic-resistant bacteria. Valve surgery usually is delayed until the patient is stable.[66] Early surgery is indicated for patients demonstrating signs of heart failure or for persistent symptomatic infection lasting longer than 5 to 7 days with appropriate antimicrobial treatment.[69] An increasing number of patients with uncomplicated IE are being discharged earlier than in the past and are continuing intravenous antimicrobial therapy at home with a surgically or peripherally implanted long-term central venous catheter.

Nursing Management

Care management for a patient with IE incorporates a variety of patient diagnoses (Box 11.14). Nursing priorities focus on timely antimicrobial administration to resolve the infection, prevent complications, provide pain medication, and individualize patient education.

Resolving the Infection

IE requires a long course (usually 4–6 weeks) of intravenous antibiotics. Treatment is begun in the hospital and continued at home with an indwelling central catheter after the patient is in a stable condition. Nursing assessment includes monitoring for complications and possible signs of worsening infection, such as persistent temperature elevation, malaise, weakness, easy fatigability, night sweats, or new emboli on hands or feet.

Preventing Complications

Complications occur in 20% to 50% of patients with IE.[69] The nursing assessment is attuned to the early detection of changes, such as shortness of breath or chest pain with hemoptysis. As valvular dysfunction accelerates, acute heart failure develops. Cardiac assessment includes auscultation of heart sounds to detect the presence of or change in a cardiac murmur. Murmurs can be caused by worsening heart failure or by pulmonary emboli. Changes in level of consciousness, visual changes, or complaints of headache should always be reported immediately because of the risk of emboli. Evaluation of liver and kidney function is essential to monitor the health of those organs because of the risk of emboli. Because of the complex and prolonged antibiotic therapy required for treating IE, adverse medication reactions are another important consideration.

Educate the Patient and Family

A patient with IE needs to know the manifestations of infection, how to take an oral temperature, and what medical procedures increase risk for recurrence of IE. A written list of all medications must be supplied (Box 11.15). It is essential to reinforce to patients the necessity to provide a comprehensive endocarditis history to their other health care providers such as the dentist or the podiatrist.[67] The known IVDA has a unique set of challenges to overcome. Multidisciplinary support for the patient to meet the challenge of opiate withdrawal and psychologic dependence is essential to prevent a relapse.

Evidence-Based Practice for Endocarditis

Evidence-based practice for management and prophylaxis for IE is summarized in Box 11.16.

VALVULAR HEART DISEASE

Description and Etiology

The term *valvular heart disease* describes structural and functional abnormalities of single or multiple cardiac valves. The result is an alteration in blood flow across the valve. The two major classifications of valvular lesions are *stenotic* and *regurgitant*. These are described in this section with reference to the specific cardiac valves involved.

Admission of patients with valvular disease to the critical care unit is generally related to surgical replacement or an exacerbation of heart failure. In the past, most valvular lesions in the United States were rheumatic in origin, and damage was a direct result of group A beta-hemolytic streptococcal pharyngitis. As a result of aggressive treatment of "strep throat," this has become a rare problem. Valve lesions now more commonly occur in patients with congenital disorders and older adults with acquired valvular disease. Older adults are more likely to present with symptoms of heart failure and degenerative valve changes that do not result from an infection.[69] These degenerative changes may also be described as myxomatous leaflet degeneration, or annular calcification.[69]

Pathophysiology
Mitral Valve Stenosis

The term *mitral valve stenosis* describes a progressive narrowing of the mitral valve orifice. The primary cause is rheumatic endocarditis, with rare occurrences related to congenital malformations. Mitral stenosis occurs in twice as many women as men.[69] Symptoms occur when the normal valve size is reduced to 2 cm^2 or less. When the valve area is reduced to less than 1 cm^2, symptoms occur at rest.[70] Narrowing is caused by aging valve tissue or by acute rheumatic valvulitis (Table 11.10). The diffuse valve leaflets fibrose and fuse, reducing mobility and thickening the chordae tendineae. As a result, the mitral valve can no longer open or close passively in response to left atrial and ventricular pressure changes. Blood flow across the valve is impeded. Mitral stenosis increases the risk of developing atrial fibrillation because of the high pressures in the left atrium that stimulate left atrial remodeling and enlargement. Development of atrial fibrillation significantly increases symptoms and may increase the need for surgical replacement of the valve.

Mitral Valve Regurgitation

Mitral valve regurgitation may result from rheumatic disease, aging of the valve, endocarditis, collagen vascular disease, or papillary muscle dysfunction (see Table 11.10). In mitral regurgitation, the valve annulus, leaflets, chordae tendineae, and papillary muscles all may be dysfunctional, or the dysfunction may be isolated to just one component of the valve. Mitral valve regurgitation results in a

QSEN ## BOX 11.16   Evidence-Based Practice

Infective Endocarditis and Infective Endocarditis Prophylaxis

Diagnosis of Infective Endocarditis

The Modified Duke Criteria are recommended to guide diagnosis of infective endocarditis (IE) (see Table 11.9). Endocarditis prophylaxis is recommended for patients with:

- Prosthetic heart valve with a history of IE
- Valve repair
- Complex cyanotic congenital heart disease
- Congenital valve malformation such as bicuspid aortic valve
- Hypertrophic cardiomyopathy with latent or resting obstruction
- Mitral valve prolapse with valvular regurgitation and/or thickened valve leaflets

Special considerations apply for patients with prosthetic valve and IE:

- Patients with a risk for IE who have unexplained fever for more than 48 hours should have at least two sets of blood cultures obtained from different sites.
- Surgical valve replacement is indicated for patients with IE of a prosthetic valve who present in heart failure.

Antimicrobial Therapy

Antimicrobial therapy administered for IE is characterized by four features:

1. It is prolonged.
2. It is bactericidal.
3. It is intravenous (IV).
4. It is high dosage.

At least two sets of blood cultures are obtained every 24–48 hours until the infection is cleared from the bloodstream. IV antimicrobial therapy is continued after hospital discharge in the home setting.

Complications From IE

- Emboli from infected heart valves occur in 22%–50% of IE cases, and 65% of embolic events involve the central nervous system. The rate of embolic events decreases significantly during and after 2–3 weeks of appropriate antimicrobial therapy.
- Acute heart failure has the greatest effect on overall prognosis.

Complications From Antibiotics

- Toxicity from the high doses of antibiotics may impair kidney function or vestibular function (balance).
- Diarrhea and colitis can be caused by a reaction to the antibiotic therapy or by overgrowth by *Clostridioides difficile*.

Indications for Surgery

- Removal of infected device
- Increase in size of valve vegetation despite appropriate antimicrobial therapy
- Mitral or aortic regurgitation with acute heart failure unresponsive to medical therapy
- One or more embolic events during the first 2 weeks of antimicrobial therapy

References

Habib G, Lancellotti P, Antunes MJ, et al. 2015 ESC guidelines for the management of infective endocarditis. the task force for the management of infective endocarditis of the European Society of Cardiology (ESC). *Eur Heart J.* 2015;36(44):3075–3128.

Nishimura RA, Otto CM, Bonow RO, et al. 2014 AHA/ACC guideline for the management of patients with valvular heart disease. *J Am Coll Cardiol.* 2014;63(22):e57.

TABLE 11.10   Valvular Dysfunction.

	Pathophysiology	Clinical Manifestations	Physical Signs
Mitral Valve Stenosis 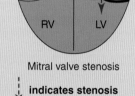 Mitral valve stenosis ¦ indicates stenosis A	Left atrium must generate more pressure to propel blood beyond lesion; rise in left atrial pressure and volume reflected retrograde into pulmonary vessels; right ventricular hypertrophy; right ventricular failure	Dyspnea on exertion; fatigue and weakness; pronounced respiratory symptoms (e.g., orthopnea, paroxysmal nocturnal dyspnea); mild hemoptysis with bronchial capillary rupture; susceptibility to pulmonary infections	• Chest radiograph: pulmonary congestion, redistribution of blood flow to upper lobes • ECG: atrial fibrillation and other atrial dysrhythmias • Auscultation: diastolic murmur, accentuated S_1, opening snap • Catheterization: elevated pressure gradient across valve; increased left atrial pressure, pulmonary artery occlusion pressure, and pulmonary artery pressure; low cardiac output
Mitral Valve Regurgitation 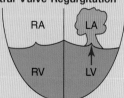 Mitral valve regurgitation indicates backward flow from a valve that is leaking or regurgitant B	LV dilation and hypertrophy; left atrial dilation and hypertrophy	Weakness and fatigue; exertional dyspnea; palpitations; severe symptoms precipitated by LV failure, with consequent low output and pulmonary congestion	• Chest radiograph: left atrial and LV enlargement, variable pulmonary congestion • ECG: P mitrale, LV hypertrophy, atrial fibrillation • Auscultation: murmur throughout systole • Catheterization: opacification of left atrium during LV injection, v waves, increased left atrial and LV pressures • Variable elevations of pulmonary pressures

TABLE 11.10 Valvular Dysfunction.—cont'd

	Pathophysiology	Clinical Manifestations	Physical Signs
Aortic Valve Stenosis Aortic valve stenosis	LV hypertrophy; progressive failure of ventricular emptying; pulmonary congestion; failure of right side of heart, with systemic venous congestion; sudden cardiac death	Exertional dyspnea; exercise intolerance; syncope; angina; heart failure (LV failure)	• Chest radiograph: poststenotic aortic dilation, calcification • ECG: LV hypertrophy • Auscultation: systolic ejection murmur • Catheterization: significant pressure gradient, increased LV end-diastolic pressure
C ↑ **indicates stenosis**			
Aortic Valve Regurgitation Aortic valve regurgitation	Increased volume load imposed on LV; LV dilation and hypertrophy	Fatigue; dyspnea and exertion; palpitations	• Chest radiograph: boot-shaped elongation of cardiac apex • ECG: LV hypertrophy • Auscultation: diastolic murmur • Catheterization: opacification of LV during aortic injection • Peripheral signs: hyperdynamic myocardial action and low peripheral resistance
D **indicates backward flow from a valve that is leaking or regurgitant**			
Tricuspid Valve Stenosis Tricuspid valve stenosis	Right atrium must generate higher pressure to eject blood beyond lesion; right atrial dilation; systemic venous engorgement; increased venous pressure	Venous distention; peripheral edema; ascites; hepatic engorgement; anorexia	• Chest radiograph: right atrial enlargement • ECG: right atrial enlargement (P pulmonale) • Auscultation: diastolic murmur • Catheterization: elevated right atrial pressure with large a waves; pressure gradient across tricuspid valve
E ↓ **indicates stenosis**			
Tricuspid Valve Regurgitation Tricuspid valve regurgitation	Right ventricular hypertrophy and dilation	Decreased cardiac output; neck vein distention; hepatic engorgement; ascites; edema; pleural effusions	• Chest radiograph: right atrial and ventricular enlargement • ECG: right ventricular hypertrophy and right atrial enlargement, atrial fibrillation • Auscultation: murmur throughout systole • Catheterization: elevated right atrial pressure and v waves
F **indicates backward flow from a valve that is leaking or regurgitant**			

ECG, Electrocardiogram; *LA,* left atrium; *LV,* left ventricular; *P mitrale,* m-shaped P waves that occur in left atrial hypertrophy and are often caused by mitral stenosis; *P pulmonale,* tall, peaked P waves that occur in right atrial hypertrophy and are often caused by chronic pulmonary disease. *RA,* right atrium; *RV,* right ventricle.

retrograde flow of blood into the left atrium with each ventricular contraction. It is always described as chronic or acute because of the very different effect on the left-sided chambers.

In chronic mitral valve regurgitation, the left atrium has dilated to accommodate the additional regurgitant volume, whereas the left ventricle has hypertrophied (increased muscle) to maintain an adequate stroke volume and cardiac output.[71] In contrast, acute mitral valve regurgitation is precipitated by chordae tendineae or papillary muscle rupture resulting from an acute MI or IE.[70] This is a medical emergency. The left atrium cannot accommodate the sudden increase in volume and pressure. An IABP and inotropic and afterload-reducing pharmacologic support are often required to increase forward output and to reduce pulmonary congestion.[71,72] After the patient's condition has stabilized, surgical replacement or repair of the incompetent valve is performed.[69] A transcatheter mitral valve repair may be considered for a patient with chronic severe MR and NYHA class III or IV symptoms. Percutaneous mitral valve repair using the MitraClip (Abbot Vascular) device provides a minimally invasive transcatheter means of mitral valve repair. This procedure has reduced severity of MR, improved symptoms, and led to reverse left ventricular remodeling.[70,73] Current clinical studies are in progress to evaluate a new transcatheter mitral valve replacement system (Medtronic Intrepid) for high-risk surgical patients.[74]

Aortic Valve Stenosis

The term *aortic valve stenosis* describes a narrowing of the aortic valve area. It can result from aging, rheumatic valvulitis, or deterioration of a congenital bicuspid valve (see Table 11.10).[70,75] The pathologic hallmarks are inflammation, fibrous valvular thickening, and tissue calcification resembling bone formation.[70] When the aortic valvular opening is reduced to less than 1.5 cm^2, the condition is classified as mild. Cardiac catheterization or Doppler echocardiography can identify a gradient of less than 25 mm Hg across the valve.[70] *Gradient* represents the difference in systolic pressure between the left ventricle and the aorta. A significant pressure difference is a diagnostic hallmark of valvular stenosis.

If the valve orifice has narrowed to 1 cm^2 or less, the gradient will be greater than 40 mm Hg, and the diagnosis will be upgraded to severe aortic valve stenosis.[70] The impedance of left ventricular ejection into the aorta results in increased left ventricular systolic pressure, left ventricular hypertrophy, and eventually left ventricular dilation.

When symptoms such as angina, dyspnea, syncope, and other indicators of heart failure develop, it is critical to intervene to prevent further damage to the left ventricle. Aortic valve replacement is usually indicated. Congenitally abnormal valves may require replacement by the fourth to sixth decades, and the degenerative changes are often tolerated until approximately 72 years of age.[70] For patients with severe aortic stenosis and high to intermediate surgical risk, percutaneous transcatheter aortic valve replacement procedures have proven safe and effective.[76,77] Studies of these percutaneous procedures have demonstrated decreased mortality, improved quality of life, and cost-effectiveness.[70,76,77]

Aortic Valve Regurgitation

Aortic regurgitation, also known as *aortic insufficiency*, may occur as a result of rheumatic fever, systemic hypertension, Marfan syndrome, syphilis, rheumatoid arthritis, aging valve tissue, discrete subaortic stenosis, or percutaneous interventions such as balloon dilation or transcatheter aortic valve replacement (see Table 11.10).[70] Aortic valve incompetence results in a reflux of blood back into the left ventricle during ventricular diastole. To accommodate this extra volume, the

left ventricle initially dilates and then enlarges in an attempt to empty more completely and to meet the needs of the peripheral circulation. Aortic valve replacement is recommended for symptomatic patients with well-preserved or moderate left ventricular dysfunction.[70]

Tricuspid Valve Stenosis

Tricuspid valve stenosis is rarely an isolated lesion (see Table 11.10). It often occurs in conjunction with mitral or aortic disease or congenital disease (Ebstein anomaly). Its origin most often is rheumatic fever or a complication of IVDA and resultant IE.[70] Tricuspid valve stenosis increases the pressure and work of the usually low-pressure right atrium, resulting in right atrial hypertrophy. The right atrium dilates in an attempt to accommodate the residual right atrial volume and the incoming venous return. As a result, systemic venous congestion occurs, the consequences of which include jugular venous congestion, liver failure, hepatomegaly, ascites, and peripheral edema.

Tricuspid Valve Regurgitation

Tricuspid valve regurgitation usually results from advanced failure of the left side of the heart that eventually affects the right side of the heart, severe PH, or as a complication of IE. Other causes include carcinoid, rheumatoid arthritis, radiation therapy, trauma, and Marfan syndrome (see Table 11.10).[70]

Pulmonary Valve Disease

Pulmonary valve disease is an uncommon disorder in adults. It is most often related to congenital anomalies and produces failure of the right side of the heart.[70] Acquired cases are most often related to carcinoid or rheumatic fever pathologies. Initial symptoms include dyspnea, and symptoms of severe heart failure occur with disease progression. Balloon valvuloplasty has proven successful for treatment of these patients,[70] although there is a high recurrence rate. More recent studies have proved percutaneous pulmonary valve and valve conduits as successful replacements for the pulmonary valve apparatus.[78]

Mixed Valvular Lesions

Many persons have *mixed valvular lesions* as an element of stenosis and regurgitation. Mixed lesions can accentuate the severity of a condition. For example, when combined, aortic stenosis and aortic regurgitation increase left ventricular volume and pressure and multiply the degree of left ventricular work.

Medical Management

Management of valvular disorders includes pharmacologic therapy to control symptoms of heart failure and cardiac surgical repair or replacement of the affected valve.[69] When surgery is not feasible, balloon dilation is a rare option selected for patients too ill to undergo a major cardiac surgical procedure.[70] Percutaneous valve devices including stent valves and mitral clips are being evaluated as a less invasive alternative.[70]

Nursing Management

Care management for a patient with valvular heart disease incorporates a variety of patient diagnoses (Box 11.17). Nursing priorities focus on achievement of adequate cardiac output, maintenance of fluid balance, and patient and family education. See Appendix A for patient care management plans specific to patients with valvular heart disease.

Cardiac Output

Low cardiac output is a common finding in patients with valvular heart disease. It can occur because of decreased forward flow through a

BOX 11.17 PRIORITY PATIENT CARE MANAGEMENT

Valvular Heart Disease

- Impaired Cardiac Output due to alterations in preload
- Impaired Cardiac Output due to alterations in afterload
- Impaired Cardiac Output due to alterations in contractility
- Impaired Cardiac Output due to alterations in heart rate or rhythm
- Activity Intolerance due to cardiopulmonary dysfunction
- Lack of Knowledge of Treatment Regime due to lack of previous exposure to information (see Box 11.18, Patient and Family Education Plan: Valvular Heart Disease)

  Patient Care Management plans are located in Appendix A.

stenotic valve, bidirectional flow across an incompetent valve, or associated heart failure. Vital signs and the effect of positive inotropic and afterload-reducing agents are assessed and documented. If the patient has hemodynamic catheters inserted, cardiac output and hemodynamic parameters are measured and evaluated. Patient care activities are carefully planned to provide adequate rest periods to prevent fatigue.

Fluid Balance

Fluid status is evaluated by auscultation of breath sounds for crackles, heart sounds for presence of S_3, daily weights to trend a "sudden weight gain," and presence of peripheral edema. The appearance of pulmonary crackles or an S_3 heart sound confirms volume overload. The jugular vein is assessed for signs of increased distention. Diuretics

BOX 11.18 PRIORITY PATIENT AND FAMILY EDUCATION

Valvular Heart Disease

Before discharge, the patient should be able to teach back the following topics:

- Pathophysiology of valvular disease
- Infection control: prophylactic antibiotics related to dental work or other invasive procedures
- Heart failure: If symptoms of heart failure are present, education is provided on fluid and sodium restriction, fluid balance, diuretic management, daily weight, and controlling breathlessness.
- Surgery: If open-heart surgery was performed, information about postsurgical recovery is provided.
- Medications: Medications may be complex, and information must be given in writing and orally:
  - Preload: purpose of diuretics, increased urine output, and control of fluid volume

- Afterload: purpose of vasodilators or angiotensin-converting enzyme inhibitors in decreasing the workload of the heart
- Heart rate: Purpose of digoxin is to control the rate in atrial fibrillation, a frequent dysrhythmia in heart failure.
- Contractility: With the exception of digoxin, no oral contractility medications are approved by US Food and Drug Administration.
- Anticoagulation: Patients with distended atria, enlarged ventricles, atrial fibrillation, or mechanical valves may be prescribed anticoagulants such as warfarin (Coumadin); risks of bleeding, importance of correct dosages, prothrombin times, international normalized ratio, and nutritional-pharmacologic interactions are emphasized.
- Follow-up care after discharge
- Symptoms to report to a health care professional

BOX 11.19 Evidence-Based Practice

Valvular Heart Disease

Class I recommendations with strong evidence are provided.

Recommendations for Detection and Surveillance of Valvular Disease by Echocardiography

- Echocardiography is noninvasive and is used for all initial diagnostic and serial follow-up evaluations.

Recommendations for Aortic Stenosis

- Echocardiography is the primary diagnostic tool.
- Coronary arteriography is used before aortic valve replacement (AVR) if coronary artery disease (CAD) is suspected.
- AVR is recommended for symptomatic patients with severe aortic stenosis; AVR can be combined with coronary artery bypass graft (CABG) surgery when CAD is present.

Recommendations for Aortic Regurgitation

- Echocardiography is the primary diagnostic tool.
- Cardiac catheterization is used if noninvasive tests are inconclusive.
- AVR is indicated for symptomatic patients with severe AR regardless of left ventricular (LV) systolic function.
- AVR is indicated for nonsymptomatic patients with severe AR with LV systolic dysfunction (ejection fraction <0.5 [50%]); AVR can be combined with CABG surgery if CAD is present.

Recommendations for Mitral Stenosis

- Echocardiography is the primary diagnostic tool.
- Anticoagulation is indicated in patients with mitral stenosis (MS) and atrial fibrillation (paroxysmal, persistent, or permanent) and in patients with MS in sinus rhythm with a prior embolic event or left atrial thrombus.
- Cardiac catheterization if noninvasive tests are inconclusive.
- Mitral valve repair (preferable) or mitral valve replacement is indicated for symptomatic (New York Heart Association functional class III or IV) moderate or severe MS if percutaneous mitral balloon valvuloplasty is contraindicated.

Recommendations for Mitral Regurgitation

- Echocardiography is the primary diagnostic tool.
- Cardiac catheterization if noninvasive tests are inconclusive or if additional hemodynamic measurements are required.
- Mitral valve repair is the operation of choice over valve replacement in most patients with chronic mitral regurgitation.

  See Box 11.16 for prophylaxis to prevent infective endocarditis for patients with valve disease and prosthetic valves.

Reference

Nishimura RA, Otto CM, Bonow RO, et al. 2014 AHA/ACC guideline for the management of patients with valvular heart disease. *J Am Coll Cardiol.* 2014;63(22):e57.

BOX 11.20 **Informatics**

Internet Resources: Cardiovascular Disorders
American Heart Association: Guidelines and Statements https://professional. heart.org/en/guidelines-and-statements
American Heart Association: Health Topics https://www.heart.org/en/ health-topics/

and vasodilators are administered to counteract excess fluid retention. The patient is weighed daily, and fluid intake and output are monitored and recorded.

Educate the Patient and Family

Education for a patient with acute or chronic heart failure caused by valvular dysfunction includes (1) information related to diet, (2) fluid restrictions, (3) the actions and side effects of heart failure medications, (4) the need for prophylactic antibiotics before undergoing any invasive procedures, and (5) when to call the health care provider to report a negative change in cardiac symptoms (see Box 11.18).

Many patients also require information about valvular heart surgery or percutaneous replacement procedures. Achieving optimal outcomes for a patient with valve disease requires contributions from a team of educated health care clinicians. Collaborative multidisciplinary priorities are listed in Box 11.19. In Chapter 12, the section on valvular surgery provides more information on surgical management.

ADDITIONAL RESOURCES

Internet resources related to cardiovascular disorders are found in Box 11.20.

REFERENCES

1. Benjamin EJ, Muntner P, Alonso A, et al. Heart disease and stroke statistics—2019 update: a report from the American Heart Association. *Circulation.* 2019;139:e56—e528.
2. Lloyd-Jones DM, Hong Y, Labarthe D, et al. Defining and setting national goals for cardiovascular health promotion and disease reduction. The American Heart Association's Strategic Impact Goal through 2020 and beyond. *Circulation.* 2010;121:586—613.
3. Vikulova DN, Grubisic M, Zhai Y, et al. Premature atherosclerotic cardiovascular disease: trends in incidence, risk factors, and sex-related differences, 2000 to 2016. *J Am Heart Assoc.* 2019;8:e1—e12.
4. Yusef S, Hawken S, Ounpuu S, et al. INTERHEART Study Investigators. Effect of potentially modifiable risk factors associated with myocardial infarction in 52 countries (The INTERHEART Study): case-control study. *Lancet.* 2004;364(9438):937.
5. Arnett DK, Blumenthal RS, Albert MA, et al. ACC/AHA guideline on the primary prevention of cardiovascular disease: a report of the American College of Cardiology/American Heart Association Task Force on Clinical Practice Guidelines. *Circulation.* 2019;140(11):e596—e646.
6. Grundy SM, Stone NJ, Bailey AL, et al. AHA/ACC/AACVPR/AAPA/ABC/ APCM/ADA/AGS/APhA/ASPC/NLA/PCNA guidelines on management of blood cholesterol: executive summary. *Circulation.* 2018;(139):e1046—e1081.
7. Arora S, Patra SK, Saini R. HDL—a molecule with multifaceted role in coronary artery disease. *Clin Chim Acta.* 2016;452:66—81.
8. Miller M, Stone NJ, Ballantyne C, et al. Triglycerides and cardiovascular disease: a scientific statement from the American Heart Association. *Circulation.* 2011;123:2292—2333.
9. Eckel RH, Jakicic JM, Ard JD, et al. 2013 Guidelines on lifestyle management to reduce cardiovascular risk. *J Am Coll Cardiol.* 2014;63(25): 2960—2984.
10. Fox CS. Update on prevention of cardiovascular disease in adults with type 2 diabetes mellitus in light of recent evidence: a scientific statement from the American Heart Association and the American Diabetes Association. *Diabetes Care.* 2015;38:1777—1803.
11. Goff DC, Lloyd-Jones DM, Bennett G, et al. ACC/AHA guideline on assessment of cardiovascular risk. A report of the American College of Cardiology/American Heart Association Task Force on Practice Guidelines. *J Am Coll Cardiol.* 2013;63(25):2935—2959.
12. Smith SC, Benjamin EJ, Bonow RO, et al. AHA/ACC secondary prevention and risk reduction therapy for patients with coronary and other atherosclerotic vascular disease. 2011 update: a guideline from the American Heart Association and American College of Cardiology Foundation. *Circulation.* 2011;24:2458.
13. Rosendorff C, Lackland DT, Allison M, et al. Treatment of hypertension in patients with coronary artery disease. A scientific statement from the American Heart Association, American College of Cardiology, and American Society of Hypertension. *Hypertension.* 2015;65:1372—1407.
14. Grundy SM. Pre-diabetes, metabolic syndrome, and cardiovascular risk. *J Am Coll Cardiol.* 2012;59(7):635—643.
15. James PA. Evidence-based guidelines for the management of high blood pressure in adults. report from the panel members appointed to the Eighth Joint National Committee (JNC8). *JAMA.* 2014;311(5):507—520.
16. Sargent RP, Shepard RM, Glantz SA. Reduced incidence of admissions for myocardial infarction associated with public smoking ban: before and after study. *BMJ.* 2004;328(7446):977.
17. Mosca L, Benjamin EJ, Berra K, et al. Effectiveness-based guidelines for the prevention of cardiovascular disease in women—2011 update: a guideline from the American Heart Association. *Circulation.* 2011;123: 1243—1262.
18. Anderson GL, Limacher M, Assaf AR, et al. Effects of conjugated equine estrogen in postmenopausal women with hysterectomy: The Women's Health Initiative randomized controlled trial. *JAMA.* 2004;291(14):1701.
19. Mehta LS, Beckie TM, DeVon HA, et al. Acute myocardial infarction in women. A scientific statement from the American Heart Association. *Circulation.* 2016;133:916—947.
20. McSweeney JC. Preventing and experiencing ischemic heart disease as a woman: state of the science. A scientific statement from the American Heart Association. *Circulation.* 2016;133:1302—1331.
21. Brown HL, Warner JJ, Gianos E, et al. Promoting risk identification and reduction of cardiovascular disease in women through collaboration with obstetricians and gynecologists. *Circulation.* 2018;137:e843—e852.
22. Soeki T, Sata M. Inflammatory biomarkers and atherosclerosis. *Int Heart J.* 2016;57(2):134—139.
23. Aydin S, Ugur K, Aydin S, Sahin I, Yardim M. Biomarkers in acute myocardial infarction: current perspectives. *Vasc Health and Risk Manag.* 2019;15:1—10.
24. Adamcova M, Popelova-Lencova O, Jirkovsky E, et al. Cardiac troponins—translational biomarkers in cardiology: theory and practice of cardiac troponin high-sensitivity assays. *Biofactors.* 2016;42(2):133—148.
25. Lupton JR, Quispe R, Kulkarni K, Martine SS, Jones SR, et al. Serum homocysteine is not independently associated with an atherogenic lipid profile: the Very Large Database of Lipids (VLDL-21) study. *Atherosclerosis.* 2016;249:59—64.
26. Fihn SD, Gardin JM, Abrams J, et al. ACCF/AHA/ACP/AATS/PCNA/ SCAI/STS guideline for the diagnosis and management of patients with stable ischemic heart disease: a report of the American College of Cardiology Foundation/American Heart Association Task Force on Practice Guidelines, and the American College of Physicians, American Association for Thoracic Surgery, Preventive Cardiovascular Nurses Association, Society for Cardiovascular Angiography and Interventions, and Society of Thoracic Surgeons. *Circulation.* 2012;126(25):e354—e471.
27. Amsterdam EA, Wenger NK, Brindis RG, et al. AHA/ACC guideline for the management of patients with non-ST elevation acute coronary syndromes. A report of the American College of Cardiology/American Heart Association Task Force on Practice Guidelines. *Circulation.* 2014;2014(130): e344—e426.
28. O'Gara PT, Kushner FG, Ascheim DD, et al. ACCF/AHA guideline for the management of ST-elevation myocardial infarction: a report of the

American College of Cardiology Foundation/American Heart Association Task Force on Practice Guidelines. *Circulation.* 2013;127(4):e362.

29. de Luna AB, Cygankiewicz I, Baranchuk A, et al. Prinzmetal angina: ECG changes and clinical considerations: a consensus paper. *Ann Noninvasive Electrocardiol.* 2014;19(5):442–453.

30. Levine GN, Bates ER, Blankenship J, et al. ACC/AHA/SCAI guideline for percutaneous coronary intervention: executive summary: a report of the American College of Cardiology Foundation/American Heart Association Task Force on Practice Guidelines and the Society for Cardiovascular Angiography and Interventions. *Circulation.* 2011;124:2574.

31. Craig TJ. AHA/ACC/HRS focused update of the 2014 AHA/ACC/HRS guideline for the management of patients with atrial fibrillation. *Circulation.* 2019;2019(140):e125–e151.

32. Novak M, Novak M, Hlinomaz O, et al. Ventricular septal rupture—a critical condition as a complication of acute myocardial infarction. *JCCM.* 2015;1(4):162–166.

33. Meris A, Amigoni M, Verma A, et al. Mechanisms and predictors of mitral regurgitation after high-risk myocardial infarction. *J Am Soc Echocardiogr.* 2012;25(5):535.

34. Bière L, Mateus V, Clerfond G, et al. Predictive factors of pericardial effusion after a first acute myocardial infarction and successful reperfusion. *Am J Cardiol.* 2015;116:497–503.

35. Kloos JA. Characteristics, complications, and treatment of acute pericarditis. *Crit Care Nurs Clin North Am.* 2015;27(4):483.

36. Krumholz HM, Merrill AR, Schone EM, et al. Patterns of hospital performance in acute myocardial infarction and heart failure 30-day mortality and readmission. *Circ Cardiovasc Qual Outcomes.* 2009;5(2):407.

37. O'Neil A, Sanderson K, Oldenburg B. Depression as a predictor of work resumption following myocardial infarction (MI): a review of recent research evidence. *Health Qual Life Outcomes.* 2010;8:95.

38. Anderson L, Oldridge N, Thompson DR, et al. Exercise-based cardiac rehabilitation for coronary heart disease Cochrane systematic review and meta-analysis. *J Am Coll Cardiol.* 2016;67:1–12.

39. Al-Khatib SM, Stevenson WG, Ackerman MJ, et al. AHA/ACC/HRS guideline for management of patients with ventricular arrhythmias and the prevention of sudden cardiac death: executive summary: a report of the American College of Cardiology Foundation/American Heart Association Task Force on Clinical Practice Guidelines and the Heart Rhythm Society. *Circulation.* 2017;2018(138):e210–e271.

40. Ong MEH, Perkins GD, Cariou A. Out of hospital cardiac arrest: prehospital management. *Lancet.* 2018;391:980–988.

41. Packer M. What causes sudden death in patients with chronic heart failure and a reduced ejection fraction? *EurHeart J.* 2019:1–7.

42. Probst V, Veltmann C, Eckardt L, et al. Long term prognosis of patients diagnosed with Brugada syndrome. results from the FINGER Brugada syndrome registry. *Circulation.* 2010;121:635–643.

43. Priori SG, Blomström-Lundqvist C, Mazzanti A, et al. ESC guidelines for the management of patients with ventricular arrhythmias and the prevention of sudden cardiac death. *Eur Heart J.* 2015;2015(36):2793–2867.

44. Ghani A, Maas AH, Delnoy PP, Ramdat Misier AR, Ottervanger JP, Elvan A. Sex based differences in cardiac arrhythmias. ICD utilization and cardiac resynchronization therapy. *Neth Heart.* 2011;19(1):35.

45. Yancy CW, Jessup M, Bozkurt B, et al. ACCF/AHA guideline for the management of heart failure. A report of the American College of Cardiology Foundation/American Heart Association Task Force on Practice Guidelines. *J Am Coll Cardiol.* 2013;62(16):e147–e239.

46. Namana V, Gupta SS, Abbasi AA, Hitesh R, Shani J, Hallander G. Right ventricular infarction. *Card Revasc Med.* 2018;19:43–50.

47. Yancy CW, Jessup M, Bozkurt B, et al. ACC/AHA/HFSA focused update of the 2013 ACCF/AHA guideline for the management of heart failure: a report of the American College of Cardiology/American Heart Association Task Force on Clinical Practice Guidelines and the Heart Failure Society of America. *Circulation.* 2017;2017(136):e137–e161.

48. Paul S, Page RL. Foundations of pharmacotherapy for heart failure with reduced ejection fraction. Evidence meets practice, part 1. *J Cardiovasc Nurs.* 2016;31(2):101–113.

49. Heo S, Shin MS, Hwang SY, et al. Sex differences in heart failure symptoms and factors associated with heart failure symptoms. *J Cardiovasc Nurs.* 2019;34(4):306–312.

50. Tanai E, Frantz S. Pathophysiology of heart failure. *Comp Physiol.* 2016;6:187–214.

51. Chow, Maisel AS, Anand I, et al. Role of biomarkers for the prevention, assessment, and management of heart failure a scientific statement from the American Heart Association. *Circulation.* 2017;135:e1054–e1091.

52. Prasad R, Pugh PJ. Drug and device therapy for patients with chronic heart failure. *Expert Rev Cardiovasc Ther.* 2012;10(3):313.

53. Singh JP, Gras D. Biventricular pacing: current trends and future strategies. *Eur Heart J.* 2012;33:305.

54. Arshad A, Moss AJ, Foster E, et al. Cardiac resynchronization therapy is more effective in women than in men: The MADIT-CRT (Multicenter Automatic Defibrillator Implantation Trial With Cardiac Resynchronization Therapy) trial. *J Am Coll Cardiol.* 2011;57:813.

55. Linde C, Ellenbogen K, McAllister FA. Cardiac resynchronization therapy (CRT): clinical trials, guidelines, and target populations. *Heart Rhythm.* 2012;9(suppl 8):S3.

56. Kavalieratos D, Gelfman LP, Tycon LE, et al. Palliative care in heart failure rationale, evidence, and future priorities. *J Am Coll Cardiol.* 2017;20(15):1919–1930.

57. Rogers JG, Patel CB, Mentz RJ, et al. Palliative care in heart failure: the PAL-HF randomized, controlled clinical trial. *JACC.* 2017;70(3):331–341.

58. Cajita MI, Cajita TR, Han HR. Health literacy and heart failure: a systematic review. *J Cardiovasc Nurs.* 2016;31(2):121–130.

59. White M, Garbez R, Carroll M, Brinker E, Howie-Esquivel J. Is "teach-back" associated with knowledge retention and hospital readmission in hospitalized heart failure patients? *J Cardiovasc Nurs.* 2013;28(2):137–146.

60. Jessup M, Drazner MH, Book W, et al. ACC/AHA/HFSA/ISHLT/ACP advanced training statement on advanced heart failure and transplant cardiology (revision of the ACCF/AHA/ACP/HFSA/ISHLT 2010 clinical competence statement on management of patients with advanced heart failure and cardiac transplant). A report of the ACC Competency Management Committee. *Circ Heart Fail.* 2017;2017(10):e000021.

61. Bozkurt B, Colvin M, Cook J, et al. Current diagnostic and treatment strategies for specific dilated cardiomyopathies: a scientific statement from the American Heart Association. *Circulation.* 2016;134:e579–e646.

62. Hensley N, Dietrich J, Nyhan D, Mitter N, Yee MS, Brady M. Hypertrophic cardiomyopathy: a review. *Anesth Analg.* 2015;120:554–569.

63. Shah M. Hypertrophic cardiomyopathy. *Cardiol Young.* 2017;27(1):s25–s30.

64. Kelkar AA, Butler J, Schelbert EB, et al. Mechanisms contributing to the progression of ischemic and nonischemic dilated cardiomyopathy: possible modulating effects of paracrine activities of stem cells. *J Am Coll Cardiol.* 2015;66(18):2038–2047.

65. Luttenberger K, DiNapoli M. Subacute bacterial endocarditis: making the diagnosis. *Nurs Practice.* 2011;36(3):31–38.

66. Bojar RM. *Manual of Perioperative Care in Adult Cardiac Surgery.* 5th ed. Hoboken, NJ: Wiley-Blackwell; 2011.

67. Laing C. Understanding infective endocarditis. *Nursing 2015 Critical Care.* 2015;10(5):6–9.

68. Baddour, Wilson WR, Bayer AS, et al. Infective endocarditis in adults: diagnosis, antimicrobial therapy, and management of complication. *Circulation.* 2015;132:1435–1485.

69. Habib G, Lancellotti P, Antunes MJ, et al. ESC guidelines for the management of infective endocarditis. The Task Force for the Management of Infective Endocarditis of the European Society of Cardiology (ESC). *Eur Heart J.* 2015;36(42):2921–2964.

70. Nishimura RA, Otto CM, Bonow RO, et al. AHA/ACC guideline for the management of patients with valvular heart disease: a report of the American College of Cardiology/American Heart Association Task Force on Practice Guidelines. *J Am Coll Cardiol.* 2014;63(22):e57–e185.

71. Reimche R, et al. Complications of infective endocarditis: the common to the devastating. *Can J Cardiol.* 2017;33(10):s211.

72. Romeo F, Acconcia MC, Sergi D, et al. The outcome of intra-aortic balloon pump support in acute myocardial infarction complicated by cardiogenic shock according to the type of revascularization: a comprehensive meta-analysis. *Am Heart J.* 2013;165:679—692.

73. Magruder JT, Crawford TC, Grimm JC, Fredi JL, Shah AS. Managing mitral regurgitation: focus on the MitraClip device. *Medical Devices.* 2016;9: 53—60.

74. Overtchouk P, Granada JF, Modine T. Transcatheter mitral valve replacement: current challenges and future perspective. *Cardiac Interventions Today.* 2019;13(3):42—46.

75. Siu SC, Silverside CK. Bicuspid aortic valve. *J Am Coll Cardiol.* 2010;55(2):2789.

76. Popma JJ, Deeb M, Yakubov SJ, et al. Transcatheter aortic-valve replacement with self-expanding valve in low-risk patients. *N Engl J Med.* 2019;380(18):1706—1715.

77. Brown DL. Expanding indications for TAVR: the preferred procedure in intermediate risk patients? *Cleve Clin J Med.* 2017;84(12 suppl 4):e10—e14.

78. Ansari MM, Cardoso R, Garcia D, et al. Percutaneous pulmonary valve implantation, present status and evolving future. *J Am Coll Cardiol.* 2015;66(20):2246—2255.

Cardiovascular Therapeutic Management

Joni L. Dirks and Julie M. Waters

PACEMAKERS

Pacemakers are electronic devices that can be used to initiate the heartbeat when the intrinsic electrical system of the heart cannot effectively generate a rate adequate to support cardiac output. Pacemakers may be used temporarily, either supportively or prophylactically, until the condition responsible for the rate or conduction disturbance resolves. The use of permanent pacemakers as a form of device-based therapy has expanded significantly.[1] Only a brief discussion of permanent pacemakers is provided, to describe similarities and differences between permanent (implanted) and temporary pacemakers. Pacemakers are also used diagnostically to elicit ventricular and supraventricular dysrhythmias during an electrophysiology study (EPS).[1-4]

This section emphasizes temporary pacemakers because the critical care nurse is responsible for preventing, assessing, and managing pacemaker malfunctions when these devices are used in the clinical setting.

Indications for Temporary Pacing

The clinical indications for instituting temporary pacemaker therapy are similar regardless of the cause of the rhythm disturbance that necessitates the placement of a pacemaker. The causes range from ischemia and electrolyte imbalances to sequelae related to acute myocardial infarction (MI) or following cardiac surgery.

Pacemaker System

A pacemaker system is a simple electrical circuit consisting of a pulse generator and a pacing lead (an insulated electrical wire) with one, two, or three electrodes.

Temporary Pacemaker Pulse Generator

The pulse generator is designed to generate an electrical current that travels through the pacing lead and exits through an electrode (exposed portion of the wire) that is in direct contact with the heart. This electrical current initiates a myocardial depolarization. The current then returns by one of several pathways to the pulse generator to complete the circuit.

Temporary Pacing Lead Systems

The pacing lead used for temporary pacing may be bipolar or unipolar. In a bipolar system, two electrodes (positive and negative) are located within the heart, whereas in a unipolar system, only one electrode (negative) is in direct contact with the myocardium. In both systems, the current flows from the negative terminal of the pulse generator, down the pacing lead to the negative electrode, and into the heart. The current is then picked up by the positive electrode (ground)

and flows back up the lead to the positive terminal of the pulse generator.[5]

Transvenous Pacing

The bipolar lead used in transvenous pacing has two electrodes on one catheter (Fig. 12.1). The distal, or negative, electrode is at the tip of the pacing lead and is in direct contact with the heart, usually inside the right atrium or right ventricle. Approximately 1 cm from the negative electrode is a positive electrode. The negative electrode is attached to the negative terminal, and the positive electrode is attached to the positive terminal of the pulse generator, either directly or by means of a bridging cable (see Fig. 12.1B).

Epicardial Pacing

An epicardial lead system is often used for temporary pacing after cardiac surgery.[6] The bipolar epicardial lead system has two separate insulated wires (one negative and one positive electrode) that are loosely secured with sutures to the cardiac chamber to be paced. Both leads are in contact with the myocardial tissue, so either wire may be used as the negative, or pacing, electrode. The remaining wire is then used as the positive, or ground, electrode.

Pacing Routes

Several routes are available for temporary cardiac pacing.

Transcutaneous Pacing

Transcutaneous cardiac pacing involves the use of two large skin electrodes, one placed anteriorly and the other posteriorly on the chest, connected to an external pulse generator. It is a rapid, noninvasive procedure that nurses can perform in the emergency setting and is recommended in the advanced cardiac life support algorithm for the treatment of symptomatic bradycardia that does not respond to atropine.[7] Improved technology related to stimulus delivery and the development of large electrode pads that help disperse the energy have helped reduce the pain associated with cutaneous nerve and muscle stimulation. Discomfort may still be an issue for some patients, particularly when higher energy levels are required to achieve capture. This route is typically used as a short-term therapy until the situation resolves or another route of pacing can be established.

Epicardial Pacing

The insertion of temporary epicardial pacing wires has become a routine procedure during many cardiac surgical cases. Ventricular and, in many cases, atrial pacing wires are loosely sewn to the epicardium. The terminal pins of these wires are pulled through the skin before the chest is closed. If both chambers have pacing wires

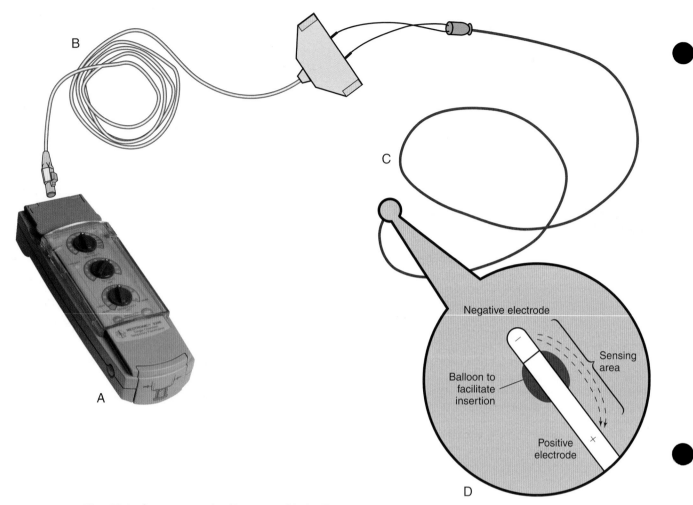

Fig. 12.1 Components of a Temporary Bipolar Transvenous Catheter. (A) Single-chamber temporary (external) pulse generator. (B) Bridging cable. (C) Pacing lead. (D) Enlarged view of pacing lead tip. (A, Reproduced with permission from Medtronic, Inc.)

attached, the atrial wires exit subcostally to the right of the sternum, and the ventricular wires exit in the same region but to the left of the sternum. These wires can be removed several days after surgery by gentle traction at the skin surface with minimal risk of bleeding.[8]

Transvenous Pacing

Temporary transvenous endocardial pacing is accomplished by advancing a pacing electrode wire through a vein, often the subclavian or internal jugular vein, and into the right atrium or right ventricle. Insertion can be facilitated through direct visualization with fluoroscopy or use of a standard electrocardiogram (ECG).

In some rare cases, the pacing wire is inserted through a special pulmonary artery catheter by means of a port that exits in the right atrium or right ventricle.

Five-Letter Pacemaker Codes

Pacemaker terminology was initially limited to *fixed-rate* and *demand* pacing and atrioventricular or *AV sequential* pacing. Although these terms are useful for understanding pacemaker function, the expansion of functional capabilities of pulse generators necessitated a more precise classification system. Table 12.1 describes the current five-letter code.[9] This code is designed to incorporate physiologic pacing.[10]

Temporary pacing is described using the letters in the first three positions of the code (see Table 12.1). The first letter refers to the cardiac chamber that is paced. The second letter designates which chamber is sensed, and the third letter indicates the pacemaker's response to the sensed event (I. Paced; II. Sensed; III. Response to sensing). Temporary pacing modes are listed in Table 12.2.

Temporary Pacemaker Settings

The controls on all external temporary pulse generators are similar. Their functions must be thoroughly understood so that pacing can be initiated quickly in an emergency situation and troubleshooting can be facilitated if problems with the pacemaker arise.

Rate Control

The *rate control* regulates the number of impulses that can be delivered to the heart per minute. The rate setting depends on the physiologic needs of the patient, but it is usually maintained between 60 and 80 beats/min. Pacing rates for overdrive suppression of tachydysrhythmias may greatly exceed these values. Some generators have special controls for overdrive pacing that allow for rates of 800 stimuli per minute. If the pacemaker is operating in a dual-chamber mode, the ventricular rate control also regulates the atrial rate.

TABLE 12.1 NASPE/BPEG Generic Code.

Position I: Chambers Paced	Position II: Chambers Sensed	Position III: Response to Sensing	Position IV: Rate Modulation	Position V: Multisite Pacing
0 = None	0 = None	0 = None	0 = None	0 = None
A = Atrium	A = Atrium	T = Triggered	R = Rate modulation	A = Atrium
V = Ventricle	V = Ventricle	I = Inhibited		V = Ventricle
D = Dual (A + V)	D = Dual (A + V)	D = Dual (T + I)		D = Dual (A + V)

BPEG, British Pacing and Electrophysiology Group; *NASPE*, North American Society of Pacing and Electrophysiology.
Modified from Bernstein AD, Daubert JC, Fletcher RD, et al. The revised NASPE/BPEG generic pacemaker code for antibradycardia, adaptive-rate and multisite pacing. *Pacing Clin Electrophysiol.* 2002;25:260.

TABLE 12.2 Examples of Temporary Pacing Modes.

Pacing Mode	Description
Asynchronous	
AOO	Atrial pacing, no sensing
VOO	Ventricular pacing, no sensing
DOO	Atrial and ventricular pacing, no sensing
Synchronous	
AAI	Atrial pacing, atrial sensing, inhibited response to sensed P waves
VVI	Ventricular pacing, ventricular sensing, inhibited response to sensed QRS complexes
DVI	Atrial and ventricular pacing, ventricular sensing; both atrial and ventricular pacing are inhibited if spontaneous ventricular depolarization is sensed
DDD	Both chambers are paced and sensed; inhibited response of pacing stimuli to sensed events in their respective chambers; triggered response to sensed atrial activity to allow for rate-responsive ventricular pacing

BOX 12.1 Determining Temporary Pacemaker Pacing Threshold

1. Adjust pacemaker rate setting so that patient is 100% paced. It may be necessary to increase the pacing rate to achieve this setting.
2. Gradually decrease the output (milliampere) setting until 1:1 capture is lost. The pacing threshold is the point at which capture is lost.
3. Slowly increase the output setting until 1:1 capture is re-established. With a properly positioned pacing electrode, the pacing threshold should be less than 1 mA.
4. Set the output setting two to three times higher than measured threshold because thresholds tend to fluctuate over time.
5. If a dual-chamber pulse generator is being used, evaluate pacing thresholds for the atrial and ventricular leads separately.

Output Control

The *output dial* regulates the amount of electrical current, measured in milliamperes (mA), which is delivered to the heart to initiate depolarization. The point at which depolarization occurs, called *threshold*, is indicated by a myocardial response to the pacing stimulus (i.e., capture). Threshold can be determined by gradually decreasing the output setting until 1:1 capture is lost. The output setting is then slowly increased until 1:1 capture is re-established; this threshold to pace is less than 1 mA with a properly positioned pacing electrode. The output is set two to three times higher than threshold because thresholds tend to fluctuate over time. Box 12.1 details the procedure for measuring pacing thresholds. Separate output controls for atrium and ventricle are used with a dual-chamber pulse generator.

Sensitivity Control

The *sensitivity control* regulates the ability of the pacemaker to detect the heart's intrinsic electrical activity. Sensitivity is measured in millivolts (mV) and determines the size of the intracardiac signal that the generator will recognize. If the sensitivity is adjusted to its most sensitive setting, a setting of 0.5 to 1 mV, the pacemaker can respond even to low-amplitude electrical signals coming from the heart. Turning the sensitivity to its least sensitive setting (i.e., adjusting the dial to a setting of 20 mV or to the area labeled *async*) results in inability of the

pacemaker to sense any intrinsic electrical activity and causes the pacemaker to function at a fixed rate. A sense indicator (often a light) on the pulse generator signals each time intrinsic cardiac electrical activity is sensed. A pulse generator may be designed to sense atrial activity or ventricular activity or both. Box 12.2 describes the procedure for measuring sensitivity. The sensitivity is set at half of the value of the sensitivity threshold to ensure that all appropriate intrinsic cardiac signals are sensed. For example, if the measured sensitivity threshold is 3.0 mV, the generator is set at 1.5 mV. The sensing ability of the pacemaker can be quickly evaluated by observing for a change in pacing rhythm in response to spontaneous depolarizations.

Atrioventricular (AV) Control

The *AV interval control* (available only on dual-chamber generators) regulates the time interval between the atrial and ventricular pacing stimuli. This interval is analogous to the P-R interval that occurs in the intrinsic ECG. Proper adjustment of this interval to between 150 and 250 ms preserves AV synchrony and permits maximal ventricular stroke volume and enhanced cardiac output. Because the AV interval is limited by the length of the cardiac cycle, modern temporary generators automatically adjust the AV delay based on the programmed heart rate.[11]

Dual-Chamber Controls

Temporary dual-chamber pacemakers have other settings that are required in the DDD mode. The *lower rate*, or *base rate*, determines the rate at which the generator will pace when intrinsic activity falls below the set rate of the pacemaker. The *upper rate* determines the fastest ventricular rate the pacemaker will deliver in response to sensed atrial activity. This setting is needed to protect the patient's heart from being

BOX 12.2 Determining Temporary Pacemaker Sensitivity Threshold

1. Set sensitivity control to its most sensitive setting.
2. Adjust the pulse generator rate to 10 beats/min less than patient's intrinsic rate (flash indicator should flash regularly).
3. Reduce the generator output to the minimal value to eliminate the risk of competing with the intrinsic rhythm.
4. Gradually increase the sensitivity value until the sense indicator stops flashing and the pace indicator starts flashing.
5. Decrease sensitivity until the sense indicator begins to flash again; this is the sensitivity threshold.
6. Adjust the sensitivity setting on the generator to half of threshold value; restore the generator output and rate to their original values.

paced in response to rapid atrial dysrhythmias. There also is an *atrial refractory period*, programmable from 150 to 500 ms, which regulates the length of time, after a sensed or paced ventricular event, during which the pacemaker cannot respond to another atrial stimulus. An emergency button is also available on most models to allow for rapid initiation of asynchronous (DOO) pacing during an emergency.

On all temporary pacemakers, an on/off switch is provided with a safety feature that prevents the accidental termination of pacing. On new generators, there is also a locking feature to prevent unintended changes to the prescribed settings.

Pacing Artifacts

All patients with temporary pacemakers require continuous ECG monitoring. The pacing artifact is the spike that is seen on the ECG tracing as the pacing stimulus is delivered to the heart. A *P wave* is visible after the pacing artifact if the atrium is being paced (Fig. 12.2A). Similarly, a *QRS complex* follows a ventricular pacing artifact (Fig. 12.2B). With dual-chamber pacing, a pacing artifact precedes both the P wave and the QRS complex (Fig. 12.2C).

Pacemaker Malfunctions

Most pacemaker malfunctions can be categorized as abnormalities of pacing or of sensing. Problems with pacing can involve failure of the pacemaker to deliver the pacing stimulus, a pacing stimulus that fails to depolarize the heart, or an incorrect number of pacing stimuli per minute.

Pacing Abnormalities

Failure to pace. Failure of the pacemaker to deliver the pacing stimulus results in disappearance of the pacing artifact even if the patient's intrinsic rate is less than the set rate on the pacer. This can occur intermittently or continuously and can be attributed to failure of the pulse generator or its battery, a loose connection between the various components of the pacemaker system, broken lead wires, or stimulus inhibition as a result of electromagnetic interference (EMI). Tightening connections, replacing the batteries or the pulse generator itself, or removing the source of EMI may restore pacemaker function.

Failure to capture. If the pacing stimulus fires but fails to initiate a myocardial depolarization, a pacing artifact will be present but will not

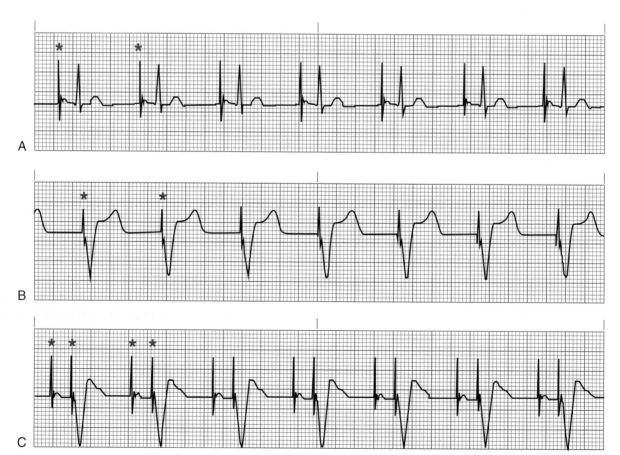

Fig. 12.2   Pacing Examples. (A) Atrial pacing. (B) Ventricular pacing. (C) Dual-chamber pacing. Each asterisk represents a pacemaker impulse.

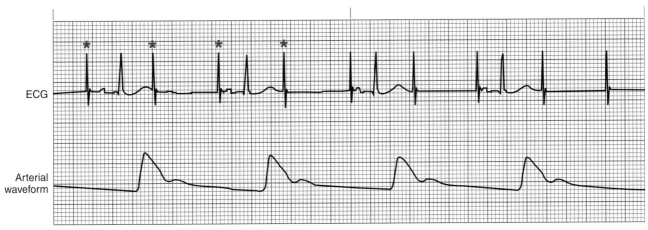

Fig. 12.3 Pacemaker Malfunction: Failure to Capture. Atrial pacing and capture occur after pacer spikes 1, 3, 5, and 7. The remaining pacer spikes fail to capture the tissue, resulting in loss of the P wave, no conduction to the ventricles, and no arterial waveform. Each asterisk represents a pacemaker impulse. *ECG,* Electrocardiogram.

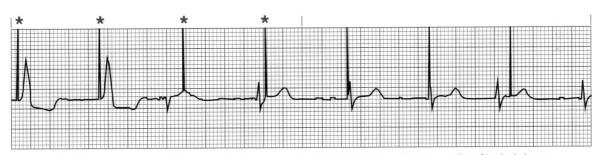

Fig. 12.4 Pacemaker Malfunction: Undersensing. After the first two paced beats, a series of intrinsic beats occurs; the pacemaker unit fails to sense these intrinsic QRS complexes. These spikes do not capture the ventricle because they occur during the refractory period of the cardiac cycle. Each asterisk represents a pacemaker impulse.

be followed by the expected P wave or QRS complex, depending on the chamber being paced (Fig. 12.3). This *loss of capture* can be attributed most often to displacement of the pacing electrode or to an increase in threshold (electrical stimulus necessary to elicit a myocardial depolarization) as a result of medications, metabolic disorders, electrolyte imbalances, or fibrosis or myocardial ischemia at the site of electrode placement. In many cases, increasing the output (mA) elicits capture. For transvenous leads, repositioning the patient on his or her left side may improve lead contact and restore capture.

Rate drift. Pacing can occur at inappropriate rates. For example, impending battery failure in a permanent pacemaker can result in a gradual decrease in the paced rate, also referred to as *rate drift.* Inappropriate stimuli from a pacemaker may result in pacemaker-mediated tachycardia; this usually is caused by sensing of inappropriate signals in a dual-chamber pacemaker that is in a trigger mode, such as DDD. The tachycardia can be terminated by placing a magnet over the generator to transiently suspend sensing.[12]

Sensing Abnormalities

Sensing abnormalities include undersensing and oversensing.

Undersensing. When the pacemaker is unable to sense spontaneous myocardial depolarizations, this is described as undersensing. This malfunction results in competition between paced complexes and the heart's intrinsic rhythm and is manifested on the ECG by pacing artifacts that occur after or are unrelated to spontaneous complexes (Fig. 12.4). Undersensing can result in the delivery of pacing stimuli into a relative refractory period of the cardiac depolarization cycle. A ventricular pacing stimulus delivered into the downslope of the T wave (R-on-T phenomenon) is a real danger with this type of pacer aberration because it may precipitate a lethal dysrhythmia. The nurse must act quickly to determine the cause and initiate appropriate interventions. The cause often can be attributed to inadequate wave amplitude (height of the P or R wave). If this is the case, the situation can be promptly remedied by increasing the sensitivity by moving the sensitivity dial toward its lowest setting. Other possible causes include inappropriate (asynchronous) mode selection, lead displacement or fracture, loose cable connections, and pulse generator failure.

Oversensing. Inappropriate sensing of extraneous electrical signals that lead to unnecessary triggering or inhibition of stimulus output is called oversensing. The source of these electrical signals can range from tall-peaked T waves to EMI in the critical care environment. Because most temporary pulse generators are programmed in demand modes, oversensing results in unexplained pauses in the ECG tracing as the extraneous signals are sensed and inhibit pacing. Moving the sensitivity dial toward 20 mV (less sensitive) often stops the pauses.

Medical Management

The physician determines the pacing route based on the patient's clinical situation. Transcutaneous pacing typically is used in emergent situations until a transvenous lead can be secured. If the patient is undergoing heart surgery, epicardial leads may be electively placed at the end of the operation. The physician places the transvenous or epicardial pacing lead or leads, repositioning them as needed to obtain adequate pacing and sensing thresholds. Decisions regarding lead placement may later limit the pacing modes available to the clinician. For example, to perform dual-chamber pacing, both atrial and ventricular leads must be placed. However, in an emergency, interventions are focused on establishing ventricular pacing, and atrial lead placement may not be feasible. After lead placement, the initial settings for output and sensitivity are determined, the pacing rate and mode are selected, and the patient's response to pacing is evaluated.

Nursing Management

Nursing priorities in the care of a patient with a temporary pacemaker are associated with several patient problems and can be combined into four primary areas: (1) preventing pacemaker malfunction, (2) protecting against microshock, (3) preventing infection, and (4) educating the patient and family.

Preventing Pacemaker Malfunction

Continuous ECG monitoring is essential to facilitate prompt recognition of and appropriate intervention for pacemaker malfunction. Proper care of the pacing system can prevent pacing abnormalities.

The temporary pacing lead and bridging cable must be properly secured to the body with tape to prevent accidental displacement of the electrode, which can result in failure to pace or sense. The external pulse generator can be secured to the patient's waist with a strap or placed in a telemetry bag for a mobile patient. If the patient is on a regimen of bed rest, the pulse generator can be suspended with twill tape from an intravenous pole mounted overhead on the ceiling. This positioning prevents tension on the lead while the patient is moved (given adequate length of bridging cable) and alleviates the possibility of accidental dropping of the pulse generator.

The nurse inspects for loose connections between the leads and pulse generator on a regular basis. Replacement batteries and pulse generators must always be available on the unit. Although the battery has an anticipated life span of 1 month, it is probably sound practice to change the battery if the pacemaker has been operating continually for several days. Newer generators provide a low-battery signal 24 hours before complete loss of battery function occurs to prevent inadvertent interruptions in pacing. The pulse generator must always be labeled with the date on which the battery was replaced.

It is important to be aware of all sources of EMI within the critical care environment that may interfere with the pacemaker's function. Sources of EMI in the clinical area include electrocautery, defibrillation current, radiation therapy, magnetic resonance imaging (MRI) scanners, and transcutaneous electrical nerve stimulation units.[13] In most cases, if EMI is suspected of precipitating pacemaker malfunction, conversion to the asynchronous mode (fixed rate) can maintain pacing until the cause of the EMI is removed.

Protecting Against Microshock

Because the pacing electrode provides a direct, low-resistance path to the heart, the nurse takes special care while handling the external components of the pacing system to avoid conducting stray electrical current from other equipment. Even a small amount of stray current transmitted through the pacing lead could precipitate a lethal dysrhythmia. The possibility of microshock can be minimized by wearing gloves when handling the pacing wires and by proper insulation of terminal pins of pacing wires when they are not in use. The latter precaution can be accomplished by the use of caps provided by the manufacturer or by improvising with a plastic syringe or section of disposable rubber glove. The wires are taped securely to the patient's chest to prevent accidental electrode displacement.

Preventing Infection

Infection at the lead insertion site is a rare but serious complication associated with temporary pacemakers. The site is carefully inspected for purulent drainage, erythema, and edema, and the patient is observed for signs of systemic infection. Site care is performed according to the institution's policies and procedures. Although most infections remain localized, endocarditis can occur in patients with endocardial pacing leads. A less common complication associated with transvenous pacing is myocardial perforation, which can result in rhythmic hiccoughs or cardiac tamponade.

Educating the Patient and Family

Teaching for a patient with a temporary pacemaker emphasizes the prevention of complications. The patient is instructed not to handle any exposed portion of the lead wire and to notify the nurse if the dressing over the insertion site becomes soiled, wet, or dislodged. The patient also is advised not to use any electrical devices brought in from home that could interfere with pacemaker functioning. Patients with temporary transvenous pacemakers need to be taught to restrict movement of the affected extremity to prevent lead displacement.

Permanent Pacemakers

More than 350,000 permanent pacemakers are implanted in an inpatient setting annually in the United States, and significantly more are implanted in outpatient areas.[14] As a result, critical care nurses are likely to encounter these devices in their clinical practice. Implanted pacemakers were originally designed to provide an adequate ventricular rate in patients with symptomatic bradycardia. Today, the goal of pacemaker therapy is to simulate, as much as possible, normal physiologic cardiac depolarization and conduction. Sophisticated generators permit rate-responsive pacing, effecting responses to sensed atrial activity (DDD), or to various physiologic sensors (body motion or minute ventilation). For patients who do not have a functional sinus node that can increase their heart rate, rate-responsive pacemakers may improve exercise capacity and quality of life.[15] The concept of physiologic pacing continues to evolve because studies have indicated that pacing initiated from the right ventricular (RV) apex, even in a dual-chamber mode, may promote heart failure in patients with permanent pacemakers.[16] Further research has been conducted to identify alternative sites for pacing and modes that can maximize intrinsic AV conduction and minimize ventricular pacing.[10]

A patient who undergoes implantation of a permanent pacemaker is usually in the hospital for less than 24 hours. Longer lengths of stay are expected for patients with serious comorbidities such as MI or cardiogenic shock. Technologic advances in the computer industry have had a major impact on permanent pacemakers. Microprocessors have allowed for the development of increasingly smaller generators despite the incorporation of more complex features. Current generators are smaller, more energy efficient, and more reliable than previous models. Newer enhancements include leadless pacemakers, which consist of a self-contained unit that is placed in the RV via the femoral vein. These devices eliminate the need for a subcutaneous pocket and transvenous leads that account for most complications associated with permanent pacemakers.[17,18] Several new generators are also compatible with MRI. A rapidly expanding role for permanent pacemakers has been the use of these devices as a type of nonpharmacologic therapy for treatment of heart failure.

Cardiac Resynchronization Therapy

Approximately one-third of patients with severe heart failure have ventricular conduction delays (prolonged QRS duration or bundle branch block). These conduction delays have been shown to create a lack of synchrony between the contractions of the left ventricle and right ventricle. The hemodynamic consequences of this dyssynchrony include impaired ventricular filling with decreased ejection fraction (EF), cardiac output, and mean arterial pressure.[19] Cardiac resynchronization therapy (CRT) uses atrial pacing plus stimulation of both the left ventricle and the right ventricle (biventricular pacing) to optimize atrial and ventricular mechanical activity. The CRT device uses three pacing leads: a lead in the right atrium, a lead in the right ventricle, and a specially designed transvenous lead that is inserted through the coronary sinus to pace the left ventricle. Because many patients with heart failure are also at risk for sudden cardiac death, biventricular pacing is available on many implantable cardioverter defibrillator (ICD) devices. Numerous clinical trials have shown that CRT improves symptoms, functional status, and mortality in patients with moderate to advanced heart failure and helps prevent progression of heart failure in patients with fewer symptoms.[20] The use of CRT has expanded to include patients requiring conventional pacing with an EF of 50% or less. The greatest benefit appears to be in patients with a confirmed left bundle branch block and a QRS duration greater than 150 ms.[21]

Medical Management

Permanent pacemakers may be implanted with the patient under local anesthesia in the cardiac catheterization laboratory. Transvenous leads usually are inserted through the cephalic or subclavian vein and positioned in the right atrium or right ventricle or both, with fluoroscopic guidance. Satisfactory lead placement is determined by testing the stimulation and sensitivity thresholds with a pacing system analyzer. The leads are then attached to the generator, which is inserted into a surgically created pocket in the subcutaneous tissue below the clavicle. Ongoing assessment of pacemaker function after discharge can now be performed remotely, using wireless technology via the Internet or a cellular network. Remote monitoring reduces the number of clinic visits and provides early detection of patient or device problems.[22]

Nursing Management

Nursing management priorities for patients after permanent pacemaker implantation include monitoring for complications related to insertion and for pacemaker malfunction. Postoperative complications are rare but include cardiac perforation and tamponade, pneumothorax, hematoma, lead displacement, and infection.[23]

The process for identification of permanent pacemaker malfunction is the same as the process described previously for temporary pacemakers. To evaluate pacemaker function, the nurse must know at least the pacemaker's programmed mode of pacing and the lower rate setting. With permanent pacemakers, settings are adjusted non-invasively through a specialized programmer that uses pulsed magnetic fields or a radio frequency (RF) signal. If a pacemaker problem is suspected, ECG strips are obtained, and the physician is notified so that the pacemaker settings can be reprogrammed as needed. If the patient experiences symptoms of decreased cardiac output, he or she may require support with temporary transcutaneous pacing until the problem is corrected.

IMPLANTABLE CARDIOVERTER DEFIBRILLATORS

An ICD is an electronic device that is used in the treatment of tachydysrhythmias. ICDs can identify and terminate life-threatening ventricular dysrhythmias. Initially, an ICD was recommended only for patients who had survived an episode of cardiac arrest caused by ventricular fibrillation (VF) or ventricular tachycardia (VT) or in whom lethal arrhythmias could be induced during EPS. This secondary prevention was supported by randomized clinical trials that found improved survival with an ICD compared with treatment with antidysrhythmic medications.[1] The use of ICDs has since expanded to primary prevention of sudden cardiac death in selected high-risk populations who have a life expectancy of 1 year or more. This includes patients with ischemic heart disease and a low left ventricular (LV) EF (less than 30%—35%) despite optimal medical management for heart failure.[24] Patients with genetic or familial conditions that predispose them to life-threatening tachyarrhythmias, such as long QT syndrome of hypertrophic cardiomyopathy, are also candidates for an ICD. At the present time, more than 80% of ICDs are implanted for primary prevention, with 60,000 implants performed in an inpatient setting in the United States each year.[14,25]

Implantable Cardioverter Defibrillator System

The ICD system consists of leads and a generator and is similar to a pacemaker but with some key differences. The leads contain not only electrodes for sensing and pacing but also integrated defibrillator coils capable of delivering a shock. The generator is larger to accommodate a more powerful battery and a high-voltage capacitor along with the microprocessor. It is surgically placed in the subcutaneous tissue of the pectoral region in the upper chest (Fig. 12.5). The early model generators could defibrillate or cardiovert only lethal dysrhythmias. The current generation of devices delivers a tiered therapy, with options for programmable antitachycardia pacing, bradycardia backup pacing, low-energy cardioversion, and high-energy defibrillation. With tiered therapy, antitachycardia pacing is used as the first line of treatment in some cases of VT. If the VT can be pace-terminated successfully, the patient will not receive a shock from the generator and may not even realize that the ICD terminated the dysrhythmia. If programmed bursts of pacing do not terminate the VT, the ICD will cardiovert the rhythm. If the dysrhythmia deteriorates into VF, the ICD is programmed to defibrillate at a higher energy. If the dysrhythmia terminates spontaneously, the device will not discharge. Occasionally, the electrical rhythm may deteriorate to asystole or a slow idioventricular rhythm; in such cases, the bradycardia backup pacing function is activated.

Many patients with ICDs have structural heart disease and may require continuous pacing or benefit from CRT. ICD product development has resulted in dual-chamber devices with leads in both atria and ventricles to provide these additional therapies. The introduction of atrial leads allows for dual-chamber pacing to optimize hemodynamic performance and atrial sensing to discriminate more accurately between atrial tachycardia and VT to decrease the incidence of inappropriate shocks. ICDs may also incorporate triple-lead systems (leads in one atrium and both ventricles) to allow for CRT and defibrillation in one device. Some studies suggest the addition of CRT may improve heart failure over time and thus reduce the number of shocks required from the ICD.[26] Other developments in ICD technology include improved diagnostic and telemetry functions, such as the ability to provide real-time electrograms obtained from the ICD electrodes or the ability to perform remote device interrogation using cellular or wireless technology.[27]

Insertion of Implantable Cardioverter Defibrillator

The ICD has progressed in both programmable functions and insertion technique. Initially, all ICDs were implanted surgically during

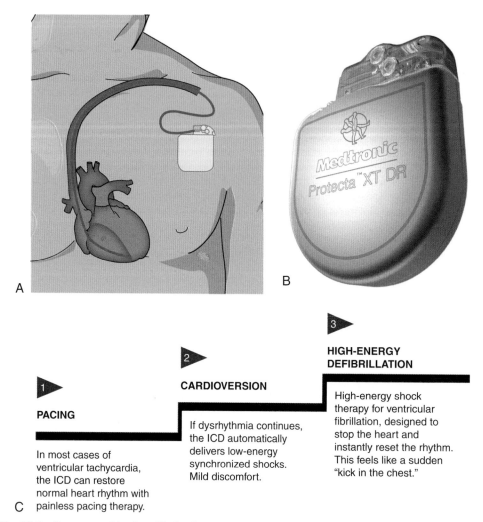

PACING

In most cases of ventricular tachycardia, the ICD can restore normal heart rhythm with painless pacing therapy.

CARDIOVERSION

If dysrhythmia continues, the ICD automatically delivers low-energy synchronized shocks. Mild discomfort.

HIGH-ENERGY DEFIBRILLATION

High-energy shock therapy for ventricular fibrillation, designed to stop the heart and instantly reset the rhythm. This feels like a sudden "kick in the chest."

Fig. 12.5 Placement of Implantable Cardioverter Defibrillator *(ICD)* With a Transvenous Lead System. (A) The generator is placed in a subcutaneous "pocket" in the pectoral region. The pacing, cardioversion, and defibrillation functions all are contained in a lead (or leads) inserted into the right atrium and ventricle. (B) Example of a dual-chamber ICD (Medtronic Gem II DR) with tiered therapy and pacing capabilities. (C) Tiered therapy is designed to use increasing levels of intensity to terminate ventricular dysrhythmias. (B, Reproduced with permission from Medtronic, Inc.)

open-heart surgery or via thoracotomy, with electrode patches attached directly to the heart. Today the majority of ICDs use transvenous leads that are positioned in the heart under fluoroscopy and then attached to a generator implanted in the tissue of the upper chest. Procedural complications are infrequent but may include hematoma, pneumothorax, cardiac tamponade, or lead dislodgment.[23] A fully subcutaneous ICD has been introduced more recently that consists of a generator implanted in the left axillary area and a single subcutaneous lead for detection of ventricular dysrhythmias and delivery of therapy. Although this device is unable to provide pacing therapies, it may provide an alternative for patients who lack vascular access and avoid complications related to transvenous lead placement.[28]

Medical Management

Medical management in a patient with an ICD begins before implantation with a thorough evaluation of the patient's risk for dysrhythmia and underlying cardiac function. Some patients may undergo EPS to determine the origin of the dysrhythmia and the effect of antidysrhythmic agents in suppressing or altering the rate of the

dysrhythmia. Further assessment of cardiac status is made to determine whether additional interventions (e.g., revascularization, CRT) are indicated to improve cardiac function. This part of the work-up may include cardiac catheterization, stress testing, and echocardiography. Based on the evaluation, decisions are made regarding the optimal implantation approach, either transvenous or subcutaneous, along with the types of therapy included, such as antitachycardia pacing, cardioversion, defibrillation, and resynchronization therapy. Current guidelines recommend that ICD implantation not be performed within 40 days of an MI or within 90 days of revascularization to allow time for ventricular recovery. In these patients an external wearable cardioverter defibrillator may be used to address the risk of sudden cardiac death during the waiting period.[24]

An electrophysiologist performs the initial programming of the device at the time of implantation. Defibrillation efficacy of the ICD may be assessed by inducing the dysrhythmia and then evaluating the ability of the device to terminate it. Although defibrillation testing was routinely performed at the time of implant with early devices, clinical trials have failed to demonstrate an improvement in shock efficacy or clinical outcomes related to this practice.[29,30] Modern ICDs are more reliable and offer higher energy levels than in the past, so some providers now omit testing and just program a high-output setting for defibrillation. Defibrillation testing is still considered a standard of care for subcutaneous ICD implants.[30]

Other adjustments in programming may be performed to decrease unnecessary shocks, including aggressive use of antitachycardia pacing and withholding shocks for supraventricular tachycardia (SVT) or nonsustained ventricular rhythms. These strategies are important, because studies indicate that the incidence of inappropriate shocks may range between 2% and 20%, resulting in unnecessary pain, reduced quality of life, and potential myocardial damage.[31] After it has been determined that the ICD functions appropriately, further follow-up can be conducted on an outpatient basis, with remote monitoring options to monitor the number of discharges and the battery life of the device.[27]

Nursing Management

If the ICD system was implanted during open-heart surgery, postoperative nursing management is similar to that for any patient undergoing cardiac surgery. If an endocardial lead system is implanted, nursing management is less intense, and the hospital stay is shorter. Nursing management priorities for a patient with an ICD focus on assessing for dysrhythmias and monitoring for complications related to insertion. In the case of a ventricular dysrhythmia, it is important to know the type of ICD implanted, how the device functions, and whether it is activated (i.e., "on"). If the patient experiences a shockable rhythm, the nurse should be prepared to defibrillate if the device has not been activated. During external defibrillation, the paddles or patches should not be placed directly over the ICD generator.[32] For recurring shocks, patients should be assessed for underlying causes such as electrolyte imbalance, ischemia, or worsening heart failure.[12] Most patients continue to take some antidysrhythmic medications to decrease the number of shocks required and to slow the rate of the tachycardia. Complications associated with a permanent ICD include infection from the implanted system, broken leads, and sensing of supraventricular tachydysrhythmias resulting in unneeded discharges.

Educating the Patient and Family

To facilitate a positive psychologic adjustment to the ICD, education of the patient and family about the device is vital. Preoperative teaching for a patient with an ICD includes information about how the device works and what to expect during the implantation procedure. After implantation, education is focused on aspects of living with an ICD. Patients need information pertaining to device follow-up, technology used for remote monitoring, and instructions about what to do if they experience a shock. Many institutions have successfully used family support groups for this patient population. Finally, because the ICD is an adjunctive treatment rather than a cure for heart failure, patients need to understand the importance of continued risk factor modification and prescribed medications.

FIBRINOLYTIC THERAPY

Fibrinolytic therapy is an important clinical intervention for patients experiencing acute ST segment elevation MI (STEMI). Before the introduction of fibrinolytic agents, medical management of acute MI was focused on decreasing myocardial oxygen demands to minimize myocardial necrosis and preserve ventricular function. Today, efforts to limit the size of the infarction are directed toward timely reperfusion of the jeopardized myocardium through restoration of blood flow in the culprit vessel (the open artery theory). Two options are available

for opening the artery: fibrinolytics and a mechanical intervention. Although mechanical catheter-based intervention has been proven to yield better outcomes when performed in a timely fashion, only 40% of US hospitals are estimated to have this capability.[33] For this reason, fibrinolytic therapy continues to play a role in the treatment of acute MI. However, after fibrinolysis is complete, transfer to a percutaneous coronary intervention (PCI)-capable hospital for early angiography and possible PCI is recommended.[34]

The use of fibrinolytic therapy is predicated on the theory that the significant event in an acute coronary syndrome (ACS, e.g., unstable angina, acute MI) is the rupture of an atherosclerotic plaque with thrombus formation (Fig. 12.6). The thrombus, which is composed of aggregated platelets bound together with fibrin strands, occludes the coronary artery, depriving the myocardium of oxygen previously supplied by that artery. The administration of a fibrinolytic agent results in lysis of the acute thrombus, resulting in recanalization, or opening, of the obstructed coronary artery and restoration of blood flow to the affected tissue. In addition to restoring perfusion, adjunctive measures (anticoagulants and antiplatelet therapy) are taken to prevent further clot formation and repeat occlusion.

ELIGIBILITY CRITERIA

Certain criteria have been developed, based on research findings, to determine the patient population that would most likely benefit from the administration of fibrinolytic therapy. For patients who present with a STEMI at a non–PCI capable hospital, the physician must determine whether the "first medical contact-to-device" time will exceed 120 minutes for any reason (e.g., time to transfer to a PCI-capable facility) and if so, then fibrinolytics are recommended.[35] Patients with recent onset of chest pain (less than 12 hours' duration) and persistent ST segment elevation (greater than 0.1 mV in two or more contiguous leads) are considered candidates for fibrinolytic therapy.[36] Patients who present with bundle branch blocks that may obscure ST segment analysis and a history suggesting acute MI are also considered candidates for therapy. The goal of therapy is to administer fibrinolytic therapy within 30 minutes after presentation ("door-to-needle") because early reperfusion yields the greatest benefit[36] (see Myocardial Infarction and Evaluation of Pre-Hospital Chest Pain in Fig. 11.3 in Chapter 11). Other common criteria for the use of fibrinolytic therapy are presented in Box 12.3.

Exclusion criteria are usually based on the increased risk of bleeding incurred from the use of fibrinolytics. Patients who have stable clots that might be disrupted by fibrinolytic therapy (recent surgery, facial or head trauma), uncontrolled hypertension, or ischemic stroke in the past 3 months are usually not considered candidates for fibrinolytic therapy.[34] At the present time, fibrinolytic therapy is not indicated for patients with unstable angina or non–ST segment elevation ACS.[37] It is believed that these conditions result from plaque rupture with the formation of only a partially occlusive thrombus. Fibrinolysis breaks up the clot and releases thrombin, and this can paradoxically increase the material necessary for further thrombosis. Instead, these patients are treated with antiplatelet agents (e.g., aspirin, clopidogrel, glycoprotein [GP] IIb/IIIa inhibitors) and antithrombin medications (e.g., heparin).

Fibrinolytic Agents

Four fibrinolytic agents are currently available for intravenous treatment of acute STEMI. All these agents stimulate lysis of the clot by converting inactive plasminogen to plasmin, an enzyme responsible for degradation of fibrin (see Fig. 12.6). The first-generation

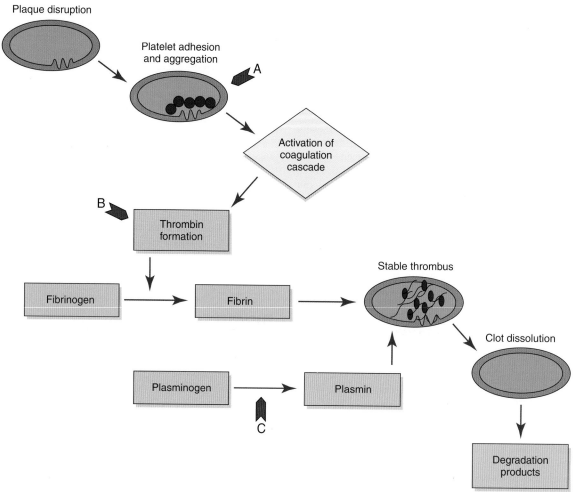

Fig. 12.6 Thrombus Formation and Site of Action of Medications Used in the Treatment of Acute Myocardial Infarction. (A) Site of action of antiplatelet agents such as aspirin, thienopyridines, and glycoprotein IIb/IIIa inhibitors. (B) Heparin bonds with antithrombin III and thrombin to create an inactive complex. (C) Fibrinolytic agents convert plasminogen to plasmin, an enzyme responsible for degradation of fibrin clots.

BOX 12.3 **Fibrinolytic Therapy Selection Criteria**

- No more than 12 hours from onset of chest pain and preferably within 30 minutes of diagnosis of ST segment elevation myocardial infarction
- ST segment elevation on electrocardiogram or new-onset left bundle branch block
- Ischemic chest pain unresponsive to sublingual nitroglycerin
- No conditions that might cause a predisposition to hemorrhage

---

fibrinolytic agents (e.g., streptokinase, urokinase) had their primary effect on circulating plasminogen. Newer fibrinolytic agents (e.g., alteplase, reteplase, tenecteplase) have a greater effect on clot plasminogen than on circulating plasminogen and are considered clot selective. Currently approved fibrinolytic agents are compared in Table 12.3. Because patients with an area of plaque disruption are still at risk for clot formation and reocclusion, fibrinolytic therapy is used in conjunction with anticoagulants and antiplatelet agents. Current guidelines recommend that anticoagulant therapy be administered for a minimum of 48 hours after reperfusion.[36]

Unfractionated heparin traditionally has been used, but low-molecular-weight heparin and fondaparinux are also acceptable options and are preferred when anticoagulation is planned for more than 48 hours after fibrinolytic therapy.[36] Antiplatelet therapy with clopidogrel is recommended for at least 14 days up to 1 year, and aspirin should be continued indefinitely.[36]

Streptokinase

Streptokinase is a fibrinolytic agent derived from beta-hemolytic streptococci, which, when combined with plasminogen, catalyzes the conversion of plasminogen to plasmin, the enzyme responsible for clot dissolution in the body. Because streptokinase is a bacterial protein, it can produce various allergic reactions, including anaphylaxis. In addition, the fibrinolytic action of streptokinase is systemic (non–clot specific) and prolonged (half-life of 20–25 minutes), increasing the risk for bleeding complications. Because of these issues, streptokinase is no longer available in the United States.

Tissue Plasminogen Activator

Tissue plasminogen activator (tPA), or alteplase (Activase), is a naturally occurring enzyme (i.e., nonantigenic) that is clot specific and has a very short half-life (3–4 minutes). It converts plasminogen to

TABLE 12.3 Pharmacologic Management.

Fibrinolytic Agents for Use in Acute Myocardial Infarction

Medication	Dosage	Actions	Special Considerations
Clot Specific			
tPA (alteplase)	IV: 100 mg total; 15 mg given as a bolus over 2 minutes followed by 50 mg IV infusion over 30 minutes then 35 mg IV infusion over 60 minutes (dose is adjusted based on weight for patients ≤67 kg)	Binds to fibrin at clot and promotes activation of plasminogen to plasmin	Anticoagulants are given concurrently. DAPT is begun with administration and continued daily.
rPA (reteplase)	IV: 10 units given as a bolus over 2 minutes, repeated in 30 minutes	Binds to fibrin at clot and promotes activation of plasminogen to plasmin	Anticoagulants are given concurrently. DAPT is begun with administration and continued daily.
Tenecteplase (TNKase)	IV: 30–50 mg based on body weight, given as a single bolus	Binds to fibrin at clot and promotes activation of plasminogen to plasmin	Anticoagulants are given concurrently. DAPT is begun with administration and continued daily.

DAPT, Dual antiplatelet therapy; *IV,* intravenous; *rPA,* recombinant plasminogen activator; *tPA,* tissue plasminogen activator.

plasmin after binding to the fibrin-containing clot. This clot-specific action results in an increased concentration and activity of plasmin at the site of the clot, where it is needed. Several different intravenous dosing regimens have been proposed and tested in the clinical setting, but accelerated-dose tPA is considered the most effective means of establishing early patency of the occluded vessel.[38]

Recombinant Plasminogen Activator

Recombinant plasminogen activator, or reteplase, is a variant of the natural human enzyme tPA. Reteplase is less fibrin selective and has a longer half-life than tPA, making it suitable for bolus administration rather than as a continuous infusion. This new-generation plasminogen activator is given as a double bolus and then followed with adjunctive therapies. In contrast to tPA, reteplase does not require weight-based dosing. Studies have shown that reteplase is as effective as tPA in the treatment of acute MI and is easier to administer.[39]

Tenecteplase

Tenecteplase (TNKase) is the newest of the fibrinolytic agents. It is a genetically engineered variant of alteplase with slower plasma clearance and better fibrin specificity. Studies have shown that tenecteplase is as effective as alteplase, and the two agents have similar rates of bleeding complications.[39] Tenecteplase requires only a single bolus injection, which may help facilitate more rapid treatment both inside and outside the hospital. Although the need for weight-based dosing is a potential disadvantage of this medication, tenecteplase is a widely used fibrinolytic agent in the United States at the present time.[40]

Outcomes of Fibrinolytic Therapy

The benefit of fibrinolytic therapy correlates with the degree of restoration of normal blood flow in the infarct-related artery. Coronary artery patency is defined by angiographic perfusion grades developed by the *Thrombolysis in Myocardial Infarction* (TIMI) study group in 1985 (Table 12.4).[41] Achievement of TIMI grade 3 flow is associated with the best long-term survival. Studies also indicate that rapid restoration of normal blood flow, within 90 minutes after treatment, results in improved LV function and reduced mortality. The three fibrin-specific fibrinolytics have been shown to achieve TIMI grade 3 flow in 50% to 60% of patients at 90 minutes.[39] Fibrinolytic

TABLE 12.4 Flow in Infarct-Related Artery as Described in the Thrombolysis in Myocardial Infarction Trial.

Perfusion Grades	Flow in the Infarct-Related Artery
TIMI 3	Normal or brisk flow through coronary artery
TIMI 2	Partial flow, slower than in normal vessels
TIMI 1	Sluggish flow with incomplete distal filling
TIMI 0	No flow beyond point of occlusion

TIMI, Thrombolysis in Myocardial Infarction Trial.
Modified from The TIMI Study Group. The thrombolysis in myocardial Infarction (TIMI) trial: phase I findings. *N Engl J Med.* 1985;312:932.

therapy continues to evolve, and medication dose ranges and regimens are subject to change when research findings are updated.

Evidence of Reperfusion

Several clinical signs may be observed after reperfusion of an artery that had been completely occluded by a thrombus, including relief of chest pain, reperfusion dysrhythmias, ST segments returning to baseline, and an early peak of cardiac biomarkers (see Fig. 11.11 in Chapter 11). Although recognition of these noninvasive markers of recanalization is important for assessing the patient's response to fibrinolytic therapy, they are less reliable than angiography in determining whether reperfusion has been successful.[42]

Pain and Reperfusion Dysrhythmias

One possible sign of reperfusion is the abrupt cessation of chest pain as blood flow is restored to the ischemic myocardium. Another potential indicator of reperfusion is the appearance of various "reperfusion dysrhythmias." A variety of dysrhythmias can occur—premature ventricular contractions, bradycardias, heart block, VT—but accelerated idioventricular rhythms have shown the best correlation with reperfusion. Reperfusion dysrhythmias are usually self-limiting or nonsustained, and aggressive antidysrhythmic therapy is not required. However, vigilant monitoring of the patient's ECG is essential, because dysrhythmias associated with ongoing ischemia could deteriorate rapidly and may necessitate emergency treatment.

ST Segment

Another noninvasive marker of recanalization is rapid return to baseline of the elevated ST segments, which indicates restoration of blood flow to previously ischemic myocardial tissue. A monitoring lead should be chosen that clearly demonstrates ST segment elevation before initiation of therapy.[43] The inability to achieve 50% resolution of the ST segment elevation within 60 to 90 minutes of administering the medication is generally considered an indication of failure of fibrinolytic therapy.[36]

Cardiac Biomarkers

Serial measurement of serum biomarkers may serve as further evidence of successful reperfusion after fibrinolytic therapy. Cardiac-specific creatine kinase and troponin increase rapidly and then decrease markedly after reperfusion of the ischemic myocardium. This phenomenon is called *washout* because it is thought to result from the rapid readmission of substances released by damaged myocardial cells into the circulation after restoration of blood flow (see Cardiac Biomarker Studies During Myocardial Infarction and Fig. 11.11 in Chapter 11).

Residual Coronary Artery Stenosis

Fibrinolytic therapy has been determined to be a successful strategy for reopening occluded coronary arteries in the setting of acute MI. It limits infarct size, salvaging myocardium and significantly reducing morbidity and mortality associated with cardiogenic shock and VF. However, residual coronary artery stenosis resulting from the atherosclerotic process remains, even after successful fibrinolysis. Subsequent prevention of reocclusion is critical to preserving myocardial function and preventing the risk of late complications. Therefore fibrinolytic therapy is recognized as an emergency procedure to restore patency until more definitive therapy can be initiated to effectively reduce the degree of stenosis. Current guidelines recommend that patients who receive fibrinolytic therapy be transferred to a facility capable of performing interventional catheter-based procedures and undergo routine angiography within the first 3 to 6 hours to allow for additional intervention as warranted.[36,44]

Nursing Management

Nursing management priorities for patients undergoing fibrinolytic therapy begin with identifying potential candidates. In many institutions, checklists are used to facilitate the rapid identification of patients who are candidates for fibrinolytics. The nurse prepares the patient for fibrinolytic therapy by starting intravenous lines and obtaining baseline laboratory values and vital signs. Throughout the administration of the fibrinolytic agent, assessment of the patient continues for clinical indicators of reperfusion and complications related to therapy.

The most common complication related to thrombolysis is bleeding, which is related to the fibrinolytic therapy itself and anticoagulation therapy that patients routinely receive to minimize the possibility of rethrombosis. The nurse must continually monitor for clinical manifestations of bleeding from hematoma or puncture sites, flank ecchymoses with any complaints of low back pain, and any changes in neurologic status. Mild gingival bleeding and oozing around venipuncture sites is common and not a cause of concern. Should serious bleeding occur, such as intracranial or internal bleeding, all fibrinolytic and antithrombotic therapies are discontinued, and volume expanders, coagulation factors, or both are administered.

In addition to accurate assessment of the patient for evidence of bleeding, nursing management priorities include preventive measures to minimize the potential for bleeding. For example, handling of the patient is limited, intramuscular injections are avoided, and additional pressure is provided to ensure hemostasis at venipuncture and arterial puncture sites. Intravenous lines are placed before lytic therapy is administered, and a heparin lock may be used for obtaining laboratory specimens during treatment.

Educating the Patient and Family

Education for the patient receiving fibrinolytic therapy includes information regarding the actions of fibrinolytic agents, with emphasis on precautions to minimize bleeding. For example, the patient is cautioned against vigorous toothbrushing and told to refrain from using straight-edge razors. Education is provided regarding ongoing risk factor management in the prevention of atherosclerotic coronary artery disease (CAD) (see Box 11.1 in Chapter 11).

CATHETER-BASED INTERVENTIONS FOR CORONARY ARTERY DISEASE

PCI has become the gold standard in the treatment of acute coronary disease and to reverse ongoing ischemia and infarction. Advances in device technology, along with more effective anticoagulant and antiplatelet regimens, have reduced complication rates and improved procedural outcomes. As a result, elective PCI is increasingly performed as a short-stay or outpatient procedure. In the setting of emergency PCI associated with acute myocardial ischemia, patients are hospitalized for a period of time depending on the cardiovascular work-up that is required.

Indications for Catheter-Based Interventions

Indications for catheter-based interventions have been considerably broadened since the initial application of percutaneous transluminal coronary angioplasty (PTCA). Current guidelines recommend that when a patient presents with a STEMI, "first medical contact-to-device" time should be less than 90 minutes for patients presenting to a PCI-capable site and less than 120 minutes for patients presenting to an outside facility who need to be transferred to a PCI-capable hospital.[36] In non–ST-elevation myocardial infarction (NSTEMI), PCI is used where there is nonocclusive but anatomically significant disease, generally greater than 70% occlusion, to revascularize the vessel, treat intractable angina, and to prevent further vessel occlusion.[45]

Percutaneous Transluminal Coronary Angioplasty

PTCA involves the use of a balloon-tipped catheter that, when advanced through an atherosclerotic lesion (atheroma), can be inflated intermittently for the purpose of dilating the stenotic area and improving blood flow through it (Fig. 12.7). The high inflation pressure of the

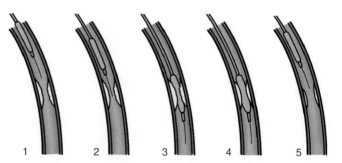

Fig. 12.7 Percutaneous Transluminal Coronary Angioplasty (PTCA). PTCA is used to open a stenotic vessel occluded by atherosclerosis.

balloon stretches the vessel wall, fractures the plaque, and enlarges the vessel lumen. After balloon deflation, the vessel exhibits some degree of elastic recoil, resulting in a residual stenosis of approximately 30%.

Although PTCA has relatively high success rates in initially opening occluded vessels, the technique by itself has major limitations, including the risk of acute vessel closure and a high frequency of restenosis. For these reasons, coronary balloon angioplasty is usually combined with stent implants. Balloon catheters now incorporate modifications of the balloon surface. Cutting balloons and scoring balloons are two types of available devices and are useful in facilitating lesion dilation. Currently, there are no trials showing any difference in recurrent restenosis between patients treated with cutting-balloon or standard-balloon angioplasty.[46] Drug-coated balloon (DCB) angioplasty adds an antiproliferative medication coating to the balloon along with an excipient to avoid drug transfer, which may help prevent restenosis. Studies are still investigating whether use of DCB angioplasty alone is a feasible strategy to avoid the potential disadvantages of stent implantation.[46,47]

Atherectomy

Initially, atherectomy focused on the excision and removal of the atherosclerotic plaque by cutting, shaving, or grinding. However, it is now accepted that the primary mechanisms of facilitating lesion dilation and stent delivery are through disruption of the calcified plaques' integrity. Management of severe coronary artery calcification relies on rotational and orbital atherectomy to prepare the lesion to facilitate stent delivery and optimal expansion.[48]

Rotational atherectomy (RA) systems (Boston Scientific) have a high-speed, rotating, diamond-coated burr that drills through the plaque, creating tiny particles (Fig. 12.8). The particulate matter is carried through the bloodstream and disposed of by the reticuloendothelial system. OA (Diamondback 360) is an eccentrically mounted crown, coated with diamonds, that rotates along the axis of the drive shaft and orbits along the vessel walls.[48] There is an increased risk of dissection, perforation, and slow/no reflow with these devices.

Thrombectomy

Thrombectomy catheters are used to decrease the risk of thrombotic emboli by removing large thrombi from the vessel before the intervention. These devices are recommended primarily for use in PCI patients with large thrombus burden.

Embolic Protection Devices

Initial devices for performing PCI were designed to optimize flow at the point of the lesion or blockage within the coronary artery. However, despite evidence of procedural success on angiography, some patients still exhibited signs of compromised distal perfusion. This "no reflow" phenomenon is believed to be caused by distal embolization of atherosclerotic plaque or thrombus at the time of the procedure.[38] Several adjunctive tools have been developed to help protect the microvasculature during PCI procedures. Embolic protection devices consist of balloons or filters that are positioned beyond the lesion to trap and remove debris that might be released during the intervention. One type of distal filter is shown in Fig. 12.9.

Coronary Stents

A major development in the field of interventional cardiology has been the coronary stent prosthesis. A stent is a metal structure that is introduced into the coronary artery over a guidewire and expanded into the vessel wall at the site of the lesion. Bare metal stents were first used to treat acute or threatened vessel closure after failed PTCA. The stent acted as a scaffold to tack dissection flaps against the vessel wall and provided mechanical support to minimize elastic recoil. Subsequent studies confirmed the clinical benefits of stents, which led to elective coronary stent placement as a primary procedure. Stent implantation was initially limited to large vessels (greater than 3 mm) with proximal, discrete lesions. Improvements in stent design and operator technique allow for deployment in smaller vessels with diffuse disease, vessels with lesions at bifurcations, and vessels with thrombus. Multiple stents may be implanted sequentially within a vessel to fully cover the area of the lesion. Numerous stents are available. They are composed of various types of metal (stainless steel, cobalt, or platinum chromium alloys) and come in a variety of configurations (mesh, coil). Although initially composed of metal alone, contemporary stents incorporate various polymer coatings and medications to improve long-term patency of the vessel. Most stents are balloon expandable (Fig. 12.10).

Drug-Eluting Stents

Drug-eluting stents (DES) were developed in an effort to minimize restenosis. These stents have polymer coatings impregnated with medications that are released slowly into the endothelium at the site of stent placement to inhibit cellular proliferation. Current DESs (second-generation everolimus-eluting stents and zotarolimus-eluting stents) have proven superior outcomes compared with first-generation stents.[49] It has been theorized that the presence of polymers may contribute to vessel inflammation and thus stent thrombosis. This has led to the development of stents with

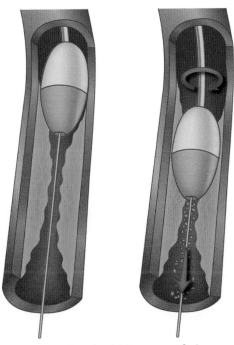

Fig. 12.8   Rotational Atherectomy Catheter.

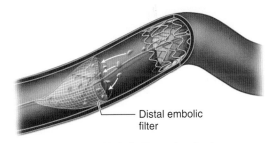

Distal embolic filter

Fig. 12.9   Embolic Protection Device.

biodegradable polymers. Bioabsorbable stents or nonmetallic "scaffolds" are another area of investigation. The idea is to create a temporary mechanical support in the vessel to prevent immediate restenosis but allow it to degrade over time and eliminate the possible long-term risks of traditional stents.[46] Even with the development of biodegradable polymer DES and stents with bioabsorbable vascular scaffolding, second-generation metallic DESs remain the most commonly used stents in PCI today.[49] Bare metal stents and DES are compared in Table 12.5.

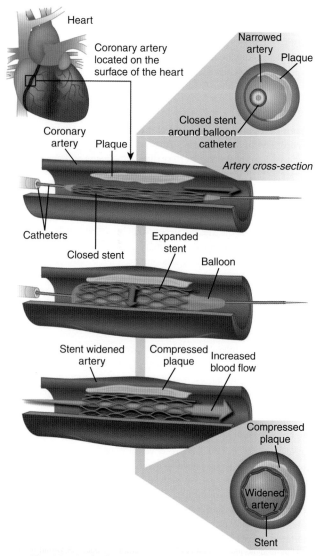

Fig. 12.10 An Intracoronary Balloon-Expandable Stent.

Stent Thrombosis Prevention

Antithrombotic therapy, including antiplatelet therapy and anticoagulation, is important to prevent stent thrombosis.[34] Because platelet activation is a complex process involving multiple pathways, combination therapy with two or more agents has proven most effective. The current standard of care for PCI typically includes dual antiplatelet therapy with aspirin and a P2Y12 inhibitor.[50] These oral agents are administered before the procedure and continued at discharge. Oral antiplatelet agents are described in Table 12.6. Cangrelor is an intravenous P2Y12 inhibitor option for patients unable to take oral antiplatelet agents or for patients scheduled for immediate surgery. Platelet inhibition occurs within 20 minutes and returns when the intravenous infusion is stopped. Although it is a seemingly ideal antiplatelet agent, both availability and cost have limited use in the United States.[50]

GPIIb/IIIa inhibitors, which are more potent intravenous antiplatelet agents, could be considered in patients who have inadequate P2Y12 receptor inhibitor loading or a large thrombus burden.[34] These medications act on the GPIIb/IIIa receptors on the platelet membrane to inhibit the final phase of platelet aggregation and prevent platelets from binding with fibrinogen. Intravenous antiplatelet agents are described in Table 12.7.

In-Stent Restenosis

Stents have been shown to decrease the incidence of restenosis compared with balloon angioplasty, most likely as a result of achieving the largest possible lumen diameter at the time of the intervention. Successful stent implantation should result in less than 10% residual stenosis and optimally as close to zero as possible. However, stents have not proved to be a cure for restenosis, as was once hoped.

Restenosis within the stent is caused by intimal hyperplasia and can occur in a diffuse pattern throughout the stent, as discrete lesions within the body of the stent, or at the stent margins. In contrast to thrombosis, restenosis is a gradual process that generally occurs within the first 6 to 12 months and manifests clinically as recurrent angina. Factors that increase the risk of in-stent restenosis include longer coronary lesions over 20 mm, and a smaller coronary artery diameter less than 3 mm; comorbidities such as acute kidney injury (AKI) or diabetes mellitus; inadequate stent expansion during the procedure; and gaps in sequential stent placement.

PCI Procedure

PCI is performed in the cardiac catheterization laboratory under fluoroscopy. Patients typically receive antiplatelet therapy (a P2Y12 inhibitor and aspirin) before beginning the procedure. An introducer catheter, or sheath, is inserted percutaneously into an artery to provide access to the coronary arteries. Access via the radial artery (transradial access) has become the preferred method, because studies show that it results in lower rates of bleeding complications, is associated with earlier ambulation, and demonstrates improved outcomes.[50] The femoral artery is still used when larger catheters are

TABLE 12.5	Comparison of Bare Metal and Drug-Eluting Stents.	
Characteristics	**Bare Metal Stent**	**Drug-Eluting Stent**
Restenosis rate (at 6 months)	15%–20%	5%–10%
Cost	$	$$$
Duration of dual antiplatelet therapy	Minimum of 1 month for non-ACS patients, at least 12 months for stents implanted for ACS	Minimum of 6 months for either non-ACS or ACS patients and longer if tolerated
Recommended lesion features	Short lesions <20 mm	Longer lesions >20 mm
	Large vessel diameter >3 mm	Small vessel diameter <3.5 mm

ACS, Acute coronary syndrome.

TABLE 12.6 Pharmacologic Management.

Oral Antiplatelet Agents

Medication	Dosage	Action	Special Considerations
COX Inhibitor			
Aspirin	81–325 mg initial dose 81 mg maintenance dose	Inhibits synthesis of thromboxane A_2 resulting in irreversible inhibition of platelet activation	Lower doses are recommended when given with other antithrombotics.
P2Y12 Inhibitors			
Clopidogrel (Plavix)	600 mg loading dose 75 mg maintenance	Irreversibly inhibits ADP P2Y12 platelet receptor to block platelet activation	Onset of action 2–4 hours Should be withheld 5–7 days before elective surgery to decrease risk of bleeding. Some patients may have a genetic resistance to clopidogrel, resulting in inadequate platelet inhibition.
Prasugrel (Effient)	60 mg loading dose 10 mg daily maintenance	Irreversibly inhibits ADP P2Y12 platelet receptor to block platelet activation	Onset of action 15–30 minutes Should be withheld 5–7 days before elective surgery to decrease risk of bleeding. Contraindicated in patients with prior TIA or stroke; not recommended in patients age >75 years.
Ticagrelor (Brilinta)	180 mg loading dose 90 mg twice daily maintenance	Reversibly inhibits ADP P2Y12 platelet receptor to block platelet activation	Onset of action 30 minutes Should be withheld 5 days before elective surgery to decrease risk of bleeding. Contraindicated in patients with history of ICH or severe hepatic impairment. Maintenance aspirin dose >100 mg reduces effectiveness.

ADP, Adenosine diphosphate; *ICH*, intracranial hemorrhage; *TIA*, transient ischemic attack.

TABLE 12.7 Pharmacologic Management.

Intravenous Antiplatelet Agents

Medication	Dosage	Action	Special Considerations
P2Y12 Inhibitor			
Cangrelor	30 mcg/kg IV bolus over 1 minute then 4 mcg/kg/min IV infusion for at least 2 hours or duration of PCI	Reversibly inhibits ADP P2Y12 platelet receptor to block platelet activation	Platelet inhibition in 20 minutes with return of platelet function with the cessation of IV infusion
GP 11b/111a Inhibitor			
Abciximab (ReoPro)	ACS: 0.25 mg/kg IV over 5 minutes followed by 0.125 mcg/kg/min (max 10 mcg/min) IV infusion for 12 hours. PCI: 0.25 mg/kg IV over 5 minutes followed by IV infusion of 10 mcg/min for 18–24 hours concluding 1 hour after PCI	Inhibits GPIIb/IIIa receptors responsible for platelet aggregation	Used concomitantly with aspirin and anticoagulants May affect platelet function for 48 hours after infusion
Eptifibatide (Integrilin)	ACS: 180 mcg/kg IV bolus, followed by continuous infusion of 2 mcg/kg/min up to 72 hours PCI: 180 mcg/kg IV bolus immediately before PCI (repeat after 10 minutes) followed by continuous infusion of 2 mcg/kg/min for 12–24 hours	Reversibly binds to GPIIb/IIIa platelet receptor and inhibits platelet aggregation	Concomitant aspirin and anticoagulants may be administered Platelet function returns to baseline within 6–8 hours Contraindicated in patients with significant kidney dysfunction
Tirofiban (Aggrastat)	ACS: 25 mcg/kg within 5 minutes, then continued at 0.15 mcg/kg/min for up to 18 hours	Reversibly binds to GPIIb/IIIa platelet receptor and inhibits platelet aggregation	Platelet function returns to baseline within 4–8 hours Dosage should be reduced in patients with kidney dysfunction

ACS, Acute coronary syndrome; *GP*, glycoprotein; *IV*, intravenous; *PCI*, percutaneous coronary intervention.

used (with ACS or cardiogenic shock) or if because of anatomic limitations the catheter cannot be advanced from the radial artery. In some cases, a venous sheath is inserted and used to perform a right heart catheterization, insert a pacing catheter, or both. A catheter with pacing capabilities may be indicated if dilation of the right coronary artery or circumflex artery is anticipated, because the blood supply to the conduction system of the heart may be interrupted, requiring emergency pacing.

The patient is systemically anticoagulated to prevent clots from forming on or in any of the catheters. Unfractionated heparin has been used traditionally, initiated with a weight-based bolus and then titrated to achieve a target-activated clotting time. Other

TABLE 12.8 Pharmacologic Management.

Anticoagulants

Medication	Dosage	Action	Special Considerations
Unfractionated Heparin			
Heparin sodium	Initial bolus 60 units/kg (maximum dose 4000 units), followed by 12 units/kg/h infusion	Enhances activity of antithrombin III, a natural anticoagulant, to prevent clot formation	Effectiveness of treatment may be monitored by aPTT or ACT Response is variable because of binding with plasma proteins Effects may be reversed with protamine sulfate Risk of developing HIT Should not be given to patients already receiving therapeutic SC enoxaparin
Low-Molecular-Weight Heparin			
Enoxaparin (Lovenox)	30 mg IV bolus, followed by 1 mg/kg SC every 12 hours For patients already on SC dosing, an additional bolus of 0.3 mg/kg is given if last dose was >8 hours before PCI	Enhances activity of antithrombin III	More predictable response than heparin because enoxaparin is not largely bound to protein No need for aPTT or ACT monitoring Lower risk of HIT than with UFH Significant reduction in dosage needed when CrCl <30 mL/min Administer within 30 minutes of initiation of fibrinolytic therapy
Direct Thrombin Inhibitors			
Bivalirudin (Angiomax)	0.75 mg/kg IV bolus, followed by infusion at 1.75 mg/kg/h during PCI	Directly inhibits thrombin	May be administered alone or in combination with GPIIb/IIIa inhibitors Produces dose-dependent increase in aPTT and ACT Coagulation times return to baseline within 1 hour after stopping infusion Dose should be reduced for patients with kidney dysfunction No reversal agent is available May be used instead of UFH for patients with HIT
Argatroban	Loading dose of 100 mcg/kg IV bolus over 1 minute, followed by infusion of 1–3 mcg/kg/min for 6–72 hours	Directly inhibits thrombin	May be used instead of UFH for patients with HIT ACT is monitored during PCI; aPTT is used during prolonged infusion Abrupt discontinuation may lead to rebound hypercoagulable state
Factor Xa Inhibitor			
Fondaparinux (Arixtra)	2.5 mg IV, followed by 2.5 mg SC once daily	Selective inhibitor of factor Xa	May be used in conjunction with fibrinolytics For PCI, must be administered with another anticoagulant (i.e., UFH) to prevent catheter thrombosis Long half-life (>17 hours) Contraindicated in patients with kidney failure

ACT, Activated clotting time; *aPTT*, activated partial thromboplastin time; *CrCl*, creatinine clearance; *GP*, glycoprotein; *HIT*, heparin-induced thrombocytopenia; *IV*, intravenous/intravenously; *MI*, myocardial infarction; *PCI*, percutaneous coronary intervention; *SC*, subcutaneous/subcutaneously; *UFH*, unfractionated heparin.

anticoagulants may be selected based on physician preference or if the patient cannot tolerate heparin. Options for anticoagulant agents are described in Table 12.8.

A special guiding catheter, designed to engage the coronary ostia, is inserted through the arterial sheath and advanced in a retrograde manner through the aorta. Nitroglycerin, calcium channel blockers, or adenosine may be given at this time to prevent coronary artery spasm and to maximize coronary vasodilation during the procedure. A guidewire is then advanced down the coronary artery and negotiated across the occluding atheroma. The balloon catheter is advanced over this guidewire and positioned across the lesion. The balloon is inflated and deflated repetitively until evidence of dilation is demonstrated on an angiogram. For lesions that do not respond well to angioplasty, additional plaque or thrombus removal may be done with an adjunctive device.

In most procedures, vessel dilation is followed by deployment of an intracoronary stent. A stent is positioned at the target site, the stent is expanded, and the catheter is removed, leaving the stent in place. Intravascular ultrasound is used by many clinicians to evaluate the vessel lumen diameter after stent deployment to ensure optimal expansion.[51] Information obtained by ultrasound provides a better estimate of residual plaque than information provided by angiography, because contrast material may surround the latticework of the stent, giving the appearance of a large lumen even when the stent is not fully open. To facilitate early sheath removal, heparin or other anticoagulants are usually discontinued immediately after the procedure. Sheaths are removed when the activated clotting time returns to normal in heparinized patients or sooner if other anticoagulants or a vascular closure device are used. If GPIIb/IIIa inhibitors were initiated during the procedure, they may be continued for 12 to 24 hours, depending on the agent used. Dual antiplatelet therapy with aspirin and a P2Y12 inhibitor (clopidogrel, prasugrel, or ticagrelor) is routinely prescribed at discharge. Recommendations for P2Y12 inhibitor administration vary based on the type of stent used (see Table 12.5), whereas aspirin is continued indefinitely.

Acute Complications

The incidence of serious cardiac complications after PCI, including coronary spasm, coronary artery dissection, and acute coronary thrombosis, has decreased significantly with improvements in technology. Stents have proved efficacious in the repair of coronary dissections, decreasing the need for emergency bypass surgery. Acute thrombosis has decreased with the established use of dual antiplatelet agents. Bleeding and complications at the site of vascular cannulation (hematoma, compromised blood flow to the involved extremity, and retroperitoneal bleeding with femoral access) occur infrequently but are associated with increased morbidity and lengthened hospitalization.[52] Other complications that can occur in the period immediately after PCI include contrast-induced kidney failure, dysrhythmias, and vasovagal response (hypotension, bradycardia, and diaphoresis) during manipulation or removal of introducer sheaths.

Nursing Management

Nursing management priorities after PCI focus on accurate assessment of the patient's condition and prompt intervention. The nurse at the bedside is in a unique position to continuously monitor for clinical manifestations of potential problems and to take quick and appropriate action to minimize the deleterious effects of complications related to the interventional catheter procedure.

Angina

It is essential that the nurse observe the patient for recurrent angina or ST segment elevation, which are clinical indicators of myocardial ischemia. Monitoring leads should be selected that will reflect ischemia in the vessels that were treated during the intervention.[43] Angina after a coronary interventional procedure may be caused by transient coronary vasospasm, or it may signal a more serious complication: acute thrombosis. In any case, the nurse must act quickly to assess for manifestations of myocardial ischemia and initiate clinical interventions as indicated. The physician usually orders intravenous nitroglycerin to be titrated to alleviate chest pain. Continued angina despite maximal vasodilator therapy usually rules out transient coronary vasospasm as the source of ischemic pain, and a return to the cardiac catheterization laboratory must be considered.

Prevention of Contrast-Induced Acute Kidney Injury

Patients undergoing PCI are exposed to significant amounts of contrast dye, with its associated nephrotoxicity. Contrast-induced acute kidney injury (CI-AKI) is one of the most common causes of kidney injury. Because there is no specific treatment for CI-AKI, protective strategies should be implemented before the procedure, especially for patients with evidence of baseline kidney impairment. First, the avoidance of unnecessary contrast administration is important to prevent CI-AKI. Whenever possible, avoid concomitant use of other nephrotoxic drugs such as nonsteroidal antiinflammatory drugs (NSAIDs) and metformin.[53] Hydrate the patient with isotonic saline

and/or sodium bicarbonate both before and after the procedure.[53] Although the strength of evidence is not strong enough for N-acetylcysteine, it is well tolerated and inexpensive and so in 2012, Kidney Disease Improving Global Outcomes (KDIGO) suggested its use for patients at risk for CI-AKI.[54]

Vascular Site Care

While the sheath is in place or after its removal, bleeding or hematoma at the insertion site may occur secondary to the effects of anticoagulation. The nurse observes the patient for bleeding or swelling at the puncture site and for changes in vital signs (hypotension, tachycardia) that could indicate hemorrhage. If a femoral approach was used, the nurse also assesses the patient for back pain, which can indicate retroperitoneal bleeding from the internal arterial puncture site.

Peripheral ischemia can also occur secondary to cannulation of the vessel, so nursing care includes frequent assessment of the adequacy of circulation to the involved extremity. After obtaining radial access, peripheral circulation may be assessed by monitoring the plethysmography waveform from a pulse oximeter probe placed on the thumb of the affected extremity.[55] The patient is instructed to keep the limb straight and minimize movement. For femoral access, the head of the bed is not elevated more than 30 degrees while the sheath is in place (to prevent dislodgment) and for a period after its removal (to prevent bleeding). For brachial or radial access, a splint may be used to prevent flexion of the arm or wrist. Additional activity restrictions vary depending on the size and location of the sheath, type of anticoagulation prescribed, methods used to achieve hemostasis, and institutional protocols. After sheath removal, direct pressure is applied to the puncture site for 15 to 30 minutes until hemostasis is achieved. If direct pressure is inadequate or the patient is at higher risk for bleeding, an external hemostatic device may be used to apply continuous pressure for 1 to 2 hours to ensure adequate hemostasis. Patients usually are allowed to resume ambulation 4 to 8 hours after the procedure or sooner if a vascular closure device is employed.[56]

Many products have been introduced to facilitate adequate hemostasis at the femoral access site after sheath removal. Active closure devices use mechanical sutures, collagen plugs, or metal clips to close the vessel when the sheath is removed. Advantages of these devices include a reduced time to hemostasis regardless of the patient's level of anticoagulation, decreased resource utilization, earlier ambulation, and increased patient and provider comfort.[56,57] Disadvantages include risk of device failure or malfunction, small risk of groin infection, potential limb ischemia, embolization, and device cost.[56] Table 12.9 compares vascular closure systems.[56]

Educating the Patient and Family

In most cases, patients undergoing elective angioplasty, atherectomy, or stent procedures are hospitalized for less than 24 hours. All patients require education about their medication regimen and about risk factor modification. Because of the short hospital stay, the nurse often has time to do little more than identify the key risk factors and initiate basic instruction. Patients are referred to local cardiac rehabilitation centers for more extensive teaching and follow-up to facilitate understanding and compliance with risk factor modification.

Another point of instruction that must be addressed is the patient's knowledge deficit related to discharge medications. Patients go home on a regimen of antiplatelet medications and medications for secondary prevention, such as lipid-lowering agents and blood pressure medications. A nitrate such as isosorbide may be prescribed to promote vasodilation, or, if the patient has demonstrated evidence of a

TABLE 12.9 Vascular Closure Devices.

Device Category	Device Name	Puncture Size, F	Comments
Active Approximators			
Clip or staple	StarClose SE	5,6	Extravascular nitinol clip over arteriotomy site
Suture	Prostar XL	8.5—10	Percutaneous braided polyester suture delivered, for procedures requiring larger sheaths
Suture	Perclose ProGlide	5—21	A suture loop is formed to close the arteriotomy.
			Two devices and a preclose technique are required for sheath sizes >8 F.
Passive Approximators			
Collagen based	Angio-Seal	5/6, 7/8	An absorbable collagen plug deployed over the arteriotomy site expands in subcutaneous tissue
Collagen based	Vascade Vascular Closure System	5—7	A low-profile disc is deployed intraluminally to abut the wall as a collagen plug is deployed extraluminally over the arteriotomy site
Sealant or gel based	MYNXGRIP	5—7	Small, semicompliant balloon is inflated intraluminally to serve as an anchor as the sealant is deployed over the arteriotomy
Sealant or gel based	Exoseal	5—7	A bioabsorbable polyglycolic acid plug is deployed extraluminally over the arteriotomy
Sealant or gel based	Closer Vascular Sealing System	5—7	Absorbable intraluminal patch and extraluminal spheres that are cinched together with absorbable stitch
Sealed or gel based	FISH CombiClose (Femoral Introducer Sheath and Hemostasis)	5—8	The introducer sheath is used to position the patch. A bioabsorbable matrix patch is deployed through the arteriotomy that straddles the arterial wall.
External Hemostasis Devices			
External compression	FemoStop	Any size	Transparent inflatable bubble placed over the puncture site and belt wrapped around patient for stabilization
	CompressAR	Any size	Hands-free stand with transparent disc that is placed over puncture site and adjusted to height
	QuickLamp	Any size	Hands-free stand with compression discs with or without calcium alginate pad, adjusted to height and amount of pressure provided

From Noori VJ, Eldrup-Jorgense J. A systematic review of vascular closure devices for femoral artery puncture sites. *J Vasc Surg.* 2018;68(3):887.

vasospastic component to the disease, calcium channel blockers may be used. It is essential that the patient clearly understands the rationale for therapy and the potential side effects of each medication. Patients also need to understand the importance of compliance with antiplatelet therapy, because premature discontinuation of these agents is associated with stent thrombosis and increased risk of death.

Percutaneous Valve Repair

Balloon Valvuloplasty

Percutaneous catheter technology has also been adapted to allow for nonsurgical interventions for valvular heart disease. Transvenous mitral commissurotomy, also known as mitral balloon valvotomy, is an accepted alternative to surgical repair for patients with mitral valve stenosis. This procedure has a limited role in aortic stenosis because it provides only short-term improvement and is associated with high morbidity and mortality. Current guidelines recommend balloon dilation for aortic stenosis only as a bridge to surgery or transcatheter valve replacement (discussed later) in patients with severe symptoms.[58]

Balloon valvuloplasty is performed in the cardiac catheterization laboratory by placing a balloon across the stenotic valve and inflating it to increase the opening size. Regurgitant flow can result, particularly after mitral valvuloplasty, and may lead to the need for emergent valve replacement if severe. The risks of balloon valvuloplasty are similar to the risks inherent in most catheterization procedures and include cardiac perforation, thromboembolic events, dysrhythmias, and vascular complications caused by the sheath. Nursing management after the procedure is similar to nursing management for other percutaneous cardiac catheter procedures.

Transcatheter Aortic Valve Replacement

Transcatheter aortic valve replacement (TAVR) is a transformational therapy for patients who have severe aortic valve stenosis. Patient inclusion criteria have been expanded from only high-risk surgical candidates to now include patients with low surgical risk.[58-60] TAVR can be done with spinal or general anesthesia in a hybrid-equipped cardiac surgery operating room. The procedure consists of positioning a bioprosthetic valve that has been loaded on a stent within the native aortic valve and then expanding the stent to anchor the valve within the aortic annulus. Different approaches are used to deploy the device; location should be checked by echocardiography (transthoracic echocardiography [TTE] or transesophageal echocardiography [TEE]), hemodynamics, and/or aortography.

Postprocedural monitoring includes mental status, telemetry, vital signs, volume status, and possible blood work.[60] Vascular access complications can be significant after TAVR, requiring close monitoring of the insertion site to detect possible bleeding, hematoma formation, or limb ischemia. Recommendations are for patients to be treated with dual antiplatelet therapy for 3 to 6 months to prevent thromboembolism and ensure that the valve is endothelialized.[60]

CARDIAC SURGERY

Nursing management of a patient undergoing cardiac surgery is demanding but exciting work that requires the talents of an experienced team of critical care nurses. This section introduces basic cardiac surgical techniques along with principles of cardiopulmonary bypass (CPB) and highlights the key points about postoperative care of adult patients who require valve replacement or coronary artery revascularization.

Coronary Artery Bypass Graft Surgery

Since its introduction almost 60 years ago, coronary artery bypass graft (CABG) surgery has proved to be safe and effective in relieving angina symptoms and improving survival in most patients. Although there has been a great deal of evolution involving less invasive techniques, improved pharmacologic therapy, and expanded education regarding lifestyle modifications, CABG surgery continues to have an important role in the treatment of CAD. Information on CAD is presented in Chapter 11, and catheter-based interventions for CAD are discussed earlier in this chapter.

Surgical revascularization has been shown to be more efficacious than PCI in patients with multivessel or left main coronary disease. Bypass surgery may allow for more complete revascularization, because it can be used on vessels that are not amenable to treatment with a percutaneous approach, such as vessels with total occlusions or excessive tortuosity. However, as medical therapy and surgical procedures continue to evolve, updated studies and evaluations are required to guide optimal treatment.

Myocardial revascularization involves the use of a conduit, or channel, designed to bypass an occluded coronary artery. Surgeons must evaluate which conduits would provide the best graft patency and long-term outcomes for their patients. The long saphenous vein graft (SVG) is the most frequently used conduit for CABG surgery. Saphenous vein grafting involves the anastomosis of an excised portion of the saphenous vein proximal to the aorta and distal to the coronary artery below the obstruction. Vein-graft harvesting can be done via either an open or endoscopic approach (Fig. 12.11).

Use of arterial conduits has dramatically improved long-term graft patency. The internal thoracic artery (ITA)—previously known as the internal mammary artery (IMA)—remains attached to its origin at the subclavian artery and is swung down and anastomosed distal to the coronary artery (Fig. 12.12). The left ITA is considered the gold standard conduit in CABG and has been shown to increase graft patency, survival, and freedom from cardiac events

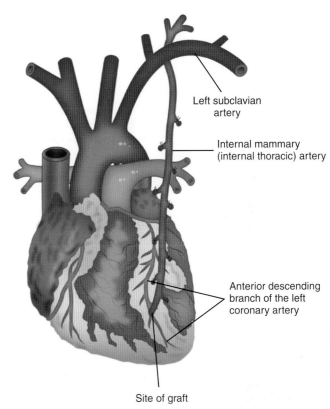

Fig. 12.12 Internal Thoracic Artery Graft.

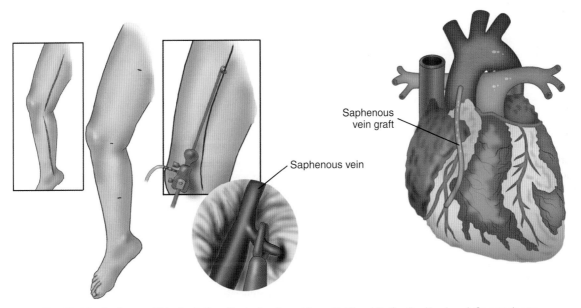

Fig. 12.11 Saphenous Vein Graft. (Leg illustration from Moser D, Riegel B. *Cardiac Nursing: A Companion to Braunwald's Heart Disease.* Philadelphia: Saunders; 2007.)

TABLE 12.10 Conduits Used for Coronary Artery Bypass Grafts.

Type of Graft	Advantages	Disadvantages
Saphenous vein	Easily harvested	Long-term patency less than arterial grafts
	Length allows for multiple grafts	Requires at least two anastomosis sites
	No anatomic limitations to graft sites	
Internal thoracic artery (ITA)	Proven patency rates	Requires extensive dissection and may not be accessible for emergency bypass
	Requires only one anastomosis	Potential increased risk of sternal wound infections with bilateral ITAs
		Anatomic limitations to bypassing some areas of the heart
Radial artery	Improved patency rates	Requires adequate collateral flow to hand through the ulnar artery
	Easily harvested	Higher rates of vasospasm require pharmacologic prophylaxis
	No anatomic limitations to graft sites	Requires two anastomosis sites

compared with SVG conduits.[61] Radial artery conduits in CABG are typically used as adjuncts to the left ITA. Graft patency has increased with improved harvesting techniques, adjunctive medication strategies (statins and antiplatelet agents), and aggressive risk factor modification such as smoking cessation. Conduits used for myocardial revascularization are compared in Table 12.10.

Valvular Surgery

Valvular disease results in various hemodynamic dysfunctions that can usually be managed medically as long as the patient remains symptom-free. There is reluctance to intervene surgically early in the course of this disease because of the surgical risks and long-term complications associated with prosthetic valve replacement. However, these consequences must be weighed against the possibility of irreversible deterioration in LV function that may develop during the compensated asymptomatic phase.

Surgical therapy for aortic valve disease consists primarily of aortic valve replacement, although repairs may be done for selected regurgitant valves. The mitral valve has a more complex anatomy, and although more technically demanding, mitral valve repair is preferred over valve replacement to avoid the complications inherent with a prosthetic valve, including the risk of thromboembolic events and the need for long-term anticoagulation. If reconstruction of the mitral valve is impossible, it is replaced.

BOX 12.4 Classification of Prosthetic Cardiac Valves

Mechanical Valves
- *Tilting-disk:* A free-floating, lens-shaped disk mounted on a circular sewing ring (Medtronic Hall)
- *Bileaflet:* Two semicircular leaflets mounted on a circular sewing ring that opens centrally (St. Jude)

Biologic or Tissue Valves (Bioprostheses)
- *Stented* (porcine xenograft or pericardial xenograft)
- *Stentless* (porcine xenograft or pericardial xenograft)
- *Homograft:* A human heart valve (aortic or pulmonic) harvested from a donated heart and cryopreserved; may or may not be mounted on a support ring

Percutaneous
- Expanded over a balloon (Edwards SAPIEN)
- Self-expandable (CoreValve)

Prosthetic Valves

The two categories of prosthetic valves are mechanical heart valves (MHV) and bioprosthetic heart valves (BHV), or tissue valves. Various valvular prostheses are described in Box 12.4.

A discussion regarding the risks and benefits of the different prosthetic valves should be had between the patient and the physician.[58]

Mechanical heart valves. MHVs are made from combinations of metal alloys, pyrolytic carbon, Dacron, and Teflon and have rigid occluding devices (Fig. 12.13). Their construction renders them highly durable, but all patients with mechanical valves require anticoagulation to reduce the incidence of thromboembolism. Because MHVs are more durable, they may be preferred for a young person who is anticipated to have a relatively long-life span ahead.

Bioprosthetic heart valves. BHVs are constructed from animal or human cardiac tissue and have flexible occluding mechanisms. Because of their low thrombogenicity, tissue valves offer the patient freedom from therapeutic anticoagulation. However, their durability is limited by their tendency toward early calcification. A BHV may be chosen for an older adult patient; the valve has a reduced longevity, but this disadvantage is offset by the older patient's shorter life expectancy.[58] For patients with medical contraindications to anticoagulation and for patients whose past compliance with medications has been questionable, a BHV may be selected. Technical considerations, such as the size of the annulus (or the anatomic ring in which the valve sits), can also influence the choice of valve; for example, a bioprosthesis may be too big for a small aortic root.

Infective endocarditis. The complication of infective endocarditis remains a significant concern due to high mortality rates. Considerations for the timing of surgery, if required, need to be made with the surgeon along with aggressive antibiotic therapy and the removal of any devices.[58]

Cardiopulmonary Bypass

CPB is a mechanical means of circulating and oxygenating a patient's blood while diverting most of the circulation from the heart and lungs during cardiac surgical procedures. The extracorporeal circuit consists of cannulas that drain off venous blood; an oxygenator that oxygenates the blood; and a pump head that propels the arterialized blood back to the ascending aorta, which has been cross-clamped to prevent the back flow of blood into the heart.

Several adjunctive strategies are used to facilitate circulation and oxygenation while the patient is on bypass (on-pump). The patient is systemically heparinized (activated clotting time >400) before initiation of bypass to prevent clotting within the bypass circuit.[62] After the

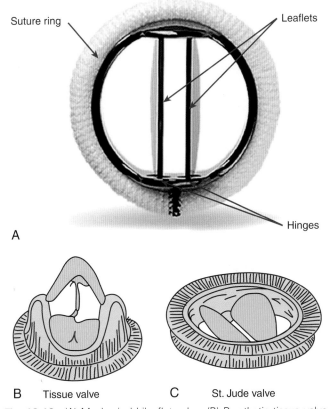

A

B   Tissue valve   C   St. Jude valve

Fig. 12.13 (A) Mechanical bileaflet valve. (B) Prosthetic tissue valve. (C) Mechanical bileaflet valve (St. Jude). (A, Courtesy St. Jude Medical.)

patient is taken off the CPB machine, protamine sulfate is given to reverse the effects of the heparin.

Rapidly stopping the heart in diastole by perfusing the coronary arteries with a potassium cardioplegic (heart-paralyzing) agent assists with intraoperative myocardial protection. The cardioplegia solution must be reinfused at regular intervals during CPB to keep the heart in an arrested state so that the surgeon can operate while the heart is stopped and to minimize myocardial oxygen requirements.

Systemic hypothermia during bypass can reduce tissue oxygen requirements to 50% of normal, which affords the major organs additional protection from ischemic injury. Lowering the body temperature to approximately 28°C (82.4°F) is accomplished through a heat exchanger incorporated into the pump. The blood is warmed back to normal body temperature before bypass is discontinued.

The technique of hemodilution is also used to enhance tissue oxygenation by improving blood flow through the systemic and pulmonary microcirculation during bypass. *Hemodilution* refers to the dilution of the patient's own (autologous) blood with the isotonic crystalloid solution used to prime the circuit. This hemodilution enhances capillary perfusion by reducing blood viscosity (stickiness) and decreasing the risk of microthrombi formation. At the completion of CPB, the large quantities of "pump blood" that remain in the bypass circuit can be collected and used for initial postoperative volume replacement.

Numerous clinical sequelae can result from CPB (Table 12.11). Knowledge of these physiologic effects allows the nurse to anticipate problems and intervene effectively in the postoperative period.

Off-Pump Coronary Artery Bypass Graft Surgery

Some surgeons may elect to perform off-pump CABG (OP-CABG) surgery with the goal of avoiding the potential complications associated with CPB and cross-clamping of the aorta. OP-CABG surgeries account

TABLE 12.11 **Physiologic Effects of Cardiopulmonary Bypass.**	
Effects	**Causes**
Intravascular fluid deficit (hypotension)	Third spacing
	Postoperative diuresis
	Sudden vasodilation (medications, rewarming)
Third spacing (weight gain, edema)	Decreased plasma protein concentration
	Increased capillary permeability
Myocardial depression (decreased cardiac output)	Hypothermia
	Increased systemic vascular resistance
	Prolonged cardiopulmonary bypass pump run
	Preexisting heart disease
	Inadequate myocardial protection
Coagulopathy (bleeding)	Systemic heparinization
	Mechanical trauma to platelets
	Decreased release of clotting factors from liver as a result of hypothermia
Pulmonary dysfunction (decreased lung mechanics and impaired gas exchange)	Decreased surfactant production
	Pulmonary microemboli
	Interstitial fluid accumulation in lungs
Hemolysis (hemoglobinuria)	Red blood cells damaged in pump circuit
Hyperglycemia (rise in serum glucose concentration)	Decreased insulin release
	Stimulation of glycogenolysis
Hypokalemia (low serum potassium concentration)	Intracellular shifts during bypass and postoperative diuresis
Hypomagnesemia (low serum magnesium concentration)	Postoperative diuresis resulting from hemodilution
Neurologic dysfunction (decreased level of consciousness, motor/sensory deficits)	Inadequate cerebral perfusion
	Microemboli to brain (air, plaque fragments, fat globules)
Hypertension (transient increase in blood pressure)	Catecholamine release and systemic hypothermia causing vasoconstriction

for less than 15% of all CABG procedures in the United States.[63] Several techniques are used to stabilize the operative area during an OP-CABG procedure. Immobilization devices that use compression or suction to create an immobile area have been developed to stabilize cardiac wall motion at the site of the anastomosis. Medications that temporarily decrease the heart rate (e.g., esmolol, diltiazem) or cause transient cardiac asystole (e.g., adenosine) may also be used to further limit cardiac motion. Although the OP-CABG procedure was developed to decrease complications associated with CPB, there is no convincing data that OP-CABG surgery is superior to on-pump CABG surgery. Long-term graft patency, complete revascularization, and overall survival may be better with conventional CABG surgery.[64]

Postoperative Management

Medical and nursing management of the postoperative cardiac surgery patient often overlaps. The physician prescribes therapeutic interventions and identifies specific hemodynamic end points to maintain adequate organ perfusion and oxygen delivery. The nurse is responsible for applying these therapies to maintain the patient's hemodynamic parameters within the desired range. In most institutions, standard protocols are used to facilitate the postoperative nursing diagnoses and management of cardiac surgical patients (Box 12.5).

Cardiovascular Support

Postoperative cardiovascular support often is indicated because of a low-output state. The most common causes of cardiac dysfunction after cardiac surgery are mechanical complications, physiologic complications, MI, and dysrhythmias. Cardiac output can be maximized by adjustments in heart rate, preload, afterload, and contractility.

Heart rate. In the presence of low cardiac output, the heart rate can be appropriately regulated via temporary pacing or medication therapy. Temporary atrial or ventricular epicardial pacing is usually instituted when the heart rate decreases to less than 60 beats/min and the patient is hypotensive, requiring a supportive rate of 80 to 100 beats/min. In the case of tachycardia, intravenous beta-blockers (esmolol) or calcium channel blockers (diltiazem) may be used in the acute postoperative period to slow supraventricular rhythms. Obtaining a 12-lead ECG to assess dysrhythmias further may also be indicated. Electrolyte disturbances such as hypokalemia, hypomagnesemia, hypocalcemia, and hypercalcemia must be closely monitored and corrected to prevent postoperative dysrhythmias.

Atrial fibrillation is the most common adverse event after cardiac surgery. It occurs in approximately 30% to 50% of patients after cardiac surgery, with a peak occurrence in the first 2 to 3 days after surgery. This rhythm may induce hemodynamic compromise, prolong hospitalization, and increase the patient's risk of stroke. Prophylactic administration of beta-blockers is recommended to decrease the incidence of atrial fibrillation and its clinical sequelae; amiodarone is an alternative for patients who have contraindications to beta-blockers.[65] Initial management of atrial fibrillation involves slowing of the ventricular rate, but if the patient is hemodynamically unstable, restoration of sinus rhythm by antiarrhythmic drugs or cardioversion is recommended.[65] Ventricular arrhythmias are uncommon, so ongoing ischemia should be suspected and investigated.

Preload. In most patients, reduced preload is the cause of low postoperative cardiac output. The most common causes of decreased preload are hypovolemia from bleeding, fluid shifts caused by the systemic inflammatory response, increased vascular capacitance with rewarming, and elevated cardiac preload requirements.[66] Appropriate volume resuscitation immediately postoperatively is one of the most important interventions and should be a first-line therapy for hemodynamic instability. To enhance preload, volume may be administered in the form of crystalloid, colloid, or packed red cells. Crystalloids are preferred for fluid resuscitation; the type of crystalloid depends on institutional preference.[66] Preload is often evaluated by intermittent pressure readings obtained from catheters placed in the right atrium or pulmonary artery. A growing body of research suggests that static indices such as central venous pressure (CVP) and pulmonary artery occlusion pressure (PAOP) have a very weak relationship with the patient's intravascular volume and are not helpful in predicting if a patient will respond to fluid resuscitation.[67] Volume resuscitation should be done in the context of the full patient picture, because excessive fluid administration can lead to adverse events.[67] Approximately 2 to 3 L of crystalloid will suffice for most patients.

Afterload. Patients who have had cardiac surgery may demonstrate postoperative hypertension. Although it is transient, postoperative hypertension can precipitate or exacerbate bleeding from the mediastinal chest tubes. The high systemic vascular resistance (SVR) (afterload) resulting from the intense vasoconstriction can increase LV workload. Vasodilator therapy with intravenous sodium nitroprusside or nitroglycerin often is used to reduce afterload, control hypertension, and improve cardiac output. Increased afterload may be partially caused by the peripheral vasoconstrictive effects of hypothermia, which can be managed with careful rewarming.

A significant percentage of patients experience hypotension after CPB secondary to peripheral vasodilation. This condition is believed to occur in part because of the systemic inflammatory response to CPB, surgical trauma, ischemia, or reperfusion. Therapy for hypotension after cardiac surgery usually includes volume loading and vasopressors. Typical vasopressor agents include norepinephrine and vasopressin in patients with excessive vasodilation. Phenylephrine should be used cautiously because it increases afterload and decreases graft flow.

Contractility. The patient's EF should also be used to inform the treatment plan. If the adjustments in heart rate, preload, and afterload

---

◉ BOX 12.5 PRIORITY PATIENT CARE MANAGEMENT

Open-Heart Surgery
- Impaired Cardiac Output due to alterations in preload
- Impaired Cardiac Output due to alterations in afterload
- Impaired Cardiac Output due to alterations in contractility
- Impaired Cardiac Output due to alterations in heart rate or rhythm
- Impaired Cardiac Output due to sympathetic blockade
- Impaired Gas Exchange due to alveolar hypoventilation
- Impaired Gas Exchange due to ventilation-perfusion mismatching or intrapulmonary shunting
- Impaired Airway Clearance due to excessive secretions or abnormal viscosity of mucus
- Activity Intolerance due to cardiopulmonary dysfunction
- Activity Intolerance due to prolonged immobility or deconditioning
- Risk for Infection
- Acute Pain due to transmission and perception of cutaneous, visceral, muscular, or ischemic impulses
- Anxiety due to threat to biologic, psychologic, or social integrity
- Impaired Sleep due to fragmented sleep
- Lack of Knowledge of Treatment Regime due to lack of previous exposure to information

(see Patient Care Management Plans located in Appendix A)

fail to produce significant improvement in cardiac output, contractility can be enhanced with positive inotropic support. There is a great deal of variability in the choice of vasoactive agents used with few data guiding decision making. Epinephrine, norepinephrine, dopamine, and dobutamine are commonly used inotropic catecholamines. Mechanical circulatory support (MCS) may also need to be added to help augment circulation (discussed later).

Mechanical Complications

Different mechanical complications after cardiac surgery include cardiac tamponade, hematomas, vasospasm of a coronary artery graft, prosthetic valve paravalvular regurgitation, and systolic anterior motion of the mitral valve. Some mechanical complications are noncardiac, such as pneumothorax, hemothorax, and endotracheal tube malposition. Identifying and intervening are important to quickly prevent any further dysfunction.

Temperature Regulation

Hypothermia can contribute to depressed myocardial contractility, vasoconstriction, and ventricular dysrhythmias in a patient who has undergone cardiac surgery. Hypothermia may also contribute to postoperative bleeding because the functioning of clotting factors is depressed. After surgery, patients may be rewarmed with the use of warm blankets or forced-air warming devices. Excessive temperature elevations must be avoided, with the goal of maintaining a target body temperature of 36°C to 37°C (96.8°F–98.6°F).

Control of Bleeding

Postoperative bleeding from the mediastinal chest tubes can be caused by inadequate hemostasis, disruption of suture lines, coagulopathy associated with CPB, residual heparin effect, clotting factor depletion, thrombocytopenia, or hypothermia, along with other less frequent factors.[68] Blood conservation strategies should be used to limit the number of transfusions, because the administration of packed red blood cells has been independently associated with increased complications and increased mortality. At the present time, blood transfusions are not recommended for a hemoglobin greater than 10 g/dL, but transfusions are reasonable in most postoperative patients whose hemoglobin is less than 7 g/dL.[69]

Although no exact definition exists for excessive bleeding, amounts greater than 200 mL/h often require further interventions. Clotting factors (fresh frozen plasma, fibrinogen, and platelets), protamine, or desmopressin may be administered. Medications used in the treatment of postoperative bleeding are described in Table 12.12. To help guide the selection of appropriate factors or medications, laboratory values such as prothrombin time/international normalized ratio, partial thromboplastin time, platelets, fibrinogen, and thrombin time are

obtained. Blood pressure drives bleeding; some recommend the systolic blood pressure should be targeted to no higher than 90 to 100 mm Hg, whereas other studies suggest there is little evidence for strict blood pressure management to reduce blood loss.[70,71] Using therapeutic positive end-expiratory pressure to reduce excessive postoperative bleeding is not well established.[69] Rewarming the patient reverses the depressed manufacture and release of clotting factors that result from hypothermia. However, persistent mediastinal bleeding, usually greater than 500 mL in 1 hour or 300 mL/h for 2 consecutive hours despite normalization of clotting studies, is an indication for reexploration of the surgical site.

Chest Tube Patency

Chest tube stripping to maintain patency of the tubes is controversial because of the high negative pressure generated by routine methods of stripping. It is believed to result in tissue damage that can contribute to bleeding. This risk must be carefully weighed against the real danger of cardiac tamponade if blood is not effectively drained from around the heart. Chest tube stripping often is advocated in instances of excessive postoperative bleeding. However, the technique of "milking" the chest tubes is advisable for routine postoperative care because this technique generates less negative pressure and decreases the risk of bleeding.

Cardiac Tamponade

Cardiac tamponade is a potentially lethal complication that may occur after surgery if blood accumulates in the mediastinal space, impairing the heart's ability to pump. Signs of tamponade include elevated and equalized filling pressures (e.g., CVP, pulmonary artery diastolic pressure, PAOP), decreased cardiac output, decreased blood pressure, jugular venous distention, pulsus paradoxus, muffled heart sounds, sudden cessation of chest tube drainage, and a widened cardiac silhouette on radiographs. A bedside echocardiogram may be done to confirm tamponade. Interventions for tamponade may include emergency sternotomy in the critical care unit or a return to the operating room for surgical evacuation of the clot.

Pulmonary Care

Mechanical ventilation is used initially to provide adequate alveolar oxygenation and ventilation in the postoperative period. Protocols that facilitate early extubation (less than 6 hours after surgery) have been implemented in most institutions and have been shown to decrease pulmonary complications after cardiac surgery.[66] Early extubation requires a multidisciplinary approach that incorporates anesthesiologists, surgeons, nurses, and respiratory therapists. Potential candidates must be identified before surgery so that the anesthetic regimen supports early extubation.

TABLE 12.12 Medications Used to Treat Postoperative Bleeding.

Medication	Dose	Action and Side Effects
Aminocaproic acid (Amicar)	Loading dose: 4–5 g over 1 hour, followed by continuous infusion of 1 g/h for 8 hours or until bleeding is controlled	Inhibits conversion of plasminogen to plasmin to prevent fibrinolysis, helping to stabilize clots
Desmopressin acetate (DDAVP)	0.3 mcg/kg IV over 20–30 minutes	Improves platelet function by increasing levels of factor VIII Side effects include facial flushing, tachycardia, headache, and hypotension
Protamine sulfate	25–50 mg IV slowly over 10 minutes	Neutralizes anticoagulant effect of heparin Can cause hypotension, bradycardia, and allergic reactions

IV, Intravenously.

After surgery, patients are evaluated for hemodynamic stability, adequate control of bleeding, normothermia, and the ability to follow commands. Once these criteria have been met, most institutions have a weaning protocol to follow that often involves a spontaneous breathing trial to evaluate the patient's readiness for extubation. Patients who exhibit hemodynamic instability or intraoperative complications or who have underlying pulmonary disease may require longer periods of mechanical ventilation. After extubation, supplemental oxygen is administered, and patients are medicated for incisional pain to facilitate aggressive pulmonary hygiene and early mobility, which is essential to help prevent postoperative complications.[72]

Neurologic Complications

The neurologic dysfunction often seen in patients who have undergone cardiac surgery has been attributed to decreased cerebral perfusion, cerebral microemboli, hypoxia, and the systemic inflammatory response. The dysfunction can range from subtle cognitive changes to signs of acute stroke. Early recognition of neurologic changes is important so that prompt initiation of therapy may prevent worsening of complications. The risk of delirium is increased in cardiac surgery patients, especially older adults, and is associated with increased mortality and reduced quality of life and cognitive function.[73] Nurses have a critical role in the prevention and recognition of delirium (see Delirium in Chapter 8).

Infection

Postoperative fever is common after CPB. However, persistent temperature elevation to greater than 101°F (38.3°C) must be investigated. Sternal wound infections and infective endocarditis are the most devastating infectious complications, but leg wound infections, pneumonia, and urinary tract infections also can occur. Infection rates are greater in patients with diabetes, malnutrition, chronic diseases, obesity, and in patients requiring emergent or prolonged surgery. Using a continuous insulin infusion to maintain blood glucose concentrations less than or equal to 180 mg/dL while avoiding hypoglycemia may reduce the incidence of adverse events, including deep sternal wound infections.[74]

Acute Kidney Injury

AKI is recognized as a significant problem after cardiac surgery because of a very complex pathogenesis. Prevention of acute injury to the kidney by avoiding renal insults is still the mainstay of management.[75] Kidney dysfunction in the postoperative period requires frequent monitoring of urine output and serum creatinine levels. Because of fluid retention, diuresis is often required to help mobilize fluids from the interstitial to the intravascular space and may be done with the administration of medications or may be allowed to occur naturally. The patient's potassium levels may be depleted with the diuresis, requiring that levels be closely monitored and replaced. See Acute Kidney Injury in Chapter 19 for more information on AKI.

Resuscitation of Patients Who Arrest After Cardiac Surgery

The incidence of cardiac arrest after cardiac surgery is relatively low. These patients have comparatively good outcomes given the high incidence of reversible causes of the cardiac arrest. Special guidelines have been developed by the Society of Thoracic Surgeons on the resuscitation of patients who arrest after cardiac surgery, focusing on the differences in this patient population.

Recommendations include: patients who arrest with VF or pulseless VT should receive three sequential attempts at defibrillation before external cardiac massage; patients with asystole or extreme bradycardia should undergo an attempt to pace if wires are available before external cardiac massage; for pulseless electrical activity, quickly reversible causes should be excluded (such as tamponade or bleeding) followed by emergency resternotomy.[76] Finally, because of the danger

---

QSEN | **BOX 12.6   Evidence-Based Practice**

Coronary Artery Bypass Graft Surgery
A summary is provided of evidence and evidence-based review recommendations for management of patients undergoing coronary artery bypass graft (CABG) surgery.

Strong Evidence to Support the Following
Coronary Artery Bypass Graft Surgery for Patients
- Emergency CABG surgery is indicated for patients with acute myocardial infarction (MI) when primary percutaneous coronary intervention (PCI) has failed or cannot be performed, coronary anatomy is suitable for CABG surgery, and persistent ischemia and/or hemodynamic instability refractory to nonsurgical therapy is present.
- Emergency CABG surgery is indicated for patients undergoing surgical repair of postinfarction mechanical complications of MI, patients with cardiogenic shock, or patients with life-threatening ventricular dysrhythmias in the presence of left main stenosis or three-vessel coronary artery disease (CAD).
- CABG surgery is indicated for patients undergoing noncoronary cardiac surgery if 50% or greater stenosis of left main or 70% or greater stenosis of other major coronary arteries.
- CABG surgery is indicated for patients with significant (50% or greater) stenosis of left main coronary artery.
- CABG surgery is indicated for patients with significant (70% or greater) stenosis in three major coronary arteries or in the proximal left anterior descending (LAD) artery plus one other major coronary artery.

- CABG surgery or PCI is indicated in patients with one or more significant (70% or greater) coronary artery stenoses with unacceptable angina despite guideline-directed medical therapy.
- Patients undergoing CABG surgery who have at least moderate aortic stenosis should undergo aortic valve replacement.
- Patients undergoing CABG surgery who have severe ischemic mitral valve regurgitation not likely to resolve with revascularization should undergo mitral valve repair or replacement.

Anesthetic Considerations
- Anesthetic management should be directed toward early postoperative extubation and accelerated recovery of low-risk to medium-risk patients.

Bypass Graft Conduits
- Internal thoracic arteries (ITAs) should be used to bypass the left anterior descending (LAD) artery when bypass of the LAD is indicated.

Antiplatelet Therapy
- Discontinuation of P2Y12 inhibitors for a few days before cardiovascular operations is recommended to reduce bleeding, especially in high-risk patients.
- For stable nonbleeding patients, aspirin should be given within 6–24 hours to optimize graft patency.

Management of Hyperlipidemia
- All patients should receive statin therapy unless contraindicated.

BOX 12.6 Evidence-Based Practice—cont'd

Blood Glucose Management

- Continuous intravenous insulin is administered to maintain early postoperative blood glucose concentration 180 mg/dL or less while avoiding hypoglycemia to reduce adverse events.

Dysrhythmia Management

- Beta-blockers should be administered for at least 24 hours before CABG surgery, reinstituted as soon as possible after surgery, and prescribed at discharge unless contraindicated to reduce the incidence and clinical sequelae of atrial fibrillation.

Angiotensin-Converting Enzyme Inhibitors and Angiotensin-Receptor Blockers

- Angiotensin-converting enzyme inhibitors and angiotensin-receptor blockers should be instituted or restarted postoperatively and continued indefinitely for patients with left ventricular ejection fraction (LVEF) 40% or less, hypertension, diabetes, or chronic kidney disease.

Smoking Cessation

- All patients who smoke should receive educational counseling and be offered smoking cessation therapy during hospitalization for CABG surgery.

Cardiac Rehabilitation

- Cardiac rehabilitation should be offered to all eligible patients after CABG surgery.

Reduction in Risk of Infection

- Antibiotics should be administered preoperatively in all patients to reduce the risk of postoperative infection.

Bleeding and Transfusions

- Aggressive attempts at blood conservation are indicated to reduce the need for red blood cell transfusions.

Moderate Evidence to Support the Following
Coronary Artery Bypass Graft Surgery for Patients

- CABG surgery is indicated in patients with multivessel CAD with recurrent angina or MI within the first 48 hours of ST segment elevation MI presentation as an alternative to a more delayed strategy.
- CABG surgery or PCI is indicated for selected patients aged 75 years or older with ST segment elevation or left bundle branch block who are suitable for revascularization regardless of the time interval from MI to the onset of shock.
- Emergency CABG surgery is indicated after failed PCI to retrieve a foreign body in a crucial anatomic location or for hemodynamic compromise in patients with impairment of the coagulation system and without previous sternotomy.
- CABG surgery is indicated in patients with significant (70% or greater) stenosis in two major coronary arteries with extensive myocardial ischemia or target vessels supplying a large area of viable myocardium.
- CABG surgery is indicated in patients with mild to moderate left ventricular systolic dysfunction (LVEF 35%–50%) and significant (70% or greater stenosis) multivessel CAD or proximal LAD stenosis with viable myocardium present.

- CABG surgery is indicated in patients with complex three-vessel CAD (SYNTAX score greater than 22) with or without involvement of the proximal LAD artery who are good candidates for CABG surgery.
- CABG surgery is preferred over PCI to improve survival in patients with multivessel CAD and diabetes mellitus, particularly if a left internal thoracic artery graft can be anastomosed to the LAD artery.
- Patients undergoing CABG surgery who have moderate ischemic mitral valve regurgitation not likely to resolve with revascularization should undergo mitral valve repair or replacement.

Hybrid Coronary Revascularization

- The planned combination of LIMA-to-LAD artery grafting and PCI of one or more non-LAD coronary arteries is reasonable for (1) limitations to CABG surgery such as heavily calcified proximal aorta or poor target vessels for CABG surgery, (2) lack of suitable graft conduits, and (3) unfavorable LAD artery for PCI.

Antiplatelet Therapy

- Clopidogrel 75 mg daily is a reasonable alternative in patients who cannot take aspirin.

Beta-Blockers

- Preoperative beta-blockers, particularly in patients with an ejection fraction greater than 30%, can reduce the risk of in-hospital mortality.
- Preoperative beta-blockers can reduce the incidence of perioperative myocardial ischemia.

Emotional Dysfunction and Psychosocial Considerations

- Cognitive-behavioral therapy or collaborative care for patients with clinical depression after CABG surgery can be beneficial to reduce objective measures of depression.

Carotid Artery Disease

- For patients with a previous transient ischemic attack or stroke and significant (50%—99%) carotid artery stenosis, carotid revascularization should be considered in conjunction with CABG surgery. Sequence and timing (staged or simultaneous) should be determined by the relative magnitude of cerebral and myocardial dysfunction.

Infection Prevention

- Leukocyte-filtered blood can be useful to reduce the rate of overall perioperative infection and in-hospital death.

Adjuncts to Myocardial Protection

- Insertion of an intraaortic balloon pump is reasonable to reduce the mortality rate in patients undergoing CABG surgery who are considered to be at high risk (e.g., LVEF less than 30% or left main CAD).
- Assessment of cardiac biomarkers in the first 24 hours after CABG surgery may be considered.

Dysrhythmia Management

- For patients who cannot take beta-blockers, amiodarone is an alternative to reduce the incidence of postoperative atrial fibrillation.
- Digoxin and nondihydropyridine calcium channel blockers can be useful to control the ventricular rate in the setting of atrial fibrillation but are not indicated for prophylaxis.

Data from Hillis LD, Smith PK, Anderson JL, et al. 2011 ACCF/AHA guideline for coronary artery bypass graft surgery: executive summary: a report of the American College of Cardiology Foundation/American Heart Association task force on practice guidelines. *Circulation.* 2011;124(23):2610; Aldea GS, Bakaeen FG, Pal J, et al. The Society of Thoracic Surgeons clinical practice guidelines on arterial conduits for coronary artery bypass grafting. *Ann Thorac Surg.* 2016;101:801; and Ferraris VA, Saha SP, Oestreich JH, et al. 2012 Update to the Society of Thoracic Surgeons guideline on use of antiplatelet drugs in patients having cardiac and noncardiac operations. *Ann Thorac Surg.* 2012;94:1761.

of extreme hypertension if a reversible cause is rapidly identified, full-dose epinephrine is not recommended unless directed by a senior physician.[76] Although there are several special caveats with this patient population, the importance of early emergency resternotomy (within 5 minutes) is also a major focus of the recommendations.[76]

Guidelines for Coronary Artery Bypass Graft Surgery

The American College of Cardiology and the American Heart Association have developed a set of clinical practice guidelines for the care of patients undergoing CABG surgery.[74] These guidelines are designed to support clinical decision making with research evidence (Box 12.6).

Educating the Patient and Family

Patient and family education includes information related to the surgical procedure, risk factor management, and prevention of atherosclerosis. Patients who have undergone valve surgery may also require information regarding the need for antibiotic prophylaxis before invasive procedures and specific instructions pertaining to their anticoagulation regimen.

Minimally Invasive Cardiac Surgery

Continuously evolving techniques have expanded the options for patients undergoing cardiac surgery. In an attempt to avoid common complications associated with traditional CABG surgery, minimally invasive direct CABG (MIDCAB) was developed. MIDCAB is performed via a left anterior mini-thoracotomy as a sternal-sparing approach. However, there are many limitations with this approach in regard to the extent of revascularization. Improvements in technology have led to endoscopic techniques coming to the forefront. Totally endoscopic coronary artery bypass (TECAB) (or robotic-assisted) is the least invasive version. The main advantage of this procedure is the avoidance of a thoracotomy or sternotomy. Robotically controlled surgical instruments are inserted through five dime-size incisions and are controlled by the surgeon from the surgical console, allowing more degrees of freedom than conventional surgical instruments.

Postoperative care of patients following TECAB is very similar to that of the standard CABG patient.[74] A few differences include the fact that early extubation may occur in the operating room. Acute pain from the telemanipulation port sites may require early initiation of patient-controlled analgesia (PCA) to assist with pain management. Because the sternum has been preserved, there are no requirements for sternal precautions, which allows for physical activity to be quickly advanced.

A hybrid operating room allows for the combination of PCI and surgical coronary artery revascularization. The goal is to combine the best of both worlds: excellent long-term patency and improved survival of the ITA grafting and minimally invasive nature of PCI.[77]

Surgical Treatment of Cardiac Dysrhythmias

Surgical techniques have assumed a more prominent role in the treatment of atrial fibrillation as surgical ablation has demonstrated effectiveness, not only in reducing atrial fibrillation but also in improving quality of life for patients. Surgical ablation of atrial fibrillation is done both concomitantly with an open or closed surgical cardiac procedure and as a stand-alone surgical atrial fibrillation ablation.[78] The surgical Cox-Maze procedure has evolved over the years but still involves a series of scars that are made in the atrial tissue to create an electrical maze that disrupts the re-entrant pathways and directs the sinus impulse through the AV node. The procedure also includes surgical isolation of the pulmonary veins, which are thought to be responsible for initiation of atrial fibrillation, and removal of the

left and right atrial appendages. The goal of treatment is not only to prevent the recurrence of atrial tachydysrhythmias but also to restore sinus rhythm and AV synchrony, if possible. Patients require continued monitoring for arrhythmias, as atrial fibrillation is common for months afterward while the scar tissue fully matures. Antiarrhythmics such as amiodarone are often continued for 2 to 3 months after surgical ablation.[79] Full anticoagulation is also common until durable rhythm restoration is established.[79]

Although future trends in the surgical management of heart disease are difficult to predict, the critical care nurse must continue to be prepared to meet the challenge of providing a high level of nursing management at the bedside. A solid knowledge base and keen assessment skills are prerequisites for the accurate anticipation of problems and prompt intervention necessary to stabilize the patient and prevent the occurrence of life-threatening complications.

MECHANICAL CIRCULATORY SUPPORT

MCS devices have become an integral part of the cardiovascular therapeutic management of patients. The primary goals of MCS are to decrease myocardial workload, maintain adequate perfusion to vital organs, reduce pulmonary congestion, augment coronary perfusion, provide circulatory support during procedures, and limit infarction size.[80] If the acute heart failure is reversible, a short duration of ventricular assistance is used to allow the myocardium time to recover. If the condition is irreversible, MCS may be used as a bridge to heart transplantation for qualified candidates or as destination therapy (DT) for patients who have no other surgical options.

Short-Term Mechanical Circulatory Support Devices

Short-term MCS devices provide hemodynamic support for the management of cardiogenic shock, decompensated heart failure, cardiopulmonary arrest, or even prophylactic insertion for high-risk invasive coronary artery procedures[80,81] (Box 12.7). Several temporary MCS devices are available, including pneumatic pumps, axial flow pumps, and centrifugal pumps (Table 12.13). Clinical evidence to guide device selection is often controversial or unavailable. Therefore it is primarily a choice of the surgeon and institutional resources. Many ventricular assist devices (VADs) cannot be placed in the critical care unit, which limits how quickly therapy can be initiated. Another consideration is that many VADs provide only single ventricular support, which would necessitate a second device in the setting of biventricular failure.

BOX 12.7   Suggested Indications for Percutaneous Mechanical Circulatory Support

- Severe heart failure in the setting of nonischemic cardiomyopathy
- Failure to wean from cardiopulmonary bypass
- Acute cardiac allograft failure
- Post-transplant right ventricular failure
- Prophylactic use for high-risk percutaneous coronary intervention
- Complications of acute myocardial infarction
- Cardiogenic shock
- Papillary muscle dysfunction or rupture with mitral regurgitation
- Refractory dysrhythmias
- Bridge to definitive therapy: cardiac transplantation or ventricular assist device

TABLE 12.13 Mechanical Circulatory Support Devices.

Type	Indications	Description
Temporary		
CentriMag	Short-term univentricular or biventricular support For central or peripheral VA-ECMO and VV-ECMO	Continuous-flow pump that produces blood flow from 0–10 L/min Blood flow is produced by rotation of a magnetically suspended impeller, eliminating contact between components Placed either through an open chest or by percutaneous methods
Impella CP and Impella 5.0	Short-term left ventricular support	Continuous-flow pump that has a percutaneously inserted catheter, allowing flows of ≥3.5 L/min or 5 L/min for the version that requires a surgical cut-down for implantation The catheter is placed retrograde across the aortic valve to pull blood from the left ventricle, which is returned to the ascending aorta
TandemHeart	Short-term left or right ventricular support	Percutaneously inserted device that provides continuous flow up to 5 L/min LVAD: Inflow is obtained from a catheter positioned in the left atrium (by a transseptal approach), and outflow is through the femoral artery RVAD: Inflow is obtained from a catheter positioned in the right atrium, and outflow is through the pulmonary artery Device allows for transport to a center for long-term therapy
Long-Term		
HeartWare	Long-term left ventricular support FDA approved for BTT and DT	A continuous-flow rotary pump with centrifugal design that produces nonpulsatile flow Its small size allows for placement above the diaphragm in the pericardial space The pump has no points of mechanical contact, which reduces damage to red blood cells
HeartMate II	Long-term left ventricular support FDA approved for BTT and DT	An electrically driven axial continuous-flow pump that produces nonpulsatile flow Anticoagulation and antiplatelet therapy are required
HeartMate 3	Long-term left ventricular support FDA approved for BTT and DT	Magnetically levitated centrifugal-flow pump that produces nonpulsatile flow Anticoagulation and antiplatelet therapy are required Improved outcomes over HeartMate II in regard to pump replacement and survival free of disabling stroke

BTT, Bridge to transplant; *DT,* destination therapy; *FDA,* US Food and Drug Administration; *LVAD,* left ventricular assist device; *RVAD,* right ventricular assist device.

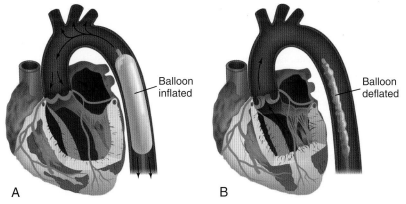

Fig. 12.14 Intraaortic Balloon Pump: Mechanisms of Action. (A) Diastolic balloon inflation augments coronary blood flow. (B) Systolic balloon deflation decreases afterload.

Intraaortic Balloon Pump

The intraaortic balloon pump (IABP) is the most commonly used temporary percutaneous circulatory assist device used in hemodynamically unstable patients. However, it is limited by its modest hemodynamic support or myocardial protection. The intraaortic balloon (IAB) catheter consists of a single sausage-shaped polyurethane balloon that is wrapped around the distal end of a vascular catheter and positioned in the descending thoracic aorta just distal to the takeoff of the left subclavian artery. "Counterpulsation" is the key mechanism for

the IABP. Its therapeutic effects are based on the hemodynamic principles of diastolic augmentation and afterload reduction.

Initially, as the balloon is inflated in diastole concurrent with aortic valve closure, the blood in the aortic arch above the level of the balloon is displaced retrograde (backward) toward the aortic root, augmenting diastolic coronary arterial blood flow and increasing myocardial oxygen supply (Fig. 12.14A). The blood volume in the aorta below the level of the balloon is propelled forward toward the peripheral vascular system, which may enhance systemic perfusion. Subsequently, the deflation of the balloon just before the opening of the aortic valve creates a potential space or vacuum in the aorta, toward which blood flows unimpeded during ventricular ejection (Fig. 12.14B). This decreased resistance to LV ejection, or decreased afterload, facilitates ventricular emptying and reduces myocardial oxygen demands. The overall physiologic effect of IABP therapy is an improvement in the balance between myocardial oxygen supply and demand. Contraindications to IABP include aortic aneurysm, significant aortic valve insufficiency, and severe peripheral vascular disease.[82]

Medical management. The IAB may be inserted in the operating room, the cardiac catheterization laboratory, or the critical care unit. The IAB catheter is usually inserted percutaneously through the femoral artery and advanced to the correct position in the descending thoracic aorta. If percutaneous catheter placement is not feasible, the catheter may be placed through surgical cut-down or by a direct thoracic approach. After insertion, the balloon is attached to the console and filled with the prescribed volume of helium, and pumping is initiated.

Nursing management. The management of the pumping console and its timing functions may be performed by the nurse caring for the patient or delegated to specially trained personnel. Multiple factors may affect the efficacy of the IABP, including position of the balloon within the aorta; balloon displacement volume; inflation and deflation timing; signal quality; the patient's cardiac function; and hemodynamic variables, which include circulating blood volume, blood pressure, and vascular resistance.[83] Clinicians need to be aware of these factors to adequately assess for and ensure optimal IABP performance.

Timing. The IABP depends on proper timing to ensure optimal hemodynamic benefits. Although systems now adjust the timing automatically, clinicians must still be aware of how to set the timing, understand the method used, and evaluate its effects. The ECG and arterial pressure tracings are constantly monitored to verify the timing and effect of balloon counterpulsation (Fig. 12.15). For counterpulsation to occur, the pump must receive a trigger signal to identify the beginning and end of the cardiac cycle. The trigger can be the R wave of the ECG, the upstroke of the arterial pressure waveform, or a pacemaker spike.

Complications. Vascular complications include lower extremity ischemia resulting from occlusion of the femoral artery by the catheter itself or by emboli caused by thrombus formation on the balloon. Evaluation of peripheral circulation remains an important nursing assessment. Signs of diminished perfusion must be reported immediately. Anticoagulation (e.g., heparin infusion) may be prescribed to decrease the incidence of thrombosis. Other vascular complications associated with IABP include acute aortic dissection and the development of pseudoaneurysms at the catheter insertion site.

Balloon complications include balloon perforation and malpositioning. A balloon leak is evidenced by a gas leak alarm from the pump console or the presence of blood in the IAB tubing. If a balloon leak is detected, pumping is stopped, and the physician is immediately notified so that the balloon can be removed. If the balloon is not promptly removed or pumping is attempted after the perforation, the IAB may become entrapped as the blood hardens within the catheter, creating a mass. If this occurs, the balloon must be surgically removed. The balloon catheter must be maintained in proper position to optimize its effectiveness and minimize complications. The balloon may migrate proximally and occlude the left subclavian artery or the carotids, or it may move distally, compromising renal and mesenteric circulation. Careful assessment of the left radial pulse, level of consciousness, urinary output, and gastrointestinal symptoms is essential along with a daily chest radiograph/x-ray. Measures to prevent accidental displacement of the balloon catheter include ensuring that the IAB is secured to the patient's skin, that the patient maintains complete bed rest with the head of the bed elevated no more than 30 degrees, and that any flexion of the involved hip is avoided.

Further complications include thrombocytopenia, which may occur as a result of mechanical destruction of the platelets by the pumping action of the balloon. Platelet counts are closely monitored, and the patient is observed for evidence of bleeding. Patients must also be monitored for signs of stroke and infections.

Weaning. Weaning from the IABP is considered after hemodynamic stability has been achieved with no, or only minimal, pharmacologic support. Weaning is accomplished by reducing the ratio of augmented to nonaugmented beats from 1:1 to 1:2 or 1:3, as tolerated. A less common weaning method involves a gradual decrease in balloon volume. To prevent thrombus formation on the balloon surface, the IABP must remain at a minimal pumping ratio (or volume) until its removal.

Educating the patient and family. Patient education for a patient with an IAB is limited to priority needs for care in the critical care unit, such as keeping the insertion leg straight to avoid kinking of the IAB catheter. Many IABP manufacturers provide helpful educational booklets designed for patients and families.

Left Atria to Aorta Assist Device

The TandemHeart device uses a continuous-flow (CF) centrifugal pump with an inflow and outflow cannula that can be configured in different ways to achieve percutaneous or minimally invasive surgical approaches.[84] Blood is pumped extracorporeally from the left atria to the iliofemoral arterial system. Increase in cardiac output and arterial blood pressure provides support for systemic perfusion. Frequently, LV contraction will virtually cease, resulting in a flat mean arterial pressure curve. Adequate RV function is required to maintain left atrial filling volumes. Complications are related to the need for anticoagulation, transseptal puncture, thrombo- or air embolism, and hemolysis. Care must be taken to prevent catheter dislodgement, which could lead to systemic desaturation or device malfunction.

Left Ventricle to Aorta Assist Device

The Impella is a nonpulsatile axial flow pump that draws blood from the LV and ejects it proximally into the ascending aorta (Fig. 12.16). Different versions are available in different sizes. The smaller device (Impella CP) can be quickly placed percutaneously, providing 3.0 to 4.0 L/min of support, whereas the larger device (Impella 5.0) requires a

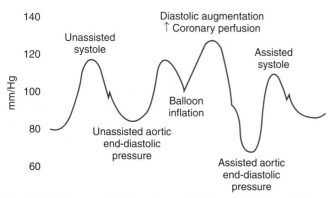

Fig. 12.15 Intraaortic Balloon Pump: Timing and Effect of Balloon Counterpulsations. Timing is adjusted by synchronizing balloon inflation with the dicrotic notch on the arterial waveform, resulting in an elevated diastolic pressure. Inflation is maintained throughout diastole to augment coronary perfusion. Deflation occurs just before the next systole, resulting in a reduced systolic pressure and decreased afterload.

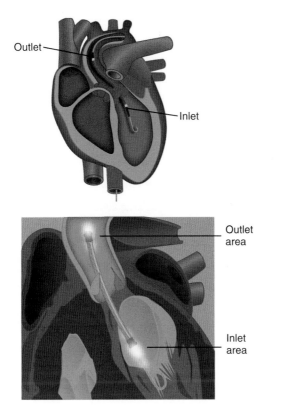

Fig. 12.16 Impella Ventricular Assist Device. Blood is pulled into the catheter from the left ventricle and returned to the ascending aorta.

surgical cut-down to provide flow rates of 5.0 L/min.[84] The Impella is contraindicated in patients with mechanical aortic valves. Monitoring for catheter migration is an import aspect of care to prevent hemolysis and ensure proper pump functioning.

Right Ventricular Assist Devices

A failing RV can be assisted by two different devices. The Impella RP catheter takes blood from the inferior vena cava and delivers it into the outlet opening in the pulmonary artery. The TandemHeart pump, along with the Protek Duo catheter, allows for right atrium-to-pulmonary artery cannulation to provide RV support.[84]

Extracorporeal Membrane Oxygenation System

Mechanical cardiopulmonary support is termed *extracorporeal membrane oxygenation* (ECMO) and is being used with increasing frequency in critical care units. The primary indication for ECMO is acute severe heart or lung failure with high mortality risk despite conventional treatment.[85] There are two types of ECMO: venoarterial (VA) and venovenous (VV). Both types provide respiratory support, but only VA-ECMO provides hemodynamic support. VA-ECMO can be initiated quickly at the bedside by either a direct right atrial cannulation (via a preexisting sternotomy) or peripherally using a percutaneous technique (Fig. 12.17).

Once the patient is connected to the ECMO circuit and hemodynamic parameters are satisfactory, vasoactive drugs can be weaned to minimal levels to allow the myocardium to rest. Anticoagulation is required for most VA-ECMO support because of the risk of venous

and arterial thromboembolization. However, consideration must also be given to the fact that bleeding is the most common complication, often requiring transfusions after placement.[85] Staff must be highly trained to maintain the ECMO circuit and monitor for other complications, such as cardiac tamponade, multiorgan failure, sepsis, limb ischemia, and pulmonary complications. Major limitations of ECMO include its limited availability, short duration of usage, required support of highly trained personnel, and complications related to vascular access. Once evidence of cardiac function has returned, weaning trials can be conducted to assess if the patient can be maintained with conventional support.

Long-Term Ventricular Assist Devices

The VAD is designed to support or replace a failing natural heart with flow assistance. The clinical use of CF left ventricular assist devices (LVADs) continues to increase with the improvement in survival rates along with quality of life in patients with heart failure.[86]

Long-term MCS devices are currently placed for two types of clinical indications. The first category, called *bridge to transplantation* (BTT), includes patients with decompensated chronic heart failure who need circulatory support until heart transplantation can be performed. The second category, called DT, includes patients with severe heart failure who are not candidates for heart transplantation and for whom all other medical options have been exhausted. There is no single ideal system, so device selection is often based on individual VAD capabilities and institutional preference (see Table 12.13). All devices consist of a blood pump, cannula, controller, and some type of power source. They differ in the mechanism by which they move blood, either through centrifugal flow or axial flow. Inlet cannulas that divert blood from the heart to the LVAD for LV support are placed in the left atrium or the LV apex, with the outlet cannula attached to the ascending aorta or femoral artery. An LVAD is used most commonly because LV failure occurs more often than RV failure. However, RV failure can happen in the immediate postoperative phase or even months after LVAD implantation, which can lead to additional clinical challenges. Another option for biventricular failure is the total artificial heart, which can be used as a BTT.

Nursing Management

Nursing management for a patient with a VAD includes monitoring for hemodynamic changes and for complications related to the device. The same interventions that are used for cardiac surgery patients to optimize cardiac output by manipulation of heart rate, preload, afterload, and contractility apply to patients with a VAD. Adequate filling volumes are essential to maintain pump flow. Afterload reduction may be needed to improve output from the unassisted ventricle when univentricular support is used. Although complication rates vary among the different models, complications common to all types of VADs include bleeding, infection, stroke, thromboembolism, respiratory failure, arrhythmias, and device failure.[83,85,87] On physical examination, patients with CF VADs may not have palpable pulses; this can make measurement of blood pressure difficult and will require an invasive arterial catheter for the initial postoperative period. An occlusive pressure obtained with a manual blood pressure cuff and Doppler at the brachial artery is the best reflection of mean arterial pressure.[88] Arterial blood gas analysis may be required, because pulse oximetry may be unreliable with little or no pulse. While in VT or VF, not all patients with an LVAD will be unconscious. Cardioversion and

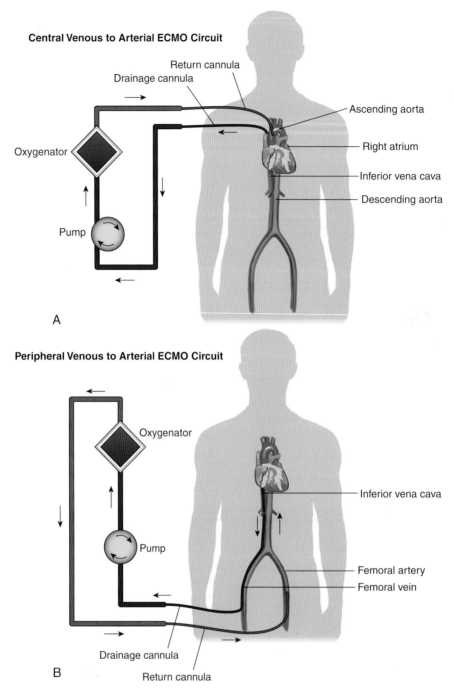

Fig. 12.17   Extracorporeal Membrane Oxygenation (ECMO). Central (A) and peripheral (B) placement of an ECMO circuit. (Modified from Hung M, Vuylsteke A, Valchanov K. Extracorporeal membrane oxygenation coming to an ICU near you. *J Intensive Care Soc.* 2012;13[1]:31−38.)

defibrillation should be performed for the same indications as other patients.[88] Nurses must often rely on basic assessments such as circulation, mentation, and urine output to determine whether the patient is receiving adequate support.

Device failure. Although the incidence of device failure continues to decrease, it is a life-threatening event because of the nature of this therapy. The two most common causes of pump failure involve failure of the driveline and power disconnection. VAD designs vary considerably, and troubleshooting methods for device failure are unique to each device. The nurse must be aware of signs of device

malfunction and patient factors (volume status, dysrhythmias, RV failure) that may affect VAD function.

Anticoagulation. Anticoagulation protocols vary with the device, individual patient, and institution. Both antiplatelet agents and warfarin are commonly used. Although bleeding is the most frequent complication, thrombotic events can also be a problem leading to stroke and device failure. Coagulation studies must be frequently monitored during support.

Infection. Patients with a VAD are at considerable risk for localized and septicemic infections. Infectious risks are posed by the presence of invasive catheters and the surgically implanted VAD. Infection is prevented by the use of strict aseptic techniques with all invasive tubing and dressing changes. Site care varies depending on institutional protocols and the type of VAD that is used. Nurses monitor patients for infection by measuring temperatures, inspecting insertion sites and incisions, and obtaining daily leukocyte counts. If an infection is suspected, pancultures (blood, urine, and sputum) are taken to guide appropriate antibiotic therapy.

Educating the patient and family. The rapid and acute nature of cardiogenic shock limits the nurse's ability to prepare patients and families for VAD insertion. Despite the critical nature of the illness, nurses explain the reason for the use of the VAD and provide information about the critical care environment and equipment. The number of patients with VADs discharged to home continues to increase. These patients and their families require education related to care of the device and reinforcement on the components of heart failure management.

CARDIOVASCULAR MEDICATIONS

Multiple medications are used in the treatment of critically ill cardiovascular patients. The critical care nurse is responsible for preparation and administration of these pharmacologic therapies and often is required to titrate the dose based on the patient hemodynamic response. The Joint Commission recently clarified criteria to enable nurses trained for critical care and procedural areas to use their clinical judgment in both titration and selection of vasoactive medications.[89] Specific parameters must be delineated in a medication order that includes the name, route, and initial/maximum rate or dose of the infusion, as well as the incremental units and time interval for increasing or decreasing the drug in response to a defined clinical measure (e.g., blood pressure, heart rate). The new regulation also provides for documentation over a specified block of time to address periods in which rapid titration of

infusions is needed to manage urgent changes in the patient's condition.

The medications used to treat cardiovascular disease are rapidly changing and expanding as more is learned about the pathophysiology of cardiac disease and as improved formulas are developed by pharmaceutical companies. The critical care nurse who has a general understanding of the mechanisms of action of the various pharmacologic classifications can readily apply this knowledge to new medications within the same classification. This section provides a concise review of medications commonly administered to support cardiovascular function in the critical care setting. The emphasis is on intravenously administered medications that are used for acute rather than long-term management of cardiovascular conditions.

Antidysrhythmic Medications

Antidysrhythmic medications comprise a diverse category of pharmacologic agents used to terminate or prevent an array of abnormal cardiac rhythms. These agents are commonly classified according to their primary effect on the action potential of cardiac cells (Fig. 12.18). The classification scheme shown in Table 12.14 is the most commonly used system. Classification of newer agents is more difficult because some of these agents have characteristics of more than one class, and others have no characteristics of the current system.

Class I

Class I agents are sodium channel blockers that decrease the influx of sodium ions through "fast" channels during phase 0 depolarization. This prolongs the absolute (effective) refractory period, decreasing the risk of premature impulses from ectopic foci. These medications also depress automaticity by slowing the rate of spontaneous depolarization of pacemaker cells during the resting phase (phase 4).

⠿ TRENDING PRIORITIES IN HEALTHCARE

Virtual Visiting

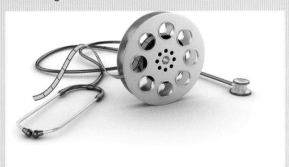

iStock.com/porcorex

Telehealth became vitally important during the COVID-19 pandemic. When families were not allowed to visit hospitals due to concerns over virus transmission, communication using video conferencing filled the void.[1,2]

Early in the pandemic, clinicians often used their own phones because there was no official way to help patients communicate with their families. Very soon, most hospitals set up official mechanisms using video tablets, either on rolling carts, handheld, or connected to the computer in the room. Nurses had to become knowledgeable about how to make the call successful in critical care.

Video conferencing in critical care is used for:
- Family and friends visiting virtually in the critical care unit, even if the patient cannot speak due to intubation, sedation, or illness

- Participation in family meetings
- Participation in rounds
- Speaking with families remotely
- During end of life, when the family cannot be physically present, video visiting allows virtual presence

Hygiene for the video tablet can be accomplished in several ways:
- Wiping down the tablet with an antimicrobial cloth after use
- Holding the tablet in a protective clear plastic pouch
- Use of an ultraviolet light sanitizer for phones and tablets
- Additional concerns using video conferencing in critical care:
  - Coordinating communication between family and the critical care team
  - Conveying empathy and concern when using video versus in person
  - Speaking clearly and making sure communication is understood
  - Involving an interpreter when the family has limited English proficiency

COVID-19 was the catalyst that introduced video conferencing and critical care virtual visits. Now, we cannot go backwards. Critical care units are retooling to allow video conferencing and virtual visiting to become a permanent part of the environment for families and friends who are not able to visit in person.

References
1. Webb H, Parson M, Hodgson LE, Daswani K. Virtual visiting and other technological adaptations for critical care. *Future Healthc J.* 2020;7(3):e93–e95.
2. Kennedy NR, Steinberg A, Arnold RM, et al. Perspectives on telephone and video communication in the intensive care unit during COVID-19. *Ann Am Thorac Soc.* 2021;18(5):838–846.

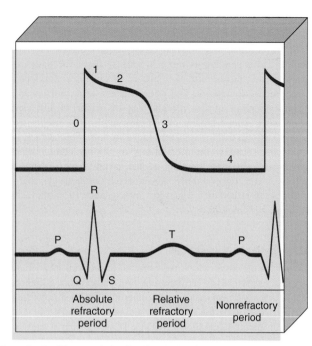

Fig. 12.18 Phases of the Cardiac Action Potential and Their Relationship to Refractory Periods of the Heart. *Phase 0*, depolarization with rapid influx of sodium. *Phase 1*, rapid repolarization with rapid efflux of potassium ions and decreased sodium conductance. *Phase 2*, plateau with slow influx of sodium and calcium ions. *Phase 3*, repolarization with continued efflux of potassium ions. *Phase 4*, resting phase with restoration of ionic balance by sodium and potassium pumps.

TABLE 12.14 Classification of Antidysrhythmic Agents.

Class	Action	Medications
I	Blocks sodium channels (stabilizes cell membrane)	
IA	Blocks sodium channels and delays repolarization, lengthening duration of the action potential	Quinidine Procainamide Disopyramide
IB	Blocks sodium channels and accelerates repolarization, shortening duration of the action potential	Lidocaine Mexiletine
IC	Blocks sodium channels and slows conduction through His-Purkinje system, prolonging QRS duration	Flecainide Propafenone
II	Blocks beta-receptors	Esmolol Metoprolol Propranolol
III	Slows repolarization and prolongs duration of the action potential	Amiodarone Dronedarone Dofetilide Ibutilide Sotalol
IV	Blocks calcium channels	Diltiazem Verapamil

TABLE 12.15 Effects of Adrenergic Receptors.

Receptor	Location	Response to Stimulation
Alpha	Vessels of skin, muscles, kidneys, and intestines	Vasoconstriction of peripheral arterioles
Beta-1	Cardiac tissue	Increased heart rate Increased conduction Increased contractility
Beta-2	Vascular and bronchial smooth muscle	Vasodilation of peripheral arterioles Bronchodilation

Class I antidysrhythmic medications can be subdivided further into three groups according to their potency as sodium channel inhibitors and their effect on phase 3 repolarization. Class IA agents—quinidine, procainamide, and disopyramide—block both the fast sodium channels and phase 3 repolarization, prolonging the action potential duration. Clinically, this may result in measurable increases in the QRS duration and lengthening of the QT interval. All class IA agents may depress myocardial contractility, with disopyramide having the most potent negative inotropic effect. Medications in class IB have only a moderate effect on sodium channels and accelerate phase 3 repolarization to shorten the action potential duration; lidocaine and mexiletine belong in this group. Class IC agents are the most potent sodium channel blockers and have little effect on repolarization. Class IC agents increase the P-R and QRS intervals. Flecainide and propafenone are included in this group. Both of these agents are proarrhythmic and have negative inotropic effects, which limits their use in patients with heart failure.[90]

Class II

Class II agents are beta-adrenergic blockers (beta-blockers). They inhibit dysrhythmias mediated by the sympathetic nervous system by competing with endogenous catecholamines for available receptor sites. As a result, spontaneous depolarization during the resting phase (phase 4) is depressed, and AV conduction is slowed. Antidysrhythmic medications in this class can be further subdivided into cardioselective agents (agents that block only beta-1-receptors) and noncardioselective agents (agents that block both beta-1- and beta-2-receptors). Knowledge of the effects of adrenergic-receptor stimulation allows for anticipation of both the therapeutic responses brought about by beta-blockade and the potential adverse

effects of these agents (Table 12.15). For example, bronchospasm can be precipitated by noncardioselective beta-blockers in a patient with chronic obstructive pulmonary disease caused by blockade of the effects of beta-2-receptors in the lungs. Beta-blockers also are negative inotropes and must be used cautiously in patients with LV dysfunction. Although numerous beta-blockers are marketed, only esmolol, metoprolol, and propranolol are available as intravenous agents for the treatment of acute dysrhythmias. Of these, esmolol (Brevibloc) offers significant advantages for critically ill patients because of its short half-life (approximately 9 minutes). It is used in the treatment of SVTs, such as AF and atrial flutter.

Class III

Class III agents include amiodarone, dronedarone, dofetilide, ibutilide, and sotalol. These agents block potassium channels to slow the rate of phase 3 repolarization, increasing the effective refractory period and the action potential duration. Although their effects on the action potential are similar, these medications differ greatly in their mechanism of action and their side effects. Intravenous amiodarone was originally approved for the treatment of serious ventricular dysrhythmias refractory to other medications. Because of its effectiveness, it is now used for both atrial and ventricular dysrhythmias.[91] Dronedarone is similar to amiodarone but has fewer extracardiac side effects. Dofetilide (Tikosyn) is a newer class III antidysrhythmic agent used for the conversion to and maintenance of normal sinus rhythm in patients with highly symptomatic atrial fibrillation or AF. Because dofetilide prolongs the refractoriness of both atrial and ventricular tissue, prolongation of the QT interval can occur and is associated with an increased risk of torsades de pointes. As a result, therapy with dofetilide is initiated in a hospital setting with mandatory ECG monitoring.[92] Ibutilide (Covert) is a short-term antidysrhythmic agent used for the rapid conversion of acute atrial fibrillation or AF to sinus rhythm. Ibutilide is administered as a 10-minute infusion in a carefully monitored clinical setting. The most serious side effect of ibutilide is its potential for inducing life-threatening dysrhythmias, especially torsades de pointes.[93] Sotalol not only blocks potassium channels but also has properties of a noncardioselective beta-blocker and should be used cautiously in patients with heart failure.

Class IV

Class IV agents are calcium channel blockers that inhibit the influx of calcium through slow calcium channels during the plateau phase (phase 2). This effect occurs primarily in tissue in which slow calcium channels predominate, primarily the sinus and AV nodes and the atrial tissue. Verapamil was the first medication in this category available as an intravenous antidysrhythmic. It depresses sinus and AV node conduction and is effective in terminating SVTs caused by AV nodal re-entry. Diltiazem (Cardizem) has become available in intravenous form and is thought to be as effective as verapamil in treating supraventricular dysrhythmias with fewer hypotensive side effects. Because accessory pathways are not affected by calcium channel blockade, both agents must be avoided when treating atrial tachycardia in patients with Wolff-Parkinson-White syndrome.[94]

Unclassified Antidysrhythmics

Adenosine (Adenocard) is an antidysrhythmic agent that remains unclassified under the current system. Adenosine occurs endogenously in the body as a building block of adenosine triphosphate. Given in intravenous boluses, adenosine slows conduction through the AV node, causing transient AV block. It is used clinically to convert SVTs and to facilitate differential diagnosis of rapid dysrhythmias. Because of its short half-life, adenosine is administered intravenously as a rapid

TABLE 12.16 Pharmacologic Management.

Selected Antidysrhythmic Agents

Medication	Dosage	Actions	Special Considerations
Adenosine	6 mg IV rapid push; if unsuccessful, repeat with 12 mg over 1–2 seconds; follow with IV fluid 10 mL flush (NS or D$_5$W)	Blocks AV node to terminate SVT, PSVT	Transient; flushing, dyspnea, hypotension
Digoxin	0.5–1 mg loading dose in divided doses; maintenance dose of 0.125–0.375 mg daily	Conversion and/or rate control in SVT, AFib, AF	Bradycardia, heart block Toxicity: CNS and GI symptoms
Diltiazem	Bolus dose of 0.25 mg/kg IV over 2 minutes, followed by infusion of 5–15 mg/h	Conversion and/or rate control in SVT, AFib, AF	Bradycardia, hypotension, AV block
Esmolol	Loading dose of 500 mcg/kg over 1 minute, followed by infusion of 50 mcg/kg/min for 4 minutes; repeat procedure every 5 minutes, increasing infusion by 25–50 mcg/kg/min to maximum of 200 mcg/kg/min	Conversion and/or rate control in SVT, AFib, AF Also used to decrease rate of sinus tachycardia	Hypotension, bradycardia, heart failure
Ibutilide	0.010–0.025 mg/kg infused over 10 minutes (may repeat once) or 1 mg diluted in 50 mL infused over 10 minutes (may repeat once)	Conversion of AFib, AF	Minimal side effects except for rare polymorphic VT (torsades de pointes)
Verapamil	5–10 mg IV over at least 2 minutes, may repeat in 15–30 minutes	Conversion and/or rate control in SVT	Hypotension, bradycardia, heart failure
Lidocaine	1–1.5 mg/kg bolus, followed by continuous infusion of 1–4 mg/min	Treatment of ventricular dysrhythmias (PVCs, VT, VF)	CNS toxicity, nausea, vomiting with repeated doses
Amiodarone	*VT/VF arrest:* 300 mg IV push; may repeat with 150 mg in 3–5 minutes (maximum dose, 2.2 g/24 h) *Pulsatile VT, AFib, AF:* 150 mg IV over 10 minutes, followed by 360 mg over 6 hours (1 mg/min); maintenance infusion of 0.5 mg/min	Treatment of atrial (AFib, AF, SVT) and ventricular (PVCs, VT, VF) dysrhythmias	Hypotension, abnormal liver function tests
Procainamide	Loading dose of 12–17 mg/kg at a rate of 20 mg/min, followed by infusion of 1–4 mg/min	Treatment of atrial (AFib, AF, SVT) and ventricular (PVCs, VT) dysrhythmias	Hypotension, GI effects Widening of QRS and Q-T lengthening

AF, Atrial flutter; *AFib,* atrial fibrillation; *AV,* atrioventricular; *CNS,* central nervous system; *D$_5$W,* 5% dextrose in water; *GI,* gastrointestinal; *IV,* intravenous/intravenously; *NS,* normal saline; *PSVT,* paroxysmal supraventricular tachycardia; *PVCs,* premature ventricular contractions; *ST,* sinus tachycardia; *SVT,* supraventricular tachycardia; *VF,* ventricular fibrillation; *VT,* ventricular tachycardia.

bolus followed by a saline flush. The bolus is delivered as centrally as possible so that the medication reaches the heart before it is metabolized. Side effects are transient, because adenosine is rapidly taken up by the cells and is cleared from the body within 10 seconds.

Magnesium is also unclassified under the present system. Although its action as an antidysrhythmic agent is not entirely understood, clinical studies suggest that it may reduce the incidence of both ventricular and supraventricular dysrhythmias in selected patient populations.[95,96] It is considered the treatment of choice in patients with torsades de pointes.[24] For acute treatment, 1 to 2 g of magnesium is administered over 1 to 2 minutes. In patients with confirmed hypomagnesemia, this bolus may be followed with repeated infusions.

Side Effects

Antidysrhythmic medications carry the risk of serious side effects, some of which can be life-threatening. The major side effects of intravenous antidysrhythmic agents are listed in Table 12.16. The most severe complication is the potential for a prodysrhythmic effect. This may result in worsening of the underlying dysrhythmia, the occurrence of a new dysrhythmia, or the development of a bradydysrhythmia. For example, torsades de pointes is a prodysrhythmia caused by many medications that prolong the QT interval on the ECG. Because the development of a prodysrhythmia is unpredictable, the nurse plays an important role in evaluating ECG changes, monitoring serum medication levels, and assessing patient symptoms. Antidysrhythmic agents may also alter the amount of energy required for defibrillation and pacing. For example, increases in the dose of an antidysrhythmic medication may increase the amount of output (mA) required to depolarize the myocardium.

Treatment of Atrial Fibrillation

More than 5 million people in the United States have atrial fibrillation, and extensive research has been done on the treatment of this disorder.[14] The goals of pharmacologic therapy for atrial fibrillation include control of symptoms—either by reestablishing and maintaining sinus rhythm, or decreasing the rapid ventricular response during episodes of atrial fibrillation—and preventing the risk of thromboembolism. Table 12.17 reviews current medications used in the treatment of atrial fibrillation. Results of several large clinical trials suggest that rate control is equivalent to restoration of sinus rhythm in terms of

TABLE 12.17 Medications Used for Atrial Fibrillation.

Treatment Goal	Classification and Medications	Special Considerations
Conversion or maintenance of sinus rhythm	**Class IA** Quinidine Procainamide (Pronestyl) Disopyramide (Norpace)	Class IA agents prolong QT intervals and may cause torsades de pointes. Rate control should be achieved before initiation of therapy.
	Class IC Flecainide (Tambocor) Propafenone (Rythmol)	Class IC agents are prodysrhythmic in patients with CAD or previous MI and should be avoided in these patients.
	Class III Amiodarone (Cordarone) Dofetilide (Tikosyn) Dronedarone (Multaq) Ibutilide (Corvert) Sotalol (Betapace)	Amiodarone and sotalol also have beta-blocking properties and may help with rate control. Treatment with dofetilide requires careful monitoring for prodysrhythmic effects. Ibutilide is an IV agent and is used for conversion only.
Control of ventricular rate	**Beta-blockers** Esmolol (Brevibloc) Metoprolol (Lopressor) Propranolol (Inderal)	IV esmolol may be used in acute settings to control ventricular rate. Oral agents are used for maintenance therapy. Beta-blockers provide good rate control during exercise.
	Calcium channel blockers Diltiazem (Cardizem) Verapamil (Isoptin)	Intravenous calcium channel blockers may be used in emergency situations, followed by oral agents for maintenance therapy.
	Digitalis compounds Digoxin (Lanoxin)	Digoxin does not effectively control rate with exercise, so it may be used in combination with other medications.
Prevention of thromboembolism	**Anticoagulants** Heparin Warfarin (Coumadin) Dabigatran (Pradaxa) Rivaroxaban (Xarelto) Apixaban (Eliquis) Edoxaban (Savaysa)	Heparin may be used in emergency situations, before cardioversion. Warfarin is used long term, with monitoring to achieve INR of 2–3. Dabigatran is an oral direct thrombin inhibitor approved to reduce risk of thromboembolism in patients with nonvalvular AFib. Dabigatran does not require routine anticoagulant monitoring. Rivaroxaban, apixaban, and edoxaban are factor Xa inhibitors approved to reduce risk of thromboembolism in patients with nonvalvular AFib. Factor Xa inhibitors do not require routine anticoagulant monitoring.
	Antiplatelet agents Aspirin	Aspirin may be used in patients with contraindications to warfarin or in low-risk patients younger than 65 years.

AFib, Atrial fibrillation; *CAD*, coronary artery disease; *INR*, international normalized ratio; *IV*, intravenous; *MI*, myocardial infarction.

mortality, with less incidence of adverse medication effects.[97] Selection of a treatment strategy should consider the patient's age, severity of symptoms, duration of the arrhythmia, and other comorbidities. Although warfarin has been the traditional choice for antithrombotic therapy, new direct-acting oral anticoagulant agents are now preferred for embolism prophylaxis in patients with nonvalvular atrial fibrillation. Dabigatran (Pradaxa) is a direct thrombin inhibitor; rivaroxaban, apixaban, and edoxaban inhibit factor Xa. These agents have advantages over warfarin because there is a rapid onset of therapeutic effect, there are fewer medication and food interactions, and there is no need for routine laboratory monitoring.[98] A potential concern regarding these newer agents is their lack of a common reversal agent, although medication-specific reversal agents are available. Idarucizumab is approved by the US Food and Drug Administration as a reversal agent for dabigatran, and andexanet alfa is approved as a reversal agent for factor Xa agents based on studies in healthy volunteers.[4]

Inotropic Medications

Critically ill patients with compromised cardiac function often require medications to enhance myocardial contractility (positive inotropes). Clinically available inotropes include cardiac glycosides, sympathomimetics, and phosphodiesterase inhibitors. These agents increase myocardial contractility, resulting in improved cardiac output, more complete emptying of the ventricles, and decreased filling pressures.

Cardiac Glycosides

Cardiac glycosides include digitalis and its derivatives. Although these medications have been used for centuries, their slow onset of action and risk of toxicity make them more appropriate for management of chronic heart failure. Because digoxin also causes slowing of the sinus rate and a decrease in AV conduction, it may be administered intravenously in the acute care setting to control supraventricular dysrhythmias.

Sympathomimetic Agents

Sympathomimetic agents stimulate adrenergic receptors, simulating the effects of sympathetic nerve stimulation. Included in this category are naturally occurring catecholamines (epinephrine, dopamine, and norepinephrine) and synthetic catecholamines (dobutamine and isoproterenol). The cardiovascular effects of these medications, which vary according to their selectivity for specific receptor sites, are often

dose dependent as well. Table 12.18 describes the cardiovascular effects of sympathomimetic agents at various dosages.

Dopamine (Intropin) is one of the most widely used medications in the critical care setting. It is a chemical precursor of norepinephrine which, in addition to both alpha-receptor and beta-receptor stimulation, can activate dopaminergic receptors in the renal and mesenteric blood vessels. The actions of dopamine are dose related, although there is some overlap in effect.[99] At low dosages of 1 to 2 mcg/kg per minute, dopamine stimulates dopaminergic receptors, causing renal and mesenteric vasodilation. The resultant increase in renal perfusion increases urinary output. However, this increase in urine output does not confer protection against the development of AKI. Moderate dosages result in stimulation of beta-1-receptors to increase myocardial contractility and improve cardiac output. At dosages greater than 10 mcg/kg per minute, dopamine predominantly stimulates alpha-receptors, resulting in vasoconstriction that often negates both the beta-adrenergic and the dopaminergic effects.

Dobutamine (Dobutrex) is a synthetic catecholamine with predominantly beta-1 adrenergic effects. It also produces some beta-2 stimulation, resulting in mild vasodilation. Dobutamine is as effective as dopamine in increasing myocardial contractility and is useful in the treatment of heart failure, especially in hypotensive patients who cannot tolerate vasodilator therapy. The usual dosage range is 2 to 20 mcg/kg per minute, titrated on the basis of hemodynamic parameters.

Epinephrine (adrenaline) is produced by the adrenal gland as part of the body's response to stress. This agent has the ability to stimulate both alpha-receptors and beta-receptors, depending on the dose administered (see Table 12.18). At doses of 1 to 2 mcg/min, epinephrine binds with beta-receptors to increase heart rate, cardiac conduction, contractility, and vasodilation, increasing cardiac output. As the dosage is increased, alpha-receptors are stimulated, resulting in increased vascular resistance and increased blood pressure. At these doses, the impact of epinephrine on cardiac output depends on the ability of the heart to pump against the increased afterload. Epinephrine accelerates the sinus rate and may precipitate ventricular dysrhythmias in the ischemic heart. Other side effects include restlessness, angina, and headache.

Norepinephrine (Levophed) is similar to epinephrine in its ability to stimulate beta-receptors and alpha-receptors, but it lacks the beta-2 effects of epinephrine. At low infusion rates, beta-1-receptors are activated to produce increased contractility, augmenting cardiac

TABLE 12.18 Physiologic Effects of Sympathomimetic Agents.

Medications	Dosage	RECEPTOR ACTIVATED[a]				CARDIOVASCULAR EFFECTS		
		Alpha	Beta-1	Beta-2	Dopa	CO	HR	SVR
Dobutamine	<5 mcg/kg/min	0	↑↑↑	↑	0	↑↑	↑	↓↓
	5–20 mcg/kg/min	0	↑↑↑	↑↑	0	↑↑↑	↑↑↑	↓↓
Dopamine	<3 mcg/kg/min	0	↑	↑	↑↑↑	0/↑	0/↑	0
	3–10 mcg/kg/min	↑↑	↑↑↑	↑	↑↑↑	↑↑↑	↑	↑
	11–20 mcg/kg/min	↑↑↑	↑↑↑	↑	↑↑	↑↑	↑↑	↑↑↑
Epinephrine	<2 mcg/min	0	↑	↑↑	0	0/↑	0/↑	↓
	2–8 mcg/min	↑↑	↑↑↑	↑↑	0	↑↑↑	↑↑	↑
	9–20 mcg/min	↑↑↑	↑↑↑	↑↑	0	↑↑	↑↑	↑↑↑
Isoproterenol	2–10 mcg/min	0	↑↑↑	↑↑↑	0	↑↑↑	↑↑↑	↓↓↓
Norepinephrine	<2 mcg/min	↑↑↑	↑↑	0	0	↑	0/↑	↑↑↑
	2–16 mcg/min	↑↑↑↑	↑↑	0	0	↓	↑	↑↑↑↑
Phenylephrine	10–100 mcg/min	↑↑↑↑	0	0	0	0	↓	↑↑↑

[a]See Table 12.15 for actions of receptors.

0, No effect; ↑, increased (number of arrows indicates degree of effect); ↓, decreased (number of arrows indicates degree of effect); *CO*, cardiac output; *HR*, heart rate; *SVR*, systemic vascular resistance.

output. At higher doses, the inotropic effects are limited by marked vasoconstriction mediated by alpha-receptors. Clinically, norepinephrine is used most often as a vasopressor to elevate blood pressure in shock states.[100]

Isoproterenol (Isuprel) is a pure beta-receptor stimulant with no alpha-adrenergic effects. It produces dramatic increases in heart rate, conduction, and contractility through beta-1 stimulation and vasodilation through beta-2 stimulation. Isoproterenol also produces vasodilation of the pulmonary arteries and bronchodilation. It greatly increases the automaticity of cardiac cells and frequently precipitates dysrhythmias, such as premature ventricular contractions and VT. These effects limit its usefulness in most patients, and it is rarely used.

Phosphodiesterase Inhibitors

Medications in this classification inhibit the enzyme phosphodiesterase, resulting in increased levels of cyclic adenosine monophosphate and intracellular calcium. Phosphodiesterase inhibitors are both inotropic agents and potent vasodilators (inodilators). Improvement in cardiac output occurs as a result of increased contractility and decreased afterload. Milrinone (Primacor), a second-generation drug in this category, is used in the treatment of patients with acute decompensated heart failure. Milrinone can cause hypotension and may induce atrial and ventricular dysrhythmias (premature ventricular contractions, VT) in some patients.[101]

Vasodilator Medications

Vasodilators are pharmacologic agents that improve cardiac performance by various degrees of arterial or venous dilation or both. The goal of vasodilator therapy may be reduction of preload, afterload, or both. Afterload reduction is accomplished by vasodilation of arterial vessels. This results in decreased resistance to LV ejection and may improve cardiac output without increasing myocardial oxygen demands. Reduction of preload is accomplished by dilation of venous vessels to increase capacitance. This results in decreased filling pressures for a failing heart. These medications may be classified into four groups on the basis of mechanism of action (Table 12.19).

Direct Smooth Muscle Relaxants

Direct-acting vasodilators include sodium nitroprusside, nitroglycerin, and hydralazine. These medications produce relaxation of vascular smooth muscle through the activation of nitric oxide, which results in decreased peripheral vascular resistance. Hypotension may occur as a result of peripheral vasodilation, and headaches may be caused by cerebral vasodilation. Compensatory mechanisms can occur in response to the decrease in blood pressure. These mechanisms include baroreceptor activation that causes reflex tachycardia and activation of the renin-angiotensin-aldosterone system with resultant sodium and water retention.

Sodium nitroprusside (Nipride) is a potent, rapidly acting venous and arterial vasodilator that is particularly suitable for rapid reduction of blood pressure in hypertensive emergencies and perioperatively. It also is effective for afterload reduction in the setting of severe heart failure. Sodium nitroprusside is administered by continuous intravenous infusion, with the dosage titrated to maintain the desired blood pressure and SVR. Prolonged administration can result in thiocyanate toxicity, manifested by nausea, confusion, and tinnitus.[102]

Intravenous nitroglycerin (Tridil) causes both arterial and venous vasodilation, but its venous effect is more pronounced. It is used in the critical care setting for the treatment of acute heart failure because it reduces cardiac filling pressures, relieves pulmonary congestion, and decreases cardiac workload and oxygen consumption. Nitroglycerin dilates the coronary arteries and is a useful adjunct in the treatment of unstable angina and acute MI. The initial dosage is 5 mcg/min, and the infusion is titrated upward to achieve the desired clinical effect: a reduction or elimination of chest pain, decreased PAOP (wedge pressure), or a decrease in blood pressure. Nitroglycerin should be avoided in patients with head injury because it can increase intracranial pressure.[103] The most common side effects of this medication are hypotension, reflex tachycardia, and headache. Nitroglycerin becomes less effective with prolonged infusions, because tolerance develops within 24 to 48 hours.[102]

Hydralazine (Apresoline) is a potent arterial vasodilator. It is not given as a continuous infusion; rather, it is administered in slow

TABLE 12.19 Pharmacologic Management.

Selected Vasodilator Agents

Medication	Dosage	Action	Special Considerations
Smooth Muscle Relaxants			
Sodium nitroprusside (Nipride, Nitropress)	0.3–10 mcg/kg/min IV infusion	Potent arterial and moderate venous dilation	May cause hypotension and reflex tachycardia, thiocyanate toxicity with prolonged infusions, or kidney dysfunction
Nitroglycerin (Tridil)	5–200 mcg/min IV infusion	Potent venodilator, with arterial effects at higher doses	May cause headache, reflex tachycardia, hypotension
Calcium Channel Blockers			
Clevidipine (Cleviprex)	1–2 mg/h IV infusion, titrated to 32 mg/h (maximum 1000 mg/24 h)	Potent arterial dilator, with no effect on venous capacitance (preload)	Hypotension, reflex tachycardia, nausea, vomiting, rebound hypertension
Nicardipine (Cardene)	5 mg/h IV, titrated to 15 mg/h	Potent arterial dilator, no effect on preload	Hypotension, headache, reflex tachycardia
ACEIs			
Enalaprilat (Vasotec)	0.625–1.25 mg IV over 5 minutes, then every 6 hours	Moderate dilation of arteries and veins	Hypotension, elevation of liver enzymes
Alpha-Adrenergic Blockers			
Labetalol (Normodyne)	20–80 mg IV bolus every 10 minutes, then 1–8 mg/min infusion	Moderate dilation of arteries and veins	Orthostatic hypotension, bronchospasm, AV block
Phentolamine (Regitine)	5 mg IV slowly every 6 hours	Moderate dilation of arteries and veins	Hypotension, tachycardia

ACEIs, Angiotensin-converting enzyme inhibitors; *AV*, atrioventricular; *IV*, intravenous/intravenously; *PO*, by mouth.

TABLE 12.20 Pharmacologic Management.

Classification of Calcium Channel Blockers

Medication	Dosage	Actions	Special Considerations
Dihydropyridines			
Nicardipine (Cardene)	5 mg/h IV, titrated to 15 mg/h	Short-term control of hypertension	Hypotension, reflex tachycardia, headache, flushing
Nifedipine (Procardia)	10–30 mg PO	Hypertension	Hypotension, reflex tachycardia, headache
Clevidipine (Cleviprex)	1–2 mg/h IV infusion, titrated to 32 mg/h	Short-term control of hypertension	Hypotension, reflex tachycardia, nausea, vomiting, rebound hypertension
Benzothiazepines			
Diltiazem (Cardizem)	Bolus dose of 0.25 mg/kg IV over 2 minutes, followed by infusion of 5–15 mg/h	Treatment of SVT, AFib, AF, angina	Bradycardia, hypotension, atrioventricular block
Phenylalkylamines			
Verapamil (Calan, Isoptin)	5–10 mg IV, may repeat in 15–30 minutes	Treatment of AFib, AF, PSVT	Hypotension, bradycardia, heart failure

AF, Atrial flutter; *AFib,* atrial fibrillation; *IV,* intravenous/intravenously; *PO,* by mouth; *PSVT,* paroxysmal supraventricular tachycardia; *SVT,* supraventricular tachycardia.

intravenous doses of 5 to 10 mg every 4 to 8 hours. Occasionally, hydralazine is given as an intermediate agent during the transition between weaning of a continuous infusion and initiation of oral antihypertensive medications. The major side effect is reflex tachycardia mediated by the sympathetic nervous system. Hydralazine has been used for treatment of preeclampsia because only minimal amounts cross the placenta, but newer guidelines recommend oral nifedipine or labetalol because of a more predictable response.[104]

Calcium Channel Blockers

Calcium channel blockers are a chemically diverse group of medications with differing pharmacologic effects based on their classification (Table 12.20). Nifedipine (Procardia), nicardipine (Cardene), and clevidipine (Cleviprex) are dihydropyridines. Medications in this group of calcium channel blockers (with the suffix "-pine") are used primarily as arterial vasodilators. These agents reduce the influx of calcium in the arterial resistance vessels. Coronary and peripheral arteries are affected. They are used in the critical care setting to treat hypertension. Nicardipine was the first available intravenous calcium channel blocker and as such could be more easily titrated to control blood pressure. Because this medication has vasodilatory effects on coronary and cerebral vessels, it has proven beneficial in treating hypertension in patients with CAD or ischemic stroke. Side effects of nicardipine are related to vasodilation and include hypotension, reflex tachycardia, flushing, and headache.

Clevidipine is a newer short-acting calcium channel blocker that allows for even more precise titration of blood pressure in the management of acute hypertension. Advantages of this agent include its short half-life (approximately 1 minute), rapid onset of action, predictable dose response, and minimal effect on heart rate.[102] It is considered a first-line agent for lowering blood pressure in acute ischemic stroke.[104] Because clevidipine is mixed in a phospholipid emulsion, it can cause allergic reactions in patients with allergies to soybeans or eggs.

Diltiazem (Cardizem) is from the benzothiazine group of calcium channel blockers. Verapamil (Calan, Isoptin) is part of the phenylalkylamine group. The different classifications account for the differing actions of these calcium channel blockers. These medications dilate coronary arteries but have little effect on the peripheral vasculature. They are used in the treatment of angina, especially angina with a vasospastic component, and as antidysrhythmics in the treatment of SVTs.

Angiotensin-Converting Enzyme Inhibitors

Angiotensin-converting enzyme inhibitors (ACEIs) produce vasodilation by blocking the conversion of angiotensin I to angiotensin II. Because angiotensin is a potent vasoconstrictor, limiting its production decreases vascular resistance. In contrast to the direct vasodilators, ACEIs do not cause reflex tachycardia or induce sodium and water retention. However, these medications may cause a profound fall in blood pressure, especially in patients who are volume depleted. Blood pressure must be monitored carefully, especially at the initiation of therapy.

ACEIs are used in patients with heart failure to decrease SVR (afterload) and PAOP (preload). Most of these agents are available only in an oral form. Enalaprilat is available in an intravenous form and may be used to decrease afterload in more emergent situations.

Angiotensin-Receptor Blockers

Angiotensin-receptor blockers prevent the vasoconstrictive effects of angiotensin II through direct blockade at the receptor site, producing hemodynamic effects similar to ACEIs. These agents may be used as an alternative in patients who cannot tolerate ACEIs because of side effects, such as cough.[105] At the present time, angiotensin-receptor blockers are available only in oral form.

Alpha-Adrenergic Blockers

Peripheral adrenergic blockers block alpha-receptors in arteries and veins, resulting in vasodilation. Orthostatic hypotension is a common side effect and may result in syncope. Long-term therapy also may be complicated by fluid and water retention.

Labetalol (Normodyne), a combined peripheral alpha-blocker and cardioselective beta-blocker, is used to decrease blood pressure in the treatment of acute stroke and other hypertensive emergencies.[103] Because the blockade of beta-1-receptors permits the decrease of blood pressure without the risk of reflexive tachycardia and increased cardiac output, labetalol is also useful in the treatment of acute aortic dissection.[104]

Phentolamine (Regitine) is a nonselective peripheral alpha-blocker that deceases blood pressure through arterial vasodilation. It is administered by slow intravenous push 1 to 5 mg every 6 hours to reduce blood pressure. Phentolamine is used only in very specific circumstances for catecholamine-induced hypertension or toxicities related to ingestion of illegal drugs (e.g., cocaine). Phentolamine is the medication of choice to control blood pressure and sweating caused by *pheochromocytoma*, an epinephrine-secreting tumor that can arise from the adrenal medulla.[104]

Phentolamine also is used to treat the *extravasation of dopamine* or other vasopressors into peripheral tissues. If this occurs, 5 to 10 mg is diluted in 10 mL normal saline and administered intradermally into the infiltrated area as soon as possible after extravasation.

Dopamine Receptor Agonists

Fenoldopam (Corlopam) is a unique type of vasodilator, a selective, specific dopamine (D1) receptor agonist. Fenoldopam is a potent vasodilator that affects peripheral, renal, and mesenteric arteries. It is administered by continuous intravenous infusion beginning at 0.01 mcg/kg per minute and titrated up to the desired blood pressure effect, with a maximum recommended dose of 1.6 mcg/kg per minute. It can be administered as an alternative to sodium nitroprusside or other antihypertensives in the treatment of hypertensive emergencies, especially in patients with AKI.[103]

Vasopressors

Vasopressors are sympathomimetic agents that mediate peripheral vasoconstriction through stimulation of alpha-receptors (see Table 12.15). This results in increased SVR and elevates blood pressure. Some of these medications (epinephrine and norepinephrine) also have the ability to stimulate beta-receptors. Vasopressors are not widely used in the treatment of critically ill cardiac patients because the dramatic increase in afterload is taxing to a damaged heart. Occasionally, vasopressors may be used to maintain organ perfusion in shock states. For example, phenylephrine (Neo-Synephrine) or norepinephrine (Levophed) may be administered as a continuous intravenous infusion to maintain organ perfusion by increasing SVR in cases of severe sepsis or septic shock.

Vasopressin, also known as antidiuretic hormone, has become popular in the critical care setting for its vasoconstrictive effects. At higher doses, vasopressin directly stimulates V1 receptors in vascular smooth muscle, resulting in vasoconstriction of capillaries and small arterioles. A one-time dose of 40 units intravenously was previously administered for treatment of cardiac arrest, but newer advanced cardiac life support guidelines suggest it offers no advantages over administration of epinephrine alone.[106] In septic shock, vasopressin levels have been reported to be lower than anticipated for a shock state. Vasopressin is a commonly used secondary infusion that may be added to the norepinephrine infusion in patients with refractory septic shock.[107] Patients must be assessed for side effects such as heart failure caused by the antidiuretic effects and monitored for increased risk of ischemia in the myocardium, spleen, and periphery. Vasopressin should be infused through a central line to avoid the risk of peripheral extravasation and resultant tissue necrosis. Placement of an arterial line is recommended in shock states to monitor blood pressure and SVR.

TABLE 12.21   Medications Used for Heart Failure.

Classification and Medications	Mechanism of Action	Effects	Special Considerations
ACEIs Captopril (Capoten) Enalapril (Vasotec) Fosinopril (Monopril) Lisinopril (Prinivil) Perindopril (Aceon) Quinapril (Accupril) Ramipril (Altace) Trandolapril (Mavik)	Interfere with RAAS by preventing conversion of angiotensin I to angiotensin II	Decrease afterload Decrease preload Reverse ventricular remodeling	Agents appear equivalent in treatment of heart failure Monitor closely for hypotension when initiating therapy May be contraindicated in patients with elevated creatinine, indicating kidney failure Side effects may include cough and life-threatening angioedema
Angiotensin-Receptor Blockers Candesartan (Atacand) Losartan (Cozaar) Valsartan (Diovan)	Interfere with RAAS by blocking effect of angiotensin II at the angiotensin II receptor site	Decrease afterload Decrease preload Reverse ventricular remodeling	Used as primary therapy or as an alternative for patients who cannot tolerate ACEIs because of side effects such as severe cough Can also be used in combination with ACEI for systolic dysfunction; monitor renal function and serum potassium levels
Angiotensin-Receptor–Neprilysin Inhibitor Valsartan/Sacubitril (Entresto)	Combines an ARB with an inhibitor of neprilysin, an enzyme that breaks down peptides with beneficial cardiovascular effects	Effects of ARBs (above) with vasodilation and natriuresis	Recommended in place of ACE or ACEI in patients with stage C heart failure and low ejection fraction to reduce mortality and morbidity Contraindicated in patients with a history of angioedema Dual treatment with an ACEI or ARB is contraindicated

TABLE 12.21 Medications Used for Heart Failure.—cont'd

Classification and Medications	Mechanism of Action	Effects	Special Considerations
Beta-Blockers Metoprolol succinate (Toprol XL) Bisoprolol (Zebeta) Carvedilol (Coreg)	Counteract SNS response activated in heart failure by blocking receptor sites Metoprolol and bisoprolol are cardioselective beta-blockers, whereas carvedilol blocks alpha- and beta-receptor sites	Slow heart rate Prevent dysrhythmias Decrease blood pressure Reverse ventricular remodeling	Not initiated during decompensated stage of heart failure Use cautiously in patients with reactive airway disease, poorly controlled diabetes, bradydysrhythmias, or heart block Carvedilol dose is increased slowly, while monitoring for symptoms caused by vasodilation such as dizziness or hypotension
Selective Sinus Node Inhibitor Ivabradine (Corlanor)		Selectively inhibits the sinoatrial node to reduce heart rate without lowering blood pressure	Recommended for class 3 heart failure patients with low ejection fraction who have a resting heart rate >70 beats/min on maximal beta-blocker therapy
Aldosterone Antagonists Spironolactone (Aldactone) Eplerenone (Inspra)	Counteract effects of aldosterone, which include sodium and water retention	Decrease preload Decrease myocardial hypertrophy	May increase serum potassium
Inotropes Digoxin (Lanoxin)	Affects Na^+,K^+-ATPase pump in myocardial cells to increase the strength of contraction	Increases contractility Increases cardiac output Prevents atrial dysrhythmias	Risk of toxicity is increased with hypokalemia

ACEI, Angiotensin-converting enzyme inhibitor; *ARB*, angiotensin-receptor blocker; *Na^+,K^+-ATPase*, sodium-potassium adenosine triphosphatase; *RAAS*, renin-angiotensin-aldosterone system; *SNS*, sympathetic nervous system.

BOX 12.8 Informatics

Internet Resources: Cardiovascular Therapeutic Management
- About Arrhythmia: https://www.heart.org/en/health-topics/arrhythmia/about-arrhythmia#.Vq7FaVKoPl4
- American Heart Association Consumer and Patient Education Materials
- Caregiver Resources: https://www.heart.org/en/health-topics/caregiver-support/resources-for-caregivers
- Devices for Arrhythmia: https://www.heart.org/en/health-topics/arrhythmia/prevention--treatment-of-arrhythmia/devices-for-arrhythmia#.Vq7GmFKoPl4
- National Heart, Lung, and Blood Institute Health Information for the Public: Heart and Vascular Diseases: www.nhlbi.nih.gov/health/resources/heart
- Prevention and Treatment of Arrhythmia: https://www.heart.org/en/health-topics/arrhythmia/prevention--treatment-of-arrhythmia#.Vq7GM1KoPl4
- Centers for Disease Control and Prevention Heart Disease Educational Material for Patients: https://www.cdc.gov/heartdisease/materials_for_patients.htm

Medication Treatment of Heart Failure

More than 6 million Americans have heart failure, making it a major chronic health issue.[14] The goals of treatment in heart failure include alleviating symptoms, slowing the progression of the disease, and improving survival. Findings from numerous randomly controlled clinical trials have resulted in guidelines for the pharmacologic treatment of heart failure.[105,108]

More information about heart failure is available in Chapter 11. Table 12.21 reviews medications currently recommended for treatment of heart failure. Types of medications that have been found to worsen heart failure should be avoided, including most antidysrhythmics, calcium channel blockers, and NSAIDs.[109]

ADDITIONAL RESOURCES

See Box 12.8 for Internet resources related to cardiovascular therapeutic management.

REFERENCES

1. Samii SM. Indications for pacemakers, implantable cardioverter-defibrillators and cardiac resynchronization devices. *Med Clin N Am.* 2015;99:795.
2. Mahida S, Derval N, Sacher F, et al. Role of electrophysiological studies in predicting risk of ventricular arrhythmia in early repolarization syndrome. *J Am Coll Cardiol.* 2015;65:151.
3. Page RL, Joglar JA, Caldwell MA, et al. ACC/AHA/HRS guideline for the management of adult patients with supraventricular tachycardia: a report of the American College of Cardiology/American Heart Association task force on clinical practice guidelines and the Heart Rhythm Society. *J Am Coll Cardiol.* 2015;2016(67):e27.
4. January CT, Wann LS, Calkins H, et al. AHA/ACC/HRS focused update of the 2014 AHA/ACC/HRS guideline for the management of patients with atrial fibrillation: a report of the American College of Cardiology/American Heart Association task force on clinical practice guidelines and the Heart Rhythm Society. *Heart Rhythm.* 2019;16:e66.
5. Sullivan BL, Bartels K, Hamilton N. Insertion and management of temporary pacemakers. *Semin CardioThorac Vasc Anesth.* 2016;20:52.
6. Schulman PM, Rozner MA. The perioperative management of implantable pacemakers and cardioverter-defibrillators. *Adv Anesthesia.* 2016;34:117.

7. Panchal AR, Bartos JA, Cabañas JG, et al. Part 3: adult basic and advanced life support: 2020 American Heart Association guidelines for cardiopulmonary resuscitation and emergency cardiovascular care. *Circulation.* 2020;142(16 suppl 2):S366−S468.

8. Elmistekawy E, Gee YY, Une D, Lemay M, Stolarik A, Rubens FD. Clinical and mechanical factors associated with the removal of temporary epicardial pacemaker wires after cardiac surgery. *J Cardiothoracic Surg.* 2016;11:8.

9. Bernstein AD, Daubert JC, Fletcher RD, et al. The revised NASPE/BPEG generic pacemaker code for antibradycardia, adaptive-rate and multi-site pacing. *Pacing Clin Electrophysiol.* 2002;25:260.

10. Vijayaraman P, Bordachar P, Ellenbogen KA. The continued search for physiological pacing: where are we now? *Am Coll Cardiol.* 2017;69:3099.

11. Ley SJ, Koulakis D. Temporary pacing after cardiac surgery. *AACN Adv Crit Care.* 2015;26(3):275.

12. Allison MG, Mallemat HA. Emergency care of patients with pacemakers and defibrillators. *Emerg Med Clin N Am.* 2015;33:653.

13. Fowler LH. Nursing management for patients postoperative cardiac implantable electronic device placement. *Crit Care Nurs Clin N Am.* 2019;31:65.

14. Benjamin EJ, Muntner P, Alonso A, et al. Heart disease and stroke statistics—2019 update: a report from the American Heart Association. *Circulation.* 2019;139:e56.

15. Mulpuro SK, Madhavan M, McLeod CJ, Cha YM, Friedman PA. Cardiac pacemakers: function, troubleshooting, and management (Part 1 of a 2-Part Series). *J Am Coll Cardiol.* 2017;69:189.

16. Slotwiner DJ, Raitt MH, Del-Carpio Munoz F, Mulpuru SK, Nasser N, Peterson PN. Impact of physiologic pacing versus right ventricular pacing among patients with left ventricular ejection fraction greater than 35%: a systematic review for the 2018 ACC/AHA/HRS guideline on the evaluation and management of patients with bradycardia and cardiac conduction delay: a report of the American College of Cardiology/American Heart Association task force on clinical practice guidelines and the Heart Rhythm Society. *Circulation.* 2019;140:e483.

17. El-Chami MF, Merchant FM, Leon AR. Leadless pacemakers. *Am J Cardiol.* 2017;119:145.

18. Leier M. Advancements in pacemaker technology: the leadless device. *Crit Care Nurs.* 2017;37(2):58.

19. Grimaldi A, Gorodeski EZ, Rickard J. Optimizing cardiac resynchronization therapy: an update on new insights and advancements. *Curr Heart Fail Rep.* 2018;15:156.

20. Chatergee NA, Singh JP. Cardiac resynchronization therapy: past, present and future. *Heart Fail Clin.* 2015;11:287.

21. Boriani G, Ziacchi M, Nesti M, et al. Cardiac resynchronization therapy: how did consensus guidelines from Europe and the United States evolve in the last 15 years? *Int J Cardiol.* 2018;261:119.

22. Freeman V, Saxon L. Remote monitoring and outcomes in pacemaker and defibrillator patients: big data saving lives? *J Am Coll Cardiol.* 2015;65(24):2612.

23. Harding ME. Cardiac implantable electronic device implantation: intraoperative, acute and remote complications. *AACN Adv Crit Care.* 2015;26(4):312.

24. Al-Khatib SM, Stevenson WG, Ackerman MJ, et al. AHA/ACC/HRS guideline for management of patients with ventricular arrhythmias and the prevention of sudden cardiac death: a report of the American College of Cardiology foundation/American Heart Association task force on clinical practice guidelines the Heart Rhythm Society. *Circulation.* 2017;2018(138):e272.

25. Swerdlow CD, Wang PJ, Zipe DP. Pacemaker and implantable cardioverter-defibrillators. In: Mann DL, ed. *Braunwald's Heart Disease.* Philadelphia: Saunders; 2019:780.

26. Galve E, Oristrell G, Acosta G, et al. Cardiac resynchronization therapy is associated with a reduction in ICD therapies as it improves ventricular function. *Clin Cardiol.* 2018;41:803.

27. Wilson D, Herweg B. New technology for implantable cardioverter defibrillators. *Card Electrophysiol Clin.* 2014;6:261.

28. Gold MR, Aasbo JD, El-Chami MF. Subcutaneous implantable cardioverter-defibrillator post-approval study: clinical characteristics and perioperative results. *Heart Rhythm.* 2017;17:8.

29. Healey JS, Hohnloser SH, Glikson M, et al. Cardioverter defibrillator implantation without induction of ventricular fibrillation: a single-blind, non-inferiority, randomized controlled trial (SIMPLE). *Lancet.* 2015;385:785.

30. Duffett S, El Hajjaji I, Manlucu J, Yee R. Implantable cardioverter defibrillator implantation with or without defibrillation testing. *Card Electrophysiol Clin.* 2018;10:119.

31. Kulkarni N, Link MS. Causes and prevention of inappropriate implantable cardioverter-defibrillator shocks. *Card Electrophysiol Clin.* 2018;10:67.

32. Jacobs I, Sunde K, Charles D, Deakin CD, et al. International Consensus on Cardiopulmonary Resuscitation and Emergency Cardiovascular Care Science with Treatment Recommendations. *Circulation.* 2010;122(16_suppl_2):S325−S337. October 2010 https://www.ahajournals.org/doi/full/10.1161/circulationaha.110.971010.

33. Langabeer JR, Henry TD, Kereiakes DJ, et al. Growth in percutaneous coronary intervention capacity relative to population and disease prevalence. *J Am Heart Assoc.* 2013;2(6):e000370.

34. Harrington DH, Stueben F, Lenahan CM. ST-Elevation myocardial infarction and non-ST-elevation myocardial infarction: medical and surgical interventions. *Crit Care Nurs Clin N Am.* 2019;31:49.

35. Promes SB, Glauser JM, Smith MD, Torbati SS, Brown MD. Clinical policy: emergency department management of patients needing reperfusion therapy for acute ST-segment elevation myocardial infarction. *Ann Emerg Med.* 2017;70(5):724.

36. O'Gara PT, Kushner FG, Ascheim DD, et al. ACCF/AHA guideline for the management of ST-elevation myocardial infarction: a report of the American College of Cardiology Foundation/American Heart Association task force on practice guidelines. *J Am Coll Cardiol.* 2013;(61):e78.

37. Amsterdam EA, Wenger NK, Brindis RG, et al. ACC/AHA guideline for the management of patients with non-ST-elevation acute coronary syndromes: a report of the American College of Cardiology/American Heart Association task force on practice guidelines. *Circulation.* 2014;2014(130):e344.

38. Thomas JL, French WJ. Current state of ST-segment myocardial infarction: evidence-based therapies and optimal patient outcomes in advanced systems of care. *Cardio Clin.* 2014;32:371.

39. Chakrabarti AK, Patel SJ, Salazar RL, et al. Newer pharmaceutical agents for STEMI interventions. *Intervent Cardiol Clin.* 2012;1(4):429.

40. Bhatt DL, Lopes RD, Harrington RA, et al. Diagnosis and Treatment of Acute Coronary Syndromes: A Review. *JAMA.* 2022;327(7):662−675.

41. The TIMI Study Group. The thrombolysis in myocardial infarction (TIMI) trial: phase I findings. *N Engl J Med.* 1985;312:932.

42. Wong GC, Welsford M, Ainsworth C, et al. Canadian Cardiovascular Society/Canadian Association of Interventional Cardiology Guidelines on the Acute Management of ST-Elevation Myocardial Infarction: Focused Update on Regionalization and Reperfusion. *Can J Cardiol.* 2019;35(2):107−132.

43. American Association of Critical Care Nurses. Ensuring accurate ST-segment monitoring. *Crit Care Nurs.* 2016;36(6):e18.

44. Welsford M, Nikolaou NI, Beygui F, et al. Part 5: acute coronary syndromes: 2015 international consensus on cardiopulmonary resuscitation and emergency cardiovascular care with treatment recommendations. *Circulation.* 2015;132(suppl 2):S146.

45. Bob-Manuel T, Ifedili I, Reed G, Ibebuogu UN, Khouzam RN. Non-ST elevation acute coronary syndromes: a comprehensive review. *Curr Probl Cardiol.* 2017;42:266.

46. Byrne RA, Stone GW, Ormiston J, Kastrati A. Coronary balloon angioplasty, stent, and scaffolds. *Lancet.* 2017;390:781.

47. Vos NS, Fagel ND, Amoroso G, et al. Paclitaxel-coated balloon angioplasty versus drug-eluting stent in acute myocardial infarction: the REVELATION Randomized Trial. *ACC Cardiovasc Interv.* 2019;12(17):1691−1699.

48. Lee MS, Gordin JS, Stone GW, et al. Orbital and rotational atherectomy during percutaneous coronary intervention for coronary artery calcification. *Cath Cardiovasc Interv.* 2018;92:61.

49. Kalra A, Rehman H, Khera S, et al. New-generation coronary stents: current data and future directions. *Curr Athero Rep.* 2017;19(14):13.

50. Widmer RJ, Pollak PM, Bell MR, Gersh BJ, Anavekar NS. The evolving face of myocardial reperfusion in acute coronary syndromes: a primer for the internist. *Mayo Clin Proc.* 2018;93(2):199.

51. Levine GN, Bates ER, Blankenship JC, et al. ACCF/AHA/SCAI guideline for percutaneous coronary intervention and executive summary. *Circulation.* 2011;124:2574.

52. Ndrepepa G, Kastrati A. Bleeding complications in patients undergoing percutaneous coronary interventions: current status and perspective. *Coron Artery Dis.* 2014;25:247.

53. Ozkok S, Ozkok A. Contrast-induced acute kidney injury: a review of practical points. *World J Nephrol.* 2017;6(3):86.

54. Kellum JA, Lameire N, Aspelin P, et al. Kidney disease: improving global outcomes: clinical practice guidelines for AKI. *J Int Soc Neph.* 2012;1(supp 2):1.

55. Bonnett C, Becker N, Hann B, Haynes A, Tremmel J. Preventing radial artery occlusion by using reserve Barbeau assessment: bringing evidence-based practice to the bedside. *Crit Care Nurs.* 2015;35:77.

56. Noori VJ, Eldrup-Jorgensen J. A systematic review of vascular closure devices for femoral artery puncture sites. *J Vasc Surg.* 2018;68(3):887.

57. Cox T, Blair L, Huntington C, Lincourt A, Sing R, Heniford BT. Systematic review of randomized controlled trials comparing manual compression to vascular closure devices for diagnostic and therapeutic arterial procedures. *Surg Tech Int.* 2015;27:32–44.

58. Nishimura RA, Otto CM, Bonow RO, et al. AHA/ACC focused update of the 2014 AHA/ACC guidelines for the management of patients with valvular heart disease. *Circulation.* 2017;2017(135):e1159.

59. Popma JJ, Deeb GM, Yakubov SJ, et al. Transcatheter aortic-valve replacement with a self-expanding valve in low-risk patients. *N Engl J Med.* 2019;380:1706–1715.

60. Otto CM, Kumbhani DJ, Alexander KP, et al. ACC expert consensus decision pathway for transcatheter aortic valve replacement in the management of adults with aortic stenosis: a report of the American College of Cardiology task force on clinical expert consensus documents. *J Am Coll Cardiol.* 2017;69(10):1313–1346.

61. Aldea GS, Bakaeen FG, Pal J, et al. The Society of Thoracic Surgeons clinical practice guidelines on arterial conduits for coronary artery bypass grafting. *Ann Thorac Surg.* 2016;101:801.

62. Shore-Lesserson L, Baker RA, Ferraris VA, et al. The Society of Thoracic Surgeons, the Society of Cardiovascular Anesthesiologist, and the American Society of Extracorporeal Technology: clinical practice guidelines-anticoagulation during cardiopulmonary bypass. *Ann Thorac Surg.* 2018;105:650.

63. Bakaeen FG, Swenson LG. Off-pump CABG fails to EXCEL in surgical revascularization of left main disease. *J Am Coll Cardiol.* 2019;74:741.

64. Benedetto U, Puskas J, Kappetein AP, et al. Off-pump versus on-pump bypass surgery for left main coronary artery disease. *J Am Coll Cardiol.* 2019;74:729.

65. O'Brien B, Burrage PS, Ngai JY, et al. Society of Cardiovascular Anesthesiologists/European Association of Cardiothoracic Anesthetists practice advisory for the management of perioperative atrial fibrillation in patients undergoing cardiac surgery. *J Cardiothorac Vasc Anesth.* 2019;33(1):12.

66. Stephens RS, Whitman GJ. Postoperative critical care of the adult cardiac surgery patient: part I: routine postoperative care. *Crit Care Med.* 2015;43:1477.

67. Kupchik N, Bridges E. Central venous pressure monitoring: what's the evidence? *Am J Nurs.* 2012;112(2):58.

68. Pereira KM, de Assis CS, Cintra HNWL, et al. Factors associated with increased bleeding in the postoperative period of cardiac surgery: a cohort study. *J Clinic Nurs.* 2019;28(5–6):850.

69. Ferraris VA, Brown JR. Society of Thoracic Surgeons Blood Conservation Guideline Task Force, et al. Update to the Society of Thoracic Surgeons and the Society of Cardiovascular Anesthesiologists blood conservation clinical practice guidelines. *Ann Thorac Surg.* 2011;91:944.

70. Stephens RS, Whitman GJ. Postoperative critical care of the adult cardiac surgical patient: part II: procedure-specific considerations, management of complications, and quality improvement. *Crit Care Med.* 2015;43:1995.

71. Demirci C, Zeman F, Schmid C, Floerchinger B. Early postoperative blood pressure and blood loss after cardiac surgery: a retrospective analysis. *Intens Crit Care Nurs.* 2017;42:122.

72. Bigeleisen PE, Goehner N. Novel approaches in pain management in cardiac surgery. *Curr Opin Anesthesiol.* 2015;28:89.

73. Barr J, Fraser GL, Puntillo K, et al. American College of Critical Care Medicine: clinical practice guidelines for the management of pain agitation, and delirium in adult patients in the intensive care unit. *Crit Care Med.* 2013;41:263.

74. Hillis LD, Smith PK, Anderson JL, et al. ACCF/AHA guidelines for coronary artery bypass surgery: a report of the American College of Cardiology Foundation/American Heart Association task force on practice guidelines. *Circulation.* 2011;124(23):e652.

75. Gaffney AM, Sladen RN. Acute kidney injury in cardiac surgery. *Curr Opin Anesthesiol.* 2015;28:50.

76. Society of Thoracic Surgeons Task Force on Resuscitation After Cardiac Surgery. The Society of Thoracic Surgeons Expert Consensus for the Resuscitation of Patients Who Arrest After Cardiac Surgery. *Ann Thorac Surg.* 2017;103(3):1005–1020.

77. Canale LS, Mick S, Mihaljevic T, Nair R, Bonatti J. Robotically assisted totally endoscopic coronary artery bypass surgery. *J Thorac Dis.* 2013;5(suppl 6):S641.

78. Calkins H, Hindricks G, Cappato R, et al. HRS/EHRA/ECAS/APHRS/SOLAECE expert consensus statement on catheter and surgical ablation of atrial fibrillation. *Heart Rhythm.* 2017;14(10):e275.

79. Badhwar V, Rankin JS, Damiano RJ, JR et al. The Society of Thoracic Surgeons 2017 clinical practice guidelines for the surgical treatment of atrial fibrillation. *Ann Thorac Surg.* 2017;103:329.

80. Rihal CS, Naidu SS, Givertz MM, et al. SCAI/ACC/HFSA/STS clinical expert consensus statement on the use of percutaneous mechanical circulatory support devices in cardiovascular care: endorsed by the American Heart Association. *J Am Coll Cardiol.* 2015;2015(65):e7.

81. Mandawat A, Rao SV. Percutaneous mechanical circulatory support devices in cardiogenic shock. *Circ Cardiovasc Interv.* 2017;10:e004337.

82. González LS, Chaney MA. Intraaortic balloon pump counterpulsation, part I: history, technical aspects, physiologic effects, contraindications, medical applications/outcomes. *Anesth Analg.* 2020;131(3):776–791.

83. González LS, Chaney MA. Intraaortic balloon pump counterpulsation part II: perioperative hemodynamic support and new directions. *Anesth Analg.* 2020;131(3):792–807.

84. Desai SR, Hwang NC. Advances in left ventricular assist devices and mechanical circulatory support. *J Cardiothoracic Vasc Anesth.* 2018;32:1193.

85. ELSO Guidelines for Patient Care, Respiratory & Cardiac Support, *Extracorporeal Life Support Organization*; version 1. Ann Arbor, MI, USA www.elso.org

86. Pinney SP, Anyanwu AC, Lala A, Teuteberg JJ, Uriel N, Mehra MR. Left ventricular assist devices for lifelong support. *J Am Coll of Card.* 2017;69(23):2845.

87. Gopinathannair R, Cornwell WK, Dukes JW, et al. Device therapy and arrhythmia management in left ventricular assist device recipients: a scientific statement from the American Heart Association. *Circulation.* 2019;139:e967.

88. Peberdy MA, Gluck JA, Ornato JP, et al. Cardiopulmonary resuscitation in adults and children with mechanical circulatory support: a scientific statement from the American Heart Association. *Circulation.* 2017;135:e1115.

89. The Joint Commission. The Joint Commission clarifies expectations for implementing medication titration orders. *Joint Comm Perspect.* 2020;40(6):7.

90. Waller JR, Waller DG. Drugs for heart failure and arrhythmias. *Medicine.* 2018;46(10):652.

91. Samarin MJ, Mobrien KM, Oliphant CS. Continuous intravenous antiarrhythmic agents in the intensive care unit: strategies for safe and effective use of amiodarone, lidocaine, and procainamide. *Crit Care Nurs Q.* 2015;38:329.

92. Sandau KE, Funk M, Auerbach A, et al. Update to practice standards for electrocardiographic monitoring in hospital settings: a scientific statement from the American Heart Association. *Circulation.* 2017;136:e273.

93. Marzlin KM. Implications of antiarrhythmic pharmacology. *AACN Adv Crit Care.* 2019;30(1):85.

94. Brubaker S, Long B, Koyfman A. Alternative treatment options for atrioventricular-nodal-reentry tachycardia: an emergency medicine review. *J Emer Med.* 2018;54(2):198.

95. Fairley JL, Zhang L, Glassford NJ, Bellomo R. Magnesium status and magnesium therapy in cardiac surgery: a systematic review and meta-analysis focusing on arrhythmia prevention. *J Crit Care.* 2017;42:69.

96. Salaminia S, Sayehmiri F, Angha P, Sayehmiri K, Motedayen M. Evaluating the effect of magnesium supplementation and cardiac arrhythmias after acute coronary syndrome: a systematic review and meta-analysis. *BMC Cardiovasc Disord.* 2018;18:129.

97. Rogers PA, Bernard ML, Madias C, Thihalolipavan S, Mark Estes 3rd NA, Morin DP. Current evidence-based understanding of the epidemiology, prevention, and treatment of atrial fibrillation. *Curr Probl Cardiol.* 2018;43:241.

98. Pickett JD. Direct oral anticoagulants in patients with nonvalvular atrial fibrillation: update and periprocedural management. *Crit Care Nurse.* 2019;39(2):54.

99. Jentzer JC, Coons JC, Link CB, Schmidhofer M. Pharmacotherapy update on the use of vasopressors and inotropes in the intensive care unit. *J Cardiovasc Pharmacol Ther.* 2015;20(3):249.

100. Stratton L, Berlin DA, Arbo JE. Vasopressors and inotropes in sepsis. *Emerg Med Clin N Am.* 2017;35:75.

101. Griffiths CL, Vestal ML, Hertel KA. Vasoactive agents in shock. *Nurs Crit Care.* 2018;13(2):6.

102. Adabeyo O, Rogers RL. Hypertensive emergencies in the emergency department. *Emerg Med Clin North Am.* 2015;33:539.

103. Braithwaite L, Reif M. Hypertensive emergencies: a review of common presentations and treatment options. *Cardiol Clin.* 2019;27:275.

104. Watson K, Broscious R, Devabhakthuni S, Noel ZR. Focused update on the pharmacologic management of hypertensive emergencies. *Curr Hypertens Rep.* 2018;20:56.

105. Yancy CW, Jessup M, Bozkurt B, et al. ACC/AHA/HFSA focused update of the 2014 ACCF/AHA guideline for the management of heart failure: a report of the American College of Cardiology/American Heart Association task force on clinical practice guidelines and the Heart Failure Society of America. *Circulation.* 2017;2017(136):e137.

106. Callaway CW, Soar J, Aibiki M, et al. Part 4: advanced life support: 2015 international consensus on cardiopulmonary resuscitation and emergency cardiovascular care science with treatment recommendations. *Circulation.* 2015;132(suppl 1):S84.

107. Gilbert BW, Reichert M, Fletcher S. Strategies for the management of sepsis. *AACN Adv Crit Care.* 2019;30:5.

108. Jackevicus CA, Page RL, Buckley LF, Jennings DL, Nappi JM, Smith AJ. Key articles and guidelines in the management of heart failure: 2018 update. *J Pharm Pract.* 2019;32:77.

109. Page RL, O'Bryant CL, Cheng D, et al. Drugs that may cause or exacerbate heart failure. A scientific statement from the American Heart Association. *Circulation.* 2016;134:e32.

13

Pulmonary Clinical Assessment and Diagnostic Procedures

Kathleen M. Stacy

HISTORY

Taking a thorough and accurate history is an essential part of the assessment process. The patient's history provides the foundation and direction for the rest of the assessment. The overall goal of the patient interview is to expose key clinical manifestations that will facilitate the identification of the underlying cause of the illness. This information then assists in the development of an appropriate management plan.

The initial presentation of the patient determines the rapidity and direction of the interview. For a patient in acute distress, the history is curtailed to just a few questions about the patient's chief complaint and precipitating events. For a patient in no obvious distress, the history focuses on five priorities areas: (1) review of the patient's present illness, (2) overview of the patient's general respiratory status, (3) examination of the patient's general health status, (4) survey of the patient's family and social background, and (5) description of the patient's current symptoms. Specific items included in each of these areas are outlined in Box 13.1.

Symptoms that are common in a patient with a pulmonary disorder include dyspnea, cough, wheezing, edema, palpitations, fatigue, chest pain, hemoptysis, and sputum abnormalities. Information is elicited regarding the location, onset and duration, characteristics, setting, aggravating and alleviating factors, associated symptoms, and efforts to treat the symptoms. If the cough is productive, the patient is asked questions about the color, amount, odor, and consistency of the sputum.[1,2]

PRIORITY CLINICAL ASSESSMENT

Four techniques are used in clinical assessment: inspection, palpation, percussion, and auscultation.

Inspection

Inspection of the patient focuses on three priorities: (1) observation of the tongue and sublingual area, (2) assessment of chest wall configuration, and (3) evaluation of respiratory effort. If possible, patients are positioned upright, with their arms resting at their sides.[3] Inspection usually begins during the interview.

Observation of the Tongue and Sublingual Area

The patient's tongue and sublingual area are observed for a blue, gray, or dark purple tint or discoloration indicating the presence of central cyanosis. *Central cyanosis* is a sign of hypoxemia, or inadequate oxygenation of the blood, and is a life-threatening condition. Central cyanosis occurs when the amount of reduced hemoglobin (unsaturated hemoglobin) exceeds 5 g/dL. The fingers and toes may also appear discolored, an indication of the presence of peripheral cyanosis.[4]

Assessment of Chest Wall Configuration

The size and shape of the patient's chest wall are assessed for an increase in the anteroposterior diameter and for structural deviations. The ratio of anteroposterior diameter to lateral diameter ranges from 1:2 to 5:7 normally.[1,2] An increase in the anteroposterior diameter is suggestive of chronic obstructive pulmonary disease (COPD).[1,2] The shape of the chest is inspected for any structural deviations. Some more frequently seen abnormalities are pectus excavatum, pectus carinatum, barrel chest, and spinal deformities. In *pectus excavatum* (funnel chest), the sternum and lower ribs are displaced posteriorly, creating a funnel or pit-shaped depression in the chest. This abnormality causes a decrease in the anteroposterior diameter of the chest and may interfere with respiratory function. In *pectus carinatum* (pigeon breast), the sternum projects forward, causing an increase in the anteroposterior diameter of the chest. The *barrel chest* also results in an increase in the anteroposterior diameter of the chest and is characterized by displacement of the sternum forward and the ribs outward. Spinal deformities, such as *kyphosis*, *lordosis*, and *scoliosis*, also may be present and can interfere with respiratory function.[5]

Evaluation of Respiratory Effort

The patient's respiratory effort is evaluated for rate, rhythm, symmetry, and quality of ventilatory movements.[1] Normal breathing at rest is effortless and regular and occurs at a rate of 12 to 20 breaths/min.[3] There are a number of abnormal respiratory patterns (Fig. 13.1). Some more commonly seen patterns in patients with pulmonary dysfunction are tachypnea, hyperventilation, and air trapping. *Tachypnea* is manifested by an increase in the rate and decrease in the depth of ventilation. *Hyperventilation* is manifested by an increase in

BOX 13.1   DATA COLLECTION

Pulmonary History

Common Pulmonary Symptoms

Cough
- Onset and duration
  Sudden or gradual
  Episodic or continuous
- Characteristics
  - Dry or wet
  - Hacking, hoarse, barking, or congested
  - Productive or nonproductive
- Sputum
  - Present or absent
  - Frequency of production
  - Appearance—color (e.g., clear, mucoid, purulent, blood-tinged, mostly bloody), foul odor, frothy
  - Amount
- Pattern
  - Paroxysmal
  - Related to time of day, weather, activities, talking, or deep breathing
  - Change over time
- Severity
  - Causes fatigue
  - Disrupts sleep or conversation
  - Produces chest pain
- Associated symptoms
  - Shortness of breath
  - Chest pain or tightness with breathing
  - Fever
  - Upper respiratory tract signs (e.g., sore throat, congestion, increased mucus production)
  - Noisy respirations or hoarseness
  - Gagging or choking
  - Anxiety, stress, or panic reactions
- Efforts made to treat
  - Prescription or nonprescription medications
  - Vaporizers
  - Effective or ineffective

Shortness of Breath or Dyspnea on Exertion
- Onset and duration
  - Sudden or gradual
  - Gagging or choking episode a few days before onset
- Pattern
  - Related to position—improves when sitting up or with head elevated; number of pillows used to alleviate problems
  - Related to activity—exercise or eating; extent of activity that produces dyspnea
  - Related to other factors—time of day, season, or exposure to something in the environment
  - Harder to inhale or harder to exhale
- Severity
  - Extent activity is limited
  - Breathing itself causes fatigue
  - Anxiety about getting enough air
- Associated symptoms
  - Pain or discomfort—exact location in respiratory tree
  - Cough, diaphoresis, swelling of ankles, or cyanosis
- Efforts made to treat
  - Prescription or nonprescription medications
  - Oxygen
  - Effective or ineffective

Chest Pain
- Onset and duration
  - Gradual or sudden
  - Associated with trauma, coughing, or lower respiratory tract infection
- Associated symptoms
  - Shallow breathing
  - Uneven chest expansion
  - Fever
  - Cough
  - Radiation of pain to neck or arms
  - Anxiety about getting enough air
- Efforts made to treat
  - Heat, splinting, or pain medication
  - Effective or ineffective

Pulmonary Risk Factors
- Tobacco use—current and past
  - Type of tobacco—cigarettes, cigars, pipes, or smokeless
  - Duration and amount—age started, inhale when smoking, amount used in the past and present
  - Pack years—number of packs per day multiplied by number of years patient has smoked
  - Efforts to quit—previous attempts and current interest
- Work environment
  - Nature of work
  - Environmental hazards—chemicals, vapors, dust, pulmonary irritants, or allergens
  - Use of protective devices
- Home environment
  - Location
  - Possible allergens—pets, house plants, plants and trees outside the home, or other environmental hazards
  - Type of heating
  - Use of air conditioning or humidifier
  - Ventilation
  - Stairs to climb

Medical History

Child
- Infectious respiratory diseases
  - Strep throat
  - Mumps
  - Tonsillitis
- Asthma
- Cystic fibrosis
- Immunizations

Adult
- Previous diagnosis of pulmonary disorders—dates of hospitalization
- Chronic pulmonary disease—date, treatment, and compliance with therapy
  - Tuberculosis
  - Bronchitis
  - Emphysema
  - Bronchiectasis
  - Asthma
  - Sinus infection
- Other chronic disorders—cardiovascular, cancer, musculoskeletal, neurologic, immune
  - Obstruction of one or both nares
  - Mouth breathing often necessary (especially at night)
  - History of nasal discharge

BOX 13.1   DATA COLLECTION—cont'd

Pulmonary History

- Compromised immune system function
- Nosebleed
- Sleep apnea
  - Obstructive
  - Central
- Previous tests
  - Allergy testing
  - Pulmonary function tests
  - Tuberculin and fungal skin tests
  - Chest radiographs

Surgical

- Thoracic trauma
- Thoracic surgery
- Nasal surgery or injury

Family History

- Tuberculosis
- Cystic fibrosis
- Emphysema
- Allergies
- Asthma
- Atopic dermatitis
- Smoking by household members
- Malignancy

Current Medication Use

- Inhalators
- Steroids
- Antibiotics
- Immunizations
  - Pneumococcal (Pneumovax)
  - Influenza

the rate and depth of ventilation. Patients with COPD often experience obstructive breathing or *air trapping*. As the patient breathes, air becomes trapped in the lungs, and ventilations become progressively shallower until the patient actively and forcefully exhales.[6]

Additional Assessment Areas

Other areas assessed are patient position, active effort to breathe, use of accessory muscles, presence of intercostal retractions, unequal movement of the chest wall, flaring of nares, and pausing midsentence to take a breath.[1,2] The presence of iatrogenic features, such as chest tubes, central venous lines, artificial airways, and nasogastric tubes, is identified, because these features may affect assessment findings.

Palpation

Palpation of the patient focuses on three priorities: (1) confirmation of the position of the trachea, (2) assessment of thoracic expansion, and

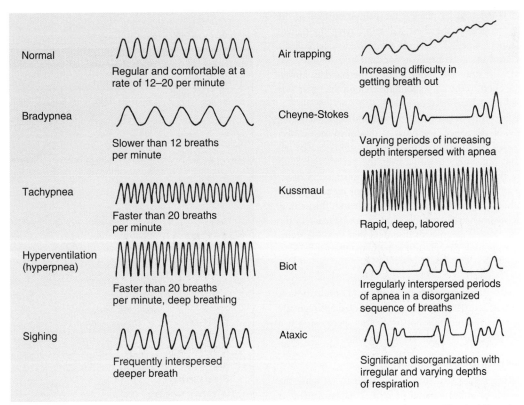

Fig. 13.1   Patterns of Respiration. (From Ball JW, Dains J, Flynn J, et al. *Seidel's Guide to Physical Examination: An Interprofessional Approach.* 9th ed. St. Louis: Elsevier; 2019.)

(3) evaluation of tactile fremitus. The thorax is assessed for any areas of tenderness, lumps, or bony deformities. The anterior, posterior, and lateral areas of the chest are evaluated in a systematic fashion.[1]

Confirmation of Position of the Trachea

The position of the patient's trachea is confirmed at midline and is assessed by placing the fingers in the suprasternal notch and moving upward.[6] Deviation of the trachea to either side may indicate a pneumothorax, unilateral pneumonia, diffuse pulmonary fibrosis, a large pleural effusion, or severe atelectasis. With atelectasis, the trachea shifts to the same side as the problem; with pneumothorax, the trachea shifts to the opposite side of the problem.[5]

Assessment of Thoracic Expansion

The patient's thoracic expansion is assessed for the degree and symmetry of movement[4] and is assessed by placing the hands on the anterolateral chest with the thumbs extended along the costal margin, pointing to the xiphoid process, or on the posterolateral chest with the thumbs on either side of the spine at the level of the 10th rib. The patient is instructed to take a few normal breaths and then a few deep breaths. Chest movement is assessed for equality, which signifies symmetry of thoracic expansion.[3,5,6] Asymmetry is an abnormal finding that can occur with pneumothorax, pneumonia, or other disorders that interfere with lung inflation. The degree of chest movement is felt to ascertain the extent of lung expansion. The thumbs should separate 3 to 5 cm during deep inspiration.[2,6] Lung expansion of a hyperinflated chest is less than expansion of a normal chest.[2,6]

Evaluation of Tactile Fremitus

The patient is assessed for tactile fremitus to identify, describe, and localize any areas of increased or decreased fremitus. Tactile fremitus refers to the palpable vibrations felt through the chest wall when the patient speaks and is assessed by placing the palmar surface of the hands against opposite sides of the chest wall and having the patient repeat the word "ninety-nine." The hands are moved systematically around the thorax until the anterior, posterior, and both lateral areas have been assessed.[5,6] If only one hand is used, the hand is moved from one side of the chest to the corresponding area on the other side of the chest until all areas have been assessed.[6]

Tactile fremitus varies from patient to patient and depends on the pitch and intensity of the voice. Fremitus is described as normal, decreased, or increased. With normal fremitus, vibrations can be felt over the trachea but are barely palpable over the periphery.[1] With decreased fremitus, there is interference with the transmission of vibrations. Examples of disorders that decrease fremitus include pleural effusion, pneumothorax, bronchial obstruction, pleural thickening, and emphysema. With increased fremitus, there is an increase in the transmission of vibrations. Examples of disorders that increase fremitus include pneumonia, lung cancer, and pulmonary fibrosis.[2]

Percussion

Percussion of the patient focuses on two priorities: (1) evaluation of the underlying lung structure and (2) assessment of diaphragmatic excursion. Although the technique is not used often, percussion is a useful method for confirming suspected abnormalities.

Evaluation of Underlying Lung Structure

The patient's underlying lung structure is evaluated to estimate the amounts of air, liquid, or solid material present. This assessment is performed by placing the middle finger of the nondominant hand on the chest wall. The distal portion, between the last joint and the nail bed, is then struck with the middle finger of the dominant hand. The hands are moved systematically and side to side around the thorax to compare similar areas until the anterior, posterior, and both lateral areas have been assessed. Five tones can be elicited: resonance, hyperresonance, tympany, dullness, and flatness. These tones are distinguished by differences in intensity, pitch, duration, and quality. Table 13.1 describes the different percussion tones and their associated conditions.[3,5]

Assessment of Diaphragmatic Excursion

The patient is assessed for diaphragmatic excursion to evaluate the movement of the diaphragm. This assessment is accomplished by measuring the difference in the level of the diaphragm on inspiration and expiration and is performed by instructing the patient to inhale and hold the breath. The posterior chest is percussed downward, over the intercostal spaces, until the dull sound produced by the diaphragm is heard. The spot is marked. The patient is then instructed to take a few breaths in and out, exhale completely, and then hold his or her breath. The posterior chest is percussed again, and the new area of dullness over the diaphragm is located and marked. The difference between the two spots is identified and measured. Normal diaphragmatic excursion is 3 to 5 cm.[6] Diaphragmatic excursion is decreased in ascites, pregnancy, hepatomegaly, and emphysema and is increased in pleural effusion and disorders that elevate the diaphragm, such as atelectasis or paralysis.[5]

Auscultation

Auscultation of the patient focuses on three priorities: (1) evaluation of normal breath sounds, (2) identification of abnormal breath sounds, and (3) assessment of voice sounds. Auscultation requires a quiet environment, proper positioning of the patient, and a bare chest.[7] Breath sounds are best heard with the patient in the upright position.[2]

TABLE 13.1	Percussion Tones	
Tone	**Description**	**Condition**
Resonance	Intensity: loud Pitch: low Duration: long Quality: hollow	Normal lung Bronchitis
Hyperresonance	Intensity: very loud Pitch: very low Duration: long Quality: booming	Asthma Emphysema Pneumothorax
Tympany	Intensity: loud Pitch: musical Duration: medium Quality: drumlike	Large pneumothorax Emphysematous blebs
Dullness	Intensity: medium Pitch: medium-high Duration: medium Quality: thudlike	Atelectasis Pleural effusion Pulmonary edema Pneumonia Lung mass
Flatness	Intensity: soft Pitch: high Duration: short Quality: extremely dull	Massive atelectasis Pneumonectomy

Evaluation of Normal Breath Sounds

The patient's breath sounds are auscultated to evaluate the quality of air movement through the lungs and to identify the presence of abnormal sounds. This assessment is performed by placing the diaphragm of the stethoscope against the chest wall and instructing the patient to breathe in and out slowly with his or her mouth open.[1] Breath sounds are assessed during both inspiration and expiration. Auscultation is done in a systematic sequence: side to side, top to bottom, posteriorly, laterally, and anteriorly (Fig. 13.2).[2] Normal breath sounds are different, depending on their location. There are three categories: vesicular, bronchovesicular, and bronchial. Fig. 13.3 describes the characteristics of normal breath sounds and their associated conditions.[1,2,7]

Abnormal Breath Sounds

Abnormal breath sounds are identified after normal breath sounds have been clearly delineated. There are three categories of abnormal breath sounds: absent or diminished breath sounds, displaced bronchial breath sounds, and adventitious breath sounds. Table 13.2 describes the various abnormal breath sounds and their associated conditions.[1,2,7]

An *absent* or *diminished breath sound* indicates that there is little or no airflow to a particular portion of the lung (a small segment or an entire lung).[7] *Displaced bronchial breath sounds* are normal bronchial sounds heard in the peripheral lung fields instead of over the trachea. This condition is usually indicative of fluid or exudate in the alveoli.[7] *Adventitious breath sounds* are extra or added sounds heard in addition to the other sounds previously discussed. They are classified as crackles, rhonchi, wheezes, and friction rubs.

Crackles, also called *rales*, are short, discrete popping or crackling sounds produced by fluid in the small airways or alveoli or by the snapping open of collapsed airways during inspiration. They can be heard on inspiration and expiration and may clear with coughing.[7] Crackles can be further classified as fine, medium, or coarse, depending on pitch.[2,3]

Rhonchi are coarse, rumbling, low-pitched sounds produced by airflow over secretions in the larger airways or narrowing of the large airways. They are heard mainly on expiration and sometimes can be cleared with coughing. Rhonchi can be further classified as bubbling, gurgling, or sonorous, depending on the characteristics of the sound.[7]

Wheezes are high-pitched, squeaking, whistling sounds produced by airflow through narrowed small airways. They are heard mainly on expiration but may be heard throughout the ventilatory cycle. Depending on their severity, wheezes can be further classified as mild, moderate, or severe.[7]

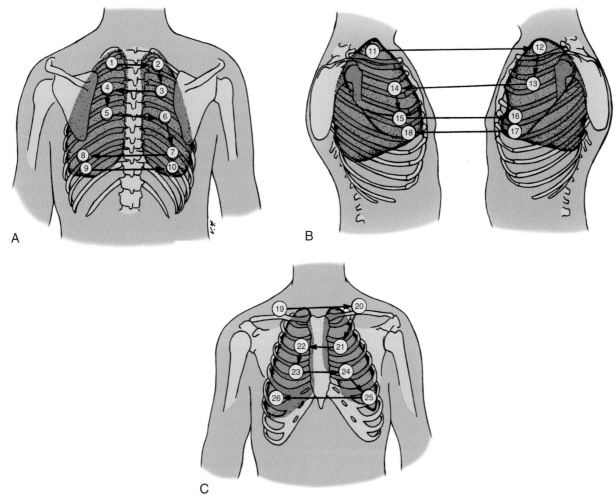

Fig. 13.2 Auscultation Sequence. (A) Posterior. (B) Lateral. (C) Anterior. (From Perry AG, Potter PA, Ostendorf WR, et al. *Clinical Nursing Skills and Techniques*. 10th ed. St. Louis: Elsevier; 2022.)

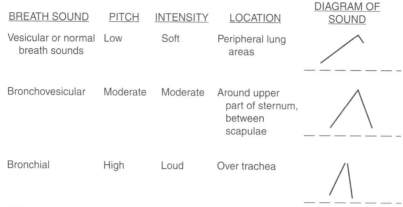

Fig. 13.3 Characteristics of Normal Breath Sounds. (From Kacmarek RM, Stoller JK, Heuer AJ, eds. *Egan's Fundamentals of Respiratory Care.* 12th ed. St. Louis: Elsevier; 2021.)

TABLE 13.2	Abnormal Breath Sounds	
Abnormal Sound	**Description**	**Condition**
Absent breath sounds	No airflow to a particular portion of the lung	Pneumothorax Pneumonectomy Emphysematous blebs Pleural effusion Lung mass Massive atelectasis Complete airway obstruction
Diminished breath sounds	Little airflow to a particular portion of the lung	Emphysema Pleural effusion Pleurisy Atelectasis Pulmonary fibrosis
Displaced bronchial sounds	Bronchial sounds heard in peripheral lung fields	Atelectasis with secretions Lung mass with exudates Pneumonia Pleural effusion Pulmonary edema
Crackles (rales)	Short, discrete popping or crackling sounds	Pulmonary edema Pneumonia Pulmonary fibrosis Atelectasis Bronchiectasis
Rhonchi	Coarse, rumbling, low-pitched sounds	Pneumonia Asthma Bronchitis Bronchospasm
Wheezes	High-pitched, squeaking, whistling sounds	Asthma Bronchospasm
Pleural friction rub	Creaking, leathery, loud, dry, coarse sounds	Pleural effusion Pleurisy

A *pleural friction rub* is a creaking, leathery, loud, dry, coarse sound produced by irritated pleural surfaces rubbing together and is usually heard best in the lower anterolateral chest area during inspiration and expiration. Pleural friction rubs are caused by inflammation of the pleura.[1,2]

Voice Sounds

Assessment of voice sounds is particularly useful in detecting lung consolidation or lung compression. Three abnormal types of voice sounds are bronchophony, whispering pectoriloquy, and egophony.[7]

Bronchophony describes a condition in which the spoken voice is heard on auscultation with higher intensity and clarity than usual. Normally, the spoken word is muffled when heard through the stethoscope. Bronchophony is assessed by placing the diaphragm of the stethoscope against the posterior side of the patient's chest and instructing the patient to say "ninety-nine." When the sound heard is clear, distinct, and loud, bronchophony is present.[7]

Whispering pectoriloquy describes a condition of unusually clear transmission of the whispered voice on auscultation. Normally, the whispered word is unintelligible when heard through the stethoscope. Whispering pectoriloquy is assessed by placing the stethoscope against the posterior side of the patient's chest and instructing the patient to whisper "one, two, three." When the sound heard is clear and distinct, whispering pectoriloquy is present.[7]

Egophony describes a condition in which the voice sounds increase in intensity and develop a nasal bleating quality on auscultation. Egophony is assessed by placing the stethoscope against the posterior side of the patient's chest and instructing the patient to say "e-e-e." When the "e" sound changes to an "a" sound, egophony is present.[1,7]

LABORATORY STUDIES

Arterial Blood Gases

Interpretation of arterial blood gas (ABG) levels can be difficult, especially if the nurse is under pressure to do it quickly and accurately. One method that can help ensure accuracy when analyzing ABG levels is to follow the same steps of interpretation each time. A specific method to be used each time that blood gas values must be interpreted is presented here (Box 13.2).

BOX 13.2 Interpretation of Arterial Blood Gases

Step 1

Look at the arterial partial pressure of oxygen (PaO$_2$) level, and answer this question: Does the PaO$_2$ level show hypoxemia?

Step 2

Look at the pH level, and answer this question: Is the pH level on the acid or alkaline side of 7.40?

Step 3

Look at the arterial partial pressure of carbon dioxide (PaCO$_2$) level, and answer this question: Does the PaCO$_2$ level show respiratory acidosis, alkalosis, or normalcy?

Step 4

Look at the bicarbonate (HCO$_3^-$) level, and answer this question: Does the HCO$_3^-$ level show metabolic acidosis, alkalosis, or normalcy?

Step 5

Look again at the pH level, and answer this question: Does the pH show a compensated or an uncompensated condition?

Steps for Interpretation of Blood Gas Levels

Step 1. Look at the PaO$_2$ level, and answer this question: Does the PaO$_2$ show hypoxemia? The PaO$_2$ is a measure of the partial pressure (P) of oxygen dissolved in arterial (a) blood plasma. Sometimes, PaO$_2$ is shortened to PO$_2$. It is reported in millimeters of mercury (mm Hg). The PaO$_2$ reflects 3% of total oxygen in the blood.[8,9]

The normal range of PaO$_2$ values for individuals breathing room air at sea level is 80 to 100 mm Hg. However, the normal range is age dependent for infants and for adults 60 years or older. The normal level for infants breathing room air is 50 to 70 mm Hg.[8] The normal level for adults 60 years or older decreases with age as changes occur in the ventilation/perfusion (V/Q) matching in the aging lung.[8,10] The correct PaO$_2$ for older adults can be ascertained as follows: 80 mm Hg (the lowest normal value) minus 1 mm Hg for every year of age more than 60 years. Using this formula, a 65-year-old individual can have a PaO$_2$ of 75 mm Hg (80 mm Hg − 5 mm Hg = 75 mm Hg) and still be within the normal range. An acceptable range for an 80-year-old person (20 years older than 60 years) is 60 mm Hg (80 mm Hg − 20 mm Hg = 60 mm Hg).

At any age, a PaO$_2$ lower than 40 mm Hg represents a life-threatening situation that necessitates immediate action.[8,9] A PaO$_2$ value less than the predicted lowest value indicates hypoxemia, which means that a lower-than-normal amount of oxygen is dissolved in plasma.[8,9]

The PaO$_2$ level is analyzed before the levels of other blood gas components. A PaO$_2$ of less than 40 mm Hg severely compromises tissue oxygenation and requires immediate administration of supplemental oxygen or mechanical ventilation or both. The test results for the PaO$_2$ level can be analyzed quickly. If the PaO$_2$ level is more than the lowest value for the patient's age, the PaO$_2$ is considered normal.

Step 2. Look at the pH level, and answer this question: Is the pH on the acid or alkaline side of 7.40? The pH is the hydrogen ion (H$^+$) concentration of plasma. Calculation of pH is accomplished by using the arterial partial pressure of carbon dioxide (PaCO$_2$) and the plasma bicarbonate level (HCO$_3^-$). The formula used is the Henderson-Hasselbalch equation.[8,9]

The normal pH of arterial blood is 7.35 to 7.45, and the mean is 7.40. If the pH level is less than 7.40, it is on the acid side of the mean. A pH level less than 7.35 is known as *acidemia*, and the overall condition is called *acidosis*. If the pH level is greater than 7.40, it is on the alkaline side of the mean. A pH level greater than 7.45 is known as *alkalemia*, and the overall condition is called *alkalosis*.[8,9]

Step 3. Look at the PaCO$_2$ level, and answer this question: Does the PaCO$_2$ show respiratory acidosis, alkalosis, or normalcy? The PaCO$_2$ is a measure of the partial pressure of carbon dioxide dissolved in arterial blood plasma, and it is reported in mm Hg. The PaCO$_2$ is the acid–base component that reflects the effectiveness of ventilation in relation to the metabolic rate.[8,9] In other words, the PaCO$_2$ value indicates whether the patient can ventilate well enough to rid the body of the carbon dioxide (CO$_2$) produced as a consequence of metabolism.

The normal range for PaCO$_2$ is 35 to 45 mm Hg. This range does not change as a person ages. A PaCO$_2$ value greater than 45 mm Hg defines *respiratory acidosis*, which is caused by alveolar hypoventilation. Hypoventilation can result from COPD, oversedation, head trauma, anesthesia, drug overdose, neuromuscular disease, or hypoventilation with mechanical ventilation.[9]

Ventilatory failure results when the PaCO$_2$ level exceeds 50 mm Hg. Acute ventilatory failure occurs when the PaCO$_2$ level is greater than 50 mm Hg and the pH level is less than 7.30. Ventilatory failure is referred to as *acute* because the pH is abnormal, not allowing enough time for the body to compensate by returning the pH to the normal range. Chronic ventilatory failure is defined as a PaCO$_2$ value greater than 50 mm Hg and a pH level greater than 7.30.[8]

A PaCO$_2$ value that is less than 35 mm Hg defines *respiratory alkalosis*, which is caused by alveolar hyperventilation. Hyperventilation can result from hypoxia, anxiety, pulmonary embolism, pregnancy, and hyperventilation with mechanical ventilation or as a compensatory mechanism for metabolic acidosis.[11]

Step 4. Look at the HCO$_3^-$ level, and answer this question: Does the HCO$_3^-$ show metabolic acidosis, alkalosis, or normalcy? Bicarbonate (HCO$_3^-$) is the acid–base component that reflects kidney function. The HCO$_3^-$ level is reduced or increased in the plasma by renal mechanisms. The normal range is 22 to 26 mEq/L.[9,11] An HCO$_3^-$ level of less than 22 mEq/L defines *metabolic acidosis*, which can result from ketoacidosis, lactic acidosis, renal failure, or diarrhea. The cumulative effect is a gain of acids or a loss of base. An HCO$_3^-$ level that is greater than 26 mEq/L defines *metabolic alkalosis*, which can result from fluid loss from the upper gastrointestinal tract (vomiting or nasogastric suction), diuretic therapy, severe hypokalemia, alkali administration, or steroid therapy.[9,11]

Step 5. Look again at the pH level, and answer this question: Does the pH show a compensated or an uncompensated condition? If the pH level is abnormal (less than 7.35 or greater than 7.45), the PaCO$_2$ value or the HCO$_3^-$ level, or both, will also be abnormal. This is an *uncompensated* condition because the body has not had enough time to return the pH to its normal range.[9,12] Box 13.3 provides two examples of uncompensated ABG values. If the pH level is within normal limits and the PaCO$_2$ value and the HCO$_3^-$ level are abnormal, the condition is *compensated* because the body has had enough time to restore the pH to within its normal range.[9,12]

BOX 13.3 Uncompensated Arterial Blood Gas Values

Example 1		Example 2	
PaO_2	90 mm Hg	PaO_2	90 mm Hg
pH	7.25	pH	7.25
$PaCO_2$	50 mm Hg	$PaCO_2$	40 mm Hg
HCO_3^-	22 mEq/L	HCO_3^-	17 mEq/L

Interpretation: Uncompensated respiratory acidosis

Interpretation: Uncompensated metabolic acidosis

BOX 13.4 Compensated Arterial Blood Gas Values

Example 1		Example 2	
PaO_2	90 mm Hg	PaO_2	90 mm Hg
pH	7.37	pH	7.42
$PaCO_2$	60 mm Hg	$PaCO_2$	48 mm Hg
HCO_3^-	38 mEq/L	HCO_3^-	35 mEq/L

Interpretation: Compensated respiratory acidosis with metabolic alkalosis. (Acidosis is considered the main disorder, and alkalosis is the compensatory response because the pH is on the acid side of 7.40.)

Interpretation: Compensated metabolic alkalosis with respiratory acidosis. (Alkalosis is considered the main disorder, and acidosis is the compensatory response because the pH is on the alkaline side of 7.40.)

Differentiating the primary disorder from the compensatory response can be difficult. The primary disorder is the abnormality that caused the pH level to shift initially and is determined according to the pH level; the primary disorder is considered the one on whichever side of 7.40 the pH level occurs.[11] Box 13.4 provides two examples of compensated ABG values. Partial compensation may be present and is evidenced by abnormal pH, $PaCO_2$, and HCO_3^- levels, indicating that the body is attempting to return the pH to its normal range.[11]

Table 13.3 summarizes the changes in the acid–base components that accompany various acid–base disorders.[11,12] In addition to the parameters previously discussed, other factors must be considered when reviewing a patient's ABG levels, including oxygen saturation, oxygen content, base excess and deficit, and anion gap analysis.

Oxygen Saturation

Oxygen saturation is a measure of the amount of oxygen bound to hemoglobin compared with the maximal capability of hemoglobin for binding oxygen. It can be assessed as a component of the ABGs (SaO_2) or can be measured noninvasively using a pulse oximeter (SpO_2).[8] Oxygen saturation is reported as a percentage or as a decimal; normal values are greater than 95% when the patient is on room air. Normally, the saturation level cannot reach 100% (on room air) because of physiologic shunting.[8] However, when supplemental oxygen is administered, oxygen saturation may approach 100% so closely that it is reported as 100%.

Proper evaluation of the oxygen saturation level is vital. For example, an SaO_2 of 97% means that 97% of the available hemoglobin is bound with oxygen. The word *available* is essential to evaluating the SaO_2 level, because the hemoglobin level is not always within normal limits, and oxygen can bind only with what is available. A 97% saturation level associated with 10 g/dL of hemoglobin does not deliver as much oxygen to the tissues as does a 97% saturation level associated with 15 g/dL of hemoglobin. Assessing only the SaO_2 level and finding it within normal limits does not ensure that the patient's oxygenation status is normal. The hemoglobin level must also be evaluated before a decision on oxygenation status can be made.[8,12]

Oxygen Content

Oxygen content (CaO_2) is a measure of the total amount of oxygen carried in the blood, including the amount dissolved in plasma (measured by the PaO_2) and the amount bound to the hemoglobin molecule (measured by the SaO_2). CaO_2 is reported in milliliters of

TABLE 13.3 Arterial Blood Gas Assessment

Disorder	pH	$PaCO_2$ (mm Hg)	HCO_3^- (mEq/L)
Respiratory Acidosis			
Uncompensated	<7.35	>45	22–26
Partially compensated	<7.35	>45	>26
Compensated	7.35–7.39	>45	>26
Respiratory Alkalosis			
Uncompensated	>7.45	<35	22–26
Partially compensated	>7.45	<35	<22
Compensated	7.41–7.45	<35	<22
Metabolic Acidosis			
Uncompensated	<7.35	35–45	<22
Partially compensated	<7.35	<35	<22
Compensated	7.35–7.39	<35	<22
Metabolic Alkalosis			
Uncompensated	>7.45	35–45	>26
Partially compensated	>7.45	>45	>26
Compensated	7.41–7.45	>45	>26
Combined (or mixed) respiratory and metabolic acidosis	<7.35	>45	<22
Combined (or mixed) respiratory and metabolic alkalosis	>7.45	<35	>26

HCO_3^-, Bicarbonate; $PaCO_2$, arterial partial pressure of carbon dioxide.

oxygen carried per 100 mL of blood. The normal value is 20 mL of oxygen per 100 mL of blood. To calculate the oxygen content, the PaO_2, the SaO_2, and the hemoglobin level are used (see Appendix B). A change in any one of these parameters affects the CaO_2.[8,12]

Base Excess and Base Deficit

Base excess and base deficit reflect the nonrespiratory contribution to acid–base balance and are reported in milliequivalents per liter (mEq/L) above or below the normal range of −2 mEq/L to +2 mEq/L. A negative base level is reported as a *base deficit*, which correlates with *metabolic acidosis*, whereas a positive base level is reported as a *base excess*, which correlates with *metabolic alkalosis*.[8,11,12]

Classic Shunt Equation and Oxygen Tension Indices

The efficiency of oxygenation can be assessed by measuring the degree of intrapulmonary shunting that occurs in a patient at any one time, using the classic shunt equation and oxygen tension indices. *Intrapulmonary shunting* (QS/QT [the portion of cardiac output not exchanging with alveolar blood divided by the total cardiac output]) refers to venous blood that flows to the lungs without being oxygenated because of nonfunctioning alveoli.[8] Other names for this condition include shunt effect, low V/Q, wasted blood flow, and venous admixture.[8,12]

Direct determination of intrapulmonary shunting requires the use of the classic shunt equation (see Appendix B), which is invasive and cumbersome. A shunt greater than 10% is considered abnormal and indicative of a shunt-producing disorder. A shunt greater than 30% is a serious and potentially life-threatening condition that requires pulmonary intervention.[8]

Often, intrapulmonary shunting is estimated by using the oxygen tension indices. One advantage to these methods is the ease of performance, although they have been found to be unreliable in critically ill patients.[8] An estimate of intrapulmonary shunting can be determined by computing the difference between the alveolar and arterial oxygen concentrations. Normally, alveolar (A) and arterial (a) PO_2 values are approximately equal. When they are not, it indicates that venous blood is passing malfunctioning alveoli and returning unoxygenated to the left side of the heart.[8] The most common oxygen tension indices used to estimate intrapulmonary shunting are the PaO_2/FiO_2 ratio, the PaO_2/PaO_2 ratio, and the A–a gradient ($P[A−a]O_2$).

PaO₂/FiO₂ Ratio

The PaO_2/FiO_2 ratio is clinically the easiest formula to calculate because this formula does not call for the computation of the alveolar PO_2. Normally, the PaO_2/FiO_2 ratio is greater than 286; the lower the value, the worse the lung function.[8,12]

PaO₂/PaO₂ Ratio

The PaO_2/PaO_2 ratio (arterial/alveolar oxygen ratio) is normally greater than 60%. The disadvantage to using this formula is that this formula calls for the computation of the alveolar PO_2 (see Appendix B), but the advantage is that this formula is unaffected by changes in the FiO_2, as long as the underlying lung condition is stable.[8,12]

Alveolar-Arterial Gradient

The A–a gradient ($P[A − a]O_2$) is normally less than 20 mm Hg on room air for patients younger than 61 years. This estimate of intrapulmonary shunting is the least reliable clinically, but it is used often in clinical decision making. A major disadvantage to using this formula is that it is greatly influenced by the amount of oxygen the patient is receiving.[8,12]

Serial determinations of the estimates of intrapulmonary shunting provide the practitioner with objective data on which to base clinical decisions.[8]

Dead Space Equation

The efficiency of ventilation can be measured using the clinical dead space (V_D/V_T) equation (see Appendix B). The formula measures the fraction of tidal volume not participating in gas exchange. A dead space value greater than 0.6 indicates a dead space–producing disorder and is considered abnormal. The major limitations to using this formula are that it requires the measurement of exhaled carbon dioxide to complete and that the work of breathing by patients must remain stable during the collection.[8,13]

Sputum Studies

Careful analysis of sputum specimens is crucial for rapid identification and treatment of pulmonary infections. The most difficult aspect of sputum examination is proper collection of the specimen. Collection of a good sputum sample requires a conscious, cooperative, and sufficiently hydrated patient.[14] When the patient has difficulty producing sputum, heated, nebulized saline may help loosen secretions for expectoration.[14] Chest physiotherapy combined with nebulization improves the success rate. Collection of a sputum specimen is best done in the morning, because a greater volume of secretions is present as a result of nighttime pooling. Brushing the teeth and rinsing the oropharyngeal airway are recommended to reduce contamination before collecting a sample.[9,14,15]

Many critically ill patients cannot cough effectively, and sputum collection by other means is required. These methods include tracheobronchial aspiration, transtracheal aspiration, and fiberoptic bronchoscopy with a protected brush catheter. Because each method has its own benefits and risks, the patient's clinical condition determines the appropriate technique.

Many critically ill patients have endotracheal or tracheostomy tubes already in place. Collecting sputum specimens from these patients requires special attention to technique (Box 13.5). Deep specimens are obtained to avoid collecting specimens that contain resident upper airway flora that may have migrated down the tube. Colonization of the lower airways with upper airway flora can occur within 48 hours of intubation.[14−16]

After a sputum specimen is obtained, the sputum is examined for volume, physical properties, mucopurulence, and color. Next, a microscopic examination is done to identify the source of the specimen. If a bacterial infection is suspected, a Gram stain is performed, followed by culture and sensitivity assessments.[14−16]

DIAGNOSTIC PROCEDURES

Table 13.4 presents an overview of the various diagnostic procedures used to evaluate the critically ill patient with pulmonary dysfunction.

Nursing Management

Nursing management of a patient undergoing a diagnostic procedure involves a variety of interventions. Priorities are directed toward (1) preparing the patient psychologically and physically for the procedure, (2) monitoring the patient's responses to the procedure, and (3) assessing the patient after the procedure. Preparing the patient includes teaching the patient about the procedure, answering any questions, and positioning the patient for the procedure. Monitoring the patient's responses to the procedure includes observing the patient for signs of pain, anxiety, or respiratory decompensation (Box 13.6)

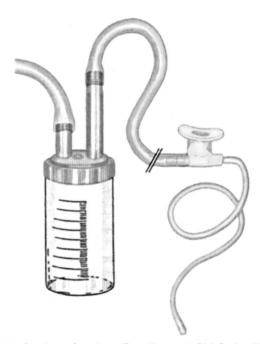

Fig. 13.4 Specimen Container. (From Kacmarek RM, Stoller JK, Heuer AJ, eds. *Egan's Fundamentals of Respiratory Care.* 12th ed. St. Louis: Elsevier; 2021.)

and monitoring vital signs, breath sounds, and oxygen saturation. Assessing the patient after the procedure includes observing for complications of the procedure and medicating the patient for any postprocedural discomfort. Any evidence of respiratory distress should be immediately reported to the physician, and emergency measure to maintain breathing must be initiated.

RESPIRATORY MONITORING

Capnography

Capnography is the measurement of exhaled carbon dioxide (CO_2) gas and is also known as *end-tidal CO_2* monitoring. Normally, alveolar and arterial carbon dioxide concentrations are equal in the presence of normal V/Q relationships. In a patient who is hemodynamically stable, the partial pressure of end-tidal CO_2 ($P_{ET}CO_2$) can be used to estimate the $PaCO_2$, with $P_{ET}CO_2$ levels 1 to 5 mm Hg less than $PaCO_2$ levels. The practitioner must determine first that a normal V/Q relationship exists before correlation of $P_{ET}CO_2$ and $PaCO_2$ can be assumed.[17] Causes of increased $P_{ET}CO_2$ include situations in which carbon dioxide production is increased, such as hyperthermia, sepsis, and seizures, or in which alveolar ventilation is decreased, such as respiratory depression. Causes of decreased $P_{ET}CO_2$ include situations in which carbon dioxide production is decreased, such as hypothermia, cardiac arrest, and pulmonary embolism, or in which alveolar ventilation is increased, such as hyperventilation.[17]

In the critical care area, continuous capnography is used for assessment and monitoring of the patient's ventilatory status in various situations, including weaning from mechanical ventilation and undergoing procedural sedation. Assessment of changes in physiologic dead space can be carried out with $P_{ET}CO_2$ monitoring, based on the degree of difference between $PaCO_2$ and $P_{ET}CO_2$. As the severity of pulmonary impairment increases, so does the disparity between $PaCO_2$ and $P_{ET}CO_2$, as indicated by an increased gradient. A gradient of greater than 5 mm Hg can be seen with underperfused alveolar-capillary units (dead space–producing situations) and nonperfused alveolar-capillary units (alveolar dead space). Increased dead space ventilation is a result of decreased pulmonary blood flow or cardiac output and lung disease. This leads to an abnormality in the transfer of carbon dioxide from the blood to the lung. The result is a $P_{ET}CO_2$ level that is lower than the $PaCO_2$ level because of the mixing of carbon dioxide between perfused and nonperfused units. The end result is an increased or widened $PaCO_2/P_{ET}CO_2$ gradient.[17]

The noninvasive measurement of $P_{ET}CO_2$ enables assessment of the adequacy of cardiopulmonary resuscitation and endotracheal tube placement. Decreased pulmonary blood flow is associated with lower $P_{ET}CO_2$ values, reflected clinically by decreased cardiac output, as in the case of cardiopulmonary resuscitation. During endotracheal intubation, a low $P_{ET}CO_2$ reading indicates that the tube is positioned in the stomach because the amount of carbon dioxide in the esophagus is expected to be low.[17]

There are three forms of capnography: mainstream, side-stream, and proximal diverting. All forms can be used in intubated patients, but side-stream and Microstream capnography can also be used in nonintubated patients, broadening the application of $P_{ET}CO_2$ monitoring. Mainstream capnography measures the carbon dioxide level directly by a sensor in the exhalation port of the ventilator tubing. During exhalation, gas passes over the sensor, and the information is transferred by an electrical cable to the display unit. The display unit produces a waveform, called a *capnogram* (Fig. 13.5), and a numeric recording ($P_{ET}CO_2$). Disadvantages to this form of capnography include the weight of the sensor on the ventilator tubing and possible obstruction of the sensor by secretions and condensation. In side-stream capnography, the carbon dioxide gas is continuously aspirated through a side port in the ventilator tubing or nasal cannula and is measured and analyzed by a side unit. Disadvantages to this form of capnography include obstruction of the sampling tube with secretions and slow response time. Proximal diverting capnography is a newer and improved version of side-stream capnography that transports gas a short distance from the airway to a site where the sensor is located, reducing the bulkiness at the airway.[17]

Capnography and $P_{ET}CO_2$ analysis have many diverse applications in the critical care area, but the practitioner must never assume that the $P_{ET}CO_2$ values reflect $PaCO_2$ values without waveform analysis. Any change in the waveform can indicate a change in the patient's pulmonary status and warrants further evaluation. Loss of the waveform may signal loss of effective respirations.[17]

TABLE 13.4 Pulmonary Diagnostic Studies

Study	Evaluation	Comments
Bronchography	Detect obstruction or malformation of the tracheobronchial tree.	Patient inspires radiopaque substance and then x-rays are taken. Inquire about possibility of pregnancy.
Chest x-ray	Detect pathologic lung condition (e.g., pneumonia, pulmonary edema, atelectasis, tuberculosis, etc.). Determine size and location of lung lesions and tumors. Verify placement of endotracheal tube, central venous catheters, and chest tubes.	Noninvasive test with minimal radiation exposure. Inquire about possibility of pregnancy. Posteroanterior (PA) and lateral films are done most commonly, but in critical care areas, anteroposterior (AP) portable films are frequently necessary because of inability to transport patient. Lateral decubitus films aid in identification of pleural effusion.
Exercise testing	Identify early disability. Differentiates between cardiac and pulmonary disease.	Monitor for changes in SpO_2 during exercise. Monitor closely for exercise-induced hypotension or ventricular dysrhythmias.
Laryngoscopy, bronchoscopy, mediastinoscopy	Obtain cytologic specimen or biopsy. Identify tumors, obstructions, secretions, or foreign bodies in tracheobronchial tree. Locate a bleeding site. May be used therapeutically to remove secretions, foreign bodies, and other contaminants.	Patient is sedated before the procedure, usually with a benzodiazepine (e.g., diazepam, midazolam). Monitor the patient for subcutaneous emphysema after study; indicates tracheal or bronchial tear. Monitor for hemoptysis; some blood in sputum is normal after biopsy, but frank hemoptysis requires immediate attention.
Lung biopsy Transthoracic needle lung biopsy Open lung biopsy	Obtain specimen for cytologic evaluation.	Transthoracic needle biopsy performed under fluoroscopy. Inquire about possibility of pregnancy. Open lung biopsy requires thoracotomy.
Magnetic resonance imaging (MRI)	Distinguishes tumors from other structures (e.g., tumor, pleural thickening, fibrosis).	Noninvasive test. Contraindicated for patients with pacemakers or implanted metallic devices.
Pulmonary angiography	Detects changes in lung tissue (e.g., masses). Diagnoses abnormalities in pulmonary vasculature including thrombi and emboli. Identifies congenital abnormalities of the circulation.	Invasive test. Inquire about possibility of pregnancy. Contrast media injected into pulmonary artery; ensure adequate hydration after study. Monitor arterial puncture point for hematoma or hemorrhage.
Pulmonary function studies • Spirometry • Ventilator mechanics • Flow-volume loop • Diffusing capacity	Measures lung volumes, capacities, and flow rates. Identifies features of restrictive or obstructive lung disease. Evaluates responsiveness to bronchodilator therapy. Aids in evaluation of surgical risk. Documents a disability or cause of dyspnea.	Noninvasive studies. Frequently repeated after bronchodilator therapy.
Sleep studies	Diagnose and differentiate between obstructive, central, and cardiac sleep apnea.	Restrict caffeine before testing. Usually done during normal sleep hours.
Thoracentesis (may include pleural biopsy)	Obtain pleural fluid and/or tissue specimen. May be used therapeutically to remove pleural fluid.	Monitor patient for indications of pneumothorax. Monitor for leakage from puncture point.
Thoracic computerized tomography (CT)	Defines lesions, masses, cavities, or shadows seen on normal chest x-rays. Evaluates tracheal or bronchial narrowing. Aids in planning radiation therapy.	X-rays are taken at different angles.
Ultrasonography	Evaluates pleural disease. Visualizes diaphragm and detects disease around diaphragm (e.g., subphrenic hematoma or abscess).	Noninvasive test.
Ventilation scan Lung perfusion scan Ventilation/perfusion scan	Diagnoses ventilation and/or perfusion abnormalities including emphysema and pulmonary emboli.	Invasive test: radioisotope inspired and injected intravascularly. Inquire about possibility of pregnancy. Nuclear scan study: assure patient that amount of radioactive material is minimal.

Modified from Dennison RD. *Pass CCRN!* 5th ed. St Louis: Elsevier; 2019.

Pulse Oximetry

Pulse oximetry is a noninvasive method for monitoring oxygen saturation (SpO_2) and is indicated in any situation in which the patient's oxygenation status requires continuous observation. A pulse oximeter consists of a microprocessor and a probe that attaches to the patient's forehead, finger, ear, toe, or nose. The probe consists of two light-emitting diodes and a photodetector. The diodes transmit red and infrared light wavelengths through the pulsating arterial vascular bed to the photodetector on the other side. The percentage of oxygen saturation is determined by the difference in absorbance of the red and infrared light caused by the difference in color between oxygen-bound (bright red) and oxygen-unbound (dark red) hemoglobin. The photodetector converts the light signals into an electric signal that is sent to the microprocessor, which converts the electric signal into a digital reading. The pulse oximeter is considered very accurate; readings vary less than 4% to 5% at a saturation level greater than 70%. However, several physiologic and technical factors limit the monitoring system.[17]

Physiologic limitations of pulse oximetry include elevated levels of abnormal hemoglobins, the presence of vascular dyes, and poor tissue perfusion. The pulse oximeter cannot differentiate between normal and abnormal hemoglobin. Elevated levels of abnormal hemoglobin falsely elevate the SpO_2. Vascular dyes such as methylene blue, indigo carmine, indocyanine green, and fluorescein interfere with pulse oximetry and can lead to falsely low readings. Poor tissue perfusion to the area with the probe leads to loss of pulsatile flow and signal failure.[17] In a critically ill patient, pulse oximetry is reliable only for monitoring the patient's oxygenation status. Pulse oximetry is an unreliable method for monitoring the patient's ventilatory status. The ability of a pulse oximeter to detect hypoventilation is accurate only when the patient is breathing room air. Because most critically ill patients require some form of oxygen therapy, pulse oximetry is an unreliable method of detecting hypercapnia and should *not* be used for this purpose.[17]

Technical limitations of pulse oximetry include bright lights, excessive motion, and incorrect placement of the probe. Bright lights may interfere with the photodetector and cause inaccurate results. The probe must be covered to limit optical interference. Excessive motion can mimic arterial pulsations and can lead to false readings. Incorrect placement of the probe can lead to inaccurate results because part of the light can reach the photodetector without having passed through blood (optical shunting). Interventions to limit these problems include using the proper probe in the appropriate spot (not using a finger probe on the ear), applying the probe according to the directions, and ensuring that the area being monitored has adequate perfusion.[17]

ADDITIONAL RESOURCES

See Box 13.7 for additional resources for the assessment and diagnosis of the patient with pulmonary dysfunction.

QSEN | **BOX 13.6** **Patient Safety**

Clinical Manifestations of Respiratory Decompensation

Inadequate Airway
Stridor
Noisy respirations
Supraclavicular and intercostal retractions
Flaring of nares
Labored breathing with use of accessory muscles

Inadequate Ventilation
Absence of air exchange at nose and mouth (breathlessness)
Minimal/absent chest wall motion
Manifestations of obstructed airway
Central cyanosis
Decreased or absent breath sounds (bilateral, unilateral)
Restlessness, anxiety, confusion
Paradoxical motion involving significant portion of chest wall
Decreased PaO_2, increased $PaCO_2$, decreased pH

Inadequate Gas Exchange
Tachypnea
Decreased PaO_2
Increased dead space
Central cyanosis
Chest infiltrates on radiographic evaluation

BOX 13.7 **Informatics** | **QSEN**

Internet Resources: Pulmonary Clinical Assessment and Diagnostic Procedures

- American Association of Critical-Care Nurses (AACN): www.aacn.org
- American Association of Respiratory Care (AARC): www.aarc.org
- American College of Chest Physicians (ACCP): www.chestnet.org/accp
- American College of Physicians (ACP): www.acponline.org
- American Lung Association: www.lung.org
- American Medical Association (AMA): www.ama-assn.org
- American Thoracic Society (ATS): www.thoracic.org
- Centers for Disease Control and Prevention (CDC): www.cdc.gov
- National Institutes for Health (NIH): www.nih.gov
- Office of Disease Prevention and Health Promotion: www.healthfinder.gov
- Respiratory Nursing Society and Interprofessional Collaborative (RNSIC): www.respiratorynursingsociety.org
- Society for Critical Care Medicine (SCCM): www.sccm.org

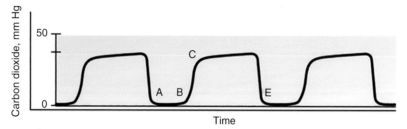

Fig. 13.5 Capnogram. Normal findings on a capnogram. *A* → *B*, indicates the baseline; *B* → *C*, the expiratory upstroke; *C* → *D*, the alveolar plateau; *D*, the partial pressure of end-tidal carbon dioxide; and *D* → *E*, the inspiratory downstroke. (From Frakes M. Measuring end-tidal carbon dioxide: clinical applications and usefulness. *Crit Care Nurse*. 2001;21[5]:23 ©2001 by the American Association of Critical-Care Nurses, All rights reserved, and Used with permission.)

REFERENCES

1. Simpson H. Respiratory assessment. *Br J Nurs.* 2006;15(9):484–488.
2. Kallet RH. Bedside assessment of the patient. In: Kacmarek RM, Stoller JK, Heuer AJ, eds. *Egan's Fundamentals of Respiratory Care.* 12th ed. St. Louis: Elsevier; 2021.
3. Reinke LF. Respiratory assessment. In: Geiger-Bronksy M, Wilson DJ, eds. *Respiratory Nursing: A Core Curriculum.* New York: Springer; 2008.
4. Smith J, Rushton M. How to perform respiratory assessment. *Nurs Stand.* 2015;30(7):34–36.
5. Fajardo E, Davis JL. History and physical examination. In: Broaddus VC, ed. *Murray and Nadel's Textbook of Respiratory Medicine.* 7th ed. Philadelphia: Elsevier; 2022.
6. Ball JW, Dains JE, Flynn JA, et al. *Seidel's Guide to Physical Examination: An Interprofessional Approach.* 9th ed. St. Louis: Elsevier; 2019.
7. Bohadana A, Izbicki G, Kraman SS. Fundamentals of lung auscultation. *N Engl J Med.* 2014;370(8):744–751.
8. Cohen Z. Gas exchange and transport. In: Kacmarek RM, Stoller JK, Heuer AJ, eds. *Egan's Fundamentals of Respiratory Care.* 12th ed. St. Louis: Elsevier; 2021.
9. Chernecky C, Berger B. *Laboratory Tests and Diagnostic Procedures.* 6th ed. St. Louis: Elsevier; 2013.
10. Yeager JJ. Laboratory and diagnostic tests. In: Meiner SE, Yeager JJ, eds. *Gerontology Nursing.* 6th ed. St. Louis: Elsevier; 2019.
11. Beachey W. Acid base balance. In: Kacmarek RM, Stoller JK, Heuer AJ, eds. *Egan's Fundamentals of Respiratory Care.* 12th ed. St. Louis: Elsevier; 2021.
12. Wettstein R, Scanlan CL. Interpretation of blood gases. In: Heuer AJ, Scanlon CL, eds. *Wilkin's Clinical Assessment in Respiratory Care.* 8th ed. St. Louis: Elsevier; 2018.
13. Mireles-Cabodevila E. Ventilation. In: Kacmarek RM, Stoller JK, Heuer AJ, eds. *Egan's Fundamentals of Respiratory Care.* 12th ed. St. Louis: Elsevier; 2021.
14. Fisher DF. Solutions, body fluids and electrolytes. In: Kacmarek RM, Stoller JK, Heuer AJ, eds. *Egan's Fundamentals of Respiratory Care.* 12th ed. St. Louis: Elsevier; 2021.
15. American Association for Clinical Chemistry. *Lab Tests Online: Bacterial Sputum Culture*; 2021. https://labtestsonline.org/understanding/analytes/sputum-culture/tab/sample/#.Vg1PEsfMrak.gmail.
16. Kallet R. Interpreting clinical and laboratory data. In: Kacmarek RM, Stoller JK, Heuer AJ, eds. *Egan's Fundamentals of Respiratory Care.* 12th ed. St. Louis: Elsevier; 2021.
17. Siegel BK, Heuer AJ, Kallet RH. Analysis and monitoring of gas exchange. In: Kacmarek RM, Stoller JK, Heuer AJ, eds. *Egan's Fundamentals of Respiratory Care.* 12th ed. St. Louis: Elsevier; 2021.

14

Pulmonary Disorders

Kathleen M. Stacy

ACUTE LUNG FAILURE

Description and Etiology

Acute lung failure (ALF),[1] also known as acute respiratory failure, is a clinical condition in which the pulmonary system fails to maintain adequate gas exchange.[1,2] It is the most common type of organ failure seen in the critical care unit, with approximately 56% of the patients in the critical care unit experiencing it.[1] One-third of patients with ALF requiring mechanical ventilation die in the hospital.[3]

ALF results from a deficiency in the performance of the pulmonary system.[2,4] It usually occurs secondary to another disorder that has altered the normal function of the pulmonary system in such a way as to decrease the ventilatory drive, decrease muscle strength, decrease chest wall elasticity, decrease the lung's capacity for gas exchange, increase airway resistance, or increase metabolic oxygen requirements.[1,5]

ALF can be classified as hypoxemic normocapnic respiratory failure (type I) or hypoxemic hypercapnic respiratory failure (type II), depending on analysis of the patient's arterial blood gases (ABGs). In type I respiratory failure, the patient presents with a low arterial oxygen pressure (PaO_2) and a normal arterial carbon dioxide pressure ($PaCO_2$); in type II respiratory failure, the patient presents with a low PaO_2 and a high $PaCO_2$.[2,4]

The causes of ALF may be classified as *extrapulmonary* or *intrapulmonary*, depending on the origin of the patient's primary disorder. Extrapulmonary causes include disorders that affect the brain, the spinal cord, the neuromuscular system, the thorax, the pleura, and the upper airways. Intrapulmonary causes include disorders that affect the lower airways and alveoli, the pulmonary circulation, and the alveolar-capillary membrane.[1,6] Table 14.1 lists the different etiologies of ALF and their associated disorders.

Pathophysiology

Hypoxemia is the result of impaired gas exchange and is the hallmark of ALF. Hypercapnia may be present, depending on the underlying cause of the problem. The main causes of hypoxemia are alveolar hypoventilation, ventilation/perfusion (V/Q) mismatching, and intrapulmonary shunting.[1,2,7] Type I respiratory failure usually results from V/Q mismatching and intrapulmonary shunting, whereas type II respiratory failure usually results from alveolar hypoventilation, which may or may not be accompanied by V/Q mismatching and intrapulmonary shunting.[2]

Alveolar Hypoventilation

Alveolar hypoventilation occurs when the amount of oxygen being brought into the alveoli is insufficient to meet the metabolic needs of the body.[6] This can be the result of increasing metabolic oxygen needs or decreasing ventilation.[5] Hypoxemia caused by alveolar hypoventilation is associated with hypercapnia and commonly results from extrapulmonary disorders.[1,2,7]

Ventilation/Perfusion Mismatching

V/Q mismatching occurs when ventilation and blood flow are mismatched in various regions of the lung in excess of what is normal. Blood passes through alveoli that are underventilated for the given amount of perfusion, leaving these areas with a lower than normal amount of oxygen. V/Q mismatching is the most common cause of hypoxemia and is usually the result of alveoli that are partially collapsed or partially filled with fluid.[1,2,7]

Intrapulmonary Shunting

Intrapulmonary shunting, the extreme form of V/Q mismatching, occurs when blood reaches the arterial system without participating in gas exchange. The mixing of unoxygenated (shunted) blood and oxygenated blood lowers the average level of oxygen present in the blood. Intrapulmonary shunting occurs when blood passes through a portion of a lung that is not ventilated. This may be the result of (1) alveolar collapse secondary to atelectasis or (2) alveolar flooding with pus, blood, or fluid.[1,2,7]

If allowed to progress, hypoxemia can result in a deficit of oxygen at the cellular level. As the tissue demands for oxygen continue and the supply diminishes, an oxygen supply/demand imbalance occurs, and tissue hypoxia develops. Decreased oxygen to the cells contributes to impaired tissue perfusion and the development of lactic acidosis and multiple-organ dysfunction syndrome.[8]

Assessment and Diagnosis

A patient with ALF may experience a variety of clinical manifestations, depending on the underlying cause and the extent of tissue hypoxia. The clinical manifestations commonly seen in patients with ALF are usually related to the development of hypoxemia, hypercapnia, and acidosis.[9] Because the clinical symptoms are so varied, they are not considered reliable in predicting the degree of hypoxemia or hypercapnia or the severity of ALF.[5]

Diagnosing and following the course of respiratory failure is best accomplished by ABG analysis. ABG analysis confirms the level of $PaCO_2$, PaO_2, and blood pH. ALF is generally accepted as being present when the PaO_2 is less than 60 mm Hg. If the patient is also experiencing hypercapnia, the $PaCO_2$ will be greater than 45 mm Hg. In patients with chronically elevated $PaCO_2$ levels, these criteria must be broadened to include a pH less than 7.35.[9]

Various additional tests are performed depending on the patient's underlying condition. These include bronchoscopy for airway surveillance or specimen retrieval, chest radiography, thoracic ultrasound,

TABLE 14.1 Etiologies of Acute Lung Failure.

Affected Area	Disorders[a]
Extrapulmonary	
Brain	Oversedation
	Central alveolar hypoventilation syndrome
	Brain trauma or lesion
	Postoperative general anesthesia depression
Spinal cord	Guillain-Barré syndrome
	Poliomyelitis
	Amyotrophic lateral sclerosis
	Spinal cord trauma or lesion
Neuromuscular system	Myasthenia gravis
	Multiple sclerosis
	Neuromuscular blocking agents
	Organophosphate poisoning
	Muscular dystrophy
	Critical illness polyneuropathy
Thorax	Massive obesity
	Chest trauma
Pleura	Pleural effusion
	Pneumothorax
	Malignancy
Upper airways	Sleep apnea
	Tracheal obstruction
	Epiglottitis
	Vocal cord paralysis
Intrapulmonary	
Lower airways and alveoli	Chronic obstructive pulmonary disease
	Asthma
	Bronchiolitis
	Cystic fibrosis
	Pneumonia
Pulmonary circulation	Pulmonary emboli
Alveolar-capillary membrane	Acute respiratory distress syndrome
	Inhalation of toxic gases
	Near-drowning

[a]Not an exhaustive list.

thoracic computed tomography (CT), and selected lung function studies.[10]

Medical Management

Medical management of a patient with ALF is aimed at treating the underlying cause, promoting adequate gas exchange, correcting acidosis, initiating nutrition support, and preventing complications. Medical interventions to promote gas exchange are aimed at improving oxygenation and ventilation.[1]

Oxygenation

Actions to improve oxygenation include supplemental oxygen administration, with either a low-flow system or a high-flow system, and the use of positive pressure ventilation.[7,11,12] The purpose of oxygen therapy is to correct hypoxemia; although the absolute level of hypoxemia varies in each patient, most treatment approaches aim to keep the arterial hemoglobin oxygen saturation greater than 90%.[5] The goal is to keep the tissues' needs satisfied but not produce hypoxemia or hyperoxemia.[11] Supplemental oxygen administration is effective in treating hypoxemia related to alveolar hypoventilation and V/Q mismatching. When intrapulmonary shunting exists, supplemental oxygen alone is ineffective. In this situation, positive pressure is necessary to open collapsed or fluid-filled alveoli and facilitate their participation in gas exchange. Positive pressure is delivered via invasive and noninvasive mechanical ventilation. To avoid intubation, positive pressure is usually administered initially noninvasively via a mask.[13] A recent study comparing low-flow oxygen, high-flow oxygen, and noninvasive ventilation found that high-flow oxygen therapy and noninvasive ventilation were superior to low-flow oxygen therapy in the treatment of hypoxemia. The study also found that high-flow oxygen therapy is better tolerated and more comfortable than noninvasive ventilation.[12] For further information on supplemental oxygen therapy and noninvasive ventilation, see Chapter 15.

Ventilation

Interventions to improve ventilation include the use of noninvasive and invasive mechanical ventilation. Depending on the underlying cause and the severity of the ALF, the patient may be treated initially with noninvasive ventilation.[13] Current guidelines recommend that patients with hypercapnic respiratory failure be given a trial on noninvasive ventilation unless the patient is rapidly deteriorating.[14] The selection of ventilatory mode and settings depends on the patient's underlying condition, severity of respiratory failure, and body size. Initially, the patient is started on volume ventilation in the assist/control mode. In a patient with chronic hypercapnia, the settings are adjusted to keep the ABG values within the parameters expected to be maintained by the patient after extubation.[15] For further information on mechanical ventilation, see Chapter 15.

Pharmacology

Medications to facilitate dilation of the airways may also be beneficial in the treatment of ALF. Bronchodilators, such as beta-2 agonists and anticholinergic agents, aid in smooth muscle relaxation and are of particular benefit to patients with airflow limitations. Methylxanthines, such as aminophylline, are no longer recommended because of their negative side effects. Steroids also are often administered to decrease airway inflammation and enhance the effects of the beta-2 agonists. Mucolytics and expectorants are also no longer used because they have been found to be of no benefit in this patient population.[16]

Sedation is necessary in many patients to assist with maintaining adequate ventilation. Sedation can be used to comfort the patient and decrease the work of breathing, particularly if the patient is fighting the ventilator. Analgesics are administered for pain control.[17,18] In some patients, sedation does not decrease spontaneous respiratory efforts enough to allow adequate ventilation. Neuromuscular paralysis may be necessary to facilitate optimal ventilation. Paralysis also may be necessary to decrease oxygen consumption in severely compromised patients.[18]

Acidosis

Acidosis may occur in a patient for many reasons. Hypoxemia causes impaired tissue perfusion, which leads to the production of lactic acid and the development of metabolic acidosis. Impaired ventilation leads to the accumulation of carbon dioxide and the development of respiratory acidosis. Once the patient is adequately oxygenated and ventilated, the acidosis should correct itself. The use of sodium bicarbonate to correct metabolic acidosis has been shown to be of minimal benefit to the patient and is no longer recommended as first-line treatment.

Bicarbonate therapy shifts the oxygen-hemoglobin dissociation curve to the left and can worsen tissue hypoxia. Sodium bicarbonate may be used if metabolic acidosis is severe (pH less than 7.2), refractory to therapy, and causing dysrhythmias or hemodynamic instability.[19]

Nutrition Support

The initiation of nutrition support is of utmost importance in the management of a patient with ALF. The goals of nutrition support are to meet the overall nutrition needs of the patient while avoiding overfeeding, to prevent nutrition delivery—related complications, and to improve patient outcomes.[20] Failure to provide the patient with adequate nutrition support leads to the development of malnutrition. Both malnutrition and overfeeding can interfere with the performance of the pulmonary system, further perpetuating ALF. Malnutrition decreases the patient's ventilatory drive and muscle strength, whereas overfeeding increases carbon dioxide production, which increases the patient's ventilatory demand, resulting in respiratory muscle fatigue.[21]

The enteral route is the preferred method of nutrition administration. If the patient cannot tolerate enteral feedings or cannot receive enough nutrients enterally, he or she will be started on parenteral nutrition. Because the parenteral route is associated with a higher rate of complications, the goal is to switch to enteral feedings as soon as the patient can tolerate them.[20,21] Nutrition support is initiated before the third day of mechanical ventilation for well-nourished patients and within 24 hours for malnourished patients.[20,21]

Complications

Patients with ALF may experience many complications, including ischemic-anoxic encephalopathy, cardiac dysrhythmias, venous thromboembolism (VTE), and stress ulcers.[22-25] Ischemic-anoxic encephalopathy results from hypoxemia, hypercapnia, and acidosis.[22] Dysrhythmias are precipitated by hypoxemia, acidosis, electrolyte imbalances, and the administration of beta-2 agonists.[23] Maintaining oxygenation, normalizing electrolytes, and monitoring medication levels facilitate the prevention and treatment of encephalopathy and dysrhythmias.[22,23] VTE is precipitated by venous stasis resulting from immobility and can be prevented through the use of intermittent pneumatic compression devices and low-dose unfractionated heparin or low—molecular-weight heparin (LMWH).[24] Stress ulcers can be prevented through the use of histamine receptor antagonists and proton pump inhibitors. However, the use of stress ulcer prophylaxis has been associated with an increased risk of ventilator-associated pneumonia (VAP).[25] In addition, the patient is at risk for the complications associated with the artificial airway, mechanical ventilation, enteral and parenteral nutrition, and vascular access devices.

Nursing Management

The patient care management plan for a patient with ALF incorporates a variety of patient problems (Box 14.1). Nursing actions are driven by the specific cause of the respiratory failure, although there are some common interventions that are appropriate for all patients with ALF. Nursing priorities focus on (1) optimizing oxygenation and ventilation, (2) providing comfort and emotional support, (3) maintaining surveillance for complications, and (4) educating the patient and family.

Optimizing Oxygenation and Ventilation

Nursing interventions to optimize oxygenation and ventilation include positioning, preventing desaturation, and promoting secretion clearance.

> ⊚ **BOX 14.1   PRIORITY PATIENT CARE MANAGEMENT**
>
> **Acute Lung Failure**
> - Impaired Gas Exchange due to alveolar hypoventilation
> - Impaired Gas Exchange due to ventilation-perfusion mismatching or intrapulmonary shunting
> - Impaired Breathing due to musculoskeletal fatigue or neuromuscular impairment
> - Anxiety due to threat to biologic, psychologic, social integrity
> - Lack of Knowledge of Treatment Regime due to lack of previous exposure to information (see Box 14.2, Priority Patient and Family Education: Acute Lung Failure)
>
> Patient Care Management Plans are located in Appendix A.

Positioning. Positioning of a patient with ALF depends on the type of lung injury and the underlying cause of hypoxemia. For patients with V/Q mismatching, positioning is used to facilitate better matching of ventilation with perfusion to optimize gas exchange.[26] Because gravity normally facilitates preferential ventilation and perfusion to the dependent areas of the lungs, the best gas exchange would take place in the dependent areas of the lungs.[26] Thus the goal of positioning is to place the least affected area of the patient's lung in the most dependent position. Patients with unilateral lung disease are positioned with the healthy lung in a dependent position.[26,27] Patients with diffuse lung disease may benefit from being positioned with the right lung down, because it is larger and more vascular than the left lung.[27,28] For patients with alveolar hypoventilation, the goal of positioning is to facilitate ventilation. These patients benefit from nonrecumbent positions such as sitting or a semierect position.[29] Elevating the head of the bed 30 to 45 degrees has also been shown to decrease the risk of aspiration; however, it also has been shown to increase the risk of pressure injuries.[30] Frequent repositioning (at least every 2 hours) is beneficial in optimizing the patient's ventilatory pattern and V/Q matching.[31]

Preventing desaturation. Numerous activities can prevent desaturation from occurring, including performing procedures only as needed, hyperoxygenating the patient before suctioning, providing adequate rest and recovery time between procedures, and minimizing oxygen consumption. Interventions to minimize oxygen consumption include limiting the patient's physical activity, administering sedation to control anxiety, and providing measures to control fever.[29] The patient is continuously monitored with a pulse oximeter to warn of signs of desaturation.

Promoting secretion clearance. Interventions to promote secretion clearance include providing adequate systemic hydration, humidifying supplemental oxygen, coughing, and suctioning. Postural drainage and chest percussion and vibration have been found to be of little benefit in critically ill patients and are not discussed here.[32,33]

To facilitate deep breathing, the patient's thorax is maintained in alignment, and the head of the bed is elevated 30 to 45 degrees. This position best accommodates diaphragmatic descent and intercostal muscle action.

Deep breathing and incentive spirometry are started as soon as possible after the patient is extubated. Deep breathing involves having the patient take a deep breath and holding it for approximately 3 seconds or longer. Incentive spirometry involves having the patient take at least 10 deep, effective breaths per hour using an incentive spirometer. These actions help prevent atelectasis and re-expand any collapsed lung tissue. The chest is auscultated during inflation to

BOX 14.2 PRIORITY PATIENT AND FAMILY EDUCATION

Acute Lung Failure

Before discharge, the patient should be able to teach back the following topics:

- Pathophysiology of disease
- Specific etiology
- Modification of precipitating factors
- Importance of taking medications
- Breathing techniques (e.g., pursed-lip breathing, diaphragmatic breathing)
- Energy conservation techniques
- Measures to prevent pulmonary infections (e.g., proper nutrition, hand-washing, immunization against *Streptococcus pneumoniae* and influenza viruses)
- Signs and symptoms of pulmonary infections (e.g., sputum color change, shortness of breath, fever)
- Cough enhancement techniques (e.g., cascade cough, huff cough, end-expiratory cough, augmented cough)

ensure that all dependent parts of the lung are well ventilated and to help the patient understand the depth of breath necessary for optimal effect. Coughing is avoided unless secretions are present because it promotes collapse of the smaller airways.

Educating the Patient and Family

Early in the patient's hospital stay, the patient and family are taught about ALF, its causes, and its treatment. Closer to discharge, patient and family education focuses on the interventions necessary for preventing the reoccurrence of the precipitating disorder (Box 14.2). If the patient smokes, he or she is encouraged to stop smoking and is referred to a smoking cessation program (Box 14.3). In addition, the importance of participating in a pulmonary rehabilitation program is stressed.

Interprofessional collaborative management of a patient with ALF is outlined in Box 14.4.

ACUTE RESPIRATORY DISTRESS SYNDROME

Description and Etiology

Acute respiratory distress syndrome (ARDS) is a systemic process that is considered to be the pulmonary manifestation of multiple-organ dysfunction syndrome.[34] It is characterized by noncardiac pulmonary edema and disruption of the alveolar-capillary membrane as a result of injury to either the pulmonary vasculature or the airways.[35] ARDS results in 75,000 patient deaths annually.[36]

Many different diagnostic criteria have been used to identify ARDS, which has led to confusion, particularly among researchers. In 2012, in an attempt to address the limitations of the existing definition of ARDS, the ARDS Definition Task Force drafted a new definition (known as the *Berlin Definition*) of ARDS.[37] This definition eliminated

BOX 14.3 Evidence-Based Practice

Smoking Cessation Guidelines

The following are the key recommendations of the updated guideline *Treating Tobacco Use and Dependence*, based on the literature review and expert panel opinion:

- Tobacco dependence is a chronic disease that often requires repeated intervention and multiple attempts to quit. Effective treatments exist, however, that can significantly increase rates of long-term abstinence.
- It is essential that clinicians and health care delivery systems consistently identify and document tobacco use status and treat every tobacco user seen in a health care setting.
- Tobacco dependence treatments are effective across a broad range of populations. Clinicians should encourage every patient willing to make a quit attempt to use the counseling treatments and medications recommended in this guideline.
- Brief tobacco dependence treatment is effective. Clinicians should offer every patient who uses tobacco at least the brief treatments shown to be effective in this guideline.
- Individual, group, and telephone counseling are effective, and their effectiveness increases with treatment intensity. Two components of counseling are especially effective, and clinicians should use these when counseling patients making a quit attempt:
  - Practical counseling (problem solving/skills training)
  - Social support delivered as part of treatment
- Numerous effective medications are available for tobacco dependence, and clinicians should encourage their use by all patients attempting to quit smoking, except when medically contraindicated or with specific populations for which there is insufficient evidence of effectiveness (e.g., pregnant women, smokeless tobacco users, light smokers, and adolescents).

- Seven first-line medications (five nicotine and two nonnicotine) reliably increase long-term smoking abstinence rates:
  - Bupropion SR
  - Nicotine gum
  - Nicotine inhaler
  - Nicotine lozenge
  - Nicotine nasal spray
  - Nicotine patch
  - Varenicline
- Clinicians also should consider the use of certain combinations of medications identified as effective in this guideline.
- Counseling and medication are effective when used by themselves for treating tobacco dependence. The combination of counseling and medication, however, is more effective than either alone. Thus clinicians should encourage all individuals making a quit attempt to use both counseling and medication.
- Telephone quitline counseling is effective with diverse populations and has broad reach. Therefore clinicians and health care delivery systems should both ensure patient access to quitlines and promote quitline use.
- If a tobacco user currently is unwilling to make a quit attempt, clinicians should use the motivational treatments shown in this guideline to be effective in increasing future quit attempts.
- Tobacco dependence treatments are both clinically effective and highly cost-effective relative to interventions for other clinical disorders. Providing coverage for these treatments increases quit rates. Insurers and purchasers should ensure that all insurance plans include the counseling and medication identified as effective in this guideline as covered benefits.

From Tobacco Use and Dependence Guideline Panel. Treating Tobacco Use and Dependence: 2008 Update. *Health and Human Services Website.* 2008. https://www.ahrq.gov/sites/default/files/wysiwyg/professionals/clinicians-providers/guidelines-recommendations/tobacco/clinicians/update/treating_tobacco_use08.pdf.

BOX 14.4 Collaborative Management of Acute Lung Failure

- Identify and treat underlying cause.
- Administer oxygen therapy.
- Intubate patient.
- Initiate mechanical ventilation.
- Administer medications:
  - Bronchodilators
  - Steroids
  - Sedatives
  - Analgesics
- Position patient to optimize ventilation/perfusion matching.
- Suction as needed.
- Provide adequate rest and recovery time between procedures.
- Correct acidosis.
- Initiate nutrition support.
- Maintain surveillance for complications:
  - Encephalopathy
  - Cardiac dysrhythmias
  - Venous thromboembolism
  - Gastrointestinal bleeding
- Provide comfort and emotional support.

BOX 14.5 Risk Factors for Acute Respiratory Distress Syndrome

Direct Injury	Indirect Injury
Aspiration	Sepsis
Near-drowning	Nonthoracic trauma
Toxic inhalation	Hypertransfusion
Pulmonary contusion	Cardiopulmonary bypass
Pneumonia	Severe pancreatitis
Oxygen toxicity	Embolism—air, fat, amniotic fluid
Transthoracic radiation	Disseminated intravascular coagulation
	Shock states

Modified from American Association of Critical-Care Nurses: AACN Practice Alert: Prevention of aspiration in adults. *Crit Care Nurse.* 2016;38(1): e20—e24 (updated 2018). ©2016 by the American Association of Critical-Care Nurses," "All rights reserved," and "Used with permission.

the term "acute lung injury" and proposed three distinct categories (mild, moderate, and severe) of ARDS based on the severity of hypoxemia. The Berlin Definition of ARDS is as follows:

- Timing: Within 1 week of known clinical insult or new or worsening respiratory symptoms
- Chest imaging: Bilateral opacities not fully explained by effusions, lobar/lung collapse, or nodules
- Origin of edema: Respiratory failure not fully explained by heart failure or fluid overload; objective assessment needed to exclude hydrostatic edema if no risk factor present
- Oxygenation: Mild (200 mm Hg less than PaO_2/fraction of inspired oxygen [FiO_2] less than or equal to 300 mm Hg with positive end-expiratory airway pressure [PEEP] or continuous positive airway pressure [CPAP] greater than or equal to 5 cm H_2O); moderate (100 mm Hg less than PaO_2/FiO_2 less than or equal to 200 mm Hg with PEEP greater than or equal to 5 cm H_2O); or severe (PaO_2/FiO_2 less than or equal to 100 mm Hg with PEEP greater than or equal to 5 cm H_2O).[37]

A wide variety of clinical conditions is associated with the development of ARDS. These are categorized as *direct* or *indirect*, depending on the primary site of injury (Box 14.5).[35,38] Direct injuries are injuries in which the lung epithelium sustains a direct insult. The SARS-CoV-2 virus is an example of a virus causing direct injury to the lung epithelium (Box 14.6). Indirect injuries are injuries in which the insult occurs elsewhere in the body and mediators are transmitted via the bloodstream to the lungs. Sepsis, aspiration of gastric contents, diffuse pneumonia, and trauma were found to be major risk factors for the development of ARDS.[36]

Pathophysiology

The progression of ARDS can be described in three phases: exudative, fibroproliferative, and resolution. ARDS is initiated with stimulation of the inflammatory-immune system as a result of a direct or indirect injury (Fig. 14.1). Inflammatory mediators are released from the site of injury, resulting in the activation and accumulation of the neutrophils, macrophages, and platelets in the pulmonary capillaries. These cellular mediators initiate the release of humoral mediators that cause damage to the alveolar-capillary membrane.[38]

Exudative Phase

Within the first 72 hours after the initial insult, the exudative phase or acute phase ensues. Once released, the mediators cause injury to the pulmonary capillaries, resulting in increased capillary membrane permeability leading to the leakage of fluid filled with protein, blood cells, fibrin, and activated cellular and humoral mediators into the pulmonary interstitium. Damage to the pulmonary capillaries also causes the development of microthrombi and elevation of pulmonary artery pressures. As fluid enters the pulmonary interstitium, the lymphatics are overwhelmed and unable to drain all the accumulating fluid, resulting in the development of interstitial edema. Fluid is then forced from the interstitial space into the alveoli, resulting in alveolar edema. Pulmonary interstitial edema also causes compression of the alveoli and small airways. Alveolar edema causes swelling of the type I alveolar epithelial cells and flooding of the alveoli. Protein and fibrin in the edema fluid precipitate the formation of hyaline membranes over the alveoli. Eventually, the type II alveolar epithelial cells are also damaged, leading to impaired surfactant production. Injury to the alveolar epithelial cells and the loss of surfactant lead to further alveolar collapse.[38,39]

Hypoxemia occurs as a result of intrapulmonary shunting and V/Q mismatching secondary to compression, collapse, and flooding of the alveoli and small airways. Increased work of breathing occurs as a result of increased airway resistance, decreased functional residual capacity (FRC), and decreased lung compliance secondary to atelectasis and compression of the small airways. Hypoxemia and the increased work of breathing lead to patient fatigue and the development of alveolar hypoventilation. Pulmonary hypertension occurs as a result of damage to the pulmonary capillaries, microthrombi, and hypoxic vasoconstriction leading to the development of increased alveolar dead space and right ventricular afterload. Hypoxemia worsens as a result of alveolar hypoventilation and increased alveolar dead space. Right ventricular afterload increases and leads to right ventricular dysfunction and a decrease in cardiac output (CO).[38]

Fibroproliferative Phase

The fibroproliferative phase begins as disordered healing and starts in the lungs. Cellular granulation and collagen deposition occur within

BOX 14.6 Coronaviruses and COVID-19

Coronaviruses

The global COVID-19 pandemic has focused the world's attention on viral infectious disease transmission and mortality risk. According to the Centers for Disease Control and Prevention, there are seven known types of infectious coronavirus.[1]

Four coronavirus types cause mild upper respiratory infections similar to the common cold and do not pose a serious health risk:[1]

- Alpha coronaviruses 229E and NK63
- Beta coronaviruses OC43 and HKU1

Three coronaviruses are known to be highly infectious for humans and associated with high mortality. Coronaviruses are present in both animals and humans, and the following three have evolved to infect humans:[1]

- MERS-CoV: a beta coronavirus that causes Middle East Respiratory Syndrome (MERS)
- SARS-CoV: a beta coronavirus that causes severe acute respiratory syndrome (SARS)
- SARS-CoV-2: a novel coronavirus that causes coronavirus disease 2019 (COVID-19).

The mortality for SARS is reported at 9.5%.[2] The mortality for MERS is much higher and is reported as 34%.[2] The absolute mortality rate for COVID-19 is still uncertain as the pandemic continues. What is known is that COVID-19 extracts a higher mortality on older adults and on those with underlying medical conditions or comorbidities. In addition, COVID-19 is more easily transmitted from person to person than either SARS or MERS.[2]

COVID-19 Clinical Features

The clinical features associated with COVID-19 are highly variable. Some individuals may contract the virus and be asymptomatic. Others may have a high temperature, cough, dyspnea, muscle aches, and extreme fatigue but can recover at home. Other individuals are so severely affected that they are admitted to a hospital or to a critical care unit.

Patients with severe COVID-19 admitted to a critical care unit often have respiratory distress and low oxygen saturation that requires high-flow oxygen, or intubation and mechanical ventilation. COVID-19 can also impair the neurologic, cardiovascular, and gastrointestinal systems.

COVID-19 Clinical Management

The clinical management of COVID-19 is highly dependent on the specific manifestations of the infection. Critical care management is individualized to signs and symptoms, and treatments evolve as new medications with proven effectiveness are approved. Examples for severe COVID-19 are use of the antiviral medication remdesivir[3] and the corticosteroid dexamethasone.[4] Many other medications are undergoing clinical trials.

COVID-19 Environmental Management

Because COVID-19 is highly transmissible, it poses unique risks for health care workers caring for patients who are positive for COVID-19. Optimal use of personal protective equipment (PPE) continues to evolve as more is learned about the virus. Environmental protection can include a negative-flow pressure room (if available) and limiting family visitors to decrease transmission. Depending on the situation, health care personnel may use N95 masks, eye goggles/face-shields, disposable protective gowns, gloves, head-covering hats, and shoe covers. There have been controversies about optimal PPE, especially due to shortages at the beginning of the pandemic. The CDC has some guidance about optimizing supply of PPE during shortages and the correct procedures for donning and doffing PPE.[5]

References

1. Centers for Disease Control and Prevention. *Coronavirus types*; 2020. https://www.cdc.gov/coronavirus/types.html.
2. Malik P, Patel K, Akrmah M, et al. COVID-19: a disease with a potpourri of histopathologic findings-a literature review and comparison to the closely related SARS and MERS. *SN Compr Clin Med.* 2021;3(12):2407–2434.
3. Beigel JH, Tomashek KM, Dodd LE, et al. Remdesivir for the treatment of Covid-19 - final report. *N Engl J Med.* 2020;383(19):1813–1826.
4. RECOVERY Collaborative Group, Horby P, Lim WS, et al. Dexamethasone in hospitalized patients with Covid-19. *N Engl J Med.* 2021;384(8):693–704.
5. Centers for Disease Control and Prevention. *Optimizing personal protective equipment (PPE) supplies*; 2020. https://www.cdc.gov/coronavirus/2019-ncov/hcp/ppe-strategy/index.html.

---

the alveolar-capillary membrane. The alveoli become enlarged and irregularly shaped (fibrotic), and the pulmonary capillaries become scarred and obliterated. This leads to further stiffening of the lungs, increasing pulmonary hypertension, and continued hypoxemia.[38,39]

Resolution Phase

Recovery occurs over several weeks as structural and vascular remodeling take place to reestablish the alveolar-capillary membrane. The hyaline membranes are cleared, and intraalveolar fluid is transported out of the alveolus into the interstitium. The type II alveolar epithelial cells multiply, some of which differentiate to type I alveolar epithelial cells, facilitating the restoration of the alveolus. Alveolar macrophages remove cellular debris.[38,39]

Assessment and Diagnosis

A patient with ARDS initially may be seen with a variety of clinical manifestations, depending on the precipitating event. As the disorder progresses, the patient's signs and symptoms can be associated with the phase of ARDS that he or she is experiencing (Table 14.2). During the exudative phase, the patient presents with tachypnea, restlessness, apprehension, and moderate increase in accessory muscle use. During

the fibroproliferative phase, the patient's signs and symptoms progress to agitation, dyspnea, fatigue, excessive accessory muscle use, and fine crackles as respiratory failure develops.[40,41]

ABG analysis shows a low PaO_2, despite increases in supplemental oxygen administration (refractory hypoxemia).[40] The $PaCO_2$ initially is low as a result of hyperventilation but eventually increases as the patient fatigues. The pH is high initially but decreases as respiratory acidosis develops.[40,41]

Initially the chest radiograph may be normal, because changes in the lungs do not become evident for up to 24 hours. As the pulmonary edema becomes apparent, diffuse, patchy interstitial and alveolar infiltrates appear. This progresses to multifocal consolidation of the lungs, which appears as a "whiteout" on the chest radiograph.[40]

Medical Management

Medical management of a patient with ARDS involves a multifaceted approach. This strategy includes treating the underlying cause, promoting gas exchange, supporting tissue oxygenation, and preventing complications. Given the severity of hypoxemia, the patient is intubated and mechanically ventilated to facilitate adequate gas exchange.[38]

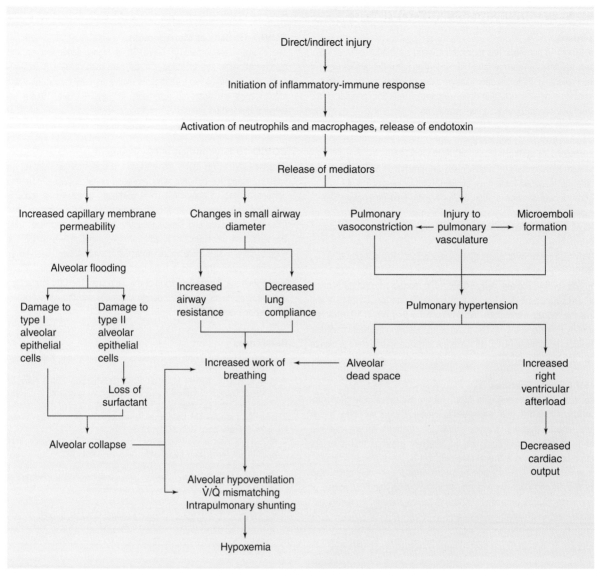

Fig. 14.1 Pathophysiology of Acute Respiratory Distress Syndrome.

Ventilation

Traditionally, patients with ARDS were ventilated with a mode of volume ventilation, such as assist/control ventilation or synchronized intermittent mandatory ventilation (SIMV), with tidal volumes adjusted to deliver 10 to 15 mL/kg. Current research indicates that this approach may have actually led to further lung injury. It is now known that repeated opening and closing of the alveoli cause injury to the lung units (atelectrauma), resulting in inhibited surfactant production, and increased inflammation (biotrauma), resulting in the release of mediators and an increase in pulmonary capillary membrane permeability. In addition, excessive pressure in the alveoli (barotrauma) or excessive volume in the alveoli (volutrauma) leads to excessive alveolar wall stress and damage to the alveolar-capillary membrane, resulting in air escaping into the surrounding spaces.[38,42] Thus several different approaches have been developed to facilitate the mechanical ventilation of patients with ARDS.

Low tidal volume. Low tidal volume ventilation uses smaller tidal volumes (6 mL/kg) to ventilate the patient in an attempt to limit the effects of barotrauma and volutrauma. The goal is to provide the maximum

tidal volume possible, while maintaining end-inspiratory plateau pressure less than 30 cm H_2O. To allow for adequate carbon dioxide elimination, the respiratory rate is increased to 20 to 30 breaths/min.[42,43]

Permissive hypercapnia. Permissive hypercapnia uses low tidal volume ventilation in conjunction with normal respiratory rates in an attempt to limit the effects of atelectrauma and biotrauma. To maintain normocapnia, the patient's respiratory rate normally would have to be increased to compensate for the small tidal volume. In ARDS, increasing the respiratory rate can lead to worsening alveolar damage. Thus the patient's carbon dioxide level is allowed to increase, and the patient becomes hypercapnic. As a general rule, the patient's $PaCO_2$ should not rise faster than 10 mm Hg per hour and overall should not exceed 80 to 100 mm Hg. Because of the negative cardiopulmonary effects of severe acidosis, the arterial pH is generally maintained at 7.20 or greater. To maintain the pH, the patient may be given intravenous sodium bicarbonate, or the respiratory rate, tidal volume, or both are increased. Permissive hypercapnia is contraindicated in patients with increased intracranial pressure, pulmonary hypertension, seizures, and heart failure.[44]

TABLE 14.2 Physiology and Signs and Symptoms of Acute Respiratory Distress Syndrome.

Physiology	Physical Examination
Exudative Phase	
Parenchymal surface hemorrhage	Restless, apprehensive, tachypneic
Interstitial or alveolar edema	Respiratory alkalosis
Compression of terminal bronchioles	PaO_2 normal
Destruction of type I alveolar cells	CXR: normal
	Chest examination: moderate use of accessory muscles, lungs clear
	Pulmonary artery pressures: elevated
	Pulmonary artery occlusion pressure: normal or low
Fibroproliferative Phase	
Destruction of type II alveolar cells	Pulmonary artery pressures: elevated
Gas exchange compromised	Increased workload on right ventricle
Increased peak inspiratory pressure	Increased use of accessory muscles
Decreased compliance (static and dynamic)	Fine crackles
Refractory hypoxemia:	Increasing agitation related to hypoxia
• Intraalveolar atelectasis	CXR: interstitial or alveolar infiltrates; elevated diaphragm
• Increased shunt fraction	Hyperventilation; hypercarbia
• Decreased diffusion	Decreased SVO_2
Decreased functional residual capacity	Widening alveolar-arterial gradient
Interstitial fibrosis	Increased work of breathing
Increased dead space ventilation	Worsening hypercarbia and hypoxemia
	Lactic acidosis (related to aerobic metabolism)
	Alteration in perfusion:
	• Increased heart rate
	• Decreased blood pressure
	• Change in skin temperature and color
	• Decreased capillary filling
	• End-organ dysfunction:
	• Brain: change in mentation, agitation, hallucinations
	• Heart: decreased cardiac output → angina, HF, papillary muscle dysfunction, dysrhythmias, MI
	• Renal: decreased urinary or GFR
	• Skin: mottled, ischemic
	• Liver: elevated SGOT, bilirubin, alkaline phosphatase, PT/PTT; decreased albumin

CXR, Chest radiograph; GFR, glomerular filtration rate; HF, heart failure; MI, myocardial infarction; PaO_2, arterial oxygen pressure; PT, prothrombin time; PTT, partial thromboplastin time; SGOT, serum glutamate oxaloacetate transaminase; SVO_2, venous oxygen saturation.
Modified from Phillips JK. Management of patients with acute respiratory distress syndrome. Crit Care Nurs Clin North Am. 1999;11(2):233–247.

Pressure control ventilation. In pressure control ventilation mode, each breath is delivered or augmented with a preset amount of inspiratory pressure as opposed to tidal volume, which is used in volume ventilation. Thus the actual tidal volume the patient receives varies from breath to breath. Pressure control ventilation is used to limit and control the amount of pressure in the lungs and decrease the incidence of volutrauma. The goal is to keep the patient's plateau pressure (end-inspiratory static pressure) lower than 30 cm H_2O. A known problem with this mode of ventilation is that as the patient's lungs get stiffer, it becomes harder and harder to maintain an adequate tidal volume, and severe hypercapnia can occur.[42,43]

Inverse ratio ventilation. Another alternative ventilatory mode that is used in managing patients with ARDS is inverse ratio ventilation (IRV), either pressure controlled or volume controlled. IRV prolongs the inspiratory time and shortens the expiratory time, thus reversing the normal inspiratory-to-expiratory ratio. The goal of IRV is to maintain a more constant mean airway pressure throughout the ventilatory cycle, which helps keep alveoli open and participating in gas exchange. It also increases FRC and decreases the work of breathing. In addition, as the breath is delivered over a longer period of time, the peak inspiratory pressure in the lungs is decreased. A major disadvantage to IRV is the development of auto-PEEP. As the expiratory phase of ventilation is shortened, air can become trapped in the lower airways, creating unintentional PEEP (or auto-PEEP), which can cause hemodynamic compromise and worsening gas exchange. Patients on IRV usually require heavy sedation with neuromuscular blockade to prevent them from fighting the ventilator.[42,43]

High-frequency oscillatory ventilation. High-frequency oscillatory ventilation is another alternative ventilatory mode that is used in patients who remain severely hypoxemic despite the treatments previously described. The goal of this method of ventilation is similar to that of IRV in that it uses a constant airway pressure to promote alveolar recruitment while avoiding overdistention of the alveoli. High-frequency oscillatory ventilation uses a piston pump to deliver very low tidal volumes (1–3 mL/breath) at very high rates or oscillations (300–900 breaths/min). Current research has failed to demonstrate that this method of ventilation provides any additional benefit over conventional ventilation and may even be harmful.[45]

Oxygen Therapy

Oxygen is administered at the lowest level possible to support tissue oxygenation. Continued exposure to high levels of oxygen can lead to oxygen toxicity, which perpetuates the entire process. The goal of oxygen therapy is to maintain an arterial hemoglobin oxygen saturation of 90% or greater using the lowest level of oxygen, preferably less than 0.50.[11]

Positive end-expiratory pressure. Because the hypoxemia that develops with ARDS is often refractory or unresponsive to oxygen therapy, it is necessary to facilitate oxygenation with PEEP. The purpose of using PEEP in a patient with ARDS is to improve oxygenation while reducing FiO_2 to less toxic levels. PEEP has several positive effects on the lungs, including opening collapsed alveoli, stabilizing flooded alveoli, and increasing FRC. Thus PEEP decreases intrapulmonary shunting and increases compliance. PEEP also has several negative effects, including (1) decreasing CO as a result of decreasing venous return secondary to increased intrathoracic pressure and (2) barotrauma as a result of gas escaping into the surrounding spaces secondary to alveolar rupture. The amount of PEEP a patient requires is determined by evaluating both arterial hemoglobin oxygen saturation and CO. In most cases, a PEEP of 10 to 15 cm H_2O is adequate. If PEEP is too high, it can result in overdistention of the alveoli, which can impede pulmonary capillary blood flow, decrease surfactant production, and worsen intrapulmonary shunting. If PEEP is too low, it allows the alveoli to collapse during expiration, which can result in more damage to alveoli.[42]

Extracorporeal and intracorporeal gas exchange. Extracorporeal and intracorporeal gas exchanges are last-resort techniques used in the treatment of severe ARDS when conventional therapy has failed. These methods allow the lungs to rest by facilitating the removal of carbon dioxide and providing oxygen external to the lungs by means of an "artificial lung," or membrane/fiber oxygenator. Extracorporeal membrane oxygenation (ECMO) and extracorporeal carbon dioxide removal are two techniques that employ this type of technology. ECMO is similar to cardiopulmonary bypass in that blood is removed from the body and pumped through a membrane oxygenator, where CO_2 is removed and O_2 is added, and then returned to the body. Extracorporeal carbon dioxide removal is a variation of ECMO in which the primary focus is removal of CO_2.[46]

Tissue Perfusion

Adequate tissue perfusion depends on an adequate supply of oxygen being transported to the tissues. An adequate CO and hemoglobin level is critical to oxygen transport. CO depends on heart rate, preload, afterload, and contractility. Various fluids and medications are used to manipulate this parameter. Newer approaches to fluid management include maintaining a very low intravascular volume (pulmonary artery occlusion pressure of 5–8 mm Hg) with fluid restriction and diuretics, while supporting the CO with vasoactive and inotropic medications. The goal is to decrease the amount of fluid leakage into the lungs.[47]

Nursing Management

The patient care management plan for a patient with ARDS incorporates a variety of patient problems (Box 14.7). Nursing priorities focus on (1) optimizing oxygenation and ventilation, (2) providing comfort and emotional support, and (3) maintaining surveillance for complications.

Optimizing Oxygenation and Ventilation

Nursing interventions to optimize oxygenation and ventilation include positioning, preventing desaturation, and promoting secretion

---

◎ BOX 14.7 PRIORITY PATIENT CARE MANAGEMENT

Acute Respiratory Distress Syndrome
- Impaired Gas Exchange due to ventilation/perfusion mismatching or intrapulmonary shunting
- Impaired Cardiac Output due to alterations in preload
- Impaired Nutritional Intake due to lack of exogenous nutrients or increased metabolic demand
- Risk for Aspiration
- Risk for Infection
- Anxiety due to biologic, psychologic, and/or social integrity
- Impaired Family Coping due to critically ill family member
- Patient Care Management plans are located in Appendix A.

---

clearance. For further discussion of these interventions, see Nursing Management of ALF earlier in this chapter. One additional nursing intervention that can be used to improve the oxygenation and ventilation of a patient with ARDS is prone positioning.

Prone positioning. Numerous studies have shown that prone positioning of a patient with ARDS results in an improvement in oxygenation. Although many theories propose how prone positioning improves oxygenation, the discovery that with ARDS there is greater damage to the dependent areas of the lungs probably provides the best explanation. It was originally thought that ARDS was a diffuse homogeneous disease that affected all areas of the lungs equally. It is now known that the dependent lung areas are more heavily damaged than the nondependent lung areas. Turning the patient prone improves perfusion to less damaged parts of lungs and improves V/Q matching and decreases intrapulmonary shunting. Prone positioning appears to be more effective when initiated during the early phases of ARDS and applied for at least 12 hours a day.[48] For more information on prone positioning, see Chapter 15.

Interprofessional collaborative management of a patient with ARDS is outlined in Box 14.8.

PNEUMONIA

Description and Etiology

Pneumonia is an acute inflammation of the lung parenchyma that is caused by an infectious agent that can lead to alveolar consolidation. Pneumonia can be classified as community-acquired pneumonia (CAP), hospital-acquired pneumonia (HAP), or VAP.[49] Pneumonia is referred to as community acquired when it occurs outside of the hospital or within 48 hours of admission to the hospital.[50] Severe CAP requires admission to the critical care unit and accounts for approximately 22% of all patients with pneumonia. The mortality for this patient group is approximately 50%, with increasing age as a major risk factor.[51] Pneumonia is referred to as hospital acquired when it occurs while the patient is in the hospital for at least 48 hours and not associated with mechanical ventilation.[49] VAP refers to development of pneumonia occurring at least 48 hours after the insertion of an artificial airway.[49] VAP is one of the most common infections acquired in the critical care unit.[52]

The spectra of etiologic pathogens of pneumonia vary with the type of pneumonia, as do the risk factors for the disease.

BOX 14.8   Collaborative Management of Acute Respiratory Distress Syndrome

- Administer oxygen therapy.
- Intubate patient.
- Initiate mechanical ventilation:
  - Permissive hypercapnia
  - Pressure control ventilation
  - Inverse ratio ventilation
  - Use positive end-expiratory pressure (PEEP)
- Administer medications:
  - Bronchodilators
  - Sedatives
  - Analgesics
  - Neuromuscular blocking agents
- Maximize cardiac output:
  - Preload
  - Afterload
  - Contractility
- Position patient prone.
- Suction as needed.
- Provide adequate rest and recovery time between procedures.
- Initiate nutrition support.
- Maintain surveillance for complications:
  - Encephalopathy
  - Cardiac dysrhythmias
  - Venous thromboembolism
  - Gastrointestinal bleeding
  - Atelectrauma
  - Biotrauma
  - Volutrauma
  - Barotrauma
  - Oxygen toxicity
- Provide comfort and emotional support.

Modified from American Association of Critical-Care Nurses: AACN Practice Alert: Preventing venous thromboembolism in adults. *Crit Care Nurse.* 2016;36(5):e20–e23. ©2016 by the American Association of Critical-Care Nurses," "All rights reserved," and "Used with permission.

Severe Community-Acquired Pneumonia

Pathogens that can cause severe CAP include *Streptococcus pneumoniae, Legionella* spp., *Haemophilus influenzae, Moraxella catarrhalis, Staphylococcus aureus, Mycoplasma pneumoniae,* respiratory viruses, *Chlamydia pneumoniae,* and *Pseudomonas aeruginosa.*[50,51] Numerous factors increase the risk for developing CAP, including alcoholism; chronic obstructive pulmonary disease; and comorbid conditions such as diabetes, malignancy, and coronary artery disease. Impaired swallowing and altered mental status also contribute to the development of CAP, because they result in an increased exposure to the various pathogens related to chronic aspiration of oropharyngeal secretions.[51] Box 14.9 presents an overview of cystic fibrosis.

Hospital-Acquired Pneumonia

Pathogens that can cause HAP include *Escherichia coli, H. influenzae,* methicillin-sensitive *S. aureus, S. pneumoniae, P. aeruginosa, Acinetobacter baumannii,* methicillin-resistant *S. aureus, Klebsiella* spp., and *Enterobacter* spp. Two of the pathogens most frequently associated with VAP are *S. aureus* and *P. aeruginosa.* Risk factors for HAP can be categorized as host-related, treatment-related, and infection control–related (Box 14.10).[53]

Ventilator-Associated Pneumonia

VAP is a misleading term, because it is not really related to mechanical ventilation but to the presence of an artificial airway. The types of pathogens that can cause VAP vary with the time of onset. Pathogens

---

BOX 14.9   Adults With Cystic Fibrosis

- Cystic fibrosis (CF) is an autosomal recessive genetic disorder characterized by altered cellular sodium and chloride ions transport, affecting the exocrine glands. This life-limiting multisystem disorder affects various body systems, including the lungs, pancreas, biliary tract, and reproductive tract.[1]
- The initial signs and symptoms of CF usually appear during childhood; however, given the variation in the severity and progression of the disorder, some patients are diagnosed as adults. The prognosis for patients with CF has significantly improved over the past several decades due to improvements in diagnosis and management. Fifty years ago, the median age of survival was 16 years. Today patients are living for 40 years or longer.[2] These improvements have also resulted in more adult patients being admitted to the critical care unit with a history of CF.
- CF's lung effects result in the airway secretions becoming thick and sticky, making them difficult to clear. Eventually, the secretions obstruct the small airways and promote infection, leading to chronic infections, tissue destruction, and ultimately the development of bronchiectasis.[3] Patients with CF often present with respiratory failure secondary to pneumonia. Patients with CF may also experience pancreatic insufficiency, chronic pancreatitis, cirrhosis, malabsorption syndrome, chronic sinusitis, and infertility. These conditions can also lead to diabetes, pneumothorax, portal hypertension, and pulmonary hypertension.[3]

- Nursing priorities for patients with pneumonia secondary to CF focus on airway clearance techniques:
- Chest physiotherapy to include:
  - Postural drainage, percussion, and vibration to mobilize lung secretions
  - Oscillating positive expiratory pressure devices (i.e., flutter valves) to promote clearance of excess secretions and reduce air trapping
  - High-frequency chest wall oscillation vests to help loosen secretions
- Breathing exercises.
- Metered-dose inhalers and ultrasonic nebulizers to administer:
  - Beta-2 adrenergic receptor agonists to dilate airways
  - Inhaled glucocorticoids to reduce lung inflammation
  - Hypertonic saline to loosen and liquefy thickened mucus
  - Mucolytics (e.g., dornase alfa [specifically for patients with CF]) to decrease mucus viscosity
  - Inhaled antibiotics to treat pulmonary infections

Additional information can be found on the CF Foundation website (www.cff.org).

References

1. Elborn JS. Cystic fibrosis. *Lancet.* 2016;388(10059):2519–2531.
2. Bergeron C, Cantin AM. Cystic fibrosis: pathophysiology of lung disease. *Semin Respir Crit Care Med.* 2019;40(6):715–726.
3. Brown SD, White R, Tobin P. Keep them breathing: cystic fibrosis pathophysiology, diagnosis, and treatment. *JAAPA.* 2017;30(5):23–27.

BOX 14.10 Risk Factors for Hospital-Acquired Pneumonia

Host-Related
- Advanced age
- Altered level of consciousness
- Chronic obstructive pulmonary disease
- Altered immune system
- Severity of illness
- Poor nutrition
- Hemodynamic compromise
- Trauma
- Smoking
- Dental plaque

Infection Control—Related
- Poor handwashing practices

Treatment-Related
- Mechanical ventilation
- Endotracheal intubation
- Unintentional extubation
- Bronchoscopy
- Nasogastric tube
- Previous antibiotic therapy
- Elevated gastric pH secondary to histamine receptor antagonists, proton pump inhibitors, and enteral feedings
- Upper abdominal surgery
- Thoracic surgery
- Supine position

associated with early-onset VAP include *Enterobacteriaceae, Candida albicans*, and *S. aureus*, whereas pathogens associated with late-onset VAP include *P. aeruginosa, Klebsiella pneumoniae*, and *E. coli*.[54]

Pathophysiology

Development of acute pneumonia implies a defect in host defenses, a particularly virulent organism, or an overwhelming inoculation event. Bacterial invasion of the lower respiratory tract can occur by inhalation of aerosolized infectious particles, aspiration of organisms colonizing the oropharynx, migration of organisms from adjacent sites of colonization, direct inoculation of organisms into the lower airway, spread of infection to the lungs from adjacent structures, spread of infection to the lung through the blood, and reactivation of latent infection (usually in the setting of immunosuppression). The most common mechanism appears to be aspiration of oropharyngeal

organisms.[55,56] Table 14.3 lists the precipitating conditions that can facilitate the development of pneumonia.

Fig. 14.2 depicts the pathophysiology of HAP. Colonization of the patient's oropharynx with infectious organisms is a major contributor to the development of HAP. The oropharynx normally has a stable population of resident flora that may be anaerobic or aerobic. When stress occurs, such as with illness, surgery, or infection, pathogenic organisms replace normal resident flora. Previous antibiotic therapy also affects the resident flora population, making replacement by pathologic organisms more likely. The pathogens are then able to invade the sterile lower respiratory tract.[53]

Disruption of the gag and cough reflexes, altered consciousness, abnormal swallowing, and artificial airways all predispose the patient to aspiration and colonization of the lungs and subsequent infection. Histamine-2 agonists, antacids, and enteral feedings also contribute to this problem, because they raise the pH of the stomach and promote bacterial overgrowth. The nasogastric tube then acts as a wick, facilitating the movement of bacteria from the stomach to the pharynx, where the bacteria can be aspirated.[53]

Infection results in pulmonary inflammation with or without significant exudates. Increased capillary permeability occurs, leading to increased interstitial and alveolar fluid. V/Q mismatching and intrapulmonary shunting occur, resulting in hypoxemia as lung consolidation progresses. Untreated pneumonia can result in ALF and initiation of the inflammatory-immune response. In addition, the patient may develop a pleural effusion. This is the result of the vascular response to inflammation, whereby capillary permeability is increased, and fluid from the pulmonary capillaries diffuses into the pleural space.[56]

Prevention of VAP is discussed in the mechanical ventilation section of Chapter 15.

Assessment and Diagnosis

The clinical manifestations of pneumonia vary with the offending pathogen. The patient may first be seen with a variety of signs and symptoms including dyspnea, fever, and cough (productive or nonproductive). Coarse crackles on auscultation and dullness to percussion may also be present.[52] Patients with severe CAP may present with confusion and disorientation, tachypnea, hypoxemia, uremia, leukopenia, thrombocytopenia, hypothermia, and hypotension.[57]

Chest radiography is used to evaluate a patient with suspected pneumonia. The diagnosis is established by the presence of a new pulmonary infiltrate. The radiographic pattern of the infiltrates varies with the organism.[53] A sputum Gram stain and culture are done to facilitate identification of the infectious pathogen. In 50% of cases, a causative agent is not identified.[53] A diagnostic bronchoscopy may be needed, particularly if the diagnosis is unclear or current therapy is not working.[52] In addition, a complete blood count with differential, chemistry panel, blood cultures, and ABGs is obtained.[53]

TABLE 14.3 Precipitating Conditions of Pneumonia.

Condition	Etiologies
Depressed epiglottal and cough reflexes	Unconsciousness, neurologic disease, endotracheal or tracheal tubes, anesthesia, aging
Decreased cilia activity	Smoke inhalation, smoking history, oxygen toxicity, hypoventilation, intubation, viral infections, aging, chronic obstructive pulmonary disease (COPD)
Increased secretion	COPD, viral infections, bronchiectasis, general anesthesia, endotracheal intubation, smoking
Atelectasis	Trauma, foreign body obstruction, tumor, splinting, shallow ventilations, general anesthesia
Decreased lymphatic flow	Heart failure, tumor
Fluid in alveoli	Heart failure, aspiration, trauma
Abnormal phagocytosis and humoral activity	Neutropenia, immunocompetent disorders, patients receiving chemotherapy
Impaired alveolar macrophages	Hypoxemia, metabolic acidosis, cigarette smoking history, hypoxia, alcohol use, viral infections, aging

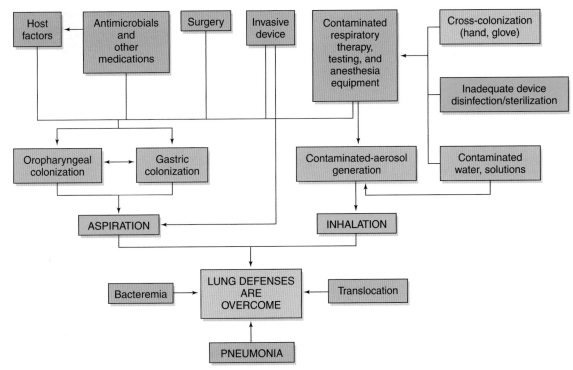

Fig. 14.2 Pathophysiology of Pneumonia. (From Tablan OC, Anderson LJ, Arden NH, Breiman RF, Butler JC, McNeil MM. Guideline for prevention of nosocomial pneumonia. The Hospital Infection Control Practices Advisory Committee, Centers for Disease Control and Prevention. *Am J Infect Control.* 1994;22[4]:247-292.)

Medical Management

Medical management of a patient with pneumonia includes antibiotic therapy, oxygen therapy for hypoxemia, mechanical ventilation if ALF develops, fluid management for hydration, nutrition support, and treatment of associated medical problems and complications. For patients having difficulty mobilizing secretions, a therapeutic bronchoscopy may be necessary.[52]

Antibiotic Therapy

Although bacterium-specific antibiotic therapy is the goal, this may not always be possible because of difficulties in identifying the organism and the seriousness of the patient's condition. The time involved obtaining cultures is balanced against the need to begin some treatment based on the patient's condition. Empiric therapy has become a generally acceptable approach. In this approach, choice of antibiotic treatment is based on the most likely etiologic organism while avoiding toxicity, superinfection, and unnecessary cost. If available, Gram stain results are used to guide choices of antibiotics. Antibiotics that offer broad coverage of the usual pathogens in the hospital or community are chosen. Failure to respond to such therapy may indicate that the chosen antibiotic regimen does not appropriately cover all the etiologic pathogens or that a new source of infection has developed.[52,53] Optimal timing for the initiation of antibiotics has been an ongoing issue. A recent systematic review concluded that in the patient with CAP, antibiotic therapy should be initiated within 4 to 8 hours of hospital arrival.[57]

Independent Lung Ventilation

In patients with unilateral pneumonia or severely asymmetric pneumonia, independent lung ventilation, an alternative mode of mechanical ventilation, may be necessary to facilitate oxygenation. As the alveoli in the affected lung become flooded with pus, the lung becomes less compliant and difficult to ventilate. This results in a shifting of ventilation to the good lung without a concomitant shift in perfusion and thus an increase in V/Q mismatching. Independent lung ventilation allows each lung to be ventilated separately, controlling the amount of flow, volume, and pressure each lung receives. A double-lumen endotracheal tube is inserted, and each lumen is usually attached to a separate mechanical ventilator. The ventilator settings are then customized to the needs of each lung to facilitate optimal oxygenation and ventilation.[58]

Nursing Management

The patient care management plan for a patient with pneumonia incorporates a variety of patient problems (Box 14.11). Nursing priorities focus on (1) optimizing oxygenation and ventilation, (2) preventing the spread of infection, (3) providing comfort and emotional support, and (4) maintaining surveillance for complications. The patient's response to antibiotic therapy is monitored for adverse effects.

Optimizing Oxygenation and Ventilation

Nursing interventions to optimize oxygenation and ventilation include positioning, preventing desaturation, and promoting secretion clearance. For further discussion of these interventions, see Nursing Management of ALF earlier in this chapter.

Preventing Spread of Infection

Prevention is directed at eradicating pathogens from the environment and interrupting the spread of organisms from person to person. Significant progress has been made in removing contaminants from the patient environment through proper disinfection of respiratory equipment and increased use of disposable supplies. Other possible environmental sources of pathogens include suctioning equipment and indwelling lines. These invasive tools must be given proper aseptic care.[59]

BOX 14.11 PRIORITY PATIENT CARE MANAGEMENT

Pneumonia
- Impaired Airway Clearance due to excessive secretions or abnormal viscosity of mucus
- Impaired Gas Exchange due to ventilation/perfusion mismatching or intrapulmonary shunting
- Impaired Nutritional Intake due to lack of exogenous nutrients or increased metabolic demand
- Risk for Aspiration
- Powerlessness due to lack of control over current situation or disease progression

Patient Care Management Plans are located in Appendix A.

BOX 14.13 Collaborative Management of Pneumonia

- Administer oxygen therapy.
- Initiate mechanical ventilation as required.
- Administer medications:
  - Antibiotics
  - Bronchodilators
- Position patient to optimize ventilation/perfusion matching.
- Suction as needed.
- Provide adequate rest and recovery time between procedures.
- Maintain surveillance for complications:
  - Acute lung failure
- Provide comfort and emotional support.

Proper hand hygiene is the most important measure available to prevent the spread of bacteria from person to person (Box 14.12). Hand hygiene is performed before and after touching a patient or their surroundings, before a procedure, and after exposure to any body fluids.[60] In addition, meticulous oral care, including suctioning of the secretions pooling above the cuff of the artificial airway, is critical to decreasing the bacterial colonization of the oropharynx.[59] Oral care is discussed further in Chapter 15.

Interprofessional collaborative management of a patient with pneumonia is outlined in Box 14.13.

ASPIRATION PNEUMONITIS

Description and Etiology

The presence of abnormal substances in the airways and alveoli as a result of aspiration is misleadingly called *aspiration pneumonia*. This term is misleading because the aspiration of toxic substances into the lung may or may not involve an infection. *Aspiration*

pneumonitis is a more accurate term because injury to the lung can result from the chemical, mechanical, or bacterial characteristics of the aspirate.[61,62]

Numerous factors have been identified that place the patient at risk for aspiration (Table 14.4). Gastric contents and oropharyngeal bacteria (see Pneumonia section earlier in this chapter) are the most common aspirates of critically ill patients.[62–64] The effects of gastric contents on the lungs vary based on the pH of the liquid. If the pH is less than 2.5, the patient will develop a severe chemical pneumonitis resulting in hypoxemia. If the pH is greater than 2.5, the immediate damage to the lungs will be lessened, but the elevated pH may have promoted bacterial overgrowth of the stomach.[62,63] Once the bacteria-laden gastric contents are aspirated into the lungs, overwhelming bacterial pneumonia can develop.[63]

Pathophysiology

The type of lung injury that develops after aspiration is determined by many factors, including the quality of the aspirate and the status of the patient's respiratory defense mechanisms.

BOX 14.12 Quality Improvement

Hand Hygiene Guidelines

The following are key recommendations of the Hand Hygiene Task Force, based on the literature review and expert panel opinion:
- Wash hands with soap and water when visibly dirty or contaminated with blood and other body fluids.
- When washing hands with soap and water, wet hands first with water, apply an amount of product recommended by the manufacturer to hands, and rub hands together vigorously for at least 15 seconds, covering all surfaces of the hands and fingers. Rinse hands with water, and dry thoroughly with a disposable towel. Use towel to turn off the faucet. Avoid using hot water, because repeated exposure to hot water may increase the risk of dermatitis.
- If hands are not visibly soiled, use an alcohol-based hand rub for routinely decontaminating hands.
- When decontaminating hands with an alcohol-based hand rub, apply product to palm of one hand and rub hands together, covering all surfaces of hands

and fingers, until hands are dry (follow the manufacturer's recommendations regarding the volume of product to use).
- Decontaminate hands before and after having direct contact with patients.
- Decontaminate hands before and after donning gloves.
- Wear gloves when contact with blood or other potentially infectious materials, mucous membranes, or nonintact skin could occur.
- Change gloves during patient care if moving from a contaminated body site to a clean body site.
- Remove gloves after caring for a patient. Do not wear the same pair of gloves for the care of more than one patient, and do not wash gloves between uses with different patients.
- Decontaminate hands after contact with inanimate objects (including medical equipment).
- Do not wear artificial fingernails or extenders when having direct contact with patients at high risk (e.g., those in critical care units or operating rooms).
- Keep natural nail tips less than one-fourth-inch long.

From Boyce JM, Pittet D; Healthcare Infection Control Practices Advisory Committee; HICPAC/SHEA/APIC/IDSA Hand Hygiene Task Force. Guideline for hand hygiene in health care settings: Recommendations of Healthcare Infection Control Practices Advisory Committee, and the HICPAC/SHEA/APIC/IDSA Hand Hygiene Task Force. Society for Healthcare Epidemiology of America/Association for Professionals in Infection Control/Infectious Diseases Society of America. *MMWR Recomm Rep.* 2002;51(RR16):1-45.

TABLE 14.4 Risk Factors for Aspiration.

Risk Factor	Rationale
Decreased LOC from either CNS problems or use of sedatives	Decreased ability to protect airway from oropharyngeal secretions and regurgitated gastric contents
	Cough and gag reflexes diminish as LOC diminishes, whether from CNS disorder or sedation
	Slowed gastric emptying
	Decreased tone of lower esophageal sphincter
Supine position	Increases probability of gastroesophageal reflux
Presence of nasogastric tube	Interferes with closure of lower esophageal sphincter
	Biofilm on tube predisposes to aspiration of pathogenic organisms
Vomiting	Sudden and forceful entry of gastric contents into oropharynx predisposes to aspiration
	Predisposes to displacement of feeding tube ports into esophagus
Feeding tube ports positioned in esophagus	Infused feedings reflux into oropharynx
Tracheal intubation	Reduction in upper airway defense related to ineffective cough, desensitization of oropharynx and larynx, disuse atrophy of laryngeal muscles, and esophageal compression by an inflated cuff
Mechanical ventilation	Positive abdominal pressure predisposes to aspiration of gastric contents, probably by increasing gastroesophageal reflux
Accumulation of subglottic secretions above endotracheal cuff	Subglottic secretions can leak around cuff into lower respiratory tract, especially when cuff is deflated
Inadequate cuff inflation of tracheal devices	Persistent low cuff pressure predisposes to aspiration of oropharyngeal secretions and refluxed gastric contents
Gastric feeding site when gastric emptying significantly impaired	Accumulation of formula and gastrointestinal secretions predisposes to gastroesophageal reflux and aspiration
High GRVs	High GRVs predispose to gastroesophageal reflux and aspiration
Bolus feedings	Volume of infused formula may exceed tolerance of patients who have poor cough and gag reflexes
Poor oral health	Colonized oropharyngeal secretions may be aspirated into respiratory tract
Advanced age	Older patients tend to have reduced swallowing ability and are more likely to have neurologic disorders that increase aspiration risks
	Strong association between advanced age and probability of developing pneumonia once aspiration has occurred
Hyperglycemia	Mild hyperglycemia can cause delayed gastric emptying by disrupting postprandial antral contractions

CNS, Central nervous system; *GRVs,* gastric residual volumes; *LOC,* level of consciousness.
From Metheny NA. Strategies to prevent aspiration-related pneumonia in tube-fed patients. *Respir Care Clin N Am.* 2006;12(4):603-617.

Acid Liquid

The aspiration of acid (pH less than 2.5) liquid gastric contents results in the development of bronchospasm and atelectasis almost immediately. Over the next 4 hours, tracheal damage, bronchitis, bronchiolitis, alveolar-capillary breakdown, interstitial edema, and alveolar congestion and hemorrhage occur.[64] Severe hypoxemia develops as a result of intrapulmonary shunting and V/Q mismatching. As the disorder progresses, necrotic debris and fibrin fill the alveoli, hyaline membranes form, and hypoxic vasoconstriction occurs, resulting in elevated pulmonary artery pressures.[63,64] The clinical course follows one of three patterns: (1) rapid improvement in 1 week, (2) initial improvement followed by deterioration and development of ARDS or pneumonia, or (3) rapid death from progressive ALF.[64]

Acid Food Particles

The aspiration of acid (pH less than 2.5), nonobstructing food particles can produce the most severe pulmonary reaction because of extensive pulmonary damage. Severe hypoxemia, hypercapnia, and acidosis occur.[63,64]

Nonacid Liquid

The aspiration of nonacid (pH greater than 2.5) liquid gastric contents is similar to acid liquid aspiration initially, but minimal structural damage occurs. Intrapulmonary shunting and V/Q mismatching usually start to reverse within 4 hours, and hypoxemia clears within 24 hours.[63,64]

Nonacid Food Particles

The aspiration of nonacid (pH greater than 2.5), nonobstructing food particles is similar to acid aspiration initially, with significant edema and hemorrhage occurring within 6 hours. After the initial reaction, the response changes to a foreign body—type reaction with granuloma formation occurring around the food particles within 1 to 5 days.[64] In addition to hypoxemia, hypercapnia and acidosis occur as a result of hypoventilation.[62,63]

Assessment and Diagnosis

Clinically patients present with signs of acute respiratory distress, and gastric contents may be present in the oropharynx. Patients have shortness of breath, coughing, wheezing, cyanosis, and signs of hypoxemia. Tachypnea, tachycardia, hypotension, fever, and crackles also are present. Copious amounts of sputum are produced as alveolar edema develops.[62,63]

ABGs reflect severe hypoxemia. Changes on chest radiography appear 12 to 24 hours after the initial aspiration, with no one pattern being diagnostic of the event. Infiltrates appear in various distribution patterns depending on the position of the patient during aspiration and the volume of the aspirate. If bacterial infection becomes established, leukocytosis and positive sputum cultures occur.[63]

Medical Management

Management of a patient with aspiration lung disorder includes both emergency and follow-up treatment. When aspiration is witnessed,

BOX 14.14 PRIORITY PATIENT CARE MANAGEMENT

Aspiration Pneumonitis
- Impaired Gas Exchange due to ventilation/perfusion mismatching or intrapulmonary shunting
- Impaired Airway Clearance due to excessive secretions or abnormal viscosity of mucus
- Risk for Infection
- Anxiety due to biologic, psychologic, and/or social integrity
- Impaired Family Coping due to critically ill family member
  Patient Care Management Plans are located in Appendix A.

emergency treatment is instituted to secure the airway and minimize pulmonary damage. The patient's head is turned to the side, and the oral cavity and upper airway is suctioned immediately to remove the gastric contents.[63,64] Direct visualization by bronchoscopy is indicated to remove large particulate aspirate or to confirm an unwitnessed aspiration event. Bronchoalveolar lavage is not recommended, because this practice disseminates the aspirate in lungs and increases damage.[64]

After airway clearance, attention is given to supporting oxygenation and hemodynamics. Hypoxemia is corrected with supplemental oxygen or mechanical ventilation with PEEP, if necessary.[63,64] Hemodynamic changes result from fluid shifts into the lungs that can occur after massive aspirations. Monitoring intravascular volume is essential, and judicious amounts of replacement fluids are instituted to maintain adequate urinary output and vital signs.[63,64]

Empiric antibiotic therapy is usually not indicated after aspiration of gastric contents. However, antibiotic therapy is considered if VAP is suspected or the aspiration event occurred in the presence of a small bowel obstruction or colonized gastric contents.[64] Corticosteroids have not been demonstrated to be of any benefit in the treatment of aspiration pneumonitis and are not recommended.[63,64]

Nursing Management

The patient care management plan for a patient with aspiration lung disorder incorporates a variety of patient problems (Box 14.14). **Nursing priorities focus on (1) optimizing oxygenation and ventilation, (2) preventing further aspiration events, (3) providing comfort and emotional support, and (4) maintaining surveillance for complications.**

Optimizing Oxygenation and Ventilation

Nursing interventions to optimize oxygenation and ventilation include positioning, preventing desaturation, and promoting secretion

clearance. For further discussion of these interventions, see Nursing Management of ALF earlier in this chapter.

Preventing Aspiration

One of the most important interventions for preventing aspiration is identifying patients at risk for aspiration (Box 14.15). Actions to prevent aspiration include confirming feeding tube placement, checking for signs and symptoms of feeding intolerance, elevating the head of the bed at least 30 to 45 degrees, feeding the patient via a small-bore feeding tube or gastrostomy tube, avoiding the use of a large-bore nasogastric tube, ensuring proper inflation of artificial airway cuffs, and frequent suctioning of the oropharynx of an intubated patient to prevent secretions from pooling above the cuff of the tube. For patients at risk for aspiration or intolerant of gastric feedings, the feeding tube is placed in the small bowel.[65]

Interprofessional collaborative management of a patient with aspiration pneumonitis is outlined in Box 14.16.

ACUTE PULMONARY EMBOLISM

Description and Etiology

A pulmonary embolism (PE) occurs when a clot (thrombotic embolus) or other matter (nonthrombotic embolus) lodges in the pulmonary arterial system, disrupting the blood flow to a region of the lungs (Fig. 14.3). Most thrombotic emboli arise from the pelvic and deep leg veins, particularly the iliac, femoral, and popliteal veins.[66] Other sources include the right ventricle, the upper extremities, and the pelvic veins. Nonthrombotic emboli arise from fat, tumors, amniotic fluid, air, and foreign bodies. This section focuses on thrombotic emboli.

Numerous predisposing factors and precipitating conditions put a patient at risk for developing a PE (Box 14.17). Of the three predisposing factors (i.e., hypercoagulability, injury to vascular endothelium, and venous stasis [Virchow triad]), endothelial injury appears to be the most significant.[66] Two of these three conditions usually must be present for thrombosis to occur. Patients in critical care units generally have one or more risk factors that predispose them to the development of a venous thrombus. A hospitalized patient has more than a 100-fold increased incidence of acute VTE compared with the general public.[67] The incidence of deep vein thrombosis (DVT) increases with age and markedly increases the patient's risk of fatal PE.

The American Heart Association has developed a classification schema for an acute PE, which stratifies patients into one of three categories: massive, submassive, or low risk. A massive PE is defined as an acute PE with sustained hypotension (systolic blood pressure less than 90 mm Hg) for more than 15 minutes, the need for inotropes not based on other causes, or signs of shock. A submassive PE is defined as an acute PE with evidence of right ventricular dysfunction or

BOX 14.15 Evidence-Based Practice

Aspiration Prevention Guidelines
The following are the key recommendations from the AACN Practice Alert: Preventing Aspiration:
1. Maintain head-of-bed elevation at an angle of 30 to 45 degrees, unless contraindicated.
2. Use sedatives as sparingly as feasible.
3. For patients receiving gastric tube feedings, assess for gastrointestinal intolerance to the feedings at 4-hour intervals.

4. For tube-fed patients, avoid bolus feedings in those at high risk for aspiration.
5. Consult with physician about obtaining a swallowing assessment before oral feedings are started for recently extubated patients who have experienced prolonged intubation.
6. Maintain endotracheal cuff pressures at an appropriate level and ensure that secretions are cleared from above the cuff before it is deflated.

Modified from American Association of Critical-Care Nurses. AACN Practice Alert: prevention of aspiration in adults. *Crit Care Nurse.* 2016;38(1):e20—e24 (updated 2018).

BOX 14.16 Collaborative Management of Aspiration Pneumonitis

- Administer oxygen therapy.
- Secure patient's airway.
- Place patient in slight Trendelenburg position.
- Turn patient to right lateral decubitus position.
- Suction patient's oropharyngeal area.
- Initiate mechanical ventilation as required.
- Maintain surveillance for complications:
  - Pneumonia
  - Acute lung failure
  - Acute respiratory distress syndrome
- Provide comfort and emotional support.

myocardial necrosis. A patient with none of these conditions is defined as low risk.[68]

Pathophysiology

A massive PE occurs with the blockage of a lobar or larger artery, resulting in occlusion of the pulmonary vascular bed. Blockage of the pulmonary arterial system has both pulmonary and hemodynamic consequences.[66] The effects on the pulmonary system are increased alveolar dead space, bronchoconstriction, and compensatory shunting.[69] Hemodynamic effects include an increase in pulmonary vascular resistance and right ventricular workload.[70,71]

Increased Dead Space

An increase in alveolar dead space occurs because an area of the lung is receiving ventilation without being perfused. The ventilation to this

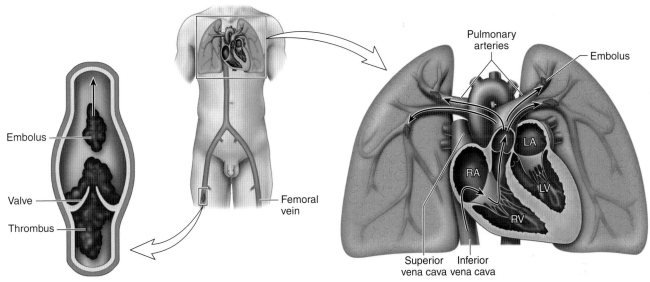

Fig. 14.3 Pathophysiology of Pulmonary Embolism. Thromboemboli travel through the right side of the heart to reach the lungs. *LA*, Left atrium; *LV*, left ventricle; *RA*, right atrium; *RV*, right ventricle.

BOX 14.17 Risk Factors for Pulmonary Thromboembolism

Predisposing Factors
- Venous stasis
  - Atrial fibrillation
  - Decreased cardiac output
  - Immobility
- Injury to vascular endothelium
  - Local vessel injury
  - Infection
  - Incision
  - Atherosclerosis
- Hypercoagulability
  - Polycythemia

Precipitating Conditions
- Previous pulmonary embolus
- Cardiovascular disease
  - Heart failure
  - Right ventricular infarction
  - Cardiomyopathy
  - Cor pulmonale

- Surgery
  - Orthopedic
  - Vascular
  - Abdominal
- Cancer
  - Ovarian
  - Pancreatic
  - Stomach
  - Extrahepatic bile duct system
- Trauma (injury or burns)
  - Lower extremities
  - Pelvis
  - Hips
- Gynecologic status
  - Pregnancy
  - Postpartum
  - Birth control pills
  - Estrogen replacement therapy

area is known as *wasted ventilation* because it does not participate in gas exchange. This effect leads to alveolar dead space ventilation and an increase in the work of breathing. To limit the amount of dead space ventilation, localized bronchoconstriction occurs.[71]

Bronchoconstriction

Bronchoconstriction develops as a result of alveolar hypocarbia, hypoxia, and the release of mediators. Alveolar hypocarbia occurs as a consequence of decreased carbon dioxide in the affected area and leads to constriction of the local airways, increased airway resistance, and redistribution of ventilation to perfused areas of the lungs. Various mediators are released from the site of the injury, either from the clot or the surrounding lung tissue, which further causes constriction of the airways. Bronchoconstriction promotes the development of atelectasis.[71]

Compensatory Shunting

Compensatory shunting occurs as a result of the unaffected areas of the lungs having to accommodate the entire CO. A situation results in which perfusion exceeds ventilation and blood is returned to the left side of the heart without participating in gas exchange. This leads to the development of hypoxemia.[71]

Hemodynamic Consequences

The major hemodynamic consequence of a PE is the development of pulmonary hypertension, which is part of the effect of a mechanical obstruction when more than 50% of the vascular bed is occluded. In addition, the mediators released at the injury site and the development of hypoxia cause pulmonary vasoconstriction, which further exacerbates pulmonary hypertension. As the pulmonary vascular resistance increases, so does the workload of the right ventricle, as reflected by an increase in pulmonary artery pressures. Consequently, right ventricular failure occurs, which can lead to decreases in left ventricular preload, CO, and blood pressure and shock.[66,67–71]

Assessment and Diagnosis

A patient with a PE may have numerous presenting signs and symptoms, with the most common being tachycardia and tachypnea. Additional signs and symptoms that may be present include dyspnea, apprehension, increased pulmonic component of the second heart sound (P_1), fever, crackles, pleuritic chest pain, cough, evidence of DVT, and hemoptysis.[66] Syncope and hemodynamic instability can occur as a result of right ventricular failure.[70]

Initial laboratory studies and diagnostic procedures that may be done include ABG analysis, D-dimer, electrocardiogram (ECG), chest radiography, and echocardiography. ABGs may show a low PaO_2, indicating hypoxemia; a low $PaCO_2$, indicating hypocarbia; and a high pH, indicating a respiratory alkalosis. The hypocarbia with resulting respiratory alkalosis is caused by tachypnea.[69] An elevated D-dimer occurs with a PE and many other disorders. A normal D-dimer does not occur with a PE and can be used to rule out a PE as the diagnosis.[66] The most common ECG finding among patients with PE is sinus tachycardia.[66] The classic ECG pattern associated with a PE, S wave in lead I and Q wave with inverted T wave in lead III, occurs in less than 20% of patients.[66] Other ECG findings associated with a PE include right bundle branch block, new-onset atrial fibrillation, T wave inversion in the anterior or inferior leads, and ST segment changes.[71] Chest x-ray findings vary from normal to abnormal and are of little value in confirming the presence of a PE. Abnormal findings include cardiomegaly, pleural effusion, elevated hemidiaphragm, enlargement of the right descending pulmonary artery (Palla sign), a wedge-shaped density above the diaphragm (Hampton hump), and the presence of atelectasis.[69] Transthoracic or transesophageal echocardiography is also useful in the identification of a PE, because it can provide visualization of any embolus in the central pulmonary arteries. In addition, it can be used for assessing the hemodynamic consequences of the PE on the right side of the heart.[71]

Differentiating a PE from other illnesses can be difficult because many clinical manifestations of a PE are found in a variety of other disorders.[67] Therefore various other tests may be necessary, including V/Q scintigraphy, pulmonary angiography, and DVT studies.[66,69,71] With the advent of more sophisticated CT scanners, spiral CT is also being used to diagnose a PE.[69–71] A definitive diagnosis of a PE requires confirmation by a high-probability V/Q scan, an abnormal pulmonary angiogram or CT scan, or strong clinical suspicion coupled with abnormal findings on lower extremity DVT studies.[69]

Medical Management

Medical management of a patient with a PE involves both prevention and treatment strategies. Prevention strategies include the use of prophylactic anticoagulation with low-dose or adjusted-dose heparin, LMWH, or oral anticoagulants. The use of pneumatic compression has also been demonstrated as an effective method of prophylaxis in low-risk patients.[24]

Treatment strategies include preventing the recurrence of a PE, facilitating clot dissolution, reversing the effects of pulmonary hypertension, promoting gas exchange, and preventing complications. Medical interventions to promote gas exchange include supplemental oxygen administration, intubation, and mechanical ventilation.[66]

Prevention of Recurrence

Interventions to prevent the recurrence of a PE include the administration of parenteral and oral anticoagulants. A parenteral anticoagulant is administered to prevent further clots from forming; however, this treatment has no effect on the existing clot. An oral anticoagulant is started, overlapping with the parenteral anticoagulant. Once the appropriate level of anticoagulation is achieved with the oral anticoagulant, the parenteral anticoagulant is discontinued. The patient remains on the oral anticoagulant for at least 3 months, depending on his or her risk for thromboembolic disease.[67]

Interruption of the inferior vena cava is reserved for patients in whom anticoagulation is contraindicated.[72] The procedure involves placement of a percutaneous venous filter (e.g., Greenfield filter) into the vena cava, usually below the renal arteries. The filter prevents further thrombotic emboli from migrating into the lungs.[73]

Clot Dissolution

The administration of fibrinolytic agents in the treatment of PE has had limited success. At the present time, fibrinolytic therapy is reserved for patients with a massive PE and concomitant hemodynamic instability. Either recombinant tissue-type plasminogen activator or streptokinase may be used. The therapeutic window for using fibrinolytic therapy is up to 14 days, although the most benefit is usually obtained when given within 48 hours.[71]

If fibrinolytic therapy is contraindicated, a pulmonary embolectomy may be performed to remove the clot. Generally, pulmonary embolectomy is performed as an open procedure while the patient is on cardiopulmonary bypass. An emerging alternative to surgical embolectomy is catheter embolectomy. It appears to be particularly useful if surgical embolectomy is unavailable or is contraindicated. It appears to be most successful when performed within 5 days of the occurrence of the PE.[72]

Reversal of Pulmonary Hypertension

To reverse the hemodynamic effects of pulmonary hypertension, additional measures may be taken, including the administration of inotropic agents and fluid. Fluids are administered to increase right ventricular preload, which would stretch the right ventricle and increase contractility, overcoming the elevated pulmonary arterial pressures. Inotropic agents also can be used to increase contractility to facilitate an increase in CO.[66,71]

Nursing Management

Prevention of PE is a major nursing focus, because most critically ill patients are at risk for this disorder. Nursing actions are aimed at preventing the development of DVT (Box 14.18), which is a major complication of immobility and a leading cause of PE. These measures include the use of pneumatic compression devices, active/passive range-of-motion exercises involving foot extension, adequate hydration, and progressive ambulation.[24]

The patient care management plan for a patient with a PE incorporates a variety of patient problems (Box 14.19). Nursing priorities focus on (1) optimizing oxygenation and ventilation, (2) monitoring for bleeding, (3) providing comfort and emotional support, (4) maintaining surveillance for complications, and (5) educating the patient and family.

Optimizing Oxygenation and Ventilation

Nursing interventions to optimize oxygenation and ventilation include positioning, preventing desaturation, and promoting secretion clearance. For further discussion of these interventions, see Nursing Management of ALF earlier in this chapter.

Monitoring for Bleeding

Patients receiving anticoagulant or fibrinolytic therapy are observed for signs of bleeding. The patient's gums, skin, urine, stool, and emesis are monitored for signs of overt or covert bleeding. In addition,

monitoring the patient's INR or activated partial thromboplastin time is critical to managing the anticoagulation therapy.

Educating the Patient and Family

Early in the patient's hospital stay, the patient and family are taught about pulmonary embolus, its causes, and its treatment (Box 14.20). Closer to discharge, the patient's education plan focuses on the interventions necessary for preventing the reoccurrence of DVT and subsequent emboli, signs and symptoms of DVT and anticoagulant complications, and measures to prevent bleeding. Patients who smoke are encouraged to stop smoking and referred to a smoking cessation program.

Interprofessional collaborative management of a patient with a pulmonary embolus is outlined in Box 14.21.

STATUS ASTHMATICUS

Description and Etiology

Asthma is a chronic obstructive pulmonary disease that is characterized by partially reversible airflow obstruction, airway inflammation, and hyperresponsiveness to a variety of stimuli.[74] Status asthmaticus is

---

◎ BOX 14.19   PRIORITY PATIENT CARE MANAGEMENT

Acute Pulmonary Embolism

- Impaired Gas Exchange due to ventilation/perfusion mismatching or intrapulmonary shunting
- Acute Pain due to transmission and perception of cutaneous, visceral, muscular, or ischemic impulses
- Anxiety due to threat to biologic, psychologic, and/or social integrity
- Powerlessness due to lack of control over current situation or disease progression
- Impaired Family Coping due to critically ill family member
- Lack of Knowledge of Treatment Regime due to lack of previous exposure to information (see Box 14.20, Priority Patient and Family Education: Acute Pulmonary Embolism)

Patient Care Management Plans are located in Appendix A.

QSEN   BOX 14.18   Quality Improvement

Prevention of Venous Thromboembolism

The following are key recommendations from the AACN Practice Alert: Preventing Venous Thromboembolism in Adults:

1. Assess all patients on admission to the critical care unit for risk factors of venous thromboembolism (VTE) and anticipate orders for VTE prophylaxis based on the risk assessment.
2. For patients at risk for VTE prophylaxis:
   - For acutely ill medical patients use low–molecular-weight heparin (LMWH), low-dose unfractionated heparin (LDUH), or fondaparinux.
   - For acutely ill general surgery patients use LMWH, LDUH, or mechanical prophylaxis (graduated compression stockings or intermittent pneumatic compression devices).
   - For critically ill patients use LMWH or LDUN.

- For patients at high risk for bleeding use mechanical prophylaxis.
- The use of mechanical prophylaxis should be anticipated in conjunction with anticoagulant-based prophylaxis regimens.

3. Review the patient's current risk factors daily during multidisciplinary rounds. Risk factors include the patient's current clinical status and response to treatment, the need for central venous access devices, and the patient's current VTE prophylaxis regimen and risk for bleeding.
4. Maximize the patient's mobility whenever possible. Implement measures to reduce the amount of time the patient is immobile. Mobilizing the patient does not negate the need for chemical prophylaxis, because the patient may still be at risk for VTE.
5. Ensure that mechanical prophylaxis devices are fitted properly and in use at all times except when being removed for cleaning and/or inspection of skin.

Modified from American Association of Critical-Care Nurses. AACN Practice Alert: preventing venous thromboembolism in adults. *Crit Care Nurse.* 2016;36(5):e20–e23.

✳ BOX 14.20 PRIORITY PATIENT AND FAMILY EDUCATION

Acute Pulmonary Embolism

Before discharge, the patient should be able to teach back the following topics:

- Pathophysiology of disease
- Specific etiology
- Modification of precipitating factors
- Measures to prevent deep vein thrombosis (DVT) (e.g., avoid tight-fitting clothes, crossing legs, and prolonged sitting or standing; elevate legs when sitting; exercise)
- Signs and symptoms of DVT (e.g., redness, swelling, sharp or deep leg pain)
- Importance of taking medications
- Signs and symptoms of anticoagulant complications (e.g., excessive bruising, discoloration of skin, changes in color of urine or stools)
- Measures to prevent bleeding (e.g., use soft-bristle toothbrush, caution when shaving)

BOX 14.21 Collaborative Management of Acute Pulmonary Embolism

- Administer oxygen therapy.
- Intubate patient.
- Initiate mechanical ventilation.
- Administer medications:
  - Fibrinolytic therapy
  - Anticoagulants
  - Bronchodilators
  - Inotropic agents
  - Sedatives
  - Analgesics
- Administer fluids.
- Position patient to optimize ventilation/perfusion matching.
- Maintain surveillance for complications:
  - Bleeding
  - Acute respiratory distress syndrome
- Provide comfort and emotional support.

a severe asthma attack that fails to respond to conventional therapy with bronchodilators, which may result in ALF.[75,76]

The precipitating cause of the attack is usually an upper respiratory infection, allergen exposure, or a decrease in antiinflammatory medications. Other factors that have been implicated include over-reliance on bronchodilators, environmental pollutants, lack of access to health care, failure to identify worsening airflow obstruction, and noncompliance with the health care regimen.[75]

Pathophysiology

An asthma attack is initiated when exposure to an irritant or trigger occurs, resulting in the initiation of the inflammatory-immune response in the airways. Bronchospasm occurs along with increased vascular permeability and increased mucus production. Mucosal edema and thick, tenacious mucus further increase airway responsiveness. The combination of bronchospasm, airway inflammation, and hyperresponsiveness results in narrowing of the airways and airflow obstruction. These changes have significant effects on the pulmonary and cardiovascular systems.[75]

Pulmonary Effects

As the diameter of the airways decreases, airway resistance increases, resulting in increased residual volume, hyperinflation of the lungs, increased work of breathing, and abnormal distribution of ventilation. V/Q mismatching occurs, which results in hypoxemia. Alveolar dead space also increases as hypoxic vasoconstriction occurs, resulting in hypercapnia.[75]

Cardiovascular Effects

Inspiratory muscle force also increases in an attempt to ventilate the hyperinflated lungs. This results in a significant increase in negative intrapleural pressure, leading to an increase in venous return and pooling of blood in the right ventricle. The stretched right ventricle causes the intraventricular septum to shift, impinging on the left ventricle. In addition, the left ventricle has to work harder to pump blood from the markedly negative pressure in the thorax to elevated pressure in systemic circulation. This leads to a decrease in CO and a fall in systolic blood pressure on inspiration (pulsus paradoxus).[75]

Assessment and Diagnosis

The patient may initially present with a cough, wheezing, and dyspnea. As the attack continues, the patient develops tachypnea, tachycardia, diaphoresis, increased accessory muscle use, and pulsus paradoxus greater than 25 mm Hg. Decreased level of consciousness, inability to speak, significantly diminished or absent breath sounds, and inability to lie supine herald the onset of ALF.[74–76]

Initial ABGs indicate hypocapnia and respiratory alkalosis caused by hyperventilation. As the attack continues and the patient starts to fatigue, hypoxemia and hypercapnia develop.[76] Lactic acidosis also may occur as a result of lactate overproduction by the respiratory muscles. The end result is the development of respiratory and metabolic acidosis.

Deterioration of pulmonary function tests despite aggressive bronchodilator therapy is diagnostic of status asthmaticus and indicates the potential need for intubation. A peak expiratory flow rate (PEFR) less than 40% of predicted or forced expiratory volume in 1 second (maximum volume of gas that the patient can exhale in 1 second) less than 20% of predicted indicates severe airflow obstruction, and the need for intubation with mechanical ventilation may be imminent.[77]

Medical Management

Medical management of a patient with status asthmaticus is directed toward supporting oxygenation and ventilation. Bronchodilators, corticosteroids, oxygen therapy, and intubation and mechanical ventilation are the mainstays of therapy.[76]

Bronchodilators

Inhaled beta-2 agonists and anticholinergics are the bronchodilators of choice for status asthmaticus. Beta-2 agonists promote bronchodilation and can be administered by nebulizer or metered-dose inhaler (MDI). Usually larger and more frequent doses are given, and the medication is titrated to the patient's response. Anticholinergics that inhibit bronchoconstriction are not very effective by themselves, but in conjunction with beta-2 agonists, they have a synergistic effect and produce a greater improvement in airflow. The routine use of xanthines is not recommended in the treatment of status asthmaticus, because they have been shown to have no therapeutic benefit.[75–77]

Many studies have focused on the bronchodilator abilities of magnesium. Although it has been demonstrated that magnesium is inferior to beta-2 agonists as a bronchodilator, it may be beneficial in patients who are refractory to conventional treatment. A bolus of 1 to 4 g of intravenous magnesium given over 10 to 40 minutes has been reported to produce desirable effects.[75-77]

Many other studies are evaluating the effects of leukotriene inhibitors such as zafirlukast, montelukast, and zileuton in the treatment of status asthmaticus. Leukotrienes are inflammatory mediators known to cause bronchoconstriction and airway inflammation. Research suggests that these agents may be beneficial as bronchodilators in patients who are refractory to beta-2 agonists.[77]

Systemic Corticosteroids

Intravenous or oral corticosteroids also are used in the treatment of status asthmaticus. Their antiinflammatory effects limit mucosal edema, decrease mucus production, and potentiate beta-2 agonists. It usually takes 6 to 8 hours for the effects of the corticosteroids to become evident.[76] The use of inhaled corticosteroids for the treatment of status asthmaticus is undecided at the present time.[75,76] Initial studies indicate they may be beneficial in certain patient populations.[76]

Oxygen Therapy

Initial treatment of hypoxemia is with supplemental oxygen. High-flow oxygen therapy is administered to keep the patient's oxygen saturation greater than 92%.[75] Another therapy currently under investigation is the use of heliox. A mixture of helium and oxygen, heliox, has a lower density and higher viscosity than an oxygen and air mixture. Heliox is believed to reduce the work of breathing and improve gas exchange because it flows more easily through constricted areas. Studies have shown that it reduces air trapping and carbon dioxide and helps relieve respiratory acidosis.[75]

Intubation and Mechanical Ventilation

Indications for mechanical ventilation include cardiac or respiratory arrest, disorientation, failure to respond to bronchodilator therapy, and exhaustion.[75-77] A large endotracheal tube (8 mm) is used to decrease airway resistance and to facilitate suctioning of secretions. Ventilating the patient with status asthmaticus can be very difficult. High inflation pressures are avoided, because they can result in barotrauma. The use of PEEP is monitored closely, because the patient is prone to developing air trapping. Patient-ventilator asynchrony also can be a major problem. Sedation and neuromuscular paralysis may be necessary to allow for adequate ventilation of the patient.[75,77]

Nursing Management

The patient care management plan for a patient with status asthmaticus incorporates a variety of patient problems (Box 14.22). Nursing priorities focus on (1) optimizing oxygenation and ventilation, (2) providing comfort and emotional support, (3) maintaining surveillance for complications, and (4) educating the patient and family. A systematic review examined the effect of severe asthma on the quality of life and found that the symptoms and activity limitations had a negative effect on the quality of life for these patients.[78]

Optimizing Oxygenation and Ventilation

Nursing interventions to optimize oxygenation and ventilation include positioning, preventing desaturation, and promoting secretion clearance. For further discussion of these interventions, see Nursing Management of ALF earlier in this chapter.

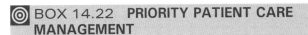

> **BOX 14.22 PRIORITY PATIENT CARE MANAGEMENT**
>
> **Status Asthmaticus**
> - Impaired Gas Exchange due to alveolar hypoventilation
> - Impaired Breathing Pattern due to musculoskeletal fatigue or neuromuscular impairment
> - Impaired Airway Clearance due to excessive secretions or abnormal viscosity of mucus
> - Anxiety due to threat to biologic, psychologic, and/or social integrity
> - Lack of Knowledge of Treatment Regime due to lack of previous exposure to information (see Box 14.23, Priority Patient and Family Education: Status Asthmaticus)
>
> Patient Care Management Plans are located in Appendix A.

Educating the Patient and Family

Early in the patient's hospital stay, the patient and family are taught about asthma, its triggers, and its treatment (Box 14.23). Closer to discharge, patient and family education focuses on the interventions necessary for preventing the recurrence of status asthmaticus, early warning signs of worsening airflow obstruction, correct use of an inhaler and a peak flowmeter, measures to prevent pulmonary infections, and signs and symptoms of a pulmonary infection. Patients who smoke are encouraged to stop smoking and referred to a smoking cessation program. In addition, the importance of participating in a pulmonary rehabilitation program is stressed.

Interprofessional collaborative management of a patient with status asthmaticus is outlined in Box 14.24.

LONG-TERM MECHANICAL VENTILATOR DEPENDENCE

Description

Long-term mechanical ventilator dependence (LTMVD) is a secondary disorder that occurs when a patient requires assisted ventilation longer than expected given the patient's underlying condition. It is the result of complex medical problems that do not allow the weaning process to take place in a normal and timely manner. Generally, the patient has failed multiple weaning attempts. A review of the literature reveals a great deal of confusion regarding an exact definition of LTMVD, particularly in regard to an actual time frame. One approach is to consider weaning as simple, difficult, or prolonged:[79]

- Short weaning: The first weaning attempt results in termination of the weaning process within 1 day either because of successful separation from the ventilator or death.
- Difficult weaning: The weaning process is completed after more than 1 day but in less than 1 week after the first separation attempt either because of successful separation from the ventilator or death.
- Prolonged weaning: The weaning process is still not terminated 7 days after the first separation attempt.
- Prolonged weaning leading to a successful separation from the ventilator after 7 days or more after the first attempt.
- Prolonged weaning without successful separation from the ventilator.

Etiology and Pathophysiology

Approximately 20% of patients requiring mechanical ventilation develop LTMVD.[80] A wide variety of physiologic and psychologic

✳ BOX 14.23   PRIORITY PATIENT AND FAMILY EDUCATION

Status Asthmaticus

Before discharge, the patient should be able to teach back the following topics:

- Pathophysiology of disease
- Specific etiology
- Early warning signs of worsening airflow obstruction (20% decrease in peak expiratory flow rate below predicted or personal best, increase in cough, shortness of breath, chest tightness, wheezing)
- Treatment of attacks
- Importance of taking prescribed medications and avoidance of over-the-counter asthma medications
- Correct use of an inhaler (with and without spacer device)

- Correct use of a peak flowmeter
- Removal or avoidance of environmental triggers (e.g., pollen; dust; mold spores; cat and dog dander; cold, dry air; strong odors; household aerosols; tobacco smoke; air pollution)
- Measures to prevent pulmonary infections (e.g., proper nutrition and hand-washing, immunization against *Streptococcus pneumoniae* and influenza viruses)
- Signs and symptoms of pulmonary infection (e.g., sputum color change, shortness of breath, fever)
- Importance of participating in pulmonary rehabilitation program

BOX 14.24   Collaborative Management of Status Asthmaticus

- Administer oxygen therapy.
- Intubate patient.
- Initiate mechanical ventilation.
- Administer medications:
  - Bronchodilators
  - Corticosteroids
  - Sedatives
- Maintain surveillance for complications:
  - Acute lung failure
- Provide comfort and emotional support.

factors contribute to the development of LTMVD. Physiologic factors include conditions that result in decreased gas exchange, increased ventilatory workload, increased ventilatory demand, decreased ventilatory drive, and increased respiratory muscle fatigue (Box 14.25).[80] Psychologic factors include conditions that result in loss of breathing pattern control, lack of motivation and confidence, and delirium

(Box 14.26).[81] The development of LTMVD also is affected by the severity and duration of the patient's current illness and any underlying chronic health problems.

Medical and Nursing Management

The goal of medical and nursing management of patients with LTMVD is successful weaning. The management of a patient with LTMVD is described within this framework. In addition, the common patient problems for this patient population are listed in Box 14.27.

Preweaning Stage

For a patient with LTMVD, the preweaning phase consists of resolving the precipitating event that necessitated ventilatory assistance and preventing the physiologic and psychologic factors that can interfere with weaning. Before any attempts at weaning, the patient is assessed for weaning readiness, an approach is determined, and a method is selected.

Weaning preparedness. The patient should be physiologically and psychologically prepared to initiate the weaning process by addressing factors that can interfere with weaning. Aggressive medical management to prevent and treat V/Q mismatching, intrapulmonary shunting, anemia, heart failure, decreased lung compliance, increased

BOX 14.25   Physiologic Factors Contributing to Long-Term Mechanical Ventilator Dependence

- Decreased gas exchange
  - Ventilation/perfusion mismatching
  - Intrapulmonary shunting
  - Alveolar hypoventilation
  - Anemia
  - Acute heart failure
- Increased ventilatory workload
  - Decreased lung compliance
  - Increased airway resistance
  - Small endotracheal tube
  - Decreased ventilatory sensitivity
  - Improper positioning
  - Abdominal distention
  - Dyspnea
- Increased ventilatory demand
  - Increased pulmonary dead space
  - Increased metabolic demands
  - Improper ventilator mode/settings

- Metabolic acidosis
- Overfeeding
- Decreased ventilatory drive
  - Respiratory alkalosis
  - Metabolic alkalosis
  - Hypothyroidism
  - Sedatives
  - Malnutrition
- Increased respiratory muscle fatigue
  - Increased ventilatory workload
  - Increased ventilatory demand
  - Malnutrition
  - Hypokalemia
  - Hypomagnesemia
  - Hypophosphatemia
  - Hypothyroidism
  - Critical illness polyneuropathy
  - Inadequate muscle rest

BOX 14.26 Psychologic Factors Contributing to Long-Term Mechanical Ventilator Dependence

- Loss of breathing pattern control
  - Anxiety
  - Fear
  - Dyspnea
  - Pain
  - Ventilator asynchrony
  - Lack of confidence in ability to breathe
- Lack of motivation and confidence
  - Inadequate trust in staff
  - Depersonalization

- Hopelessness
- Powerlessness
- Depression
- Inadequate communication
- Delirium
  - Sensory overload
  - Sensory deprivation
  - Sleep deprivation
  - Pain
  - Medications

airway resistance, acid–base disturbances, hypothyroidism, abdominal distention, and electrolyte imbalances should be initiated. In addition, interventions to decrease the work of breathing should be implemented, such as replacing a small endotracheal tube with a larger tube or a tracheostomy, suctioning airway secretions, administering bronchodilators, optimizing the ventilator settings and trigger sensitivity, initiating early mobilization, and positioning the patient in straight alignment with the head of the bed elevated at least 30 degrees. Enteral nutrition is started, and the patient's nutrition state optimized. Physical therapy is initiated, because increased mobility facilitates weaning. A means of communication should be established with the patient. Sedatives can be administered to provide anxiety control, but it is critical to avoid respiratory depression.

Weaning readiness. Although various methods for assessing weaning readiness have been developed, none has proven to be very accurate in predicting weaning success in a patient with LTMVD. Because so many variables can affect the patient's ability to wean, any assessment of weaning readiness should incorporate these variables. Cardiac function, gas exchange, pulmonary mechanics, nutrition status, electrolyte and fluid balance, and motivation are considered when making the decision to wean. This assessment is ongoing to reflect the dynamic nature of the process.[81,82]

Weaning approach. Although weaning patients requiring short-term mechanical ventilation is a relatively simple process that can usually be accomplished with a nurse and respiratory therapist, weaning a patient with LTMVD is a much more complex process that usually requires a multidisciplinary team approach. Multidisciplinary weaning teams that use a coordinated and collaborative approach to weaning have demonstrated improved patient outcomes and decreased weaning times. The team ideally consists of a physician, nurse, respiratory therapist, dietitian, physical therapist, social worker or case manager,

and clinical nurse specialist. Additional members, if possible, include an occupational therapist, a speech therapist, and a discharge planner. Working together, the team members develop a comprehensive plan of care for the patient that is efficient, consistent, progressive, and cost-effective.[83] Several studies have demonstrated successful weaning through the use of nurse and respiratory therapist–managed protocols.[84]

Weaning method. Various weaning methods are available, and no one method has consistently proven to be superior to the others. These methods include T-tube (T-piece), CPAP, pressure support ventilation (PSV), and SIMV. One multicenter study lends evidence to support the use of PSV for weaning over T-tube or SIMV weaning. Often these weaning methods are used in combination with each other, such as SIMV with PSV, CPAP with PSV, or SIMV with CPAP.[80]

Weaning Process Stage

For a patient with LTMVD, the weaning process phase consists of initiating the weaning method selected and minimizing the physiologic and psychologic factors that can interfere with weaning. It is imperative that the patient not become exhausted during this phase, because this can result in a setback in the weaning process. During this phase, the patient is assessed for weaning progress and signs of weaning intolerance.[81]

Weaning initiation. Ideally, weaning is initiated in the morning while the patient is rested. Before starting the weaning process, the patient is given an explanation of how the process works and a description of the sensations to expect and is reassured that he or she will be closely monitored and returned to the original ventilator mode and settings if any difficulty occurs. This information is reinforced with each weaning attempt.

T-tube and CPAP weaning are accomplished by removing the patient from the ventilator and placing the patient on a T-tube or placing the patient on CPAP mode for a specified duration of time, known as a weaning trial, for a specified number of times per day. When the weaning trial is over, the patient is placed on the assist-control mode or similar mode and allowed to rest to prevent respiratory muscle fatigue. The duration of time spent weaning is gradually increased, as is the frequency, until the patient is able to breathe spontaneously for 24 hours. If PSV is used in conjunction with CPAP, the PSV is initially set to provide the patient with an assisted tidal volume of 10 to 12 mL/kg, and this is gradually weaned until a level of 6 to 8 cm H_2O of pressure support is achieved. Weaning with SIMV and PSV is accomplished by gradually decreasing the number of breaths or the amount of pressure support the patient receives by a specified amount until the patient is able to breathe spontaneously for 24 hours.[81]

BOX 14.27 PRIORITY PATIENT CARE MANAGEMENT

Long-Term Mechanical Ventilation Dependence
- Impaired Ventilatory Weaning due to physical, psychosocial, or situational factors
- Risk for Aspiration
- Impaired Nutritional Intake due to lack of exogenous nutrients or increased metabolic demand
- Risk for Infection
- Relocation Stress due to transfer out of intensive care unit

Patient Care Management Plans are located in Appendix A.

Weaning progress. Weaning progress can be evaluated using various methods. Evaluation of weaning progress when using a weaning method that gradually withdraws ventilatory support, such as SIMV or PSV, can be accomplished by measuring the percentage of the minute ventilation requirement that is provided by the ventilator. If the percentage steadily decreases, weaning is progressing. Evaluation of weaning progress when using a weaning method that removes ventilatory support, such as T-tube or CPAP, can be accomplished by measuring the amount of time the patient remains free from support. If the time steadily increases, weaning is progressing.

Weaning intolerance. Once the weaning process has begun, the patient is continuously assessed for signs of intolerance. When present, these signs indicate when to place the patient back on the ventilator or to return the patient to the previous ventilator settings. Commonly used indicators include dyspnea; accessory muscle use; restlessness; anxiety; change in facial expression; changes in heart rate and blood pressure; rapid, shallow breathing; and discomfort.[81] See the patient management plan "Impaired Ventilatory Weaning" in Appendix A for specific interventions to manage these issues.

Facilitative therapies. Additional therapies may be needed to facilitate weaning in a patient who is having difficulty making weaning progress. These therapies include ventilatory muscle training and biofeedback. Inspiratory muscle training is used to enhance the strength and endurance of the respiratory muscles. Biofeedback can be used to promote relaxation and assist in the management of dyspnea and anxiety.

Weaning Outcome Stage

Two outcomes are possible for a patient with LTMVD: weaning completed and incomplete weaning.

Weaning completed. Weaning is deemed successful when a patient is able to breathe spontaneously for 24 hours without ventilatory support. When this occurs, the patient may be extubated or decannulated at any time, although this is not necessary for weaning to be considered successful.

Incomplete weaning. Weaning is deemed incomplete when a patient has reached a plateau (5 days at the same ventilatory support level without any changes) in the weaning process despite managing the physiologic and psychologic factors that impede weaning. Thus the patient is unable to breathe spontaneously for 24 hours without full or partial ventilatory support. Once this occurs, the patient is placed in a subacute ventilator facility or discharged home on a ventilator with home care nursing follow-up.

ADDITIONAL RESOURCES

See Box 14.28 for additional resources for the management of the patient with pulmonary dysfunction.

REFERENCES

1. MacSweeney R, McAuley DF, Matthay MA. Acute lung failure. *Semin Respir Crit Care Med*. 2011;32(5):607–625. https://doi.org/10.1055/s-0031-1287870.
2. Lamba TS, Sharara RS, Singh AC, Balaan M. Pathophysiology and classification of respiratory failure. *Crit Care Nurs Q*. 2016;39(2):85–93. https://doi.org/10.1097/CNQ.0000000000000102.
3. Wright BJ. Lung-protective ventilation strategies and adjunctive treatments for the emergency medicine patient with acute respiratory failure. *Emerg Med Clin N Am*. 2014;32(4):871–887. https://doi.org/10.1016/j.emc.2014.07.012.
4. Balk R, Bone RC. Classification of acute respiratory failure. *Med Clin North Am*. 1983;67(3):551–556.

5. Weinberger SE, Cockrill BA, Mandel J. Classification and pathophysiologic aspects of respiratory failure. In: Weinberger SE, Cockrill BA, Mandel J, eds. *Principles of Pulmonary Medicine*. 7th ed. Philadelphia: Elsevier; 2019.
6. Hocker S. Primary acute neuromuscular respiratory failure. *Neurol Clin*. 2017;35(4):707–721. https://doi.org/10.1016/j.ncl.2017.06.007.
7. Broaddus CV, Gomez A. In: Broaddus VC, ed. *Murray and Nadel's Textbook of Respiratory Medicine*. 7th ed. Philadelphia: Elsevier; 2022.
8. Siela D, Kidd M. Oxygen requirements for acutely and critically ill patients. *Crit Care Nurse*. 2017;37(4):58–70. https://doi.org/10.4037/ccn2017627.
9. Hill NS, Garpestad E, Schumaker GL. Acute ventilatory failure. In: Broaddus VC, ed. *Murray and Nadel's Textbook of Respiratory Medicine*. 7th ed. Philadelphia: Elsevier; 2022.
10. Dakin J, Griffiths M. The pulmonary physician in critical care 1: pulmonary investigations for acute respiratory failure. *Thorax*. 2002;57(1):79–85.
11. O'Driscoll BR, Smith R. Oxygen use in critical illness. *Respir Care*. 2019;64(10):1293–1307. https://doi.org/10.4187/respcare.07044 (epub ahead of print).
12. Zhao H, Wang H, Sun F, Lyu S, An Y. High-flow nasal cannula oxygen therapy is superior to conventional oxygen therapy but not to noninvasive mechanical ventilation on intubation rate: a systematic review and meta-analysis. *Crit Care*. 2017;21(1):184. https://doi.org/10.1186/s13054-017-1760-8.
13. Bello G, Ionescu Maddalena A, Giammatteo V, Antonelli M. Noninvasive options. *Crit Care Clin*. 2018;34(3):395–412. https://doi.org/10.1016/j.ccc.2018.03.007.
14. Rochwerg B, Brochard L, Elliot MW, et al. Official ERS/ATS clinical practice guidelines: noninvasive ventilation for acute respiratory failure. *Eur Respir J*. 2017;50(2):1602426. https://doi.org/10.1183/13993003.02426-2016.
15. Pham T, Brochard LJ, Slutsky AS. Mechanical ventilation: state of the art. *Mayo Clin Proc*. 2017;92(9):1382–1400. https://doi.org/10.1016/j.mayocp.2017.05.004.
16. Brand J, Arrowsmith JE. Respiratory system: applied pharmacology. *Anaesth Intensive Care Med*. 2017;18(12):609–613. https://doi.org/10.1016/j.mpaic.2017.09.001.
17. Devlin JW, Skrobik Y, Gélinas C, et al. Clinical practice guidelines for the prevention and management of pain, agitation/sedation, delirium, immobility, and sleep disruption in adult patients in the ICU. *Crit Care Med*. 2018;46(9):e825–e873. https://doi.org/10.1097/CCM.0000000000003299.

18. DeBacker J, Hart N, Fan E. Neuromuscular blockade in the 21st century management of the critically ill patient. *Chest*. 2017;151(3):697–706. https://doi.org/10.1016/j.chest.2016.10.040.

19. Reddy AJ, Lam SW, Bauer SR, Guzman JA. Lactic acidosis: clinical implications and management strategies. *Cleve Clin J Med*. 2015;82(9):615–624. https://doi.org/10.3949/ccjm.82a.14098.

20. McClave SA, Taylor BE, Martindale RG, et al. Guidelines for the provision and assessment of nutrition support therapy in the adult critically ill patient: Society of Critical Care Medicine (SCCM) and American Society for Parenteral and Enteral Nutrition (ASPEN). *J Parenter Enteral Nutr*. 2016;40(2):159–211. https://doi.org/10.1177/0148607115621863.

21. Patel JJ, Hurt RT, McClave SA, Martindale RG. Critical care nutrition: where's the evidence? *Crit Care Clin*. 2017;33(2):397–412. https://doi.org/10.1016/j.ccc.2016.12.006.

22. Girard TD, Dittus RS, Ely EW. Critical illness brain injury. *Annu Rev Med*. 2016;67:497–513. https://doi.org/10.1146/annurev-med-050913-015722.

23. van der Jagt, Miranda DR. Beta-blockers in intensive care medicine: potential benefit in acute brain injury and acute respiratory distress syndrome. *Recent Pat Cardiovasc Drug Discov*. 2012;7(2):141–151.

24. Kahn SR, Lim W, Dunn AS, et al. Prevention of VTE in nonsurgical patients: antithrombotic therapy and prevention of thrombosis, 9th ed, American College of Chest Physicians Evidence-Based Clinical Practice Guidelines. *Chest*. 2012;141(suppl 2):e195S–e226S. https://doi.org/10.1378/chest.11-2296.

25. Reintam Balser A, Jakob SM, Starkopf J. Gastrointestinal failure in the ICU. *Curr Opin Crit Care*. 2016;22(2):128–141. https://doi.org/10.1097/MCC.0000000000000286.

26. Mezidi M, Guérin C. Effects of patient positioning on respiratory mechanics in mechanically ventilated ICU patients. *Ann Transl Med*. 2018;6(19):384. https://doi.org/10.21037/atm.2018.05.50.

27. Johnson KL, Meyenburg T. Physiological rationale and current evidence for therapeutic positioning of critically ill patients. *AACN Adv Crit Care*. 2009;20(3):228–242. https://doi.org/10.1097/NCI.0b013e3181add8db.

28. Marklew A. Body positioning and its effect on oxygenation—a literature review. *Nurs Crit Care*. 2006;11(1):16–22. https://doi.org/10.1111/j.1362-1017.2006.00141.x.

29. Cosenza JJ, Norton LC. Secretion clearance: state-of-the-art from a nursing perspective. *Crit Care Nurse*. 1986;6(4):23–39.

30. Metheny NA, Frantz RA. Head-of-bed elevation in critically ill patients: a review. *Crit Care Nurse*. 2013;33(3):53–66. https://doi.org/10.4037/ccn2013456.

31. Krishnagopalan S, Johnson EW, Low LL, Kaufman LJ. Body positioning of intensive care patients: clinical practice versus standards. *Crit Care Med*. 2002;30(11):2588–2592.

32. Stiller K. Physiotherapy in intensive care: an updated systematic review. *Chest*. 2013;144(3):825–847. https://doi.org/10.1378/chest.12-2930.

33. Stickland SL, Rubin BK, Drescher GS, et al. AARC clinical practice guideline: effectiveness of nonpharmacologic airway clearance therapies in hospitalized patients. *Respir Care*. 2013;58(12):2187–2193. https://doi.org/10.4187/respcare.02925.

34. Del Sorbo L, Slutsky AS. Acute respiratory distress syndrome and multiple organ failure. *Curr Opin Crit Care*. 2011;17(1):1–6. https://doi.org/10.1097/MCC.0b013e3283427295.

35. Derwall M, Martin L, Rossaint R. The acute respiratory distress syndrome: pathophysiology, current clinical practice, and emerging therapies. *Expert Rev Respir Med*. 2018;12(12):1021–1029. https://doi.org/10.1080/17476348.2018.1548280.

36. Fan E, Brodie D, Slutsky AS. Acute respiratory distress syndrome: advances in diagnosis and treatment. *J Am Med Assoc*. 2018;319(7):698–710. https://doi.org/10.1001/jama.2017.21907.

37. The ARDS Definition Task Force. Acute respiratory distress syndrome: the Berlin definition. *J Am Med Assoc*. 2012;307(23):2526–2533. https://doi.org/10.1001/jama.2012.5669.

38. Dechert RE, Hass CF, Ostwani W. Current knowledge of acute lung injury and acute respiratory distress syndrome. *Crit Care Nurs Clin N Am*. 2012;24(3):377–401. https://doi.org/10.1016/j.ccell.2012.06.006.

39. Kaku S, Nguyen CD, Htet NN, et al. Acute respiratory distress syndrome: etiology, pathogenesis, and summary of management. *J Intensive Care Med*. 2020;35(8):723–737. https://doi.org/10.1177/0885066619855021.

40. Przybysz TM, Heffner AC. Early treatment of severe acute respiratory distress syndrome. *Emerg Med Clin North Am*. 2016;34(1):1–14. https://doi.org/10.1016/j.emc.2015.08.001.

41. Cannon JW, Gutsche JT, Brodie D. Optimal strategies for severe acute respiratory distress syndrome. *Crit Care Clin*. 2017;33(2):259–275. https://doi.org/10.1016/j.ccc.2016.12.010.

42. Chiumello D, Brioni M. Severe hypoxemia: which strategy to choose. *Crit Care*. 2016;20(1):132. https://doi.org/10.1186/s13054-016-1304-7.

43. Mauri T, Lazzeri M, Bellani G, Zanella A, Grasselli G. Respiratory mechanics to understand ARDS and guide mechanical ventilation. *Physiol Meas*. 2017;38(12):R390–H303. https://doi.org/10.1088/1361-6579/aa9052.

44. Barnes T, Zochios V, Parhar K. Re-examining permissive hypercapnia in ARDS: a narrative review. *Chest*. 2018;154(1):185–195. https://doi.org/10.1016/j.chest.2017.11.010.

45. Goligher EC, Munshi L, Adhikari NKJ, et al. High-frequency oscillation for adult patients with acute respiratory distress syndrome: a systematic review and meta-analysis. *Ann Am Thorac Soc*. 2017;14(suppl 4):S289–S296. https://doi.org/10.1513/AnnalsATS.201704-341OT.

46. Combes A, Pesenti A, Ranieri VM. Fifty years of research in ARDS. Is extracorporeal circulation the future of acute respiratory distress syndrome management? *Am J Respir Crit Care Med*. 2017;195(9):1161–1170. https://doi.org/10.1164/rccm.201701-0217CP.

47. Gattinoni L, Cressoni M, Brazzi L. Fluids in ARDS: from onset through recovery. *Curr Opin Crit Care*. 2014;20(4):373–377. https://doi.org/10.1097/MCC.0000000000000105.

48. Munshi L, Del Sorbo L, Adhikari NKJ, et al. Prone position for acute respiratory distress syndrome. A systematic review and meta-analysis. *Ann Am Thorac Soc*. 2017;14(suppl 4):S280–S288. https://doi.org/10.1513/AnnalsATS.201704-343OT.

49. Kalil AC, Metersky ML, Klompas M, et al. Management of adults with hospital-acquired and ventilator-associated pneumonia: 2016 clinical practice guidelines by the Infectious Diseases Society of America and the American Thoracic Society. *Clin Infect Dis*. 2016;63(5):e61–e111. https://doi.org/10.1093/cid/ciw353.

50. Rider AC, Frazee BW. Community-acquired pneumonia. *Emer Med Clin North Am*. 2018;36(4):665–683. https://doi.org/10.1016/j.emc.2018.07.001.

51. Prina E, Raznzani OT, Torres A. Community-acquired pneumonia. *Lancet*. 2015;386(9998):1097–1108. https://doi.org/10.1016/S0140-6736(15)60733-4.

52. Spalding MC, Cripps MW, Minshall CT. Ventilator-associated pneumonia: new definitions. *Crit Care Clin*. 2017;33(2):277–292. https://doi.org/10.1016/j.ccc.2016.12.009.

53. Lanks CW, Musani AL, Hsia DW. Community-acquired pneumonia and hospital-acquired pneumonia. *Med Clin North Am*. 2019;103(3):487–501. https://doi.org/10.1016/j.mcna.2018.12.008.

54. Lau ACW, So HM, Tang SL, et al. Prevention of ventilator associated pneumonia. *Hong Kong Med J*. 2015;21(1):61–68.

55. Mandell LA, Niederman MS. Aspiration pneumonia. *N Engl J Med*. 2019;380(7):651–663. https://doi.org/10.1056/NEJMra1714562.

56. Henig O, Kaye KS. Bacterial pneumonia in older adults. *Infect Dis Clin North Am*. 2017;31(4):689–713. https://doi.org/10.1016/j.idc.2017.07.015.

57. Lee LS, Giesler DL, Gellad WF, Fine MJ. Antibiotic therapy for adults hospitalized with community-acquired pneumonia: a systematic review. *J Am Med Assoc*. 2016;315(6):593–602. https://doi.org/10.1001/jama.2016.0115.

58. Minhas JS, Halligan K, Dargin JM. Independent lung ventilation in the management of ARDS and bronchopleural fistula. *Heart Lung*. 2016;45(3):258–260. https://doi.org/10.1016/j.hrtlng.2016.02.007.

59. Osman MF, Askari R. Infection control in the intensive care unit. *Surg Clin North Am*. 2014;94(6):1175–1194. https://doi.org/10.1016/j.suc.2014.08.011.

60. Bolon MK. Hand hygiene: an update. *Infect Dis Clin North Am*. 2016;30(3):591–607. https://doi.org/10.1016/j.idc.2016.04.007.

61. Hu X, Lee JS, Pianosi PT, Ryu JH. Aspiration-related pulmonary syndromes. *Chest*. 2015;147(3):815–823. https://doi.org/10.1378/chest.14-1049.

62. Paintal HS, Kuschner WG. Aspiration syndromes: 10 clinical pearls every physician should know. *Int J Clin Pract*. 2007;61(5):846–852. https://doi.org/10.1111/j.1742-1241.2007.01300.x.

63. Marik PE. Pulmonary aspiration syndrome. *Curr Opin Pulm Med*. 2011;17(3):148–154. https://doi.org/10.1097/MCP.0b013e32834397d6.

64. Lee AS, Ryu JH. Aspiration pneumonia and related syndromes. *Mayo Clin Proc.* 2018;93(6):752–762. https://doi.org/10.1016/j.mayocp.2018.03.011.

65. Schallom M, Orr J, Metheny N, Pierce J. Gastroesophageal reflux in critically ill patients. *Dimens Crit Care Nurs.* 2013;32(2):69–77. https://doi.org/10.1097/DCC.0b013e318280836b.

66. Doherty S. Pulmonary embolism: an update. *Aust Fam Physician.* 2017;46(11):816–820.

67. Kearon C, Akl EA, Ornelas J, et al. Antithrombotic therapy for VTE disease: CHEST guideline and expert panel report. *Chest.* 2016;149(2):315–352. https://doi.org/10.1016/j.chest.2015.11.026.

68. Jaff MR, McMurtry MS, Archer SL, et al. Management of massive and submassive pulmonary embolism, iliofemoral deep vein thrombosis, and chronic thromboembolic pulmonary hypertension: a scientific statement from the American Heart Association. *Circulation.* 2011;123(16):1788–1830. https://doi.org/10.1161/CIR.0b013e318214914f.

69. Tonelli AR, Dweik RA, Arroliga AC. Pulmonary vascular disease. In: Kacmarek RM, Stoller JK, Heuer AJ, eds. *Egan's Fundamentals of Respiratory Care.* 12th ed. St. Louis: Elsevier; 2021.

70. Essien EO, Rali P, Mathai SC. Pulmonary embolism. *Med Clin North Am.* 2019;103(3):549–564. https://doi.org/10.1016/j.mcna.2018.12.013.

71. Petriş AO, Konstantinides S, Tint D, Cimpoeşu D, Pop C. Therapeutic advances in emergency cardiology: acute pulmonary embolism. *Am J Ther.* 2019;26(2):e248–e256. https://doi.org/10.1097/MJT.0000000000000917.

72. Javed QA, Sista AK. Endovascular therapy for acute severe pulmonary embolism. *Int J Cardiovasc Imaging.* 2019;35(8):1443–1452. https://doi.org/10.1007/s10554-019-01567-z.

73. Olaf M, Coony R. Deep venous thrombosis. *Emerg Med Clin North Am.* 2017;35(4):743–770. https://doi.org/10.1016/j.emc.2017.06.003.

74. Trevor JL, Chipps BE. Severe asthma in primary care: identification and management. *Am J Med.* 2018;131(5):484–491. https://doi.org/10.1016/j.amjmed.2017.12.034.

75. Mannam P, Siegel MD. Analytic review: management of life-threatening asthma in adults. *J Intensive Care Med.* 2010;25(1):3–15. https://doi.org/10.1177/0885066609350866.

76. Mims JW. Asthma: definitions and pathophysiology. *Int Forum Allergy Rhinol.* 2015;5(suppl 1):S2–S6. https://doi.org/10.1002/alr.21609.

77. Castillo JR, Peters SP, Busse WW. Asthma exacerbations: pathogenesis, prevention, and treatment. *J Allergy Clin Immunol Pract.* 2017;5(4):918–927. https://doi.org/10.1016/j.jaip.2017.05.001.

78. Likhar N, Mothe RK, Esam H, Badgujar L, Kanukula A, Dang A. The impact of severe asthma on the quality of life: a systematic review. *Value Health.* 2015;18(7):A710. https://doi.org/10.1016/j.jval.2015.09.2673.

79. Béduneau G, Pham T, Schortgen F, et al. Epidemiology of weaning outcome according to a new definition. The WIND study. *Am J Respir Crit Care Med.* 2017;195(6):772–783. https://doi.org/10.1164/rccm.201602-0320OC.

80. Navalesi P, Frigerio P, Patzlaff A, Häußermann S, Henseke P, Kubitschek M. Prolonged weaning: from the intensive care unit to home. *Rev Port Pneumol.* 2014;20(5):264–272. https://doi.org/10.1016/j.rppnen.2014.04.006.

81. Cairo J. Weaning and discontinuation from mechanical ventilation. In: Cairo J, ed. *Pilbeam's Mechanical Ventilation, Physiological and Clinical Applications.* 7th ed. St Louis: Elsevier; 2020.

82. Ward D, Fulbrook P. Nursing strategies for effective weaning of the critically ill mechanically ventilated patient. *Crit Care Nurs Clin North Am.* 2016;28(4):499–512. https://doi.org/10.1016/j.cnc.2016.07.008.

83. White V, Curry J, Botti M. Multidisciplinary team developed and implemented protocols to assist mechanical ventilation weaning: a systematic review of literature. *Worldviews Evid Based Nurs.* 2011;8(1):51–59. https://doi.org/10.1111/j.1741-6787.2010.00198.x.

84. Borges LGA, Savi A, Teixeira C, et al. Mechanical ventilation weaning protocol improves medical adherence and results. *J Crit Care.* 2017;41:296–302. https://doi.org/10.1016/j.jcrc.2017.07.014.

15

Pulmonary Therapeutic Management

Kathleen M. Stacy

OXYGEN THERAPY

Normal cellular function depends on the delivery of an adequate supply of oxygen to the cells to meet their metabolic needs. The goal of oxygen therapy is to provide a sufficient concentration of inspired oxygen to permit full use of the oxygen-carrying capacity of the arterial blood; this ensures adequate cellular oxygenation, provided that the cardiac output and hemoglobin concentration are adequate.[1,2]

Principles of Therapy

Oxygen is an atmospheric gas that must also be considered a medication because, similar to most other medications, it has detrimental as well as beneficial effects. Oxygen is one of the most commonly used and misused medications. As a medication, oxygen must be administered for a good reason and in a proper, safe manner.[1] Oxygen is usually ordered in liters per minute (L/min), as a concentration of oxygen expressed as a percentage (e.g., 40%), or as a fraction of inspired oxygen (FiO_2; e.g., 0.4).

The primary indication for oxygen therapy is hypoxemia.[3] The amount of oxygen administered depends on the pathophysiologic mechanisms affecting the patient's oxygenation status. In most cases, the amount required should provide an arterial partial pressure of oxygen (PaO_2) of greater than 60 mm Hg or an arterial hemoglobin saturation (SaO_2) of greater than 90% during rest and exercise.[2] The concentration of oxygen given to an individual patient is a clinical judgment based on the many factors that influence oxygen transport, such as hemoglobin concentration, cardiac output, and arterial oxygen tension.[2]

After oxygen therapy has begun, the patient is continuously assessed for level of oxygenation and the factors affecting it. The patient's oxygenation status is evaluated several times daily until the desired oxygen level has been reached and has stabilized. If the desired response to the amount of oxygen delivered is not achieved, the oxygen supplementation is adjusted, and the patient's condition is reevaluated. It is important to use this dose-response method so that the lowest possible level of oxygen is administered that will still achieve a satisfactory PaO_2 or SaO_2.[2,3]

Methods of Delivery

Oxygen therapy can be delivered by many different devices (Table 15.1). Common problems with these devices include system leaks and obstructions, device displacement, and skin irritation. These devices are classified as low-flow, reservoir, or high-flow systems.[3]

Low-Flow Systems

A low-flow oxygen delivery system provides supplemental oxygen directly into the patient's airway at a flow of 8 L/min or less. Because this flow is insufficient to meet the patient's inspiratory volume requirements, this method of oxygen delivery results in a variable FiO_2 as the supplemental oxygen is mixed with room air. The patient's ventilatory pattern affects the FiO_2 of a low-flow system: as this pattern changes, differing amounts of room air gas are mixed with the constant flow of oxygen. A nasal cannula is an example of a low-flow device.[3]

Reservoir Systems

A reservoir system incorporates some type of device to collect and store oxygen between breaths. When the patient's inspiratory flow exceeds the oxygen flow of the oxygen delivery system, the patient is able to draw from the reservoir of oxygen to meet his or her inspiratory volume needs. Less mixing of the inspired oxygen occurs with room air than in a low-flow system. A reservoir oxygen delivery system can deliver a higher FiO_2 than a low-flow system. Examples of reservoir systems are simple face masks, partial rebreathing masks, and nonrebreathing masks.[3]

High-Flow Systems

With a high-flow system, the oxygen flows out of the device and into the patient's airways in an amount sufficient to meet all inspiratory volume requirements. This type of system is not affected by the patient's ventilatory pattern. A high-flow system uses either an air-entrainment system or a blending system to mix air and oxygen to achieve the desired FiO_2. An air-entrainment mask is an example of a high-flow system that delivers precisely controlled oxygen at the lower FiO_2 range.[3]

One newer high-flow system is the high-flow nasal cannula. With this system, warmed and humidified oxygen is delivered to the patient via a nasal cannula using a blending system. This system has been shown to improve oxygenation and ventilation and decrease the work of breathing in a patient with acute lung failure. A high-flow nasal cannula also is more comfortable and better tolerated than similar therapies.[4]

Complications of Oxygen Therapy

Oxygen, similar to most medications, has adverse effects and complications resulting from its use. The adage "if a little is good, a lot is better" does not apply to oxygen. The lung is designed to handle a concentration of 21% oxygen, with some adaptability to higher concentrations, but adverse effects and oxygen toxicity can result if a high concentration is administered for too long.[5]

Oxygen Toxicity

The most detrimental effect of breathing a high concentration of oxygen is the development of oxygen toxicity. Oxygen toxicity can occur in any patient who breathes oxygen concentrations of greater than

TABLE 15.1   Oxygen Therapy Systems.

Category	Device	Flow	FiO$_2$ Range (%)	FiO$_2$ Stability	Advantages	Disadvantages	Best Use
Low-flow	Nasal cannula	0.25–8 L/min (adults) ≤2 L/min (infants)	22–45	Variable	Use on adults, children, infants; easy to apply; disposable, low cost; well tolerated	Unstable, easily dislodged; high flows uncomfortable; can cause dryness or bleeding; polyps, deviated septum may block flow	Stable patient needing low FiO$_2$; home care patient requiring long-term therapy
	Nasal catheter	0.25–8 L/min	22–45	Variable	Use on adults, children, infants; good stability; disposable, low cost	Difficult to insert; high flows increase back-pressure; needs regular changing; polyps, deviated septum may block insertion; may provoke gagging, air swallowing, aspiration	Procedures in which cannula is difficult to use (bronchoscopy); long-term care for infants
	Transtracheal catheter	0.25–4 L/min	22–35	Variable	Lower oxygen usage/cost; eliminates nasal/skin irritation; improved compliance; increased exercise tolerance; increased mobility; enhanced image	High cost; surgical complications; infection; mucous plugging; lost tract	Home care or ambulatory patients who need increased mobility or who do not accept nasal oxygen
Reservoir	Reservoir cannula	0.25–4 L/min	22–35	Variable	Lower oxygen usage/cost; increased mobility; less discomfort because of lower flows	Unattractive, cumbersome; poor compliance; must be regularly replaced; breathing pattern affects performance	Home care or ambulatory patients who need increased mobility
	Simple mask	5–12 L/min	35–50	Variable	Use on adults, children, infants; quick, easy to apply; disposable, inexpensive	Uncomfortable; must be removed for eating; prevents radiant heat loss; blocks vomitus in unconscious patients	Emergencies; short-term therapy requiring moderate FiO$_2$
	Partial rebreathing mask	6–10 L/min (prevent bag collapse on inspiration)	35–60	Variable	Same as simple mask; moderate to high FiO$_2$	Same as simple mask; potential suffocation hazard	Emergencies; short-term therapy requiring moderate to high FiO$_2$
	Nonrebreathing mask	6–10 L/min (prevent bag collapse on inspiration)	55–70	Variable	Same as simple mask; high FiO$_2$	Same as simple mask; potential suffocation hazard	Emergencies; short-term therapy requiring high FiO$_2$
	Nonrebreathing circuit (closed)	3× V$_E$ (prevent bag collapse on inspiration)	21–100	Fixed	Full range of FiO$_2$	Potential suffocation hazard; requires 50 psi air or oxygen; blender failure common	Patients requiring precise FiO$_2$ at any level (21%–100%)

TABLE 15.1 Oxygen Therapy Systems.—cont'd

Category	Device	Flow	FiO$_2$ Range (%)	FiO$_2$ Stability	Advantages	Disadvantages	Best Use
High-flow	Air-entrainment mask	Varies; should provide output flow >60 L/min	24–50	Fixed	Easy to apply; disposable, inexpensive; stable, precise FiO$_2$	Limited to adult use; uncomfortable, noisy; must be removed for eating; FiO$_2$ >0.40 not ensured; FiO$_2$ varies with back-pressure	Unstable patients requiring precise low FiO$_2$
	Air-entrainment nebulizer	10–15 L/min input; should provide output flow of at least 60 L/min	28–100	Fixed	Provides temperature control and extra humidification	FiO$_2$ <28% or >0.40 not ensured; FiO$_2$ varies with back-pressure; high infection risk	Patients with artificial airways requiring low to moderate FiO$_2$
	Blending system (open)	Should provide output flow of at least 60 L/min	21–100	Fixed	Full range of FiO$_2$	Requires 50 psi air + oxygen; blender failure or inaccuracy common	Patient with high V$_E$ who needs high FiO$_2$
	High-flow cannula system	Up to 40 L/min (depending on system)	35–90	Variable or fixed depending on system and input flow	Wide range of FiO$_2$ and relative or absolute humidity; use on adults, children, infants	FiO$_2$ not ensured depending on input flow and patient breathing pattern; infection risk	Patients of all ages with high or variable V$_E$ who need supplemental oxygen, positive pressure, or humidity

FiO$_2$, Fraction of inspired oxygen; *V$_E$*, minute volume.

Modified from Kacmarek RM, Stoller JK, Heuer AJ, eds. *Egan's Fundamentals of Respiratory Care.* 12th ed. St. Louis: Elsevier; 2021.

50% for longer than 24 hours. Oxygen toxicity is most likely to develop in patients who require intubation, mechanical ventilation, and high oxygen concentrations for extended periods.[3]

Hyperoxia, or the administration of higher-than-normal oxygen concentrations, produces an overabundance of oxygen free radicals. These radicals are responsible for the initial damage to the alveolar–capillary membrane. Oxygen free radicals are toxic metabolites of oxygen metabolism. Normally, enzymes neutralize the radicals, preventing any damage from occurring. During the administration of high levels of oxygen, the large number of oxygen free radicals produced exhausts the supply of neutralizing enzymes. Damage to the lung parenchyma and vasculature occurs, resulting in the initiation of acute respiratory distress syndrome (ARDS).[2,5]

Many clinical manifestations are associated with oxygen toxicity. The first symptom is substernal chest pain that is exacerbated by deep breathing. A dry cough and tracheal irritation follow. Eventually, definite pleuritic pain occurs on inhalation, followed by dyspnea. Upper airway changes may include a sensation of nasal stuffiness, sore throat, and increased pressure sensation in the ears. Chest radiographs and pulmonary function tests show no abnormalities until symptoms are severe. Complete, rapid reversal of these symptoms occurs as soon as normal oxygen concentrations are restored.[5]

Carbon Dioxide Retention

In patients with severe chronic obstructive pulmonary disease (COPD), carbon dioxide (CO$_2$) retention may occur as a result of administration of oxygen in high concentrations. Numerous theories have been proposed for this phenomenon. One states that the normal stimulus to breathe (i.e., increasing CO$_2$ levels) is muted in patients with COPD and that decreasing oxygen levels become the stimulus to breathe. If hypoxemia is corrected by the administration of oxygen, the stimulus to breathe is abolished; hypoventilation develops, resulting in a further increase in the arterial partial pressure of carbon dioxide (PaCO$_2$).[2,3] Another theory is that the administration of oxygen abolishes the compensatory response of hypoxic pulmonary vasoconstriction. This results in an increase in perfusion of underventilated alveoli and the development of dead space, producing ventilation/perfusion ($\dot{V}/\dot{Q}$) mismatch. As alveolar dead space increases, so does CO$_2$ retention.[2,3] One further theory states that the increase in CO$_2$ is related to the ratio of deoxygenated to oxygenated hemoglobin (Haldane effect). Deoxygenated hemoglobin carries more CO$_2$ compared with oxygenated hemoglobin. Administration of oxygen increases the proportion of oxygenated hemoglobin, which causes increased release of CO$_2$ at the lung level.[5] Because of the risk of CO$_2$ accumulation, all patients who are chronically hypercapnic require careful low-flow oxygen administration.[3]

Absorption Atelectasis

Another adverse effect of high concentrations of oxygen is absorption atelectasis. Breathing high concentrations of oxygen washes out the nitrogen that normally fills the alveoli and helps hold them open (residual volume). As oxygen replaces the nitrogen in the alveoli, the alveoli start to shrink and collapse. This occurs because oxygen is absorbed into the bloodstream faster than it can be replaced in the alveoli, particularly in areas of the lungs that are minimally ventilated.[3]

Nursing Management

Nursing priorities for the patient receiving oxygen focus on (1) ensuring the oxygen is being administered as ordered and (2) observing for complications of the therapy. Confirming that the oxygen therapy device is properly positioned and replacing it after removal is important. During meals, an oxygen mask is changed to a nasal cannula if the patient can tolerate one. A patient receiving oxygen therapy is also transported with the oxygen. In addition, oxygen saturation is periodically monitored using a pulse oximeter.

ARTIFICIAL AIRWAYS

Pharyngeal Airways

Pharyngeal airways are used to maintain airway patency by keeping the tongue from obstructing the upper airway. The two types of pharyngeal airways are oropharyngeal and nasopharyngeal airways. Complications of these airways include trauma to the oral or nasal cavity, obstruction of the airway, laryngospasm, gagging, and vomiting.[6,7]

Oropharyngeal Airway

An oropharyngeal airway is made of plastic and is available in various sizes. The proper size is selected by holding the airway against the side of the patient's face and ensuring that it extends from the corner of the mouth to the angle of the jaw. If the airway is improperly sized, it will occlude the airway.[6,7] An oral airway is placed by inserting a tongue depressor into the patient's mouth to displace the tongue downward and then passing the airway into the patient's mouth, slipping it over the patient's tongue.[7] When properly placed, the tip of the airway lies above the epiglottis at the base of the tongue. An oropharyngeal airway is used only in an unconscious patient who has an absent or diminished gag reflex.[6,7]

Nasopharyngeal Airway

A nasopharyngeal airway is usually made of plastic or rubber and is available in various sizes. The proper size is selected by holding the airway against the side of the patient's face and ensuring that the nasopharyngeal airway extends from the tip of the nose to the ear lobe.[6,7] A nasal airway is placed by lubricating the tube and inserting it midline along the floor of the naris into the posterior pharynx.[7] When properly placed, the tip of the airway lies above the epiglottis at the base of the tongue.[6,7]

Endotracheal Tubes

An endotracheal tube (ETT) is the most commonly used artificial airway for providing short-term airway management. Indications for endotracheal intubation include maintenance of airway patency, protection of the airway from aspiration, application of positive-pressure ventilation, facilitation of pulmonary hygiene, and use of high oxygen concentrations.[8] An ETT may be placed through the orotracheal route via direct laryngoscopy or video laryngoscopy or the nasotracheal route via blind nasal intubation.[9] In most situations involving emergency placement, the orotracheal route is used, because this route is simpler and allows the use of a larger diameter ETT. Nasotracheal intubation provides greater patient comfort over time and is preferred in patients with a jaw fracture.[8] The advantages of orotracheal and nasotracheal intubation are presented in Table 15.2.

ETTs are available in various sizes, which are based on the inner diameters of the tubes, and have a radiopaque marker that runs the length of the tube. On one end of the tube is a cuff that is inflated with the use of the pilot balloon. Because of the high incidence of cuff-related problems, low-pressure, high-volume cuffs are preferred. On the other end of the tube is a 15-mm adapter that facilitates connection of the tube to a manual resuscitation bag (MRB), T-tube, or ventilator (Fig. 15.1).[10,11]

Rapid Sequence Intubation

Rapid sequence intubation (RSI) is a seven-step process that is often used to intubate a critically ill patient. This method is considered safer for the patient, because it decreases the risk of aspiration.[12,13]

Step 1: preparation. Before intubation, the necessary equipment is gathered and organized to facilitate the procedure. Readily available equipment includes a suction system with catheters and tonsil suction, an MRB with a mask connected to 100% oxygen, a laryngoscope handle with assorted blades, ETTs in various sizes, and a stylet. Before the procedure is started, all equipment is inspected to ensure that the equipment is in working order. The patient is prepared for the procedure, if possible, with an intravenous catheter in place and monitored with a pulse oximeter.[12-14]

Step 2: preoxygenation. Once everything is ready, the patient is preoxygenated with 100% oxygen for 3 to 5 minutes via a tight-fitting face mask. If the patient is unable to maintain adequate spontaneous ventilations, assisted ventilations are initiated with an MRB. The goal is to avoid positive-pressure ventilation, if possible, because this intervention increases the chances of gastric distention and the risk of aspiration.[12-14]

Step 3: pretreatment. While the patient is being preoxygenated, the patient is pretreated with adjunct medications to decrease the physiologic response to intubation. These medications include lidocaine,

TABLE 15.2 Advantages of Orotracheal, Nasotracheal, and Tracheostomy Tubes.

Orotracheal Tubes	Nasotracheal Tubes	Tracheostomy Tubes
Easier access	Easily secured and stabilized	Easily secured and stabilized
Avoids nasal and sinus complications	Reduces risk of unintentional extubation	Reduces risk of unintentional decannulation
Allows for larger diameter tube, which facilitates	Well tolerated by patient	Well tolerated by patient
• Work of breathing	Enables swallowing and oral hygiene	Enables swallowing, speech, and oral hygiene
• Suctioning		
• Fiberoptic bronchoscopy		
	Facilitates communication	Avoids upper airway complications
	Avoids need for bite block	Allows for larger diameter tube, which facilitates:
		• Work of breathing
		• Suctioning
		• Fiberoptic bronchoscopy

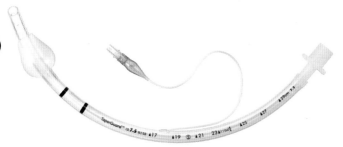

Fig. 15.1 Endotracheal Tube. (Image used by permission from Nellcor Puritan Bennett, LLC, Boulder, CO.)

fentanyl, and atropine. A very low dose of a paralytic agent may be administered to prevent fasciculations. The use of these medications depends on the patient's underlying condition. If possible, pretreatment occurs 3 minutes before the next step.[12-14]

Step 4: paralysis with induction. A sedative agent and a paralytic agent are administered in "rapid sequence" to achieve induction and paralysis. Various sedative agents, including etomidate, midazolam, ketamine, and propofol, are used to facilitate rapid loss of consciousness. Induction dosages for these medications are usually slightly higher than the typical dosages used for sedation. The two most commonly administered neuromuscular blocking agents used to facilitate skeletal muscle relaxation are succinylcholine and rocuronium.[12-14]

Step 5: protection and positioning. The procedure is initiated by positioning the patient with the neck flexed and head slightly extended in the "sniff" position. The oral cavity and pharynx are suctioned, and any dental devices are removed.

Step 6: placement of endotracheal tube. The ETT is inserted into the trachea (Fig. 15.2), and placement is confirmed.[12,13] Each intubation attempt is limited to 30 seconds to prevent hypoxemia. After the ETT is inserted, the patient is assessed for bilateral breath sounds and chest movement. The absence of breath sounds is indicative of esophageal intubation, whereas breath sounds heard over only one side of the chest is indicative of a mainstem intubation. A disposable end-tidal CO_2 detector is used to initially verify correct airway placement, after which the cuff of the tube is inflated and the tube is secured. Finally, a chest radiograph is obtained to confirm placement. The tip of the ETT should be approximately 3 to 4 cm above the carina when the patient's head is in the neutral position.[8]

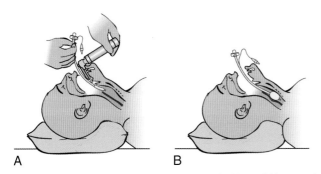

Fig. 15.2 Insertion of Tube with Laryngoscope in Place. (A) Insert tube with the tip initially against the right buccal mucosa so that a clear view of the vocal cords can be maintained at all times. As it advances, watch the tube pass through the cord. (B) Tube is correctly placed when the tip is 2 to 3 cm beyond the vocal cords. (From Fowler GC, ed. *Pfenninger and Fowler's Procedures for Primary Care*. 4th ed. Philadelphia: Elsevier; 2020.)

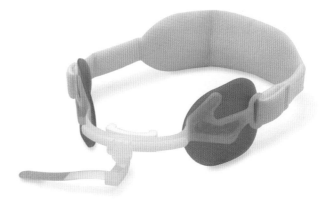

Fig. 15.3 Commercial Tube Holder. Anchor Fast oral endotracheal tube fastener. (Courtesy of Hollister Incorporated, Libertyville, Illinois.)

Step 7: postintubation management. After final adjustment of the ETT position is complete, the level of insertion (marked in centimeters on the side of the tube) at the teeth is noted. The ETT is then secured to the patient's face using tape or a commercial tube holder (Fig. 15.3). Securing the tube stabilizes it to prevent movement and potential dislodgment.[8]

Complications

Numerous complications can occur during the intubation procedure, including nasal and oral trauma, pharyngeal and hypopharyngeal trauma, vomiting with aspiration, and cardiac arrest.[15] Tracheal rupture is a rare and often fatal complication that is associated with emergent intubation.[16] Hypoxemia and hypercapnia can also occur, resulting in bradycardia, tachycardia, dysrhythmias, hypertension, and hypotension.[8,15]

Several complications can occur while the ETT is in place, including nasal and oral inflammation and ulceration, sinusitis and otitis, laryngeal and tracheal injuries, and tube obstruction and displacement. Other complications can occur days to weeks after the ETT is removed, including laryngeal and tracheal stenosis and a cricoid abscess (Box 15.1). Delayed complications usually require some form of surgical intervention.[17,18]

Tracheostomy Tubes

A tracheostomy tube is the preferred method of airway maintenance in a patient who requires long-term intubation. Although no ideal time to perform the procedure has been identified, it is commonly accepted that if a patient has been intubated or is anticipated to be intubated for longer than 7 days, a tracheostomy should be performed.[19] A tracheostomy is also indicated in several other situations such as the presence of an upper airway obstruction secondary to trauma, tumors, or swelling and the need to facilitate airway clearance secondary to spinal cord injury, neuromuscular disease, or severe debilitation.[20,21]

A tracheostomy tube provides the best route for long-term airway maintenance, because this route avoids the oral, nasal, pharyngeal, and laryngeal complications associated with an ETT. The tube is shorter, has a wider diameter, and is less curved than an ETT; the resistance to airflow is less; and breathing is easier. Additional advantages of a tracheostomy tube include ease with secretion removal, increased patient acceptance and comfort, capability of the patient to eat and talk if possible, and easier ventilator weaning.[8,20] See Table 15.2 for a list of the advantages of a tracheostomy tube.

Tracheostomy tubes are made of plastic or metal and may have one or two lumens. Single-lumen tubes consist of the tube; a built-in cuff,

BOX 15.1   Complications of Endotracheal Tubes

Complications	Causes	Prevention and Treatment
Tube obstruction	Patient biting tube Tube kinking during repositioning Cuff herniation Dried secretions, blood, or lubricant Tissue from tumor Trauma Foreign body	**Prevention:** Place bite block. Sedate patient PRN. Suction PRN. Humidify inspired gases. **Treatment:** Replace tube.
Tube displacement	Movement of patient's head Movement of tube by patient's tongue Traction on tube from ventilator tubing Self-extubation	**Prevention:** Secure tube to upper lip. Sedate patient PRN. Ensure that only 2 inches of tube extend beyond lip. Support ventilator tubing. **Treatment:** Replace tube.
Sinusitis and nasal injury	Obstruction of paranasal sinus drainage Pressure necrosis of nares	**Prevention:** Avoid nasal intubations. Cushion nares from tube and tape or ties. **Treatment:** Remove all tubes from nasal passages. Administer antibiotics.
Tracheoesophageal fistula	Pressure necrosis of posterior tracheal wall, resulting from overinflated cuff and rigid nasogastric tube	**Prevention:** Inflate cuff with minimal amount of air necessary. Monitor cuff pressures every 8 hours. **Treatment:** Position cuff of tube distal to fistula. Place gastrostomy tube for enteral feedings. Place esophageal tube for secretion clearance proximal to fistula.
Mucosal lesions	Pressure at tube and mucosal interface	**Prevention:** Inflate cuff with minimal amount of air necessary. Monitor cuff pressures every 8 hours. Use appropriate size tube. **Treatment:** May resolve spontaneously. Perform surgical intervention.
Laryngeal or tracheal stenosis	Injury to area from end of tube or cuff, resulting in scar tissue formation and narrowing of airway	**Prevention:** Inflate cuff with minimal amount of air necessary. Monitor cuff pressures every 8 hours. Suction area above cuff frequently. **Treatment:** Perform tracheostomy. Place laryngeal stent. Perform surgical repair.
Cricoid abscess	Mucosal injury with bacterial invasion	**Prevention:** Inflate cuff with minimal amount of air necessary. Monitor cuff pressures every 8 hours. Suction area above cuff frequently. **Treatment:** Perform incision and drainage of area. Administer antibiotics.

PRN, As needed.

which is connected to a pilot balloon for inflation purposes; and an obturator, which is used during tube insertion. Double-lumen tubes consist of the tube with the attached cuff, the obturator, and an inner cannula that can be removed for cleaning and then reinserted or, if disposable, replaced by a new sterile inner cannula. The inner cannula can be removed quickly if the cannula becomes obstructed, making the system safer for patients with significant secretion problems. Single-lumen tubes provide a larger internal diameter for airflow, so airflow resistance is reduced, and the patient can ventilate through the tube with greater ease. Plastic tracheostomy tubes also have a 15-mm adapter on the end (Fig. 15.4).[20,21]

Tracheostomy Procedure

A tracheostomy tube is inserted by an open procedure or a percutaneous procedure. An open procedure is usually performed in the operating room, whereas a percutaneous procedure can be done at the patient's bedside.[21,22]

Complications

Numerous complications can occur during the tracheostomy procedure, including misplacement of the tracheal tube, hemorrhage, laryngeal nerve injury, pneumothorax, pneumomediastinum, and cardiac arrest.[17,21,23] Several complications can occur while the tracheostomy tube is in place, including stomal infection, hemorrhage, tracheomalacia, tracheoesophageal fistula, tracheoinnominate artery fistula, and tube obstruction and displacement.[21,23] Many complications can occur days to weeks after the tracheostomy tube is removed, including tracheal stenosis and tracheocutaneous fistula (Box 15.2). Delayed complications usually require some form of surgical intervention.[23]

Nursing Management

Nursing management of a patient with an endotracheal or tracheostomy tube requires some additional measures to address the effects associated with tube placement on the respiratory and other body systems. Nursing priorities for the patient with an artificial airway

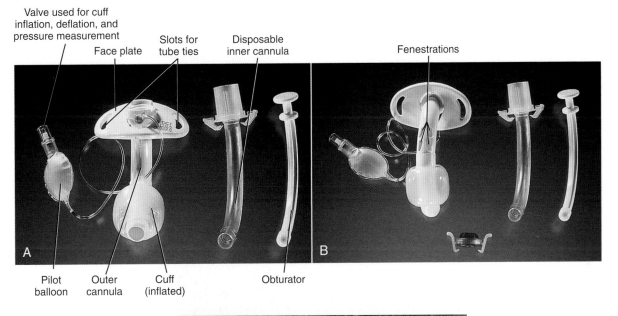

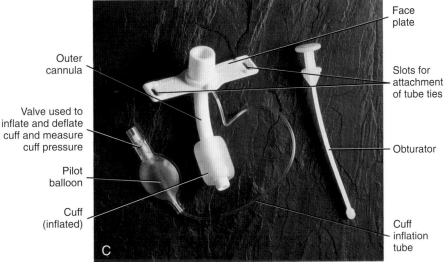

Fig. 15.4 Tracheostomy Tubes. (A) Dual-lumen cuffed tracheostomy tube with disposable inner cannula. (B) Dual-lumen cuffed fenestrated tracheostomy tube. (C) Single-lumen cannula cuffed tracheostomy tube. (From Ignatavicius DD, Workman ML, Rebar C, Heimgartner M, eds. *Medical-Surgical Nursing: Concepts for Interprofessional Collaborative Care.* 9th ed. St. Louis: Elsevier; 2018.)

BOX 15.2   Complications of Tracheostomy Tubes

Complications	Causes	Prevention and Treatment
Hemorrhage	Vessel opening after surgery Vessel erosion caused by tube	**Prevention:** Use appropriate size tube. Treat local infection. Suction gently. Humidify inspired gases. Position tracheal window not lower than third tracheal ring. **Treatment:** Pack lightly. Perform surgical intervention.
Wound infection	Colonization of stoma with hospital flora	**Prevention:** Perform routine stoma care. **Treatment:** Remove tube, if necessary. Perform aggressive wound care and débridement. Administer antibiotics.
Subcutaneous emphysema	Positive-pressure ventilation Coughing against tight, occlusive dressing or sutured or packed wound	**Prevention:** Avoid suturing or packing wound closed around tube. **Treatment:** Remove any sutures or packing, if present.
Tube obstruction	Dried blood or secretions False passage into soft tissues Opening of cannula positioned against tracheal wall Foreign body Tissue from tumor	**Prevention:** Suction PRN. Humidify inspired gases. Use tube with removable inner cannula. Position tube so that opening does not press against tracheal wall. **Treatment:** Remove or replace inner cannula. Replace tube.
Tube displacement	Patient movement Coughing Traction on ventilatory tubing	**Prevention:** Use commercial tube holder. Use tubes with adjustable neck plates for patients with short necks. Support ventilatory tubing. Sedate patient PRN. Restrain patient PRN. **Treatment:** Cover stoma and manually ventilate patient by mouth. Replace tube.
Tracheal stenosis	Injury to area from end of tube or cuff, resulting in scar tissue formation and narrowing of airway	**Prevention:** Inflate cuff with minimal amount of air necessary. Monitor cuff pressures every 8 hours. **Treatment:** Perform surgical repair.
Tracheoesophageal fistula	Pressure necrosis of posterior tracheal wall, resulting from overinflated cuff and rigid nasogastric tube	**Prevention:** Inflate cuff with minimal amount of air necessary. Monitor cuff pressures every 8 hours. **Treatment:** Perform surgical repair.
Tracheoinnominate artery fistula	Direct pressure from elbow of cannula against innominate artery Placement of tracheal stoma below fourth tracheal ring High-lying innominate artery	**Prevention:** Position tracheal window not lower than third tracheal ring. **Treatment:** Hyperinflate cuff to control bleeding. Remove tube and replace with ETT, and apply digital pressure through stoma against sternum. Perform surgical repair.
Tracheocutaneous fistula	Failure of stoma to close after removal of tube	**Treatment:** Perform surgical repair.

ETT, Endotracheal tube; *PRN,* as needed.

focus on (1) providing humidification, (2) managing the cuff, (3) suctioning, (4) establishing a method of communication, and (5) providing oral hygiene. Because the tube bypasses the upper airway system, warming and humidifying the air must be performed by external means. Because the cuff of the tube can cause damage to the walls of the trachea, proper cuff inflation and management are imperative. In addition, the normal defense mechanisms are impaired, and secretions may accumulate; thus suctioning may be needed to promote secretion clearance. Because the tube does not allow airflow over the vocal cords, developing a method of communication is also very important. Last, observing the patient to ensure proper placement of the tube and patency of the airway is essential.

Patient safety is of paramount importance when caring for a patient with an artificial airway, because loss of the tube can result in loss of the patient's airway. In the event of unintentional extubation or decannulation, the patient's airway is opened with the head tilt–chin lift maneuver and maintained with an oropharyngeal or nasopharyngeal airway. If the patient is not breathing, he or she is manually ventilated with an MRB and face mask with 100% oxygen. In the case of a tracheostomy, the stoma is covered to prevent air from escaping through it. If the tracheostomy remains open, consideration is given to ventilating the patient through the stoma instead of the mouth.

One study examined patients' perception of ETT-related discomforts. Of the patients, 46% reported remembering having the ETT while in the critical care unit. Most of these patients found the discomfort associated with the ETT and the inability to speak very stressful. In addition, some patients continued to have problems with hoarseness, sore throat, and voice changes days to months later.[24]

Humidification

Humidification of air normally is performed by the mucosal layer of the upper respiratory tract. When this area is bypassed, as occurs with ETT and tracheostomy tubes or when supplemental oxygen is used, humidification by external means is necessary. Various humidification devices add water to inhaled gas to prevent drying and irritation of the respiratory tract, to prevent undue loss of body water, and to facilitate secretion removal.[25,26] The humidification device provides inspired gas conditioned (heated) to body temperature and saturated with water vapor.[27]

Cuff Management

Because the cuff of the ETT or tracheostomy tube is a major source of the complications associated with artificial airways, proper cuff management is essential. To prevent the complications associated with cuff design, only low-pressure, high-volume cuffed tubes are used in clinical practice.[8,10] Even with these tubes, cuff pressures can be generated that are high enough to lead to tracheal ischemia and injury. Proper cuff inflation techniques and cuff pressure monitoring are critical components of the care of a patient with an artificial airway.[8,10]

Cuff pressure monitoring. Cuff pressures are monitored at a minimum of every shift with a cuff pressure manometer. Cuff pressures are maintained within 20 to 30 cm H_2O, because greater pressures decrease blood flow to the capillaries in the tracheal wall and lesser pressures increase the risk of aspiration. Pressures greater than 30 cm H_2O should be reported to the physician. Cuffs are not routinely deflated, because this increases the risk of aspiration.[8]

Foam cuff tracheostomy tubes. One tracheostomy tube on the market has a cuff made of foam that is self-inflating. The cuff is deflated during insertion, after which the pilot port is opened to atmospheric pressure (room air), and the cuff self-inflates. After inflation, the

foam cuff conforms to the size and shape of the patient's trachea, reducing the pressure against the tracheal wall. The pilot port can be left open to atmospheric pressure or attached to the mechanical ventilator tubing, allowing the cuff to inflate and deflate with the cycling of the ventilator. Routine maintenance of a foam cuff tracheostomy tube includes aspirating the pilot port every 8 hours to measure cuff volume, to remove any condensation from the cuff area, and to assess the integrity of the cuff. Removal is accomplished by deflating the cuff; this can be complicated if the plastic sheath covering the foam is perforated. If perforation occurs, the foam may not be deflatable, because the air cannot be totally aspirated.[23]

Subglottic secretion removal. The cuff has also been implicated in the development of ventilator-associated pneumonia (VAP). Fluids can leak around the cuff into the airway, resulting in microaspiration. Bacteria-laden oral secretions trickle down the larynx and pool above the cuff of the artificial airway. These secretions are referred to as *subglottic secretions.* Subglottic secretions can then leak into the lower airways around the cuff via the longitudinal folds that form in the cuff as it accommodates to the shape of the airway, when an underinflated cuff fails to form a proper seal in the airway, or in the event of inadvertent movement of the ETT within the airway. The use of established cuff inflation techniques, monitoring of cuff pressures, using an appropriate method of tube stabilization, and oral hygiene are important interventions for preventing this problem.[28] Deep oropharyngeal suctioning to remove subglottic secretions is performed at least every 12 hours and before deflating the cuff or moving the tube.[29]

Specialized tubes are available to allow for the continuous removal of subglottic secretions. These tubes have an additional lumen, with an opening above the cuff, which is connected to continuous (-20 to -30 cm H_2O) suction.[10] These tubes are recommended for patients who are expected to be intubated for longer than 48 to 72 hours.[10] One issue with these tubes is that the aspiration lumen can become clogged, and a small amount of air needs to be injected into the aspiration port every few hours.

Suctioning

Suctioning is often required to maintain a patent airway in a patient with an ETT or tracheostomy tube. Suctioning is a sterile procedure that is performed only when the patient needs it and not on a routine schedule.[30,31] Indications for suctioning include the presence of coarse crackles over the trachea on auscultation,[30] coughing, visible secretions in the airway, a sawtooth pattern on the flow-volume loop on the ventilator monitor,[30,31] increased peak airway pressures on the ventilator, decreasing oxygenation saturation, and acute respiratory distress.[31] Complications associated with suctioning include hypoxemia, atelectasis, bronchospasms, dysrhythmias, increased intracranial pressure, and airway trauma.[31]

There are two different methods for suctioning based on the type of catheter. The open suction method requires disconnecting the patient from the ventilator and inserting a single-use, disposable, suction catheter into the artificial airway. The closed suction method requires a sterile, closed tracheal suction system (CTSS) and allows the patient to remain on the ventilator when suctioned. The closed method is preferable, because the evidence suggests that this method appears to limit the hypoxemia associated with suctioning.[13,31]

There are two different techniques for suctioning depending on how deeply the suction catheter is inserted into the trachea: shallow suctioning and deep suctioning. For shallow suctioning, the suction catheter is inserted to the end of the ETT or tracheostomy tube, and then the suction is applied. For deep suctioning, the suction catheter is inserted until resistance is met, the catheter is pulled back approximately 1 cm, and then suction is applied.[13,31] Evidence suggests that shallow suctioning is as effective as deep suctioning for secretion removal and is associated with fewer complications.[13]

Complications. Hypoxemia can result because the oxygen source is disconnected from the patient or the oxygen is removed from the patient's airways when the suction is applied. Atelectasis is thought to occur when the suction catheter is larger than one half of the diameter of the ETT. Excessive negative pressure occurs when suction is applied, promoting collapse of the distal airways. Bronchospasms are the result of stimulation of the airways with the suction catheter. Cardiac dysrhythmias, particularly bradycardias, are attributed to vagal stimulation. Airway trauma occurs with impaction of the catheter in the airways and excessive negative pressure applied to the catheter.[8,31]

Suctioning protocol. Many protocols regarding suctioning have been developed. Several practices have been found to be helpful in limiting the complications of suctioning. Hypoxemia can be minimized by hyperoxygenating the patient with 100% oxygen for 30 to 60 seconds before suctioning and for at least 60 seconds after suctioning.[31] Recently the practice of routine hyperoxygenation has been called into question, because hyperoxygenation is not without risk, and there is limited evidence to support this practice. It has been suggested that hyperoxygenation should be limited to patients known to desaturate and those on high levels of oxygen or positive end-expiratory pressure (PEEP).[32] Atelectasis can be avoided by using a suction catheter with an external diameter of less than one half of the internal diameter of the ETT.[31,32] Using 150 mm Hg or less of suction decreases the chances of hypoxemia, atelectasis, and airway trauma.[32] Limiting the duration of each suction pass to 10 to 15 seconds also helps minimize hypoxemia, airway trauma, and cardiac dysrhythmias.[13,31,32] The process of applying intermittent (instead of continuous) suction has been shown to be of no benefit.[33] The instillation of normal saline to help remove secretions has not been proved to be of any benefit, and it may contribute to the development of hypoxemia and lower airway colonization resulting in VAP.[13,31,34]

Closed tracheal suction system. One device to facilitate the suctioning of a patient on a ventilator is the CTSS (Fig. 15.5). This device consists of a suction catheter in a plastic sleeve that attaches directly to the ventilator tubing. The CTSS allows the patient to be suctioned while remaining on the ventilator. Advantages of the CTSS include maintenance of oxygenation and PEEP during suctioning, reduction of hypoxemia-related complications, and protection of staff members from the patient's secretions.[35] The CTSS is convenient to use, requiring only one person to perform the procedure.

Concerns related to the CTSS include autocontamination, inadequate removal of secretions, and increased risk of unintentional extubation resulting from the extra weight of the system on the ventilator tubing. Autocontamination has been shown not to be an issue if the catheter is cleaned properly after every use. Inadequate removal of secretions may or may not be a problem, and further investigation is required to settle this issue.[32] Although recommendations for changing the catheter vary, one study indicated that the catheter could be changed on an as-needed basis without increasing the incidence of VAP.[36]

Communication

Impaired communication is a major stressor for a patient with an artificial airway. This stress is related to the inability to speak, insufficient explanations from staff members, inadequate understanding, fear of being unable to communicate, and difficulty with communication

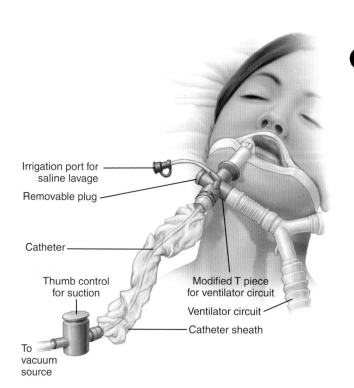

Fig. 15.5 Closed Tracheal Suction System. (Modified from Sills JR. *Entry-Level Respiratory Therapist Exam Guide.* St. Louis: Mosby; 2000.)

methods.[37] Many interventions can facilitate communication for a patient with an ETT or tracheostomy tube. These include establishing an environment that fosters communication, performing a complete assessment of the patient's ability to communicate, anticipating the patient's needs, teaching the patient and family how to communicate, using a variety of methods to communicate, and facilitating the patient's ability to communicate by providing the patient with his or her eyeglasses or hearing aid.[38]

Methods to facilitate communication in this patient population include the use of verbal and nonverbal language and various devices to assist the patient on short-term and long-term ventilator assistance. Nonverbal communication may include the use of sign language, gestures, lip reading, pointing, facial expressions, or eye blinking. Simple devices include pencil and paper; Magic Slates; magnetic boards with plastic letters; picture, alphabet, or symbol boards; and flash cards. More sophisticated devices include typewriters, computers, talking ETT and tracheostomy tubes, and external handheld vibrators. Regardless of the method selected, the patient must be taught how to use the device.[38]

Passy-Muir valve. The Passy-Muir valve is a device used to assist a mechanically ventilated patient with a tracheostomy to speak. This one-way valve opens on inhalation, allowing air to enter the lungs through the tracheostomy tube, and closes on exhalation, forcing air over the vocal cords and out the mouth, permitting the patient to speak (Fig. 15.6). Before the valve can be placed on a tracheostomy tube, the cuff must be deflated to allow air to pass around the tube, and the tidal volume of the ventilator must be increased to compensate for the air leak. In addition to aiding communication, the Passy-Muir valve can assist a ventilator-dependent patient with relearning normal breathing patterns. The valve is contraindicated in patients with laryngeal or pharyngeal dysfunction, excessive secretions, or poor lung compliance.

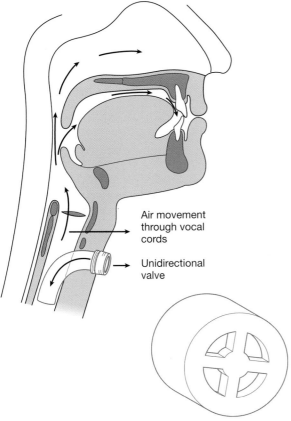

Fig. 15.6 Passy-Muir Valve. (Redrawn from Manzano JL, Lubillo S, Henríquez D, Martín JC, Pérez MC, Wilson DJ. Verbal communication of ventilator dependent patients. *Crit Care Med*. 1992;21[4]:512–517; with permission.)

Air movement through vocal cords

Unidirectional valve

Oral Hygiene

Patients with artificial airways are extremely susceptible to developing VAP because of microaspiration of subglottic secretions. These secretions are full of micro-organisms from the patient's mouth. Because the cuff of the artificial airway does not form a tight seal in the patient's airway, these secretions seep around the cuff into the patient's lungs, promoting the development of VAP.[39] Although bacteria are normally present in a patient's mouth, increased amounts of bacteria and more resistant bacteria are present in critically ill patients. Decreased salivary flow, poor mucosal status, and dental plaque all contribute to this problem.[40]

Proper oral hygiene has been shown to decrease the incidence of VAP.[41–43] No evidence-based protocol exists for oral care at the present time. Research studies are lacking, particularly with regard to frequency and effectiveness of different procedures. However, most experts agree that oral care should consist of brushing the patient's teeth with a soft toothbrush to reduce plaque, brushing the patient's tongue and gums with a foam swab to stimulate the tissue,[40] and performing deep oropharyngeal suctioning to remove any secretions that have pooled above the patient's cuff.[39] In addition, chlorhexidine solution should be applied to the inside of the mouth to decrease the prevalence of oropharyngeal organisms. To be effective, chlorhexidine should be applied with a sponge swab to the teeth, tongue, and inside of the oral cavity. To have the greatest effect, 2% chlorhexidine should be applied four times daily.[44] This procedure has been shown to reduce oral colonization of bacteria and to decrease the incidence of VAP in patients undergoing mechanical ventilation.[45] A sample oral care protocol is outlined in Box 15.3.

Extubation and Decannulation

An artificial airway is removed when it is no longer needed. Extubation, the process of removing an ETT, is a simple procedure that can be done at the bedside.[46] Before the cuff of an ETT or tracheostomy tube is deflated in preparation for removal, it is important to ensure that secretions are cleared from above the tube cuff. Complications of extubation include sore throat, stridor, hoarseness, odynophagia, vocal cord immobility, pulmonary aspiration, and cough.[46] Decannulation is the process of removing a tracheostomy tube. This is also a simple process that can be performed at the bedside. After removal of the tracheostomy tube, the stoma is usually covered with a dry dressing with the expectation that it will close within several days.[18,47,48] Difficulty removing the tracheostomy tube because of a tight stoma is usually the only complication associated with decannulation.[47]

INVASIVE MECHANICAL VENTILATION

Indications

Mechanical ventilation is the process of using an apparatus to facilitate the transport of oxygen and CO_2 between the atmosphere and the alveoli for the purpose of enhancing pulmonary gas exchange.

BOX 15.3   Sample Oral Care Protocol

Standard of Care

1. The oral cavity is assessed initially and daily by the registered nurse (RN).
2. Unconscious patients and patients with artificial airways (endotracheal or tracheostomy tubes) are provided oral care every 4 hours and as needed.
3. Patients with cuffed artificial airways have oropharyngeal and subglottic secretions suctioned at least every 12 hours and before repositioning of the tube or deflation of the cuff.

Procedure

1. Set up suction equipment.
2. Position patient's head to the side, or place patient in semi-Fowler position.
3. Provide suction, as needed, to patients with an artificial airway to remove any oropharyngeal and subglottic secretions (secretions that migrate down the tube and settle on top of the cuff).

4. Brush teeth using a suction toothbrush, small amounts of water, and alcohol-free antiseptic oral rinse.
   - Brush for approximately 1–2 minutes.
   - Exert gentle pressure while moving in short horizontal or circular strokes.
5. Gently brush surface of tongue.
6. Use suction swab to clean the teeth and tongue if brushing causes discomfort or bleeding.
   - Place swab perpendicular to gum line, applying gentle mechanical action for 1–2 minutes.
   - Turn swab in clockwise rotation to remove mucus and debris.
7. Swab mouth (teeth, tongue, and oral cavity) with 15 mL of 0.12% chlorhexidine every 6 hours.
8. Apply mouth moisturizer inside mouth.
9. Apply lip balm, if needed.

TRENDING PRIORITIES IN HEALTHCARE

Internal Disaster Preparedness

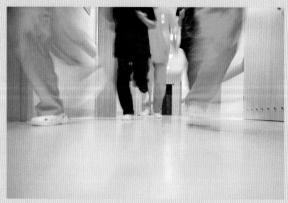

iStock.com/gpointstudio

Internal disasters preparedness is needed to respond to events that may significantly impact normal hospital operations. Some examples of internal disasters include electrical power outages,[1] total or partial interruption to water supply,[2] and oxygen pipeline failure.[3]

Electrical Power Supply

Hospitals are dependent on electricity for powered medical equipment and devices, lighting, alarms, and temperature regulation systems.[1] Emergency and standby power are required to respond to power outages with distribution of power prioritized to life-safety systems that protect the lives of the building occupants.[1]

Water Supply

Hospitals utilize water for patient and health care worker hygiene, food and drink preparation, proper functioning and maintenance of medical equipment and devices, and sprinkler and sanitary systems.[2] Alternative means of providing water (e.g., prepackaged water or water storage tanks) are required to respond to total or partial interruptions to water supply with consideration of need for essential care activities and consumption as well as for equipment and sanitary purposes.[2]

Oxygen Supply

Hospitals provide oxygen to patients in need of supplemental amounts of inspired oxygen, during procedures and as a component of therapies delivered through medical equipment and devices. Early detection of low oxygen supply alarm systems may alert hospital personnel to utilize backup sources (e.g., full reserve portable oxygen tanks) to provide supplemental oxygen until oxygen supply is restored.[3]

Overall preparedness for internal disasters includes performing a vulnerability assessment, preparing policies and procedures, and planning for the unexpected with mock events[1–3]:

- Performing a vulnerability assessment
  - What hospital systems are supplied by the emergency and standby power supply?
  - What is the hospital's overall water usage? What is the minimum water supply needed for essential care activities and consumption? What is the minimum water supply needed for equipment and sanity purposes?
  - What is the minimum number of oxygen tanks needed to supply the daily rate of oxygen consumption?
- Preparing policies and procedures
  - Ensure roles and responsibilities are clearly delineated
- Planning for the unexpected with mock events
  - Evaluate adherence to policies and procedures

For additional information about preparing for internal hospital disasters, check out the following websites:

- Centers for Medicare & Medicaid Services—https://www.cms.gov/Medicare/Provider-Enrollment-and-Certification/SurveyCertEmergPrep/Emergency-Prep-Rule
- The Joint Commission—https://www.jointcommission.org/resources/patient-safety-topics/emergency-management/
- National Fire Protection Association—https://www.nfpa.org/

References

1. *Healthcare Facilities and Power Outages: Guidance for State, Local, Tribal, Territorial, and Private Sector Partners*; 2019. www.fema.gov/sites/default/files/2020-07/healthcare-facilities-and-power-outages.pdf.
2. *Emergency Water Supply Planning Guide for Hospitals and Healthcare Facilities*; 2019. www.cdc.gov/healthywater/emergency/pdf/emergency-water-supply-planning-guide-2019-508.pdf.
3. Mostert L, Coetzee AR. Central oxygen pipeline failure. *South Afr J Anaesth Analg.* 2014;20(5):214–217.

Mechanical ventilation is indicated for physiologic and clinical reasons. Physiologic objectives include supporting cardiopulmonary gas exchange (alveolar ventilation and arterial oxygenation), increasing lung volume (end-expiratory lung inflation and functional residual capacity), and reducing the work of breathing. Clinical objectives include reversing hypoxemia and acute respiratory acidosis, relieving respiratory distress, preventing or reversing atelectasis and respiratory muscle fatigue, permitting sedation and neuromuscular blockade, decreasing oxygen consumption, reducing intracranial pressure, and stabilizing the chest wall.[49–52]

Use of Mechanical Ventilators

Types of Ventilators

The two main types of ventilators available at the present time are (1) positive-pressure ventilators and (2) negative-pressure ventilators. Negative-pressure ventilators are applied externally to the patient and decrease the atmospheric pressure surrounding the thorax to initiate inspiration. They generally are not used in the critical care environment. Positive-pressure ventilators use a mechanical drive mechanism to force air into the patient's lungs through an ETT or tracheostomy tube.[51]

Ventilator Mechanics

To properly ventilate the patient, the ventilator must complete four phases of ventilation: (1) change from exhalation to inspiration, (2) inspiration, (3) change from inspiration to exhalation, and (4) exhalation. The ventilator uses four different variables to begin, sustain, and terminate each of these phases. These variables are described in terms of *volume, pressure, flow,* and *time.*[51,53,54]

Trigger. The phase variable that initiates the change from exhalation to inspiration is called the *trigger.* Breaths may be pressure triggered or flow triggered, depending on the sensitivity setting of the ventilator and the patient's inspiratory effort, or they may be time triggered, depending on the rate setting of the ventilator. A breath that is initiated by the patient is known as a *patient-triggered* or *patient-assisted* breath, whereas a breath that is initiated by the ventilator is known as a *machine-triggered* or *machine-controlled* breath.[51,53]

A *time-triggered breath* is a machine-controlled breath that is initiated by the ventilator after a preset length of time has elapsed and is controlled by the rate setting on the ventilator (e.g., a rate of 10 breaths/min yields 1 breath every 6 seconds). *Flow-triggered* and *pressure-triggered* breaths are patient-assisted breaths that are initiated by decreased flow or pressure, respectively, within the breathing circuit. Flow triggering (also known as *flow-by*) is controlled by adjusting the flow-sensitivity setting of the ventilator, whereas pressure triggering is controlled by adjusting the pressure-sensitivity setting. Many ventilators offer the various types of triggers in combination. For example, a breath may be time triggered and flow triggered, depending on the patient's ability to interact with the ventilator and initiate a breath.[51,53]

Limit. The variable that maintains inspiration is called the *limit* or *target.* Inspiration can be pressure limited, flow limited, or volume limited. A *pressure-limited breath* is one in which a preset pressure is attained and maintained during inspiration. A *flow-limited breath* is one in which a preset flow is reached before the end of inspiration. A *volume-limited breath* is one in which a preset volume is delivered during the inspiration. However, the limit variable does not end inspiration; it only sustains it.[51,53]

Cycle. The variable that ends inspiration is called the *cycle.* The classification of positive-pressure ventilators is based on this variable: volume-cycled, pressure-cycled, flow-cycled, and time-cycled ventilators. Volume-cycled ventilators are designed to deliver a breath until a preset volume is delivered. Pressure-cycled ventilators deliver a breath until a preset pressure is reached within the patient's airways. Flow-cycled ventilators deliver a breath until a preset inspiratory flow rate is achieved. Time-cycled ventilators deliver a breath over a preset time interval.[51,53]

Baseline. The variable that is controlled during exhalation is called the *baseline.* Pressure is almost always used to adjust this variable. The patient exhales to a certain baseline pressure that is set on the ventilator. The baseline variable may be set at zero (i.e., atmospheric pressure) or above atmospheric pressure (i.e., PEEP).[51,53]

Modes of Ventilation

The term *ventilator mode* refers to how the machine ventilates the patient. Selection of a particular mode of ventilation determines how much the patient will participate in his or her own ventilatory pattern. The choice depends on the patient's situation and the goals of treatment. The mode is determined by the combination of phase variables selected. Many modes are available (Table 15.3), and some may be used in conjunction with others.[49-52,54] Because brands of ventilators vary in their ability to perform certain functions, not all modes are available on all ventilators.[53-55]

Ventilator Settings

Settings on the ventilator allow the ventilator parameters to be individualized to the patient and allow selection of the desired ventilation mode (Table 15.4). Each ventilator has a patient-monitoring system that allows all aspects of the patient's ventilatory pattern to be assessed, monitored, and displayed.[49,52-54,56]

Complications

Mechanical ventilation is often lifesaving, but, similar to other interventions, it is not without complications. Some complications are preventable, whereas others can be minimized but not eradicated. Physiologic complications associated with mechanical ventilation include ventilator-induced lung injury, cardiovascular compromise, gastrointestinal disturbances, patient-ventilator dyssynchrony, and VAP.

Ventilator-Induced Lung Injury

Mechanical ventilation can cause two different types of injury to the lungs: (1) air leaks and (2) biotrauma.[57] Air leaks related to mechanical ventilation are the result of excessive pressure in the alveoli (barotrauma), excessive volume in the alveoli (volutrauma), or shearing caused by repeated opening and closing of the alveoli (atelectrauma).[58] Barotrauma, volutrauma, and atelectrauma can lead to excessive alveolar wall stress and damage to the alveolar-capillary membrane, resulting in air leakage into the surrounding spaces. The air then travels out through the hilum and into the mediastinum (pneumomediastinum), pleural space (pneumothorax), subcutaneous tissues (subcutaneous emphysema), pericardium (pneumopericardium), peritoneum (pneumoperitoneum), and retroperitoneum (pneumoretroperitoneum). The resultant disorders vary from fairly benign to potentially lethal—the most lethal of which is a pneumothorax or pneumopericardium resulting in cardiac tamponade.[59]

Barotrauma, volutrauma, and atelectrauma can also cause the release of cellular mediators and initiation of the inflammatory-immune response. This type of ventilator-induced injury is known as *biotrauma.*[60] Biotrauma can result in the development of ARDS.[61] To limit ventilator-induced lung injury, the plateau pressure (pressure needed to inflate the alveoli) is kept at less than 32 cm H_2O, PEEP is used to avoid end-expiratory collapse and reopening, and the tidal volume is set at 6 to 10 mL/kg.[57,60]

Cardiovascular Compromise

Positive-pressure ventilation increases intrathoracic pressure, which decreases venous return to the right side of the heart. Impaired venous return decreases preload, which results in a decrease in cardiac output. As a secondary consequence, hepatic and renal dysfunction may occur. Positive-pressure ventilation impairs cerebral venous return. In patients with impaired autoregulation, positive-pressure ventilation can result in increased intracranial pressure.[62]

Gastrointestinal Disturbances

Gastrointestinal disturbances can occur as a result of positive-pressure ventilation. Gastric distention occurs when air leaks around the ETT or tracheostomy tube cuff and overcomes the resistance of the lower esophageal sphincter. Vomiting can occur as a result of pharyngeal stimulation from the artificial airway.[9] These problems can be prevented by inserting a nasogastric tube and ensuring appropriate cuff inflation. Hypomotility and constipation may occur as a result of immobility and the administration of paralytic agents, analgesics, and sedatives.

Patient-Ventilator Dyssynchrony

Because the ventilatory pattern is normally initiated by the establishment of negative pressure within the chest, the application of positive pressure can lead to patient difficulties in breathing while on the ventilator. To achieve optimal ventilatory assistance, the patient should breathe in synchrony with the machine. The selected mode of ventilation, the settings, and the type of ventilatory circuitry used can increase the work of breathing and lead to breathing out of synchrony with the ventilator. Patient-ventilator dyssynchrony can result in decreased effectiveness of mechanical ventilation, the development of auto-PEEP, and psychologic distress. Patients who are not breathing in synchrony with the ventilator appear to be fighting or "bucking" the

TABLE 15.3 Modes of Mechanical Ventilation.

Mode of Ventilation	Clinical Application	Nursing Implications
Continuous mandatory (volume or pressure) ventilation (CMV), also known as assist/control (AC) ventilation: Delivers gas at preset tidal volume or pressure (depending on selected cycling variable) in response to patient's inspiratory efforts and initiates breath if patient fails to do so within preset time.	Volume-controlled (VC) CMV is used as primary mode of ventilation in spontaneously breathing patients with weak respiratory muscles. Pressure-controlled (PC) CMV is used in patients with decreased lung compliance or increased airway resistance, particularly when patient is at risk for volutrauma.	Hyperventilation can occur in patients with increased respiratory rates. Sedation may be necessary to limit number of spontaneous breaths. Patient on VC-CMV is monitored for volutrauma. Patient on PC-CMV is monitored for hypercapnia.
Pressure-regulated volume control ventilation (PRVCV): Variation of CMV that combines volume and pressure features; delivers preset tidal volume using lowest possible airway pressure; airway pressure will not exceed preset maximum pressure limit.	PRVCV is used in patients with rapidly changing pulmonary mechanics (airway resistance and lung compliance), limiting potential complications.	
Pressure-controlled inverse ratio ventilation (PC-IRV): PC-CMV mode in which inspiratory-to-expiratory (I:E) time ratio is >1:1.	PC-IRV is used in patients with hypoxemia refractory to PEEP; longer inspiratory time increases functional residual capacity and improves oxygenation by opening collapsed alveoli, and shorter expiratory time induces auto-PEEP that prevents alveoli from recollapsing.	Requires sedation and/or pharmacologic paralysis because of discomfort. Increased intrathoracic pressure can result in excessive air trapping and decreased cardiac output.
Intermittent mandatory (volume or pressure) ventilation (IMV), also known as synchronous intermittent mandatory ventilation (SIMV): Delivers gas at preset tidal volume or pressure (depending on selected cycling variable) and rate, while allowing patient to breathe spontaneously; ventilator breaths are synchronized to patient's respiratory effort.	VC-IMV is used as primary mode of ventilation in many clinical situations and as weaning mode. PC-IMV is used in patients with decreased lung compliance or increased airway resistance when the need to preserve the patient's spontaneous efforts is important.	May increase work of breathing and promote respiratory muscle fatigue. Patient is monitored for hypercapnia, particularly with PC-IMV.
Adaptive support ventilation (ASV): Ventilator automatically adjusts settings to maintain 100 mL/min/kg of minute ventilation; pressure support.	ASV is a computerized mode of ventilation that increases or decreases ventilatory support based on patient needs; can be used with any patient requiring volume-controlled ventilation.	Not intended as a weaning mode. Adapts to changes in patient position.
Continuous positive airway pressure (CPAP): Positive pressure applied during spontaneous breaths; patient controls rate, inspiratory flow, and tidal volume.	CPAP is spontaneous breathing mode used in patients to increase functional residual capacity and improve oxygenation by opening collapsed alveoli at end expiration; it is also used for weaning.	Side effects include decreased cardiac output, volutrauma, and increased intracranial pressure. No ventilator breaths are delivered in PEEP or CPAP mode unless used with CMV or IMV.
Airway pressure release ventilation (APRV): Two different levels of CPAP (inspiratory and expiratory) are applied for set periods of time, allowing spontaneous breathing to occur at both levels.	APRV is spontaneous breathing mode used to maintain alveolar recruitment without imposing additional peak inspiratory pressures that could lead to barotrauma.	Patient needs to be monitored for hypercapnia.
Pressure support ventilation (PSV): Preset positive pressure used to augment patient's inspiratory efforts; patient controls rate, inspiratory flow, and tidal volume.	PSV is spontaneous breathing mode used as primary mode of ventilation in patients with stable respiratory drive to overcome any imposed mechanical resistance (e.g., artificial airway). PSV can also be used with IMV to support spontaneous breaths.	Patient is monitored for hypercapnia. Advantages include reduced patient work of breathing and improved patient-ventilator synchrony.
Volume-assured pressure support ventilation (VAPSV), also known as pressure augmentation (PA): Variation of PSV with set tidal volume to ensure that patient receives minimum tidal volume with each pressure support breath.	VAPSV is spontaneous breathing mode used to treat acute respiratory illness and to facilitate weaning.	Advantages include increased patient comfort, decreased work of breathing, decreased respiratory muscle fatigue, and promotion of respiratory muscle conditioning.
Neurally adjusted ventilatory assist (NAVA): Partial ventilatory support mode that uses electrical activity of diaphragm to control patient-ventilator interaction.	NAVA delivers assisted breath in proportion to and in synchrony with patient's respiratory effort.	Requires esophageal catheter (similar to nasogastric tube) that measures electrical signal to diaphragm.
Independent lung ventilation (ILV): Each lung is ventilated separately.	ILV is used in patients with unilateral lung disease, bronchopleural fistulas, or bilateral asymmetric lung disease.	Requires double-lumen ETT, two ventilators, sedation, and pharmacologic paralysis.

TABLE 15.3   Modes of Mechanical Ventilation.—cont'd

Mode of Ventilation	Clinical Application	Nursing Implications
High-frequency ventilation (HFV): Delivers small volume of gas at rapid rate. • High-frequency positive-pressure ventilation (HFPPV): Delivers 60—100 breaths/min • High-frequency jet ventilation (HFJV): Delivers 100—600 cycles/min • High-frequency oscillation (HFO): Delivers 900—3000 cycles/min	HFV is used in situations in which conventional mechanical ventilation compromises hemodynamic stability, in patients with bronchopleural fistulas, during short-term procedures, and with diseases that create risk of volutrauma.	Patients require sedation and/or pharmacologic paralysis. Inadequate humidification can compromise airway patency. Assessment of breath sounds is difficult.

ETT, Endotracheal tube; *PEEP,* positive end-expiratory pressure.

TABLE 15.4   Ventilator Settings.

Parameter	Description	Typical Settings
Respiratory rate or frequency	Number of breaths ventilator delivers per minute	6—20 breaths/min
V_T	Volume of gas delivered to patient during each ventilator breath	6—10 mL/kg 4—8 mL/kg in ARDS
Oxygen concentration (FiO$_2$)	FiO$_2$ delivered to patient	May be set between 21% and 100%; adjusted to maintain PaO$_2$ level >60 mm Hg or SpO$_2$ level >92%
PEEP	Positive pressure applied at end of expiration of ventilator breaths	3—5 cm H$_2$O
PS	Positive pressure used to augment patient's inspiratory efforts	5—10 cm H$_2$O
Inspiratory flow rate and time	Speed with which V_T is delivered	40—80 L/min Time: 0.8—1.2 seconds
I:E ratio	Ratio of duration of inspiration to duration of expiration	1:2 to 1:1.5 unless inverse ratio ventilation is desired
Sensitivity	Determines amount of effort patient must generate to initiate a ventilator breath; it may be set for pressure triggering or flow triggering	Pressure trigger: 0.5—1.5 cm H$_2$O below baseline pressure Flow trigger: 1—3 L/min below baseline flow
High-pressure limit	Regulates maximal pressure ventilator can generate to deliver V_T; when pressure limit is reached, ventilator terminates breath and spills undelivered volume into atmosphere	10—20 cm H$_2$O above peak inspiratory pressure

ARDS, Acute respiratory distress syndrome; *FiO$_2$,* fraction of inspired oxygen; *I:E,* inspiratory to expiratory; *PaO$_2$,* arterial oxygen pressure; *PEEP,* positive end-expiratory time; *PS,* pressure support; *SpO$_2$,* oxygen saturation as measured by pulse oximetry; *V$_T$,* tidal volume.

ventilator. To minimize this problem, the ventilator is adjusted to accommodate the patient's spontaneous breathing pattern and to work with the patient. If this is not possible, the patient may need to be sedated or pharmacologically paralyzed.[63—65]

Ventilator-Associated Pneumonia

VAP is a type of hospital-acquired pneumonia that refers to the development of pneumonia 48 to 72 hours after endotracheal intubation.[66] A great potential for the development of pneumonia exists after placement of an artificial airway, because the tube bypasses or impairs many of the normal defense mechanisms of the lung. After an artificial airway has been placed, contamination of the lower airways follows within 24 hours. This results from many factors that directly and indirectly promote airway colonization. The use of respiratory therapy devices (e.g., ventilators, nebulizers, intermittent positive-pressure breathing machines) also can increase the risk of pneumonia.[53,67] The severity of the patient's illness, increased age, and the presence of ARDS or malnutrition significantly increase the likelihood that an infection will ensue. Therapeutic measures such as nasogastric intubation and gastric alkalization with enteral feedings or medications facilitate the development of pneumonia. Nasogastric tubes promote aspiration by acting as a wick for stomach contents, whereas enteral feedings, antacids, histamine inhibitors, and proton pump inhibitors increase the pH level of the stomach, promoting the growth of bacteria that can then be aspirated (Fig. 15.7).[68] Additional information on managing a patient with pneumonia is provided in Chapter 14. Prevention of VAP is crucial; strategies to prevent VAP are listed in Box 15.4.

Semirecumbency. Positioning of a patient who requires mechanical ventilation is very important. Semirecumbent positioning (elevation of the head of the bed 30—45 degrees) reduces the incidence of gastroesophageal reflux and subsequent aspiration of oropharyngeal secretions and decreases the incidence of VAP. The head of the patient's bed is elevated to 30 to 45 degrees at all times unless contraindicated (e.g., hemodynamic instability, presence of intraaortic balloon pump, physician's order to the contrary). However, this intervention increases the risk of skin shear on the coccyx, and extra surveillance is mandatory for prevention of pressure injuries.[69,70]

Sedation vacation. Many patients receiving mechanical ventilation require sedation to ameliorate symptoms of anxiety and stress associated with critical illness. However, the prolonged use of sedation has been shown to contribute to the development of complications, including oversedation, prolonged mechanical ventilation, and delirium. To decrease the incidence of these complications, the concept of a "sedation vacation" has been developed. A "sedation vacation" is simply the daily interruption of sedation to evaluate the

Pathogenesis of VAP

Common Sources of VAP Pathogens:
- ☐ Aspiration
- ☐ Intubation Procedure
- ☐ Biofilm Formation
- ☐ Contaminated Secretions
- ☐ Contaminated Respiratory Equipment

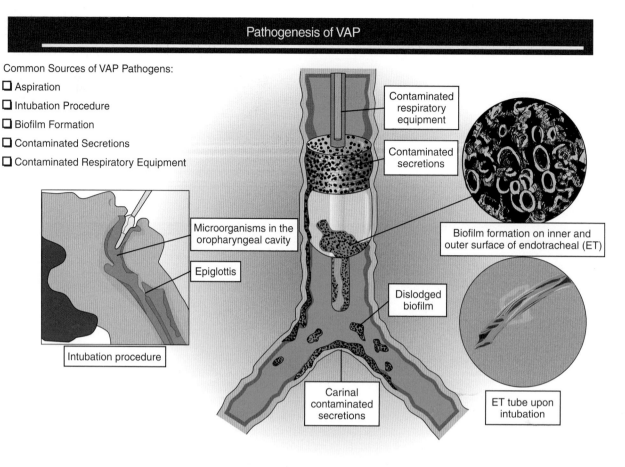

Contaminated respiratory equipment

Contaminated secretions

Biofilm formation on inner and outer surface of endotracheal (ET)

Microorganisms in the oropharyngeal cavity

Epiglottis

Dislodged biofilm

Intubation procedure

Carinal contaminated secretions

ET tube upon intubation

Fig. 15.7 Pathogenesis of Ventilator-Associated Pneumonia (VAP). (Redrawn from Sachdev G, Napolitano LM. Postoperative pulmonary complications: pneumonia and acute respiratory failure. *Surg Clin North Am.* 2012;92[2]:321–344.)

QSEN

BOX 15.4 Evidence-Based Practice

Prevention of Ventilator-Associated Pneumonia
- Use noninvasive positive-pressure ventilation when possible.
- Avoid or minimize the use of sedation.
- Conduct a spontaneous awakening trial daily unless contraindicated.
- Conduct a spontaneous breathing trial daily unless contraindicated.
- Initiate early mobilization and exercise.
- Begin intermittent or continuous subglottic secretion removal.

- Elevate the head of the bed 30–45 degrees.
- Change ventilator circuits only when visibly soiled.
- Perform routine oral care with chlorhexidine.
- Consider administration of prophylactic probiotics.
- Consider selective decontamination of the oropharynx and/or the digestive tract.

Modified from Klompas M, Branson R, Eichenwald EC, et al. Strategies to prevent ventilator-associated pneumonia in acute care hospitals: 2014 update. *Infect Control Hosp Epidemiol.* 2014;35(8):915–936.

---

patient and his or her need for continued sedation and mechanical ventilation. Not every patient is a candidate for this procedure. Contraindications include hemodynamic instability, increased intracranial pressure, ongoing agitation, seizures, alcohol withdrawal, and use of neuromuscular blocking agents. If the patient is able to tolerate being off the sedation for more than 4 hours (this number varies depending on the protocol being used), the sedation is discontinued. Signs of intolerance include ongoing agitation, increased respiratory rate, decreasing oxygen saturation, cardiac dysrhythmias, and signs of respiratory distress.[71]

Other measures to reduce incidence of ventilator-associated pneumonia. Studies have shown that use of an ETT with a polyurethane cuff may decrease the incidence of VAP. A traditional ETT has a polyvinyl low-

pressure, high-volume cuff. When the cuff is inflated, folds form in the cuff, allowing fluids and air to leak around the cuff and into the lungs; this is why subglottic secretion removal is so important. Polyurethane cuffs are much thinner than the traditional polyvinyl cuffs and do not form folds when they are inflated. No leakage of fluids into the lungs occurs.[67,72,73] In addition, some evidence suggests that the shape of the cuff may also affect this issue. A taper-shaped cuff appears to be better for preventing fluid leakage compared with a cylindrical cuff commonly found on most tubes.[74]

Another meta-analysis found limited evidence to support the use of silver-coated ETTs to reduce the incidence and delay the onset of VAP compared with a regular ETT.[75] The silver-coated tube decreases the incidence of VAP by preventing bacterial colonization and biofilm formation. Biofilm is formed when bacteria cling to the inner lumen of the ETT and then secrete an exopolysaccharide substance. This substance forms a gelatinous matrix that allows bacteria to thrive on a nonbiologic surface.[72,73]

Weaning

Weaning is the withdrawal of the mechanical ventilator and the reestablishment of spontaneous breathing. In the past weaning was the gradual withdrawal of mechanical ventilation; however, newer approaches use a more abrupt discontinuation and transition to spontaneous breathing.[76] Weaning is begun only after the original process for which ventilator support was required has been corrected and patient stability has been achieved. Other factors to consider when weaning are length of time on ventilator, sleep deprivation, and nutritional status. Major factors that affect the patient's ability to wean include the ability of the lungs to participate in ventilation and respiration, cardiovascular performance, and psychologic readiness.[76] This discussion focuses on weaning of a patient from short-term (3 days or less) mechanical ventilation. Management of weaning in a patient on long-term mechanical ventilation is discussed in Chapter 14.

Readiness to Wean

Patients are screened every day for their readiness to be weaned. The screen includes an evaluation of the patient's level of consciousness, physiologic and hemodynamic stability, adequacy of oxygenation and ventilation, spontaneous breathing capability, and respiratory rate and pattern.[76] Parameters that may be assessed are presented in Table 15.5.

The rapid shallow breathing index (RSBI) can predict weaning success. To calculate an RSBI, the patient's respiratory rate and minute ventilation are measured for 1 minute during spontaneous breathing. The measured respiratory rate is then divided by the tidal volume (expressed in liters). An RSBI of less than 105 is considered predictive of weaning success. If the patient is receiving sedation, the medication is discontinued at least 1 hour before the RSBI is measured. If the patient meets criteria for weaning readiness and has an RSBI of less than 105, a spontaneous breathing trial (SBT) can be performed.[77] One study showed that implementation of a weaning program that incorporated daily SBTs had a positive effect on extubation rates and no effect on reintubation rates.[78] Fig. 15.8 outlines one approach commonly used in the critical care setting.

Weaning Trial

After the patient's readiness to be weaned has been established, the patient is prepared for a weaning trial.[79] The patient is positioned upright to facilitate breathing and suctioned to ensure airway patency. The process is explained to the patient, and the patient is offered reassurance and diversional activities. The patient is assessed immediately before the start of the trial and frequently during the weaning period for signs of weaning intolerance (Box 15.5).[76,77,79]

Numerous methods can be used for conducting a weaning. The three main methods that are used are (1) SBT, (2) pressure support ventilation (PSV) trial, and synchronized intermittent mandatory ventilation (SIMV) trial.[76] The method selected depends on the patient, his or her pulmonary status, and length of time on the ventilator. Regardless of the method selected, evidence shows that using a standardized approach decreases weaning time and length of stay in the critical care unit.[80]

Spontaneous breathing trials. An SBT can be done with the patient either on or off the ventilator. One method is to remove the patient

TABLE 15.5 Conventional Weaning Parameters.

Parameters	Weanable Values	Normal Ranges
NIF (cm H_2O)	< −20	< −50
VC (mL/kg)	> 10	> 65–75
V_T (mL/kg)	< 5	> 5–7
RR (breaths/min)	< 32	12–20
V_E (L/min)	> 10	> 10
RSBI (RR/V_T)	< 105	< 40

NIF, Negative inspiratory force; *RR*, respiratory rate; *RSBI*, rapid shallow breathing index; *VC*, vital capacity; *V$_E$*, minute ventilation; *V$_T$*, tidal volume.
From Benjamin IJ, ed. *Andreoli and Carpenter's Cecil Essentials of Medicine*. 9th ed. Philadelphia: Elsevier; 2016.

from the ventilator, placing him or her on a T-piece oxygen delivery system via the ETT or tracheostomy tube, and have the patient breathe spontaneously. Another method is to leave the patient on the ventilator and discontinue the mandatory breaths. When this is done, continuous positive airway pressure (CPAP) may be added to prevent atelectasis and improve oxygenation, or pressure support may be added to augment inspiration.[77,79,81] One recommendation for the initial SBT for patients who have been mechanically ventilated for longer than 24 hours is the addition of 5 to 8 cm H_2O of pressure support.[82] A single daily SBT usually lasts from 30 minutes to 2 hours. During the weaning process, the patient is observed closely for respiratory muscle fatigue. If the trial is successful, extubation is considered. If the trial is unsuccessful, a period of rest is provided before another trial is attempted.[76,77,79] If the patient has been receiving mechanical ventilation for longer than 24 hours and is at high risk for extubation failure, the patient should be extubated and placed on noninvasive ventilation (NIV).[82]

Synchronized intermittent mandatory ventilation trials. The goal of SIMV weaning is the gradual transition from ventilatory support to spontaneous breathing. SIMV weaning is initiated by placing the ventilator in the SIMV mode and slowly decreasing the rate, usually one to three breaths at a time, until a rate of zero or near-zero is reached. An arterial blood gas (ABG) sample is usually obtained 30 minutes after the trial. This method of weaning can increase the work of breathing, and the patient must be closely monitored for signs of respiratory muscle fatigue.[76]

Pressure support ventilation trials. PSV weaning consists of placing the patient on the pressure support mode and setting the pressure support at a level that facilitates the patient's achieving a spontaneous tidal volume of 10 to 12 mL/kg. PSV augments the patient's spontaneous breaths with a positive pressure boost during inspiration. During the weaning process, the level of pressure support is gradually decreased in increments of 3 to 6 cm H_2O, while the tidal volume is maintained at 10 to 15 mL/kg until a level of 5 cm H_2O is achieved. If the patient is able to maintain adequate spontaneous respirations at this level, extubation is considered. PSV also can be used with SIMV weaning to help overcome the resistance in the ventilator system.[76]

Nursing Management

Nursing priorities for the patient requiring invasive mechanical ventilation focus on (1) evaluating the patient for patient-related complications and (2) monitoring the patient for ventilator-related complications.

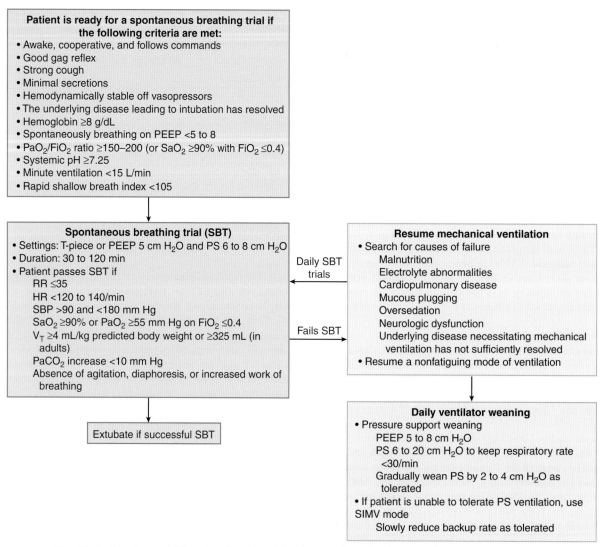

Patient is ready for a spontaneous breathing trial if the following criteria are met:
- Awake, cooperative, and follows commands
- Good gag reflex
- Strong cough
- Minimal secretions
- Hemodynamically stable off vasopressors
- The underlying disease leading to intubation has resolved
- Hemoglobin ≥8 g/dL
- Spontaneously breathing on PEEP <5 to 8
- PaO_2/FiO_2 ratio ≥150–200 (or SaO_2 ≥90% with FiO_2 ≤0.4)
- Systemic pH ≥7.25
- Minute ventilation <15 L/min
- Rapid shallow breath index <105

Spontaneous breathing trial (SBT)
- Settings: T-piece or PEEP 5 cm H_2O and PS 6 to 8 cm H_2O
- Duration: 30 to 120 min
- Patient passes SBT if
    RR ≤35
    HR <120 to 140/min
    SBP >90 and <180 mm Hg
    SaO_2 ≥90% or PaO_2 ≥55 mm Hg on FiO_2 ≤0.4
    V_T ≥4 mL/kg predicted body weight or ≥325 mL (in adults)
    $PaCO_2$ increase <10 mm Hg
    Absence of agitation, diaphoresis, or increased work of breathing

Daily SBT trials

Fails SBT

Extubate if successful SBT

Resume mechanical ventilation
- Search for causes of failure
    Malnutrition
    Electrolyte abnormalities
    Cardiopulmonary disease
    Mucous plugging
    Oversedation
    Neurologic dysfunction
    Underlying disease necessitating mechanical ventilation has not sufficiently resolved
- Resume a nonfatiguing mode of ventilation

Daily ventilator weaning
- Pressure support weaning
    PEEP 5 to 8 cm H_2O
    PS 6 to 20 cm H_2O to keep respiratory rate <30/min
    Gradually wean PS by 2 to 4 cm H_2O as tolerated
- If patient is unable to tolerate PS ventilation, use SIMV mode
    Slowly reduce backup rate as tolerated

Fig. 15.8 Weaning and Liberation Algorithm. Weaning and liberation from mechanical ventilators. FiO_2, Fraction of inspired oxygen; *HR*, heart rate; $PaCO_2$, partial pressure of arterial carbon dioxide; PaO_2, partial pressure of arterial oxygen; *PEEP*, positive end-expiratory pressure; *PS*, pressure support; *RR*, respiratory rate; SaO_2, arterial oxygen saturation; *SBP*, systolic blood pressure; *SIMV*, synchronized intermittent mandatory ventilation; V_T, tidal volume. (Modified from MacIntyre NR, Cook DJ, Ely EW Jr, et al. Evidence-based guidelines for weaning and discontinuing ventilatory support. *Chest.* 2001;120[6 suppl]:375S–395S. [From Goldman L, Scharfer AI, eds. *Goldman-Cecil Medicine.* 26th ed. Philadelphia: Elsevier; 2020.])

Patient Assessment

Assessment of a patient requiring mechanical ventilation focuses on the pulmonary system, placement of the ETT or tracheostomy tube, and monitoring for the development of subcutaneous emphysema and dyssynchrony with the ventilator. Bedside evaluation of vital capacity, minute ventilation, ABG values, and other pulmonary function tests may be warranted, according to the patient's condition. The use of pulse oximetry can facilitate continuous, noninvasive assessment of oxygenation. The use of capnography may facilitate continuous noninvasive assessment of ventilation. Static and dynamic compliance are also monitored to assess for changes in lung compliance (see Appendix B).[83]

Symptom Management

Patients requiring mechanical ventilation may present with a variety of disturbing symptoms, including anxiety, pain, shortness of breath, confusion and agitation, and sleep disturbances. These symptoms are often managed with sedation and analgesic medications. As discussed earlier, these medications could contribute to prolonged mechanical ventilation and delirium. Nonpharmacologic interventions have been shown to be of benefit to these patients. These interventions include promoting a healing environment, promoting sleep, and interventions to lessen anxiety (e.g., music therapy, guided imagery, nursing presence, and animal-assisted therapy). Nursing activities to promote a healing environment include minimizing noise levels, ensuring the patient has access to natural light, establishing a method of communication with the patient, and providing the patient with explanations of what is occurring around them.[84] Referral to a complementary and alternative therapy specialist (if one is available) is also appropriate.

ABCDEF Bundle

Another bundle that has been proposed is the Awakening and Breathing Coordination, Delirium Monitoring, Early Mobility, and Family Engagement and Empowerment (ABCDEF) bundle. This

BOX 15.5 Weaning Intolerance Indicators

- Decrease in level of consciousness
- Systolic blood pressure increased or decreased by 20 mm Hg
- Diastolic blood pressure greater than 100 mm Hg
- Heart rate increased by 20 beats/min
- Premature ventricular contractions greater than 6 per minute, couplets, or runs of ventricular tachycardia
- Changes in ST segment (usually elevation)
- Respiratory rate greater than 30 breaths/min or less than 10 breaths/min
- Respiratory rate increased by 10 breaths/min
- Spontaneous tidal volume less than 250 mL
- $PaCO_2$ increased by 5–8 mm Hg and/or pH less than 7.30
- SpO_2 less than 90%
- Use of accessory muscles of ventilation
- Complaints of dyspnea, fatigue, or pain
- Paradoxical chest wall motion or chest abdominal asynchrony
- Diaphoresis
- Severe agitation or anxiety unrelieved by reassurance

PaCO₂, Arterial carbon dioxide pressure; *SpO₂*, oxygen saturation as measured by pulse oximetry.

bundle focuses on enhancing communication between team members in the critical care unit, standardizing patient care processes, and decreasing the incidence of delirium and prolonged weakness associated with critical illness.[85] The ABCDEF bundle activities are presented in Box 15.6. To facilitate the implementation of the ABCDEF bundle, the patient must be allowed to sleep.

Ventilator Assessment

Assessment of the ventilator includes a review of all the ventilator settings and alarms. A clear understanding of the alarms and their related problems is important (Box 15.7). Peak inspiratory pressure, exhaled tidal volume, and ABGs are also monitored.

Patient Safety

Several measures are required to maintain a trouble-free ventilator system. These include maintaining a functional MRB connected to oxygen at the bedside, ensuring that the ventilator tubing is free of water, positioning the ventilator tubing to avoid kinking, maintaining the patency of ventilator tubing and connections, changing ventilator tubing per hospital policy, and monitoring the temperature of the inspired air. If the ventilator malfunctions, the patient is removed from the ventilator and ventilated manually with an MRB. Alarms should be sufficiently audible with respect to distance and competing noise within the unit.

NONINVASIVE VENTILATION

NIV is an alternative method of ventilation that uses a mask instead of an ETT to deliver the therapy. Advantages of this type of ventilation include decreased frequency of hospital-acquired pneumonia; increased comfort; and the noninvasive nature of the procedure, which allows easy application and removal. NIV is indicated in type I and type II acute lung failure, cardiogenic pulmonary edema, and other situations in which intubation is not an option. Contraindications to NIV include hemodynamic instability; dysrhythmias; apnea; uncooperativeness; intolerance of the mask; recent upper airway or esophageal surgery; and inability to maintain a patent airway, clear secretions, or properly fit the mask.[86]

NIV can be applied with a full-face, nasal, or face mask and ventilator or with a bilevel positive airway pressure (BiPAP) machine (Respironics, Inc., Murrysville, PA). One study found that a full-face mask is better tolerated than a nasal mask and associated with a diminished incidence of pressure injuries.[87] This type of ventilation uses a combination of PSV and PEEP supplied by a ventilator, or inspiratory and expiratory positive airway pressure supplied by a BiPAP machine to assist the spontaneously breathing patient with ventilation. On inspiration, the patient receives PSV or inspiratory positive airway pressure to increase tidal volume and minute ventilation, resulting in increased alveolar ventilation, a decreased $PaCO_2$ level, relief of dyspnea, and reduced accessory muscle use. On expiration, the patient receives PEEP or expiratory positive airway pressure to increase functional residual capacity, resulting in an increased PaO_2 level. Humidified supplemental oxygen is administered to maintain a clinically acceptable PaO_2 level, and timed breaths may be added, if necessary.[88]

Nursing Management

Nursing interventions for the patient with noninvasive mechanical ventilation focus on evaluating the patient for patient-related complications and monitoring the patient for ventilator-related complications. Routine assessment of these patients includes monitoring for patient-related and ventilator-related complications. As with invasive mechanical ventilation, the patient must be closely monitored. Respiratory rate, accessory muscle use, and oxygenation status are continually assessed to ensure that the patient is tolerating this method of ventilation. Continuous pulse oximetry is also used.[88,89]

The key to ensuring adequate ventilatory support is a properly fitted mask. A nasal mask, face mask, or full-face mask may be used, depending on the patient. A properly fitted mask minimizes air leakage and discomfort for the patient. Transparent dressings placed over the pressure points of the face help minimize air leakage and prevent facial pressure injuries caused by the mask.[89] The BiPAP machine is able to compensate for air leaks.[88]

The patient is positioned with the head of the bed elevated at 45 degrees to minimize the risk of aspiration and to facilitate breathing. Insufflation of the stomach is a complication of this mode of therapy and places the patient at risk for aspiration. The patient is closely monitored for gastric distention, and a nasogastric tube is placed for decompression, as necessary. Patients are often very anxious and have high levels of dyspnea before the initiation of noninvasive mechanical ventilation. After adequate ventilation has been established, anxiety and dyspnea are usually sufficiently relieved. Heavy sedation is avoided, but if it is needed, it would constitute the need for intubation and invasive mechanical ventilation. It is important to spend 30 minutes with the patient after initiation of NIV, because the patient needs reassurance and must learn how to breathe on the machine.[88] The patient who requires NIV with a face mask should never be restrained. The patient must be able to remove the mask if it becomes displaced or the patient vomits. A displaced mask can force the patient's bottom jaw inward and occlude the patient's airway.

POSITIONING THERAPY

Positioning therapy can help match ventilation and perfusion through the redistribution of oxygen and blood flow in the lungs, which improves gas exchange. On the basis of the concept that preferential blood flow occurs to the gravity-dependent areas of the lungs, positioning therapy is used to place the least damaged portion of the lungs into a dependent position. The least damaged portions of the lungs

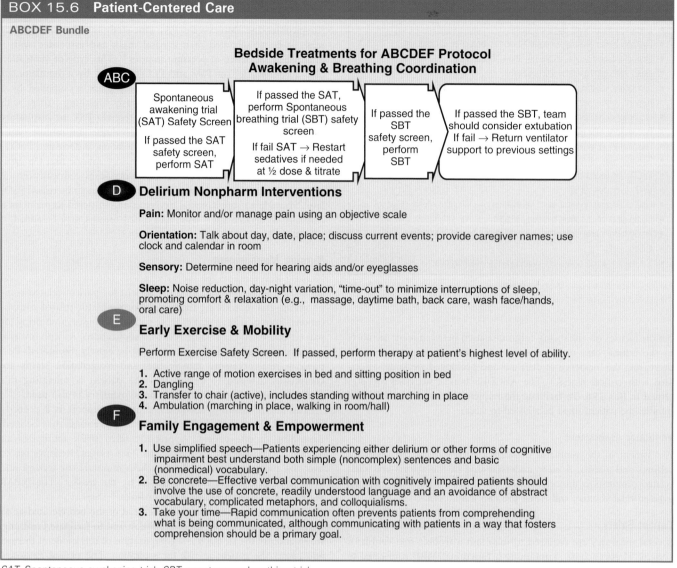

QSEN BOX 15.6 Patient-Centered Care

ABCDEF Bundle

Bedside Treatments for ABCDEF Protocol
Awakening & Breathing Coordination

ABC

Spontaneous awakening trial (SAT) Safety Screen

If passed the SAT safety screen, perform SAT

If passed the SAT, perform Spontaneous breathing trial (SBT) safety screen

If fail SAT → Restart sedatives if needed at ½ dose & titrate

If passed the SBT safety screen, perform SBT

If passed the SBT, team should consider extubation
If fail → Return ventilator support to previous settings

D Delirium Nonpharm Interventions

Pain: Monitor and/or manage pain using an objective scale

Orientation: Talk about day, date, place; discuss current events; provide caregiver names; use clock and calendar in room

Sensory: Determine need for hearing aids and/or eyeglasses

Sleep: Noise reduction, day-night variation, "time-out" to minimize interruptions of sleep, promoting comfort & relaxation (e.g., massage, daytime bath, back care, wash face/hands, oral care)

E Early Exercise & Mobility

Perform Exercise Safety Screen. If passed, perform therapy at patient's highest level of ability.

1. Active range of motion exercises in bed and sitting position in bed
2. Dangling
3. Transfer to chair (active), includes standing without marching in place
4. Ambulation (marching in place, walking in room/hall)

F Family Engagement & Empowerment

1. Use simplified speech—Patients experiencing either delirium or other forms of cognitive impairment best understand both simple (noncomplex) sentences and basic (nonmedical) vocabulary.
2. Be concrete—Effective verbal communication with cognitively impaired patients should involve the use of concrete, readily understood language and an avoidance of abstract vocabulary, complicated metaphors, and colloquialisms.
3. Take your time—Rapid communication often prevents patients from comprehending what is being communicated, although communicating with patients in a way that fosters comprehension should be a primary goal.

SAT, Spontaneous awakening trial; *SBT,* spontaneous breathing trial.

Modified from ICU Delirium and Cognitive Impairment Study Group. Bedside treatments for ABCDE protocol. http://www.icudelirium.org/docs/ABCDEF_Pocket_Reference.pdf.

receive preferential blood flow, resulting in less ($\dot{V}/\dot{Q}$) mismatch. Two approaches to position therapy are (1) prone positioning and (2) rotation therapy.

Prone Positioning

Prone positioning is a therapeutic modality that is used to improve oxygenation in patients with ARDS.[90-92] It involves turning the patient completely over onto his or her stomach in the face-down position. Although numerous theories have been proposed to explain how prone positioning improves oxygenation, the discovery that ARDS causes greater damage to the dependent areas of the lungs probably provides the best explanation. It was originally thought that ARDS was a diffuse, homogeneous disease that affected all areas of the lungs equally. It is now known that the dependent lung areas are more heavily damaged than the nondependent lung areas. Turning the patient to the prone position improves perfusion to the less damaged areas of the lungs, improves ($\dot{V}/\dot{Q}$) match, and

decreases intrapulmonary shunting. Prone positioning can be used to facilitate the mobilization of secretions and provide pressure relief. Prone positioning is contraindicated in patients with increased intracranial pressure, hemodynamic instability, spinal cord injuries, or abdominal surgery. Patients who are unable to tolerate the face-down position are also not appropriate candidates for this type of therapy.[90-92]

No standard has been established for the length of time a patient should remain in the prone position. A review of the research on this subject revealed a wide variation ranging from 12 to 20 hours.[92] The therapy is considered successful if the patient has an improvement in PaO_2 of greater than 10 mm Hg within 30 minutes of being placed in the prone position.[93] The positioning schedule (length of time in the prone position and frequency of turning) is usually based on the patient's tolerance of the procedure, the success of the procedure in improving the patient's PaO_2, and whether the patient is able to sustain improvements in PaO_2 when turned back

BOX 15.7 Troubleshooting Ventilator Alarms

Problem	Causes	Interventions
Low exhaled V_T	Altered settings; any condition that triggers high- or low-pressure alarm; patient stops spontaneous respirations; leak in system preventing V_T from being delivered; cuff insufficiently inflated; leak through chest tube; airway secretions; decreased lung compliance; spirometer disconnected or malfunctioning	Check settings; evaluate patient, check respiratory rate; check all connections for leaks; suction patient's airway; check cuff pressure; calibrate spirometer.
Low inspiratory pressure	Altered settings; unattached tubing or leak around ETT; ETT displaced into pharynx or esophagus; poor cuff inflation or leak; tracheoesophageal fistula; peak flows that are too low; low V_T; decreased airway resistance resulting from decreased secretions or relief of bronchospasm; increased lung compliance resulting from decreased atelectasis; reduction in pulmonary edema; resolution of ARDS; change in position	Reset alarm; reconnect tubing; modify cuff pressures; tighten humidifier; check chest tube; adjust peak flow to meet or exceed patient demand and correct for patient's V_T; reposition or change ETT.
Low exhaled minute volume	Altered settings; leak in system; airway secretions; decreased lung compliance; malfunctioning spirometer; decreased patient-triggered respiratory rate resulting from medications, sleep, hypocapnia, alkalosis, fatigue, change in neurologic status	Check settings; assess patient's respiratory rate, mental status, work of breathing; evaluate system for leaks; suction airway; assess patient for changes in disease state; calibrate spirometer.
Low PEEP/CPAP pressure	Altered settings; increased patient inspirator/flows; leak; decreased expiratory flows from ventilator	Check settings and correct; observe for leaks in system; if unable to correct problem, increase PEEP settings.
High respiratory rate	Increased metabolic demand; medication administration; hypoxia; hypercapnia; acidosis; shock; pain; fear; anxiety	Evaluate ABGs; assess patient; calm and reassure patient.
High-pressure limit	Improper alarm setting; airway obstruction resulting from patient fighting ventilator (holding breath as ventilator delivers V_T); patient circuit collapse; tubing kinked; ETT in right mainstem bronchus or against carina; cuff herniation; increased airway resistance resulting from bronchospasm, airway secretions, plugs, and coughing; water from humidifier in ventilator tubing; decreased lung compliance resulting from tension pneumothorax, change in patient position, ARDS, pulmonary edema, atelectasis, pneumonia, or abdominal distention	Reset alarms; clear obstruction from tubing; unkink and reposition patient off of tubing; empty water from tubing; check breath sounds; reassure patient and sedate if necessary; check ABGs for hypoxemia; observe for abdominal distention that would put pressure on diaphragm; check cuff pressures; obtain chest radiograph and evaluate for ETT position, pneumothorax, and pneumonia; reposition ETT; give bronchodilator therapy.
Low-pressure oxygen inlet	Improper oxygen alarm setting; oxygen not connected to ventilator; dirty oxygen intake filter	Correct alarm setting; reconnect or connect oxygen line to 50-psi source; clean or replace oxygen filter.
I:E ratio	Inspiratory time longer than expiratory time; use of an inspiratory phase that is too long with a fast rate; peak flow setting too low, whereas rate too high; machine too sensitive	Change inspiratory time or adjust peak flow; check inspiratory phase, or hold; check machine sensitivity.
Temperature	Sensor malfunction; overheating resulting from too low or no gas flow; sensor picking up outside airflow (from heater, open door or window, air conditioner); improper water levels	Test or replace sensor; check gas flow; protect sensor from outside source that would interfere with readings; check water levels.

ABGs, Arterial blood gases; *ARDS*, acute respiratory distress syndrome; *CPAP*, continuous positive airway pressure; *ETT*, endotracheal tube; *I:E*, inspiratory to expiratory; *PEEP*, positive end-expiratory pressure; V_T, tidal volume.
Modified from Flynn JBM, Bruce NP. *Introduction to Critical Care Nursing Skills*. St. Louis: Mosby; 1993.

to the supine position. Prone positioning is discontinued when the patient no longer demonstrates a response to the position change.[93]

The biggest limitation to prone positioning is the actual mechanics of turning the patient. Numerous methods have been discussed in the literature, including manually turning the patient and positioning with pillows to support the patient and use of the RotoProne therapy system (ArjoHuntleigh, Malmö, Sweden).[90] Regardless of the method used, the abdomen must be allowed to hang free to facilitate diaphragmatic descent.

Before the patient is turned to the prone position, his or her eyes are lubricated and taped closed, tubes and drains are secured, and the procedure is explained to the patient and family (Box 15.8). A team is organized to implement the turning procedure, and one member is positioned at the head of the bed to maintain the patient's airway. Complications of the procedure include dislodgment or obstruction of

tubes and drains, hemodynamic instability, massive facial edema, pressure injuries (Box 15.9), aspiration, and corneal ulcerations.[90,92]

Rotation Therapy

Automated turning beds to provide rotation therapy are often used in the critical care setting. Kinetic therapy and continuous lateral rotation therapy (CLRT) are two forms of rotation therapy. The patient is continuously turned from side to side with a rotation of 40 degrees or greater (kinetic therapy) or with a rotation of less than 40 degrees (CLRT).[94] Two types of beds can perform this type of therapy: (1) an oscillation bed, in which the mattress inflates and deflates to provide rotation, and (2) a kinetic bed, in which the entire platform of the bed rotates.[95]

Rotation therapy is thought to improve oxygenation through better matching of ventilation to perfusion and to prevent pulmonary

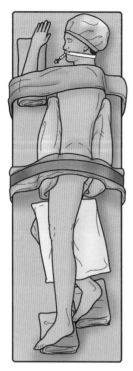 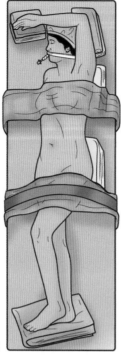

A **B**

Fig. 15.9 Positions for Thoracotomy Incisions. (A) Lateral position for posterolateral incision. (B) Semilateral position for axillary or anterolateral position. (From Rothrock JC, McEwen DR, eds. Alexander's Care of the Patient in Surgery. 16th ed. St. Louis: Elsevier; 2019.)

Complications of the procedure include dislodgment or obstruction of tubes, drains, and lines; hemodynamic instability; and pressure injuries. Lateral rotation does not replace manual repositioning to prevent pressure injuries.[99] Repositioning changes the relationship of the patient's posterior surface to the mattress. This gives the skin a chance to reperfuse and to ventilate. Repositioning shifts weight-bearing points. To prevent pressure injuries, the patient is positioned 30 degrees from the surface of the mattress regardless of the degree of rotational turn. One study found that patients receiving rotational therapy still developed pressure injuries of the sacrum, occiput, and heels.[100]

THORACIC SURGERY

The term *thoracic surgery* refers to numerous surgical procedures that involve opening the thoracic cavity (thoracotomy), the organs of respiration, or both. Indications for thoracic surgery range from tumors and abscesses to repair of the esophagus and thoracic vessels.[101] Table 15.6 describes various thoracic surgical procedures and their indications. This discussion focuses only on the surgical procedures that involve the removal of lung tissue.

Preoperative Care

Before surgery, a complete evaluation of the patient is needed to determine the appropriateness of surgery as a treatment and to determine whether lung tissue can be removed without jeopardizing respiratory function. This is especially important when a lobectomy or pneumonectomy is being considered. When resection is being undertaken for tumor treatment, preoperative care includes evaluation of the type and extent of the tumor and the physical condition of the patient.[102]

The evaluation of the patient's physical status focuses on the adequacy of cardiopulmonary function. The preoperative evaluation includes pulmonary function tests to determine the patient's ability to manage with less lung tissue. Cardiac function is also evaluated. Uncontrolled dysrhythmias, acute myocardial infarction, severe chronic heart failure, and unstable angina all are contraindications to surgery.[103,104]

Surgical Considerations

The type and location of surgery dictate the type of surgical approach that is used (Fig. 15.9). The most common approach is the posterolateral thoracotomy, which allows for exposure of both the lung and

complications associated with bed rest and mechanical ventilation.[96,97] However, to achieve such benefits, rotation must be aggressive, and the patient must be turned at least 40 degrees per side, with a total arc of at least 80 degrees, for at least 18 hours a day.[97,98] CLRT has been shown to be of minimal pulmonary benefit to critically ill patients.[94] Kinetic therapy decreases the incidence of VAP, particularly in patients with neurologic problems and in patients who have undergone surgery.[98] In one study, kinetic therapy decreased the incidence of VAP and lobar atelectasis in medical, surgical, and trauma patients.[97]

QSEN

BOX 15.8 Safety

ABCDEFG of Prone Positioning

		Before Prone Positioning	After Prone Positioning
A	Attachments	Disconnect attachments such as ECG electrodes, oxygen saturation probe, end-tidal carbon dioxide probe, temperature probe, and noninvasive blood pressure cuff.	Reattach the disconnected attachments.
B	Bedding	Keep another bed sheet ready for replacement.	Check the bedding for any inappropriate item that might hurt, for example, an inappropriate fold in the sheet, bumps, needle caps.
C	Catheters	The horizontal movement should be to the side with central venous catheters, detach infusions if necessary. Be careful with dialysis and arterial catheters. Ensure adequate slack in infusion lining.	Check position, reattach infusions.
D	Dependent regions	Pad dependent regions which are common sites of pressure sores, such as forehead, chin, and knee, with adhesive pads.	Padding may get displaced while rotating; ensure position after prone positioning.
E	Endotracheal tube	Mark the position of the endotracheal tube. Secure the tube throughout the movement. Ensure adequate slack in the ventilator tubings.	Confirm position by noting down the mark.
F	Foley Catheter	Foley catheter with the urine bag should be detached from the side of the bed and should be kept between the legs.	Attach on either side.
G	Genitals	Genitals need special attention, as these can be an ignored site of pressure sores.	

From Baldi, M, Sehgal IS, Dhooria S, Agarwal R. Prone positioning? Remember ABCDEFG. *Chest.* 2017;151(5):1184–1185.

BOX 15.9   Quality Improvement

Prevention of Hospital-Acquired Pressure Injury in the Prone Patient

Patients undergoing prone positioning are at risk for several complications, including hospital-acquired pressure injuries. Once the patient is placed in the prone position, they may remain there for 18 hours or longer, depending on the proning protocol. Sustained periods in this position place the patient at risk of pressure damage. Areas at high risk include the patient's head (i.e., forehead, nose, cheeks, and chin), torso (i.e., clavicle, breasts, iliac crests, ischium, symphysis pubis, and genitalia), and arms and legs (i.e., shoulders, elbows, knees, feet, and toes).[1]

Assessment is vital in preventing pressure injuries, particularly watching for uneven pressure redistribution. The patient's skin should be assessed regularly and before turning either supine or prone. It is important to document a comprehensive skin assessment at regular intervals. The patient's skin should be kept clean and moisturized.

If manually proning the patient, a pressure redistribution surface (e.g., mattress or overlay) should be used along with positioning devices to offload pressure to high-risk areas. While in the prone position, minor position adjustments can be performed. The patient's arms and head should be placed in the freestyle swim position. In this position, one arm is placed at the patient's side, and the other is placed next to the head. The patient's head is then turned toward the arm. The position of the patient's arms and head is routinely alternated at least every 4 hours, allowing for pressure relief. Additional prophylactic measures that can be taken include the application of[1]:

- Soft silicone multilayered form dressings to the high-risk pressure areas
- Thin foam dressings under medical devices
- Liquid skin sealants on the face to protect from excessive moisture and oral secretions
- Foam positioning devices to offload pressure to the patient's head and feet

It is essential to follow the manufacturer's instructions when using positioning devices, dressings, and other products. For more information about pressure injuries, check out the National Pressure Injury Advisory Panel (NPIAP) website (www.npiap.com).

Reference

1. National Pressure Injury Advisory Panel. *Pressure injury prevention: PIP tips for prone positioning,* 2020. https://cdn.ymaws.com/npiap.com/resource/resmgr/online_store/posters/npiap_pip_tips_-_proning_202.pdf.

---

the mediastinum. Other approaches that are used include anterolateral thoracotomy and median sternotomy.[101]

Special care is taken to avoid drainage of blood or secretions into the unaffected lung during surgery, because such an occurrence could cause hypoxemia and cardiac dysfunction. A double-lumen ETT is used during surgery to protect the unaffected lung from secretions and necrotic tumor fragments. To decrease the incidence of hypoxemia during the procedure, 5 to 10 cm H_2O of PEEP is maintained to the deflated lung. In addition, the deflated lung is intermittently ventilated during the procedure.[105]

Complications and Medical Management

Many complications are associated with a lung resection, including acute lung failure, bronchopleural fistula, hemorrhage, cardiovascular disturbances, and mediastinal shift.

Acute Lung Failure

In the postoperative period, acute lung failure may result from atelectasis or pneumonia. Atelectasis can occur as a result of anesthesia, the surgical procedure, immobilization, and pain. Treatment is aimed at correcting the underlying problems and supporting gas exchange. Supplemental oxygen and mechanical ventilation with PEEP may be necessary.[106]

Bronchopleural Fistula

Development of a postoperative bronchopleural fistula is a major cause of mortality after a lung resection. A bronchopleural fistula develops when the suture line fails to secure occlusion of the bronchial stump and an opening develops into the pleural space.[107] This can result from an imperfect stump closure, perforation of the stump (e.g., with a suction catheter), high pressure within the airways (e.g., caused by mechanical ventilation), or infection.[108] During surgery, careful attention is given to isolating and closing the bronchus in an attempt to secure a lasting seal with subsequent stump healing.[101] In addition, early extubation is encouraged to eliminate the possibility of perforation of the stump and high airway pressures.[108] Clinical manifestations of a bronchopleural fistula include shortness of breath and coughing up serosanguineous sputum. Immediate surgery is usually necessary to close the stump and prevent flooding of the remaining lung with fluid from the residual space. If this occurs, the patient is placed with the operative side down (remaining lung up), and a chest tube is inserted to drain the residual space.[101]

Hemorrhage

Hemorrhage is an early, life-threatening complication that can occur after a lung resection and can result from bronchial or intercostal artery bleeding or disruption of a suture or clip around a pulmonary vessel.[108] Excessive chest tube drainage can signal the presence of this complication. During the immediate postoperative period, chest tube drainage is measured every 15 minutes; this frequency is decreased as the patient stabilizes. If chest tube drainage is greater than 100 mL/h, fresh blood is noted, or a sudden increase in drainage occurs, hemorrhage should be suspected.

Cardiovascular Disturbances

Cardiovascular complications after thoracic surgery include dysrhythmias and pulmonary edema. Resections of a large lung area or a pneumonectomy may be followed by an increase in central venous pressure. With the loss of one lung, the right ventricle must empty its stroke volume into a vascular bed that has been reduced by 50%. This means a higher pressure system is created, which increases right ventricular workload and precipitates right ventricular failure. Depending on previous heart function, acute decompensation of both ventricles can result. Measures are aimed at supporting cardiac function and avoiding intravascular volume excess. These measures include optimizing preload, afterload, and contractility with vasoactive agents.[108]

Postoperative Nursing Management

Nursing care of a patient who has had thoracic surgery incorporates many patient problems (Box 15.10). Nursing priorities focus on (1) optimizing oxygenation and ventilation, (2) preventing atelectasis, (3)

TABLE 15.6 Thoracic Surgeries.

Procedure	Definition	Indications
Pneumonectomy	Removal of entire lung with or without resection of mediastinal lymph nodes	Malignant lesions Unilateral tuberculosis Extensive unilateral bronchiectasis Multiple lung abscesses Massive hemoptysis Bronchopleural fistula
Lobectomy	Resection of one or more lobes of lung	Lesions confined to single lobe Pulmonary tuberculosis Bronchiectasis Lung abscesses or cysts Trauma
Segmental resection	Resection of bronchovascular section of lung lobe	Small peripheral lesions Bronchiectasis Congenital cysts or blebs
Wedge resection	Removal of small wedge-shaped section of lung tissue	Small, peripheral lesions (without lymph node involvement) Peripheral granulomas Pulmonary blebs
Bronchoplastic reconstruction (also called *sleeve resection*)	Resection of lung tissue and bronchus with end-to-end reanastomosis of bronchus	Small lesions involving carina or major bronchus without evidence of metastasis May be combined with lobectomy
Lung volume reduction surgery	Resection of most damaged portions of lung tissue, allowing more normal chest wall configuration	Severe emphysema
Bullectomy	Resection of large bulla (airspace that is >1 cm in diameter that formed as a result of pulmonary tissue destruction)	Severe emphysema with large bullae compressing surrounding tissue

TABLE 15.6 Thoracic Surgeries.—cont'd

Procedure	Definition	Indications
Open lung biopsy	Resection of small portion of lung for biopsy	Failure of closed lung biopsy Removal of small lesions
Decortication	Removal of fibrous membrane from pleural surface of lung.	Fibrothorax resulting from hemothorax or empyema
Drainage of empyema	Drainage of pus in pleural space	Acute and chronic infections
Partial rib resection	Removal of one or more ribs to allow healing of underlying lung tissue	Chronic empyemic infections
Video-assisted thoracoscopy (VATS)	Endoscopic procedure performed through small incisions in chest	Evaluation of pulmonary, pleural, mediastinal, or pericardial conditions Biopsy of lung, pleural, or mediastinal lesions Recurrent spontaneous pneumothorax Evacuation of emphysema, hemothorax, pleural effusion, or pericardial effusion Blebectomy or bullectomy Pleurodesis Sympathectomy Closure of bronchopleural fistula Lysis of adhesions

---

BOX 15.10 PRIORITY PATIENT CARE MANAGEMENT

Thoracic Surgery

- Impaired Breathing due to decreased lung expansion
- Impaired Gas Exchange due to ventilation-perfusion mismatching or intrapulmonary shunting
- Impaired Gas Exchange due to alveolar hypoventilation
- Acute Pain due to transmission and perception of cutaneous, visceral, muscular, or ischemic impulses
- Anxiety due to threat to biologic, psychologic, or social integrity
Patient Care Management plans are located in Appendix A.

---

maintaining the chest tube system, (4) assisting the patient to return to an adequate activity level, (5) providing comfort and emotional support, and (6) maintaining surveillance for complications.

Optimizing Oxygenation and Ventilation

Nursing interventions to optimize oxygenation and ventilation include positioning, preventing desaturation during procedures, and promoting secretion clearance.

Prevent Atelectasis

Nursing interventions to prevent atelectasis include proper patient positioning and early ambulation, deep-breathing exercises, incentive spirometry, and pain management. The goal is to promote maximal lung ventilation and prevent hypoventilation.

Patient positioning and early ambulation. When positioning the patient, the nurse considers the surgical incision site and the type of surgery. After a lobectomy, the patient is turned onto the nonoperative side to promote ($\dot{V}/\dot{Q}$) matching. When the good lung is dependent and blood flow is greater to the area with better ventilation, ($\dot{V}/\dot{Q}$) matching is better. ($\dot{V}/\dot{Q}$) mismatching results when the affected lung is positioned down because of the increase in blood flow to an area with less ventilation. The patient is turned frequently to promote secretion removal but should have the affected lung dependent as little as possible. A patient who has had a pneumonectomy is positioned supine or on the operative side during the initial period. Turning onto the operative side promotes splinting of the incision and facilitates deep-breathing exercises. Tilting the patient slightly toward the unaffected side is possible, but the surgeon should indicate when free side-to-side positioning is safe.

When sitting at the bedside or ambulating, patients must be encouraged to keep the thorax in straight alignment while they breathe deeply. This position best accommodates diaphragmatic descent and intercostal muscle action. The sitting or standing position provides enhanced ventilation to areas of the lung that are dependent in the supine position, accommodating maximal inflation and promoting gas exchange. Ambulation is essential in restoring lung function and is initiated as soon as possible.

Deep breathing and incentive spirometry. Deep breathing and incentive spirometry are performed regularly by patients who have undergone a thoracotomy. Deep breathing involves having the patient take a deep breath and holding the breath for approximately 3 seconds or longer. Incentive spirometry involves having the patient take at least 10 deep, effective breaths per hour using an incentive spirometer. These activities help reexpand collapsed lung tissue, promoting early resolution of the pneumothorax in patients with partial lung resections. The chest is auscultated during inflation to ensure that all dependent parts of the lung are well ventilated and to help the patient understand the depth of breath necessary for optimal effect. Coughing, which is encouraged only when secretions are present, assists in mobilizing secretions for removal.[109]

Pain management. Pain can be a significant problem after thoracic surgery. Pain can increase the workload of the heart, precipitate hypoventilation, and inhibit mobilization of secretions. Clinical manifestations of pain include tachypnea, tachycardia, elevated blood pressure, facial grimacing, splinting of the incision, hypoventilation, moaning, and restlessness. Several alternatives for pain management after thoracic surgery can be used. The two most common methods are systemic opioid administration and epidural opioid administration. Opioids can be administered intravenously or via patient-controlled analgesia. In addition, the patient is assisted with splinting the incision with a pillow or blanket when deep breathing and coughing. Splinting stabilizes the area and reduces pain when moving, deep breathing, or coughing.[106] See Chapter 7 for in-depth discussion of pain management.

Maintaining the Chest Tube System

Chest tubes are placed after most thoracic surgery procedures to remove air and fluid. The drainage initially appears bloody, becoming serosanguineous and then serous over the first 2 to 3 days postoperatively. Approximately 100 to 300 mL of drainage occurs during the first 2 hours postoperatively, which decreases to less than 50 mL/h over the next several hours. Routine stripping of chest tubes is not recommended, because excessive negative pressure can be generated in the chest. If blood clots are present in the drainage tubing or an obstruction is present, the chest tubes may be carefully milked. The chest tube may be placed to suction or water seal.[110]

During auscultation of the lungs, air leaks are evaluated. In the early phase, an air leak is commonly heard over the affected area, because the pleura have not yet tightly sealed. As healing occurs, this leak should disappear. An increase in an air leak or the appearance of a new air leak warrants prompt investigation of the chest drainage system to discover whether air is leaking into the system from outside or whether the leak is originating from the incision. Increased air leaks not related to the thoracic drainage system may indicate disruption of sutures.[108]

Assisting the Patient to Return to Adequate Activity Level

Within a few days after surgery, range-of-motion exercises for the shoulder on the operative side are performed. The patient frequently splints the operative side and avoids shoulder movement because of pain. If immobility is allowed, stiffening of the shoulder joint can result. This is referred to as *frozen shoulder* and may require physical therapy and rehabilitation to regain satisfactory range of motion of the shoulder joint.

The patient is usually able to sit in a chair the day after surgery. Activity is systematically increased, with attention to the patient's activity tolerance. With adequate pulmonary function before surgery and a surgical approach designed to preserve respiratory function, full return to previous activity levels is possible. This may take 6 months to 1 year, depending on the tissue resected and the patient's general condition.[101]

PULMONARY PHARMACOLOGY

Numerous pharmacologic agents are used in the care of a critically ill patient with pulmonary dysfunction. Table 15.7 reviews these agents and the special considerations necessary for administering them.

TABLE 15.7 Pharmacologic Management: Pulmonary Disorders.

Medication	Dosage	Actions	Special Considerations
NMBAs			
Vecuronium (Norcuron)	Loading dose: 0.08–0.1 mg/kg IV IV infusion: 0.8–1.2 mcg/kg/min	Used to paralyze patient to decrease oxygen demand and avoid ventilator dyssynchrony	*Boxed Warning From FDA:* Risk of anaphylactic and anaphylactoid-type adverse reactions, including fatalities reported in association with use of neuromuscular blockers.
Pancuronium (Pavulon)	Loading dose: 0.06–0.1 mg/kg IV IV infusion: 0.02–0.04 mg/kg/h		Administer sedative and analgesic agents concurrently, because NMBAs have no sedative or analgesic properties.
Rocuronium (Zemuron)	Loading dose: 0.6–1.2 mg/kg IV IV infusion: 10–12 mcg/kg/min		Evaluate level of paralysis q4h using peripheral nerve stimulator.
Atracurium (Tracrium)	Loading dose: 0.30–0.50 mg/kg IV IV infusion: 4–12 mcg/kg/min		Protect patients from environment because they are unable to respond.
Cisatracurium (Nimbex)	Loading dose: 0.15–0.2 mg/kg IV IV infusion: 0.5–10.2 mcg/kg/min		Prolonged muscle paralysis may occur after discontinuation of paralytic agent.
Mucolytics			
Acetylcysteine (Mucomyst)	Nebulizer, 20% solution: 3–5 mL tid–qid Nebulizer, 10% solution: 6–10 mL tid–qid	Used to decrease viscosity and elasticity of mucus by breaking down disulfide bonds within mucus	May be administered with a bronchodilator because medication can cause bronchospasms and inhibit ciliary function. Treatment considered effective when bronchorrhea develops and coughing occurs. Antidote for acetaminophen overdose.
Beta-2 Agonists			
Epinephrine (Adrenalin)	Nebulizer, 1% solution: 2.5–5 mg (0.25–0.5 mL) qid	Used to relax bronchial smooth muscle and dilate airways to prevent bronchospasms	May cause skeletal muscle tremors.
Racemic epinephrine	Nebulizer, 2.25% solution: 5.625–11.25 mg (0.25–0.5 mL) qid		Higher doses may cause tachycardia, palpitations, increased blood pressure, dysrhythmias, and angina.

TABLE 15.7 Pharmacologic Management: Pulmonary Disorders.—cont'd

Medication	Dosage	Actions	Special Considerations
Isoetharine 1% (Bronkosol)	Nebulizer, 1% solution: 2.5—5 mg (0.25—0.5 mL) qid		May increase serum glucose and decrease serum potassium levels.
Terbutaline	MDI, 340 mcg/puff: 1—2 puffs qid		Treatment considered effective when breath sounds improve and dyspnea is lessened.
	MDI, 200 mcg/puff: 2 puffs q4—6 h		Only approximately 10% of administered dose reaches the site of action within the lungs.
Metaproterenol (Alupent, Metaprel)	Nebulizer, 5% solution: 15 mg (0.3 mL) tid-qid		
	MDI, 650 mcg/puff: 2—3 puffs tid-qid		
Albuterol (Proventil, Ventolin)	Nebulizer, 5% solution: 2.5 mg (0.5 mL) tid—qid		
	MDI, 90 mcg/puff: 2 puffs tid—qid		
Levalbuterol (Xopenex)	Nebulizer: 0.63 mg q6—8 h		
Anticholinergic Agents			
Ipratropium (Atrovent)	Nebulizer, 0.02% solution: 0.5 mg (2.5 mL) q6—8 h	Used to block constriction of bronchial smooth muscle and reduce mucus production	There are relatively few adverse effects, because systemic absorption is poor.
Xanthines			
Theophylline	Loading dose: 4.6 mg/kg IV IV infusion: 0.4—0.8 mg/kg/h	Used to dilate bronchial smooth muscle and reverse diaphragmatic muscle fatigue	Administer loading dose over 30 minutes. Monitor serum blood levels; therapeutic level is 10—20 mg/dL.
Aminophylline	Loading dose: 5.7 mg/kg IV IV infusion: 0.5—1 mg/kg/h		Administer with caution to patients with cardiac, renal, or hepatic disease. Signs of toxicity include central nervous system excitation, seizures, confusion, irritability, hyperglycemia, headache, nausea, hypotension, and dysrhythmias.
Inhaled Corticosteroids			
Beclomethasone (Vanceril, Beclovent)	MDI, 42 mcg/puff: 2 puffs tid—qid	Used to decrease airway inflammation and enhance effectiveness of beta-agonists	Suppresses inflammatory response and interferes with ability to fight infection.
Flunisolide (AeroBid)	MDI, 250 mcg/puff: 2 puffs bid		Oral candidiasis is a side effect that can be minimized by having patients rinse their mouths after treatment.
Triamcinolone (Azmacort)	MDI, 100 mcg/puff: 2 puffs tid—qid		

FDA, US Food and Drug Agency; *IV,* intravenous/intravenously; *MDI,* metered-dose inhaler, *NMBAs,* neuromuscular blocking agents; *qid,* four times a day; *tid,* three times a day.
Data from Gold Standard.

BOX 15.11 Informatics

Internet Resources: Pulmonary Therapeutic Management
- American Association of Critical-Care Nurses (ACCN): www.aacn.org/
- American Association of Respiratory Care (AARC): www.aarc.org/
- American College of Chest Physicians (ACCP): www.chestnet.org/
- American College of Physicians (ACP): www.acponline.org/
- American College of Surgeons (ACS): www.facs.org/
- American Holistic Nurses Association (AHNA): www.ahna.org/
- American Lung Association: www.lung.org/
- American Medical Association (AMA): www.ama-assn.org/
- American Thoracic Society (ATS): www.thoracic.org/
- Centers for Disease Control and Prevention (CDC): www.cdc.gov/
- Critical Illness, Brain Dysfunction, and Survivorship (CIBS) Center: www.icudelirium.org/index.html
- National Heart, Lung, and Blood Institute: www.nhlbi.nih.gov/
- Respiratory Nursing Society and Interprofessional Collaborative (RNSIC): www.respiratorynursingsociety.org/
- Society for Critical Care Medicine (SCCM): www.sccm.org/Home

ADDITIONAL RESOURCES

See Box 15.11 for Internet resources pertaining to pulmonary disorders and therapeutic management.

REFERENCES

1. Rolfe S, Paul F. Oxygen therapy in adult patients. Part 1: understanding the relevant physiology and pathophysiology. *Br J Nurs.* 2018;27(14):798—804. Available from: https://doi.org/10.12968/bjon.2018.27.14.798.
2. Rolfe S, Paul F. Oxygen therapy in adult patients. Part 2: promoting safe and effective practice in patients' care and management. *Br J Nurs.* 2018;27(17):988—995. Available from: https://doi.org/10.12968/bjon.2018.27.17.988.
3. Heuer AJ. Medical gas therapy. In: Kacmarek RM, Stoller JK, Heuer AJ, eds. *Egan's Fundamentals of Respiratory Care.* 12th ed. St. Louis: Elsevier; 2021.
4. Wang J, Lee KP, Chong SL, Loi M, Lee JH. High flow nasal cannula in the emergency department: indications, safety and effectiveness. *Expert Rev Med Devices.* 2018;15(12):929—935. Available from: https://doi.org/10.1080/17434440.2018.1548276.
5. Allardet-Servent J, Sicard G, Metz V, Chiche L. Benefits and risks of oxygen therapy during acute medical illness: just a matter of dose. *Rev Med*

Interne. 2019;40(10):670—676. Available from: https://doi.org/10.1016/j.revmed.2019.04.003.

6. Barnes TA. Emergency cardiovascular life support. In: Kacmarek RM, Stoller JK, Heuer AJ, eds. *Egan's Fundamentals of Respiratory Care.* 12th ed. St. Louis: Elsevier; 2021.

7. Myatra SN. Airway management in the critically ill. *Curr Opin Crit Care.* 2021;27(1):37—45. Available from: https://doi.org/10.1097/MCC.0000000000000791.

8. LaVita CJ. Airway management. In: Kacmarek RM, Stoller JK, Heuer AJ, eds. *Egan's Fundamentals of Respiratory Care.* 12th ed. St. Louis: Elsevier; 2021.

9. Mechlin MW, Hurford WE. Emergency tracheal intubation: techniques and outcomes. *Respir Care.* 2014;59(6):881—894. Available from: https://doi.org/10.4187/respcare.02851.

10. Haas CF, Eakin RM, Konkle MA, Blank R. Endotracheal tubes: old and new. *Respir Care.* 2014;59(6):933—955. Available from: https://doi.org/10.4187/respcare.02868.

11. Colice GL. Technical standards for tracheal tubes. *Clin Chest Med.* 1991;12(3):433—448.

12. Higgs A, McGrath BA, Goddard C, et al. Guidelines for the management of tracheal intubation in critically ill adults. *Br J Anaesth.* 2018;120(2):323—352. Available from: https://doi.org/10.1016/j.bja.2017.10.021.

13. Scott JA, Heard SO, Zayaruzny M, Walz JM. Airway management in critical illness: an update. *Chest.* 2020;157(4):877—887. Available from: https://doi.org/10.1016/j.chest.2019.10.026.

14. Smith TL, Van Meter J. Maximizing success with rapid sequence intubations. *Adv Emerg Nurs J.* 2018;40(3):183—193. Available from: https://doi.org/10.1097/TME.0000000000000204.

15. Kabrhel C, Thomsen TW, Setnick GS, Walls RM. Videos in clinical medicine. Orotracheal intubation. *N Engl J Med.* 2007;356(17):e15. Available from: https://doi.org/10.1056/NEJMvcm063574.

16. Schaeffer C, Galas T, Teruzzi B, Sudrial J, Allou N, Martinet O. Iatrogenic tracheal rupture caused by endotracheal intubation: a case report. *J Emerg Med.* 2018;55(1):e15—e18. Available from: https://doi.org/10.1016/j.jemermed.2018.02.014.

17. Pacheco-Lopez PC, Berkow LC, Hillet AT, Akst LM. Complications of airway management. *Respir Care.* 2014;59(6):1006—1021. Available from: https://doi.org/10.4187/respcare.02884.

18. Tikka T, Hilmi OJ. Upper airway tract complications of endotracheal intubation. *Br J Hosp Med.* 2019;80(8):441—447. Available from: https://doi.org/10.12968/hmed.2019.80.8.441.

19. Adly A, Youssef TA, El-Begermy MM, Younis HM. Timing of tracheostomy in patients with prolonged endotracheal intubation: a systematic review. *Eur Arch Oto-Rhino-Laryngol.* 2018;275(3):679—690. Available from: https://doi.org/10.1007/s00405-017-4838-7.

20. Cheung NH, Napolitano LM. Tracheotomy: epidemiology, indications, timing, technique, and outcomes. *Respir Care.* 2014;59(6):895—919. Available from: https://doi.org/10.4187/respcare.02971.

21. Hess DR, Altobelli NP. Tracheostomy tubes. *Respir Care.* 2014;59(6):956—973. Available from: https://doi.org/10.4187/respcare.02920.

22. Lerner AD, Yarmua L. Percutaneous dilational tracheostomy. *Clin Chest Med.* 2018;39(1):211—222. Available from: https://doi.org/10.1016/j.ccm.2017.11.009.

23. Bontempo LJ, Manning SL. Tracheostomy emergencies. *Emerg Med Clin North Am.* 2019;37(1):109—119. Available from: https://doi.org/10.1016/j.emc.2018.09.010.

24. Samuelson KA. Adult intensive care patients' perception of endotracheal tube-related discomforts: a prospective evaluation. *Heart Lung.* 2011;40(1):49—55. Available from: https://doi.org/10.1016/j.hrtlng.2009.12.009.

25. American Association for Respiratory Care, Restrepo RD, Walsh BK. Humidification during invasive and noninvasive mechanical ventilation: 2012. *Respir Care.* 2012;57(5):782—788. Available from: https://doi.org/10.4187/respcare.01766.

26. Fink J, Ari A. Humidity and bland aerosol therapy. In: Kacmarek RM, Stoller JK, Heuer AJ, eds. *Egan's Fundamentals of Respiratory Care.* 12th ed. St. Louis: Elsevier; 2021.

27. Branson RK, Gomaa D, Rodriquez D. Management of the artificial airway. *Respir Care.* 2014;59(6):974—990. Available from: https://doi.org/10.4187/respcare.03246.

28. Rouzé A, Martin-Loeches I, Nseir S. Airway devices in ventilator-associated pneumonia pathogenesis and prevention. *Clin Chest Med.* 2018;39(4):775—783. Available from: https://doi.org/10.1016/j.ccm.2018.08.001.

29. Browne JA, Evans D, Christmas LA, Rodriguez M. Pursuing excellence: development of an oral hygiene protocol for mechanically ventilated patients. *Crit Care Nurs Q.* 2011;34(1):25—30. Available from: https://doi.org/10.1097/CNQ.0b013e318204809b.

30. Sole ML, Bennett M, Ashworth S. Clinical indicators for endotracheal suctioning in adult patients receiving mechanical ventilation. *Am J Crit Care.* 2015;24(4):318—324. Available from: https://doi.org/10.4037/ajcc2015794.

31. American Association for Respiratory Care. AARC clinical practice guidelines. Endotracheal suctioning of mechanically ventilated patients with artificial airways 2010. *Respir Care.* 2010;55(6):758—764.

32. Chaseling W, Baliss SL, Armstrong L, et al. *Suctioning an Adult ICU Patient With an Artificial Airway.* 2nd ed. Chatswood, NSW, Australia: Agency for Clinical Innovation NSW Government; 2014.

33. Czarnik RE, Stone KS, Everhart CC Jr, Preusser BA. Differential effects of continuous versus intermittent suction on tracheal tissue. *Heart Lung.* 1991;20(2):144—151.

34. Wang CH, Tsai JC, Chen SF, et al. Normal saline instillation before suctioning: a meta-analysis of randomized controlled trials. *Aust Crit Care.* 2017;30(5):260—265. Available from: https://doi.org/10.1016/j.aucc.2016.11.001.

35. Coppadoro A, Bellani G, Foti G. Non-pharmacological interventions to prevent ventilator-associated pneumonia: a literature review. *Respir Care.* 2019;64(12):1586—1595. Available from: https://doi.org/10.4187/respcare.07127.

36. Jelic S, Cunningham JA, Factor P. Clinical review: airway hygiene in the intensive care unit. *Crit Care.* 2008;12(2):209. Available from: https://doi.org/10.1186/cc6830.

37. Jenabzadeh NE, Chlan L. A nurse's experience being intubated and receiving mechanical ventilation. *Crit Care Nurse.* 2011;31(6):51—54. Available from: https://doi.org/10.4037/ccn2011182.

38. Ten Hoorn S, Elbers PW, Girbes AR, Tuinman PR. Communicating with conscious and mechanically ventilated critically ill patients: a systematic review. *Crit Care.* 2016;20(1):333. Available from: https://doi.org/10.1186/s13054-016-1483-2.

39. Mao Z, Gao L, Wang G, et al. Subglottic secretion suction for preventing ventilator-associated-associated pneumonia: an updated meta-analysis and trial sequential analysis. *Crit Care.* 2016;20(1):353. Available from: https://doi.org/10.1186/s13054-016-1527-1.

40. Andrews T, Steen C. A review of oral preventative strategies to reduce ventilator-associated pneumonia. *Nurs Crit Care.* 2013;18(3):116—122. Available from: https://doi.org/10.1111/nicc.12002.

41. Haghighi A, Shafipour V, Bagheri-Nesami M, Gholipour Baradari A, Yazdani Charati J. The impact of oral care on oral health status and prevention of ventilator-associated pneumonia in critically ill patients. *Aust Crit Care.* 2017;30(2):69—73. Available from: https://doi.org/10.1016/j.aucc.2016.07.002.

42. Zhao T, Wu X, Zhang Q, Li C, Worthington HV, Hua F. Oral hygiene care for critically ill patients to prevent ventilator-associated pneumonia. *Cochrane Database Syst Rev.* 2020;12(12):CD008367. Available from: https://doi.org/10.1002/14651858.CD008367.pub4.

43. Galhardo LF, Ruivo GF, Santos FO, et al. Impact of oral care and antisepsis on the prevalence of ventilator-associated pneumonia. *Oral Health Prev Dent.* 2020;18(1):331—336. Available from: https://doi.org/10.3290/j.ohpd.a44443.

44. Villar CC, Pannuti CM, Nery DM, Morillo CM, Carmona MJ, Romito GA. Effectiveness of intraoral chlorhexidine protocols in the prevention of ventilator-associated pneumonia: meta-analysis and systemic review. *Respir Care.* 2016;61(9):1245—1259. Available from: https://doi.org/10.4187/respcare.04610.

45. Malhan N, Usman M, Trehan N, et al. Oral care and ventilator-associated pneumonia. *Am J Ther.* 2019;26(5):604–607. Available from: https://doi.org/10.1097/MJT.0000000000000878.

46. Artime CA, Hagberg CA. Tracheal extubation. *Respir Care.* 2014;59(6):991–1005. Available from: https://doi.org/10.4187/respcare.02926.

47. O'Connor HH, White AC. Tracheostomy decannulation. *Respir Care.* 2010;55(8):1076–1081.

48. Credland N. How to remove a tracheostomy tube. *Nurs Stand.* 2015;30(9):34–35. Available from: https://doi.org/10.7748/ns.30.9.34.s43.

49. Pham T, Brochard LJ, Slutsky AS. Mechanical ventilation: state of the art. *Mayo Clin Proc.* 2017;92(9):1382–1400. Available from: https://doi.org/10.1016/j.mayocp.2017.05.004.

50. Walter JM, Corbridge TC, Singer BD. Invasive mechanical ventilation. *South Med J.* 2018;111(12):746–753. Available from: https://doi.org/10.14423/SMJ.0000000000000905.

51. Spiegel R, Mallemat H. Emergency department treatment of the mechanically ventilated patient. *Emerg Med Clin North Am.* 2016;34(1):63–75. Available from: https://doi.org/10.1016/j.emc.2015.08.005.

52. Chatburn RL, Volsko TA. Mechanical ventilators. In: Kacmarek RM, Stoller JK, Heuer AJ, eds. *Egan's Fundamentals of Respiratory Care.* 12th ed. St. Louis: Elsevier; 2021.

53. Cairo JM. How a breath is delivered. In: Cairo JM, ed. *Pilbeam's Mechanical Ventilation: Physiological and Clinical Applications.* 7th ed. St. Louis: Elsevier; 2020.

54. Hess DR, Kacmarek RM. Ventilator mode classification. In: *Essentials of Mechanical Ventilation.* 4th ed. New York: McGraw Hill; 2019. Available from: https://doi.org/10.14423/SMJ.0000000000000905.

55. Mireles-Cabodevila E, Hatipoglu U, Chatburn RL. A rationale framework for selecting modes of ventilation. *Respir Care.* 2013;58(2):348–366. Available from: https://doi.org/10.4187/respcare.01839.

56. Kacmarek RM. Initiating and adjusting invasive ventilatory support. In: Kacmarek RM, Stoller JK, Heuer AJ, eds. *Egan's Fundamentals of Respiratory Care.* 12th ed. St. Louis: Elsevier; 2021.

57. Gattinoni L, Protti A, Caironi P, Carlesso E. Ventilator-induced lung injury: the anatomical and physiological framework. *Crit Care Med.* 2010;38(suppl 10):S539–S548. Available from: https://doi.org/10.1097/CCM.0b013e3181f1fcf7.

58. Cruz FF, Ball L, Rocco PRM, Pelosi P. Ventilator-induced lung injury during controlled ventilation in patient with acute respiratory distress syndrome: less is probably better. *Expert Rev Respir Med.* 2018;12(5):403–414. Available from: https://doi.org/10.1080/17476348.2018.1457954.

59. Wahla AS, Khan FZ. Development of massive pneumopericardium after intubation and positive pressure ventilation. *J Coll Physicians Surg Pak.* 2012;22(6):401–402.

60. Terragni P, Ranieri VM, Brazzi L. Novel approaches to minimize ventilator-induced lung injury. *Curr Opin Crit Care.* 2015;21(1):20–25. Available from: https://doi.org/10.1097/MCC.0000000000000172.

61. Dreyfuss D, Ricard JD, Gaudry S. Did studies on HFOV fail to improve ARDS survival because they did not decrease VILI? On the potential validity of a physiological concept enounced several decades ago. *Intensive Care Med.* 2015;41(12):2076–2086. Available from: https://doi.org/10.1007/s00134-015-4062-0.

62. Marini JJ, Prodhan P. Cardiopulmonary interactions. In: Cheifetz I, MacIntyre N, Marini JJ, eds. *Mechanical Ventilation: Essentials for Current Adult and Pediatric Practice.* Mount Prospect, IL: Society of Critical Care Medicine; 2017.

63. Davies JD, Kneyber MCJ. Optimizing patient-ventilator synchrony in adult and pediatric populations. In: Cheifetz I, MacIntyre N, Marini JJ, eds. *Mechanical Ventilation: Essentials for Current Adult and Pediatric Practice.* Mount Prospect, IL: Society of Critical Care Medicine; 2017.

64. Cawley MJ. Advanced modes of mechanical ventilation: introduction for the critical care pharmacist. *J Pharm Pract.* 2019;32(2):186–198. Available from: https://doi.org/10.1177/0897190017734766.

65. Grossbach I, Chlan L, Tracy MF. Overview of mechanical ventilator support and management of patient- and ventilator-related responses. *Crit Care Nurse.* 2011;31(3):30–45. Available from: https://doi.org/10.4037/ccn2011595.

66. Spalding MC, Cripps MW, Minshall CT. Ventilator-associated pneumonia: new definitions. *Crit Care Clin.* 2017;33(2):277–292. Available from: https://doi.org/10.1016/j.ccc.2016.12.009.

67. Mietto C, Pinciroli R, Patel N, Berra L. Ventilator associated pneumonia: evolving definitions and preventive strategies. *Respir Care.* 2013;58(6):990–1003. Available from: https://doi.org/10.4187/respcare.02380.

68. Kallet RH. The vexing problem of ventilator-associated pneumonia: observations on pathophysiology, public policy, and clinical science. *Respir Care.* 2015;60(10):1495–1508. Available from: https://doi.org/10.4187/respcare.03774.

69. Schallom M, Dykeman B, Metheny N, Kirby J, Pierce J. Head-of-bed elevation and early outcomes of gastric reflux, aspiration and pressure ulcers: a feasibility study. *Am J Crit Care.* 2015;24(1):57–66. Available from: https://doi.org/10.4037/ajcc2015781.

70. Grap MJ, Munro CL, Wetzel PA, et al. Backrest elevation and tissue interface pressure by anatomical location during mechanical ventilation. *Am J Crit Care.* 2016;25(3):e56–e63. Available from: https://doi.org/10.4037/ajcc2016317.

71. Berry E, Zecca H. Daily interruptions of sedation: a clinical approach to improve outcomes in critically ill patients. *Crit Care Nurse.* 2012;32(1):43–51. Available from: https://doi.org/10.4037/ccn2012599.

72. Ramirez P, Bassi GL, Torres A. Measures to prevent nosocomial infections during mechanical ventilation. *Curr Opin Crit Care.* 2012;18(1):86–92. Available from: https://doi.org/10.1097/MCC.0b013e32834ef3ff.

73. Coppadoro A, Bittner E, Berra L. Novel preventive strategies for ventilator-associated pneumonia. *Crit Care.* 2012;16(2):210.

74. Rouzé A, Jaillette E, Poissy J, Préau S, Nseir S. Tracheal tube design and ventilator-associated pneumonia. *Respir Care.* 2017;62(10):1316–1323. Available from: https://doi.org/10.4187/respcare.05492.

75. Tokmaji G, Vermeulen H, Müller MC, Kwakman PH, Schultz MJ, Zaat SA. Silver-coated endotracheal tubes for the prevention of ventilator-associated pneumonia in critically ill patients. *Cochrane Database Syst Rev.* 2015;2015(8):CD009201. Available from: https://doi.org/10.1002/14651858.CD009201.pub2.CD009201.

76. Kacmarek RM. Discontinuing ventilatory support. In: Kacmarek RM, Stoller JK, Heuer AJ, eds. *Egan's Fundamentals of Respiratory Care.* 12th ed. St. Louis: Elsevier; 2021.

77. Penuelas O, Thille AW, Esteban A. Discontinuation of ventilator support: new solutions to old dilemmas. *Curr Opin Crit Care.* 2015;21(1):74–81. Available from: https://doi.org/10.1097/MCC.0000000000000169.

78. Robertson TE, Sona C, Schallom L, et al. Improved extubation rates and earlier liberation from mechanical ventilation with implementation of a daily spontaneous-breathing trial protocol. *J Am Coll Surg.* 2008;206(3):489–495. Available from: https://doi.org/10.1016/j.jamcollsurg.2007.08.022.

79. Ward D, Fulbrook P. Nursing strategies for effective weaning of the critically ill mechanically ventilated patient. *Crit Care Nurs Clin North Am.* 2016;28(4):499–512. Available from: https://doi.org/10.1016/j.cnc.2016.07.008.

80. Blackwood B, Alderdice F, Burns KE, Cardwell CR, Lavery G, O'Halloran P. Protocolized versus non-protocolized weaning for reducing the duration of mechanical ventilation in critically ill adult patients. *Cochrane Database Syst Rev.* 2010;(5):CD006904. Available from: https://doi.org/10.1002/14651858.CD006904.pub3.CD006904.

81. McConville JF, Kress JP. Weaning patients from the ventilator. *N Engl J Med.* 2012;367(23):2233–2239. Available from: https://doi.org/10.1056/NEJMra1203367.

82. Schmidt G, Girard TD, Kress JP, et al. Official executive summary of an American Thoracic Society/American College of Chest Physicians clinical practice guideline: liberation from mechanical ventilation in critically ill adults. *Am J Respir Crit Care Med.* 2017;195(1):115–119. Available from: https://doi.org/10.1164/rccm.201610-2076ST.

83. Grasselli G, Brioni M, Zanella A. Monitoring respiratory mechanics during assisted ventilation. *Curr Opin Crit Care.* 2020;26(1):11–17. Available from: https://doi.org/10.1097/MCC.0000000000000681.

84. Tracy MF, Chlan L. Nonpharmacological interventions to management common symptoms in patient receiving mechanical ventilation. *Crit*

Care Nurse. 2011;31(3):19−28. Available from: https://doi.org/10.4037/ccn2011653.

85. ABCDEF (A2F) overview. Critical illness, brain dysfunction, and survivorship. *CIBS Center.* 2019. www.icudelirium.org/medicalprofessionals.html.

86. Bello G, Ionescu Maddalena A, Giammatteo V, Antonelli M. Noninvasive options. *Crit Care Clin.* 2018;34(3):395−412. Available from: https://doi.org/10.1016/j.ccc.2018.03.007.

87. Schallom M, Cracchiolo L, Falker A, et al. Pressure ulcer incidence in patients wearing nasal-oral versus full-face noninvasive ventilation masks. *Am J Crit Care Nurs.* 2015;24(4):349−357. Available from: https://doi.org/10.4037/ajcc2015386.

88. Williams PF. Noninvasive ventilation. In: Kacmarek RM, Stoller JK, Heuer AJ, eds. *Egan's Fundamentals of Respiratory Care.* 12th ed. St. Louis: Elsevier; 2021.

89. Alqahtani JS, Al Ahmari MD. Evidence based synthesis for prevention of noninvasive ventilation related facial pressure ulcers. *Saudi Med J.* 2018;39(5):443−452. Available from: https://doi.org/10.15537/smj.2018.5.22058.

90. Scholten EL, Beitler JR, Prisk GK, Malhotra A. Treatment of ARDS with prone positioning. *Chest.* 2017;151(1):215−224. Available from: https://doi.org/10.1016/j.chest.2016.06.032.

91. Kallet RH. A comprehensive review of prone position in ARDS. *Respir Care.* 2015;60(11):1660−1687. Available from: https://doi.org/10.4187/respcare.04271.

92. Athota KP, Millar D, Branson RD, Tsuei BJ. A practical approach to the use of prone therapy in acute respiratory distress syndrome. *Expert Rev Respir Med.* 2014;8(4):453−463. Available from: https://doi.org/10.1586/17476348.2014.918850.

93. Wright AD, Flynn M. Using the prone position for ventilated patients with respiratory failure: a review. *Nurs Crit Care.* 2011;16(1):19−27. Available from: https://doi.org/10.1111/j.1478-5153.2010.00425.x.

94. Goldhill DR, Imhoff M, McLean B, Waldmann C. Rotational bed therapy to prevent and treat respiratory complications: a review and meta-analysis. *Am J Crit Care.* 2007;16(1):50−61.

95. Stiller K. Physiotherapy in intensive care: an updated systematic review. *Chest.* 2013;144(3):825−847. Available from: https://doi.org/10.1378/chest.12-2930.

96. Kang SY, DiStefano MJ, Yehia F, Koszalka MV, Padula WV. Critical care beds with continuous lateral rotation therapy to prevent ventilator-associated pneumonia and hospital-acquired pressure injury: a cost-effective analysis. *J Patient Saf.* 2021;17(2):149−155. Available from: https://doi.org/10.1097/PTS.0000000000000582.

97. Ahrens T, Kollef M, Stewart J, Shannon W. Effect of kinetic therapy on pulmonary complications. *Am J Crit Care.* 2004;13(5):376−383.

98. Collard HR, Saint S, Matthay MA. Prevention of ventilator-associated pneumonia: an evidence-based systematic review. *Ann Intern Med.* 2003;138(6):494−501.

99. Powers J, Daniels D. Turning points: implementing kinetic therapy in the ICU. *Nurs Manage.* 2004;35(5 suppl 1−7):1−8.

100. Wanless S, Aldridge M. Continuous lateral rotation therapy—a review. *Nurs Crit Care.* 2012;17(1):28−35.

101. Moewen DR. Thoracic surgery. In: Rothrock JC, McEwen DR, eds. *Alexander's Care of the Patient in Surgery.* 16th ed. St. Louis: Elsevier; 2019.

102. Keogy BF, Alexander D. Preoperative assessment for thoracic surgery. *Anaesth Intensive Care Med.* 2015;16(2):59−62.

103. Davies AN, Saravanan P. Tests of pulmonary function before thoracic surgery. *Anaesth Intensive Care Med.* 2014;15(11):495−498.

104. von Groote-Bidlingmaier F, Koegelenberg CF, Bolliger CT. Functional evaluation before lung resection. *Clin Chest Med.* 2011;32(4):773−787. Available from: https://doi.org/10.1016/j.ccm.2011.08.001.

105. Liu Z, Liu X, Huang Y, Zhao J. Intraoperative mechanical ventilation strategies in patients undergoing one-lung ventilation: a meta-analysis. *SpringerPlus.* 2016;5(1):1251. Available from: https://doi.org/10.1186/s40064-016-2867-0.

106. Sachdev G, Napolitano LM. Postoperative pulmonary complications: pneumonia and acute respiratory failure. *Surg Clin North Am.* 2012;92(2):321−344. Available from: https://doi.org/10.1016/j.suc.2012.01.013.

107. Keshishyan S, Revelo AE, Epelbaum O. Bronchoscopic management of prolonged air leak. *J Thorac Dis.* 2017;9(suppl 10):S1034−S1046. Available from: https://doi.org/10.21037/jtd.2017.05.47.

108. Soll C, Hahnloser D, Frauenfelder T, Russi EW, Weder W, Kestenholz PB. The postpneumonectomy syndrome: clinical presentation and treatment. *Eur J Cardio Thorac Surg.* 2009;35(2):319−324. Available from: https://doi.org/10.1016/j.ejcts.2008.07.070.

109. Vines DL, Gardner DD. Airway clearance therapy (ACT). In: Kacmarek RM, Stoller JK, Heuer AJ, eds. *Egan's Fundamentals of Respiratory Care.* 12th ed. St. Louis: Elsevier; 2021.

110. Sasa RI. Evidence-based update on chest tube management. *Am Nurse Today.* 2019;14(4):10−14.

16

Neurologic Clinical Assessment and Diagnostic Procedures

Darlene M. Burke

HISTORY

Common to all neurologic assessments is the need to obtain a comprehensive history. An adequate neurologic history includes information about the patient's normal baseline status, manifestation of neurologic symptoms, events preceding the onset of symptoms, precipitating factors, progression of symptoms, current medication use, substance use and/or abuse, and familial occurrences (Box 16.1).[1,2] The ideal historian for recounting this information is someone who is able to provide a detailed description and chronology of events. If the patient is incapable of serving as the historian, family members or significant others who frequently interact with the patient should be queried. The information obtained from the history often informs the priorities of the physical examination.[2]

PRIORITY CLINICAL ASSESSMENT

The assessment helps establish baseline data regarding the patient's condition. The neurologic evaluation of a critically ill patient comprises five major components: (1) level of consciousness, (2) motor function, (3) pupillary function, (4) respiratory function, and (5) vital signs. A complete neurologic examination requires assessment of all five components.[3]

Level of Consciousness

Assessment of the level of consciousness is the most important aspect of the neurologic examination. In most situations, a patient's level of consciousness deteriorates before any other neurologic changes are noticed. These deteriorations often are subtle and must be monitored carefully. Arousal and awareness are the fundamental constituents of consciousness and should be evaluated and documented repeatedly for trend analysis.[2] Documenting a brief description of the applied stimulus and arousal pattern is preferred to using terms that categorize the level of consciousness.[4]

Evaluation of Arousal

Assessment of the arousal component of consciousness is an evaluation of the reticular activating system and its connection to the thalamus and the cerebral cortex. Arousal is the lowest level of consciousness, and observation centers on the patient's ability to respond to verbal or noxious stimuli in an appropriate manner.[5] To stimulate the patient, the nurse begins with verbal stimuli in a normal tone. Eye opening in response to name is an indication that the patient's reticular activating center (brainstem) functioning is intact. However, it does not provide evidence that the patient is awake or aware.[2] If the patient does not respond, the nurse increases the stimuli by talking very loudly to the patient. If there is still no response, the nurse further increases the stimuli by gently shaking the patient.

If previous attempts to arouse the patient are unsuccessful, noxious stimuli are employed using central stimulation techniques.[4] Central stimulation produces an overall body response and is more reliable than peripheral stimulation.[4] Two common central stimulation techniques are the *sternal rub* and the *trapezius muscle pinch*. A sternal rub is conducted by applying pressure to the center of the sternum with the knuckles of a clenched fist.[3] A trapezius muscle squeeze involves pitching or squeezing the trapezius muscle located at the angle of the shoulder and the neck muscle.[4] If the patient does not respond to verbal stimulus but moves spontaneously in a purposeful manner, the patient is *localizing*. Painful stimulus is not required if spontaneous localization has been observed. Localizing is purposeful and intentional movement intended to eliminate a noxious stimulus, whereas *withdrawal* is a smaller movement used to get away from noxious stimulus.[2] The symmetry and pattern of the motor response to noxious stimuli and associated neurologic symptoms are documented for all patients suspected of having a neurologic dysfunction.[4]

Appraisal of Awareness

If a patient is arousable, an assessment of awareness should follow. As a higher level function, awareness means that the cerebral cortex is working in conjunction with the reticular activating system (arousal) and that the patient can interact with and interpret their environment.[2] Appraisal of awareness is concerned with assessment of the patient's orientation to person, place, time, and situation and requires the patient to give appropriate answers to various questions.[5] Changes in the patient's answers that indicate increasing degrees of confusion and disorientation may be the first sign of neurologic deterioration.[1]

BOX 16.1 DATA COLLECTION

Neurologic History

Common Neurologic Symptoms

- Fainting
- Dizziness
- Blackouts
- Seizures
- Headache
- Memory loss
- Weakness
- Paralysis
- Tremors or other involuntary movements
- Pain
- Numbness
- Tingling
- Speech disturbances
- Vision disturbances

Events Preceding Onset of Symptoms

- Travel
- Animal contact
- Falls
- Infection
- Dental problems or procedures
- Sinus or middle ear infections
- Prodromal symptoms
- Food or medications ingested

Progression of Symptoms

- Initial onset
- Evolution
- Frequency
- Severity
- Duration
- Associated activities or aggravating factors

Family History

- Stroke (arteriovenous malformation, aneurysm)
- Diabetes mellitus
- Hypertension
- Seizures
- Tumors
- Headaches
- Emotional problems or depression

Medical History

Child

- Birth injuries, congenital defects, encephalitis, meningitis, bedwetting, fainting, seizures, trauma

Adult

- Diabetes; hypertension; cardiovascular, pulmonary, kidney, liver, or endocrine disease; tuberculosis; tropical infection; sinusitis; visual problems; tumors; psychiatric disorders

Surgical History

- Neurologic, ear-nose-throat, dental, eye surgery

Traumatic History

- Motor vehicle accidents; falls; blows to head, neck, or back; being knocked unconscious

Allergies

- Medications, food, environment

Patient Profile

- Personal habits
- Use of alcohol, recreational drugs, over-the-counter medications, smoking, dietary habits, sleeping patterns, elimination patterns, exercise habits
- Recent life changes
- Living conditions
- Working conditions
- Exposure to toxins, chemicals, fumes; occupational duties
- General temperament

Current Medication Use

- Sedatives, tranquilizers
- Anticonvulsants
- Psychotropics
- Anticoagulants
- Antibiotics
- Calcium channel blockers
- Beta-blockers
- Nitrates
- Oral contraceptives

Glasgow Coma Scale

Introduced in 1974, the Glasgow Coma Scale (GCS) is the most widely recognized tool for assessing level of consciousness.[6] The scored scale is based on evaluation of three categories: (1) eye opening, (2) verbal response, and (3) best motor response (Table 16.1). The three components can be scored separately or combined in a sum score ranging from 3 to 15; a score of 7 or less usually indicates coma. Reliability of the sum score is less than that of the components of the GCS.[7] The GCS has additional shortcomings, which include inconsistent interobserver reliability, concerns over its ability to predict the extent of the brain damage, the impracticality of verbal response assessment in intubated patients or in patients with dysphasia, the exclusion of brainstem functions from the GCS, and the inability to detect subtle changes in

neurologic status.[8] The GCS also is a poor indicator of lateralization of neurologic deterioration.[9] *Lateralization* involves decreasing motor response on one side or unilateral changes in pupillary reaction.

Full Outline of UnResponsiveness Score

The Full Outline of UnResponsiveness (FOUR) score may be a suitable alternative or complementary tool for the GCS.[10] The FOUR score has been compared with the GCS and was found to have equivalent interrater reliability and a similar if not higher predication of mortality and poor neurologic outcome in general critical care unit population, traumatic brain injury (TBI) patients, and stroke patients.[8] It is a 17-point scale used to assess four domains of the neurologic functions: eye responses, motor responses, brainstem reflexes, and breathing pattern (Fig. 16.1).[11] Each of the domains carries five parameters with total

TABLE 16.1 Glasgow Coma Scale.

Category	Score	Response
Eye opening	4	Spontaneous: Eyes open spontaneously without stimulation
	3	To speech: Eyes open with verbal stimulation but not necessarily to command
	2	To pain: Eyes open with noxious stimuli
	1	None: No eye opening regardless of stimulation
Verbal response	5	Oriented: Accurate information about person, place, time, reason for hospitalization, and personal data
	4	Confused: Answers not appropriate to questions, but use of language is correct
	3	Inappropriate words: Disorganized, random speech, no sustained conversation
	2	Incomprehensible sounds: Moans, groans, and incomprehensible mumbles
	1	None: No verbalization despite stimulation
Best motor response	6	Obeys commands: Performs simple tasks on command; able to repeat performance
	5	Localizes to pain: Organized attempt to localize and remove painful stimuli
	4	Withdraws from pain: Withdraws extremity from source of painful stimuli
	3	Abnormal flexion: Decorticate posturing spontaneously or in response to noxious stimuli
	2	Extension: Decerebrate posturing spontaneously or in response to noxious stimuli
	1	None: No response to noxious stimuli; flaccid

points ranging from 0 to 4, with a potential sum score ranging from 0 to 16. The FOUR score is applicable for both traumatic and non-traumatic brain injuries.[8]

Motor Function

Assessment of motor function provides valuable information about the patient with neurologic dysfunction and includes assessing the patient's muscle size and tone; muscle strength; response to peripheral, tactile stimuli; and abnormal motor responses.[2] Each side of the body is assessed individually and compared with the other.[10]

Evaluation of Muscle Size and Tone

Initially, muscles are inspected for size and shape. The presence of atrophy is noted. Muscle tone is assessed by evaluating opposition to passive movement. The patient is instructed to relax the extremity while the nurse performs passive range-of-motion movements and evaluates the degree of resistance. Muscle tone is appraised for signs of flaccidity (no resistance), hypotonia (little resistance), hypertonia (increased resistance), spasticity, or rigidity.[12] If tone is absent in an unconscious patient, the hand is lifted approximately 30 cm above the bed and carefully dropped while protecting the limb from injury. The test is repeated with all extremities. Typically, the lower the level of consciousness, the closer to flaccid the limb(s) will be. An asymmetric examination may indicate a lesion in the contralateral hemisphere or brainstem.[2]

Estimation of Muscle Strength

Having the patient perform movements against resistance assesses muscle strength. The strength of the movement is graded on a six-point scale (Box 16.2). The patient is asked to extend both arms with the palms turned upward and to hold that position with the eyes closed. If the patient has a weaker side, that arm will drift downward and pronate. The lower extremities are tested by asking the patient to push and pull the feet against resistance or to elevate the legs.[12]

Peripheral Tactile Response

Peripheral reflex response is response to tactile stimuli peripherally and usually elicits a reflex response rather than a central or brain response.[2] The nurse should apply stimuli in a progressive manner using the least noxious stimuli necessary to elicit a response. Each extremity is assessed individually. If there is no response to light or firm pressure, the nurse must use noxious stimuli. The typical technique for peripheral noxious stimuli involves pressure on the nail beds for asserting a peripheral stimulus.[2]

Abnormal Motor Responses

Patients may experience abnormal motor responses spontaneously or to stimuli. If the patient is incapable of comprehending and following a simple command, noxious stimuli are necessary to determine motor responses. The stimulus is applied to each extremity separately to allow evaluation of individual extremity function. The *triple-flexion response* is a withdrawal of the limb in a straight line with flexion of the wrist-elbow-shoulder or the ankle-knee-hip. This response is considered a spinal reflex and is not an indication of brain involvement in the movement. The triple-flexion response is common in patients with severe neurologic dysfunction.[2] *Decorticate (flexor) posturing* is seen when there is involvement of a cerebral hemisphere and the brainstem (Fig. 16.2A). It is characterized by adduction of the shoulder and arm, elbow flexion, and pronation and flexion of the wrist while the legs extend. *Decerebrate (extensor) posturing* is seen with severe metabolic disturbances or upper brainstem lesions (see Fig. 16.2B). It is characterized by extension and pronation of the arm(s) and extension of the legs.[2] Additionally, it is possible for the patient to exhibit abnormal flexion on one side of the body and extension on the other (see Fig. 16.2C).[3] Onset of posturing or a change from abnormal flexion to abnormal extension requires immediate health care provider notification.

Pupillary Function

Assessment of pupillary function focuses on three areas: (1) estimation of pupil size and shape, (2) evaluation of pupillary reaction to light, and (3) assessment of eye movements. Pupillary function is an extension of the autonomic nervous system. Parasympathetic control of the pupil occurs through innervation of the oculomotor nerve (CN III), which exits from the brainstem in the midbrain area. When the parasympathetic fibers are stimulated, the pupil constricts. Sympathetic control originates in the hypothalamus and travels down the entire length of the brainstem. When the sympathetic fibers are

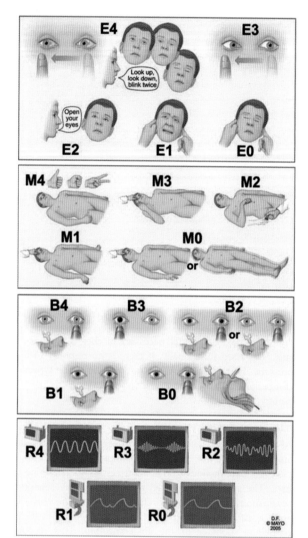

Fig. 16.1 Description of Full Outline of UnResponsiveness (FOUR) Score. Eye response: *E4*, Eyelids open or opened, tracking, or blinking to command; *E3*, eyelids open but not tracking; *E2*, eyelids closed but open to loud voice; *E1*, eyelids closed but open to pain; *E0*, eyelids remain closed with pain. Motor response: *M4*, thumbs-up, fist, or peace sign; *M3*, localizing to pain; *M2*, flexion response to pain; *M1*, extension response to pain; *M0*, no response to pain or generalized myoclonus status. Brainstem reflexes: *B4*, pupil and corneal reflexes present; *B3*, one pupil wide and fixed; *B2*, pupil or corneal reflexes absent; *B1*, pupil and corneal reflexes absent; *B0*, absent pupil, corneal, and cough reflex. Respiration pattern: *R4*, not intubated, regular breathing pattern; *R3*, not intubated, Cheyne-Stokes breathing pattern; *R2*, not intubated, irregular breathing; *R1*, breathes above ventilatory rate; *R0*, breathes at ventilator rate or apnea. (From Iyer VN. Validity of the FOUR Score Coma Scale in the medical intensive care unit. *Mayo Clin Proc.* 2009;84[8]:694-701).

BOX 16.2   Muscle Strength Grading Scale

0/5	No movement or muscle contraction
1/5	Trace contraction
2/5	Active movement with gravity eliminated
3/5	Active movement against gravity
4/5	Active movement with some resistance
5/5	Active movement with full resistance

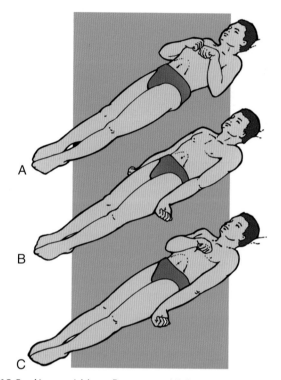

Fig. 16.2 Abnormal Motor Responses. (A) Decorticate posturing. (B) Decerebrate posturing. (C) Decorticate posturing on right side and decerebrate posturing on left side of body.

stimulated, the pupil dilates. Pupillary changes provide a valuable assessment tool because of pathway locations. The oculomotor nerve lies at the junction of the midbrain and the tentorial notch. Any increase of pressure that exerts force down through the tentorial notch compresses the oculomotor nerve. Oculomotor nerve compression results in a dilated, nonreactive pupil. Sympathetic pathway disruption occurs with involvement in the brainstem. Loss of sympathetic control leads to pinpoint, nonreactive pupils. Control of eye movements occurs with interaction of three cranial nerves: (1) oculomotor (CN III),

(2) trochlear (CN IV), and (3) abducens (CN VI). The pathways for these cranial nerves provide integrated function through the internuclear pathway of the medial longitudinal fasciculus (MLF), located in the brainstem. The MLF provides co-ordination of eye movements with the vestibular nerve (CN VIII) and the reticular formation.[13]

Estimation of Pupil Size and Shape

Diameter of the pupil is documented in millimeters with the use of a pupillometer to reduce the subjectivity of description. Most people have pupils of equal size, between 2 and 5 mm. Change or inequality in pupil size (anisocoria), especially in patients who previously have not shown this discrepancy, is a significant neurologic sign.[14] It may indicate impending danger of herniation and should be reported immediately. With the location of CN III at the notch of the tentorium, pupil size and reactivity play a key role in the physical assessment of intracranial pressure (ICP) changes and herniation syndromes. Changes in pupil size occur for other reasons in addition to CN III compression. Large pupils can result from the instillation of cycloplegic agents such as atropine or scopolamine. Extremely small pupils can indicate opioid overdose.[15]

Pupil shape is included in the assessment of pupils. Although the pupil is normally round, an irregularly shaped or oval pupil may be observed in patients who have undergone eye surgery. Initial stages of CN III compression from elevated ICP can cause the pupil to have an oval shape.[3]

Evaluation of Pupillary Reaction to Light

The pupillary light reflex depends on optic nerve (CN II) and oculomotor nerve (CN III) function (Fig. 16.3).[12] The technique for evaluation of the pupillary light response involves use of a narrow-beamed bright light shone into the pupil from the outer canthus of the eye. If the light is shone directly onto the pupil, glare or reflection of the light may prevent the assessor's proper visualization. Pupillary reaction to light is identified as brisk, sluggish, or nonreactive or fixed.[3] Each pupil is evaluated for direct light response and for consensual response. The consensual pupillary response is constriction in response to a light shone into the opposite eye.[3] This reflex occurs as a result of the crossing of nerve fibers at the optic chiasm.[3] Evaluation of consensual response is necessary to rule out optic nerve dysfunction as a cause for lack of a direct light reflex. Because the optic nerve is the afferent pathway for the light reflex, shining a light into a blind eye produces neither a direct light response in that eye nor a consensual response in the opposite eye. A consensual response in a blind eye produced by shining a light into the opposite eye demonstrates an intact oculomotor nerve. Oculomotor compression associated with transtentorial herniation affects the direct light response and the consensual response in the affected pupil.[3,13]

Assessment of Eye Movement

In a conscious patient, the function of the three cranial nerves of the eye and their MLF innervation can be assessed by asking the patient to follow a finger through the full range of eye motion. If the eyes move together into all six fields, extraocular movements are intact (Fig. 16.4).[3,13]

In an unconscious patient, assessment of ocular function and innervation of the MLF is performed by eliciting the doll's eye reflex. If the patient is unconscious as a result of trauma, the nurse must ascertain the absence of cervical injury before performing this examination. To assess the oculocephalic reflex, the nurse holds the patient's eyelids open and briskly turns the head to one side and observes the eye movement and then briskly turns the head to the other side and observes the eye movement again. If the eye movement deviates to the opposite direction in which the head is turned, the doll's eye reflex is present, and the oculocephalic reflex arc is intact (Fig. 16.5A). If the oculocephalic reflex arc is not intact, the reflex is absent. This lack of response, in which the eyes remain midline and move with the head, indicates significant brainstem injury (see Fig. 16.5C). The reflex may also be absent in severe metabolic coma. An abnormal oculocephalic reflex is present when the eyes rove or move in opposite directions from each other (see Fig. 16.5B). An abnormal oculocephalic reflex indicates some degree of brainstem injury.[3,13]

The oculovestibular reflex is performed by a health care provider often as one of the final physical assessments of brainstem function. After confirmation that the tympanic membrane is intact, the patient's head is raised to a 30-degree angle, and 20 to 100 mL of ice water is injected into the external auditory canal. The normal eye movement response is a conjugate, slow, tonic nystagmus, deviating toward the irrigated ear and lasting 30 to 120 seconds. This response indicates brainstem integrity. Rapid nystagmus returns the eye position back to the midline only in a conscious patient with cortical functioning (Fig. 16.6).[3,10] An abnormal response is disconjugate eye movement, which indicates a brainstem lesion, or no response,

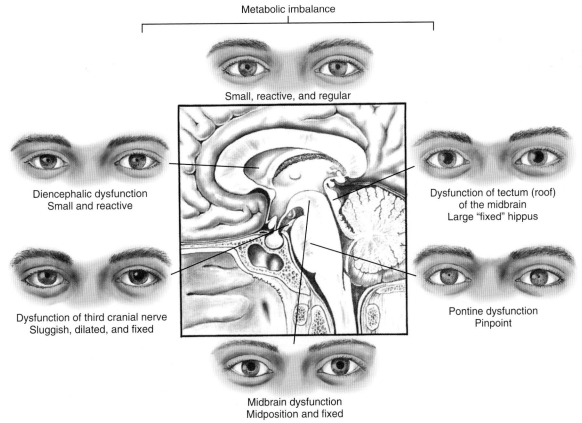

Metabolic imbalance

Small, reactive, and regular

Diencephalic dysfunction
Small and reactive

Dysfunction of tectum (roof)
of the midbrain
Large "fixed" hippus

Dysfunction of third cranial nerve
Sluggish, dilated, and fixed

Pontine dysfunction
Pinpoint

Midbrain dysfunction
Midposition and fixed

Fig. 16.3 Abnormal Pupillary Responses.

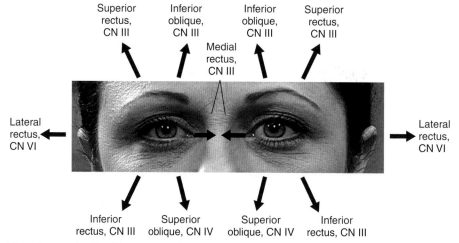

Fig. 16.4 Extraocular Eye Movements. (From Ball JW, Dains JE, Flynn JA, et al., eds. *Seidel's Guide to Physical Examination: An Interprofessional Approach.* 9th ed. St. Louis: Elsevier; 2019.)

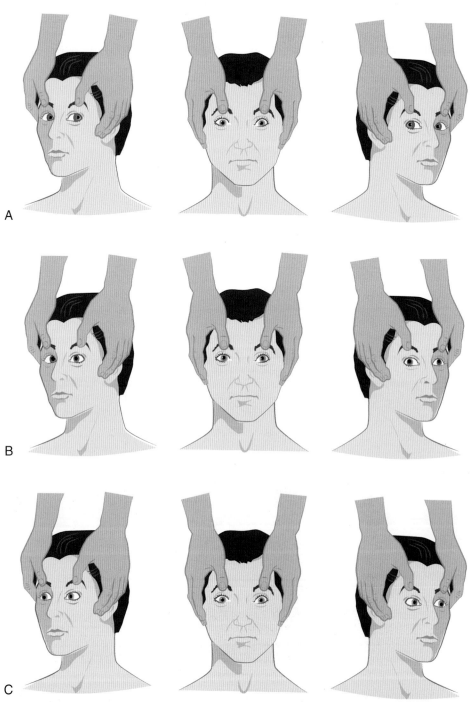

Fig. 16.5 Oculocephalic Reflex (Doll's Eye Reflex). (A) Normal. (B) Abnormal. (C) Absent.

Respiratory Function

Assessment of respiratory function focuses on two areas: (1) observation of respiratory pattern and (2) evaluation of airway status. The activity of respiration is a highly integrated function that receives input from the cerebrum, brainstem, and metabolic mechanisms. Correlations exist among altered levels of consciousness, the level of brain or brainstem injury, and the patient's respiratory pattern. Under the influence of the cerebral cortex and the diencephalon, three brainstem centers control respirations. The lowest center, the *medullary respiratory center*, sends impulses through the vagus nerve to innervate muscles of inspiration and expiration. The *apneustic* and *pneumotaxic centers of the pons* are responsible for the length of inspiration and expiration and the underlying respiratory rate.[3,10]

Observation of Respiratory Pattern

Changes in respiratory patterns assist in identifying the level of brainstem dysfunction or injury (Table 16.2). Evaluation of the respiratory pattern must include assessment of the effectiveness of gas exchange in maintaining adequate oxygen and carbon dioxide levels. Hypoventilation is common in patients with altered level of consciousness. Alterations in oxygenation or carbon dioxide levels can result in further neurologic dysfunction. ICP increases with hypoxemia or hypercapnia.[3,10]

Evaluation of Airway Status

Evaluation of respiratory function in a patient with a neurologic deficit must include assessment of airway maintenance and secretion control. Cough, gag, and swallow reflexes responsible for protection of the airway may be absent or diminished.[16]

Vital Signs

Assessment of vital signs focuses on two areas: (1) evaluation of blood pressure and (2) observation of heart rate and rhythm. As a result of the brain and brainstem influences on cardiac, respiratory, and body temperature functions, changes in vital signs could be signs of deterioration in neurologic status.[3]

Evaluation of Blood Pressure

A common manifestation of intracranial injury is systemic hypertension. Cerebral autoregulation, responsible for the control of cerebral blood flow (CBF), frequently is lost with any type of intracranial injury. After cerebral injury, the body often is in a hyperdynamic state (increased heart rate, blood pressure, and cardiac output) as part of a compensatory response. With the loss of autoregulation as blood pressure increases, CBF and cerebral blood volume increase, and ICP increases. Control of systemic hypertension is necessary to stop this

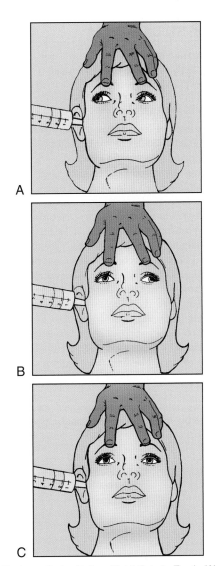

Fig. 16.6 Oculovestibular Reflex (Cold Caloric Test). (A) Normal. (B) Abnormal. (C) Absent.

which indicates little or no brainstem function. The oculovestibular reflex may be temporarily absent in reversible metabolic encephalopathy. This test is an extremely noxious stimulation and may produce a decorticate or decerebrate posturing response in a comatose patient. In a conscious patient, this procedure may produce nausea, vomiting, or dizziness.[3,13]

TABLE 16.2	Respiratory Patterns.	
Pattern of Respiration	**Description of Pattern**	**Significance**
Cheyne-Stokes breathing	Rhythmic crescendo and decrescendo of rate and depth of respiration; includes brief periods of apnea	Usually seen with bilateral deep cerebral lesions or some cerebellar lesions
Central neurogenic hyperventilation	Very deep, very rapid respirations with no apneic periods	Usually seen with lesions of midbrain and upper pons
Apneustic breathing	Prolonged inspiratory and/or expiratory pause of 2–3 seconds	Usually seen in lesions of middle to lower pons
Cluster breathing	Clusters of irregular, gasping respirations separated by long periods of apnea	Usually seen in lesions of lower pons or upper medulla
Ataxic respirations	Irregular, random pattern of deep and shallow respirations with irregular apneic periods	Usually seen in lesions of medulla

cycle, but caution must be exercised. The mean arterial pressure (MAP) must be maintained at a level sufficient to produce adequate CBF in the presence of elevated ICP. Attention must also be paid to the pulse pressure, because widening of this value may occur in the late stages of intracranial hypertension.[16,17]

Observation of Heart Rate and Rhythm

The medulla and the vagus nerve provide parasympathetic control to the heart. When stimulated, this lower brainstem system produces bradycardia. Sympathetic stimulation increases the rate and contractility. Various intracranial pathologies and abrupt ICP changes can produce bradycardia, premature ventricular contractions, QT interval changes, and myocardial damage.[18]

Cushing triad. Cushing triad is a set of three clinical manifestations (systolic hypertension with widening pulse pressure, bradycardia, and bradypnea) related to pressure on the medullary area of the brainstem. These signs may occur in response to intracranial hypertension or a herniation syndrome. The appearance of Cushing triad is a late finding that may be absent in patients with severe neurologic deterioration. Once this pattern of vital signs occurs, it may be too late to completely reverse intracranial hypertension.[4]

Neurologic Changes Associated With Intracranial Hypertension

Assessment of a patient for signs of increasing ICP is an important responsibility of the critical care nurse. Increasing ICP can be identified by changes in level of consciousness, pupillary reaction, motor response, vital signs, and respiratory patterns (Fig. 16.7).[10,19]

LABORATORY STUDIES

The major laboratory study performed in a patient with neurologic dysfunction is analysis of cerebrospinal fluid (CSF) obtained by a lumbar puncture (LP) or a ventriculostomy.[3,4]

Cerebrospinal Fluid Analysis

LP is an important tool for diagnosing brain pathology.[20] The main purpose of an LP is to obtain CSF for laboratory analysis (Table 16.3). CSF opening pressure also may be obtained.

An LP involves the introduction of a 25-gauge hollow needle into the subarachnoid space at L3 to L4 or L4 to L5, using aseptic technique.[20] For the procedure, a patient is most commonly placed in a flexed lateral recumbent position and must remain still. If the patient is not fully alert and co-operative, the nurse may need to assist the patient in maintaining the position necessary for the LP. Collection of up to 30 mL of CSF is passively withdrawn and placed in designated laboratory specimen containers. The nurse must monitor the patient's neurologic and respiratory status during and after the procedure and compare the findings to the patient's preprocedure baseline. Conditions representing (potential) contraindications for LP are the risk for cerebral herniation including space-occupying lesion with mass effect, abnormal ICP caused by increased CSF pressure and Arnold–Chiari malformation, increased bleeding risk (thrombocytopenia, coagulopathies, anticoagulant medications), and local infections at the puncture site. Before the procedure is initiated, the patient's coagulation status and platelet count should be assessed for abnormalities.[20-22] Also, a CT or MRI scan should be obtained prior to an LP if the

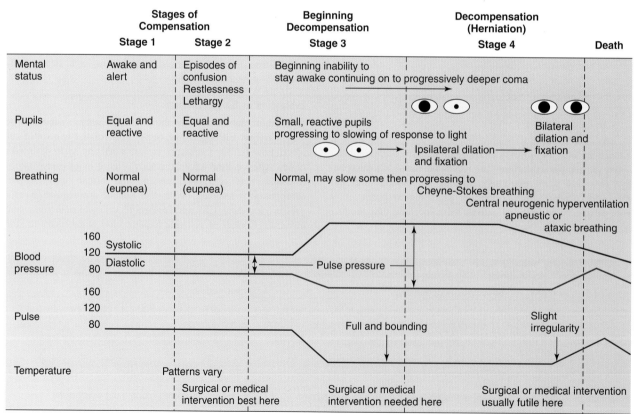

Fig. 16.7 Signs and Symptoms of Intracranial Hypertension. Clinical correlates of compensated and decompensated phases of intracranial hypertension. (From Beare PG, Myers JL, eds. *Principles and Practice of Adult Health Nursing.* 3rd ed. St. Louis: Mosby; 1998.)

TABLE 16.3 Analysis of Cerebrospinal Fluid.

Characteristic	Normal Findings	Abnormal Findings	Possible Causes and Comments
Pressure	<200 mm H_2O	<60 mm H_2O	Faulty needle placement Dehydration Spinal block along subarachnoid space Block of foramen magnum Hydrocephalus
		>200 mm H_2O	Muscle tension Abdominal compression Brain tumor Subdural hematoma Brain abscess Brain cyst Cerebral edema (any cause)
Color	Clear, colorless	Cloudy or turbid	Cloudy as a result of microorganisms (e.g., WBCs) Turbid as a result of increased cell count
		Yellow (xanthochromic) Smoky	Breakdown of RBCs with RBC pigments, high protein count RBCs
Blood	None	Red blood cells: Blood tinged Grossly bloody	Traumatic tap: Bloody in first sample Traumatic tap: Bloody in all samples
Volume	150 mL	Increase	Hydrocephalus
Specific gravity	1.007	Increase	Infection, presence of cells or protein
WBCs	0–5 cells/mm^3	<500 cells/mm^3	Bacterial or viral infections of meninges, neurosyphilis, subarachnoid hemorrhage, infarction, abscess, tuberculous meningitis, metastatic lesions
		>500 cells/mm^3	Purulent infection
Glucose	50–75 mg/dL or 60%–70% of blood glucose	<40 mg/dL	Bacterial meningitis, tuberculosis, parasitic, fungal carcinomatous, subarachnoid hemorrhage
		>80 mg/dL	May not be of neurologic significance
Chloride	700–750 mg/dL	Decreased (<625 mg/dL)	Meningeal infection, tuberculosis meningitis, hypochloremia
		Increased (>800 mg/dL)	May not be of neurologic significance; correlated with blood levels of chloride and not routine; done only on request
Culture and sensitivity	No organisms present	Neisseria or Streptococcus	Identify organisms to begin therapy; Gram stain for some cultures may take several weeks
Serology for syphilis	Negative	Positive	Syphilis
Protein[a]	15–50 mg/dL	Increased (>60 mg/dL)	Bacterial meningitis, brain tumors (benign and malignant), complete spinal block, ALS, Guillain-Barré syndrome, subarachnoid hemorrhage, infarction, CNS trauma, CNS degenerative diseases, herniated disk, DM with polyneuropathy
		Decreased (<10 mg/dL)	May not be of neurologic significance
Osmolality	295 mOsm/L	Increased	Protein, WBCs, microorganisms, RBCs
Lactate	10–20 mg/dL	Increased	Bacterial, seizure activity, fungal meningitis, CNS trauma, coma related to toxic or metabolic causes

[a]Blood in CSF will increase the protein level.

ALS, Amyotrophic lateral sclerosis; *CNS*, central nervous system; *CSF*, cerebrospinal fluid; *DM*, diabetes mellitus; *RBC*, red blood cell; *WBC*, white blood cell.

From Barker E. *Neuroscience Nursing: A Spectrum of Care*. 3rd ed. St. Louis: Mosby; 2008.

patient has an abnormal clinical neurologic examination, papilledema, reduced level of consciousness, previous central nervous system (CNS) disease, or experienced recent seizures. An intracranial space–occupying lesion with mass effect and a posterior fossa mass can lead to brain herniation during an LP.[20]

DIAGNOSTIC PROCEDURES

Table 16.4 presents an overview of the various diagnostic procedures used to evaluate the patient with neurologic dysfunction.

Nursing Management

The nursing management of a patient undergoing a diagnostic procedure involves a variety of interventions. Nursing priorities are directed toward (1) preparing the patient psychologically and physically for the procedure, (2) monitoring the patient's responses to the procedure, and (3) assessing the patient after the procedure. Preparation includes teaching the patient about the procedure, answering questions, and transporting and positioning the patient for the procedure. During the procedure, the nurse observes the patient for signs of pain, anxiety, or hemorrhage and monitors vital signs. After the

TABLE 16.4 Neurological Diagnostic Studies.

Study	Purposes	Comments
Angiography	Visualizes extracranial and intracranial vasculature. Identifies aneurysm, AVM, vasospasm, and vascular tumors. Detects arterial occlusion and allows delivery of intraarterial therapy to restore blood flow.	May cause local hematoma, vasospasm, vessel occlusion, allergic reaction to contrast media, and transient or permanent neurological dysfunction Prior to test Keep patient NPO for 4 hours and provide sedation before the study. Check for allergy to iodine. Evaluate renal function. After the test Ensure hydration postprocedure (contrast medium used). • Maintain bed rest for 8–12 hours. • Monitor arterial puncture point for hemorrhage or hematoma. • Monitor neurovascular status of affected limb. • Monitor for indications of systemic emboli. • Re-evaluate renal function. Contraindicated in intracranial hypertension
Cisternogram	Views CSF flow. Identifies hydrocephalus. Evaluates CSF leakage through a dural tear. Evaluates abnormality of structures at the base of the brain and upper cervical cord region.	
CT computerized axial tomography (CAT)	Views intracranial structures: size, shape, location, shifts. Differentiates between tumors, hemorrhage, and infarction. Identifies hydrocephalus, brain edema, infectious processes, trauma, aneurysm, hematoma, AVM, brain atrophy, and subacute and old brain infarction. Evaluates arterial system if CT angiography studies performed.	Patient must be co-operative. Contrast media may be used; contrast media may be used after a noncontrast CT. • Check for allergy to iodine or seafood before study. • Patient will be NPO for 4–8 hours before the study. • Sedation may be given. • Monitor for signs of allergic reaction. • Encourage fluid intake. • Evaluate renal function when contrast media used.
Digital subtraction angiography: brain, spine	Visualizes the vasculature, especially carotid and larger cerebral arteries. Evaluates occlusive vascular disease. Identifies tumors, aneurysms, AVM, vascular abnormalities.	May be done IV or intraarterially. • If IV, is less invasive with fewer complications than cerebral angiography • If intraarterially, care as for angiogram • Contrast media are used. • Check for allergy to iodine, seafood before study. • Patient will be NPO for 4–8 hours before the study. • Monitor for signs of allergic reaction. • Encourage fluid intake.
Electroencephalography	Differentiates epilepsy from mass lesion. Detects focus of seizure activity. Evaluates drug intoxication. Evaluates electrical function of the brain, which may be abnormal in the presence of cerebrovascular alterations. Localizes tumor, abscess, and other mass lesions. May be used in designation of brain death.	Stimulants, anticonvulsants, tranquilizer, and antidepressants may be withheld for 24–48 hours before the study. Hair shampooed before and after study.
Electromyography; nerve conduction velocity studies	Detects muscle disease. Identifies peripheral neuropathies, nerve compression. Identifies nerve regeneration and muscle recovery.	Patient must be co-operative. Contraindicated in patients taking anticoagulants, with bleeding disorders or skin infection. May be uncomfortable for patient.
Electronystagmography	Detects nystagmus, which may aid in identification of cerebellar or vestibular problem.	
Evoked potential studies	Evaluates electrical potentials (responses) of brain to external stimuli; evaluates sensory and somatosensory neurologic pathways. Identifies neuromuscular disease, cerebrovascular disease, spinal cord injury, traumatic brain injury, peripheral nerve disease, and tumors. Determines prognosis in traumatic brain injury. Contributes to diagnosis of multiple sclerosis and brainstem injury.	Hair shampooed before and after study.

TABLE 16.4 Neurological Diagnostic Studies.—cont'd

Study	Purposes	Comments
Isotope ventriculography	Visualizes CSF circulation system.	No CSF withdrawn May cause meningeal irritation and aseptic meningitis.
Lumbar puncture or cisternal puncture	Obtains CSF for analysis. Measures CSF opening pressure (roughly equivalent to intracranial pressure for most patients if done recumbent and no blockage is present).	Cisternal puncture is higher risk but may be used if scar tissue prevents LP. Patient must be co-operative. Contraindicated in patients with intracranial hypertension because herniation may occur. Contraindicated in bleeding disorders and in patients receiving anticoagulants. Patient kept flat for 4—8 hours to prevent headache. May cause headache, low back pain, meningitis, abscess, CSF leak, or puncture of spinal cord.
Magnetic resonance angiography/magnetic resonance imaging	As for CT Visualizes tissue state (diffusion and perfusion) so that early ischemic changes are apparent (CT cannot visualize most early changes). Identifies vascular lesions, tissue abnormalities, hemorrhage, infarction, epileptic foci, and multiple sclerosis. Identifies patency of large veins and venous sinuses. Identifies brainstem abnormalities. Identifies type, location, and extent of brain injury.	Patient must be co-operative. Contraindicated in patients with any implanted metallic device, including pacemakers. Tends to overestimate degree of stenosis.
Magnetic resonance spectroscopy (also known as nuclear magnetic resonance [NMR] spectroscopy)	Measures biochemical changes in the brain tissue. Detects abnormal changes as in brain tumors, epilepsy, stroke, and traumatic brain injury.	Patient must be co-operative. Contraindicated in patients with any implanted metallic device, including pacemakers.
Myelography	Visualizes spinal subarachnoid space. Detects spinal cord lesions and cord or nerve root compression. Detects pressure on spinal nerve roots.	If done with oil-based iophendylate (Pantopaque), patient must lie flat for 4—8 hours after study. May cause headache, nerve root irritation, allergic reaction, or adhesive arachnoiditis. If done with water-soluble metrizamide (Amipaque), patient should have head of bed elevated. May cause headache, nausea, vomiting, backache and neck ache, chest pain, seizures, hallucinations, speech disorders, dysrhythmias, or allergic reaction. Encourage fluid intake with either type of dye.
Nerve conduction velocity studies	Identifies peripheral neuropathies and nerve compression.	Needle electrodes are used.
Oculoplethysmography (OPG)	Indirectly measures ocular artery pressure. Reflects adequacy of cerebrovascular blood flow in the carotid artery.	Contraindicated in patients who have undergone eye surgery within the last 6 months, who have had lens implants or cataracts, or who have had retinal detachment. May cause conjunctival hemorrhage, corneal abrasions, or transient photophobia.
Pneumoencephalography	Visualizes ventricular system and subarachnoid space. Identifies intracranial tumors. Identifies brain atrophy.	Care as for LP Contraindicated in patients with intracranial hypertension. May cause headache, nausea, vomiting, autonomic dysfunction, herniation, subdural hematoma, air embolus, or seizures. Keep patient flat for 12—24 hours after the study.
Positron emission tomography or single-photon emission computed tomography	Evaluates oxygen and glucose metabolism. Measures cerebral blood flow, which may be altered by traumatic brain injury, seizure, ischemia, stroke, or neoplasm. Also used to evaluate dementia, depression, schizophrenia, and Alzheimer's disease.	Patient must be co-operative. Contraindicated in pregnant and breastfeeding patients.
Radioisotope brain scan	Identifies tumors, cerebrovascular disease, infarction, trauma, infectious processes, and seizures.	Generally replaced by CT scan Reassure patient that amount of radioactive material is minimal. Patient must be co-operative. Contraindicated in pregnant and breastfeeding patients.

Continued

TABLE 16.4   Neurological Diagnostic Studies.—cont'd

Study	Purposes	Comments
Regional cerebral blood flow (xenon [133Xe] inhalation)	Evaluates blood flow to the cerebral cortex material. Identifies cerebrovascular disease. Detects regions of increased or decreased perfusion. Determines presence of collateral blood flow. Evaluates the effect of vasospasm on tissue perfusion.	Assure patient that amount of radioactive material is minimal. Contraindicated in pregnant and breastfeeding patients.
Skull x-rays	Detects skull fracture, facial fracture, tumor, bone erosion, cranial anomalies, air-fluid level in sinuses, abnormal intracranial calcification, and radiopaque foreign bodies.	Linear and basal fractures frequently missed by routine x-rays Contraindicated in pregnant patients.
Somatosensory evoked potentials (SSEP)	Evaluates neural pathways involving spinal cord, brainstem, thalamus, and cerebral cortex. Useful in diagnosis of multiple sclerosis, brain tumor, and spinal cord injury. Useful in determination of brain death.	
Somnography	Records electroencephalogram (EEG) during sleep. Evaluates sleep and sleep disorders.	
Spinal cord arteriography	Differentiates between spinal AVM, angioma, tumor, and ischemia.	As for angiogram May cause thrombosis of spinal vessels and allergy to contrast agent.
Spine x-rays	Detects vertebral dislocation or fracture, degenerative disease, tumor, bone erosion, or calcification. Identifies structural spinal deficits and rules out associated cervical spine injuries.	Care must be taken to prevent fracture displacement and spinal cord injury. C1—C2 view best obtained via open mouth; C6—C7 best obtained with arms pulled down.
Suboccipital puncture	Obtains CSF for analysis. Measures CSF pressure. Rarely performed but may be useful when LP is contraindicated.	May cause trauma to the medulla.
Transcranial Doppler	Measures blood flow velocity through the cerebral arteries. Identifies vasospasm, emboli, vascular stenosis, and brain death.	Quality of findings and interpretation vary with user. Transtemporal window required (lacking in 14% of general population).
Ventriculography	Obtains CSF for analysis. Measures CSF pressure. Is used especially when intracranial hypertension contraindicates LP.	May cause meningeal irritation, seizures, herniation, intracerebral or intraventricular hemorrhage.

AVM, Arteriovenous malformation; *CSF,* cerebrospinal fluid; *CT,* computed tomography; *IV,* intravenous; *LP,* lumbar puncture; *NPO,* nothing by mouth.
From Dennison RD. *Pass CCRN!* 5th ed. St Louis: Elsevier; 2019.

procedure, the nurse observes for complications of the procedure and medicates the patient for any postprocedure discomfort. Any evidence of increasing ICP should be immediately reported to the physician, and emergency measures to decrease ICP must be initiated.

NEUROLOGIC MONITORING

Intracranial Pressure Monitoring

ICP monitoring is recommended as a part of protocol-driven care in patients who are at risk of elevated ICP based on clinical or imaging features.[23] In general, indications for ICP monitoring include TBI, intracranial hemorrhage, subarachnoid hemorrhage (SAH), hydrocephalus, hepatic failure with encephalopathy, acute ischemic stroke with large infarction, and meningitis.[24] A contraindication for ICP monitoring is coagulopathy.[24] The normal range for ICP in adults is generally 5 to 15 mm Hg,[25,26] and the threshold for intracranial hypertension is considered to be an ICP greater than 20 mm Hg.[23] It is recommended that ICP monitoring be used in conjunction with other intracranial monitoring devices to enhance clinical decision making.[23]

Both noninvasive and invasive methods of monitoring ICP are available. Noninvasive techniques of measuring ICP include transcranial Doppler (TCD), tympanic membrane displacement, optic nerve sheath diameter, CT/MRI, and pupillometry.[26] Noninvasive techniques do not have the complications related to invasive techniques. However, the noninvasive techniques have yet to measure ICP accurately enough to be used as alternatives to invasive measurement.[26] Pupillometry is discussed later in this chapter.

Types of Intracranial Pressure Monitoring Devices

There are several different invasive methods of ICP monitoring. Depending on the location and type of brain injury and the monitoring technique, ICP monitoring can be undertaken in different intracranial anatomic locations: intraventricular, intraparenchymal, epidural, subdural, and subarachnoid (Fig. 16.8).[26] The most commonly used ICP monitoring devices utilize the intraventricular and intraparenchymal locations.

Intraventricular catheter monitoring device. The most common method for placement of an intraventricular catheter is a coronal burr hole approach at Kocher point, with the tip of the catheter placed in the third ventricle. Once CSF flow is visualized, the catheter can be

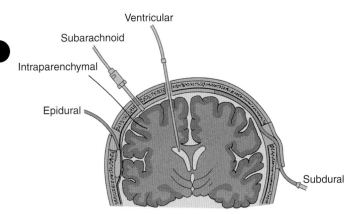

Fig. 16.8 Intracranial Pressure Monitoring Sites. (From Lewis SL, Bucher L, Heitkemper MM, et al., eds. *Medical-Surgical Nursing: Assessment and Management of Clinical Problems.* 10th ed. St. Louis: Elsevier; 2017.)

transduced to obtain an opening ICP. The mean opening pressure has significant prognostic implications and influences medical management strategies.[27] The catheter is then tunneled through the skin, sutured in place, and connected to an external drainage system.[27] The combination of a ventriculostomy with a closed drainage system is also known as an external ventricular drain (EVD). The underlying condition of the patient and the ICP are considered in determining the prescribed level of the EVD drainage point. Drainage can be continuous at a set level, fixed volume per desired time, or as needed according to ICP elevations.[27] An EVD requires repeated zeroing and leveling so that the pressure transducer is in line with the foramen of Monro (which falls at the level of the external auditory meatus of the ear when the patient is supine). Decreased CSF drainage also requires frequent nursing interventions.[24]

Drawbacks of ICP monitoring by open EVD include undetected increases in ICP above thresholds and less reliable assessment of cerebrovascular autoregulation.[28] Complications with this device include inadvertent catheter placement, postprocedural hemorrhage, and ventriculostomy-associated infections.[25,27,29] The use of imaging guidance systems may improve the likelihood of optimal placement.[29] The risk of infection may be decreased by using an antibiotic-impregnated catheter.[25] Nevertheless, further research is needed regarding the ideal method of placement for intracranial monitoring devices, the timing of deep vein thrombosis (DVT) prophylaxis as it relates to hemorrhage, and infection prophylaxis.[29]

Intraparenchymal microsensor monitoring device. ICP monitors inserted into brain parenchyma utilize fiberoptic, strain gauge, or pneumatic technologies. Fiberoptic devices transmit light via a fiberoptic cable toward a displaceable mirror. Changes in ICP move the mirror, and the differences in intensity of the reflected light are translated to an ICP value.[24,26] Another parameter that may be measured with the fiberoptic transducer-tipped catheters is brain temperature.[24] With strain gauge device technology, ICP is calculated when ICP bends the transducer and changes the level of resistance.[26] Pneumatic sensor technology measures ICP by using a small balloon in the distal end of the catheter to register changes in pressure.[26] Pneumatic sensors also allow for quantitative measurement of intracranial compliance.[26]

The accuracy of the devices depends on their placement relative to the site of injury. The catheter can be easily placed via a cranial access device, via a burr hole, or during a craniotomy. However, the device may not be a good gauge of global ICP if pockets of increased ICP arise

secondary to focal brain injuries.[27] Additional disadvantages of intraparenchymal microsensor devices are that microtransducer systems can encounter drift when used for more than 5 days, in vivo calibration and CSF drainage are impossible, and transducer-tipped catheters are not MRI compatible.[24,27,30] An error message or loss of waveform on the ICP monitor may indicate a broken catheter or malposition of the catheter.[24,26]

Combination intraventricular/fiberoptic catheter. The intraventricular/fiberoptic catheter combines the capability of EVD of CSF with monitoring of ICP. This hybrid device can be used to monitor ICP intermittently or continuously and to drain CSF intermittently or continuously.[31] There are advantages and disadvantages to using the combination catheter. A disadvantage is that the catheter can be zeroed only before insertion. However, because the transducer is in the tip of the fiberoptic catheter, there is no external strain gauge transducer and no repetitive zeroing and leveling of a transducer with the anatomic reference point for the foramen of Monro.[31] An advantage of the catheter is that it allows for CSF drainage. To prevent underdrainage or overdrainage of CSF, attention must be paid to the level of the reference point of the drip chamber to the anatomic reference point for the foramen of Monro and the setting of the pressure level at the top of the graduated burette (drip chamber).[31] Consequences of CSF underdrainage include headache, neurologic deterioration, hydrocephalus, increased ICP, secondary neuronal injury, herniation, and death.[31] Consequences of CSF overdrainage include headache, subdural hematoma, pneumocephalus, ventricular collapse, herniation, and death.[31]

Intracranial Pressure Waves

ICP waveform analysis provides information that may identify patients with decreased adaptive capacity who are at risk for increases in ICP and decreases in cerebral perfusion pressure (CPP).[32] ICP pulse waveform is observed on a continuous, real-time pressure display, and it corresponds to each heartbeat.[32] The waveform arises primarily from pulsations of the major intracranial arteries but also receives retrograde venous pulsations.[32] Although a systolic and diastolic component to the ICP waveform is evident, ICP is read as a mean value.[24]

Normal intracranial pressure waveform. The normal ICP wave has three or more defined peaks (Fig. 16.9). The first peak (P1) is called the *percussion wave.* Originating from the pulsations of the choroid plexus, it has a sharp peak which is generally consistent in its amplitude. The second peak (P2) is called the *tidal wave.* The tidal wave varies more in shape and amplitude, ending on the dicrotic notch. The P2 portion of the pulse waveform has been most directly linked to the state of decreased compliance. When the P2 component is equal to or higher than P1, decreased compliance occurs (Fig. 16.10). Immediately after the dicrotic notch is the third wave (P3), which is called the *dicrotic wave.* After the dicrotic wave, the pressure usually tapers down to the diastolic position unless retrograde venous pulsations add a few more peaks.[32] In performing basic checks of whether

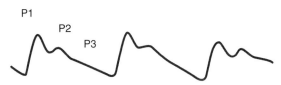

Fig. 16.9 Normal Intracranial Pressure Waveform. (From Bader MK, Littlejohns LR. *AANN Core Curriculum for Neuroscience Nursing.* 4th ed. St. Louis: Mosby; 2004.)

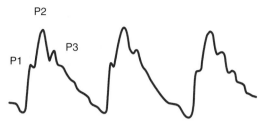

Fig. 16.10 Abnormal Intracranial Pressure Waveform. (From Bader MK, Littlejohns LR. *AANN Core Curriculum for Neuroscience Nursing.* 4th ed. St. Louis: Mosby; 2004.)

the ICP signal is truly representative of the ICP, it is important to ensure that there is an oscillating pressure curve with the progressively decreasing P1, P2, and P3 notches present, indicating propagation of the cardiac pulse pressure signal.[26] Loss of the ICP waveform may indicate blockage, loose system connections, or possibly transducer failure. A numeric value without a corresponding waveform is of no value.[24]

Abnormal intracranial pressure waveforms. A, B, and C pressure waves are not true waveforms (Fig. 16.11). Rather, they are the graphically displayed trend data of ICP over time. These waves reflect spontaneous alterations in ICP associated with respiration, systemic blood pressure, and deteriorating neurologic status.

Also called *plateau waves* because of their distinctive shape, A waves are the most clinically significant of the three types. They usually occur in an already elevated baseline ICP (>20 mm Hg) and are characterized by sharp increases in ICP of 30 to 69 mm Hg, which plateau for 2 to 20 minutes and then return to baseline. The cause of A waves is unknown, but they may result from vasodilation and increased CBF, decreased venous outflow (and increased cerebral blood volume), fluctuations in arterial partial pressure of carbon dioxide ($PaCO_2$) (and changes in cerebral blood volume), or decreased CSF absorption. B waves often precede A waves. Plateau waves are considered significant because of the reduced CPP associated with ICP, in the range of 50 to 100 mm Hg. Transient signs of intracranial hypertension, such as a decreased level of consciousness, bradycardia, pupillary changes, or respiratory changes, may accompany these waves. Sustained increases in ICP associated with plateau waves may result in permanent cell damage from ischemia.[32]

B waves are sharp, rhythmic oscillations with a sawtooth appearance that occur every 30 seconds to 2 minutes and can increase the ICP from 5 to 70 mm Hg. They are a normal physiologic phenomenon

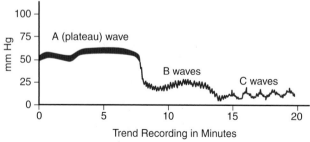

Fig. 16.11 Intracranial Pressure Waves. Composite diagram of A waves (plateau waves), B waves (sawtooth waves), and C waves (small rhythmic waves). (From Barker E. *Neuroscience Nursing: A Spectrum of Care.* 3rd ed. St. Louis: Mosby; 2008.)

that can occur in any patient, but they are amplified in states of low intracranial compliance. B waves appear to reflect fluctuations in cerebral blood volume.[32]

C waves are small, rhythmic waves that occur every 4 to 8 minutes at normal levels of ICP. They are related to normal fluctuations in respiration and systemic arterial pressure.[32]

Pupillometry

Automated infrared pupillometry enables the quantitative assessment of basic fundamental neurologic tests, such as pupillary symmetry and reactivity, using a handheld pupillometer and the Neurological Pupil index (NPi).[33] The pupillometer is a handheld infrared system that automatically tracks and analyzes pupil dynamics over a 3-second period.[24] A detachable headrest facilitates the correct and consistent placement of the pupillometer in front of the eye. The device has been specifically designed to minimize possible interobserver variability in the pupillary evaluation.[24] The NPi classifies pupil reactivity using an algorithm. An inverse relationship between decreasing pupil reactivity and increasing ICP has been identified with the use of pupillometry and the NPi.[24,33] Pupillometry is used to trend increased ICP in patients with TBI, aneurysmal SAH, or intracerebral hemorrhage.[33]

Cerebral Perfusion Pressure Monitoring

Measurement of ICP allows for an estimation of CPP. CPP is the difference between MAP and ICP and is the driving force responsible for adequate brain perfusion and oxygenation.[24] It is calculated as the difference between the incoming MAP and the opposing ICP on the arteries: (CPP = MAP − ICP). CPP is related to CBF and is modifiable through its relationship with MAP and ICP.[25] Following a significant increase in ICP, CPP decreases resulting in inadequate brain tissue perfusion and oxygenation. The consequent ischemia induces further cytotoxic edema, resulting in even higher ICP.[34] Adequate CPP provides some protection against secondary ischemia; however, the requisite CPP for each patient is unknown. Evidence-based guidelines such as the Brain Trauma Foundation Guidelines for the Management of Severe Traumatic Brain Injury support a CPP range of 60 to 70 mm Hg for adults.[35] The CPP threshold may vary from patient to patient depending on such factors as variation of how the MAP is measured, autoregulatory status, and intracranial compliance.[23] Cerebral autoregulation is the intrinsic ability of the cerebral vessels to constrict and dilate as needed to maintain adequate cerebral perfusion.[30] Intracranial compliance is defined as a change in ICP in relationship to the change in intracranial volume. It is likely that a CPP threshold exists on an individual basis and that optimal CPP can be identified by multimodality monitoring.[25]

Cerebral autoregulation is impaired with brain injury, and the CBF becomes passively dependent on the systemic blood flow.[30] The cerebral blood vessels are no longer able to react to maintain CPP in response to a change in blood pressure.[30] Continuous bedside monitoring of autoregulatory efficiency is possible through online calculation of derived indices such as the pressure reactivity index and may be useful in broad targeting of cerebral perfusion management goals and prognostication in acute brain injury.[25]

Cerebral Blood Flow Monitoring

CBF monitoring provides an understanding of the perfusion status of the brain. Tools used in the clinical and research setting for the assessment of CBF are TCD, transcranial color-coded duplex sonography (TCCS), thermal diffusion flowmetry (TDF), and laser Doppler flowmetry (LDF).

Transcranial Doppler

TCD is an established technique for assessing cerebral hemodynamics in real time. CBF velocity is measured through cranial windows (thinned areas) of the skull. Three areas commonly used are (1) the temporal bone (transtemporal), (2) the eye (transorbital), and (3) the foramen magnum (transoccipital). Depending on the angle of the Doppler probe, flow velocities can be measured in the anterior, middle, or posterior cerebral arteries and the vertebral and basilar arteries.[36] Sound waves emitted by the probe are reflected by the red blood cells moving inside the vessels, and this reflection is captured by the transducer. The obtained signal is proportional to the velocity of the blood.[37]

The noninvasive technique and portability of the equipment allow frequent bedside monitoring of flow velocity and of vascular diameter. Use of serial TCD studies for the detection of cerebral vasospasm greatly reduces the need for cerebral angiograms to verify and follow post-SAH vasospasm.[36] Additional uses of TCD include identification of intracranial lesions in a patient with stroke, evaluation of flow-velocity changes during carotid endarterectomy, and detection of reduced CBF and impaired autoregulation associated with increased ICP in patients with TBI.[36]

There are limitations associated with the use of TCD. Its accuracy is operator dependent. Correct location and angle of the probe are essential. Patient age, female sex, and other factors affecting bone thickness can make exploration through the temporal window difficult or impossible for 10% of patients.[36] Because only the larger basal arteries can be studied with this technique, the values express an estimation of the global CBF. Because of the low penetration of the sound waves, it is not possible to examine the diameter of the artery. Consequently, the given values are not absolute flow parameters, but they are rather relative speed values.[37] A normal TCD study does not completely rule out the presence of vasospasm, because vasospasm may not be evident in the particular vessel examined. TCD results should always be evaluated in conjunction with clinical assessment findings and other diagnostic modalities.[36] Additionally, TCD may take 15 to 90 minutes to complete, and the patient must remain still for the duration of the study.[36]

Transcranial Color-Coded Duplex Sonography

TCCS is a method of TCD recording that displays a two-dimensional, color-coded image. TCCS can detect narrowing or occlusion of cerebral arteries, screen for vasospasm, and monitor changes in intracranial dynamics.[23] Arteriovenous malformations also can be detected with TCCS.[38] Current recommendations for TCCS include predicting (1) angiographic vasospasm after aneurysmal SAH, (2) delayed ischemic neurologic deficits caused by vasospasm after aneurysmal SAH, and (3) vasospasm after traumatic SAH.[23]

Thermal Diffusion Flowmetry

TDF is an invasive technique that uses thermal clearance to provide an estimation of brain perfusion.[37] It allows the quantitative measurement of regional CBF, which is considered an important upstream monitoring parameter indicative of tissue viability.[37] TDF has been used to diagnose delayed cerebral ischemia in patients with SAH. For the procedure, a thermal diffusion regional CBF microprobe is placed 20 to 25 mm below the cortical surface via a small burr hole and is secured by tightening a metal bolt. When the microprobe is in place, the nurse attaches it to an umbilical cord and monitor to begin calibration.[39] The microprobe includes a heated distal thermistor and a proximal thermistor. The distal thermistor measures blood flow via heat transfer to the capillaries. A microprocessor then converts this information into a measure of CBF in mL per 100 g per minute, which is represented as the K value on the monitor. As a general rule, mean thermal diffusion regional CBF values range from 18 to 25 mL/100 g per minute.[39]

It is important to consider that CBF values measured by thermal diffusion regional CBF vary depending on the placement of the probe.[39] Another important consideration with the use of TDF is that the monitor provides CBF parameters only within a temperature range of 25°C to 39.5°C.[39] Therefore patient cooling should be considered if the temperature of the brain is greater than 38.5°C.[36] Other considerations with the use of TDF are that the probe can be viewed on CT or with radiography and is not compatible with MRI. Also, because the TDF monitor does not operate on battery power, the probe must be disconnected from the umbilical cord and secured to the patient's head dressing before patient transport. Additionally, if the probe is used in conjunction with a microdialysis catheter, the two catheters must be separated by 2 mm for accurate results.[39]

Laser Doppler Flowmetry

LDF is an invasive indirect technique that provides continuous red blood cell velocity in the cerebral capillaries and thus real-time monitoring of microcirculation.[24,37] It has been used to map microvascular blood flow intraoperatively and to help manage severe TBI and aneurysmal SAH vasospasm.[24] The laser diffusion flowmetry probe is either inserted into the brain parenchyma or placed on the cerebral cortex. In contrast to TDF, LDF does not quantify CBF absolutely but provides a measure of relative change in flow. Several limitations affect the usefulness of LDF. The main drawback is that the small volume of brain wherein the flow is assessed reflects only local microcirculation. Movement artifacts from the patient or from the probe can result in inaccurate values. Finally, the CBF is only assessed by qualitative means.[24]

Cerebral Oxygenation and Metabolic Monitoring

Maintenance of adequate brain tissue oxygenation and key brain energy substrates is a critical objective in the management of critically ill patients with neurologic disorders. The following methods may be used in the critical care unit to monitor the patient's cerebral oxygenation status and cerebral metabolic state.

Partial Brain Tissue Oxygen Pressure

Maintenance of cerebral oxygenation is essential for critically ill patients with neurologic disorders and is important in minimizing secondary hypoxic and ischemic brain damage following acute brain injury.[40]

Partial brain parenchymal oxygen tension ($PbtO_2$) uses a device similar to pulse oximetry that allows continuous monitoring of regional tissue oxygenation and, in particular, areas of high ischemic risk.[24,40] The device consists of a monitoring probe on the end of a catheter, which is inserted into the brain parenchyma and attached to a bedside monitor. The probe may be inserted into the damaged portion of the brain to measure regional oxygenation or inserted into the undamaged portion of the brain to measure global oxygenation. Placement of the catheter itself causes some microtrauma, and values obtained in that area may not be valid from 30 minutes up to 2 hours after placement.[24]

Normal $PbtO_2$ is estimated to be 23 to 35 mm Hg.[23] A $PbtO_2$ threshold of less than 20 mm Hg represents compromised brain oxygen and is a threshold at which to consider intervention.[23] $PbtO_2$ values below 20 mm Hg carry a high risk of poor outcomes, whereas a $PbtO_2$ of less than 10 mm Hg for more than 10 minutes carries a higher risk of death.[37] Observational studies suggest a potential benefit when PbtO$_2$-guided therapy is added to a management protocol for severe TBI.[23] However, it is recommended that brain oxygen monitors be used with clinical indicators and other monitoring modalities for accurate prognostication.[23] Drawbacks related to PbtO$_2$ monitoring include the requirement for a brain CT scan to confirm the positioning of the electrode and typical risks of any invasive brain monitoring (infections, bleeding, etc.).[37]

Retrograde Jugular Bulb Oxygen Saturation

Oxygen levels in the cerebral venous outflow may inversely correlate with global brain oxygen consumption. Therefore oxygen saturation in the jugular bulb (SjvO$_2$) may be used for indirect estimation of cerebral oxygen consumption.[37]

Sampling and measuring SjvO$_2$ intermittently or continuously using fiberoptic oximetry requires the tip of the catheter to be placed retrograde through the internal jugular and into the jugular bulb.[37] Normal SjvO$_2$ is 55% to 70%.[24] SjvO$_2$ of less than 50% represents global cerebral ischemia, and SjvO$_2$ of greater than 75% represents an absolute or relative global hyperemia that exceeds the brain's metabolic demand. Both SjvO$_2$ less than 50% and SjvO$_2$ greater than 75% have been associated with unfavorable outcomes.[24] Indications for SjvO$_2$ monitoring include risk for global hypoxia, severe TBI, and aneurysmal SAH.[24]

A limitation of SjvO$_2$ monitoring is that it cannot detect focal ischemia. Also, SjvO$_2$ readings are affected by the position and movement of the patient's head and the monitoring system requires frequent calibration.[41] Technical difficulties and inaccuracies with SjvO$_2$ monitoring can also include catheter misplacement, contamination with extracerebral blood when the catheter abuts the blood vessel wall, and thrombosis occurring around the catheter tip.[23]

Near-Infrared Spectroscopy

Brain oxygenation also can be assessed using transcranial near-infrared spectroscopy (NIRS).[24] A noninvasive monitor of cerebral oxygenation, NIRS quantifies the relative concentrations of oxygenated and deoxygenated hemoglobin through reliance on the transmission and absorption of near-infrared light as it passes through tissue.[25,42] NIRS has many potential advantages over other monitoring techniques. It is a noninvasive technique, has high temporal and spatial resolution, and provides simultaneous measurements over multiple regions of interest.[25] Algorithms based on multiple detectors (spatially resolved NIRS) can provide data that give a value of the regional saturation of O$_2$ (rSO$_2$).[37] The main shortcomings associated with NIRS are the unknown contribution to the signal from extracranial tissues and that the given values are relative. In the critical care unit setting, scalp and facial traumas may prevent the application of the optodes, and brain lesions, like intraparenchymal hematomas, may lead to unpredictable values.[37]

Cerebral Microdialysis

Cerebral microdialysis is a tool for investigating the metabolic status of the injured brain at the bedside. A catheter with a 10-mm semipermeable distal membrane is inserted into the brain parenchyma (ideally placed in the frontal lobe) via twist drill hole or transcranial bolt.[39,43] Here substances in the extracellular fluid surround the semipermeable membrane at the tip of the catheter. Following diffusion, the dialysate can be analyzed hourly for glucose, lactate, pyruvate (as indicators of hypoxia and ischemia) and interstitial glycerol (as an indicator of lipolysis and/or cell damage) with the goal of detecting neurochemical changes indicative of primary and secondary brain injury.[44] The ratio of lactate to pyruvate, a product from glucose metabolism, can yield information that is more valuable than looking only at lactate.[43] Monitoring cerebral microdialysis is recommended in patients with TBI or SAH who are at risk for cerebral ischemia, hypoxia, energy failure, and glucose deprivation.[23,37,43]

Continuous Electroencephalography Monitoring

Continuous electroencephalography (cEEG) has the advantage of being noninvasive and carries the potential to detect alterations in brain physiology at a reversible stage; thus triggering treatment before permanent brain injury occurs.[45] The main applications of cEEG are diagnosing nonconvulsive status epilepticus, monitoring and guiding the treatment of status epilepticus, and detecting delayed cerebral ischemia from vasospasm in SAH patients.[45] In 10% to 20% of comatose patients with poor-grade SAH, nonconvulsive seizures may be detected on continuous EEG.[46] However, as most epileptic abnormalities can be captured using a 2-hour recording, cEEG for 24 hours or more may be more appropriately used in high-risk patients (comatose and prior seizures).[45]

Clinically unrecognized electrographic seizures and periodic epileptiform discharges are often frequent and associated with poor outcome in patients with severe brain injury from different etiologies, including TBI, ischemic and hemorrhagic strokes, and CNS infection. EEG sensitivity to ischemia allows its use in situations where cerebral perfusion is at risk. Changes over time can trigger focused neurologic examination, imaging studies, and early treatment.[47]

There are several challenges related to cEEG implementation, including the requirement for continuous access to technicians and neurophysiologists for interpretation and difficulties in data storage.[45] Other drawbacks to the use of cEEG are that it is expensive, labor intensive, and subject to artifact from the critical care unit environment.[47] More recently, EEG training courses have improved the accuracy of quantitative EEG reading by general intensivists.[45] Also, the development of spectral analysis (quantitative EEG) and software enabling artifact elimination have made cEEG use in the critical care unit more practical and reliable.

BOX 16.3   Informatics   **QSEN**

Internet Resources: Neurologic Clinical Assessment and Diagnostic Procedures

- American Academy of Neurology: www.aan.com
- American Association of Critical-Care Nurses: www.aacn.org
- American Association of Neurological Surgeons: www.aans.org
- American Association of Neuroscience Nurses: www.aann.org
- American College of Physicians: www.acponline.org
- American College of Surgeons: www.facs.org
- American Medical Association: www.ama-assn.org
- American Stroke Association: www.stroke.org
- National Institutes of Health: www.nih.gov
- Society for Critical Care Medicine: www.sccm.org
- Society for Neuroscience: www.sfn.org

ADDITIONAL RESOURCES

See Box 16.3 for Internet resources pertaining to neurologic disorders and therapeutic management.

REFERENCES

1. Jankovic J, Mazziotta JC, Newman NJ, Pomeroy SL. Diagnosis of neurological disease. In: Jankovic J, Mazziotta JC, Pomeroy SL, Newman NJ, eds. *Bradley and Daroff's Neurology in Clinical Practice*. 8th ed. Philadelphia: Elsevier; 2022.
2. Chamberlain D, Kuzmiuk L. Neurological assessment and monitoring. In: Aitken L, Marshall A, Chaboyer W, eds. *ACCCN's Critical Care Nursing*. 4th ed. St. Louis: Elsevier; 2019.
3. Barker E. The neurologic assessment. In: Barker E, ed. *Neuroscience Nursing: A Spectrum of Care*. 3rd ed. St. Louis: Mosby; 2008.
4. Restrepro RD. Neurologic assessment. In: Heuer AJ, Scanlan CL, eds. *Wilkins' Clinical Assessment in Respiratory Care*. 8th ed. St. Louis: Elsevier; 2018.
5. Odiari EA, Sekhon N, Han JY, et al. Stabilizing and managing patients with altered mental status and delirium. *Emerg Med Clin North Am*. 2015;33(4):753–764. https://doi.org/10.1016/j.emc.2015.07.004.
6. Teasdale G, Jennett W. Assessment of coma and impaired consciousness—a practical scale. *Lancet*. 1974;2(7872):81–84.
7. Le Roux P, Menon DK, Citerio G, et al. Consensus summary statement of the international multidisciplinary consensus conference on multimodality monitoring in neurocritical care: a statement for healthcare professionals from the Neurocritical Care Society and the European Society of Intensive Care Medicine. *Neurocrit Care*. 2014;21(suppl 2):S1–S26. https://doi.org/10.1007/s12028-014-0041-5.
8. Ramazani J, Hosseini M. Comparison of full outline of unresponsiveness score and Glasgow coma scale in medical intensive care unit. *Ann Card Anaesth*. 2019;22(2):143–148. https://doi.org/10.4103/aca.ACA_25_18.
9. Kornbluth J, Bhardwaj A. Evaluation of coma: a critical appraisal of popular scoring systems. *Neurocrit Care*. 2011;14(1):134–143. https://doi.org/10.1007/s12028-010-9409-3.
10. Berger JR, Price R. Stupor and coma. In: Jankovic J, Mazziotta JC, Pomeroy SL, Newman NJ, eds. *Bradley and Daroff's Neurology in Clinical Practice*. 8th ed. Philadelphia: Elsevier; 2022.
11. Iyer VN. Validity of the FOUR Score Coma Scale in the medical intensive care unit. *Mayo Clin Proc*. 2009;84(8):694–701. https://doi.org/10.1016/S0025-6196(11)60519-3.
12. Ball JW, Dains JE, Flynn JA, et al. Neurologic system. In: Ball JW, Dains JE, Flynn JA, eds. *Seidel's Guide to Physical Examination: An Interprofessional Approach*. 9th ed. St. Louis: Elsevier; 2019.
13. Thurtell MJ, Rucker JC. Pupillary and eyelid abnormalities. In: Jankovic J, Mazziotta JC, Pomeroy SL, Newman NJ, eds. *Bradley and Daroff's Neurology in Clinical Practice*. 8th ed. Philadelphia: Elsevier; 2022.
14. Rasulo FA, Togni T, Romagnoli S. Essential noninvasive multimodality neuromonitoring for the critically ill patient. *Crit Care*. 2020;24(1):100. https://doi.org/10.1186/s13054-020-2781-2.
15. Rollins MD, Feiner JR, Lee JM, Shah S, Larson M. Pupillary effects of high-dose opioid quantified with infrared pupillometry. *Anesthesiology*. 2014;121(5):1037–1044. https://doi.org/10.1097/ALN.0000000000000384.
16. Ignatavicius DD. Critical care of patients with neurologic emergencies. In: Ignatavicius DD, Workman ML, Rebar CR, Heimgartner NM, eds. *Medical-Surgical Nursing: Concepts for Interprofessional Collaborative Care*. 10th ed. St. Louis: Elsevier; 2021.
17. Marehbian J, Muehlschlegel S, Edlow BL, Hinson HE, Hwang DY. Medical management of the severe traumatic brain injury. *Neurocrit Care*. 2017;27(3):430–446. https://doi.org/10.1007/s12028-017-0408-5.
18. Silvani A, Calandra-Buonaura G, Dampney RA, Cortelli P. Brain-heart interactions: physiology and clinical implications. *Philos Trans A Math Phys Eng Sci*. 2016;374(2067):20150181. https://doi.org/10.1098/rsta.2015.0181.
19. Marcoline E, Stretz C, DeWitt KM. Intracranial hemorrhage and intracranial hypertension. *Emeg Med Clin North Am*. 2019;37(3):529–544. https://doi.org/10.1016/j.emc.2019.04.001.
20. Engelborghs S, Niemantsverdriet E, Struyfs H, et al. Consensus guidelines for lumbar puncture in patients with neurological diseases. *Alzheimers Dement (Amst)*. 2017;8:111–126. https://doi.org/10.1016/j.dadm.2017.04.007.
21. Sladky JH, Piwinski SE. Lumbar puncture technique and lumbar drains. *Atlas Oral Maxillofac Surg Clin North Am*. 2015;23(2):169–176. https://doi.org/10.1016/j.cxom.2015.05.005.
22. Euerle BD. Spinal puncture and cerebrospinal fluid examination. In: Roberts JR, ed. *Roberts and Hedges' Clinical Procedures in Emergency Medicine and Acute Care*. 7th ed. Philadelphia: Elsevier; 2019.
23. Le Roux P, Menon DK, Citerio G, et al. Consensus summary statement of the international multidisciplinary consensus conference on multimodality monitoring in neurocritical care: a statement for healthcare professionals from the Neurocritical Care Society and the European Society of Intensive Care Medicine. *Neurocrit Care*. 2014;21(suppl 2):S1–S26. https://doi.org/10.1007/s12028-014-0081-x.
24. Blisset PA. Hemodynamic and intracranial monitoring in neurocritical care. In: Lough ME, ed. *Hemodynamic Monitoring: Evolving Technologies and Clinical Practice*. St. Louis: Elsevier; 2016.
25. Kirkman MA, Smith M. Intracranial pressure monitoring, cerebral perfusion pressure estimation, and ICP/CPP-guided therapy: a standard of care or optional extra after brain injury. *Br J Anesth*. 2014;112(1):3–46. https://doi.org/10.1093/bja/aet418.
26. Raboel PH, Barteck J, Andresen M, Bellander BM. Intracranial pressure monitoring: invasive versus non-invasive methods—a review. *Crit Care Res Pract*. 2012;2012:950393. https://doi.org/10.1155/2012/950393.
27. Muralidharan R. External ventricular drains: management and complications. *Surg Neurol Int*. 2015;6(suppl 6):S271–S274. https://doi.org/10.4103/2152-7806.157620.
28. Hockel K, Schuhmann MU. ICP monitoring by open extraventricular drainage: common practice but not suitable for advanced neuromonitoring and prone to false negativity. *Acta Neurochir Suppl*. 2018;126:281–286. https://doi.org/10.1007/978-3-319-65798-1_55.
29. Tavakoli S, Peitz G, Ares W, Hafeez S, Grandhi R. Complications of invasive intracranial pressure monitoring devices in neurocritical care. *Neurosurg Focus*. 2017;43(5):1–9. https://doi.org/10.3171/2017.8.FOCUS17450.
30. Slazinski T. Intraventricular/fiberoptic catheter insertion (assist), monitoring, nursing care, troubleshooting, and removal. In: Wiegand DL, ed. *AACN Procedure Manual for High Acuity, Progressive, and Critical Care*. 7th ed. St. Louis: Elsevier; 2017.
31. Slazinski T. Intracranial bolt and fiberoptic catheter insertion (assist), intracranial pressure monitoring, care, troubleshooting, and removal. In: Wiegand DL, ed. *AACN Procedure Manual for Critical Care*. 7th ed. St. Louis: Elsevier; 2017.
32. Elwishi M, Dinsmore J. Monitoring the brain. *BJA Education*. 2019;19(2):54–59. https://doi.org/10.1016/j.bjae.2018.12.001.
33. Lussier BL, Olson DM, Aiyagari V. Automated pupillometry in neurocritical care: research and practice. *Curr Neurol Neurosci Rep*. 2019;19(10):71. https://doi.org/10.1007/s11910-019-0994-z.
34. Rabba C. Intercranial pressure monitoring. In: Prabhakar H, ed. *Neuromonitoring Techniques: Quick Guide for Clinicians and Residents*. London: Academic Press; 2018.
35. Carney N, Totten AM, O'Reilly C, et al. *Guidelines for the Management of Severe Traumatic Brain Injury. 17. Cerebral Perfusion Thresholds. Brain Trauma Foundation*; 2016. https://braintrauma.org/uploads/03/12/Guidelines_for_Management_of_Severe_TBI_4th_Edition.pdf.
36. Bouzat P, Oddo M, Payen JF. Transcranial Doppler after traumatic brain injury: is there a role? *Curr Opin Crit Care*. 2014;20(2):153–160. https://doi.org/10.1097/MCC.0000000000000071.
37. Rasulo F, Matta B, Varanini N. Cerebral blood flow monitoring. In: Prabhakar H, ed. *Neuromonitoring Techniques: Quick Guide for Clinicians and Residents*. London: Academic Press; 2018.
38. Marshall SA, Nyquist P, Ziai WC. The role of transcranial Doppler ultrasonography in the diagnosis and management of vasospasm after aneurysmal subarachnoid hemorrhage. *Neurosurg Clin N Am*. 2010;21(2):291–303. https://doi.org/10.1016/j.nec.2009.10.010.
39. Cecil S, Chen PM, Callaway SE. Traumatic brain injury: advanced multimodal neuromonitoring from theory to practice. *Crit Care Nurse*. 2011;31(2):25–36. https://doi.org/10.4037/ccn2010226.
40. Peacock SH, Tomlinson AD. Multimodal neuromonitoring in neurocritical care. *AACN Adv Crit Care*. 2018;29(2):183–194. https://doi.org/10.4037/aacnacc2018632.
41. Chaikittisilpa N, Vavilala MS, Lele AV. Jugular venous oximetry. In: Prabhakar H, ed. *Neuromonitoring Techniques: Quick Guide for Clinicians and Residents*. London: Academic Press; 2018.

42. Murkin JM, Arango M. Near-infrared spectroscopy as an index of brain and tissue oxygenation. *Br J Anesth.* 2009;103(suppl 1):i3—i13.

43. McLawhorn M, James ML. Cerebral microdialysis. In: Prabhakar H, ed. *Neuromonitoring Techniques: Quick Guide for Clinicians and Residents.* London: Academic Press; 2018.

44. Grüne F, Klimek M. Cerebral blood flow and its autoregulation—when will there be some light in the black box? *Br J Anaesth.* 2017;119(6):1077—1079. https://doi.org/10.1093/bja/aex355.

45. Vulliemoz S, Perrig S, Pellise D, et al. Imaging compatible electrodes for continuous electroencephalogram monitoring in the intensive care unit.

J Clin Neurophysiol. 2009;26(4):236—243. https://doi.org/10.1097/WNP.0b013e3181af1c95.

46. Diringer MN, Bleck TP, Claude Hemphill J 3rd, et al. Critical care management of patients following aneurysmal subarachnoid hemorrhage: recommendations from the Neurocritical Care Society's multidisciplinary consensus conference. *Neurocrit Care.* 2011;15(2):211—240. https://doi.org/10.1007/s12028-011-9605-9.

47. Kubota Y, Nakamoto H, Egawa S, Kawamata T. Continuous EEG monitoring in ICU. *J Intensive Care.* 2018;6:39. https://doi.org/10.1186/s40560-018-0310-z.

17

Neurologic Disorders and Therapeutic Management

Kathleen M. Stacy

STROKE

Stroke is a descriptive term for the sudden onset of acute neurologic deficit persisting for more than 24 hours and caused by the interruption of blood flow to the brain. Stroke is the fifth leading cause of death in the United States, preceded by heart disease, cancer, preventable injuries, and chronic respiratory disease. Each year, approximately 795,000 people have a stroke; 610,000 of strokes annually are first attacks, and 185,000 are recurrent attacks.[1]

Strokes are classified as ischemic and hemorrhagic. Hemorrhagic strokes can be further categorized as subarachnoid hemorrhages (SAHs) and intracerebral hemorrhages (ICHs). Approximately 87% of all strokes are ischemic, 10% are ICHs, and 3% are SAHs.[1] Although less common, hemorrhagic strokes (ICHs and SAHs) have a higher mortality rate compared with ischemic strokes.[1] In 2015 the annual cost for care and loss of productivity was estimated to be $45.5 billion.[1]

The national concern for the incidence and effects of stroke is illustrated by the inclusion of emergent stroke care in the American Heart Association guidelines for basic and advanced life support. Major public education programs, stroke appraisal screening programs, development of stroke centers, and algorithms for stroke management are based on the success that these same approaches have had with coronary artery disease.

Ischemic Stroke

Description and Etiology

Ischemic stroke results from interruption of blood flow to the brain and accounts for 88% of all strokes.[2] The interruption can be the result of a thrombotic or embolic event. Thrombosis can form in large vessels (large-vessel thrombotic strokes) or small vessels (small-vessel thrombotic strokes). Embolic sources include the heart (cardioembolic strokes) and atherosclerotic plaques in larger vessels (atheroembolic strokes). In 25% of cases, the underlying cause of the stroke is unknown (cryptogenic strokes).[3]

Strokes are preventable. Most thrombotic strokes are the result of the accumulation of atherosclerotic plaque in the vessel lumen, especially at the bifurcations or curves of the vessel. The pathogenesis of cerebrovascular disease is identical to the pathogenesis of coronary vasculature. The greatest risk factor for ischemic stroke is hypertension.[2] Other risk factors are dyslipidemia, diabetes, smoking, and carotid atherosclerotic disease.[1] Common sites of atherosclerotic plaque are the bifurcation of the common carotid artery, the origins of the middle and anterior cerebral arteries, and the origins of the vertebral arteries.[2] Ischemic strokes resulting from vertebral artery dissection have been reported after chiropractic manipulation of the cervical spine.[4]

An embolic stroke occurs when an embolus from the heart or lower circulation travels distally and lodges in a small vessel, obstructing the blood supply. At least 20% of ischemic strokes are attributed to a cardioembolic phenomenon.[2] The most common cause of cardiac emboli is atrial fibrillation. It is responsible for approximately 50% of all cardiac emboli.[5] Other sources of cardiac emboli are from mitral stenosis, mechanical valves, atrial myxoma, endocarditis, and recent myocardial infarction.[5] Researchers hypothesize that a patent foramen ovale or atrial septal aneurysms may be the cause of cryptogenic stroke.[3]

Pathophysiology

Ischemic stroke is a cerebral hemodynamic insult. When cerebral blood flow (CBF) is reduced to a level insufficient to maintain neuronal viability, ischemic injury occurs. In focal stroke, an area of hypoperfused tissue, the ischemic penumbra, surrounds a core of ischemic cells. The ischemic penumbra can be salvaged with return of blood flow. However, sustained anoxic insult initiates a chain of biochemical events leading to apoptosis, or cellular death.[6]

The phenomenon of a focal ischemic stroke is identical to myocardial infarction, which is why the term *brain attack* is used in public education strategies. Often, a history of transient ischemic attacks, brief episodes of neurologic symptoms that last less than 24 hours, offers a warning that stroke is likely to occur. Sudden onset indicates embolism as the final insult to flow.[2] The size of the stroke depends on the size and location of the occluded vessel and the availability of collateral blood flow. Global ischemia results when severe hypotension or cardiopulmonary arrest provokes a transient decrease in blood flow to all areas of the brain.[6]

Cerebral edema sufficient to produce clinical deterioration develops in 10% to 20% of patients with ischemic stroke and can result in intracranial hypertension. The edema results from a loss of normal metabolic function of the cells and peaks at 4 days.[2] This process is commonly the cause of death during the first week after a stroke.[7] Secondary hemorrhage at the site of the stroke lesion, known as *hemorrhagic conversion*, and seizures are the two other major acute neurologic complications of ischemic stroke.[7]

Assessment and Diagnosis

The characteristic sign of an ischemic stroke is the sudden onset of focal neurologic signs persisting for more than 24 hours.[2] These signs usually occur in combination. Table 17.1 lists common patterns of

TABLE 17.1   Stroke Syndromes Secondary to Occlusion or Stenosis.

Location/Vessel	Area of Brain Infarcted	Signs and Symptoms Noted
Anterior and Central Circulation		
Note: The internal carotid artery enters the circle of Willis and supplies the lateral anterior and central portions of the cerebral hemispheres through the middle cerebral artery and the paramedial frontal lobe superior to the corpus callosum through the anterior cerebral artery; penetrating branches serve the deeper layers of the hemispheres.		
Internal carotid	If collateral circulation is intact, there is commonly no infarction; if infarcted, it is in the same area of the middle cerebral artery	• Arterial pressure may be low in the retina • Bruits over the internal carotid artery • Possible retinal emboli • History of transient ischemic attacks (TIAs) • Positive noninvasive studies
Middle cerebral artery (MCA) (most common area); either stem or branches of MCA	Cortical motor area (face, arm, leg) and/or posterior limb, internal capsule, corona radiata	• **Motor:** contralateral hemiparesis or hemiplegia, greater in face and arm than leg
	Cortical sensory area (face, arm, leg) and/or posterior limb of internal capsule	• **Sensation:** contralateral loss in same distribution as motor loss
	Broca area and deep fibers in the dominant hemisphere	• **Speech:** expressive (motor) disorder with anomia (left hemisphere most commonly affected) with nonfluent aphasia and some comprehension defects
	Broca area and deep fibers in the nondominant hemisphere	• **Speech:** dysarthria
	Optic radiations deep in the temporal lobe	• **Vision:** contralateral homonymous hemianopsia or quadranopsia
	Location not known	• **Motor:** mirror movements • **Respirations:** Cheyne-stokes respirations, contralateral hyperhidrosis, occasional mydriasis
	Posterior limb or internal capsule and adjacent corona radiate	• **Motor:** pure motor hemiplegia
	Penetrating branches of MCA (lenticulostriate branches) into the basal nuclei	• **Motor:** varying degrees of contralateral weakness of face, arm, or leg • **Sensory:** little or no loss; if present, contralateral following the motor distribution • **Speech:** transcortical sensory aphasia (communicating pathways are interrupted) • **Perception:** transient visual and sensory neglect on the left if a right lesion
Anterior cerebral artery (ACA) (least common)	Proximal segment: corona radiata (rarely)	• **Motor:** when present, a mild contralateral hemiparesis, greater in leg; with bilateral occlusion of ACA, cerebral paraplegia in both legs can occur
	Main stem (complete occlusion is uncommon; thus areas affected differ and collateral circulation may alleviate signs or symptoms); medial aspect of frontal lobes, caudate nucleus, and corpus callosum are supplied by the ACA	• **Motor:** contralateral paralysis or paresis (greater in foot and thigh); mild upper extremity weakness • **Sensory:** mild contralateral lower extremity deficiency with loss of vibratory and/or position sense, loss of two-point discrimination • **Speech:** may have transcortical motor and sensory aphasia if left hemisphere • Frontal lobe releasing signs (grasp, snout, root, and suck reflexes) • Apraxia
Posterior Circulation		
Note: The posterior circulation includes the posterior cerebral artery, the vertebral arteries, and the basilar artery; the anatomic territory covered includes the posterior aspects of the hemispheres, the central areas of the thalamus and midbrain, and the brainstem; occlusion of the vessels is most commonly by emboli; effects of infarct in these vessels and their penetrating vessels can be specific or devastatingly global; many complex syndromes have been identified.		
Vertebral arteries	Medulla and spinal cord tracts, anterior spinal artery and penetrating branches (medial medullary syndrome)	• **Motor:** contralateral hemiparesis (face spared) and/or impaired contralateral proprioception; flaccid weakness or paralysis of the tongue and/or dysarthria
Basilar artery (three sets of branches)	Midline structures of pons (paramedian branches); three general areas of infarction are common: (1) medial	• **Motor:** contralateral hemiparesis or hemiplegia, ipsilateral lower motor neuron facial palsy, "locked-in syndrome"

TABLE 17.1 Stroke Syndromes Secondary to Occlusion or Stenosis.—cont'd

Location/Vessel	Area of Brain Infarcted	Signs and Symptoms Noted
	inferior pontine syndrome, (2) medial midpontine syndrome, and (3) medial superior pontine syndrome	• **Sensory:** contralateral loss of vibratory sense, sense of position with dysmetria, loss of two-point discrimination, impaired rapid alternating movements • **Visual:** inferior pontine: diplopia; impaired abduction of ipsilateral eye: internuclear ophthalmoplegia; medial superior: diplopia, internuclear ophthalmoplegia, skewed deviation
	Corticospinal and corticobulbar tracts in pons, sensory tracts of medial and lateral lemnisci, vestibular nuclei, inferior and middle cerebellar peduncles, cranial nerve nuclei and/or fibers, cerebellar connections in tectum, descending sympathetic pathways, central brainstem, pontine tegmentum (vertebrobasilar syndrome)	• **Motor:** upper motor neuron type of weakness: paralysis in combinations involving face, tongue, throat, and extremities; dysphagia, facial weakness, dysmetria, ataxia (either trunk or extremities), weak mastication muscles • **Sensation:** combinations of impaired sensation (vibratory, two-point, position sense, pain, temperature), facial hypesthesia, anesthesia of cranial nerve V
Posterior cerebral artery (PCA)	Central territory (thalamic area, dentatothalamic tract, cerebral peduncle, red nucleus, subthalamic nucleus, and cranial nerve III)	• **Motor:** contralateral hemiplegia with possible dysmetria, dyskinesia, hemiballism or choreoathetosis, dystaxia, cerebellar ataxia, and tremor; contralateral upper motor neuron palsy; several syndromes are associated: (1) Weber: cranial nerve III palsy and contralateral hemiplegia; (2) thalamoperforate syndrome: superior crossed cerebellar ataxia or inferior crossed cerebellar ataxia with cranial nerve III palsy (Claude syndrome); (3) decerebrate attacks • **Sensory:** contralateral sensory loss of all modalities without agraphia • **Function:** prosopagnosia (inability to recognize familiar faces), topographic disorientation, memory deficits, alexia, inability to read, color anomia • **Level of consciousness:** in bilateral PCA syndromes, coma with absent doll's eyes reflex or loss of alertness may occur; if tegmentum of midbrain near hypothalamus and third ventricle is damaged, akinetic mutism may occur

Small Vessel Disease

Note: Small penetrating vessels in brain parenchyma that supply areas near the basal ganglia are most vulnerable to infarction, although any small vessels can occlude deep in the brain and cause injury, producing neurologic signs or symptoms; such infarcts are commonly called *lacunes* (small pit or hollow), a term that is changing in meaning; they can be caused by emboli but are most commonly associated with microatheromas; although they can be found in otherwise healthy people, those with concurrent atherosclerosis, arterial hypertension, and/or diabetes have a higher incidence of this type of infarct.

	Internal capsule, most commonly	• **Motor:** contralateral hemiparesis on a single side, with equal deficit in face, arm, and leg; often unaccompanied by detectable signs of sensory, visual, and speech loss, depending on location; old term is *pure motor stroke*, although evidence suggests that other neurologic signs are present but overlooked because of low intensity
	Thalamus, most commonly	• **Sensory:** complete or partial loss in face, arm, trunk, and leg that appears exactly midline; may be accompanied by pain, hyperesthesias, and uncomfortable sensations (hemisensory stroke)
	Pons	Dysarthria, clumsy hand
	Pons, midbrain, capsule or parietal white matter	Hemiparesis, ataxia on same side

Modified from Barker E. *Neuroscience Nursing*. St Louis: Mosby; 1994.

neurologic symptoms associated with an ischemic stroke. Hemiparesis, aphasia, and hemianopia are common. Changes in the level of consciousness (LOC) usually occur only with brainstem or cerebellar involvement, seizure, hypoxia, hemorrhage, or elevated intracranial pressure (ICP). These changes may be exhibited as stupor, coma, confusion, and agitation. The reported frequency of seizures in patients with ischemic stroke is approximately 11%. If seizures occur, they are usually seen within the first 2 weeks of an insult.[7]

The National Institutes of Health Stroke Scale (NIHSS) is often used as the basis of the focused neurologic examination.[8] The score ranges from 0 to 42 points; the higher the score, the more neurologically impaired the patient is. A change of four points on the scale indicates significant neurologic change. The components of the NIHSS include LOC; LOC questions; LOC commands; gaze; visual fields; face, arm, and leg strength; sensation; limb ataxia; and language function. A copy of the NIHSS with complete instructions is available at www. ninds.nih.gov/sites/default/files/nih_stroke_scale_booklet_508c.pdf.

Confirmation of the diagnosis of ischemic stroke is the first step in the emergent evaluation of these patients. Differentiation from intracranial hemorrhage is vital. In most instances, noncontrast computed tomography (CT) scanning is the method of choice for this purpose, and it is considered the most important initial diagnostic study. In addition to excluding intracranial hemorrhage, CT can assist in identifying early neurologic complications and the cause of the insult. Magnetic resonance imaging (MRI) can demonstrate infarction of cerebral tissue earlier than CT and is an appropriate alternative to a noncontrast CT scan for excluding ICH.[8]

Because of the strong correlation between acute ischemic stroke and heart disease, 12-lead electrocardiography and continuous cardiac monitoring are suggested to detect a cardiac cause or coexisting condition. A chest radiograph is obtained if lung disease is suspected. However, obtaining these studies should not delay the administration of fibrinolysis.[8] Echocardiography is valuable in identifying a cardioembolic phenomenon when a sufficient index of suspicion warrants its use.[2] Laboratory studies to evaluate hematologic and renal function, coagulation, electrolyte and glucose levels, and troponin are also recommended. Arterial blood gas analysis is performed if hypoxia is suspected. A lumbar puncture may be performed if a SAH is suspected and the CT scan is normal.[8]

Medical Management

Rapid diagnosis of stroke and initiation of treatment are important to maximize recovery, prevent recurrence of stroke, and prevent complications (Box 17.1). Definitive management of a patient with an ischemic stroke focuses on revascularization of the affected area of the brain with either fibrinolytic therapy or mechanical thrombectomy before neurons die of ischemia.[8] The goal is to reverse or minimize the effects of stroke.

Fibrinolytic therapy with intravenous recombinant tissue plasminogen activator (rtPA) is recommended within 3 hours of onset of ischemic stroke to facilitate dissolution of the clot.[8] The exclusion criteria for patients who should be considered for fibrinolysis are

---

BOX 17.2 Exclusion Criteria for Intravenous Recombinant Tissue Plasminogen Activator

- Age ≤18 years of age
- Onset of symptoms <3 or 4.5 hours (see text for more information)
- Stroke in previous 3 months
- Intracranial or intraspinal surgery in previous 3 months
- Severe head trauma in previous 3 months
- Subarachnoid hemorrhage
- Intracranial hemorrhage—acute and prior history
- Intracranial neoplasm
- Aortic arch dissection
- Infective endocarditis
- Gastrointestinal malignancy
- Gastrointestinal hemorrhage in previous 21 days
- Uncontrolled severe hypertension
- Active internal bleeding
- Coagulopathy (platelets <100,000/mm^3, INR >1.7, aPTT >40 seconds, or PT >15)
- Low—molecular-weight heparin within previous 24 hours

aPTT, Activated partial thromboplastin time; *INR*, international normalized ratio; *PT*, prothrombin time.
Data from Powers WJ, Rabinstein AA, Ackerson T, et al. Guidelines for the early management of patients with acute ischemic stroke: 2019 update to the 2018 guidelines for the early management of acute ischemic stroke: a guideline for healthcare professionals from the American Heart Association/American Stroke Association. *Stroke.* 2019;50(12):e344—e418.

---

listed in Box 17.2. The time frame for rtPA can be extended to 4.5 hours, with some additional exclusions including patients older than 80 years of age, patients taking oral anticoagulants, patients with a baseline NIHSS score greater than 25, patients with evidence of ischemic injury involving more than one-third of the middle cerebral artery territory, and patients with a history of both stroke and diabetes.[8] The diagnosis must be confirmed with CT scan before rtPA administration.[8]

The most common fibrinolytic agent used is alteplase. The recommended dosage is 0.9 mg/kg, up to a maximum dosage of 90 mg; 10% of the total dose is administered as an initial intravenous bolus, and

---

QSEN

BOX 17.1 Teamwork and Collaboration

Acute Stroke Teams

Given the short time available to restore blood flow to the brain after a stroke, an organized approach must be taken to provide the patient with the best chance of a positive outcome. To meet this challenge, many health care organizations have developed acute stroke teams. An acute stroke team comprises transdisciplinary health care professionals with the experience and training in the definitive management of a patient experiencing a stroke. The goal of the team is to reduce in-hospital delays in obtaining appropriate medical care for these patients.

Members will vary depending on the health care organization; however, the acute stroke team usually includes an emergency room physician, a neurologist, an interventional radiologist, a pharmacist, a laboratory technician, and one or more registered nurses. The team is available 24 hours a day and is notified via a specialized notification system (e.g., "Stroke Code"). The acute stroke team is responsible for stabilizing the patient, performing initial testing to determine the type of stroke, and initiating the selected treatment regimen to help the patient achieve the best possible functional outcome.[1]

Teamwork and collaboration are essential for the success of these teams. As they come together with a common shared goal, they often have to learn how to work together as a team. Many teams use crew resource management tools to facilitate team development. Crew resource tools focus on the nonclinical aspects of the team, including team communication, team leadership, and team organization. Many teams use ongoing stroke-specific simulation training to enhance team knowledge and cohesiveness.[2]

References

1. Tahtali D, Bohmann F, Rostek P, Wagner M, Steinmetz H, Pfeilschifter W. Setting up a stroke team algorithm and conducting simulation-based training in the emergency department—a practical guide. *J Vis Exp.* 2017;(119):55138. https://doi.org/10.3791/55138.
2. Willems LM, Kurka N, Bohmann F, Rostek P, Pfeilschifter W. Tools for your stroke team: adapting crew-resource management for acute stroke care. *Pract Neurol.* 2019;19(1):36—42. https://doi.org/10.1136/practneurol-2018-001966.

the remaining 90% is administered by intravenous infusion over 60 minutes.[8] Tenecteplase can be considered as an alternative in patients with minor neurologic impairment and without major intracranial occlusions. The recommended dosage is 0.4 mg/kg administered as a single intravenous bolus.[8] Bleeding, especially intracranial hemorrhage, is the major risk and complication of rtPA therapy. In contrast to fibrinolytic protocols for acute myocardial infarction, subsequent therapy with anticoagulant or antiplatelet agents is not recommended after rtPA administration in ischemic stroke. Patients receiving fibrinolytic therapy for stroke should not receive aspirin, heparin, warfarin, ticlopidine, or any other antithrombotic or antiplatelet medications for at least 24 hours after treatment.[8]

Mechanical thrombectomy is a newer therapy recommended in the treatment of ischemic stroke in selected patients.[9] Current guidelines recommend that the device be employed within 6 hours of the onset of symptoms; under certain circumstances the treatment window can be increased to 24 hours.[8,9] A mechanical thrombectomy is the endovascular retrieval of a thrombus from a large intracranial vessel with a catheter. Although there are several different types of devices available, current guidelines recommend the use of a stent retrieval system. A stent retrieval system uses a self-expanding stent that can be deployed and retrieved. When the device is deployed into a cerebral vessel across a thrombus, it pushes the thrombus against the vessel wall, re-establishing blood flow to the area downstream from the clot. The thrombus is then ensnared in the struts of the stent and the stent is retrieved.[9,10]

The major barriers to effective application of definitive therapy for ischemic stroke are prehospital and in-hospital delays. To help decrease delays, the public needs to be educated about stroke symptoms and activation of the emergency medical system. Emergency medical system responders need adequate education and training on managing a patient with an acute ischemic stroke, focusing on stabilization and transport of the patient quickly to the emergency department. The receiving hospital should ideally have certification for primary stroke treatment and have expert staff and the infrastructure to care for a patient with complex stroke.[8,11]

Other emergent care of a patient with ischemic stroke must include airway protection and ventilatory assistance to maintain adequate tissue oxygenation.[8] Supplemental oxygen should be provided to maintain oxygen saturation great than 94%.[8] Hypertension is often present in the early period as a compensatory response, and in most cases, blood pressure must not be lowered. For patients who have not received fibrinolytic therapy, antihypertensive therapy is considered only if the diastolic blood pressure is greater than 120 mm Hg or the systolic blood pressure is greater than 220 mm Hg.[8] Criteria are different for patients who have received rtPA. Their blood pressure is maintained at less than 180/105 mm Hg to prevent intracranial hemorrhage. Intravenous labetalol or nicardipine is used to achieve blood pressure control. If these agents are ineffective, nitroprusside should be considered.[8] Body temperature and glucose levels also must be normalized.[8]

Medical management also includes the identification and treatment of acute complications such as cerebral edema or seizure activity. Prophylaxis for these complications is not recommended. However, deep vein thrombosis (DVT) prophylaxis should be initiated to decrease the risk of pulmonary embolism.[8]

Subarachnoid Hemorrhage
Description and Etiology
SAH is due to bleeding into the subarachnoid space.[12] Cerebral aneurysm rupture accounts for approximately 80% of all cases of spontaneous nontraumatic SAH.[12] Other causes of SAH include arteriovenous malformations (AVMs), moyamoya, vasculitis, amyloid angiopathy, and intracranial artery dissections.[12–15] Known risk factors for SAH include prior history or family history of SAH, hypertension, smoking, heavy alcohol use, and sympathomimetic drugs such as cocaine.[12–15]

An aneurysm is an outpouching of the wall of a blood vessel that results from weakening of the wall of the vessel (Table 17.2).[13] Most aneurysms are congenital—the cause of which is unknown. Other causes include traumatic injury (that stretches and tears the muscular middle layer of the arterial vessel), infectious material (most often from infectious vegetation on valves of the left side of the heart after bacterial endocarditis) that lodges against a vessel wall and erodes the muscular layer, atherosclerosis, radiation, neoplasms, and connective tissue disorders.[16] The overall prevalence of cerebral aneurysm ranges from 0.5% to 6.0% depending on the patient population.[12] SAH is associated with a 30-day mortality rate of 45%, with 25% of the patients dying within 24 hours of the insult.[12]

AVM rupture is responsible for approximately 6% of all SAHs.[16] An AVM is a tangled mass of arterial and venous blood vessels that shunt blood directly from the arterial side into the venous side, bypassing the capillary system. AVMs may be small, focal lesions or large, diffuse lesions that occupy almost an entire hemisphere. They are always congenital, although the exact embryonic cause for these malformations is unknown. They also occur in the spinal cord and the

TABLE 17.2 Classification of Aneurysms.	
Types of Aneurysms	**Characteristics**
Berry or saccular	Most common type, usually congenital; appears at a bifurcation in anterior circulation, primarily at the base of the brain or circle of Willis and its branches; grows from the base of the arterial wall with a neck or stem; contains blood; thinned dome is usually the site of rupture
Giant or fusiform	Can have an irregular shape and be >2.5 cm and atherosclerotic; involves mainly the internal carotid or vertebrobasilar artery; rarely ruptures; has no stem; may act like a space-occupying lesion in the brain; difficult to manage
Mycotic	Rare form; usually occurs from septic emboli, usually results from bacterial infection, which weakens the vessel wall, causing dilation involving distal branches of the middle cerebral arteries
Dissecting	May occur during angiography; caused by trauma, syphilis, arteriosclerosis, or when blood is forced between layers of the arterial wall; intima is pulled away from the medial layer, allowing blood to enter
Traumatic	Sometimes called a *pseudoaneurysm*, which may resolve after trauma
Charcot-Bouchard	Small aneurysm that can be seen in the area of the basal ganglia or brainstem in individuals with a history of hypertension; chronic hypertension causes fibrinoid necrosis in the penetrating and subcortical arteries, weakening arterial walls and causing formation of small aneurysmal outpouching

renal, gastrointestinal, and integumentary systems.[16] Small, superficial AVMs are seen as port-wine stains of the skin. In contrast to SAH from an aneurysm in middle-aged patients, SAH from an AVM usually occurs in the second to fourth decades of life.[16,17] Hemorrhage from AVM rupture has a better chance of survival and is associated with an overall mortality rate of 10% to 15%.[17]

Pathophysiology

The pathophysiologies of the two most common causes of SAH, cerebral aneurysm and AVM, are distinctly different.

Cerebral aneurysm. As an individual with a congenital cerebral aneurysm gets older, blood pressure increases, and more stress is placed on the poorly developed thin vessel wall. Ballooning of the vessel occurs, giving the aneurysm a berrylike appearance. Most cerebral aneurysms are saccular or berrylike, with a stem or neck. Aneurysms are usually small, are 2 to 7 mm in diameter, and often occur at the base of the brain on the circle of Willis.[12] Fig. 17.1 illustrates the usual distribution between the vessels. Most cerebral aneurysms occur at the bifurcation of blood vessels.[12]

The aneurysm becomes clinically significant when the vessel wall becomes so thin that it ruptures, sending arterial blood at a high pressure into the subarachnoid space. For a moment after the aneurysm ruptures, ICP is thought to approach mean arterial pressure, and cerebral perfusion decreases.[16] In other situations, the unruptured aneurysm expands and places pressure on surrounding structures. This is particularly true with posterior communicating artery aneurysms, because they put pressure on the oculomotor nerve (cranial nerve III), causing ipsilateral pupil dilation and ptosis.[16]

Arteriovenous malformation. The pathophysiologic features of an AVM are related to the size and location of the malformation. One or more cerebral arteries, also known as *feeders*, supply an AVM. These

feeder arteries tend to enlarge over time and increase the volume of blood shunted through the malformation and increase the overall mass effect. Large, dilated, tortuous draining veins develop as a result of increasing arterial blood flow being delivered at a higher than normal pressure. Normal vascular flow has a mean arterial pressure of 70 to 80 mm Hg, a mean arteriole pressure of 35 to 45 mm Hg, and a mean capillary pressure that decreases from 35 to 10 mm Hg as it connects with the venous side. Lack of this capillary bridge allows blood with a mean pressure of 35 to 45 mm Hg to flow into the venous system. In contrast to arteries, veins have no muscular layer and become extremely engorged and rupture easily. Some patients with AVMs also have cerebral atrophy, which is the result of chronic ischemia secondary to the shunting of blood through the AVM and away from normal cerebral circulation.[16]

Assessment and Diagnosis

A patient with a SAH characteristically has an abrupt onset of pain, described as the "worst headache of my life." A brief loss of consciousness, nausea, vomiting, focal neurologic deficits, photophobia, and a stiff neck may accompany the headache.[12–15] The SAH may result in coma or death.

The patient's history may reveal one or more incidences of sudden onset of headache with vomiting in the weeks preceding a major SAH. These are small "warning leaks" of an aneurysm in which small amounts of blood ooze from the aneurysm into the subarachnoid space. The presence of blood is an irritant to the meninges, particularly the arachnoid membrane, and the irritation causes headache, stiff neck, and photophobia. These warning leaks seldom are detected because the condition is not severe enough for the patient to seek medical attention. If a neurologic deficit such as third cranial nerve palsy develops before aneurysm rupture, medical intervention is sought, and the aneurysm may be surgically secured before the devastation of a rupture can occur. Symptoms of unruptured AVM, such as headaches with dizziness or syncope or fleeting neurologic deficits, also may be found in the history.[12–14]

Diagnosis of SAH is based on clinical presentation, CT findings, and lumbar puncture results. Noncontrast CT is the cornerstone of definitive SAH diagnosis.[18] In 93% of the cases, CT demonstrates blood in the subarachnoid space if performed within the first hours of the hemorrhage.[19] On the basis of the appearance and the location of the SAH, diagnosis of the cause—aneurysm or AVM—may be made from the CT scan. MRI is not routinely used, but it may provide greater sensitivity for detecting the areas of SAH clot and the potential location of the bleed.[19]

If the initial CT finding is negative, a lumbar puncture is performed to obtain cerebrospinal fluid (CSF) for analysis. CSF after SAH appears bloody and has a red blood cell count greater than 1000 cells/mm³. If the lumbar puncture is performed more than 12 hours after the SAH, the CSF fluid may appear xanthochromic (dark amber) because the blood products have started to break down.[19] Cloudy CSF usually indicates some type of infectious process, such as bacterial meningitis, not SAH.[16]

After the SAH has been documented, cerebral digital subtraction angiography or CT angiography is necessary to identify the exact cause of the hemorrhage.[19] If a cerebral aneurysm rupture is the cause, angiography is essential for identifying the exact location of the aneurysm in preparation for surgery. After the aneurysm has been located, it is graded using the Hunt and Hess classification scale.[20] This scale categorizes the patient on the basis of the severity of the neurologic deficits associated with the hemorrhage (Box 17.3).[13–15] If AVM rupture is the cause, angiography is necessary to identify the feeding arteries and draining veins of the malformation.[16]

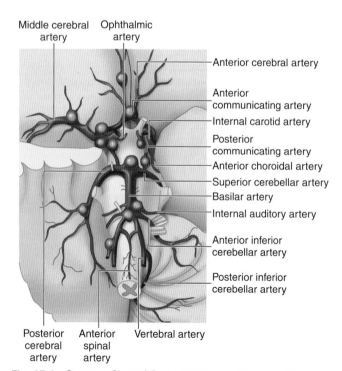

Fig. 17.1 Common Sites of Berry Aneurysms. The size of the aneurysm in the drawing is proportional to the frequency of occurrence at the various sites. (From Goldman L, Schafer AI, eds. *Goldman-Cecil Medicine*. 26th ed. Philadelphia: Elsevier; 2020.)

BOX 17.3 Hunt and Hess Classification of Subarachnoid Hemorrhage

- *Grade I:* Asymptomatic or minimal headache and slight nuchal rigidity
- *Grade II:* Moderate to severe headache, nuchal rigidity, but no neurologic deficit other than cranial nerve palsy
- *Grade III:* Drowsiness, confusion, or mild focal deficit
- *Grade IV:* Stupor, moderate to severe hemiparesis, possible early decerebrate rigidity, and vegetative disturbances
- *Grade V:* Deep coma, decerebrate rigidity, moribund appearance

From Hunt WE, Hess RM. Surgical risks as related to time of intervention in the repair of intracranial aneurysms. *J Neurosurg.* 1968;28:14–20.

Medical Management

SAH is a medical emergency, and time is of the essence. Preservation of neurologic function is the goal, and early diagnosis is crucial. Initial treatment must always support vital functions. Airway management and ventilatory assistance may be necessary.[13] If intubation is required, rapid-sequence induction is recommended using a combination of rocuronium, fentanyl, and propofol.[15] A ventriculostomy may be performed to control ICP if the patient's LOC is depressed.[13,21] After initial intervention has provided the necessary support for vital physiologic functions, medical management of acute SAH is aimed primarily at prevention and treatment of the complications of SAH, which may produce further neurologic damage and death.

Rebleeding. After initial stabilization, the focus of medical management is directed toward the prevention of rebleeding. Rebleeding is the occurrence of a second SAH in an unsecured aneurysm or, less commonly, an AVM. The majority of rebleeding episodes occurs during the first 6 hours after the first bleed. The mortality rate associated with rebleeding is approximately 20% to 60%.[19]

Historically, conservative measures to prevent rebleeding have included blood pressure control and SAH precautions (see Nursing Management). An elevation in blood pressure is a normal compensatory response to maintain adequate cerebral perfusion after a neurologic insult. In the belief that hypertension contributes to rebleeding, continuous intravenous antihypertensive medications, such as nicardipine, clevidipine, or labetalol, are used to maintain a systolic blood pressure less than 160 mm Hg.[13,18,19] Evidence suggests that rebleeding has more to do with variations or fluctuations in blood pressure than it does with maintaining blood pressure below an absolute value.[19] This is why the administration of continuous intravenous antihypertensive medications is preferred over intermittent administration of antihypertensive medications. Individualized guidelines must be determined based on the clinical condition and preexisting blood pressure values of the patient.[19] It is important that the patient's blood pressure is not kept too low, because this increases the risk for a cerebral infarction.[15] Antifibrinolytic medications may also be administered on a short-term basis (less than 72 hours) to prevent rebleeding.[13,19]

Definitive management of a ruptured cerebral aneurysm or AVM should be performed as early as possible. Early intervention eliminates the risk of rebleeding and allows more aggressive therapy to be used in the postoperative period for the treatment of vasospasm.[18] The two primary approaches used for treating a ruptured cerebral aneurysm are endovascular coiling and surgical clipping.[12,14] The two primary approaches used for treating a ruptured AVM are surgical resection and embolization.[17]

Endovascular coiling of aneurysms. Endovascular coiling involves placement of one or more detachable coils into an aneurysm to produce an endovascular thrombus (Fig. 17.2). This method is preferred over surgical clipping.[12] There are several different methods available. A microcatheter is inserted into the femoral artery and is advanced into the affected cerebral artery. Once the microcatheter is in place at the base of the aneurysm, tiny platinum coils are threaded through a microcatheter and pushed into the aneurysm, where they conform to the shape of the aneurysm. Once the aneurysm is filled in with coils, blood flow into the aneurysm is obstructed and a thrombus forms, occluding the aneurysm and preventing future bleeding. Recovery is usually shorter and easier.[22]

Surgical clipping of aneurysms. If endovascular coiling is not available or the aneurysm is not appropriate for coiling, then surgical clipping is necessary. The surgical procedure involves a craniotomy to expose and isolate the area of aneurysm. A clip is placed over the neck of the aneurysm to eliminate the area of weakness (Fig. 17.3).[16] This is a technically difficult procedure that requires the skill of an experienced neurosurgeon. It is not uncommon, particularly in early surgery, for the clot to break away from the aneurysm as it is surgically exposed. Extensive hemorrhage into the craniotomy site results, and cessation of the hemorrhage often causes increased neurologic deficits. Deficits also may occur as a result of surgical manipulation to gain access to the site of the aneurysm. Early surgery allows the neurosurgeon to flush out the excess blood and clots from the basal cisterns (reservoir of CSF around the base of the brain and circle of Willis) to reduce the risk of vasospasm. Careful consideration of the patient's clinical situation is necessary in determining the optimal time for surgery.

Surgical resection of arteriovenous malformations. Management of AVM has traditionally involved surgical excision or conservative management of symptoms such as seizures and headache. The decision for surgical excision depends on the location and size of the AVM. Some malformations are located so deep in the cerebral structures (thalamus or midbrain) that attempts to remove the AVM would cause severe neurologic deficits. History of a previous hemorrhage and the patient's age and overall condition are also considered when making the decision regarding surgical intervention.[17]

Surgical excision of large AVMs includes the risk of reperfusion bleeding. As feeding arteries of the AVM are clamped off, the arterial blood that usually flowed into the AVM is diverted into the surrounding circulation. In many cases, the surrounding tissue has been in a state of chronic ischemia, and the arterial vessels feeding these areas are maximally dilated. As arterial blood begins to flow at a higher volume and pressure into these dilated arteries, blood may seep from the vessels. Evidence of reperfusion bleeding in the operating room is an indication that no more arterial blood can be diverted from the AVM without risk of serious ICH. In the postoperative phase, low blood pressure is maintained to prevent further reperfusion bleeding. For large AVMs, two to four stages of surgery may be required over 6 to 12 months.[17]

Embolization of arteriovenous malformations. Embolization is used to secure an AVM that is surgically inaccessible because of size, location, or medical instability of the patient. Although there are a variety of interventional neuroradiology techniques used for embolization, all techniques use a percutaneous transfemoral approach in a manner like angiography. Under fluoroscopy, the catheter is threaded up to the internal carotid artery. Specially developed microcatheters are then manipulated into the area of the vascular anomaly, and embolic materials are placed endovascularly. Three embolization techniques are used, depending on the underlying pathologic derangement.[23]

The first type of embolization is used for an AVM. Small polymeric silicone (Silastic) beads or glue is slowly introduced into the vessels

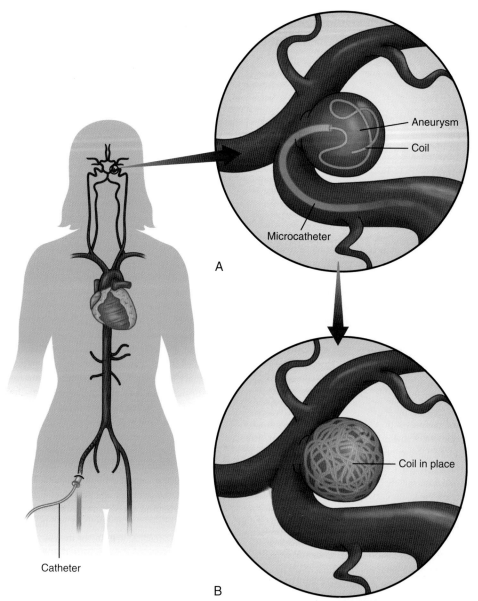

A

B

Fig. 17.2 Endovascular Occlusion of a Posterior Communicating Artery Aneurysm. (A) Insertion of the microcatheter into the aneurysm through the right femoral artery, aorta, and left carotid artery. (B) Occlusion of the aneurysm with coils.

feeding the AVM. Blood flow carries the material to the site, and embolization is achieved. This procedure may be used in combination with surgery. One to three sessions of embolization of the feeding vessels are performed to reduce the size of the lesion before a craniotomy is performed for total excision. The primary risk of this procedure is lodging of the embolic substance in a vessel that feeds normal tissue, which creates an embolic stroke with the immediate onset of neurologic symptoms.[23]

Delayed cerebral ischemia. Delayed cerebral ischemia (DCI) is a disabling complication of SAH that occurs in up to 30% of patients within 2 weeks after the hemorrhage that is not associated with the initial bleed or other complications. It presents as a new focal neurologic impairment or deterioration in LOC lasting for more than 1 hour and is associated with poor clinical outcomes. DCI is thought to occur as a result of arterial vasospasm, microthrombosis, inflammation, microcirculation dysfunction, and cortical ischemia.[24,25]

The presence or absence of cerebral vasospasm significantly affects the outcome of aneurysmal SAH. This complication does not occur with SAH resulting from AVM rupture. Cerebral vasospasm is a narrowing of the lumen of the cerebral arteries, possibly in response to subarachnoid blood clots coating the outer surface of the blood vessels. Because aneurysms usually occur at the circle of Willis, the major vessels responsible for feeding the cerebral circulation are affected by vasospasm. Depending on the arterial vessels involved in the vasospasm reaction, decreased arterial flow occurs in large areas of the cerebral hemispheres.[26] The onset of vasospasm is usually 3 to 10 days after the initial hemorrhage.[25] The three recommended treatments for the management of vasospasm are normovolemic-induced hypertension, oral nimodipine, and transluminal cerebral angioplasty.

Normovolemic-induced hypertension. Normovolemic-induced hypertension therapy involves increasing the patient's blood pressure and cardiac output with vasoactive medications. The increase in pressure

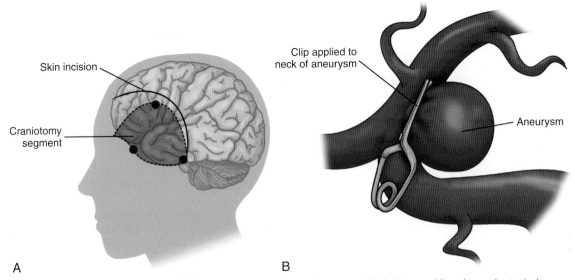

Fig. 17.3 Clipping of a Posterior Communicating Artery Aneurysm. (A) *Solid curved line* shows the typical skin incision, and *dashed lines* show the craniotomy location. (B) Application of the clip to the aneurysm.

forces blood through the vasospastic area at higher pressures. The first step is to ensure that the patient is not hypovolemic, normal saline should be administered to maintain euvolemia. Next, intravenous norepinephrine, dopamine, or phenylephrine is administered to augment the patient's blood pressure as needed. Blood pressure is raised slowly, based on the patient's clinical response, up to a maximum systolic target of 220 mm Hg or mean arterial target of 140 mm Hg. Once the desired response is achieved, the therapy is continued for 24 to 48 hours.[24,25]

The obvious deterrent to the use of normovolemic-induced hypertension is the risk of rebleeding in an unsecured aneurysm. Surgical clipping or endovascular coiling of the aneurysm before starting the therapy is preferred. Cerebral edema, elevated ICP, heart failure, and electrolyte imbalance are also risks of hemodynamic augmentation therapy. Careful monitoring of the patient's neurologic status, hemodynamic parameters, ICP, and serum electrolytes is necessary.[26]

Nimodipine. Nimodipine is strongly recommended to reduce the poor outcomes associated with vasospasm. The exact nature of the effect of nimodipine is unclear, but the use of the medication has demonstrated consistently positive effects on outcome without any demonstrable effect on the incidence or severity of vasospasm.[18,25] A dose of 60 mg of nimodipine is given orally every 4 hours for 21 days. Nimodipine may produce hypotension, especially when administered concurrently with other antihypertensive agents.[25]

Cerebral angioplasty. Cerebral angioplasty is used when pharmacologic management of cerebral vasospasm has failed. It is performed only when CT or MRI provides evidence that infarction has not occurred. An interventional neuroradiologist performs the procedure, and the patient is placed under procedural sedation. The technique of cerebral angioplasty is very similar to the technique used in the coronary vasculature. Risks include intimal perforation or rupture; cerebral artery thrombosis or embolism; recurrence of stenosis; and severe, diffuse vasospasm unresponsive to therapy. Hemorrhage at the femoral site also may occur. This procedure is recommended when conventional therapy is unsuccessful.[18,25]

Hyponatremia. Hyponatremia develops in up to 50% of patients with SAH as a result of central salt-wasting syndrome of inappropriate

secretion of antidiuretic hormone (SIADH). It usually occurs during the same period as vasospasm, several days after the initial hemorrhage.[19] Sodium is replenished with isotonic fluids in patients with SAH; the use of fluid restriction to treat hyponatremia is associated with a poor outcome.[12,25]

Hydrocephalus. Hydrocephalus is a complication that occurs in approximately 30% of patients after SAH,[12] with 20% of patients developing acute symptomatic hydrocephalus within days after the initial event.[19] Blood that has circulated in the subarachnoid space and has been absorbed by the arachnoid villi may obstruct the villi and reduce the rate of CSF absorption. Over time, increasing volumes of CSF in the intracranial space produce communicating hydrocephalus and increased ICP. In 30% of patients, hydrocephalus will resolve spontaneously. Treatment consists of placing a drain to remove CSF. This can be accomplished by inserting an external ventricular drain or a lumbar drain.[15,19]

Intracerebral Hemorrhage
Description and Etiology

ICH is bleeding directly into cerebral tissue.[27] ICH destroys cerebral tissue, causes cerebral edema, and increases ICP. The source of intracerebral bleeding is usually a small artery, but it also can occur secondary to rupture of an AVM or aneurysm, a brain tumor, or cerebral infarct.[27] The most common cause of spontaneous ICH is chronic hypertension,[27,28] and this section concentrates on spontaneous hypertensive ICH.

Spontaneous ICH accounts for at least 15% of all strokes.[27,28] The likelihood of death or disability is higher with ICH than with ischemic stroke or SAH. The mortality rate for hemorrhagic stroke is 50% within 1 month. Only 20% of patients with ICH return to a functional life at 6 months.[29] The key risk factors for ICH are age and hypertension.[27,28]

ICH is most often caused by rupture of a cerebral vessel resulting from a long-standing history of hypertension.[27] Risk factors include cigarette smoking, anticoagulation or fibrinolytic therapy, coagulation disorders, drug and alcohol abuse, diabetes, chronic kidney disease, and older age.[27,30] Often, on questioning, a patient with a hypertensive hemorrhage admits to having discontinued antihypertensive medication 2 to 3 weeks before the hemorrhage. Cerebral amyloid angiopathy is a major cause in older adults.[28]

Pathophysiology

The pathophysiology of ICH is caused by continued elevated blood pressure exerting force against smaller arterial vessels that have become damaged from arteriosclerotic changes. Eventually, these arteries break, and blood bursts from the vessels into the surrounding cerebral tissue, creating a hematoma. ICP rises precipitously in response to the increase in overall intracranial volume.[30]

Assessment and Diagnosis

Initial assessment usually reveals a critically ill patient who often is unconscious and requires ventilatory support. History from a relative or significant other describes a sudden onset of focal deficit often accompanied by severe headache, nausea, vomiting, and rapid neurologic deterioration. Signs and symptoms vary depending on the location of the ICH.[30] Approximately 50% of patients sustain early loss of consciousness, a key feature that differentiates ICH from ischemic stroke. More than one-half of patients with ICH present with a smooth progression of neurologic symptoms, an uncommon finding in cases of ischemic stroke or SAH.[31] One-third of patients have maximal symptoms at onset. Assessment of vital signs usually reveals a severely elevated blood pressure (200/100–250/150 mm Hg). Signs of increased ICP are often present by the time the patient arrives in the emergency department. Diagnosis is established easily with CT. Angiography is recommended only in patients considered surgical candidates and if a clear cause of hemorrhage is not evident.[29–31]

Medical Management

ICH is a medical emergency. Initial management requires attention to airway, breathing, and circulation. Intubation is usually necessary. Anticoagulant medications should be reversed, and coagulopathies should be corrected. Blood pressure management must be based on individual factors. Reduction in blood pressure is usually necessary to decrease ongoing bleeding, but lowering blood pressure too much or too rapidly may compromise cerebral perfusion pressure (CPP), especially in a patient with elevated ICP. National guidelines recommend that in patients presenting with systolic blood pressure between 150 mm Hg and 220 mm Hg, lowering the systolic blood pressure to 140 mm Hg is safe and can be effective for improving functional outcomes.[31]

Increased ICP is common with ICH and is a major contributor to mortality. Recommended management includes mannitol, when indicated; hyperventilation; and neuromuscular blockade with sedation. Steroids are avoided. CPP must be maintained at greater than 70 mm Hg.[29]

The goal for fluid management is euvolemia. Body temperature is maintained at less than 38.5°C by using acetaminophen or cooling blankets. Euglycemia, a blood glucose level less than 140 mg/dL, is maintained by using insulin therapy, but hypoglycemia should be avoided. Use of short-acting benzodiazepines or propofol is recommended to treat agitation or hyperactivity. Pneumatic compression devices are used to decrease the risk of pulmonary embolism. Prophylactic anticonvulsant therapy is sometimes used.[27,31]

The benefit of surgical treatment for spontaneous ICH is unclear. Recommendations for surgical removal of the clot depend on the size and location of the hematoma, the patient's ICP, and other neurologic symptoms.[31] Medical treatment is recommended if the hemorrhage is small (less than 10 cm) or neurologic deficit is minimal.[31] Likewise, surgery offers no improvement in outcome for patients with a Glasgow Coma Scale (GCS) score of 4 or less. Surgical evacuation of the clot is recommended for patients with cerebellar hemorrhage greater than 3 cm with neurologic deterioration or hydrocephalus with brainstem compression and for young patients with moderate or large lobar hemorrhage with clinical deterioration.[31] Numerous techniques are being investigated to lessen the risk of brain damage associated with craniotomy for ICH.

Interprofessional collaborative management of a patient with ICH is outlined in Box 17.4.

BOX 17.4   Evidence-Based Practice   QSEN

Spontaneous Intracerebral Hemorrhage Management Guidelines

The following are class 1 recommendations from the American Heart Association and American Stroke Association. Class 1 recommendations are conditions for which evidence and general agreement exist that the procedure or treatment is useful and effective:

- A baseline severity score should be performed as part of the initial evaluation of patients with ICH.
- Rapid neuroimaging with CT or MRI is recommended to distinguish ischemic stroke from ICH.
- Patients with a severe coagulation factor deficiency or severe thrombocytopenia should receive appropriate factor replacement therapy or platelets, respectively.
- Patients with ICH whose INR is elevated because of VKA should have their VKA withheld, should receive therapy to replace vitamin K–dependent factors and correct the INR, and should receive IV vitamin K.
- Patients with ICH should receive intermittent pneumatic compression for prevention of venous thromboembolism beginning the day of hospital admission.
- Initial monitoring and management of patients with ICH should take place in a critical care unit or a dedicated stroke unit with physician and nursing neuroscience acute care expertise.
- Blood glucose levels should be monitored, and hyperglycemia and hypoglycemia should be avoided.
- Patients with clinical seizures should be treated with antiseizure medications.
- Patients with a change in mental status who are found to have electrographic seizures on EEG should be treated with antiseizure medications.
- A formal screening procedure for dysphagia should be performed in patients before the initiation of oral intake to reduce risk of pneumonia.
- Given the potentially serious nature and complex pattern of evolving disability and the increasing evidence for efficacy, it is recommended that all patients with ICH have access to multidisciplinary rehabilitation.
- Patients with cerebellar hemorrhage who are deteriorating neurologically or who have brainstem compression, hydrocephalus, or both from ventricular obstruction should undergo surgical removal of the hemorrhage as soon as possible.

CT, Computed tomography; *EEG,* electroencephalography; *ICH,* intracerebral hemorrhage; *INR,* international normalized ratio; *IV,* intravenous; *MRI,* magnetic resonance imaging; *VKA,* vitamin K antagonists.

Modified from Hemphill JC 3rd, Greenberg SM, Anderson CS, et al. Guidelines for the management of spontaneous intracerebral hemorrhage: a guideline for healthcare professionals from the American Heart Association/American Stroke Association. *Stroke.* 2015;46(7): 2032–2060.

Nursing Management

The patient care management plan for a patient with stroke incorporates a variety of problems (Box 17.5). Nursing priorities focus on (1) monitoring for changes in neurologic and hemodynamic status, (2) maintaining surveillance for complications, (3) providing comfort and emotional support, and (4) educating the patient and family.

Monitoring for Changes in Neurologic and Hemodynamic Status

The goal of frequent assessments is early recognition of neurologic or hemodynamic deterioration. Close monitoring of the patient's neurologic signs and vital signs is essential and requires almost continuous observation. Automatic noninvasive devices such as a blood pressure cuff and a pulse oximeter are helpful. Seizure activity must be identified and treated immediately. It is essential that all personnel working with the patient be aware of the desired hemodynamic and neurologic parameters set by the physician and that the physician be notified at the first sign of any changes.[31,32]

Maintaining Surveillance for Complications

A patient with stroke should be monitored closely for signs of bleeding, vasospasm, and increased ICP. Other complications of stroke include aspiration, malnutrition, pneumonia, DVT, pulmonary embolism, pressure injuries, contractures, and joint abnormalities.[16,32] Nursing measures to prevent these complications are well known.

Additional complications that may be seen in a patient with stroke are related to the area of the brain that has been damaged. Damage to the temporoparietal area can create various disturbances that affect the patient's ability to interpret sensory information. Damage to the dominant hemisphere (usually left) produces problems with speech and language and abstract and analytic skills. Damage to the nondominant hemisphere (usually right) produces problems with spatial relationships. The resulting deficits include agnosia, apraxia, and visual field defects. Perceptual deficits are not as readily noticeable as motor deficits, but they may be more debilitating and may lead to inability to perform skilled or purposeful tasks.[33] The patient also may experience impaired swallowing.[7,8]

Bleeding and vasospasm. In a patient with a cerebral aneurysm, sudden onset of, or an increase in, headache and nausea and vomiting, increased blood pressure, and changes in respiration herald the onset of rebleeding. The first indication of vasospasm is usually the appearance of new focal or global neurologic deficits.[13,14]

SAH precautions must be implemented to prevent any stress or straining that could potentially precipitate rebleeding. Precautions include blood pressure control; bed rest; a dark, quiet environment; and stool softeners. Short-acting analgesics and sedatives are used to relieve pain and anxiety. The patient must be kept calm. Limb restraints cause straining and must be avoided. The head of the bed should always be elevated to 35 to 45 degrees. The patient is taught to avoid any activities that correspond to performance of the Valsalva maneuver, such as pushing with the legs to move up in bed, straining for a bowel movement, or holding his or her breath during procedures or discomfort. DVT precautions are routinely implemented. Caregivers collaborate with the patient and family to establish a visitation plan to meet patient and family needs. Often, family members at the bedside can assist the patient to remain calm.

Increased intracranial pressure. Numerous signs and symptoms of increased ICP can be observed. A change in the LOC is the most sensitive indicator. Others include unequal pupil size, decreased pupillary response to light, headache, projectile vomiting, altered breathing patterns, Cushing triad (bradycardia, systolic hypertension, and bradypnea), diminished brainstem reflexes, papilledema, and abnormal extension (decerebrate posturing) or flexion (decorticate posturing).

Impaired swallowing. Normal swallowing occurs in four phases that are controlled by the cranial nerves. Damage to the brain, brainstem, or cranial nerves may result in various swallowing deficits that could place the patient at risk for aspiration. A patient with stroke is observed for signs of dysphagia, including drooling; difficulty handling oral secretions; absence of gag, cough, or swallowing reflexes; moist, gurgling voice quality; decreased mouth and tongue movements; and the presence of dysarthria. A speech therapy consultation is initiated if any of these signs are present, and the patient must not be orally fed. In the absence of these warning signs, the patient may be fed, as ordered by the physician, although he or she must be continually monitored for signs of aspiration.[31,32]

Educating the Patient and Family

Rehabilitation starts in the critical care area, with a multidisciplinary team designing and implementing an individualized plan for maximizing the patient's potential for neurologic rehabilitation. Early in the patient's hospital stay, the patient and family must be taught about

---

◎ BOX 17.5 PRIORITY PATIENT CARE MANAGEMENT

Stroke

- Ineffective Tissue Perfusion due to decreased cerebral blood flow
- Unilateral Neglect due to perceptual disruption
- Impaired Verbal Communication due to cerebral speech center injury
- Impaired Swallowing due to neuromuscular impairment, fatigue, and limited awareness
- Disturbed Body Image due to actual change in body structure, function, or appearance
- Lack of Knowledge of Treatment Regime due to lack of previous exposure to information (see Box 17.6, Priority Patient and Family Education for Stroke)

Patient Care Management plans are located in Appendix A.

❋ BOX 17.6 PRIORITY PATIENT AND FAMILY EDUCATION

Stroke

Before discharge, the patient should be able to teach back the following topics:

- Pathophysiology of disease
- Specific cause
- Risk factor modification
- Importance of taking medications
- Activities of daily living
- Measures to prevent injuries of impaired limbs
- Measures to compensate for residual deficits
- Basic rehabilitation techniques
- Importance of participating in neurologic rehabilitation program or support group

Additional information for the patient can be found at the American Stroke Association website (www.stroke.org).

stroke, its causes, and its treatment (Box 17.6). Closer to discharge, teaching focuses on the interventions necessary for preventing the recurrence of the event and on maximizing the patient's rehabilitation potential. The patient's family must be encouraged to participate in the patient's care; learn how to feed, dress, and bathe the patient; and learn some basic rehabilitation techniques. The importance of participating in a neurologic rehabilitation program, support group, or both must be stressed.

Interprofessional collaborative management of a patient with stroke is outlined in Box 17.7.

TRENDING PRIORITIES IN HEALTHCARE

Evidence-Based Hospital Design

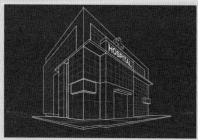

(iStock.com/stock_shoppe.)

Many hospitals are redesigning the health care environment to promote patient safety, enhance the patient experience, increase health care personnel satisfaction, and adhere to current federal, state, and local regulations.[1] To accomplish these goals, hospital architects and designers are using evidence to provide recommendations that have shown to be successful in meeting these goals. The overall objective is to transform the built environment to improve the quality of health care.[2]

Two current recommendations for remodeling a patient room are implementing single patient private rooms and designing same-handed rooms.[1] Same-handed rooms use a strategy that standardizes everything in the room so that all the units' rooms are identical. The following are some evidence-based recommendations for redesigning a patient room[3]:

- Use a barn-style door rather than a swing door.
- Position the door so the patient's head can be viewed from the entryway.
- Position patient monitors so they can be viewed from the entryway.
- Place the staff sink inside the room, next to the door.
- Place hand sanitizer dispensers near the entryway in view of the patient.
- Place personal protective equipment near the entryway.
- Allocate space for waste containers near the door.
- Allocate space for medical equipment storage within the room.

- Place lighting controls near the room entryway.
- Locate patient bed so the patient can:
  - See out of the window
  - View the entryway
  - Communicate with visitors in the family area
  - View the television comfortably
  - View the whiteboard.
- Provide space near the bed for a patient recliner and the IV pole.
- Provide a privacy barrier(s) that allows patient privacy from the hallway and the family seating area.
- Position the clock so it is visible to the patient and the staff.
- Provide night lighting in the patient room and bathroom.
- Provide a cord support system to keep all cords off the floor.
- Provide the patient control of the:
  - Lightening
  - Environment controls
  - Window coverings.

This is not an all-inclusive list, and as more rooms are designed, more evidence is being collected for what works and what does not. Evidence-based health care design is an ever-evolving field.

For more information about evidence-based health care design, check out The Center for Health Design (www.healthdesign.org).

References

1. Brambilla A, Rebecchi A, Capolongo S. Evidence based hospital design. a literature review of the recent publications about the EBD impact of built environment on hospital occupants' and organizational outcomes. *Ann Ig.* 2019;31(2):165–180.
2. The Center for Health Design. *Resources from the Center for Health Design;* 2020. www.healthdesign.org/sites/default/files/FINAL-WEB-CHD482_2019_ResourceGuide_v2.pdf.
3. Lavender SA, Sommerich CM, Sanders EB, et al. Developing evidence-based design guidelines for medical/surgical hospital patient rooms that meet the needs of staff, patients, and visitors. *HERD.* 2020;13(1):145–178.

BOX 17.7 Collaborative Management of Stroke

- Distinguish the cause of the stroke:
  - Ischemic
  - Subarachnoid hemorrhage
  - Cerebral aneurysm
  - Arteriovenous malformation
  - Intracerebral bleed
- Implement treatment according to cause of bleed:
  - Ischemic
  - Fibrinolytic therapy
  - Blood pressure control
  - Subarachnoid hemorrhage
  - Surgical aneurysm clipping or arteriovenous malformation (AVM) excision
  - Embolization
  - Intracerebral bleed
  - Blood pressure control

- Protect patient's airway.
- Provide ventilatory assistance, as required.
- Perform frequent neurologic assessments.
- Maintain surveillance for complications:
  - Cerebral edema and intracranial hypertension
  - Cerebral vasospasm and ischemia
  - Rebleeding
  - Impaired swallowing
  - Neurologic deficits
  - Hyponatremia
  - Hydrocephalus
- Provide comfort and emotional support.
- Design and implement appropriate rehabilitation program.
- Educate patient and family.

COMA

Description and Etiology

Normal consciousness requires awareness and arousal. Awareness is the combination of cognition (mental and intellectual) and affect (mood) that can be construed based on the patient's interaction with the environment. Alterations of consciousness may be the result of deficits in awareness, arousal, or both. The four discrete disorders of consciousness are (1) coma, (2) vegetative state, (3) minimally conscious state, and (4) locked-in syndrome. Coma is characterized by the absence of both wakefulness and awareness, whereas a *vegetative state* is characterized by the presence of wakefulness with the absence of awareness. In a *minimally conscious state*, wakefulness is present, and awareness is severely diminished but not absent. *Locked-in syndrome* is characterized by the presence of wakefulness and awareness, but with quadriplegia and the inability to communicate verbally; thus the patient appears to be unconscious.[34] Box 17.8 lists the disorders of consciousness in descending order of wakefulness.

Coma is the deepest state of unconsciousness; arousal and awareness are lacking.[34,35] The patient cannot be aroused and does not demonstrate any purposeful response to the surrounding environment.[35] Coma is a symptom rather than a disease, and it occurs as a result of some underlying process.[35] The incidence of coma is difficult to ascertain because a wide variety of conditions can induce coma.[35] This state of unconsciousness is commonly encountered in the critical care unit, and it is the focus of the following discussion.

The causes of coma can be divided into two general categories: structural or surgical and metabolic or medical. Structural causes of coma include ischemic stroke, ICH, trauma, and brain tumors.[35] Metabolic causes of coma include drug overdose, infectious diseases, endocrine disorders, and poisonings.[35] The three most common causes of nontraumatic coma are stroke, anoxia, and poisonings.[35] Coma demands immediate attention, resulting in a high percentage of admissions to all hospital services.[36] Box 17.9 lists the possible causes of coma.

BOX 17.9 Causes of Coma

Structural or Surgical Coma	Metabolic or Medical Coma
• Trauma	• Infection
• Epidural hematoma	• Meningitis
• Subdural hematoma	• Encephalitis
• Diffuse axonal injury	• Metabolic encephalopathy
• Brain contusion	• Metabolic conditions
• Intracerebral hemorrhage	• Hypoglycemia
• Subarachnoid hemorrhage	• Hyperglycemia
• Posterior fossa hemorrhage	• Hyperosmolar states
• Supratentorial hemorrhage	• Uremia
• Hydrocephalus	• Hepatic encephalopathy
• Ischemic stroke	• Hypertensive encephalopathy
• Tumor	• Hypoxic encephalopathy
• Other causes	• Hyponatremia
	• Hypercalcemia
	• Myxedema
	• Intoxication
	• Opioid overdose
	• Alcohol
	• Poisonings
	• Psychogenic causes

Pathophysiology

Consciousness involves arousal, or wakefulness, and awareness. Neither of these functions is present in a patient in coma. Ascending fibers of the reticular activating system (RAS) in the pons, hypothalamus, and thalamus maintain arousal as an autonomic function. Neurons in the cerebral cortex are responsible for awareness. Diffuse dysfunction of both cerebral hemispheres and diffuse or focal dysfunction of the RAS can produce coma.[35,37] Structural causes usually produce compression or dysfunction in the area of the ascending RAS, whereas most medical causes lead to general dysfunction of both cerebral hemispheres.[35,37] Trauma, hemorrhage, and tumor can damage the ascending RAS, leading to coma. Destruction of large regions of bilateral cerebral hemispheres can be the result of seizures or viral agents. Toxic drugs, toxins, or metabolic abnormalities can suppress cerebral function.[35,37]

Assessment and Diagnosis

The clinical diagnosis of the comatose state is readily established by assessment of the LOC. However, determining the full nature and cause of coma requires a thorough history and physical examination. A medical history is essential, because events immediately preceding the change in the LOC can often provide valuable clues to the origin of the coma. When limited information is available and the coma is profound, the response of the patient to emergent treatment may provide clues to the underlying diagnosis; for example, a patient who becomes responsive with the administration of naloxone can be presumed to have ingested some type of opiate.[35]

Detailed serial neurologic examinations are essential for all patients in coma. Assessment of pupillary size and reaction to light (normal, sluggish, or fixed), extraocular eye movements (normal, asymmetric, or absent), motor response to pain (normal, decorticate, decerebrate, or flaccid), and breathing pattern yields important clues for determining whether the cause of coma is structural or metabolic.[35]

BOX 17.8 Continuum of Descending States of Consciousness

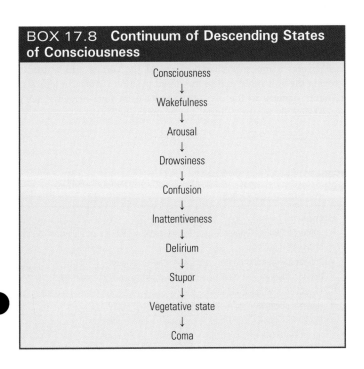

Consciousness
↓
Wakefulness
↓
Arousal
↓
Drowsiness
↓
Confusion
↓
Inattentiveness
↓
Delirium
↓
Stupor
↓
Vegetative state
↓
Coma

The areas of the brainstem that control consciousness and pupillary responses are anatomically adjacent. The sympathetic and parasympathetic nervous systems control pupillary dilation and constriction, respectively. The anatomic directions of these pathways are known, and changes in pupillary responses can help identify where a lesion may be located. For example, if damage occurs in the midbrain region, pupils will be slightly enlarged and unresponsive to light. Lesions that compress the third nerve result in a fixed and dilated pupil on the same side as the neurologic insult. Pupillary responses are usually preserved when the cause of coma is metabolic in origin. Pupillary light responses are often the key to differentiating between structural and metabolic causes of coma.[38]

Areas of the brainstem adjacent to areas responsible for consciousness also control oculomotor eye movement. The ability to maintain conjugate gaze requires preservation of the internuclear connections of cranial nerves III, VI, and VIII via the medial longitudinal fasciculus.[37] As with pupillary responses, structural lesions that impinge on these pathways cause oculomotor dysfunction such as a dysconjugate gaze. Deficits in extraocular eye movements usually accompany a structural cause.[38,39]

Focal or asymmetric motor deficits usually indicate structural lesions.[35] Abnormal motor movements may also help pinpoint the location of a lesion. Decorticate posturing (abnormal flexion) can be seen with damage to the diencephalon. Decerebrate posturing (abnormal extension) can be seen with damage to the midbrain and pons. Flaccid posturing is an ominous sign and can be seen with damage to the medulla.[38]

Abnormal breathing patterns may also assist in differentiating structural from metabolic causes of coma. Cheyne-Stokes respirations are seen in patients with cerebral hemispheric dysfunction or metabolic suppression. Central neurogenic hyperventilation, or Kussmaul breathing, occurs with metabolic acidosis or damage to the midbrain and upper pons. Apneustic breathing may occur with damage to the pons, hypoglycemia, and anoxia. Ataxic breathing occurs with damage to the medulla. Agonal breathing occurs with failure of the respiratory centers in the medulla.[38]

In addition to physical assessment, laboratory studies and diagnostic procedures are done. Structural causes of coma are usually readily apparent with CT or MRI.[35] Laboratory studies are also used to identify metabolic or endocrine abnormalities.[35] An electroencephalogram should be obtained to search for sleep patterns, particularly rapid eye movement sleep and slow-wave sleep. A positron emission tomography scan may also be helpful in detecting consciousness.[40] Occasionally, the cause of coma is never clearly determined.

Medical Management

The goal of medical management of a patient in coma is identification and treatment of the underlying cause of the condition. Initial medical management includes emergency measures to support vital functions and prevent further neurologic deterioration. Protection of the airway and ventilatory assistance are often needed. Administration of thiamine (at least 100 mg), glucose, and an opioid antagonist is suggested when the cause of coma is not immediately known. Thiamine is administered before glucose because Wernicke encephalopathy, the coma produced by thiamine deficiency, can be precipitated by a glucose load.[35]

A patient who remains in coma after emergent treatment requires supportive measures to maintain physiologic body functions and prevent complications. Intubation for continued airway protection and nutrition support is essential. Fluid and electrolyte management is often complex because of alterations in the neurohormonal system.

Anticonvulsant therapy may be necessary to prevent further ischemic damage to the brain.[39]

The health care team and the patient's family make decisions jointly regarding the level of medical management to be provided. Family members require informational support in terms of the probable cause of coma and the prognosis for recovery of consciousness and function. Prognosis depends on the cause of coma and the length of time unconsciousness persists. Only 15% of patients in nontraumatic coma make a satisfactory recovery.[35] Metabolic coma usually has a better prognosis compared with coma caused by a structural lesion, and traumatic coma usually has a better outcome compared with nontraumatic coma.[35] However, regardless of the cause or duration of coma, outcome for an individual cannot be predicted with 100% accuracy.[41]

Nursing Management

The patient care management plan for a patient in coma incorporates a variety of patient problems (Box 17.10) and is directed by the specific cause of coma, although some common interventions are used. The patient in coma totally depends on the health care team. Nursing priorities focus on (1) monitoring for changes in neurologic status and clues to the origin of coma, (2) supporting all body functions, (3) maintaining surveillance for complications, (4) providing comfort and emotional support, and (5) initiating rehabilitation measures. Measures to support body functions include promoting pulmonary hygiene, maintaining skin integrity, initiating range-of-motion exercises, managing bowel and bladder functions, and ensuring adequate nutrition support.

Eye Care

The blink reflex is often diminished or absent in a patient in coma. The eyelids may be flaccid and may depend on body positioning to remain in a closed position, and edema may prevent complete closure. Loss of these protective mechanisms results in drying and ulceration of the cornea, which can lead to permanent scarring and blindness.

Two interventions that are commonly used to protect the eyes are instilling saline or methylcellulose lubricating drops and taping the eyelids in the shut position. Evidence suggests that an alternative technique may be more effective in preventing corneal epithelial breakdown. In addition to instilling saline drops, a polyethylene film is taped over the eyes, extending beyond the orbits and eyebrows. The film creates a moisture chamber around the cornea and assists in keeping the eyes moist and in the closed position. This technique also prevents damage to the eyes that results from tape or gauze being placed directly on the delicate skin of the eyelids.[42]

◎ **BOX 17.10 PRIORITY PATIENT CARE MANAGEMENT**

Coma

- Impaired Airway Clearance due to excessive secretions or abnormal viscosity of mucus
- Impaired Breathing due to decreased lung expansion
- Impaired Nutritional Intake due to lack of exogenous nutrients and increased metabolic demand
- Risk for Aspiration
- Impaired Family Coping due to critically ill family member

Patient Care Management plans are located in Appendix A.

BOX 17.11 Collaborative Management of Coma

- Identify and treat the underlying cause.
- Protect the airway.
- Provide ventilatory assistance, as required.
- Support circulation, as required.
- Initiate nutrition support.
- Provide eye care.
- Protect skin integrity.
- Initiate range-of-motion exercises.
- Maintain surveillance for complications:
  - Infections
  - Metabolic alterations
  - Cardiac dysrhythmias
  - Temperature alterations
- Provide comfort and emotional support.
- Plan for the rehabilitation program.

Interprofessional collaborative management of a patient in coma is outlined in Box 17.11.

INTRACRANIAL HYPERTENSION

Pathophysiology

The intracranial space comprises three components: (1) brain substance (80%), (2) CSF (10%), and (3) blood (10%). Under normal physiologic conditions, the mean ICP is maintained at less than 15 mm Hg.[43–45] Essential to understanding the pathophysiology of ICP, the Monro-Kellie hypothesis proposes that an increase in volume of one intracranial component must be compensated by a decrease in one or more of the other components so that total volume remains fixed. This compensation, although limited, includes displacing CSF from the intracranial vault to the lumbar cistern, increasing CSF absorption, and compressing the low-pressure venous system.[45,46] Pathophysiologic alterations that can elevate ICP are outlined in Table 17.3.

Volume-Pressure Curve

When capable of compliance, the brain can tolerate significant increases in intracranial volume without much increase in ICP. However, the amount of intracranial compliance has a limit. After this limit has been reached, a state of decompensation with increased ICP results. As the ICP increases, the relationship between volume and pressure changes and small increases in volume may cause major elevations in ICP (Fig. 17.4).[43,44] The exact configuration of the volume-pressure curve and the point at which the steep increase in pressure occurs vary among patients. The configuration of this curve is also influenced by the cause and the rate of volume increases within the intracranial vault; for example, neurologic deterioration occurs more rapidly in a patient with an acute epidural hematoma than in a patient with a meningioma of the same size. Regardless of how fast the pressure increases, intracranial hypertension occurs when ICP is greater than 20 mm Hg.[43,44]

Cerebral Blood Flow and Autoregulation

CBF corresponds to the metabolic demands of the brain and is normally 50 mL/100 g of brain tissue/min. Although the brain makes up

TABLE 17.3 Mechanisms of Intracranial Pressure Elevation.

Pathophysiology	Examples
Disorders of CSF	
Overproduction of CSF	Choroid plexus tumors (papilloma or carcinoma)
Communicating hydrocephalus	Obstructed arachnoid villi Old subarachnoid hemorrhage
Noncommunicating hydrocephalus	Posterior fossa tumor obstructing aqueduct Aqueductal stenosis
Interstitial edema	Any of above
Disorders of Intracranial Blood Flow	
Intracranial hemorrhage	Epidural hematoma Subdural hematoma Intraparenchymal hematoma
Vasospasm	Subarachnoid hemorrhage
Vasodilation	Elevated $PaCO_2$
Increasing cerebral blood volume	Hypoxia
Disorders of Brain Substance	
Expanding mass lesion with local vasogenic edema	Brain tumor Abscess Brain injury Ischemic stroke
Ischemic brain injury with cytotoxic edema	Anoxic brain injury Hypoxic encephalopathy
Increased cerebral metabolic rate increasing CBF	Seizures Hyperthermia

CBF, Cerebral blood flow; *CSF,* cerebrospinal fluid; *PaCO₂,* arterial partial pressure of carbon dioxide.

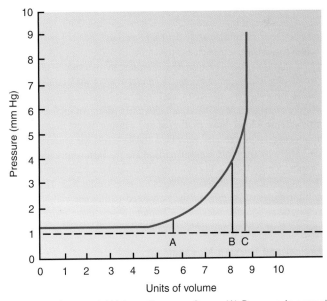

Fig. 17.4 Intracranial Volume-Pressure Curve. (A) Pressure is normal and increases in intracranial volume are tolerated without increases in intracranial pressure. (B) Increases in volume may cause increases in pressure. (C) Small increases in volume may cause larger increases in pressure.

only 2% of body weight, it requires 15% to 20% of the resting cardiac output and 15% of the body's oxygen demands. The normal brain has a complex capacity to maintain constant CBF, despite wide ranges in systemic arterial pressure—an effect known as *autoregulation*. A mean arterial pressure of 50 to 150 mm Hg does not alter CBF when autoregulation is functioning. Outside the limits of this autoregulation, CBF becomes passively dependent on the perfusion pressure.[45]

Factors other than arterial blood pressure that affect CBF are conditions that result in acidosis, alkalosis, and changes in metabolic rate. Conditions that cause acidosis (e.g., hypoxia, hypercapnia, ischemia) result in cerebrovascular dilation. Conditions causing alkalosis (e.g., hypocapnia) result in cerebrovascular constriction. Normally, a reduction in metabolic rate (e.g., from hypothermia or barbiturates) decreases CBF, and increases in metabolic rate (e.g., from hyperthermia) increase CBF.[46]

Arterial blood gases exert a profound effect on CBF. Carbon dioxide, which affects the pH of the blood, is a potent vasoactive substance. Carbon dioxide retention (hypercapnia) leads to cerebral vasodilation, with increased cerebral blood volume, whereas hypocapnia leads to cerebral vasoconstriction and a reduction in cerebral blood volume. However, prolonged hypocapnia, especially at an arterial partial pressure of carbon dioxide ($PaCO_2$) levels less than 20 mm Hg, can lead to cerebral ischemia. Low arterial partial pressure of oxygen (PaO_2) levels, especially less than 40 mm Hg, lead to cerebral vasodilation, which increases the intracranial blood volume and can contribute to increased ICP. High PaO_2 levels have not been shown to affect CBF in either direction.[46]

Assessment and Diagnosis

The numerous signs and symptoms of increased ICP include decreased LOC, Cushing triad (bradycardia, systolic hypertension, and widening pulse pressure), diminished brainstem reflexes, papilledema, decerebrate posturing (abnormal extension), decorticate posturing (abnormal flexion), unequal pupil size, projectile vomiting, decreased pupillary reaction to light, altered breathing patterns, and headache.[47] Patients may exhibit one or all of these symptoms, depending on the underlying cause of the elevation in ICP. One of the earliest and most important signs of increased ICP is a decrease in the LOC. This change must be reported immediately to the physician.[46,47]

In a patient with suspected intracranial hypertension, a monitoring device may be placed within the cranium to quantify ICP. Under normal physiologic conditions, the mean ICP is maintained at less than 15 mm Hg. The device is used to monitor serial ICPs and assist with the management of intracranial hypertension. An increase in ICP can decrease blood flow to the brain, causing brain damage. The monitoring device can also provide a sterile access for draining excess CSF. The four sites for monitoring ICP are the intraventricular space, the subarachnoid space, the epidural space, and the parenchyma. Each site has advantages and disadvantages for monitoring ICP. The type of monitor chosen depends on the suspected pathologic condition and the physician's preferences.[45-48] Chapter 16 provides a more detailed discussion of ICP monitoring.

Medical and Nursing Management

After intracranial hypertension is documented, therapy must be prompt to prevent secondary insults (Fig. 17.5). Although the exact pressure level denoting intracranial hypertension is uncertain, most current evidence suggests that ICP generally must be treated when it exceeds 20 mm Hg.[46] All therapies are directed toward reducing the volume of one or more of the components (e.g., blood, brain, CSF) that lie within the intracranial vault. A major goal of therapy is to

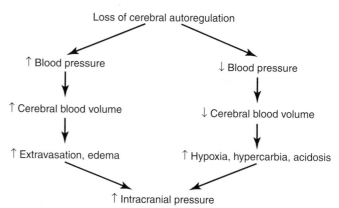

Fig. 17.5 Loss of Pressure Autoregulation.

determine the cause of the elevated pressure and, if possible, to remove the cause.[47] In the absence of a surgically treatable mass lesion, intracranial hypertension is treated medically. Nurses play an important role in rapid assessment and implementation of appropriate therapies for reducing ICP.

Positioning and Other Nursing Activities

Positioning of the patient is a significant factor in the prevention and treatment of intracranial hypertension. Head elevation has long been advocated as a conventional nursing intervention to control ICP, presumably by increasing venous return; however, this may decrease CPP. Close monitoring of ICP and CPP should be done with positioning, customizing positioning to maximize CPP and minimize ICP.[45]

Positions that impede venous return from the brain cause elevations in ICP. Obstruction of jugular veins or an increase in intrathoracic or intraabdominal pressure is communicated as increased pressure throughout the open venous system, impeding drainage from the brain and increasing ICP. Positions that decrease venous return from the head (e.g., Trendelenburg, prone, extreme flexion of the hips, and angulation of the neck) must be avoided if possible. If changes to positions such as Trendelenburg are necessary to provide adequate pulmonary care, critical care nurses must closely monitor ICP and vital signs.

Some routine nursing activities affect ICP and may be harmful. Use of positive end-expiratory pressures greater than 20 cm H_2O, coughing, suctioning, tight tracheostomy tube ties, and Valsalva maneuver have been associated with increases in ICP. Cumulative increases in ICP have been reported when care activities are performed one after another. Conversely, family contact and gentle touch have been associated with decreases in ICP.

Hyperventilation

Controlled hyperventilation has been an important adjunct of therapy for patients with increased ICP. The rationale employed in hyperventilation is that if $PaCO_2$ can be reduced from its normal level of 35 to 40 mm Hg to a range of 25 to 30 mm Hg in a patient with intracranial hypertension, vasoconstriction of cerebral arteries, reduction of CBF, and increased venous return will result. This practice is being reexamined. Additional research has indicated that severe or prolonged hyperventilation can reduce cerebral perfusion and lead to cerebral ischemia and infarction.[49] The current trend is to maintain $PaCO_2$ levels on the lower side of normal (35 mm Hg ± 2) by carefully monitoring arterial blood gas measurements and by adjusting ventilator settings.[45-48]

Although hypoxemia must be avoided, excessively high levels of oxygen offer no benefits, and increasing inspired oxygen concentrations to greater than 60% may lead to toxic changes in lung tissue. The use of pulse oximetry has led to greater awareness of the circumstances, such as pain and anxiety, which can cause oxygen desaturation and elevate ICP.

Temperature Control

Directly proportional to body temperature, cerebral metabolic rate increases 7% per 1°C of increase in body temperature.[46,47] This fact is significant because as the cerebral metabolic rate increases, blood flow to the brain must increase to meet the tissue demands. To avoid the increase in blood volume associated with an increased cerebral metabolic rate, nurses must prevent hyperthermia in a patient with a brain injury. Antipyretics and cooling devices must be used when appropriate while the source of the fever is being determined.[46,47]

Blood Pressure Control

Maintenance of arterial blood pressure in the high-normal range is essential in patients with brain injury. Inadequate perfusion pressure decreases the supply of nutrients and oxygen requirements for cerebral metabolic needs. However, a blood pressure that is too high increases cerebral blood volume and may increase ICP.[46] Fig. 17.5 shows the relationship between blood pressure and ICP.

Control of systemic hypertension may require nothing more than the administration of a sedative agent. Small, frequent doses may be sufficient to blunt noxious stimuli and prevent them from triggering increases in blood pressure. When sedation proves inadequate in controlling systemic arterial hypertension, antihypertensive agents are used. Care must be taken in choosing these agents because many of the peripheral vasodilators (e.g., nitroprusside, nitroglycerin) also are cerebral vasodilators. All antihypertensives are believed to cause some degree of cerebral vasodilation. To reduce this vasodilating effect, concurrent treatment with beta-blockers (e.g., metoprolol, labetalol) may be beneficial.[46]

Systemic hypotension should be treated aggressively with fluids to maintain a systolic blood pressure greater than 90 mm Hg. Crystalloids, colloids, and blood products can be used, depending on the patient's condition. Studies have demonstrated a positive effect on ICP and CPP with hypertonic saline.[50,51] If fluids fail to adequately elevate the patient's blood pressure, the use of inotropic agents may be necessary.

Seizure Control

The incidence of posttraumatic seizures in patients with head injury has been estimated to be 15% to 20%. Because of the risk of a secondary ischemic insult associated with seizures, many physicians prescribe anticonvulsant medications prophylactically. Seizures cause metabolic requirements to increase, which results in elevation of CBF, cerebral blood volume, and ICP, even in paralyzed patients. If blood flow cannot match demand, ischemia develops, cerebral energy stores are depleted, and irreversible neuronal destruction occurs.[45] Fast-acting, short-duration agents such as lorazepam may be indicated for breakthrough seizures until therapeutic medication levels can be achieved.[52]

Cerebrospinal Fluid Drainage

CSF drainage for intracranial hypertension may be used with other treatment modalities (Figs. 17.6 and 17.7). CSF drainage is accomplished by the insertion of a pliable catheter into the anterior horn of the lateral ventricle (ventriculostomy), preferably on the nondominant

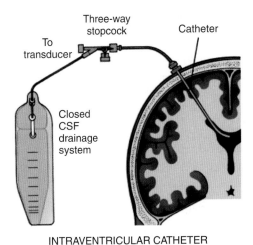

INTRAVENTRICULAR CATHETER

Fig. 17.6 Intermittent Drainage System. Intermittent drainage involves draining cerebrospinal fluid (CSF) through a ventriculostomy when intracranial pressure exceeds the upper pressure parameter set by the physician. Intermittent drainage is achieved by opening the three-way stopcock to allow CSF to flow into the drainage bag for brief periods (30–120 seconds) until the pressure is below the upper pressure parameter. (From Barker E, ed. *Neuroscience Nursing: A Spectrum of Care.* 3rd ed. St. Louis: Mosby; 2008.)

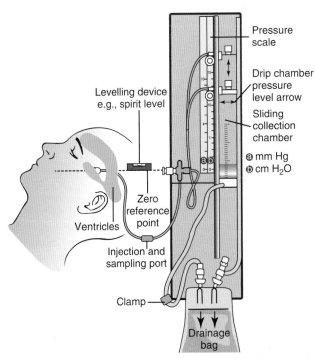

Fig. 17.7 Continuous Drainage System. Continuous drainage involves placing the drip chamber of the drainage system at a specified level above the foramen of Monro (usually 15 cm). The system is left open to allow continuous drainage of cerebrospinal fluid into the chamber (which drains into a collection bag) against a pressure gradient that prevents excessive drainage and ventricular collapse.

side. This drainage can help support the patient through periods of cerebral edema by controlling spikes in ICP. A major advantage of ventriculostomy is its dual role as a monitoring device and a treatment modality.[53] Care should be taken to avoid infection. However, cleansing ointment such as bacitracin or povidone is not recommended. Ventriculitis occurs in 10% to 20% of patients with a ventriculostomy.[54]

Hyperosmolar Therapy

Osmotic diuretics and hypertonic saline have also been used to reduce increased ICP. In the presence of an intact blood–brain barrier, hyperosmolar therapy is used to draw water from brain tissue into the intravascular compartment. The direction of flow is from the hypoconcentrated tissue to the hyperconcentrated cerebral vasculature. If the situation becomes reversed and the tissue becomes hyperconcentrated in relation to the cerebral vasculature, a rebound phenomenon may occur. These agents have little direct effect on edematous cerebral tissue situated in an area of a defective blood–brain barrier; instead, they require an intact blood–brain barrier for osmosis to occur.[50]

The most widely used osmotic diuretic is mannitol, a large-molecule agent that is retained almost entirely in the extracellular compartment and has little of the rebound effect observed with other osmotic diuretics. Administration of mannitol increases CBF and induces cerebral vasoconstriction as part of the brain's autoregulatory response to keep blood flow constant.[50,55]

Perhaps the most common difficulty associated with the use of osmotic agents is the provocation of electrolyte disturbances. Careful attention must be paid to body weight and fluid and electrolyte stability. Serum osmolality must be kept between 300 and 320 mOsm/L. Hypernatremia and hypokalemia often are associated with repeated administration of osmotic agents. Central venous pressure readings must be monitored to prevent hypovolemia. Smaller doses of mannitol simplify fluid and electrolyte management, and their use is encouraged whenever possible.[50]

Hypertonic 3% saline can also be used to treat increased ICP. Hypertonic saline has been found to be equally as effective as mannitol for reducing increased ICP.[55] Adverse effects include electrolyte abnormalities, hypotension, pulmonary edema, acute kidney injury, hemolysis, central pontine myelinolysis, coagulopathy, and dysrhythmias.

Control of Metabolic Demand

Any treatment modality that increases the incidence of noxious stimulation to the patient carries with it the potential for increasing ICP. Noxious stimuli include pain, the presence of an endotracheal tube, coughing, suctioning, repositioning, bathing, and many other routine nursing interventions. Agents used to reduce metabolic demands include the use of benzodiazepines such as midazolam and lorazepam, intravenous sedative-hypnotics such as propofol, opioids such as fentanyl and morphine, and neuromuscular blocking agents such as vecuronium and atracurium. These agents may be administered separately or in combination via continuous drip or as an intravenous bolus on an as-needed basis.

The preferred treatment regimen begins with the administration of benzodiazepines for sedation and opioids for analgesia. If these agents fail to blunt the patient's response to noxious stimuli, propofol or a neuromuscular blocking agent is added. The use of these medications is recommended only in patients who have an ICP monitor in place, because sedatives, opioids, and neuromuscular blocking agents affect the reliability of neurologic assessment. The use of neuromuscular blocking agents without sedation is not recommended, because these agents can cause skeletal muscle paralysis and because they have no analgesic effect and do not adequately protect the patient from pain and the physiologic responses that can occur from pain-producing

procedures.[46] If these agents fail to control ICP, barbiturate therapy is considered.

Barbiturate therapy. Barbiturate therapy is a treatment protocol developed for the management of uncontrolled intracranial hypertension that has not responded to the conventional treatments previously described.[46] The most commonly used medication in high-dose barbiturate therapy is pentobarbital. The goal is a reduction of ICP to 15 to 20 mm Hg while a mean arterial pressure of 70 to 80 mm Hg is maintained. Patients are maintained on high-dose barbiturate therapy until ICP has been controlled within the normal range for 24 hours. Barbiturates must never be stopped abruptly; they are tapered slowly over approximately 4 days. Despite the theoretical reasons for barbiturate use, clinical trials of its use have not shown improved outcome.[52]

Complications of high-dose barbiturate therapy can be disastrous unless a specific and organized approach is used. The most common complications are hypotension, hypothermia, and myocardial depression. If any complications occur and are allowed to persist unchecked, they may cause secondary insults to an already damaged brain. Hypotension, the most common complication, results from peripheral vasodilation and can be compounded in an already dehydrated patient who has received large doses of an osmotic diuretic to control ICP. Careful monitoring of fluid status by central venous pressure or a pulmonary artery catheter can help prevent this complication. Myocardial depression results from cardiac muscle suppression and can be avoided by frequent monitoring of fluid status, cardiac output, and serum medication levels. If an adequate cardiac output cannot be maintained in the presence of normothermia, barbiturates must be reduced, regardless of serum levels.[55,56]

Interprofessional collaborative management of intracranial hypertension in a patient is outlined in Box 17.12.

Herniation Syndromes

The goal of neurologic evaluation, ICP monitoring, and treatment of increased ICP is to prevent herniation. Herniation of intracerebral contents results in the shifting of tissue from one compartment of the brain to another and places pressure on cerebral vessels and vital function centers of the brain. If unchecked, herniation rapidly causes death as a result of the cessation of CBF and respirations.[52]

Supratentorial Herniation

The four types of supratentorial herniation syndrome are (1) uncal; (2) central, or transtentorial; (3) cingulate; and (4) transcalvarial (Fig. 17.8) (Table 17.4).

Uncal herniation. Uncal herniation is the most common herniation syndrome. In uncal herniation, a unilateral, expanding mass lesion,

---

BOX 17.12   Collaborative Management of Intracranial Hypertension

- Position patient to achieve maximal ICP reduction.
- Reduce environmental stimulation.
- Maintain normothermia.
- Control ventilation to ensure normal PaCO$_2$ level (35 mm Hg ± 2).
- Administer diuretic agents, anticonvulsants, sedation, analgesia, paralytic agents, and vasoactive medications to ensure CPP >70 mm Hg.
- Drain cerebrospinal fluid for ICP >20 mm Hg.

CPP, Cerebral perfusion pressure; *ICP,* intracranial pressure; *PaCO$_2$,* arterial partial pressure of carbon dioxide.

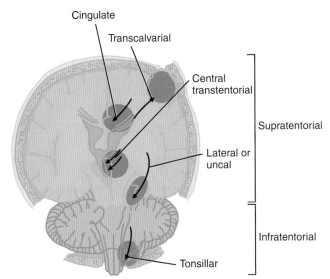

Fig. 17.8 Types of Intracranial Herniation. (From Linton AD, ed. *Introduction to Medical-Surgical Nursing.* 6th ed. St. Louis: Elsevier; 2016.)

usually of the temporal lobe, increases ICP, causing lateral displacement of the tip of the temporal lobe (uncus). Lateral displacement pushes the uncus over the edge of the tentorium, puts pressure on the oculomotor nerve (cranial nerve III) and the posterior cerebral artery ipsilateral to the lesion, and flattens the midbrain against the opposite side. Clinical manifestations of uncal herniation include ipsilateral pupil dilation, decreased LOC, respiratory pattern changes leading to respiratory arrest, and contralateral hemiplegia leading to abnormal flexion (decorticate) or abnormal extension (decerebrate) posturing. If no intervention occurs, uncal herniation results in fixed and dilated pupils, flaccidity, and respiratory arrest.[52]

Central herniation. In central, or transtentorial, herniation, an expanding mass lesion of the midline, frontal, parietal, or occipital lobe results in downward displacement of the hemispheres, basal ganglia, and diencephalon through the tentorial notch. Central herniation often is preceded by uncal and cingulate herniation. Clinical manifestations of central herniation include loss of consciousness; small, reactive pupils progressing to fixed, dilated pupils; respiratory changes leading to respiratory arrest; and abnormal flexion (decorticate) posturing progressing to flaccidity. In the late stages, uncal and central herniation syndromes affect the brainstem similarly.[52]

Cingulate herniation. Cingulate herniation occurs when an expanding lesion of one hemisphere shifts laterally and forces the cingulate gyrus under the falx cerebri. Cingulate herniation occurs often. When a lateral shift is observed on CT scan, cingulate herniation has occurred. Little is known about the effects of cingulate herniation, and no accompanying clinical manifestations exist to assist in its diagnosis. Cingulate herniation is not in itself a life-threatening condition, but if the expanding mass lesion that caused cingulate herniation is not controlled, uncal or central herniation will follow.[52]

Transcalvarial herniation. Transcalvarial herniation is the extrusion of cerebral tissue through the cranium. In the presence of severe cerebral edema, transcalvarial herniation occurs through an opening from a skull fracture or craniotomy site.[52]

Infratentorial Herniation

The two infratentorial herniation syndromes are upward transtentorial herniation and downward cerebellar herniation.

Upward transtentorial herniation. Upward transtentorial herniation occurs when an expanding mass lesion of the cerebellum causes protrusion of the vermis (central area) of the cerebellum and the midbrain upward through the tentorial notch. Compression of the third cranial nerve and diencephalon occurs. Blockage of the central aqueduct and distortion of the third ventricle obstruct CSF flow. Deterioration progresses rapidly.[52]

Downward cerebellar herniation. Downward cerebellar herniation occurs when an expanding lesion of the cerebellum exerts pressure downward, sending the cerebellar tonsils through the foramen magnum. Compression and displacement of the medulla oblongata occur, rapidly resulting in respiratory and cardiac arrest.[52]

CRANIOTOMY

Types of Surgery

A craniotomy is performed to gain access to portions of the central nervous system (CNS) inside the cranium, usually to allow removal of a space-occupying lesion such as a brain tumor (Table 17.5). Common procedures include tumor resection or removal, cerebral decompression, evacuation of hematoma or abscess, and clipping or removal of an aneurysm or AVM. Most patients who undergo craniotomy for tumor resection or removal do not require care in a critical care unit. Patients who do require such care usually need intensive monitoring or are at greater risk for complications because of underlying

TABLE 17.4 Herniation Syndromes.		
Herniation	**Pathophysiology**	**Presentation**
Uncal subtype: Kernohan notch	• Parasympathetic fibers of cranial nerve III compression • Pyramidal tract compression • Compression of cerebral peduncle in uncal herniation • Secondary condition caused by primary injury on opposite hemisphere	• Ipsilateral fixed and dilated pupil • Contralateral motor paralysis • Ipsilateral hemiplegia/hemiparesis, called Kernohan sign • False localizing sign
Central transtentorial	• Midline lesion with compression of midbrain	• Bilateral nonresponsive midpoint pupils, bilateral Babinski, increased muscular tone
Cerebellotonsillar	• Cerebellar tonsil herniation through foramen magnum	• Pinpoint pupils, flaccid paralysis, sudden death
Upward posterior fossa/transtentorial	• Cerebellar and midbrain movement upward through tentorial opening	• Pinpoint pupils, downward conjugate gaze, irregular respirations • Death

From Long G, Koyfman A. Secondary gains: advances in neurotrauma management. *Emerg Med Clin North Am.* 2018;36(1):107–133. https://doi.org/10.1016/j.emc.2017.08.007.

TABLE 17.5   Types of Brain Tumors Occurring in Adults.

Type	Pathology
Gliomas	
Astrocytomas (grades I–III)	Nonencapsulated, tend to infiltrate brain tissue; arise in any part of brain connective tissue;
Glioblastoma multiforme (also called astrocytoma grade IV)	infiltrate primarily cerebral hemisphere tissue; not well outlined, so difficult to excise
Oligodendroglioma (grades I–III)	completely; grow rapidly—most patients live months to years after diagnosis; tumors
Ependymoma (grades I–IV)	assigned grades I–IV, with IV being most malignant
Medulloblastoma	
Tumors From Support Structures	
Meningiomas	Arise from meningeal coverings of brain; usually benign but may undergo malignant changes; usually encapsulated and surgical cure possible; recurrence possible
Neuromas (acoustic neuroma, schwannoma)	Arise from Schwann cells inside auditory meatus on vestibular portion of cranial nerve VIII; usually benign but may undergo cellular change and become malignant; will regrow if not completely excised; surgical resection often difficult because of location
Pituitary adenoma	Arise from various tissues; surgical approach usually successful; recurrence possible
Developmental (Congenital) Tumors	
Dermoid, epidermoid, craniopharyngioma	Arise from embryonic tissue in various sites in brain; success of surgical resection depends on location and invasiveness
Angiomas	Arise from vascular structures; usually difficult to resect
Metastatic Tumors	
	Cancer cells spreading to brain via circulatory system; surgical resection difficult; even with treatment, prognosis poor; survival beyond 1–2 years uncommon

From Monahan FD, Sands J, Neighbors M, et al., eds. *Phipps' Medical-Surgical Nursing: Health and Illness Perspective.* 8th ed. St. Louis: Mosby; 2007.

cardiopulmonary dysfunction or the surgical approach used.[57] Box 17.13 provides definitions of common neurosurgical terms.

Preoperative Care

Protection of the integrity of the CNS is a major priority of care for a patient awaiting a craniotomy. Optimal arterial oxygenation, hemodynamic stability, and cerebral perfusion are essential for maintaining adequate cerebral oxygenation. Management of seizure activity is essential for controlling metabolic needs.

Detailed assessment and documentation of the patient's preoperative neurologic status are imperative for accurate postoperative evaluation. Attention is focused on identifying and describing the nature and extent of any preoperative neurologic deficits. When pituitary surgery is planned, a thorough evaluation of endocrine function is necessary to prevent major intraoperative and postoperative complications.[58]

Trends in health care demand judicious use of routine preoperative studies. Depending on the type of surgery to be performed and the general health of the patient, preoperative screening may include a complete blood cell count; tests for blood urea nitrogen, creatinine, and fasting blood sugar; chest radiography; and electrocardiography. A blood type and crossmatch may also be ordered.[59]

Preoperative teaching is necessary to prepare the patient and family for what to expect in the postoperative period. A description of the intravascular lines and intracranial catheters used during the postoperative period allows the family to focus on the patient and not be overwhelmed by masses of tubing. Some or all the patient's hair is shaved off in the operating room, and a large, bulky, turban-like craniotomy dressing is applied. Most patients experience some degree of postoperative eye or facial swelling and periorbital ecchymosis. An explanation of these temporary changes in appearance helps alleviate the shock and fear many patients and families experience in the immediate postoperative period.[59]

All patients who undergo craniotomy require instruction to avoid activities known to provoke sudden changes in ICP. These activities include bending, lifting, straining, and the Valsalva maneuver. Patients commonly elicit the Valsalva maneuver during repositioning in bed by holding their breath and straining with a closed epiglottis. This is prevented effectively by teaching the patient to continue to breathe deeply through the mouth during all position changes.[59]

Patients undergoing transsphenoidal surgery require preparation for the sensations associated with nasal packing. Patients often awaken with alarm because of the inability to breathe through the nose. Preoperative instruction in mouth breathing and avoidance of coughing, sneezing, or blowing of the nose facilitates postoperative cooperation.[58]

The psychosocial issues associated with the prospect of neurosurgery cannot be overemphasized. Few procedures are as threatening as procedures involving the brain or spinal cord. For some patients, the

BOX 17.13   Operative Terms

- *Burr hole:* Hole made into the cranium using a special drill
- *Craniotomy:* Surgical opening of the skull
- *Craniectomy:* Removal of a portion of the skull without replacing it
- *Cranioplasty:* Plastic repair of the skull
- *Supratentorial:* Above the tentorium, separating the cerebrum from the cerebellum
- *Infratentorial:* Below the tentorium; includes the brainstem and the cerebellum; an infratentorial surgical approach may be used for temporal or occipital lesions
- *Stereotactic:* Minimally invasive surgical intervention that uses a three-dimensional coordinate system to localize a specific area of the brain for ablation, biopsy, dissection, or radiosurgery

fear of permanent neurologic impairment may be as ominous as or more ominous than the fear of death. Steps to meet the needs of the patient and the family include collaboration with religious and social services personnel, patient-controlled visitation, and provision of as much privacy as the patient's condition permits. The patient and family must be provided with the opportunity to express their fears and concerns jointly and apart from each other.[51]

Surgical Considerations

Although the emphasis in the surgical approach for most other types of surgery is to gain adequate exposure of the surgical site, the neurosurgeon must select a route that also produces the least amount of disruption to the intracranial contents. Neural tissue is unforgiving. A significant portion of neurologic trauma and postoperative deficits is related to the surgical pathway through the brain tissue, rather than to the procedure performed at the site of pathology. Depending on the location of the lesion and the surgical route chosen, a transcranial or a transsphenoidal approach is used to open the skull.

Transcranial Approach

In the transcranial approach, a scalp incision is made, and a series of burr holes is drilled into the skull to form an outline of the area to be opened (Fig. 17.9). A special saw is used to cut between the holes. In most cases, the bone flap is left attached to the muscle to create a hinge effect. In some cases, the bone flap is removed completely and placed in the abdomen for later retrieval and implantation, or discarded and replaced with synthetic material. Next, the dura mater is opened and retracted. After the intracranial procedure, the dura mater and the bone flap are closed, the muscles and scalp are sutured, and a turban-like dressing is applied.[57]

Transsphenoidal Approach

The transsphenoidal approach is the technique of choice for removal of a pituitary tumor without extension into the intracranial vault (Fig. 17.10).[58,59] This approach involves creating a microsurgical entrance into the cranial vault through the nasal cavity. The sphenoid sinus is entered to reach the anterior wall of the sella turcica. The sphenoid bone and the dura mater are then opened to gain intracranial access. After removal of the tumor, the surgical bed is packed with a small section of adipose tissue grafted from the patient's abdomen or thigh. After closure of the intranasal structures, nasal splints and soft packing or nasal tampons impregnated with antibiotic ointment are placed in the nasal cavities. Occasionally, epistaxis balloons are used instead. A nasal drip pad or mustache-type dressing is placed at the base of the nose to catch surgical drainage.[57]

The patient may be placed in the supine, prone, or sitting position for a craniotomy procedure. A skull clamp connected to skull pins is used to position and secure the patient's head throughout the operation. During a transsphenoidal approach or a transcranial approach into the infratentorial area, the patient's head is elevated during surgery. This position places the patient at risk for an air embolism. Air can enter the vascular system through the edges of the dura mater or a

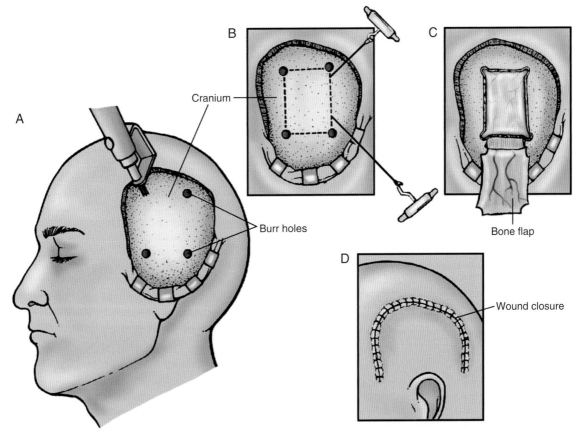

Fig. 17.9 Craniotomy Procedure. (A) Burr holes are drilled into skull. (B) Skull is cut between burr holes with a surgical saw. (C) Bone flap is turned back to expose cranial contents. (D) After surgery, bone flap is replaced, and wound is closed. (From Monahan FD, Sands J, Neighbors M, et al., eds. *Phipps' Medical-Surgical Nursing: Health and Illness Perspective.* 8th ed. St. Louis: Mosby; 2007.)

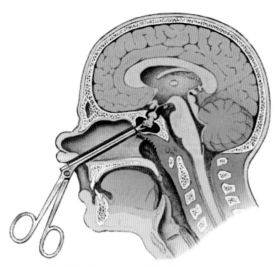

Fig. 17.10 Transsphenoidal Hypophysectomy.

venous opening. Continuous monitoring of the patient's heart sounds by Doppler signal allows immediate recognition of this complication. If air embolism occurs, an attempt may be made to withdraw the embolus from the right atrium through a central line. Flooding the surgical field with irrigation fluid and placing a moistened sterile surgical sponge over the surgical site creates an immediate barrier to any further air entrance.[57]

Postoperative Medical Management

Definitive management of a postoperative neurosurgical patient varies depending on the underlying reason for the craniotomy. During the initial postoperative period, management is usually directed toward the prevention of complications. Complications associated with a craniotomy include intracranial hypertension, surgical hemorrhage, fluid imbalance, CSF leak, and DVT.

Intracranial Hypertension

Postoperative cerebral edema is expected to peak 48 to 72 hours after surgery. If the bone flap is not replaced at the time of surgery, intracranial hypertension will produce bulging at the surgical site. Close monitoring of the surgical site is important so that integrity of the incision can be maintained. Management of intracranial hypertension after craniotomy is usually accomplished through CSF drainage, patient positioning, and steroid administration.[60]

Surgical Hemorrhage

Surgical hemorrhage after a transcranial procedure can occur in the intracranial vault and manifests as signs and symptoms of increasing ICP. Hemorrhage after a transsphenoidal craniotomy may be evident from external drainage, the patient's complaint of persistent postnasal drip, or excessive swallowing. Loss of vision after pituitary surgery indicates an evolving hemorrhage. Postoperative hemorrhage requires surgical reexploration.[60]

Fluid Imbalance

Fluid imbalance in a patient after craniotomy usually results from a disturbance in production or secretion of antidiuretic hormone (ADH). ADH is secreted by the posterior pituitary (neurohypophysis) gland. It stimulates the renal tubules and collecting ducts to retain water in response to low circulating blood volume or increased serum osmolality. Inoperative trauma or postoperative edema of the pituitary

gland or hypothalamus can result in insufficient ADH secretion. The outcome is unabated renal water loss even when blood volume is low and serum osmolality is high. This condition is known as *diabetes insipidus* (DI). The polyuria associated with DI is often more than 200 mL/h. Urine specific gravity of 1.005 or less and elevated serum osmolality provide evidence of insufficient ADH. The loss of volume may provoke hypotension and inadequate cerebral perfusion. DI is usually self-limiting, and fluid replacement is the only required therapy. However, in some cases, it may be necessary to administer vasopressin intravenously to control the loss of fluid.[61]

SIADH commonly occurs with neurologic insult and results from excessive ADH secretion. SIADH manifests as inappropriate water retention with hyponatremia in the presence of normal renal function. Urine specific gravity is elevated, and urine osmolality is greater than serum osmolality. The dangers associated with SIADH include circulating volume overload and electrolyte imbalance, both of which may impair neurologic functioning. SIADH is usually self-limiting, with the mainstay of treatment being fluid restriction.[61]

Cerebrospinal Fluid Leak

Leakage of CSF results from an opening in the subarachnoid space, as evidenced by clear fluid draining from the surgical site. When this complication occurs after transsphenoidal surgery, it is evidenced by excessive, clear drainage from the nose or persistent postnasal drip.[62] To differentiate CSF drainage from postoperative serous drainage, a specimen is tested for glucose content. A CSF leak is confirmed by glucose values of 30 mg/dL or greater. Management of a patient with a CSF leak includes bed rest and head elevation. Lumbar puncture or placement of a lumbar subarachnoid catheter may be used to reduce CSF pressure until the dura mater heals. The risk of meningitis associated with CSF leak often necessitates surgical repair to reseal the opening.[63]

Deep Vein Thrombosis

Patients who have undergone neurosurgery are at particularly high risk for development of DVT. Research has demonstrated that these patients have a variety of additional risk factors, including preoperative leg weakness, longer preoperative and postoperative stay in the critical care unit, longer operative procedure time, prone positioning on frames with flexion of the hips or knees, longer time in the postanesthesia care unit, more days on bed rest, lengthy operative procedures, and delay of postoperative mobility and activity.[64,65] Clinical manifestations of DVT include leg or calf pain and erythema, warmth, and swelling of the affected limb. However, a patient with a DVT is often asymptomatic, and the diagnosis is not made until the patient experiences a pulmonary embolus.[66] The primary treatment for DVT is prophylaxis. After neurosurgery, sequential (intermittent) pneumatic compression sleeves are effective in reducing the incidence of DVT. Effectiveness is enhanced when these devices are initiated in the preoperative period. Low—molecular-weight heparin may also be used prophylactically in high-risk patients when the risk of bleeding has decreased.[67]

Postoperative Nursing Management

The patient care management plan for a patient after neurosurgery incorporates a variety of patient problems (Box 17.14). As in preoperative care, the primary goal of postcraniotomy nursing management is protection of the integrity of the CNS. **Nursing priorities focus on (1) preserving adequate CPP, (2) promoting arterial oxygenation, (3) providing comfort and emotional support, (4) maintaining surveillance for complications, (5) initiating early rehabilitation,**

BOX 17.14 PRIORITY PATIENT CARE MANAGEMENT

Craniotomy

Decreased Intracranial Adaptive Capacity due to failure of normal intracranial compensatory mechanisms

Ineffective Tissue Perfusion due to decreased cerebral blood flow

Acute Pain due to transmission and perception of cutaneous, visceral, muscular, or ischemic impulses

Disturbed Body Image due to actual change in body structure, function, or appearance

Lack of Knowledge of Treatment Regime due to lack of previous exposure to information (See Box 17.15, Priority Patient and Family Education for Craniotomy)

Patient Care Management plans are located in Appendix A.

and (6) educating the patient and family. Frequent neurologic assessment is necessary to evaluate accomplishment of these objectives and to identify problems and quickly intervene if complications do arise. A ventriculostomy often is placed to facilitate ICP monitoring and CSF drainage.

Preserve Cerebral Perfusion

Nursing interventions to preserve cerebral perfusion include patient positioning, fluid management, and avoidance of postoperative vomiting and fever.

Positioning. Patient positioning is an important component of care after craniotomy. The head of the bed should always be elevated to 30 to 45 degrees to reduce the incidence of hemorrhage, facilitate venous drainage, and control ICP. Other positioning measures to control ICP include always maintaining the patient's head in a neutral position and avoiding neck or hip flexion. These rules of positioning must be followed throughout all nursing activities, including linen changes and transporting the patient for diagnostic evaluation. Most patients after craniotomy can be turned from side to side within these restrictions, using pillows for support, except in some cases of extensive tumor removal, cranioplasty, and when the bone flap is not replaced. Specific orders from the surgeon must be obtained in these instances. A patient with an infratentorial incision may be restricted to only a very small pillow under the head to prevent strain on the incision. Avoidance of anterior or lateral neck flexion also protects the integrity of this type of incision.

Fluid management. Fluid management is another important component of postcraniotomy care. Hourly monitoring of fluid intake and output facilitates early identification of fluid imbalance. Urine specific gravity must be measured if DI is suspected. Fluid restriction may be ordered as a routine measure to lessen the severity of cerebral edema or as treatment for the fluid and electrolyte imbalances associated with SIADH.[61]

Avoidance of vomiting and fever. Postoperative vomiting must be avoided to prevent sharp spikes in ICP and possibly surgical hemorrhage. Antiemetics are administered as soon as nausea is apparent. Early nutrition in the patient is beneficial. If the patient is unable to eat, enteral hyperalimentation delivered through a feeding tube is the preferred method of nutrition support and can be initiated 24 hours after surgery. Postoperative fever may also adversely affect ICP and increase the metabolic needs of the brain. Acetaminophen is administered orally, rectally, or through a feeding tube. External cooling measures such as a hypothermia blanket may be necessary.

Promote Arterial Oxygenation

Routine pulmonary care is used to maintain airway clearance and prevent pulmonary complications. To prevent dangerous elevations in ICP, this care measure must be performed using proper technique and at time intervals that are adequately spaced from other patient care activities. If pulmonary complications arise, consideration must be given to maintaining adequate oxygenation during repositioning. It may be necessary to restrict turning to only the side that places the good lung down.

Provide Comfort and Emotional Support

Pain management in patients after craniotomy primarily involves control of headache. Traditionally small doses of intravenous opioids are used with a goal of starting oral analgesics as soon as can be tolerated. Nonopioid analgesics may be used as an adjunct medication. Because opioid analgesics cause constipation, administration of stool softeners and initiation of a bowel program are important components of postcraniotomy care. Constipation is hazardous because straining to have a bowel movement can create significant elevations in blood pressure and ICP. However, newer approaches are being evaluated because of the side effects of opioid analgesics. Intraoperative dexmedetomidine, preoperative and postoperative gabapentin and acetaminophen, and scalp blocks are just some of the alternative pain modalities being researched.[68]

Maintain Surveillance for Complications

Following neurosurgery, patients are at risk for infection, corneal abrasions, and injury from falls or seizures.

Infection. After neurosurgery, patients are at risk for a variety of infections, including meningitis, cerebral abscesses, bone flap infections, and subdural empyema.[69] Care of the incision and surgical dressings is specific to the institution and the physician. The rule of thumb for a craniotomy dressing is to reinforce it as needed and change it only on a physician's order. A drain is often left in place to facilitate decompression of the surgical site. If a ventriculostomy is present, it is treated as a component of the surgical site. All drainage devices must be secured to the dressing to prevent unintentional displacement with patient movement. Sterile technique is required to prevent infection. Postoperatively, infection should be suspected if the patient exhibits signs of mental status changes, headache, fever, and purulent drainage and swelling around the incision site.[69]

Corneal abrasions. Routine eye care may be necessary to prevent corneal drying and ulceration. Periorbital edema interferes with normal blinking and eyelid closure, which are essential to adequate corneal lubrication. Saline drops are instilled to maintain lubrication. If the patient remains in a comatose state, covering the eyes with a polyethylene film extending over the orbits and eyebrows may be beneficial.[42]

Injury. After craniotomy, the patient may experience periods of altered mentation. Protection from injury may require the use of restraint devices. The side rails of the bed must be padded to protect the patient from injury. Having a family member stay at the bedside or the use of music therapy is often helpful to keep the patient calm during periods of restlessness. In rare circumstances, continuous sedation with or without neuromuscular blockade may be necessary to control patient activity and metabolic needs on a short-term basis.

Initiate Early Rehabilitation

Increased activity, including ambulation, is begun as soon as tolerated by the patient in the postoperative period. Rehabilitation measures and discharge planning may begin in the critical care unit, but discussion is

✳ BOX 17.15 PRIORITY PATIENT AND FAMILY EDUCATION

Craniotomy

Before discharge, the patient should be able to teach back the following topics:

Before Surgery
- Pathophysiology and expected outcome of underlying disease
- Need for critical care management after surgery
- Routine preoperative surgical care

After Surgery
- Routine postoperative surgical care

- Discharge medications—purpose, dosage, and side effects
- Incisional care
- Signs and symptoms of infection
- Signs and symptoms of increased intracranial pressure
- Measures to compensate for residual deficits
- Basic rehabilitation techniques
- Importance of participating in neurologic rehabilitation program

Additional information for the patient can be found at the National Brain Tumor Society website (www.braintumor.org).

TABLE 17.6   Neurologic Pharmacology.

Medication	Dosage	Action	Special Considerations
Anticonvulsants			
Phenytoin (Dilantin)	Loading dose: 10–20 mg/kg IV	Prevents influx of sodium at cell membrane	Monitor serum levels closely; therapeutic level is 10–20 mg/L (if hypoalbuminuria, monitor free phenytoin serum levels: therapeutic level of 0.1–0.2 mg/L)
	Maintenance dose: 100 mg q6–8 hours IV		Infuse phenytoin no faster than 50 mg/min; administer with normal saline only because it precipitates with other solutions
Fosphenytoin (Cerebyx)	Loading dose: 15–20 mg/kg IV	Prevents influx of sodium at cell membrane	Monitor serum levels closely; therapeutic level is 10–20 mg/L
	Maintenance dose: 4–6 mg/kg/ 24 hours IV		Dosage, concentration, and infusion rate of fosphenytoin expressed as FE
Barbiturates			
Phenobarbital	Loading dose: 6–8 mg/kg IV	Produces CNS depression and reduces spread of epileptic focus	May depress cardiac and respiratory function
	Maintenance dose: 1–3 mg/kg/ 24 hours IV		Administer phenobarbital at a rate of 60 mg/min; monitor serum level closely; therapeutic level is 15–40 mcg/mL
Pentobarbital	Loading dose: 3–10 mg/kg over 30 min	Induces barbiturate coma	Monitor serum level of pentobarbital closely; therapeutic level for coma is 15–40 mg/L
	Maintenance dose: 0.5–3 mg/kg/ hours IV		
Osmotic Diuretics			
Mannitol	1–2 g/kg IV	Treats cerebral edema by pulling fluid from extravascular space into intravascular space; requires intact blood–brain barrier	Side effects include hypovolemia and increased serum osmolality
			Monitor serum osmolality and notify physician if >310 mOsm/L
			Warm and shake before administering to ensure crystals are dissolved
Calcium Channel Blockers			
Nimodipine (Nimotop)	60 mg q4h NG or PO for 21 days	Decreases cerebral vasospasm	Side effects include hypotension, palpitations, headache, and dizziness
			Monitor blood pressure frequently when implementing therapy
Local Anesthetics			
Lidocaine	50–100 mg IV or 2 mL of 4% solution	Blunts effects of tracheal stimulation on intracranial pressure	Must be administered not longer than 5 minutes before suctioning
Fibrinolytics			
tPA	0.9 mg/kg total, with 10% of dose administered as IV bolus over 1 minute and 90% of dose administered as continuous IV infusion over 1 hour	Converts plasminogen to plasmin to dissolve clot	Treatment must start within 4.5 hours of onset of symptoms
			Do not exceed 90 mg
			Do not use anticoagulants during the first 24 hours
			Monitor patient for bleeding

CNS, Central nervous system; *FE*, phenytoin sodium equivalents; *IV*, intravenous/intravenously; *NG*, nasogastric; *PO*, by mouth; *tPA*, tissue-type plasminogen activator.

Data from Gold Standard (www.clinicalkey.com).

BOX 17.16 Informatics

Internet Resources: Neurologic Disorders and Therapeutic Management

- American Academy of Neurology (AAN): www.aan.com
- American Association of Critical-Care Nurses (AACN): www.aacn.org
- American Association of Neurological Surgeons (AANS): www.aans.org
- American Association of Neuroscience Nurses (AANN): www.aann.org
- American College of Physicians (ACP): www.acponline.org
- American College of Surgeons (ACS): www.facs.org
- American Medical Association (AMA): www.ama-assn.org
- American Stroke Association: www.stroke.org
- National Institutes of Health (NIH): www.nih.gov
- Society for Critical Care Medicine (SCCM): www.sccm.org
- Society for Neuroscience (SNF): www.sfn.org

beyond the scope of this chapter. Transfer to a general care or rehabilitation unit is usually accomplished as soon as the patient is deemed stable and free of complications.

Educate the Patient and Family

Preoperatively, the patient and family should be taught about the precipitating event necessitating the craniotomy and its expected outcome (Box 17.15). The severity of the disease and the need for critical care management postoperatively must be stressed. As the patient moves toward discharge, teaching focuses on medication instructions, incisional care including the signs of infection, and the signs and symptoms of increased ICP. If the patient has neurologic deficits, teaching focuses on the interventions to maximize the patient's rehabilitation potential, and the patient's family members must be encouraged to participate in the patient's care and to learn some basic rehabilitation techniques. The importance of participating in a neurologic rehabilitation program must be stressed.

PHARMACOLOGIC AGENTS

Many pharmacologic agents are used in the care of patients with neurologic disorders. Table 17.6 reviews the various agents used and any special considerations necessary for administering them.

ADDITIONAL RESOURCES

See Box 17.16 for Internet resources pertaining to neurologic disorders and therapeutic management.

REFERENCES

1. Virani SS, Alonso A, Aparicio HJ, et al. Heart disease and stroke statistics-2021 update: a report from the American Heart Association. *Circulation.* 2021;143(8):e254—e743. https://doi.org/10.1161/CIR.0000000000000950.
2. Biller J, Schneck MJ, Ruland S. Ischemic cerebrovascular disease. In: Jankovic J, Massiotta JC, Pomeroy SL, Newman NJ, eds. *Bradley and Daroff's Neurology in Clinical Practice.* 8th ed. Philadelphia: Elsevier; 2022.
3. Mac Grory B, Flood SP, Apostolidou E, Yaghi S. Cryptogenic stroke: diagnostic workup and management. *Curr Treat Options Cardiovasc Med.* 2019;21(11):77. https://doi.org/10.1007/s11936-019-0786-4.
4. Swait G, Finch R. What are the risks of manual treatment of the spine? A scoping review for clinicians. *Chiropr Man Therap.* 2017;25:37. https://doi.org/10.1186/s12998-017-0168-5.
5. O'Carroll CB, Barrett KM. Cardioembolic stroke (1, Cerebrovascular Disease) *Continuum.* 2017;23(1, Cerebrovascular Disease):111—132. https://doi.org/10.1212/CON.0000000000000419.
6. Boss BJ, Huether SE. Disorders of central and peripheral nervous system and the neuromuscular junction. In: McCance KL, Huether SE, eds. *Pathophysiology: The Biologic Basis for Disease in Adults and Children.* 8th ed. St. Louis: Elsevier; 2019.
7. Bustamante A, García-Berrocoso T, Rodriguez N, et al. Ischemic stroke outcome: a review of the influence of post-stroke complications within the different scenarios of stroke care. *Eur J Intern Med.* 2016;29:9—21. https://doi.org/10.1016/j.ejim.2015.11.030.
8. Powers WJ, Rabinstein AA, Ackerson T, et al. Guidelines for the early management of patients with acute ischemic stroke: 2019 update to the 2018 guidelines for the early management of acute ischemic stroke: a guideline for healthcare professionals from the American Heart Association/American Stroke Association. *Stroke.* 2019;50(12):e344—e418. https://doi.org/10.1161/STR.0000000000000211.
9. Pratit P, Yavagal D, Khadelwal P. Hyperacute management of ischemic stroke. *J Am Coll Cardiol.* 2020;75(15):1844—1856. https://doi.org/10.1016/j.jacc.2020.03.006.
10. Sacks D, Baxter B, Campbell BCV, et al. Multisociety consensus quality improvement revised consensus statement for endovascular therapy of acute ischemic stroke. *J Vasc Interv Radiol.* 2018;29(4):441—453. https://doi.org/10.1016/j.jvir.2017.11.026.
11. White CJ. Acute stroke intervention: the role of interventional cardiologists. *J Am Coll Cardiol.* 2019;73(12):1491—1493. https://doi.org/10.1016/j.jacc.2018.12.071.
12. Long B, Koyfman A, Runyon MS. Subarachnoid hemorrhage: updates in diagnosis and management. *Emerg Med Clin North Am.* 2017;35(4):803—824. https://doi.org/10.1016/j.emc.2017.07.001.
13. Abraham MK, Chang WW. Subarachnoid hemorrhage. *Emerg Med Clin North Am.* 2016;34(4):901—916. https://doi.org/10.1016/j.emc.2016.06.011.
14. Wilson SE, Ashcraft S, Troiani L. Aneurysmal subarachnoid hemorrhage: management by the advanced practice provider. *J Nurse Pract.* 2019;15(8):553—558.
15. Boling B, Groves TR. Management of subarachnoid hemorrhage. *Crit Care Nurse.* 2019;39(5):58—67. https://doi.org/10.4037/ccn2019882.
16. Szeder V, Tateshima S, Jahan J, et al. Intracranial aneurysms and subarachnoid hemorrhage. In: Jankovic J, Massiotta JC, Pomeroy SL, Newman NJ, eds. *Bradley and Daroff's Neurology in Clinical Practice.* 8th ed. Philadelphia: Elsevier; 2022.
17. Lawton MT, Rutledge WC, Kim H, et al. Brain arteriovenous malformations. *Nat Rev Dis Primers.* 2015;1:15008. https://doi.org/10.1038/nrdp.2015.8.
18. Connolly ES, Jr., Rabinstein AA, Carhuapoma JR, et al. Guidelines for the management of aneurysmal subarachnoid hemorrhage: a guideline for healthcare professionals from the American Heart Association/American Stroke Association. *Stroke.* 2012;43(6):1711—1737. https://doi.org/10.1161/STR.0b013e3182587839.
19. Muehlschlegel S. Subarachnoid hemorrhage. *Continuum.* 2018;25(6):1623—1657. https://doi.org/10.1212/CON.0000000000000679.
20. Hunt WE, Hess RM. Surgical risks as related to time of intervention in the repair of intracranial aneurysms. *J Neurosurg.* 1968;28(1):14—20.
21. Marcolini E, Hine J. Approach to the diagnosis and management of subarachnoid hemorrhage. *West J Emerg Med.* 2019;20(2):203—211. https://doi.org/10.5811/westjem.2019.1.37352.
22. Bowles E. Cerebral aneurysm and aneurysmal subarachnoid haemorrhage. *Nurs Stand.* 2014;28(34):52—59. https://doi.org/10.7748/ns2014.04.28.34.52.e8694.
23. Ellis JA, Lavine SD. Role of embolization for cerebral arteriovenous malformations. *Methodist Debakey Cardiovasc J.* 2014;10(4):234—239. https://doi.org/10.14797/mdcj-10-4-234.
24. Francoeur CL, Mayer SA. Management of delayed cerebral ischemia after subarachnoid hemorrhage. *Crit Care.* 2016;20(1):277. https://doi.org/10.1186/s13054-016-1447-6.

25. Rouanet C, Sampaio G. Aneurysmal subarachnoid hemorrhage: current concepts and updates. *Arq Neuropsiquiatr.* 2019;77(11):806–814. https://doi.org/10.1590/0004-282X20190112.

26. Baggott CD, Aagaard-Kienitz B. Cerebral vasospasm. *Neurosurg Clin N Am.* 2014;25(3):497–528. https://doi.org/10.1016/j.nec.2014.04.008.

27. Alerhand S, Lay C. Spontaneous intracerebral hemorrhage. *Emerg Med Clin North Am.* 2017;35(4):825–845. https://doi.org/10.1016/j.emc.2017.07.002.

28. Schrag M, Kirshner H. Management of intracerebral hemorrhage: JACC focus seminar. *J Am Coll Cardiol.* 2020;75(15):1819–1831. https://doi.org/10.1016/j.jacc.2019.10.066.

29. Godoy DA, Piñero GR, Koller P, Masotti L, Di Napoli M. Steps to consider in the approach and management of critically ill patient with spontaneous intracerebral hemorrhage. *World J Crit Care Med.* 2015;4(3):213–229. https://doi.org/10.5492/wjccm.v4.i3.213.

30. Mayer SA. Hemorrhagic cerebrovascular disease. In: Goldman L, Schafer AI, eds. *Goldman-Cecil Medicine.* 26th ed. St. Louis: Elsevier; 2020.

31. Hemphill JC 3rd, Greenberg SM, Anderson CS, et al. Guidelines for the management of spontaneous intracerebral hemorrhage: a guideline for healthcare professionals from the American Heart Association/American Stroke Association. *Stroke.* 2015;46(7):2032–2060. https://doi.org/10.1161/STR.0000000000000069.

32. Amatangelo MP, Thomas SB. Priority nursing interventions caring for the stroke patient. *Crit Care Nurs Clin North Am.* 2020;32(1):67–84. https://doi.org/10.1016/j.cnc.2019.11.005.

33. Grow WA. The cerebral cortex. In: Haines DE, Mihailoff GA, eds. *Fundamental Neuroscience for Basic and Clinical Applications.* Philadelphia: Elsevier; 2018.

34. Eapen BC, Georgekutty J, Subbarao B, Bavishi S, Cifu DX. Disorders of consciousness. *Phys Med Rehabil Clin N Am.* 2017;28(2):245–258. https://doi.org/10.1016/j.pmr.2016.12.003.

35. Traub SJ, Wijdicks EF. Initial diagnosis and management of coma. *Emerg Med Clin North Am.* 2016;34(4):777–793. https://doi.org/10.1016/j.emc.2016.06.017.

36. Horsting MW, Franken MD, Meulenbelt J, van Klei WA, de Lange DW. The etiology and outcome of non-traumatic coma in critical care: a systematic review. *BMC Anesthesiol.* 2015;15:65. https://doi.org/10.1186/s12871-015-0041-9.

37. Edlow JA, Rabinstein A, Traub SJ, Wijdicks EF. Diagnosis of reversible causes of coma. *Lancet.* 2014;384(9959):2064–2076. https://doi.org/10.1016/S0140-6736(13)62184-4.

38. Boss BJ, Huether SE. Alteration in cognitive systems, cerebral hemodynamics, and motor function. In: McCance KL, Huether SE, eds. *Pathophysiology: The Biologic Basis for Disease in Adults and Children.* 8th ed. St. Louis: Elsevier; 2019.

39. Hocker S, Rabinstein AA. Management of the patient with diminished responsiveness. *Neurol Clin.* 2012;30(1):1–9. https://doi.org/10.1016/j.ncl.2011.09.009.

40. Kondziella D, Bender A, Diserens K, et al. European Academy of Neurology guideline on the diagnosis of coma and other disorders of consciousness. *Eur J Neurol.* 2020;27(5):741–756. https://doi.org/10.1111/ene.14151.

41. Bruno MA, Vanhaudenhuyse A, Thibaut A, Moonen G, Laureys S. From unresponsive wakefulness to minimally conscious PLUS and functional locked-in syndromes: recent advances in our understanding of disorders of consciousness. *J Neurol.* 2011;258(7):1373–1384. https://doi.org/10.1007/s00415-011-6114-x.

42. Nikseresht T, Abdi A, Khatony A. Effectiveness of polyethylene cover versus polyethylene cover with artificial tear drop to prevent dry eye in critically ill patients: a randomized controlled clinical trial. *Clin Ophthalmol.* 2019;13:2203–2210.

43. Robinson JD. Management of refractory intracranial pressure. *Crit Care Nurs Clin North Am.* 2016;28(1):67–75. https://doi.org/10.1016/j.cnc.2015.09.004.

44. Oswal A, Toma AK. Intracranial pressure and cerebral haemodynamics. *Anesthesia and Intensive Care Medicine.* 2017;18(5):259–263. https://doi.org/10.1016/j.mpaic.2017.03.002.

45. Blissitt PA. Hemodynamic and intracranial dynamic monitoring in neurocritical care. In: Lough ME, ed. *Hemodynamic Monitoring: Evolving Technologies and Clinical Practice.* 1st ed. St Louis: Elsevier; 2016.

46. Perez-Barcena J, Llompart-Pou JA, O'Phelan KM. Intracranial pressure monitoring and management of intracranial hypertension. *Crit Care Clin.* 2014;30(4):735–750. https://doi.org/10.1016/j.ccc.2014.06.005.

47. Latorre JG, Greer DM. Management of acute intracranial hypertension: a review. *Neurol.* 2009;15(4):193–207. https://doi.org/10.1097/NRL.0b013e31819f956a.

48. Bhatia A, Gupta AK. Neuromonitoring in the intensive care unit. I. Intracranial pressure and cerebral blood flow monitoring. *Intens Care Med.* 2007;33(7):1263–1271. https://doi.org/10.1007/s00134-007-0678-z.

49. Curley G, Kavanagh BP, Laffey JG. Hypocapnia and the injured brain: more harm than benefit. *Crit Care Med.* 2010;38(5):1348–1359. https://doi.org/10.1097/CCM.0b013e3181d8cf2b.

50. Farrokh S, Cho SM, Suarez JI. Fluids and hyperosmolar agents in neurocritical care: an update. *Curr Opin Crit Care.* 2019;25(2):105–109. https://doi.org/10.1097/MCC.0000000000000585.

51. Abdelmalik PA, Draghic N, Ling GSF. Management of moderate and severe brain injury. *Transfusion.* 2019;59(S2):1529–1538. https://doi.org/10.1111/trf.15171.

52. Long G, Koyfman A. Secondary gains: advances in neurotrauma management. *Emerg Med Clin North Am.* 2018;36(1):107–133. https://doi.org/10.1016/j.emc.2017.08.007.

53. Hepburn-Smith M, Dynkevich I, Spektor M. Establishment of an external ventricular drain best practice guideline: the quest for a comprehensive, universal standard for external ventricular drain care. *J Neurosci Nurs.* 2016;48(1):54–65. https://doi.org/10.1097/JNN.0000000000000174.

54. Atkinson RA, Fikrey L, Vail A, Patel HC. Silver-impregnated external-ventricular-drain-related cerebrospinal fluid infections: a meta-analysis. *J Hosp Infect.* 2016;92(3):263–272. https://doi.org/10.1016/j.jhin.2015.09.014.

55. Stevens RD, Shoykhet M, Cadena R. Emergency neurological life support: intracranial hypertension and herniation. *Neurocrit Care.* 2015;23(suppl 2):S76–S82. https://doi.org/10.1007/s12028-015-0168-z.

56. Sacco TL, Delibert SA. Management of intracranial pressure: part 1: pharmacologic interventions. *Dimens Crit Care Nurs.* 2018;37(3):120–129. https://doi.org/10.1097/DCC.0000000000000293.

57. Murphy MP, Whitmore DM. Neurosurgery. In: Rothrock JC, McEwen DR, eds. *Alexander's Care of the Patient in Surgery.* 16th ed. St. Louis: Elsevier; 2019.

58. Miller BA, Ioachimescu AG, Oyesiku NM. Contemporary indications for transsphenoidal pituitary surgery. *World Neurosurg.* 2014;82(suppl 6):S147–S151. https://doi.org/10.1016/j.wneu.2014.07.037.

59. Yuan W. Managing the patient with transsphenoidal pituitary tumor resection. *J Neurosurg Nurs.* 2013;45(2):101–107. https://doi.org/10.1097/JNN.0b013e3182828e28.

60. Fugate JE. Complications of neurosurgery. *Continuum.* 2015;21(5 Neurocritical Care):1425–1444. https://doi.org/10.1212/CON.0000000000000227.

61. Hannon MJ, Finucane FM, Sherlock M, Agha A, Thompson CJ. Clinical review: disorders of water homeostasis in neurosurgical patients. *J Clin Endocrinol Metab.* 2012;97(5):1423–1433. https://doi.org/10.1210/jc.2011-320107.

62. Ausiello JC, Bruce JN, Freda PU. Postoperative assessment of the patient after transsphenoidal pituitary surgery. *Pituitary.* 2008;11(4):391–401. https://doi.org/10.1007/s11102-008-0086-6.

63. Daele JJ, Goffart Y, Machiels S. Traumatic, iatrogenic, and spontaneous cerebrospinal fluid (CSF) leak: endoscopic repair. *B-ENT.* 2011;7(suppl 17):47–60.

64. Ganau M, Prisco L, Cebula H, et al. Risk of deep vein thrombosis in neurosurgery: state of the art on prophylaxis protocols and best clinical practices. *J Clin Neurosci.* 2017;45:60–66. https://doi.org/10.1016/j.jocn.2017.08.008.

65. Schneck MJ. Venous thromboembolism in neurologic disease. *Handb Clin Neurol.* 2014;119:289–304. https://doi.org/10.1016/B978-0-7020-4086-3.00020-5.

66. O'Brien A, Redley B, Wood B, Botti M, Hutchinson AF. STOPDVTs: development and testing of a clinical assessment tool to guide nursing assessment of postoperative patients for deep vein thrombosis. *J Clin Nurs*. 2018;27(9–10):1803–1811. https://doi.org/10.1111/jocn. 14329.

67. Anderson DR, Morgano GP, Bennett C, et al. American Society of Hematology 2019 guidelines for management of venous thromboembolism: prevention of venous thromboembolism in surgical hospitalized patients.

Blood Adv. 2019;3(23):3898–3944. https://doi.org/10.1182/bloodadvances. 2019000975.

68. Ban VS, Bhoja R, McDonagh DL. Multimodal analgesia for craniotomy. *Curr Opin Anaesthesiol*. 2019;32(5):592–599. https://doi.org/10.1097/ACO. 0000000000000766.

69. Dashti SR, Baharvahdat H, Spetzler RF, et al. Operative intracranial infection following craniotomy. *Neurosurg Focus*. 2008;24(6):E10. https:// doi.org/10.3171/FOC/2008/24/6/E10.

18

Kidney Clinical Assessment and Diagnostic Procedures

Kimberly Sanchez

HISTORY

The history begins with a description of the chief complaint or primary problem stated in the patient's own words. A description of the chief complaint includes the onset, location, duration, and factors or strategies that lessen or aggravate the problem.[1]

Predisposing factors for acute kidney dysfunction are obtained during the history, including the use of over-the-counter medicines, recent infections requiring antibiotic therapy, antihypertensive medicines, and any diagnostic procedures performed using radiopaque contrast dye.[2] Nonsteroidal antiinflammatory drugs (NSAIDs, e.g., ibuprofen), antibiotics (especially aminoglycosides), antihypertensives (especially medicines that block angiotensin),[3] and iodine-based dyes may cause an acute or chronic decline in kidney function. A history of recent onset of nausea and vomiting or appetite loss caused by taste changes (uremia often causes a metallic taste) may provide clues to the rapid onset of kidney problems.[2] Symptoms that indicate rapid fluid volume gains are explored. For example, weight gains of more than 1 kg/day, sleeping on additional pillows, and sitting in a chair to sleep are signals of volume overload and potential cardiac stress related to kidney dysfunction. Fluid volume overload and edema are frequent findings in severe critical illness related to systemic inflammation, fluid loss from capillaries, volume administration, and acute kidney injury (AKI).[4] Box 18.1 summarizes the information gained from a kidney history.

PRIORITY CLINICAL ASSESSMENT

Inspection

Bleeding

Visual inspection related to the kidneys focuses on the patient's flank and abdomen. Kidney trauma is suspected if a purplish discoloration is present on the flank (Grey-Turner sign) or near the posterior 11th or 12th ribs. Bruising, abdominal distention, and abdominal guarding may also signal kidney trauma or a hematoma around a kidney. Individuals who have experienced a traumatic injury should be carefully assessed for signs of kidney trauma.[1]

Volume

Inspection is especially helpful in looking for signs of volume depletion or overload that may signal or lead to kidney problems. Fluid volume assessment begins with an inspection of the patient's jugular neck veins. The supine position facilitates normal jugular venous distention. An absence of distention (flat neck veins) indicates hypovolemia. Assessment continues with the head of the bed elevated 45 to 90 degrees.[1] Fluid overload exists when the neck veins remain distended more than 2 cm above the sternal notch when the bed is at 45 degrees.[2]

Inspection of the veins of the hand may be helpful in assessing volume status and is performed by observing for venous distention when the hand is held in the dependent position. Venous filling that takes longer than 5 seconds suggests hypovolemia. When the hand is elevated, the distention should disappear within 5 seconds. If distention does not disappear within 5 seconds after the hand is elevated, fluid overload is suspected.

Assessment of skin turgor provides additional data for identifying fluid-related problems. To assess turgor, the skin over the forearm is picked up and released. Normal elasticity and fluid status allow an almost immediate return to shape after the skin is released. In the presence of fluid volume deficit, the skin remains raised and does not return to its normal position for several seconds. Because of the loss of skin elasticity in older persons, skin turgor assessment may not be an accurate fluid assessment measure for this age group.[5]

Inspection of the oral cavity provides clues to fluid volume status. When a fluid volume deficit exists, the mucous membranes of the mouth become dry. However, mouth breathing and some medicines (e.g., antihistamines) can also dry the mucous membranes temporarily. The most accurate way to assess the oral cavity is to inspect the mouth using a tongue blade and light. Dryness of the oral cavity is more indicative of fluid volume deficit than complaints of a dry mouth.

Edema

Edema is the presence of excess fluid in the interstitial space, and it can be a sign of volume overload. In the presence of volume excess, edema may develop in the lungs and in dependent areas of the body, such as

BOX 18.1 DATA COLLECTION

Kidney History
Common Kidney-Related Symptoms
- Dyspnea
- Peripheral-dependent edema
- Nocturia
- Nausea
- Metallic taste in mouth
- Loss of appetite
- Headache
- Rapid weight gain
- Itching
- Dry, scaly skin
- Weakness, fatigue
- Cognitive function changes
- Mental status changes

Patient Profile
- Use of over-the-counter medications, herbs, vitamins, and dietary supplements
- Illicit drug use
- Change in employment caused by illness
- Financial problems resulting from illness (financial cost, time off work)
- Sexual function (decreased libido, amenorrhea)

Risk Factors
- Family history
- Hypertension
- Diabetes mellitus
- Prior acute kidney injury

Medical History
Child
- Nephrotic syndrome, streptococcal infection, hypoplastic kidneys, obstructive uropathy

Adult
- Frequent urinary tract infections
- Calculi
- Vasculitis
- Use of iodine-based radiographic contrast media
- Use of nonsteroidal antiinflammatory medications

Family History
- Hypertension
- Diabetes mellitus
- Polycystic kidney disease
- Kidney disease
- Chronically swollen extremities

Current Medication Use
- Nonsteroidal antiinflammatory medications
- Antibiotics
- Antihypertensives
- Diuretics

Past Kidney Studies
- Urinalysis with proteinuria
- Creatinine clearance
- Kidney-ureter-bladder (KUB) radiograph
- Intravenous pyelogram
- Kidney ultrasound
- Renal arteriography
- Kidney biopsy

---

the feet and legs of an ambulatory person or the sacrum of an individual confined to bed. However, edema does not always indicate fluid volume overload. A loss of albumin from the vascular space can cause peripheral edema despite hypovolemia or normal fluid states. A critically ill patient may have a low serum albumin level (hypoalbuminemia) because of inadequate nutrition after surgery, a burn, or a head injury and may exhibit edema as a result of the loss of plasma oncotic pressure and not as a result of volume overload. Edema also may signal circulatory difficulties. An individual who is fluid balanced but who has poor venous return may experience pedal edema after prolonged sitting in a chair with the feet dependent. Similarly, an individual with heart failure may experience edema because the left ventricle is unable to pump blood effectively through the vessels. A key feature that distinguishes edema resulting from excess volume or hypoalbuminemia from circulatory compromise is that the edema does not reverse with elevation of the extremity.

Edema can be assessed by applying fingertip pressure on the swollen area over a bony prominence, such as the ankles, pretibial areas (shins), and sacrum. If the indentation made by the fingertip does not disappear within 15 seconds, pitting edema exists. Pitting edema indicates increased interstitial volume, and it usually is not evident until significant weight gain has occurred. Edema also may appear in the hands and feet, around the eyes, and in the cheeks. In patients confined to a wheelchair or bed, dependent areas such as the feet and sacrum are most likely to demonstrate edema. One way of

measuring the extent of edema is by using a subjective scale of 1 to 4, with 1 indicating only minimal pitting and 4 indicating severe pitting (Table 18.1).[1] Other scales for assessing and measuring edema also can be used (see Table 10.2).

Auscultation

Auscultation of the kidneys yields virtually no useful information. However, the renal arteries are auscultated for a bruit, a blowing or swishing sound that resembles a cardiac murmur (Fig. 18.1). The examiner listens for bruits above and to the left and right of the umbilicus.[1] A renal artery bruit usually indicates stenosis, which may lead to acute or chronic kidney dysfunction secondary to compromised blood flow to one or both kidneys. A bruit over the upper portion of the abdominal aorta may indicate an aneurysm or a stenotic area that can decrease blood flow to the kidneys.

TABLE 18.1 Pitting Edema Scale

Rating	Approximate Equivalent
+1	2-mm depth
+2	4-mm depth (lasting up to 15 seconds)
+3	6-mm depth (lasting up to 60 seconds)
+4	8-mm depth (lasting longer than 60 seconds)

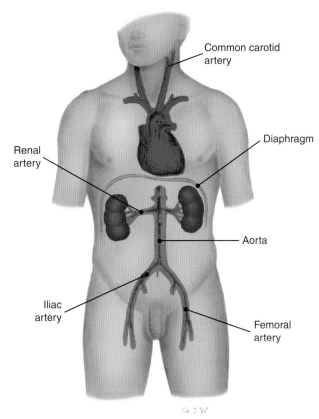

Common carotid artery

Diaphragm

Renal artery

Aorta

Iliac artery

Femoral artery

G J W

Fig. 18.1 Sites for Auscultation of Bruits.

Heart

Auscultation of the heart requires assessing the rate and rhythm and listening for extra sounds. Fluid overload is often accompanied by a third or fourth heart sound, which is best heard with the bell of the stethoscope.[1] Increased heart rate alone provides little information about fluid volume, but combined with a low blood pressure, it may indicate hypovolemia. The heart is auscultated for the presence of a pericardial friction rub. A rub can best be heard at the third intercostal space to the left of the sternal border while the patient leans slightly forward.[1] A pericardial friction rub indicates pericarditis that can occur with uremia (elevated blood urea) in kidney failure.

Blood Pressure

Blood pressure and heart rate changes are very useful in assessing fluid volume deficit.[3] In stable critically ill patients or in patients on a telemetry unit, orthostatic vital sign measurements provide clues to blood loss, dehydration, unexplained syncope, and the effects of some antihypertensive medications. A decrease in systolic blood pressure of 20 mm Hg or more, a decrease in diastolic blood pressure of 10 mm Hg or more, or an increase in pulse rate of more than 15 beats/min from lying to sitting or from sitting to standing indicates orthostatic hypotension. Box 18.2 describes how to assess for orthostatic hypotension. The decrease in blood pressure occurs because insufficient preload is available immediately as the patient changes position. The heart rate increases in an attempt to maintain cardiac output and circulation. Orthostatic hypotension produces subjective feelings of weakness, dizziness, or faintness. Orthostatic hypotension occurs with hypovolemia, prolonged bed rest, or as a side effect of medications that affect blood volume or blood pressure.

Lungs

Lung assessment is essential in gauging fluid status. Crackles indicate fluid overload. Dyspnea with mild exertion, dyspnea at night that prevents sleeping in a supine position (orthopnea), or dyspnea that awakens the individual from sleep (paroxysmal nocturnal dyspnea) may indicate pooling of fluid in the lungs. Shallow, gasping breaths with periods of apnea reflect severe acid–base imbalances. See Chapter 13 for further information on auscultation of the lungs.

Palpation

Although rarely performed in critically ill patients, palpation of the kidneys in stable patients provides information about the size and shape of the kidneys. Palpation of the kidneys is done through the bimanual capturing approach. Capturing is accomplished by placing one hand posteriorly under the flank of a supine patient with the examiner's fingers pointing to the midline and placing the opposite hand just below the rib cage anteriorly.[1,2] The patient is asked to inhale deeply while pressure is exerted to bring the hands together (Fig. 18.2). As the patient exhales, the examiner may feel the kidney between the hands. After each kidney is palpated in this manner, the two kidneys should be compared for size and shape. Each kidney should be firm and smooth, and the two organs should be of equal size. The examiner is usually unable to palpate a normal left kidney. The right kidney is more easily palpated because of its lower position, caused by

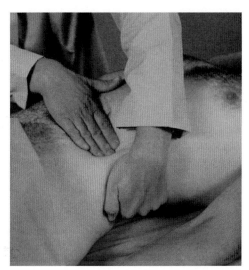

Fig. 18.2 Palpation of the Kidney. (From Barkauskas V, Baumann L, Darling-Fisher C. *Health and Physical Assessment*. 3rd ed. St. Louis: Mosby; 2002.)

downward displacement by the liver. Problems should be suspected if a mass (cancer) or an irregular surface (polycystic kidneys) is palpated, a size difference is detected, the kidney extends significantly lower than the rib cage on either side, or there is evidence of recent blunt trauma.[1]

Percussion

Percussion is performed to detect pain in the area of a kidney or to determine excess accumulation of air, fluid, or solids around the kidneys. Percussion of the kidneys also provides information about kidney location, size, and possible problems. Similar to palpation, percussion of the kidneys is not a routine part of a nursing assessment in critical care.

Kidneys

Percussion of a kidney is performed with the patient in a side-lying or sitting position, with the examiner's hand placed over the costo-vertebral angle (lower border of the rib cage on the flank).[1] Striking the back of the hand with the opposite fist produces a dull thud, which is normal. Pain may indicate infection (e.g., urinary tract infection that has extended into the kidneys) or injury resulting from trauma. Traumatic injury to the kidneys should be assessed in the presence of a penetrating abdominal wound, blunt abdominal trauma, or a fractured pelvis or ribs.

Abdomen

Observation and percussion of the abdomen may help in assessing fluid status. Percussing the abdomen with the patient in the supine position generally yields a dull sound (solid bowel contents or fluid) or a hollow sound (gaseous bowel).[1]

Ascites, or excess fluid accumulation and distention of the abdominal cavity, is an important observation in determining fluid overload. Differentiating ascites from distortion caused by solid bowel contents is accomplished by producing a fluid wave. A fluid wave is elicited by exerting pressure to the abdominal midline while one hand is placed on the right or left flank.[1] Tapping the opposite flank produces a wave in the accumulated fluid that can be felt under the hands (Fig. 18.3). Other signs of ascites include a protuberant, rounded

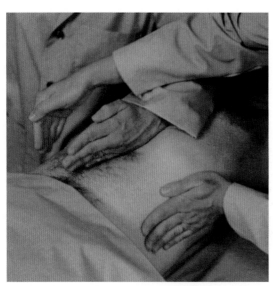

Fig. 18.3   Test for the Presence of a Fluid Wave. (From Barkauskas V, Baumann L, Darling-Fisher C. *Health and Physical Assessment*. 3rd ed. St. Louis: Mosby; 2002.)

abdomen and abdominal striae.[1] Individuals with kidney failure may have ascites caused by volume overload, which forces fluid into the abdomen as a result of increased capillary hydrostatic pressures. However, ascites may or may not represent fluid volume excess. Severe ascites in patients with compromised liver function may result from decreased plasma proteins. The ascites occurs because the increased vascular pressure associated with liver dysfunction forces fluid and plasma proteins from the vascular space into the interstitial space and abdominal cavity. Although the patient may exhibit marked edema, the intravascular space is volume depleted, and the patient is hypovolemic.

LABORATORY STUDIES

There is no single or ideal laboratory test or marker that detects a decrease in kidney function. Laboratory tests used to detect and diagnose kidney dysfunction have limitations, but when reviewed daily for changes or trends, they provide valuable information concerning the status of the kidneys.[6] AKI must be identified as early as possible because it is associated with significant mortality in critically ill patients.[7]

Blood Urea Nitrogen

Blood urea nitrogen (BUN) is a byproduct of protein and amino acid metabolism. The normal value for BUN is 5 to 20 mg/dL; this value is increased when kidney function deteriorates. With kidney dysfunction, the BUN is elevated because of a decrease in the glomerular filtration rate (GFR) and resulting decrease in urea excretion. Elevations in the BUN can be correlated with the clinical manifestations of uremia; as BUN increases, symptoms of uremia become more pronounced.[2] However, a decrease in the GFR with an increase in the BUN also may be caused by hypovolemia and dehydration, nephrotoxic medications, or a sudden hypotensive episode. In these cases, the increase in BUN is caused by a decreased GFR in the presence of normal kidney function. BUN is also increased by changes in protein metabolism that occur with excessive protein intake and catabolism. A catabolic state may occur with starvation (or chronic poor nutrition in a critically ill patient), severe infection, surgery, or trauma. The BUN level also may be elevated as the result of hematoma resorption, gastrointestinal bleeding, excessive licorice ingestion, or steroid or tetracycline therapy. A decrease in the BUN level may indicate volume overload, liver damage, severe malnutrition (as a result of depleted protein stores), use of phenothiazines, or pregnancy.

Creatinine

Creatinine is a byproduct of muscle and normal cell metabolism, and it appears in serum in amounts generally proportional to the body muscle mass. The normal serum creatinine level is approximately 0.5 to 1.2 mg/dL; this value is slightly higher in men than women. Creatinine is freely filtered by the glomerulus and minimally resorbed or secreted in the tubules.[2] Creatinine levels are fairly constant and are affected by fewer factors than BUN levels. As a result, the serum creatinine level is a more sensitive and specific indicator of kidney function than BUN.

Creatinine excess occurs most often in patients with kidney failure resulting from impaired excretion. However, the body's production and release of creatinine may vary during muscle wasting in acute illness, leading to a falsely low serum level of creatinine. Elevated levels of creatinine are seen in muscle growth disorders such as acromegaly, with traumatic skeletal muscle injury, and with some medications that decrease creatinine removal (e.g., trimethoprim, cimetidine) in the absence of kidney dysfunction. Malnutrition can result in transient increases in creatinine levels, as the rapid muscle catabolism associated with malnutrition releases increased amounts of creatinine into the circulation.

Blood Urea Nitrogen-to-Creatinine Ratio

Another useful diagnostic parameter in kidney disease is the ratio of BUN to creatinine. The usual ratio of BUN to creatinine is 10:1, and a change in the ratio may indicate kidney dysfunction. For example, if BUN and creatinine levels are elevated and maintained at an approximate ratio of 10:1, the disorder is intrarenal, or affecting the tubules of the kidneys. If the ratio of BUN to creatinine levels is greater than 10:1, the cause is most likely prerenal (e.g., hypovolemia). In prerenal kidney failure, the creatinine is excreted by functioning tubules, but the urea nitrogen is retained because of the poor GFR and hemoconcentration, leading to the increased ratio. In the diagnosis of prerenal kidney failure, the ratio is a more useful indicator of kidney function than the separate tests of BUN and creatinine.[5]

Creatinine Clearance

The urine creatinine clearance is a measure of how well the kidneys remove creatinine. Because of the relatively constant rate at which creatinine is produced and the nearly complete removal of creatinine by normal kidneys, the ability of the kidneys to remove (clear) creatinine from the blood is an indication of how well the glomeruli and tubules are working. Measuring the creatinine clearance, the amount of creatinine in the excreted urine and the amount of creatinine in the blood over 24 hours, provides a reliable and accurate estimate of glomerular filtration and of kidney function.[2] The normal value for creatinine clearance is 110 to 120 mL/min; values less than 50 mL/min indicate significant kidney dysfunction. The creatinine clearance is traditionally measured using a 12-hour or 24-hour urine collection and blood sample. Newer methods use a random, smaller volume urine specimen and blood sample.

Creatinine clearance can also be estimated from the serum creatinine level (Box 18.3), a method commonly used in the critical care

unit. The estimated or calculated creatinine clearance is widely used to determine changes in medication dosing with kidney dysfunction because of the many medications excreted by the kidneys.

Osmolality

The serum osmolality reflects the concentration or dilution of vascular fluid and measures the dissolved particles in the serum. The normal serum osmolality is 275 to 295 mOsm/L.[3] An elevated osmolality level indicates hemoconcentration or dehydration, and a decreased osmolality level indicates hemodilution or volume overload. When the serum osmolality level increases, antidiuretic hormone (ADH) is released from the posterior pituitary gland and stimulates increased water resorption in the kidney tubules. This expands the vascular space, returns the serum osmolality level back to normal, and results in more concentrated urine and an elevated urine osmolality level. The opposite occurs with a decreased serum osmolality level, which inhibits the production of ADH. The decreased ADH results in increased excretion of water in the tubules, producing dilute urine with a low osmolality, and returns the serum osmolality level back to normal. Sodium accounts for 85% to 95% of the serum osmolality value; doubling the serum sodium level gives an estimate of the serum osmolality level in healthy individuals. Other particles in the serum can increase the osmolality and need to be considered in patients with common comorbid conditions.

A more precise estimation of serum osmolality can be calculated from this formula:

$$2 \times Na(mEq/L) + BUN/3(mg/dL) + Glucose/18(mg/dL)$$

The calculated serum osmolality level is a useful tool while awaiting full laboratory results.

Measured serum osmolality is a useful parameter in determining fluid balance and fluid replacement therapy for critically ill patients. Serum osmolality is also a useful parameter in determining disorders of ADH secretion that may occur in critically ill patients. A decreased serum osmolality level may indicate syndrome of inappropriate ADH secretion, or too much ADH, whereas an elevation of the serum osmolality level may indicate diabetes insipidus, or too little ADH.

Anion Gap

The *anion gap* is a calculation of the difference between the measurable extracellular plasma cations (sodium and potassium) and the measurable anions (chloride and bicarbonate).[3] In plasma, sodium is the predominant cation, and chloride is the predominant anion.

Extracellular potassium concentration in plasma is so small that it is generally ignored, leaving this equation for calculation of the anion gap:

$$Na^+ - (Cl^- + HCO^{-3})$$

The normal anion gap is 8 to 16 mEq/L, a range that has been verified in a healthy population of adults.[8] The "gap" represents the unmeasurable ions present in the extracellular fluid (phosphates, sulfates, ketones, lactate). An increased anion gap level usually reflects overproduction or decreased excretion of acid products and indicates metabolic acidosis; a decreased anion gap indicates metabolic alkalosis.

Acute and chronic kidney failure can increase the anion gap because of retention of acids and altered bicarbonate resorption. The anion gap is also increased in diabetic ketoacidosis caused by ketone production. The measurement of the anion gap is a rapid method for identifying acid–base imbalance but cannot be used to pinpoint the source of the acid–base disturbance specifically.

BOX 18.3 Creatinine Clearance Calculations[a]

Measured: 24-Hour Urine
(Urine creatinine × Volume of urine)/Serum creatinine

Estimated: Adults—Cockcroft-Gault Formula
[(140 − Age) × Body weight (kg)] / [72 × Plasma creatinine (mg/dL)]
For women, multiply the result by 0.85.

Estimated: Adults—Modification of Diet in Renal Disease (MDRD) Formula
186 × Plasma creatinine − 1.154 × Age in years − 0.203
For women, multiply the result by 0.742.
For African Americans, multiply the result by 1.210.[b]

Estimated: Children
<10 kg: 0.45 × Height (cm)/Serum creatinine (mg/dL)
10-70 kg: 0.55 × Height (cm)/Serum creatinine (mg/dL)
>70 kg: [1.55 × Age (y)] + [0.5 × Height (cm)/Serum creatinine (mg/dL)]

[a]Online calculators available from the National Kidney Foundation at http://www.kidney.org/professionals.
[b]Both risk factor assessments apply for African American women. The number would be multiplied by both 0.742 (woman) and 1.210 (African American).

Hemoglobin and Hematocrit

The hemoglobin and hematocrit levels can indicate increases or decreases in intravascular fluid volume.

An increase in the hematocrit value often indicates a fluid volume deficit, which results in hemoconcentration. Conversely, a decreased hematocrit value can indicate fluid volume excess because of the dilutional effect of the extra fluid load. Decreases also can result from blood loss, liver damage, or hemolytic reactions. A decreased hematocrit level may indicate the anemia of kidney failure or may reflect fluid volume overload. If the hematocrit value is decreasing but the hemoglobin concentration remains constant, the cause is fluid volume overload. Decreased hematocrit values and hemoglobin concentrations indicate a true loss of RBCs. Anemia is a frequent finding in patients with kidney failure, complicating management in critical illness.

Urinalysis

Analysis of the urine provides excellent information about the patient's kidney function and condition relative to fluids and electrolytes. Specific tests and abnormal indications are presented in Table 18.2. In a critically ill patient, a routine urinalysis specimen may be obtained to rule out the presence of urinary protein or glucose. A sterile urine culture may be obtained if a urinary tract infection is suspected.

DIAGNOSTIC PROCEDURES

Weight Monitoring

One of the most important assessments of kidney and fluid status is the patient's weight. In the critical care unit, weight is monitored for each patient every day and is an important vital sign measurement. Significant fluctuations in body weight over a 1- to 2-day period indicate fluid gains and losses. Rapid weight gains or losses of more than 1 kg/day usually indicate fluid rather than nutritional factors; 1 L of fluid equals 1 kg, or approximately 2.2 lb.

Whenever possible, the patient is weighed during admission to the critical care unit. It is important to document whether the current weight differs significantly from the weight 1 to 2 weeks before admission to the hospital. The patient is weighed daily for comparison with the previous day's weight. The weight is obtained at the same time each day, with the patient wearing the same amount of clothing and using the same scale.

Intake and Output Monitoring

Similar to patient weight, intake and output are monitored for all patients in the critical care unit. Intake and output can be compared with the patient's weight to evaluate fluid gains or losses more accurately.[9] Urinary output plus insensible fluid losses (perspiration, stool, and water vapor from the lungs) can vary by 750 to 2400 mL/day. When intake exceeds output (e.g., excessive intravenous fluid, decreased urine output), a positive fluid balance exists. With impaired kidney function, the positive fluid balance results in fluid volume overload. Conversely, if output exceeds intake (e.g., fever, increased respiration, profuse sweating, vomiting, diarrhea, gastric suction, diuretic therapy), a negative fluid balance exists, and volume deficit results. During a 24-hour period, fever can increase skin and respiratory losses by 75 mL/1°F increase in temperature.

Individuals with AKI often exhibit a decrease in urine output, or oliguria (less than 0.5 mL/kg per hour in adults; less than 1 mL/kg per hour in infants and young children). However, there may be a normal or only slightly decreased urine output that reflects water removal without solute removal in the early phases of AKI. Although urine output is a sensitive indicator, kidney function cannot be accurately determined by urine output alone. For additional information on AKI, see Chapter 19.

Abnormal output of body fluids creates fluid imbalances and causes electrolyte and acid–base disturbances. For example, gastrointestinal suction or loss by diarrhea can result in fluid deficit, sodium and potassium deficits, and metabolic acidosis from excessive loss of bicarbonate. In maintaining daily records of intake and output, all gains or losses must be recorded. A standard list of the fluid volume held in various containers (e.g., milk cartons, juice containers) expedites this process. Discussions about the importance of accurate recording of intake and output with the patient and family or friends are necessary and can improve the accuracy of assessment of intake and output volumes.

Hemodynamic Monitoring

Body fluid status is indirectly reflected in cardiovascular hemodynamic values.[10] A central venous catheter may be inserted to measure the CVP, which represents the filling pressure of the right atrium and is a measurement of right ventricular preload. A normal CVP is 2 to 5 mm Hg. Traditionally the CVP has been used to assess volume status in critical illness, although this practice has now been called into question as discussed under Central Venous Pressure Monitoring in Chapter 10.

Mean arterial pressure (MAP) is regulated by cardiac output and systemic vascular resistance (SVR) and represents an averaged blood pressure within the arterial system. Changes in cardiac output or SVR inevitably result in corresponding MAP changes. For example, an increase in SVR during the early stages of hypovolemic shock leads to elevation of the MAP. Ongoing fluid losses eventually lead to decreased cardiac output, which leads to a reduction in MAP. The net effect of a decreased MAP on the kidneys is a reduction in effective blood flow, which can lead to AKI.

Imaging Studies

Although laboratory assessment is used most often in diagnosing kidney problems in critically ill patients, imaging studies can confirm or clarify causes of particular disorders. Imaging assessment includes the use of ultrasound and radiologic techniques. Ultrasound is a noninvasive imaging technique that is available in most hospitals. Kidney ultrasound is especially useful in determining the size, shape, and contour of the kidneys; the presence of masses or cysts; and the presence of renal artery stenosis.[11] Radiologic assessment ranges from basic to more complex (Table 18.3) and provides information about abnormal masses, abnormal fluid collections, obstructions, vascular supply alterations, and other disorders of the kidneys and urinary tract.[11] Some radiologic studies require the use of a contrast agent or injection of a radiopaque dye.

Because contrast agents used in radiology are potentially nephrotoxic, a thorough evaluation of the patient history is vital to avoid contrast-induced kidney injury. Patients with the highest risk have preexisting kidney injury; have a creatine above 1.5 mg/dL; are older than 75 years; take medications such as NSAIDs, diuretics, angiotensin-converting enzyme inhibitors, angiotensin II receptor blockers; and receive a large contrast load.[11] To prevent contrast-induced nephrotoxicity, adequate hydration before and after the test and careful monitoring of kidney function are always indicated.

Kidney Biopsy

The increase in kidney imaging has led to an increase in the detection of kidney tumors, some benign and some cancerous. Kidney biopsy is

TABLE 18.2   Urinalysis Results

Test	Normal	Possible Causes for High Urine Values	Possible Causes for Low Urine Values
pH	4.5–8.0	Alkalosis (high PH)	Acidosis (low pH)
			Intrarenal AKI
Specific gravity	1.003–1.030[a]	Volume deficit, dehydration (concentrated urine)	Volume overload: dilute urine with normal kidneys
		Glycosuria	Diabetes insipidus (SG <1.005)
		Proteinuria	
		Prerenal AKI (SG >1.020)	
Osmolality	300–1200	Volume deficit/dehydration (concentrated urine)	Volume overload/dilute urine with normal kidney function
	mOsm/kg	Prerenal AKI (urine osmolality >serum osmolality)	Intrarenal AKI (urine osmolality <serum osmolality)
		SIADH (urine osmolality >serum osmolality)	Diabetes insipidus (urine osmolality <serum osmolality)
Protein	30–150 mg/24 h[b]	Trauma	Negative for protein is normal
		Infection	
		Intrarenal AKI	
		Glomerulonephritis	
Glucose	Absent	Diabetes mellitus	Negative for glucose is normal
Ketones	Absent	DKA	Negative for ketones is normal
		Starvation	
Sodium	40–220 mEq/24 h	High-sodium diet	Adrenal gland(s) release excess aldosterone
		Intrarenal AKI	Dehydration or diarrhea
Creatinine	1–2 g/24 h	Large muscle mass	Kidney failure, as kidneys cannot excrete creatinine
Urea	6–17 g/24 h	AKI	
Bilirubin	Absent	Liver failure	Negative for bilirubin is normal
Myoglobin	Absent	Crush injury	Negative for myoglobin is normal
		Rhabdomyolysis	
Urobilinogen	0.5–1.0 mg/dL	Hemolysis	Biliary tract obstruction
RBCs	0–5[c]	Crush injury	Negative for RBCs is normal
		Trauma	
		Infection	
		Intrarenal AKI	
		Renal artery thrombosis	
		Coagulopathy	
WBCs	0–5[c]	UTI/CAUTI	Negative for WBCs is normal
		Infection	
		Inflammation	
Leukocyte esterase	Absent	UTI/CAUTI	Negative for leukocyte esterase is normal
		Infection	
Nitrites	Absent	UTI/CAUTI	Negative for nitrates is normal
		Infection	
Bacteria	Absent	UTI/CAUTI	Negative for bacteria is normal, with the exception of
		Infection	asymptomatic bacteriuria[d]
		Pyelonephritis	
		Asymptomatic bacteriuria[d]	
Casts	Few to none	Glomerular disease	Negative for casts is normal
Epithelial cells	<15–20[c]	Glomerular disease	A small number of epithelial cells is normal
		Nephrotic syndrome	

[a]Adult value; newborn value is slightly lower at 1.001–1.020.
[b]Higher values usually apply for persons after strenuous exercise and are transient; lower values at rest.
[c]Cells per high-power field. The number of epithelial cells may be described quantitatively as the number visible in the microscope field, or qualitatively as low, moderate, or high in a urine sample.
[d]Asymptomatic bacteriuria (ASB) describes one or multiple species of bacteria in the urine ($\geq 10^5$ colony-forming units [CFU]/mL or $\geq 10^8$ CFU/L), without signs or symptoms associated with urinary tract infection (UTI).
AKI, Acute kidney injury; CAUTI, catheter-associated urinary tract infection; DKA, diabetic ketoacidosis; RBC, red blood cell; SG, specific gravity; SIADH, syndrome of inappropriate antidiuretic hormone; UTI, urinary tract infection; WBC, white blood cell.

TABLE 18.3	Kidney Imaging Tests
Test	**Comments**
KUB radiograph	Flat-plate radiograph of abdomen; determines position, size, and structure of kidneys, urinary tract, and pelvis; useful for evaluating the presence of calculi and masses; usually followed by additional tests
IVP	Intravenous injection of contrast agent with radiography; allows visualization of internal kidney tissues
Angiography	Injection of contrast agent into arterial blood perfusing kidneys; allows visualization of renal blood flow; may also visualize stenosis, cysts, clots, trauma, and infarctions
CT	Radioisotope is administered by intravenous route and absorbed by kidneys; scintillation photography is performed in several planes; spiral or helical CT allows rapid imaging; density of image helps evaluate kidney vessels, perfusion, tumors, cysts, stones/calculi, hemorrhage, necrosis, and trauma
Ultrasound	High-frequency sound waves are transmitted to kidneys and urinary tract and image is viewed on oscilloscope; noninvasive; identifies fluid accumulation or obstruction, cysts, stones/calculi, and masses; useful for evaluating kidney before biopsy
MRI	Scanner produces three-dimensional images in response to application of high-energy radiofrequency waves to tissues; produces clear images; density of image may indicate trauma, cysts, masses, malformation of vessels or tubules, stones/calculi, and necrosis

CT, Computed tomography; *IVP,* intravenous pyelogram; *KUB,* kidney-ureter-bladder; *MRI,* magnetic resonance imaging.

the definitive tool for diagnosing disease processes involving the parenchyma of the kidney. Percutaneous needle biopsy involves inserting a needle through the flank to obtain a specimen of cortical and medullary kidney tissue.

Some small tumors are amenable to ablation. An open biopsy is a surgical procedure and is rarely done in critically ill patients. Biopsy is the last choice for diagnostic assessment in critically ill patients because of the periprocedural risks of bleeding, hematoma, and infection.

ADDITIONAL RESOURCES

See Box 18.4 for Internet resources related to kidney clinical assessment and diagnostic procedures.

QSEN

BOX 18.4   Informatics

Internet Resources: Kidney Clinical Assessment and Diagnostic Procedures
- National Kidney Foundation: https://www.kidney.org/
- National Institute of Diabetes and Digestive and Kidney Diseases: https://www.niddk.nih.gov/
- International Society of Nephrology: https://www.theisn.org/
- American Society of Nephrology: https://www.asn-online.org/
- American Nephrology Nurses Association: https://www.annanurse.org/

REFERENCES

1. Ball J, Dains J, Flynn J, Solomon B, Stewart R. *Seidel's Guide to Physical Examination.* 9th ed. St. Louis: Elsevier; 2019.
2. American Association of Nephrology Nurses Association (ANNA). *Core Curriculum for Nephrology Nursing.* 6th ed. Pitman, NJ: American Nephrology Nurses Association; 2015.
3. Nelson DA, Marks ES, Deuster PA, O'Connor FG, Kurina LM. Association of nonsteroidal anti-inflammatory drug prescriptions with kidney disease among active young and middle-aged adults. *JAMA Netw Open.* 2019;2(2):e187896.
4. Ekinci C, Karabork M, Siriopol D, Dincer N, Covic A, Kanbay M. Effects of volume overload and current techniques for the assessment of fluid status in patients with renal disease. *Blood Purif.* 2018;46:34−47.
5. Morley JE. Dehydration, hypernatremia, and hyponatremia. *Clin Geriatr Med.* 2015;31(3):389−399.
6. Kashani K, Rosner MH, Ostermann M. Creatinine: from physiology to clinical application. *Eur J Intern Med.* 2020;72:9−14.
7. Ronco C, Bellomo R, Kellum JA. Acute kidney injury. *Lancet.* 2019;394:1949−1964.
8. Farwell WR, Taylor EN. Serum anion gap, bicarbonate and biomarkers of inflammation in healthy individuals in a national survey. *Can Med Assoc J.* 2010;182:137.
9. Davies A, Srivastava S, Seligman W, et al. Prevention of acute kidney injury through accurate fluid balance monitoring. *BMJ Open Qual.* 2017;6(2):e000006.
10. Giglio M, Dalfino L, Puntillo F, Brienza N. Hemodynamic goal-directed therapy and postoperative kidney injury: an updated meta-analysis with trial sequential analysis. *Crit Care.* 2019;23:232.
11. Wymer DC, Wymer DT. Kidney imaging techniques. In: Lerna EV, Sparks MA, Toff JM, eds. *Nephrology Secrets.* 4th ed. Philadelphia: Elsevier; 2019.

19

Kidney Disorders and Therapeutic Management

Kimberly Sanchez

ACUTE KIDNEY INJURY

Description and Etiology

Acute kidney injury (AKI) describes the spectrum of acute-onset kidney disorders that can range from mild impairment of kidney function through acute kidney failure that requires renal replacement therapy (dialysis). AKI is characterized by a sudden increase in creatinine and an abrupt decline in urine output signaling a decrease in glomerular filtration rate (GFR) and retention of products in the blood that are normally excreted by the kidneys.[1] AKI disrupts electrolyte balance, acid–base homeostasis, and fluid volume equilibrium. A transition to use of the word *kidney* rather than *renal* reflects a trend in the nephrology literature that emphasizes the vulnerability of the kidney during critical illness.

Typically, a patient is not admitted to the critical care unit with a diagnosis of AKI alone; there is always coexisting hemodynamic, cardiac, pulmonary, or neurologic compromise. More than 50% of critically ill patients may have AKI in addition to a primary illness.[1,2] High-risk diagnoses include heart failure, shock, respiratory failure, and sepsis.[2] One-third of patients were mechanically ventilated, and half were on vasopressors at the time of AKI diagnosis.[2] Critical care patients with AKI have a higher mortality and more complications.[3] Mortality associated with AKI ranges from 10% to over 50% and is influenced by kidney recovery, with higher mortality associated with nonrecovery of the kidney.[1] The kidneys recover within 7 days in almost two-thirds of AKI cases[1]; if the kidneys do not recover, a diagnosis of kidney failure increases risk of death to 47%.[1] The most common causes of AKI were sepsis (40%), hypovolemia (34%), drug or medication related (14%), and cardiogenic shock (13%).[2] The picture of AKI in the modern critical care unit has changed to encompass patients with kidney injury who also have multisystem dysfunction that complicates their clinical course.[4]

Types of Acute Kidney Injury

Traditionally, AKI was classified by the location of the insult relative to kidney anatomy: prerenal (before), intrarenal (within), and postrenal (after). This classification is no longer commonly used, although it remains a useful way to describe the relationship between anatomy and functional insults to the kidney. The risk and susceptibility for the development of AKI are presented in Box 19.1. An overview of the possible outcomes of AKI is presented in Fig. 19.1.

Prerenal Acute Kidney Injury

Any condition that decreases blood flow, blood pressure, or kidney perfusion before arterial blood reaches the renal artery that supplies the kidney may be anatomically described as *prerenal AKI*. When arterial hypoperfusion secondary to low cardiac output, hemorrhage, vasodilation, thrombosis, or other cause reduces the blood flow to the kidney, glomerular filtration decreases, and consequently urine output decreases. This is a major reason the critical care nurse monitors urine output on an hourly basis. Initially, in prerenal states, the integrity of the kidney's nephron structure and function may be preserved. If normal perfusion and cardiac output are restored quickly, the kidney recovers with no permanent injury. However, if the prerenal insult is not corrected, GFR declines, blood urea nitrogen (BUN) concentration rises (prerenal azotemia), and the patient develops oliguria and is at risk for significant kidney damage.[5] Oliguria, defined as urine output less than 400 mL/day or urine output less than 0.5 mL/kg per hour, with an elevated serum creatinine, is a classic finding in AKI. Prerenal azotemia is associated with a lower mortality rate than other forms of AKI.

Intrarenal Acute Kidney Injury

Any condition that produces an ischemic or toxic insult directly at parenchymal nephron tissue places the patient at risk for development of intrarenal AKI. Ischemic damage may be caused by prolonged hypotension or low cardiac output. Toxic injury reaction may occur in response to substances that damage the kidney tubular endothelium, such as some antimicrobial medications and the contrast dye used in radiologic diagnostic studies. The insult may involve the glomeruli and the tubular epithelium. When the internal filtering structures are pathologically affected, the condition was previously known as *acute tubular necrosis*, but the newer term of *AKI* is now used.[5,6]

Postrenal Acute Kidney Injury

Any obstruction that hinders the flow of urine from beyond the kidney through the remainder of the urinary tract may lead to postrenal AKI. This is an uncommon cause of kidney failure in critically ill patients. When monitoring of the urine output reveals a sudden decrease in the patient's urine output from the urinary catheter, a blockage may be responsible. Sudden development of anuria (urine output less than 100 mL/24 h) should prompt verification that the urinary catheter is not occluded.

Assessment and Diagnosis

Measurement of kidney function is indirect, and the diagnosis of AKI is predominantly derived from changes in urine output and elevation of serum creatinine level, with the understanding that changes in these values reflect a decline in the GFR.

BOX 19.1 Acute Kidney Injury: Risk and Susceptibility

Critical Illness
- Sepsis
- Burns
- Trauma
- Diabetes mellitus
- Chronic kidney disease
- Advanced age

Prerenal Acute Kidney Injury Risk
- Prolonged hypotension (sepsis, vasodilation)
- Prolonged low cardiac output (heart failure, cardiogenic shock)
- Prolonged volume depletion (dehydration, hemorrhage)
- Renovascular thrombosis (thromboemboli)

Intrarenal Acute Kidney Injury Risk
- Kidney ischemia (advanced stage of prerenal acute kidney injury)
- Endogenous toxins (rhabdomyolysis, tumor lysis syndrome)
- Exogenous toxins (radiocontrast dye, nephrotoxic medications)
- Infection (acute glomerulonephritis, interstitial nephritis)

Postrenal Acute Kidney Injury Risk
- Obstruction (urethra, prostate, or bladder)
- Rare as a cause of acute kidney injury in critical care

Physical Assessment

Physical signs and symptoms are used to assess fluid balance. Signs that suggest extracellular fluid depletion include thirst, decreased skin turgor, and lethargy. Signs that imply intravascular fluid volume overload include pulmonary congestion, increasing heart failure, and rising blood pressure. A patient with untreated AKI is edematous. The following factors contribute to this state:

- Fluid retention caused by inadequate urine output
- Low serum albumin levels that create a lower oncotic pressure in the vasculature, causing more fluid to seep out into the interstitial spaces and cause peripheral edema
- Inflammation associated with AKI or a coexisting nonrenal disease that increases vascular permeability, facilitating fluid movement from the vessels into interstitial spaces

In critical illness, even though there is peripheral edema, and the patient may have gained 8 to 10 L of fluid over his or her "dry-weight" baseline, the patient may remain "intravascularly dry" and hemodynamically unstable because the retained fluid is not inside a vascular compartment and cannot contribute to maintenance of hemodynamic stability. A patient with AKI is assessed frequently for pitting edema over bony prominences and in dependent body areas.

Hemodynamic Monitoring

Hemodynamic monitoring is important for the analysis of fluid volume status in a critically ill patient with AKI. Hemodynamic monitoring includes surveillance of changes in vital signs, including cardiac output. The range of monitoring devices has expanded, and assessment may be continuous or intermittent and be invasive, minimally invasive, or noninvasive, as described in Chapter 10.

Daily Weight

A less "high-tech" but important monitoring method is a daily weight. The daily weight, combined with accurate intake and output monitoring, is a powerful indicator of fluid gains or losses over 24 hours. A 1-kg weight gain over 24 hours represents 1000 mL (1 L) of additional fluid retention.

Laboratory Studies

Both serum and urine laboratory values can be used to assess whether the AKI is at a prerenal stage or has already affected intrarenal function. The differences between prerenal and intrarenal laboratory values are listed in Table 19.1.

Serum creatinine. Creatinine is a by-product of muscle metabolism that is formed nonenzymatically from creatine in muscles. Creatinine

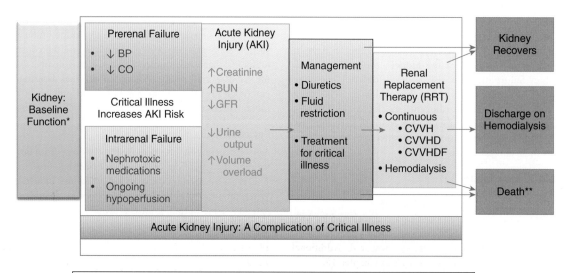

Fig. 19.1 Acute Kidney Injury in Critical Care Illness. *AKI,* Acute kidney injury; *BP,* blood pressure; *BUN,* blood urea nitrogen; *CO,* cardiac output; *CVVH,* continuous venovenous hemofiltration; *CVVHD,* continuous venovenous hemofiltration dialysis; *CVVHDF,* continuous venovenous hemodiafiltration; *GFR,* glomerular filtration rate.

TABLE 19.1 Initial Laboratory Urinalysis Findings in Acute Kidney Injury.[a]

Assessment	Prerenal[b]	Intrarenal[c]	Postrenal[d]
Urine volume	Normal	Oliguria or nonoliguria	Oliguria to anuria
Urine specific gravity	>1.020	1.010	1.000—1.010
Urine osmolality (mOsm/kg)	>350	<300	300—400
Urine sodium (mEq/L)	<20	>30	20—40
FENa (%)	<1%	>2%—3%	1%—3%
BUN/Cr ratio[e]	20:1	Ischemic: 20:1	10:1
		Toxic: 10:1	
Urine microscopy (sediment)	Normal	Dark granular casts, hyaline casts, kidney epithelial cells	Normal

[a]Results of urine laboratory tests are valid only in the absence of diuretics.
[b]Urine in prerenal failure is concentrated, with low sodium.
[c]Urine in intrarenal failure shows kidney damage because the nephron cannot concentrate urine or conserve sodium, and evidence of kidney damage (casts) is seen.
[d]Urine test results in postrenal failure vary because findings initially depend on the hydration status of the patient rather than the status of the kidney.
[e]The BUN/serum creatinine ratio is a blood test.
Anuria, Urine volume less than 100 mL/24 h; *BUN,* blood urea nitrogen; *Cr,* creatinine; *FENa,* fractional excretion of sodium; *oliguria,* urine volume of 100—400 mL/24 h; *polyuria,* urine volume excessive over 24 hours.

is completely excreted when kidney function is normal. Consequently, when the kidneys are not working, the serum creatinine level rises. Even small increases in serum creatinine will represent a significant decline in GFR. Serum creatinine level is assessed daily to follow the trend of kidney function and to determine whether it is stable, improving, or worsening.

Creatinine clearance. If the patient is making sufficient urine, urinary creatinine clearance can be measured. A normal urinary creatinine clearance rate is 120 mL/min, but this value decreases with kidney failure. Critical care patients with severe AKI manifest elevated serum creatinine and may be oliguric. Consequently, the urinary creatinine clearance rate is rarely measured during critical illness.

Blood urea nitrogen. The BUN level is an unreliable indicator of kidney injury as an individual test. The BUN concentration is changed by protein intake, blood in the gastrointestinal tract, and cell catabolism, and it is diluted by fluid administration. A BUN-to-creatinine ratio may be calculated to determine the cause of AKI (see Table 19.1). The BUN-to-creatinine ratio is most useful in diagnosing prerenal AKI (often described as prerenal azotemia), in which the BUN level is greatly elevated relative to the serum creatinine value, although critically ill patients can be developing AKI before changes in this ratio are evident. The term *azotemia* is used to describe an acute increase in the BUN level often associated with prerenal AKI.[7] *Uremia* is another term used to describe an elevated BUN value.

Serum electrolytes. When AKI is suspected, the degree of injury is assessed using blood analysis. Electrolytes in the serum become increasingly elevated as AKI progresses. Table 19.2 lists normal serum electrolyte values. Abnormal changes in serum electrolytes and clinical findings associated with AKI are listed in Table 19.3.

Urine electrolytes. Electrolyte levels in urine are also altered by AKI, although these values are not predictive of outcome in critical illness. Consequently, urinary electrolytes are rarely measured. Additional urinalysis results are summarized in Table 18.2 in Chapter 18.

Fractional excretion of sodium. The fractional excretion of sodium (FENa) in the urine can be measured early in the course of AKI to differentiate between prerenal AKI and interrenal AKI (parenchymal). An FENa value less than 1% (in the absence of diuretics) suggests prerenal compromise, because resorption of almost all of the filtered

TABLE 19.2 Normal Serum Electrolyte Values.

Electrolyte	Normal Value
Sodium	135—145 mEq/L
Potassium	3.5—4.5 mEq/L
Chloride	98—108 mEq/L
Calcium	8.5—10.5 mg/dL or 4.5—5.8 mEq/L
Phosphorus	2.7—4.5 mg/dL
Magnesium	1.5—2.5 mEq/L
Bicarbonate	24—28 mEq/L

sodium is an appropriate response to decreased perfusion to the kidneys. If diuretics are administered, the test is not helpful. An FENa value greater than 2% implies that the kidney cannot concentrate the sodium and that the damage is intrarenal (AKI). FENa values do not have any predictive benefit in critical illness and are rarely measured.

Urinary sodium is measured in milliequivalents per liter. Interpretation of results is similar to the FENa. A urinary sodium concentration less than 10 mEq/L (low) suggests a prerenal condition. A urinary sodium level greater than 40 mEq/L (in the presence of elevated serum creatinine and the absence of a high sodium load) suggests that intrarenal damage has occurred. As with other urinalysis tests, the use of diuretics invalidates any results because diuretics alter resorption of water and produce dilute urine, with test results not reflecting actual kidney function.

Acidosis

Acidosis (pH less than 7.35) is one of the trademarks of a severe acute kidney insult. Metabolic acidosis occurs as a result of the accumulation of waste products in the bloodstream and tissues. The acid waste products consist of strong negative ions (anions), elevated serum phosphorus levels (hyperphosphatemia), and other normally unmeasured ions (e.g., sulfate, urate, lactate) that decrease the serum pH. A low serum albumin concentration, which often occurs in AKI, has a slight alkalinizing effect, but it is not enough to offset the metabolic acidosis. Respiratory compensation and mechanical ventilatory

TABLE 19.3 Serum Electrolytes in Acute Kidney Failure.

Electrolyte Disturbance	Serum Value	Clinical Findings
Potassium		
Hypokalemia	<3.5 mEq/L	Muscular weakness
		Cardiac irregularities on EDG
		Abdominal distention and flatulence
		Paresthesia
		Decreased reflexes
		Anorexia
		Dizziness, confusion
		Increased sensitivity to digitalis
Hyperkalemia	>4.5mEq/L	Irritability and restlessness
		Anxiety
		Nausea and vomiting
		Abdominal cramps
		Weakness
		Numbness and tingling (fingertips and circumoral)
		Cardiac irregularities on ECG
Sodium		
Hyponatremia	<135 mEq/L	Disorientation
		Muscle twitching
		Nausea, vomiting, Abdominal cramps
		Headaches, dizziness
		Seizures, postural hypotension
		Cold, clammy skin
		Decreased skin turgor
		Tachycardia
		Oliguria
Hypernatremia	>145 mEq/L	Extreme thirst
		Dry, sticky mucous membranes
		Altered mentation
		Seizures (later stages)
Calcium		
Hypocalcemia	<8.5 mg/dL or <4.5 mEq/L	Irritability
		Muscular tetany, muscle cramps
		Decreased cardiac output (decreased contractions)
		Bleeding (decreased ability to coagulate)
		Changes on ECG
		Positive Chvostek or Trousseau signs
Hypercalcemia	>10.5 mg/dL >5.8 mEq/L	Deep bone pain
		Excessive thirst
		Anorexia

TABLE 19.3 Serum Electrolytes in Acute Kidney Failure.—cont'd

Electrolyte Disturbance	Serum Value	Clinical Findings
		Lethargy, weakened muscles
Magnesium		
Hypomagnesemia	<1.4 mEq/L	Choroid athetoid muscle activity
		Facial tics, spasticity
		Cardiac dysrhythmias
Hypermagnesemia	>2.5 mEq/L	CNS depression
		Respiratory depression
		Lethargy
		Coma
		Bradycardia
		Changes on ECG
Phosphorus		
Hypophosphatemia	<3.0 mg/dL	Hemolytic anemias
		Depressed white blood cell function
		Bleeding (decreased platelet aggregation)
		Nausea, vomiting
		Anorexia
Hyperphosphatemia	>4.5 mg/dL	Tachycardia
		Nausea, diarrhea, Abdominal cramps
		Muscle weakness, flaccid paralysis
		Increased reflexes
Chloride		
Hypochloremia	<98 mEq/L	Hyperirritability
		Tetany or muscular excitability
		Slow respirations
Hyperchloremia	>108 mEq/L	Weakness, lethargy
		Deep, rapid breathing
		Possible unconsciousness (later stages)
Albumin		
Hypoalbuminemia	<3.8 g/dL	Muscle wasting
		Peripheral edema (fluid shift)
		Decreased resistance to infection
		Poorly healing wounds

CNS, Central nervous system; *ECG,* electrocardiogram.

support are rarely sufficient to reverse the metabolic acidosis. Acidosis in AKI is complex, as evidenced by the fact that many patients with AKI maintain a normal anion gap; the reasons for this are unknown. Anion gap measurement is discussed in Chapter 18.

Diagnostic Criteria

Rifle criteria. The definition of AKI has been standardized by a multinational group of nephrologists using the acronym *RIFLE: r*isk, injury, *failure, loss,* and *end-*stage renal disease.[4] The RIFLE system classifies AKI in three categories of increasing severity (R, I, F) and two outcome criteria (L, E) based on GFR status reflected by the change in urine output or loss of kidney function (Table 19.4).[1,7] If AKI is superimposed on a kidney that is already compromised, the term *chronic* may be added to the RIFLE criteria to denote the cause as acute-on-chronic kidney failure.

Acute Kidney Injury Network criteria. The Acute Kidney Injury Network (AKIN) diagnostic criteria are listed in Box 19.2.[1,7] These criteria are similar to the criteria proposed by the RIFLE group (see Table 19.4). Both groups indicate that in an acutely ill patient, small changes in the serum creatinine level and urine output may signal important declines in GFR and kidney function.[7] The severity of kidney injury is described in stages from 1 to 3, using serum creatinine level, urine output, use of renal replacement therapy, and estimated GFR (eGFR) (Table 19.5).[1]

Priority diagnostic assessments and priority nursing interventions for AKI are displayed in Fig. 19.2.

At-Risk Disease States and Acute Kidney Injury

Many patients come into the critical care unit with disease states that predispose them to the development of AKI.[7] Many others already have kidney damage but are unaware of this condition.

Heart Failure and Acute Kidney Injury

There is a strong association between kidney failure and heart failure. Heart-kidney interactions have been categorized into five types under the term *cardiorenal syndrome (CRS)*[8]:

- Type 1 CRS: Acute heart failure that results in AKI
- Type 2 CRS: Chronic heart failure that results in AKI
- Type 3 CRS: AKI that results in acute heart failure
- Type 4 CRS: Chronic kidney disease (CKD) that results in chronic heart failure
- Type 5 CRS: A systemic condition that damages both the heart and kidney; examples include amyloidosis, sepsis, and liver cirrhosis[8]

Several risk factors for atherosclerotic cardiovascular disease also affect the kidneys, notably hypertension and diabetes. Maintenance of blood pressure below 130/80 mm Hg and blood glucose within the normal range decreases the risk of developing both CKD and the atherosclerotic cardiac diseases such as coronary artery disease and peripheral artery disease. A treatment challenge often encountered in CRS is *diuretic resistance* to loop diuretics.[8]

BOX 19.2 Diagnostic Criteria for Acute Kidney Injury (AKI)

AKI is defined by any one of the following:
- Serum creatinine increases by $\geq$0.3 mg/dL within 48 hours.
- Serum creatinine increases by $\geq$1.5 mg/dL from baseline within 7 days.
- Urine volume decreases to <0.5 mL/kg/h for 6 hours.

Respiratory Failure and Acute Kidney Injury

There is a significant association between kidney failure and respiratory failure.[9] Positive-pressure ventilation reduces blood flow to the kidney, which can lower the GFR and decrease urine output. These effects are intensified with the addition of positive end-expiratory pressure.[9] Patients with chronic lung conditions such as chronic obstructive pulmonary disease have a 41% increased risk of death if they also have AKI.[10] Management recommendations for patients with lung disease and AKI include lung protective ventilation, a conservative fluid management strategy, and early recognition and treatment of pulmonary infections.[11]

Sepsis and Acute Kidney Injury

Sepsis causes almost half of cases of AKI in critically ill patients.[12] Sepsis and septic shock create hemodynamic instability and reduce perfusion to the kidney. In severely septic patients, inflammation increases vascular permeability, and much of this fluid may move into the third space (interstitial space). In septic shock, vasopressors are used after volume resuscitation. Vasopressors raise blood pressure and increase systemic vascular resistance, but they also may raise the vascular resistance within the kidney microvasculature.

Trauma and Acute Kidney Injury

Traumatically injured patients often have a different demographic profile than other critical care populations. This is because patients with a traumatic injury are always emergency admissions, are often younger and male, and may have fewer coexisting illnesses.

Rhabdomyolysis. Trauma patients with major crush injuries have an elevated risk of kidney failure because of the release of creatine and myoglobin from damaged muscle cells, a condition called

TABLE 19.4 RIFLE Criteria for Acute Kidney Dysfunction.

RIFLE	Serum Creatinine Criteria[a]	Urine Output Criteria
*R*isk	Serum Cr increased 1.5 times above normal *or* Serum Cr increased $\geq$0.3 mg/dL	UO <0.5 mL/kg/h for 6 hours
*I*njury	Serum Cr increased 2 times above normal	UO <0.5 mL/kg/h for 12 hours
*F*ailure	Serum Cr increased 3 times above normal *Or* Serum Cr $\geq$4 mg/dL *Or* Serum Cr acute rise $\geq$0.5 mg/dL	UO <0.3 mL/kg/h for 24 hours *or* anuria for 12 hours (oliguria)
*L*oss	Persistent AKI—complete loss of kidney function for >4 weeks	
*E*SKD	End-stage kidney disease	

[a]All serum creatinine references are based on changes from baseline.
AKI, Acute kidney injury; *Cr,* creatinine; *UO,* urine output.
Data from Kellum JA, Bellomo R, Ronco C. Definition and classification of acute kidney injury. *Nephron Clin Pract.* 2008;109(4):c182–c187; Ronco C, Bellomo R, Kellum JA. Acute kidney injury. *Lancet.* 2019;394(10212):1949–1964.

TABLE 19.5 Acute Kidney Injury Stages.

	Serum Creatinine[a]	Urine Output	RRT
AKI Stage 1	Serum Cr rises 1.5 times above baseline *Or* Serum Cr increases by 0.3 mg/dL	Output less than 0.5 mL/kg/h for 6—12 hours	
AKI Stage 2	Serum Cr rises 2.0—3.0 times above baseline	Output less than 0.5 mL/kg/h for >12 hours	
AKI Stage 3	Serum Cr rises above 4.0 mg/dL	Output less than 0.3 mL/kg/h for >24 hours *Or* Anuria for 12 hours	RRT initiated

[a]All serum creatinine references are based on changes from baseline.
AKI, Acute kidney injury; *Cr,* creatinine; *RRT,* renal replacement therapy.
Data from Kellum JA, Lameire N, Aspelin P, et al.; Kidney Disease: Improving Global Outcomes (KDIGO) Acute Kidney Injury Work Group. KDIGO clinical practice guideline for acute kidney injury. *Kidney Int Suppl.* 2012;2:1—138; Ronco C, Bellomo R, Kellum JA. Acute kidney injury. *Lancet.* 2019;394(10212):1949—1964.

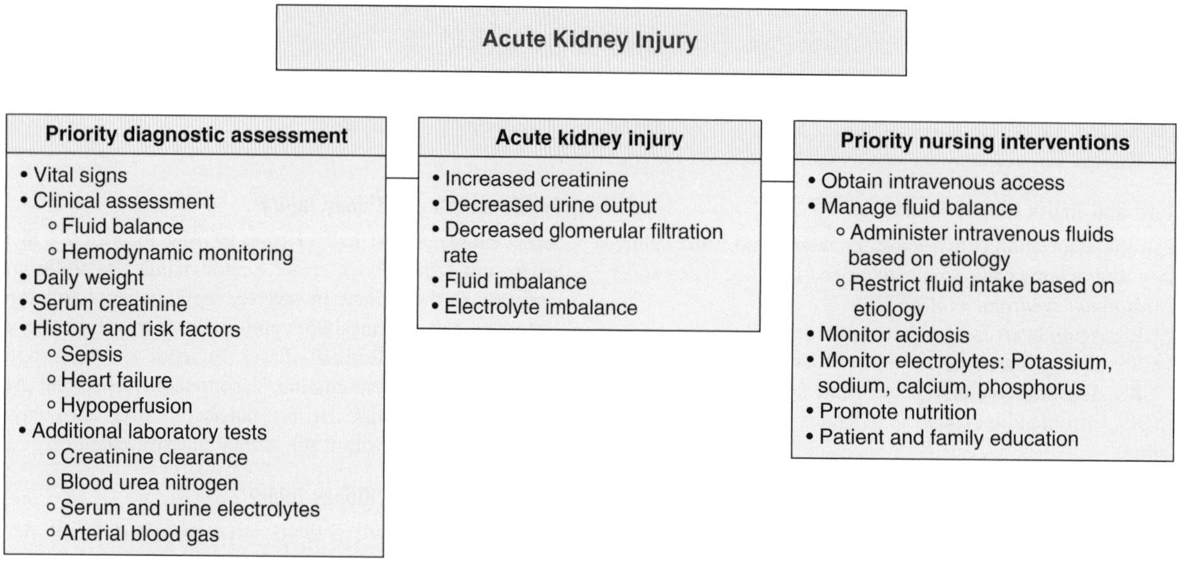

Acute Kidney Injury

Priority diagnostic assessment
- Vital signs
- Clinical assessment
  - Fluid balance
  - Hemodynamic monitoring
- Daily weight
- Serum creatinine
- History and risk factors
  - Sepsis
  - Heart failure
  - Hypoperfusion
- Additional laboratory tests
  - Creatinine clearance
  - Blood urea nitrogen
  - Serum and urine electrolytes
  - Arterial blood gas

Acute kidney injury
- Increased creatinine
- Decreased urine output
- Decreased glomerular filtration rate
- Fluid imbalance
- Electrolyte imbalance

Priority nursing interventions
- Obtain intravenous access
- Manage fluid balance
  - Administer intravenous fluids based on etiology
  - Restrict fluid intake based on etiology
- Monitor acidosis
- Monitor electrolytes: Potassium, sodium, calcium, phosphorus
- Promote nutrition
- Patient and family education

Fig. 19.2 Priority Diagnostic Assessments and Priority Nursing Interventions for Acute Kidney Injury.

rhabdomyolysis.[13] Myoglobin in large quantities is toxic to the kidney. A major goal of treatment is to prevent rhabdomyolysis-induced AKI. Large volumes of crystalloid are administered early in the course of treatment to hydrate the kidneys. It is important to trend the serum potassium levels. Life-threatening hyperkalemia can occur as cell lysis permits intracellular potassium to be released into the bloodstream.

The level of creatine kinase (CK), a marker of systemic muscle damage, increases in patients with rhabdomyolysis. One trauma service reported that of 2083 critical care trauma admissions, 85% had elevated CK levels, and 10% developed AKI resulting from rhabdomyolysis.[14] A CK level of 5000 units/L was the lowest abnormal value in patients who developed AKI associated with rhabdomyolysis.[14]

Crystalloid volume resuscitation is the primary treatment for preservation of kidney function and prevention of AKI in rhabdomyolysis.[15] Most treatment measures are empiric and may include intravenous (IV) fluids alkalinized by the addition of sodium bicarbonate and increased urine output by IV administration of the diuretic mannitol.[15] A bicarbonate and mannitol regimen is believed to prevent acidosis and hyperkalemia, both of which are common complications of rhabdomyolysis. Close attention is paid to hourly urine output that can be dark brown or tea-colored, CK levels, serum creatinine levels,

serum potassium levels, and any signs of compartment syndrome in all patients admitted with this diagnosis.

Contrast-Induced Nephrotoxic Injury and Acute Kidney Injury

More than 1 million radiologic studies or procedures that involve use of IV radiopaque contrast medium are performed every year. Patients most at risk of contrast-induced nephropathy (CIN) are patients with preexisting CKD, an elevated baseline serum creatinine level, and dehydration. The clinical definition of CIN is an increase in serum creatinine concentration of 0.5 mg/dL or more, or a 25% increase from the patient's baseline within 3 days of contrast medium exposure, without an alternative clinical explanation for development of AKI.[16] The effects of contrast-induced AKI are linked to increased mortality compared with similar patients who did not have contrast-induced kidney injury.[16]

High-molecular-weight contrast medium is a potential cause of nephrotoxicity. A recommended strategy to prevent CIN involves use of a lower quantity of contrast medium and use of nonionic low-osmolar or iso-osmolar contrast media that is less nephrotoxic.[16] Patients with preexisting kidney failure or a low estimated eGFR are at highest risk.[17]

The best method of prevention is aggressive hydration with IV normal saline during and after the procedure. After diagnostic intravascular catheterization procedures, an alert patient is asked to drink up to a liter of water before and after the procedure to protect the kidney. Avoiding dehydration is vital.[16]

Medications. Strategies such as the addition of sodium bicarbonate and adjunctive use of *N*-acetylcysteine have not shown benefit in research studies and are no longer recommended.[18]

Potentially nephrotoxic medications are always stopped before the procedure. Metformin, a medication that decreases insulin resistance in type 2 diabetes, has been associated with lactic acidosis in rare instances. For patients with elevated serum creatinine, metformin is stopped the day before any procedure involving contrast medium and not started again for 48 hours when serum creatinine has returned to baseline.

The mainstay measures to protect the kidney from contrast-induced AKI are to use the smallest possible dose of low-osmolar or iso-osmolar contrast, stop all nephrotoxic medications, provide vigorous fluid volume expansion, and avoid repeat contrast media injections within 48 hours.[16]

Medical Management

Treatment goals for patients with AKI focus on prevention, compensation for the deterioration of kidney function, and regeneration of kidney functional capacity. Key treatment areas include prevention strategies, electrolyte balance, fluid resuscitation, and nutrition.

Prevention

The only truly effective remedy for AKI is prevention. Effective prevention requires assessment of the patient's risk for AKI. Knowledge of the most common causes of AKI in critically ill patients is essential for prevention strategies to be enacted. The critical care team collaborates closely with the clinical pharmacist to avoid medications with nephrotoxic side effects in patients with AKI or CKD. Nonsteroidal antiinflammatory medications for pain relief are avoided in patients with elevated creatinine levels. The use of intravascular contrast dye is preferably avoided or delayed until the patient is fully rehydrated.

Electrolyte Balance

Potassium. Hyperkalemia is a risk in all phases of kidney failure.[19] Electrolyte levels require frequent observation, especially in the critical phases of AKI when potassium can quickly reach levels of 6.0 mEq/L or higher. Specific electrocardiogram changes are associated with hyperkalemia, including peaked T waves, a widening of the QRS interval, and ultimately ventricular tachycardia or fibrillation.[20] If hyperkalemia is identified, all potassium supplements are stopped. Acute hyperkalemia can be treated temporarily by emergent IV administration of insulin and glucose. An infusion of 50 mL of 50% dextrose accompanied by 10 units of IV regular insulin forces potassium out of the serum and into the cells.[20] The blood glucose should be carefully monitored after the dextrose and insulin are administered. The IV insulin dose may be decreased to 5 units if hypoglycemia is a concern.[20] The patient may also experience hyperglycemia from the 50% dextrose.[20]

In nonemergency situations, other options to lower serum potassium include aerosolized beta-2 agonists (albuterol) and IV loop diuretics (if the patient is making urine).[20] To treat smaller increases in serum potassium, nonabsorbable potassium-binding resins may be used. The binding resins can be administered orally, through a nasogastric (NG) tube, or rectally to treat hyperkalemia. Cation exchange resins use either sodium (Kayexalate) or calcium (Sorbisterit, Calcium Resonium, Argamate) and exchange the cation for potassium

across the gastrointestinal wall. The potassium is contained in the lower gastrointestinal tract and is eliminated with the stool. If the patient is oliguric and nonresponsive to diuretics, emergency dialysis is instituted.[20] Potassium-binding resins and dialysis are the only permanent methods of potassium removal to manage hyperkalemia.[20]

Sodium. Alterations in sodium level are an expected finding in kidney failure. Both hypernatremia (elevated serum sodium) and hyponatremia (low serum sodium) are associated with increased mortality with kidney failure.[21]

Calcium and Phosphorus. Serum calcium levels are reduced (hypocalcemia) in kidney failure. This reduction results from multiple factors, including hyperphosphatemia.[22] Chronically elevated serum phosphorus levels (above 5.5 mg/dL) are associated with higher mortality rates for patients with kidney failure.[23] Calcium and phosphorus levels are regulated by a complex physiologic feedback mechanism involving parathyroid hormone and fibroblast growth factor.[22,23] Normally, parathyroid hormone helps calcium be resorbed back into the bloodstream at the proximal tubule and distal nephron, and it promotes excretion of phosphorus by the kidney to maintain homeostasis. In kidney failure, this mechanism is nonfunctional; the serum phosphorus level rises, and the serum calcium level falls. Consequently, patients with kidney failure with elevated phosphate levels must take oral phosphate-binder medications to control serum phosphorus.[22,23]

Calcium Replacement. Most calcium in the bloodstream is bound to protein. Calcium levels can be measured in two ways: total calcium or ionized calcium. Protein-calcium binding confounds the measurement of accurate calcium levels. In the past, calculations were used to estimate the amounts of protein-bound versus unbound calcium, but these calculations have been shown to produce inaccurate results. The metabolically active, non–protein-bound portion is known as *ionized calcium* and is the preferred method of measurement.[24] Without adequate levels of serum calcium, a compensatory mechanism "steals" calcium from bones, making patients with kidney failure more vulnerable to fractures. Maintaining adequate calcium stores in the body is important and is achieved by administration of calcium supplements and vitamin D.[22]

Dietary Phosphorus–Binding Medications. A second method used in tandem with calcium supplements to achieve normal calcium levels is to reduce the level of phosphorus in the bloodstream. Phosphorus is present in many foods, especially foods with a high protein content such as meat, fish, and dairy.[23] Phosphorus is also present in many food additives and some carbonated beverages.[23] After eating these foods, free phosphorus passes from the gastrointestinal tract into the bloodstream and raises the serum level. Medications that bind dietary phosphorus in the gastrointestinal tract are administered orally or by feeding tube. The binding agent must be taken at the same time as a meal. After the dietary phosphorus is bound to the binding substance in the bowel, it is eliminated from the intestine with stool. This lowers the serum phosphorus level.

The types of dietary phosphorus binders used have changed over the years. The original binders were aluminum salts (aluminum hydroxide) that bound dietary phosphorus effectively in the gastrointestinal tract but conferred aluminum toxicity because some of the aluminum metal was also absorbed. For this reason, aluminum binders have been abandoned. The second-generation dietary phosphorus–binding agents use calcium salts including calcium carbonate or calcium acetate to bind dietary phosphorus in the gastrointestinal tract. Calcium-based medications are safer, but elevated serum calcium levels and calcium deposits in other areas of the body (extraosseous calcification) are a problem.

A third generation of nonabsorbable dietary phosphorus—binding medications is available. These are non—aluminum-based and non—calcium-based and include sevelamer hydrochloride and lanthanum carbonate.[23] These medications have a better safety profile and are frequently prescribed to lower serum phosphorus levels in patients with CKD.

Fluid Resuscitation

Prerenal failure is caused by decreased perfusion and flow to the kidney. It is often associated with trauma, hemorrhage, hypotension, and major fluid losses. If contrast dye is used, aggressive fluid resuscitation with normal saline (NaCl) is recommended. The objectives of volume replacement are to replace fluid and electrolyte losses and to prevent ongoing loss. Maintenance IV fluid therapy is initiated when oral fluid intake is inadvisable. Maintenance fluids are calculated with consideration for individual body surface area. Adults require approximately 1500 mL/m^2 per 24 hours; fever, burns, and trauma significantly increase fluid requirements. Other important criteria when calculating fluid volume replacement include baseline metabolism, environmental temperature, and humidity. The rate of replacement depends on cardiopulmonary reserve, adequacy of kidney function, urine output, fluid balance, ongoing loss, and type of fluid replaced.

Crystalloids and colloids. Crystalloids and colloids are two different types of IV fluids used for volume management in critically ill patients. These IV solutions are used on all types of patients, not just patients with acute kidney failure. Adequacy of IV fluid replacement depends on strict, ongoing evaluation and frequent adjustment. Frequent monitoring of serum electrolyte levels is required, and strictly regulated intake and output are correlated with daily weight records. In septic shock, hemodynamic readings are taken frequently. After a fluid challenge, a merely minimal increase in central venous pressure implies that additional fluid replacement is required. Continued decreases in central venous pressure, pulmonary artery occlusion pressure, and cardiac index indicate ongoing volume losses.

Which IV fluid to select to successfully resuscitate hemodynamically unstable patients has been a controversial topic in critical care. The debate often centers on the differences between crystalloid and colloid solutions.

Crystalloids. Crystalloid solutions are in widespread use for IV maintenance infusion and replacement therapy. Crystalloid fluids include 0.9% sodium chloride solution (0.9% NaCl), often referred to as *normal saline solution*; half-normal saline solution (0.45% NaCl); and balanced crystalloid solutions such as lactated Ringer solution, Normasol, or Plasmalyte (Table 19.6).[25,26] Balanced crystalloid solutions are avoided in kidney failure because they contain potassium.

Studies have evaluated patient outcomes after infusion of a balanced crystalloid solution compared with normal saline. Although the differences are small, there was lower mortality at 28 days for balanced crystalloid solutions.[27,28] A noncrystalloid solution that is infused in small volumes in cardiac conditions to limit sodium intake is dextrose (5%) in water (D$_5$W) (see Table 19.6).

Colloids. Colloids are solutions containing oncotically active particles that are used to expand intravascular volume to achieve and maintain hemodynamic stability. Albumin (5% and 25%) and hydroxyethyl starch (HES) are examples of colloid solutions (see Table 19.6). Colloids expand intravascular volume, and this effect can last 24 hours. Debate as to whether colloids or crystalloid fluids are most effective for volume resuscitation and survival has been studied in many clinical trials. Current study results suggest that there is little difference in short- or long-term outcomes between IV crystalloid or colloid in critical care patients or after major abdominal surgery.[29—31]

Intravenous fluid volume. Controversy continues as to whether routine fluid replacement should be restrictive or liberal after trauma, major surgery, and sepsis.[32,33] Different medical and surgical teams often manage patients' fluid requirements very differently, because the research is not yet conclusive. The critical care nurse may find that patients with similar diagnoses have different fluid requirements depending on the philosophy of the medical team.

Fluid restriction in kidney failure. Fluid restriction constitutes a large part of medical management once AKI is established. Fluid restriction is used to prevent circulatory overload and the development of interstitial edema when the kidneys cannot remove excess volume. The fluid requirements are calculated on the basis of daily urine volumes and insensible losses. Obtaining daily weight measurements and keeping accurate intake and output records is essential. Patients with kidney failure are usually restricted to 1 L of fluid per 24 hours if the urine output is 500 mL or less. Insensible losses range from 500 to 750 mL/day.

Fluid removal. Acute kidney failure results in retention of water, solutes, and potential toxins in the circulation, and prompt measures are needed to decrease their levels. Diuretics are used to stimulate urine output in the early stages of AKI. Renal replacement therapy (hemodialysis or hemofiltration) is another choice, particularly if volume overload exacerbates pulmonary edema or heart failure.

Nutrition

Diet or nutritional supplementation for a patient with AKI in the critical care unit is designed to account for the diminished excretory capacity of the kidney. The recommended energy intake is between 20 and 30 kcal/kg per day, with 1.2 to 1.5 g/kg of protein per day to control azotemia (increased BUN level). Oral nutrition is preferred, and if the patient cannot eat, enteral nutrition is recommended over parenteral (IV) nutrition. Fluids are limited, and monitoring of blood glucose levels is recommended. The electrolytes potassium, sodium, and phosphorus are strictly limited.

Nursing Management

The patient care management plan for a patient with AKI incorporates a variety of patient problems (Box 19.3). The nurse plays a significant role in monitoring fluid and electrolyte balance, preventing catheter-associated urinary tract infections (CAUTIs), and educating the patient and family.

Fluid Balance

Intravascular fluid balance is often assessed on an hourly basis for a critically ill patient who has hemodynamic lines inserted. Hemodynamic values (heart rate, blood pressure, central venous pressure, pulmonary artery occlusion pressure, cardiac output, and cardiac index) and daily weight measurements are correlated with intake and output. Urine output is measured hourly by means of a urinary catheter and drainage bag throughout all phases of AKI, particularly in response to diuretics. Any fluid removed with dialysis is included in the daily fluid balance. Recognition of the clinical signs and symptoms of fluid overload is important. Excess fluid moves from the vascular system into the peripheral tissues (dependent edema), abdomen (ascites), and lungs (crackles, pulmonary edema, and pulmonary effusions); around the heart (pericardial effusions); and into the brain (increased intracranial swelling).

Electrolyte Balance

Hyperkalemia, hypocalcemia, hyponatremia, hyperphosphatemia, and acid—base imbalances occur during AKI (see Table 19.3). Clinical manifestations of these electrolyte imbalances must be prevented, and

TABLE 19.6 Frequently Used Intravenous Solutions.

Solution	Electrolytes	Indications
Crystalloids[a]		
Dextrose in water (D₅W), isotonic	None	Maintain volume Replace mild loss Provide minimal calories
Normal saline solution (0.9% NaCl)	Sodium: 154 mEq/L Chloride: 154 mEq/L Osmolality: 308 mEq/L	Maintain volume Replace mild loss
Half-normal saline solution (0.45% NaCl)	Sodium: 77 mEq/L Chloride: 77 mEq/L	Free water replacement Correct mild hyponatremia Free water and electrolyte replacement (fluid- and electrolyte-restricted conditions)
Lactated Ringer solution	Sodium: 130 mEq/L Potassium: 4 mEq/L Calcium: 2.7 mEq/L Chloride: 107 mEq/L Lactate: 27 mEq/L pH: 6.5	Fluid and electrolyte replacement (contraindicated for patients with kidney or liver disease or in lactic acidosis)
Normosol/Plasmalyte	Sodium: 140 mEq/L Potassium: 5 mEq/L Magnesium: 3 mEq/L Chloride: 98 mEq/L Acetate: 27 Gluconate: 23 Osmolality: 295	
Colloids		
5% Albumin (Albumisol)	Albumin: 50 g/L Sodium: 130–160 mEq/L Potassium: 1 mEq/L Osmolality: 300 mOsm/L Osmotic pressure: 20 mm Hg pH: 6.4–7.4	Volume expansion Moderate protein replacement Achievement of hemodynamic stability in shock states
25% Albumin (salt-poor)	Albumin: 240 g/L Globulins: 10 g/L Sodium: 130–160 mEq/L Osmolality: 1500 mOsm/L pH: 6.4–7.4	Concentrated form of albumin sometimes used with diuretics to move fluid from tissues into vascular space for diuresis
Hetastarch	Sodium: 154 mEq/L Chloride: 154 mEq/L Osmolality: 310 mOsm/L Colloid osmotic pressure: 30–35 mm Hg	Synthetic polymer (6% solution) used for volume expansion Hemodynamic volume replacement after cardiac surgery, burns, sepsis
LMWD	Glucose polysaccharide molecules with average molecular weight of 40,000; no electrolytes	Volume expansion and support (contraindicated for patients with bleeding disorders)
HMWD	Glucose polysaccharide molecules with average molecular weight of 70,000; no electrolytes	Used prophylactically in some cases to prevent platelet aggregation; available in saline and glucose solutions

[a]For crystalloid solutions that contain electrolytes, specific concentrations of electrolytes and pH vary according to the manufacturer.
HMWD, High–molecular-weight dextran; *LMWD*, low–molecular-weight dextran.

their associated side effects must be controlled. The more likely imbalances are hyperkalemia and hypocalcemia, which can result in life-threatening cardiac dysrhythmias. Dilutional hyponatremia may develop as fluid overload worsens in patients with oliguria. Monitoring the serum sodium level is important to prevent this complication. Hyperphosphatemia results in severe pruritus. Nursing care is directed at soothing the itching by performing frequent skin care with emollients, discouraging scratching, and administering phosphate-binding medications. The acid–base imbalances that occur with AKI are monitored by arterial blood gas analyses. The goal of treatment is to maintain the pH within the normal range.

Catheter-Associated Urinary Tract Infection

A urinary catheter may be inserted to facilitate accurate urine measurement. Many critically ill patients have an indwelling urinary drainage catheter inserted to record hourly urine output accurately. However, any indwelling catheter is a potential source for infection and prevention of infection is paramount, as described in Box 19.4.

Acute Kidney Injury
- Ineffective Tissue Perfusion due to decreased kidney blood flow
- Hypervolemia due to renal dysfunction
- Anxiety due to threat to biologic, psychologic, or social integrity
- Impaired Cardiac Output due to alterations in preload
- Risk for Infection
- Disturbed Body Image due to functional dependence on life-sustaining technology
- Lack of Knowledge of Treatment Regime due to lack of previous exposure to information (see Box 19.5, Patient and Family Education Plan for Acute Kidney Injury)

Patient Care Management plans are located in Appendix A.

Critically ill patients who have a protracted illness have a significant risk of contracting a CAUTI, especially if the catheter is required for several days. Additionally, critically ill patients who have developed a CAUTI risk higher mortality and longer lengths of stay. A critical care patient with AKI is at risk for infectious complications and should have the catheter removed as soon as clinically feasible.

Urinary catheter management. When the patient no longer makes large quantities of urine and is hemodynamically stable, the catheter must be removed. After removal, if the patient cannot void urine spontaneously, intermittent urinary catheterizations are performed to avoid catheter reinsertion. Frist, a bladder scanner is used to estimate quantity of urine in the bladder. Then, an intermittent urinary catheterization, colloquially called a *straight cath*, is performed and involves insertion of a small catheter into the bladder using sterile technique. After urine drainage, this catheter is immediately removed. This procedure allows the patient's bladder to be emptied, but the catheter does not remain in place. After removal, if the patient voids urine spontaneously, external urine collection options are available to avoid catheter reinsertion. For males, the condom catheter is used. For females, there are external female collection systems that wick away voided urine via an external tube connected to wall suction.[34] Often, performing intermittent urinary catheterizations and use of external urine collection options are nurse-led interventions.[35]

Educate the Patient and Family

Accurate and uncomplicated information must be provided to the patient and family about AKI, including its prognosis, treatment, and possible complications. Education of the patient and family can be challenging, because elevations of BUN and creatinine levels can negatively affect the level of consciousness. Sleep-rest disorders and emotional upset often occur as complications of AKI and can disrupt short-term memory. Encouraging the patient and family to voice concerns, frustrations, or fears and allowing the patient to control some aspects of the acute care environment and treatment also are essential (Box 19.5).

CHRONIC KIDNEY DISEASE

Clinical practice guidelines for the management of end-stage kidney disease categorize kidney dysfunction into five stages. The estimated incidence of chronic kidney failure in the United States is 14%.[36] Because of the large numbers of adults with kidney dysfunction (diagnosed or not), kidney function must be assessed on all critically ill patients at risk for fluid and electrolyte imbalance. The GFR associated with each stage and the population estimates for each stage of kidney dysfunction are shown in Table 19.7. The number of older adults with CKD is increasing in tandem with increases in diabetes and hypertension in the US population.[36]

Preventing Anemia

Anemia is an expected side effect of kidney failure that occurs because the kidney no longer produces the hormone erythropoietin. As a result, bone marrow is not stimulated to produce erythrocytes (red blood cells). Additionally, the normal erythrocyte survival of 80 to 120 days is decreased in patients with CKD on dialysis to 70 to 80 days, increasing their risk for anemia. Care is taken to prevent blood loss in patients with AKI, and blood withdrawal is minimized as much as possible. Irritation of the gastrointestinal tract from metabolic waste accumulation is expected, and stress ulcer prophylaxis must be prescribed. Gastrointestinal bleeding remains a possibility. Stool, NG tube drainage, and emesis are routinely tested for occult blood.

Erythropoiesis-Stimulating Medications

Anemia associated with CKD may be treated pharmacologically by the administration of recombinant human erythropoietin. Three medications are approved by the US Food and Drug Administration (FDA) for treatment of CKD-associated anemia in the United States: epoetin alfa (Procrit, Epogen), darbepoetin alfa (Aranesp), and methoxy polyethylene glycol–epoetin beta. These agents stimulate erythrocyte production by bone marrow. Adjunctive treatments include administration of iron supplements, vitamin B_{12}, vitamin B_6, and folate. Erythropoietin has been shown to prevent anemia and reduce blood transfusions before dialysis, but it does not slow the progression of kidney disease.[37]

RENAL REPLACEMENT THERAPY: DIALYSIS

Two types of renal replacement therapy are available for the treatment of AKI: intermittent hemodialysis (IHD) therapy and continuous renal replacement therapy (CRRT).

Hemodialysis

Hemodialysis roughly translates as "separating from the blood" (Fig. 19.3). Indications and contraindications for hemodialysis are listed in Box 19.6. As a treatment, hemodialysis separates and removes from the blood the excess electrolytes, fluids, and toxins by means of a hemodialyzer (Fig. 19.4). Hemodialysis is efficient in removing solutes. Because levels of electrolytes, toxins, and fluids increase between treatments, hemodialysis occurs on a regular basis. Traditional hemodialysis treatments last 3 to 4 hours.

Hemodialyzer

Hemodialysis works by circulating blood outside the body through synthetic tubing to a dialyzer, which consists of hollow-fiber tubes. The dialyzer is sometimes described as an artificial kidney (Figs. 19.3 and 19.5). While the blood flows through the membranes, which are semipermeable, a fluid (dialysate bath) bathes the membranes and, through osmosis and diffusion, performs exchanges of fluid, electrolytes, and toxins from the blood to the bath, where toxins and dialysate then pass out of the artificial kidney. The blood and the dialysate bath are shunted in opposite directions (countercurrent flow) through the dialyzer to match the osmotic and chemical gradients at the most efficient level for effective dialysis.

BOX 19.4 Safety

Prevention of Catheter-Associated Urinary Tract Infections

1. Avoid Unnecessary Use of Indwelling Urinary Catheters

Critical Care Indications

- Accurate measurements of urinary output
- Prolonged immobilization (e.g., potentially unstable thoracic or lumbar spine, multiple traumatic injuries such as pelvic fractures)

Perioperative Indications

- Urologic or genitourinary tract surgery
- Prolonged duration of surgery (catheters inserted for this reason should be removed in the postanesthesia care unit)
- Large-volume infusions or diuretics administered during surgery
- Intraoperative monitoring of urinary output

Other Indications

- Acute urinary retention or bladder outlet obstruction
- Assist in healing of open sacral or perineal wounds in incontinent patients
- Improve comfort for end-of-life care if needed

2. Insert Urinary Catheters Using Aseptic Technique

Hand Hygiene

- Wash hands thoroughly before or after any patient care activity.
- Use gloves when touching catheter site or meatus.

Sterile Technique and Sterile Equipment

- Use standard supply kits that contain all necessary items: sterile gloves, drape, sponges, antiseptic solution for cleaning meatus, and single-use packet of lubricant jelly for insertion.
- Use as small a catheter as possible to minimize urethral trauma.
- Allow only a single attempt to insert urinary catheter.
- Use new catheter if second attempt at catheterization is required.

3. Adopt Evidence-Based Standards for Maintenance of Urinary Catheters

Maintenance of Closed Drainage System

- Maintain sterile closed drainage system.
- Maintain unobstructed urine flow (avoid dependent loops).
- Keep drainage bag below the level of the bladder at all times.
- Do not allow drainage bag to touch the floor.

- Empty collection bag regularly, using a separate container for each patient.
- Do not allow drainage spigot to touch the collection container.
- Do not break the system to collect a urine sample. Collect from sampling port in the tubing drainage system, disinfecting the port and aspirating using aseptic technique.
- Avoid catheter irrigation except in the case of an obstructed catheter; use a bladder ultrasound scan to determine whether there is urine in the bladder.
- Routine scheduled replacement of catheters is not recommended.

Catheter Securement and Hygiene

- Keep urinary catheter secured to prevent catheter movement and urethral friction.
- Do not clean periurethral area with antiseptics. Urethral cleaning during a bath is appropriate.

4. Review Need for the Indwelling Urinary Catheter Daily and Remove Catheter Promptly

Documentation and Monitoring

- Document when catheter was inserted.
- Nurses and physicians should review the need for the urinary catheter for every patient every day.

Hospital Strategies to Ensure Early Removal of an Indwelling Urinary Catheter

- Ensure clinicians are aware that longer duration of catheter use increases catheter-associated urinary tract infection (CAUTI) risk. This awareness can be reinforced by:
  - Alerts in computerized ordering systems
  - Automatic stops on catheter orders at 24 hours, 48 hours, or 72 hours, depending on the clinical situation
  - Development of standardized nursing protocols that allow nurses to remove urinary catheters if predetermined criteria are met

Know Your Own CAUTI Data

- Each critical care unit should ensure that all nurses and physicians are aware of their unit/patient statistics on CAUTI per 1000 catheter days.
- Publicize strategies used to prevent CAUTI.

Data from Gould CV, Umscheid CA, Agarwa RK, et al. Guideline for prevention of catheter associated urinary tract infections 2009. *Centers for Disease Control and Prevention.* 2009. http://www.cdc.gov/hicpac/pdf/cauti/cautiguideline2009final.pdf; Norrick B. NHSN catheter associated urinary tract surveillance in 2019. *Centers for Disease Control and Prevention; National Center for Emerging and Zoonotic Infectious Diseases.* 2019. https://www.cdc.gov/nhsn/pdfs/training/2019/cauti-508.pdf.

BOX 19.5 PRIORITY PATIENT AND FAMILY EDUCATION

Acute Kidney Injury

Before discharge, the patient should be able to teach back the following topics:

- Pathophysiology of acute kidney injury as a sudden decline in kidney function that caused an acute buildup of toxins in the blood.
- Explain level of kidney function after discharge from the hospital (if known).
- Explain diet and fluid restrictions.
- Emphasize need for exercise and rest.
- Describe medications and adverse effects.
- Explain need for ongoing follow-up with health care professional.
- Explain purpose of dialysis and importance of regular treatments.

Ultrafiltration

To remove fluid, a positive hydrostatic pressure is applied to the blood, and a negative hydrostatic pressure is applied to the dialysate bath. The two forces together, called *transmembrane pressure*, pull the excess fluid from the blood. The difference between the two values, expressed in millimeters of mercury, represents the transmembrane pressure and results in fluid extraction, known as *ultrafiltration*, from the vascular space.

Anticoagulation

Heparin or sodium citrate is added to the system just before the blood enters the dialyzer to anticoagulate the blood within the dialysis tubing. Without an anticoagulant, the blood clots because its passage through the foreign tubular substances of the dialysis machine activates the clotting mechanism. Heparin can be administered

TABLE 19.7 Decreased Kidney Function by Stage in Adult US Population.

Stage[a]	Population Affected[a]	Glomerular Filtration Rate and Diagnosis[a]	Percentage Who Know They Have Kidney Dysfunction (%)[b]
1	9 million (3.3%)	Normal; persistent albuminuria	40.5
2	5.3 million (3.0%)	60–89; persistent albuminuria	29.3
3	7.6 million (4.3%)	30–59	22.0
4	400,000 (0.2%)	15–29	44.5
5	300,000 (0.2%)	<15: ESKD	100

[a]Data from Coresh J, Astor BC, Greene T, Eknoyan G, Levey AS. Prevalence of chronic kidney disease and decreased kidney function in the adult US population: Third National Health and Nutrition Examination Survey. *Am J Kidney Dis.* 2003;41(1):1.

[b]Data from Nickolas TL, Frisch GD, Opotowsky AR, Arons R, Radhakrishnan J. Awareness of kidney disease in the US population: findings from the National Health and Nutrition Examination Survey (NHANES) 1999 to 2000. *Am J Kidney Dis.* 2004;44(2):185.

ESKD, End-stage kidney disease; *GFR,* glomerular filtration rate (mL/min/1.73 m² of body surface area).

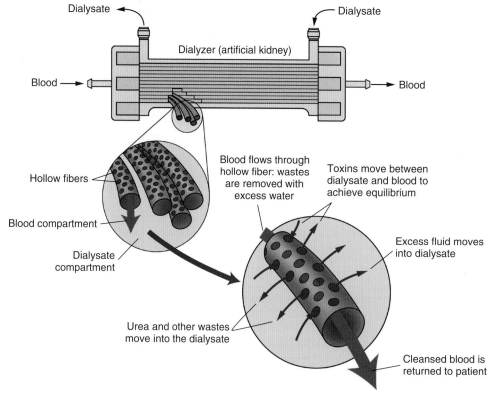

Fig. 19.3 Hemodialyzer.

by bolus injection or intermittent infusion. It has a short half-life, and its effects subside within 2 to 4 hours. If necessary, the effects of heparin are easily reversed with the antidote protamine sulfate. When there is concern about the development of heparin-induced thrombocytopenia, alternative anticoagulants can be used. Citrate can be infused as an anticoagulant by intermittent bolus or continuous infusion.

Vascular Access

Hemodialysis requires access to the bloodstream. Various types of temporary and permanent devices are in clinical use. It is important for patient safety to be able to recognize these different vascular access devices and to care for them properly. This section discusses temporary vascular access catheters used in the acute care hospital environment and permanent methods used for long-term hemodialysis.

Temporary vascular access. Subclavian and *femoral* veins are catheterized when short-term access is required or when a graft or fistula vascular access is nonfunctional in a patient requiring immediate hemodialysis. Subclavian and femoral catheters are routinely inserted at the bedside. Most temporary catheters are venous lines only. Blood flows out toward the dialyzer and flows back to the patient through the same catheterized vein. A dual-lumen venous catheter is most commonly used. It has a central partition running the length of the catheter. The outflow catheter section pulls the blood flow through openings that are proximal to the inflow openings on the opposite side (Fig. 19.5). This design helps prevent dialyzing the same blood just returned to the area (recirculation), which would severely reduce the efficiency of the procedure. A silicone rubber dual-lumen catheter with a polyester cuff designed to decrease catheter-related infections is also available.

BOX 19.6 Indications and Contraindications for Hemodialysis

Indications
- Blood urea nitrogen level greater than 90 mg/dL
- Serum creatinine level of 9 mg/dL
- Hyperkalemia
- Medication toxicity
- Intravascular and extravascular fluid overload
- Metabolic acidosis
- Symptoms of uremia
- Pericarditis
- Gastrointestinal bleeding
- Changes in mentation
- Contraindications to other forms of dialysis

Contraindications
- Hemodynamic instability
- Inability to anticoagulate
- Lack of access to circulation

Permanent vascular access. The common feature in permanent vascular access devices is a conduit connection between the arterial circulation and the venous circulation.

Arteriovenous fistula. The arteriovenous fistula is created by surgically exposing a peripheral artery and vein, creating a side-by-side opening in the artery and the vein to join the two vessels together. The high arterial flow creates a swelling of the vein, or a pseudoaneurysm, at which point (when healed) a large-bore needle can be inserted to obtain arterial outflow to the dialyzer. Inflow is accomplished through a second large-bore needle inserted into a peripheral vein distal to the fistula (Fig. 19.6A). Fistulas are the preferred mode of access because of the durability of blood vessels, relatively few complications, and less need for revision compared with other access methods. An initial disadvantage of a fistula is the time required for development of sufficient arterial flow to enlarge the new access. The minimum reported length of time before a fistula can be cannulated for dialysis is 14 days, but the time lag for many patients can be longer. Ideally, the fistula should be established 6 months before the requirement for hemodialysis to ensure it is useable for dialysis when required.

In caring for a patient with a fistula, there are some important nursing priorities to ensure the ongoing viability of the vascular access and safety of the limb (Table 19.8). The critical care nurse frequently assesses the quality of blood flow through the fistula. A patent fistula has a thrill when palpated gently with the fingers and has a bruit if auscultated with a stethoscope. The extremity should be pink and warm to the touch. No blood pressure measurements, IV infusions, or laboratory phlebotomy procedures are performed on the arm with the fistula.

The arteriovenous fistula is the preferred long-term access for hemodialysis. It provides the most favorable long-term patency for hemodialysis access if patients require long-term hemodialysis.

Arteriovenous grafts. Arteriovenous grafts connect a vein and artery to allow vascular access for dialysis in chronic kidney failure. The graft is a tube made of synthetic material that is surgically implanted inside the limb. The area is surgically opened, and an artery and a vein are located. A tunnel is created in the tissue where the graft is placed. Anastomoses are made with the graft ends connected to the

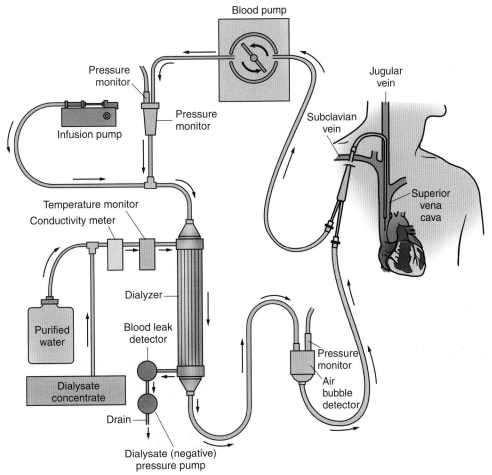

Fig. 19.4 Components of a Hemodialysis System.

Double-Lumen Catheter

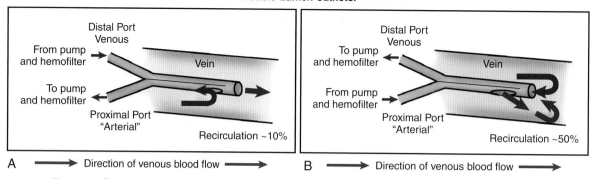

Fig. 19.5   Temporary Dialysis Venous Access Catheter. (A) Reduced recirculation from pump and hemofilter connection to proximal port as blood pulled through opening that is proximal to the openings on the opposite site (where blood is being returned from the pump and hemofilter). (B) Increased recirculation from pump and hemofilter connection to distal port as blood pulled through opening that is distal to the openings on the opposite side (where blood is being returned from the pump and hemofilter).

artery and vein. The blood is allowed to flow through the graft, and the surgical area is closed. The graft creates a raised area that looks like a large peripheral vein just under the skin (Fig. 19.6B). Two large-bore needles are used for outflow from and inflow to the graft during dialysis. For grafts and fistulas, firm pressure must be applied to stop any bleeding after needle removal at the end of the hemodialysis treatment (see Table 19.8).

Tunneled catheters. While waiting for the fistula or graft to mature to be ready for access, some patients with CKD may have a tunneled, cuffed catheter placed in either the internal or the external jugular vein. The cuff and tunneling are physical barriers to reduce central venous line infections. Modern catheters are made of silicone or Silastic elastomers, making them more pliable than temporary catheters.

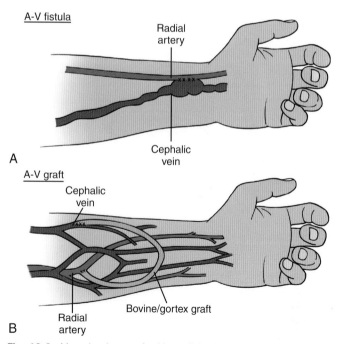

Fig. 19.6   Vascular Access for Hemodialysis. (A) Arteriovenous *(A-V)* fistula between the vein and artery. (B) Internal synthetic graft connects the artery and vein.

Medical Management

Medical management involves the decision to place a vascular access device and then to choose the most appropriate type and location for each patient. Patients in the critical care setting who require vascular access for hemodialysis typically use a temporary hemodialysis catheter. The exact quantity of fluid and solute removal to be achieved by hemodialysis is determined individually for each patient by clinical examination and review of all relevant laboratory results.

Nursing Management

A non–critical care nurse who is specially trained in dialysis manages the IHD. The dialysis nurse typically comes to the patient's bedside with the hemodialysis machine. During the acute phase of treatment, hemodialysis occurs daily. The frequency is reduced to 3 days per week as the patient becomes hemodynamically stable. The essential role of the critical care nurse during dialysis is to monitor the patient's hemodynamic status and ensure the patient remains hemodynamically stable. A patient with AKI on hemodialysis depends on a viable venous access catheter. When not in use, the catheter is "heparin-locked" to preserve patency. The critical care nurse provides education about the disease process and treatment plan to the patient and family.

Continuous Renal Replacement Therapy

CRRT is a continuous mode of dialysis that has been used for more than 40 years and has many similarities to hemodialysis.[38] CRRT is monitored by the critical care nurse, and it may continue over many days. The venous blood is circulated through a highly porous hemofilter. As with traditional hemodialysis, access and return of blood are achieved through a large venous catheter (venovenous). The CRRT system allows the continuous removal of fluid from the plasma. The patient's blood flow is 100 to 200 mL/min, and the dialysate flow ranges from 20 to 30 mL/kg per minute. The fluid removal rate varies depending on the particular CRRT method used and removal of solutes (urea, creatinine, and electrolytes), as listed in Table 19.9. The removed fluid is described as *ultrafiltrate*. In an ideal situation, the hydrostatic pressure exerted by a mean arterial pressure greater than 70 mm Hg would propel a continuous flow of blood through the hemofilter to remove fluid and solute. However, because many critically ill patients are hypotensive and cannot provide adequate flow through the hemofilter, an electric roller pump "milks" the tubing to augment flow. If large amounts of fluid are to be removed, IV replacement solutions are infused. Indications and contraindications for CRRT are listed in Box 19.7.

TABLE 19.8 Complications and Nursing Management of Arteriovenous Fistula or Graft.

Type	Complications	Nursing Management
Fistula	Thrombosis	Teach patients to avoid wearing constrictive clothing on limbs containing access.
	Infection	Teach patients to avoid sleeping on or bending accessed limb for prolonged periods.
	Pseudoaneurysm	Use aseptic technique when cannulating access.
	Vascular steal syndrome	Avoid repetitious cannulation of one segment of access.
	Venous hypertension	Offer comfort measures, such as warm compresses and ordered analgesics, to lessen pain
	Carpal tunnel syndrome	of vascular steal.
	Inadequate blood flow	Teach patients to develop blood flow in fistulas through exercises (squeezing a rubber ball) while applying mild impedance to flow just distal to the access (at least once per day for 10–15 minutes).
		Avoid too-early cannulation of new access.
Graft	Bleeding	Teach patients to avoid wearing constrictive clothing on accessed limbs.
	Thrombosis	Avoid repeated cannulation of one segment of access.
	False aneurysm formation	Use aseptic technique when cannulating access.
	Infection	Monitor for changes in arterial or venous pressure while patients are on dialysis.
	Arterial or venous stenosis	Provide comfort measures to reduce pain of vascular steal (e.g., warm compresses,
	Vascular steal syndrome	analgesics as ordered).

TABLE 19.9 Comparison of Continuous Renal Replacement Therapy Modes.

Type	Ultrafiltration Rate	Fluid Replacement	Mode of Solute Removal	Indication
SCUF	100–300 mL/h	None	None	Fluid removal
CVVH	500–800 mL/h	Predilution or postdilution, calculating hourly net loss	Convection	Fluid removal, moderate solute removal
CVVHD	500–800 mL/h	Predilution or postdilution, subtracting dialysate, then calculating hourly net loss	Diffusion	Fluid removal, maximum solute removal
CVVHDF		Predilution or postdilution, subtracting dialysate, then calculating hourly net loss	Convection and diffusion	Maximal fluid removal, maximal solute removal

CVVH, Continuous venovenous hemofiltration; *CVVHD,* continuous venovenous hemodialysis; *CVVHDF,* continuous venovenous hemodiafiltration; *SCUF,* slow continuous ultrafiltration.

BOX 19.7 Indications and Contraindications for Continuous Renal Replacement Therapy

Indications
- Need for large fluid volume removal in hemodynamically unstable patient
- Hypervolemic or edematous patients unresponsive to diuretic therapy
- Patients with multiple-organ dysfunction syndrome
- Ease of fluid management in patients requiring large daily fluid volume
- Replacement for oliguria
- Administration of total parenteral nutrition
- Contraindication to hemodialysis and peritoneal dialysis
- Inability to be anticoagulated

Contraindications
- Hematocrit greater than 45%
- Terminal illness

Controversy exists about when CRRT should be started, the optimal dialysis dose, which patients can derive the greatest benefit, and when CRRT should be discontinued. The debate over the optimal "dose" of dialysis is likely to continue because, although clinical trials have not shown a difference in mortality between critically ill patients receiving intensive or nonintensive dialysis regimens, the amount of dialysis in the research studies was greater than that normally achieved in clinical practice.[39]

Because controlled removal and replacement of fluid is possible over many hours or days with CRRT, hemodynamic stability is maintained. This makes CRRT highly advantageous for use in hemodynamically unstable patients with multisystem problems. Several modes of CRRT are used in critical care units; a partial list follows:
- Slow continuous ultrafiltration (SCUF)
- Continuous venovenous hemofiltration (CVVH)
- Continuous venovenous hemodialysis (CVVHD)
- Continuous venovenous hemodiafiltration (CVVHDF)

The decision about which type of therapy to initiate is based on clinical assessment, metabolic status, severity of uremia, whether a particular treatment modality is available at that institution, and other factors.

Continuous Renal Replacement Therapy Terminology

In CRRT, solutes are removed from the blood by diffusion or convection.[40] Both processes remove fluid, and the two methods remove molecules of different sizes.

Diffusion. Diffusion describes the movement of solutes along a concentration gradient from a high concentration to a low concentration across a semipermeable membrane. This is the main mechanism used in hemodialysis. Solutes such as creatinine and urea cross the dialysis membrane from the blood to the dialysis fluid compartment.

Convection. Convection occurs when a pressure gradient is set up so that the water is pushed or pumped across the dialysis filter and carries the solutes from the bloodstream with it. This method of solute removal is known as *solvent drag*, and it is commonly used in CRRT.

Absorption. The filter attracts solute, and molecules attach (adsorb) to the dialysis filter. The size of solute molecules is measured in daltons. The different sizes of molecules that can be removed by convection or diffusion methods are shown in Table 19.9. Tiny molecules such as urea and creatinine are removed by diffusion and convection (all methods). As the molecular size increases beyond 500 daltons, convection is the more efficient method (Table 19.10).

Ultrafiltrate volume. The fluid that is removed each hour is not called *urine*; it is known as *ultrafiltrate*.

Replacement fluid. Typically, some of the ultrafiltrate is replaced through the CRRT circuit by a sterile replacement fluid. The replacement fluid can be added before the filter (prefilter dilution) or after the filter (postfilter dilution).[39] The purpose is to increase the volume of fluid passing through the hemofilter and improve solute convection.

Anticoagulation. Because the blood outside the body is in contact with artificial tubing and filters, the coagulation cascade and complement cascades are activated. To prevent the hemofilter from becoming obstructed by clotting, or clotting off, low-dose anticoagulation must be used.[39] The dose should be low enough to have no effect on the patient's anticoagulation parameters. Systemic anticoagulation is not the goal. Typical anticoagulant choices include unfractionated heparin and sodium citrate.[39] Citrate is an effective prefilter anticoagulant, which has the side effect that it chelates (binds to and removes) calcium from the blood. Consequently, ionized calcium levels are verified, and calcium is replaced per protocol when sodium citrate is the anticoagulant.

Modes of Continuous Renal Replacement

Because of the design of the CRRT machine, it is impossible to look at the outside and follow the flow of blood and, if used, dialysate. Each of the CRRT modes is described in the following sections, and diagrams clarify the mode of CRRT that is used.

Slow continuous ultrafiltration. SCUF slowly removes fluid (100–300 mL/h) through a process of ultrafiltration (Fig. 19.7A). This consists of a movement of fluid across a semipermeable membrane. SCUF has minimal effect on solute removal. However, SCUF is an uncommon clinical choice, because it requires both arterial and venous access for effective functioning, and the circuit is more likely to thrombose (clot off) than other CRRT methods that use higher flows. Because small amounts of fluid are gently removed, initially it was hoped that SCUF would be a suitable choice for edematous patients with acute heart failure and diminished perfusion to the kidneys that were unresponsive to diuretics. Currently, intermittent ultrafiltration using a peripheral venous catheter is more likely to be used to remove excess volume from patients with acute decompensated heart failure when the kidneys are unresponsive to diuretics.

Continuous venovenous hemofiltration. CVVH is indicated when the patient's clinical condition warrants removal of significant volumes of fluid and solutes. Fluid is removed by ultrafiltration in volumes of 5 to 20 mL/min or up to 7 to 30 L/24 h. Removal of solutes such as urea, creatinine, and other small non–protein-bound toxins is accomplished by convection. The replacement fluid rate of flow

through the CRRT circuit can be altered to achieve desired fluid and solute removal without causing hemodynamic instability. Replacement fluid can be added via a prehemofilter replacement fluid (Fig. 19.7B) or posthemofilter replacement fluid.

As with other CRRT systems, the blood outside the body is anticoagulated, and the ultrafiltrate is drained off by gravity or by the addition of negative-pressure suction into a large drainage bag. Because large volumes of fluid may be removed in CVVH, some of the removed ultrafiltrate volume must be replaced hourly with a continuous infusion (replacement fluid) to avoid intravascular dehydration. Replacement fluids may consist of standard solutions of bicarbonate, potassium-free lactated Ringer solution, acetate, or dextrose. Electrolytes such as potassium, sodium, calcium chloride, magnesium sulfate, and sodium bicarbonate may be added. The formula used to calculate the volume removed from the patient follows along with an example:

$$\text{Ultrafiltrate in bag} + \text{Other output}-$$
$$(\text{CVVH replacement fluid} + \text{IV/oral/NG intake}) = \text{Output}$$
$$1000\,\text{mL} - 800\,\text{mL} = 200\,\text{mL/h output}$$

Continuous Venovenous Hemodialysis. CVVHD is technically similar to traditional hemodialysis, and it removes solute by diffusion because of a slow (15–30 mL/min) countercurrent drainage flow on the membrane side of the hemofilter (Fig. 19.7C). Blood and fluid move by countercurrent flow through the hemofilter. *Countercurrent* means the blood flows in one direction, and the dialysate flows in the opposite direction. As with other types of CRRT and hemodialysis, although arterial access is always possible, venovenous vascular access is the most common choice.

CVVHD is indicated for patients who require large-volume removal for severe uremia or critical acid–base imbalances or for patients who are resistant to diuretics. A mean arterial pressure of at least 70 mm Hg is desirable for effective volume removal and dialysis, and it is most effective when used over days, not hours. The use of replacement fluid is optional and depends on the patient's clinical condition and plan of care. The critical care nurse is responsible for calculating the hourly intake and output, identifying fluid trends, and replacing excessive losses. This therapy is ideal for hemodynamically unstable patients in the critical care setting because they do not experience the abrupt fluid and solute changes that can accompany standard hemodialysis treatments.

Continuous venovenous hemodiafiltration. Another CRRT option is CVVHDF, which combines two of the previously described methods (CVVH and CVVHD) to achieve maximal fluid and solute removal. A strong transmembrane pressure is applied to the hemofilter to push water across the filter, and a negative pressure is applied at the other side to pull fluid across the membrane and produce large volumes of ultrafiltrate and to create a "solvent drag" (CVVH method). The blood and the dialysate are circulated in a countercurrent flow pattern to remove fluid and solutes by diffusion (hemodialysis method). CVVHDF can remove large volumes of fluid and solute because it uses diffusion gradients and convection.

TABLE 19.10	Size of Molecules Cleared by Continuous Renal Replacement Therapy.		
Type of Molecule	**Size of Molecule**	**Solutes**	**Solute Removal Method**
Small	<500 daltons	Urea, creatinine	Convection, diffusion
Middle	500–5000 daltons	Vancomycin	Convection better than diffusion
Low-molecular-weight (small) proteins	5000–50,000 daltons	Cytokines, complement	Convection or absorption onto hemofilter
Large proteins	>50,000 daltons	Albumin	Minimal removal

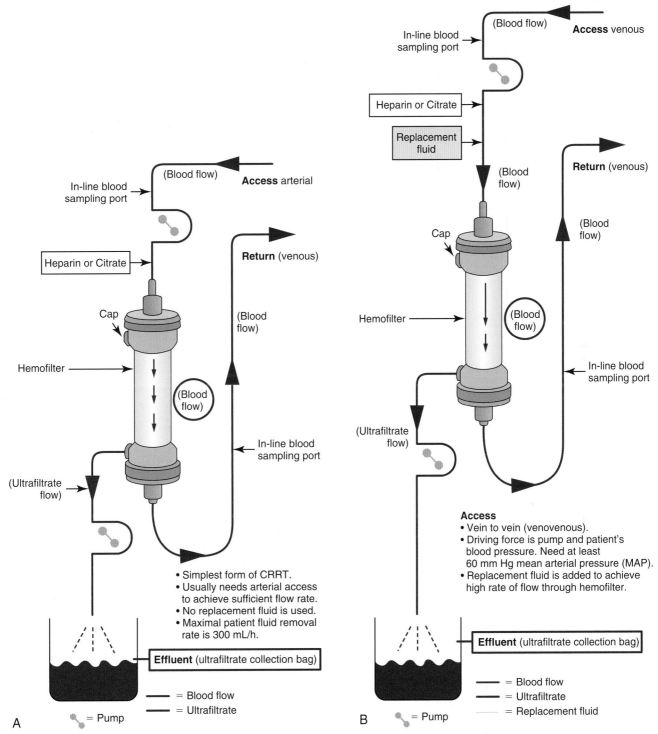

Fig. 19.7 Continuous Renal Replacement Therapy *(CRRT)* Systems. (A) Slow continuous ultrafiltration. (B) Continuous venovenous hemofiltration.

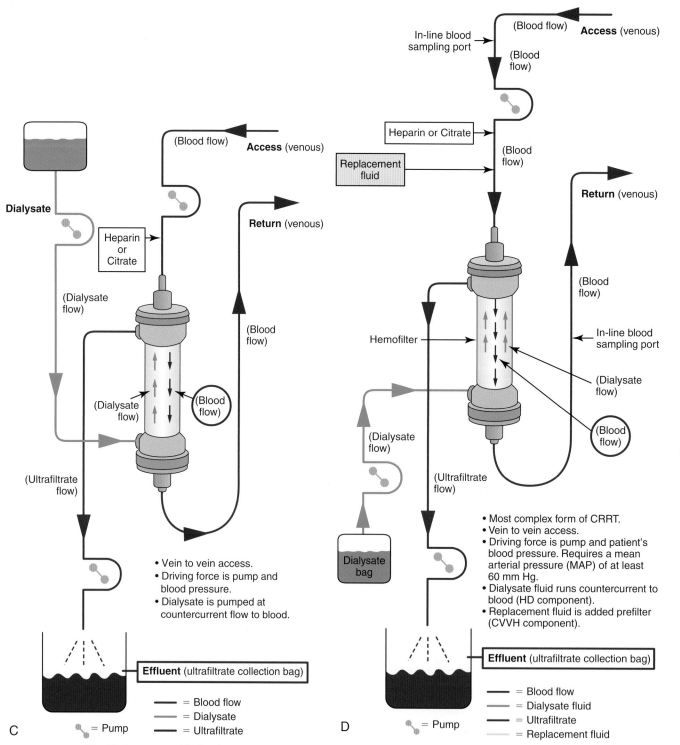

Fig. 19.7, cont'd. (C) Continuous venovenous hemofiltration dialysis. (D) Continuous venovenous hemo-diafiltration *(CVVH).*

Complications

Potential problems associated with CRRT and appropriate nursing interventions are listed in Box 19.8. Complications are often related to the rate of flow through the system. If the patient becomes hypotensive or the access lines remain kinked, the ultrafiltration rate decreases. This can lead to increased clot formation within the hemofilter. As the surface of the hemofilter becomes more clotted, it does not provide effective fluid or solute clearance, and CRRT is stopped; a new CRRT circuit must then be set up. The most common reasons for interruption in CRRT are clotting and patient clinical issues.

The critical care nurse monitors the pressures displayed on the CRRT machine screen to monitor the positive pressure of fluid going into the hemofilter (inflow) and the pressures coming out of the hemofilter to ensure that resistance to the negative-pressure pull of the

QSEN

BOX 19.8 Safety

Complications Associated With Continuous Renal Replacement Therapy

Problem	Cause	Clinical Manifestations	Nursing Management
Decreased ultrafiltration rate	Hypotension Dehydration Kinked lines Bending of catheters Clotting of filter	Ultrafiltration rate decreased Minimal flow through blood lines	Observe filter and arteriovenous system Control blood flow Control coagulation time Position patient on back Lower height of collection container
Filter clotting	Obstruction Insufficient heparinization	Ultrafiltration rate decreased, despite height of collection container being lower	Control anticoagulation (heparin/citrate) Maintain continuous system anticoagulation Call physician Remove system Prime catheters with anticoagulated solution Prime new system; connect it Start predilution with 1000 mL saline 0.9% solution/h Do not use three-way stopcocks
Hypotension	Increased ultrafiltration rate Blood leak Disconnection of one of lines	Bleeding Call physician	Control amount of ultrafiltration Control access sites Clamp lines
Fluid and electrolyte changes	Too much or too little removal of fluid Inappropriate replacement of electrolytes Inappropriate dialysate	Changes in mentation ↑ or ↓ CVP ↑ or ↓ PAOP ECG changes ↑ or ↓ BP and heart rate Abnormal electrolyte levels	Observe for: • Changes in CVP or PAOP • Changes in vital signs • ECG change resulting from electrolyte abnormalities Monitor output values every hour Control ultrafiltration
Bleeding	System disconnection ↑ Heparin dose	Oozing from catheter insertion site or connection	Monitor ACT no less than once every hour (heparin) Adjust heparin dose within specifications to maintain ACT Monitor serum calcium if using citrate as an anticoagulant Observe dressing on vascular access for blood loss Observe for blood in filtrate (filter leak)
Access dislodgment or infection	Catheter or connections not secured Break in sterile technique Excessive patient movement	Bleeding from catheter site or connections Inappropriate flow or infusion Fever Drainage at catheter site	Observe access site at least once every 2 hours Ensure that clamps are available within easy reach at all times Observe strict sterile technique when dressing vascular access

ACT, Activated coagulation time; *BP,* blood pressure; *CRRT,* continuous renal replacement therapy; *CVP,* central venous pressure; *ECG,* electrocardiogram; *PAOP,* pulmonary artery occlusion pressure; ↑, increased; ↓, decreased.

fluid across the hemofilter membrane has not developed. Other patient-related complications include fluid and electrolyte alterations, bleeding because of anticoagulation, or problems with the access site such as dislodgment or infection.

Medical Management

The choice of the method of blood purification to treat AKI is a medical decision. There is no clinical or research consensus about whether IHD or CRRT is the most beneficial, and no difference in outcomes has been shown in clinical research trials.[39,41] Age, sex, and preexisting chronic conditions are of little help in determining whether to select IHD or CRRT. Often the acute clinical diagnosis, physician's preference, availability of the CRRT machine, and knowledgeable nurses and physicians at the hospital are the deciding factors.[42]

The current trend is to start IHD or CRRT earlier rather than later in the course of AKI, especially for hemodynamically unstable patients.[39,41] There is no definitive number at which renal replacement therapy is initiated. The threshold to begin treatment is based on an increasing serum creatinine and the patient's illness, especially organ failure. If the patient has severe electrolyte imbalance or fluid overload, even earlier intervention may be required. Another concern is to determine the correct dose of CRRT for an individual patient. One estimate is to aim for a solute removal of 20 to 25 mL/kg/h of CRRT effluent generation.[1] If the patient is receiving antibiotics or other medications normally filtered by the kidneys, the dosages may need to be adjusted to account for loss in the CRRT effluent.

Another challenge is when to stop CRRT, or rather how to determine that the kidneys have recovered sufficiently to produce urine and effective solute clearance.[1] One recommendation is a urine output of 500 mL/day.[1]

Nursing Management

Critical care nurses play a vital role in monitoring patients receiving CRRT. In many critical care units, the CRRT system is set up by the dialysis staff but is run on a 24-hour basis by critical care nurses with additional training. Complications may be related to the CRRT circuit, the CRRT pump, or the patient (Box 19.9). The critical care nurse monitors fluid intake and output, prevents or detects potential complications (e.g., bleeding, hypotension), identifies trends in electrolyte laboratory values, supervises safe operation of the CRRT equipment, and provides patient and family education about the patient's condition and the use of CRRT.

KIDNEY PHARMACOLOGY

The first step is to stop all nephrotoxic medications. Second, if medications are eliminated through the kidneys, it is important to decrease the frequency of administration (e.g., from every 6 hours to every 12 or 24 hours) or to decrease the dose and to monitor the concentration by measuring serum medication levels.

Diuretics

Diuretics are used to stimulate urinary output in a patient with fluid overload and functioning kidneys. Care must be taken to prevent the creation of secondary electrolyte abnormalities (Table 19.11). Diuretics reduce volume overload and are helpful for symptoms such as pulmonary edema, but they have not been shown to prevent AKI. Diuretics are used in many patients other than those with incipient kidney failure.

Loop Diuretics

Loop diuretics include furosemide (Lasix), bumetanide (Bumex), and torsemide. Furosemide is the most commonly used diuretic in critical care patients. It may be administered orally, as an IV bolus, or as a continuous IV infusion. Electrolyte abnormalities are common, and close monitoring of serum potassium, magnesium, and sodium is essential. Loop diuretics block the Na-K-2Cl transporter in the nephron on the ascending limb of the loop of Henle, where most sodium is reabsorbed[43,44] (Fig. 19.8). This diuresis is also a *natriuresis*, because sodium is excreted in the urine.[44] Diuretic resistance can develop over time in patients with chronic heart failure or kidney failure who were taking loop diuretics at home before they were admitted to the hospital. The higher diuretic medication dosages are a reflection of diuretic resistance.[43,44]

Thiazide Diuretics

Diuretics from different classes may be prescribed in combination. A thiazide diuretic such as chlorothiazide (Diuril) or metolazone (Zaroxolyn) may be administered and followed by a loop diuretic to take advantage of the fact that these medications work on different parts of the nephron (see Fig. 19.8). Creatinine clearance affects the efficacy of thiazide diuretics. Metolazone is an effective diuretic in kidney injury to

---

⚙ TRENDING PRIORITIES IN HEALTHCARE

Greening of Health Care Organizations: Recycling Plastics

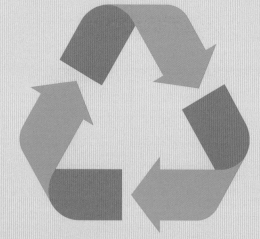

(iStock.com/MariaTkach.)

Recycling has become a way of life at home but not necessarily in health care organizations. While the bottles and cans used by the staff during their breaks may go into a blue recycling bucket, the recycling usually stops there. According to the Healthcare Plastics Recycling Council (HRPC), health care organizations generate about 14,000 tons of waste every day. This waste ends up in landfills or incinerators. HRPC estimates that up to 25% of that waste is plastic packaging and plastic products.[1] Common plastics that could be recycled include sterilization wrap (i.e., blue wrap), irrigation bottles, basins, pitchers, trays, flexible primary packaging (e.g., pouches, blister packs), and flexible clear packaging (e.g., shrink wrap, plastic bags).

Often recycling programs start at a grassroots level, with the staff approaching leadership about "greening" the health care organization. It is important to engage everyone to support a recycling program, including the hospital's waste hauler. CleanRiver listed six steps to starting a recycling program:

1. Start with your waste hauler.
2. Conduct a waste audit.
3. Opt for sustainable suppliers and packaging.
4. Start composting.
5. Keep your recycling program consistent.
6. Educate and communicate with hospital personal about the new recycling program.[2]

It is time for health care organizations to step up and develop a proposal and business case for recycling. Start with one item at a time and expand the program as milestones are achieved.

For additional information about sustainability programs for health care organizations, check out the following websites:

- CleanRiver—www.cleanriver.com
- Global Green and Healthy Hospitals—https://www.greenhospitals.net/
- Healthcare Packaging—www.healthcarepackaging.com
- Healthcare Plastics Recycling Council—www.hprc.org/hospitals
- Plastics Today—www.plasticstoday.com
- Practice Greenhealth—www.practicegreenhealth.org
- Roadrunner Smart Recycling—www.roadrunnerwm.com/
- Sustainability Roadmap for Hospitals—www.sustainabilityroadmap.org/
- Waste 360—www.waste360.com

References

1. Healthcare Plastics Recycling Council. Solutions for hospitals, 2020. https://www.hprc.org/hospitals.
2. CleanRiver. 6 simple steps to start a hospital recycling program; 2018. https://cleanriver.com/6-steps-to-start-a-hospital-recycling-program/.

QSEN BOX 19.9 **Safety**

Complications of Continuous Renal Replacement Therapy

Circuit
- Air embolism
- Clotted hemofilter
- Poor ultrafiltration
- Blood leaks
- Broken filter
- Recirculation or disconnection
- Access failure
- Catheter dislodgment

Pump
- Circuit pressure alarm
- Decreased inflow pressure
- Decreased outflow pressure
- Increased outflow resistance
- Air bubble detector alarm
- Power failure
- Mechanical dysfunction

Patient
- Code or emergency situation
- Dehydration
- Hypotension
- Electrolyte imbalances
- Acid–base imbalances
- Blood loss or hemorrhage
- Hypothermia
- Infection

TABLE 19.11 Pharmacologic Management Kidney Disorders.

Medication	Dosage	Action	Special Considerations
Diuretics			
Loop Diuretics			
Furosemide (Lasix)	20–80 mg/day	Acts on loop of Henle to inhibit sodium and chloride resorption (natriuresis)	Ototoxicity if administered too rapidly or with other ototoxic medications. Caution with sulfa allergy.
Bumetanide (Bumex)	0.5–2 mg/day		Monitor intake and output; hydration; monitor for hypotension. Titrate to maintenance, may increase by 20–40 mg orally at 6–8-hour intervals after the previous dose; this individual dose may be given once or twice daily; maximum 600 mg/day orally. Caution with sulfa allergy.
Thiazide Diuretics			
Chlorothiazide (Diuril)	500–1000 mg/once or twice/day PO/IV	Inhibits sodium, chloride resorption in distal tubule	Enhanced with low-sodium diet; 500–1000 mg PO once or twice daily; may also give intermittently (alternate days or 3–5 days per week). Use IV only when patient cannot take by mouth; caution with sulfa allergy. Synergistic effect with loop diuretics.
Metolazone (Zaroxolyn)	2.5–10 mg/day PO initial dose May increase to 20 mg/day with edema	Inhibits sodium, chloride resorption in distal tubule	Effective to creatinine clearance of 10 mL/min.
Osmotic Diuretics			
Mannitol	0.25–1.0 g/kg IV infusion as 15%–20% solution over 30–90 minutes	Increases urine output because of higher plasma osmolality	Often used in head injury to decrease cerebral edema.
		Increases flow of water from tissues, causing increased GFR	Can be used to promote urinary secretion of toxic substances.
		Increases serum sodium, potassium levels	Mannitol may crystallize at low temperatures; use in-line 5-micron IV filter with >15% (>15 g/100 mL) solutions.
Potassium-Sparing Diuretics			
Spironolactone (Aldactone)	25–50 mg/day	Exerts effects on collecting duct; retains potassium, increases sodium diuresis	Weak diuretic effect. Potassium supplements not required; monitor for hyperkalemia. Used as an aldosterone blocker to treat heart failure.
Vaptans			
Conivaptan (Vaprisol)	Loading dose: 20 mg IV as 30-minute infusion Continuous IV infusion: 20 mg over 24 hours After first day, can be increased to 40 mg/24 h Maximum infusion is 4 days	Blocks V2 aquaporin channels in collecting tubules	Used only in hyponatremia with hypervolemia. Monitor volume status and serum sodium frequently.

BP, Blood pressure; *ECG*, electrocardiogram; *GFR*, glomerular filtration rate; *GI*, gastrointestinal; *IV*, intravenous/intravenously; *PO*, by mouth.

a creatinine clearance of 10 mL/min. A normal creatinine clearance is 120 mL/min. Sometimes a thiazide diuretic is added to a loop diuretic to compensate for the development of loop diuretic resistance.[44]

Osmotic Diuretics

Osmotic diuretics, such as mannitol, are prescribed to increase urine output and decrease fluid overload. It is important to use an in-line 5-micron filter when administering this IV medication. Mannitol is commonly administered to patients with brain injury and increased intracranial pressure. More information on the use of mannitol in patients with neurologic disorders can be found in Chapter 17. Mannitol is filtered by the glomerulus, is not absorbed by the nephron, and works in the proximal tubule and the descending section of the loop of Henle via aquaporin water channels (see Fig. 19.8).

Carbonic Anhydrase Inhibitor Diuretics

Only one carbonic anhydrase inhibitor acts as a diuretic, and it is used in very specific clinical circumstances. Acetazolamide (Diamox) acts on the proximal tubule, where it inhibits the carbonic anhydrase enzyme, allowing more bicarbonate (HCO_3^-) to be released into the filtrate and resulting in an alkaline diuresis (see Fig. 19.8). Acetazolamide is administered to treat the metabolic alkalosis that sometimes occurs after aggressive diuresis with loop diuretics.[45] Acid–base balance and serum bicarbonate levels are typically monitored when acetazolamide is used to treat metabolic alkalosis.

Potassium-Sparing Diuretics

Spironolactone (Aldactone) is a "potassium-sparing" diuretic. Spironolactone inhibits the aldosterone mineralocorticoid receptor in the late distal tubule and collecting duct of the kidneys, causing potassium to be retained and sodium to be excreted (see Fig. 19.8). At high dosages, it has a diuretic action, although that is rarely the rationale behind its use today. Spironolactone is most often administered as an aldosterone antagonist in the management of heart failure.

Vaptans

A newer class of medications collectively described as *vaptans* inhibit the effect of antidiuretic hormone (vasopressin) on the V2 aquaporin channels in the collecting ducts of the kidney (see Fig. 19.8). Blockage of the aquaporin channels renders the collecting ducts impermeable, resulting in solute-free water excretion, or aquadiuresis.[46] Vaptans are used to correct symptomatic hypervolemic hyponatremic (dilutional) states. The clinical intent is to eliminate water and retain sodium.[46] These medications must not be administered for hypovolemic hyponatremia or anuria. Conditions that can cause dilutional hyponatremia include syndrome of inappropriate antidiuretic hormone secretion (described in Chapter 23), liver cirrhosis with ascites, and heart failure. Only two vaptans are approved by the FDA for use in the United States. Conivaptan (Vaprisol), which is administered intravenously, is approved for short-term use in the hospital only. Tolvaptan (Samsca) is available only as an oral medication.[46]

Dopamine

Low-dose dopamine (2 to 3 mcg/kg per minute), previously known as *renal-dose dopamine*, is commonly infused to stimulate blood flow to the kidney. Dopamine is effective in increasing urine output in the short-term, but tolerance of the dopamine renal receptor to the medication is theorized to develop in critically ill patients who are most at risk for AKI. Low-dose dopamine does not prevent onset of AKI, decrease the need for dialysis, or reduce mortality. At this point, the support for routine use of low-dose dopamine for the prevention of AKI remains anecdotal only. Low-dose dopamine infusions may have other therapeutic uses, such as increasing urine output, in combination with furosemide in patients with heart failure.

Acetylcysteine

Acetylcysteine (Mucomyst, Mucosil) is an *N*-acetyl derivative of the amino acid l-cysteine. It has been used for many years as a mucolytic agent to assist with expectoration of thick pulmonary secretions. It is

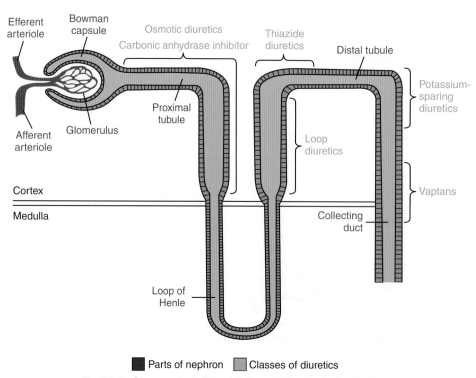

Fig. 19.8 Pharmacologic Site of Action of Diuretics in the Nephron.

also commonly prescribed for patients with mildly elevated serum creatinine levels before a radiologic study using contrast dye. In research trials, the addition of acetylcysteine to normal saline hydration did not reduce the incidence of contrast-induced AKI.

Dietary Phosphorus Binders

Many patients with kidney failure are prescribed a dietary phosphorus—binding medication (see earlier section Dietary Phosphorus—Binding Medications). Many dietary phosphorus binders are available, and some important issues concern all of them. The dietary phosphorus binder must be taken at the time of the meal. If it is taken 2 hours later, it will increase only the level of the binding substance (e.g., calcium) in the bloodstream and will not lower the serum phosphorus level. Related issues, such as the quantity of phosphorus in the diet, should be discussed with a clinical nutritionist (dietitian).

ADDITIONAL RESOURCES

Refer to Box 19.10 for Internet resources related to kidney disorders and therapeutic management.

QSEN | **BOX 19.10 INFORMATICS**

Internet Resources: Kidney Disorders and Therapeutic Management
- American Kidney Fund: https://www.kidneyfund.org/
- National Health Service: https://www.nhs.uk/conditions/acute-kidney-injury/
- Urology Care Foundation: https://www.urologyhealth.org/urology-a-z/k/kidney-(renal)-failure

---

REFERENCES

1. Ronco C, Bellomo R, Kellum JA. Acute kidney injury. *Lancet.* 2019;394(10212):1949—1964.
2. Hoste EA. Epidemiology of acute kidney injury in critically ill patients: the multinational AKI-EPI study. *Intensive Care Med.* 2015;41(8):1411—1423.
3. Legrand M, Hollinger A, Vieillard-Baron A, et al. The French and euRopean Outcome reGistry in ICUs (FROG-ICU) Investigators. One-year prognosis of kidney injury at discharge from the ICU: a multicenter observational study. *Crit Care Med.* 2019;47(12):e953—e961.
4. Bellomo R, Ronco C, Mehta RL, et al. Acute kidney injury in the ICU: from injury to recovery: reports from the 5th Paris International Conference. *Ann Intensive Care.* 2017;7(1):49.
5. Makris K, Spanou L. Acute kidney injury: definition, pathophysiology and clinical phenotypes. *Clin Biochem Rev.* 2016;37(2):85—98.
6. Moore PK, Hsu RK, Liu KD. Management of acute kidney injury: core curriculum 2018. *Am J Kidney Dis.* 2018;72(1):136—148.
7. Kellum JA, Lameire N, Aspelin P, et al. Kidney Disease: Improving Global Outcomes (KDIGO) Acute Kidney Injury Work Group. KDIGO clinical practice guideline for acute kidney injury. *Kidney Int Suppl.* 2012;2(2):1—138.
8. Rangaswami J, Bhalla V, Blair JEA, et al. The American Heart Association Council on the Kidney in Cardiovascular Disease and Council on Clinical Cardiology. Cardiorenal syndrome: classification, pathophysiology, diagnosis, and treatment strategies: a scientific statement from the American Heart Association. *Circulation.* 2019;139(16):e840—e878.
9. Husain-Syed F, Slutsky AS, Ronco C. Lung-kidney cross-talk in the critically ill patient. *Am J Respir Crit Care Med.* 2016;194(4):402—414.
10. Navaneethan SD, Schold JD, Huang H, et al. Mortality outcomes of patients with chronic kidney disease and chronic obstructive pulmonary disease. *Am J Nephrol.* 2016;43(1):39—46.
11. Joannidis M, Forni LG, Klein SJ, et al. Lung-kidney interactions in critically ill patients: consensus report of the Acute Disease Quality Initiative (ADQI) 21 Workgroup. *Intensive Care Med.* 2020;46(4):654—672.
12. Bellomo R, Kellum JA, Ronco C, et al. Acute kidney injury in sepsis. *Intensive Care Med.* 2017;43(6):816—828.
13. Perkins ZB, Haines RW, Prowle JR. Trauma-associated acute kidney injury. *Curr Opin Crit Care.* 2019;25(6):565—572.
14. Parekh R, Care DA, Tainter CR. Rhabdomyolysis: advances in diagnosis and treatment. *Emerg Med Pract.* 2012;14(3):1—15; quiz 15.
15. Zimmerman JL, Shen MC. Rhabdomyolysis. *Chest.* 2013;144(3):1058—1065.
16. Lambert P, Chaisson K, Horton S, et al. The Northern New England Cardiovascular Disease Study Group. Reducing acute kidney injury due to contrast material: how nurses can improve patient safety. *Crit Care Nurse.* 2017;37(1):13—26.
17. Helgason D, Long TE, Helgadottir S, et al. Acute kidney injury following coronary angiography: a nationwide study of incidence, risk factors and longterm outcomes. *J Nephrol.* 2018;31(5):721—730.
18. Siew ED, Liu KD. Contrast-induced acute kidney injury in the PRESERVE Trial: lessons learned. *Clin J Am Soc Nephrol.* 2018;13(6):949—951.
19. Palmer BF, Clegg DJ. Hyperkalemia across the continuum of kidney function. *Clin J Am Soc Nephrol.* 2018;13(1):155—157.
20. Dépret F, Peacock WF, Liu KD, Rafique Z, Rossignol P, Legrand M. Management of hyperkalemia in the acutely ill patient. *Ann Intensive Care.* 2019;9(1):32.
21. Woitok BK, Funk GC, Walter P, Schwarz C, Ravioli S, Lindner G. Dysnatremias in emergency patients with acute kidney injury: a cross-sectional analysis. *Am J Emerg Med.* 2020;38(12):2602—2606.
22. Hill Gallant KM, Spiegel DM. Calcium balance in chronic kidney disease. *Curr Osteoporos Rep.* 2017;15(3):214—221.
23. Vervloet MG, Sezer S, Massy ZA, et al. The ERA-EDTA Working Group on Chronic Kidney Disease-Mineral and Bone Disorders, the European Renal Nutrition Working Group. The role of phosphate in kidney disease. *Nat Rev Nephrol.* 2017;13(1):27—38.
24. Aberegg SK. Ionized calcium in the ICU: should it be measured and corrected? *Chest.* 2016;149(3):846—855.
25. Friederich A, Martin N, Swanson MB, Faine BA, Mohr NM. Normal saline solution and lactated Ringer's solution have a similar effect on quality of recovery: a randomized controlled trial. *Ann Emerg Med.* 2019;73(2):160—169.
26. Duffy RA, Foroozesh MB, Loflin RD, et al. Normal saline versus Normosol-R in sepsis resuscitation: a retrospective cohort study. *J Intensive Care Soc.* 2019;20(3):223—230.
27. Semler MW, Self WH, Wanderer JP. The SMART investigators and the pragmatic critical care resource group, et al. Balanced crystalloids versus saline in critically ill adults. *N Engl J Med.* 2018;378(9):829—839.
28. Hammond DA, Lam SW, Rech MA, et al. Balanced crystalloids versus saline in critically ill adults: a systematic review and meta-analysis. *Ann Pharmacother.* 2020;54(1):5—13.
29. Lewis SR, Pritchard MW, Evans DJ, et al. Colloids versus crystalloids for fluid resuscitation in critically ill people. *Cochrane Database Syst Rev.* 2018;8(8):CD000567.
30. Heming N, Lamothe L, Jaber S, et al. Morbidity and mortality of crystalloids compared to colloids in critically ill surgical patients: a subgroup analysis of a randomized trial. *Anesthesiology.* 2018;129(6):1149—1158.
31. Joosten A, Delaporte A, Mortier J, et al. Long-term impact of crystalloid versus colloid solutions on renal function and disability-free survival after major abdominal surgery. *Anesthesiology.* 2019;130(2):227—236.
32. Myles PS, Bellomo R, Corcoran T, et al. The Australian and New Zealand College of Anaesthetists Clinical Trials Network, and the Australian and New Zealand Intensive Care Society Clinical Trials Group. Restrictive versus liberal fluid therapy for major abdominal surgery. *N Engl J Med.* 2018;378(24):2263—2274.
33. Meyhoff TS, Møller MH, Hjortrup PB, Cronhjort M, Perner A, Wetterslev J. Lower versus higher fluid volumes during initial management of sepsis—a systematic review with meta-analysis and trial sequential analysis. *Chest.* 2020;157(6):1478—1496.
34. Beeson T, Davis C. Urinary management with an external female collection device. *J Wound Ostomy Continence Nurs.* 2018;45(2):187—189.

35. Durant DJ. Nurse-driven protocols and the prevention of catheter-associated urinary tract infections: a systematic review. *Am J Infect Control.* 2017;45(12):1331−1341.

36. National Institute of Diabetes and Digestive and Kidney Diseases (NIDDK). Kidney disease statistics for the United States. https://www.niddk.nih.gov/health-information/health-statistics/kidneydisease. Accessed October 4, 2020.

37. Cody JD, Hodson EM. Recombinant human erythropoietin versus placebo or no treatment for the anaemia of chronic kidney disease in people not requiring dialysis. *Cochrane Database Syst Rev.* 2016;1:CD003266.

38. Ronco C. Continuous renal replacement therapy: forty-year anniversary. *Int J Artif Organs.* 2017;40(6):257−264.

39. Ronco C, Ricci Z, De Backer D, et al. Renal replacement therapy in acute kidney injury: controversy and consensus. *Crit Care.* 2015;19:146.

40. Neri M, Villa G, Garzotto F, et al. Nomenclature for renal replacement therapy in acute kidney injury: basic principles. *Crit Care.* 2016;20(1):318.

41. Villa G, Ricci Z, Ronco C. Renal replacement therapy. *Crit Care Clin.* 2015;31(4):839−848.

42. Murugan R, Ostermann M, Peng Z, et al. Net ultrafiltration prescription and practice among critically ill patients receiving renal replacement therapy: a multinational survey of critical care practitioners. *Crit Care Med.* 2020;48(2):e87−e89.

43. Masella C, Viggiano D, Molfino I, et al. Diuretic resistance in cardio-nephrology: role of pharmacokinetics, hypochloremia, and kidney remodeling. *Kidney Blood Press Res.* 2019;44(5):915−927.

44. Ellison DH. Clinical pharmacology in diuretic use. *Clin J Am Soc Nephrol.* 2019;14(8):1248−1257.

45. Wongboonsin J, Thongprayoon C, Bathini T, et al. Acetazolamide therapy in patients with heart failure: a meta-analysis. *J Clin Med.* 2019;8(3):349.

46. Berl T. Vasopressin antagonists. *N Engl J Med.* 2015;372(23):2207−2216.

Gastrointestinal Clinical Assessment and Diagnostic Procedures

Jacqueline Fitzgerald Close

HISTORY

Taking a thorough and accurate history is extremely important to the assessment process. The patient's history provides the foundation and direction for the rest of the assessment. The overall goal of the patient interview is to expose key clinical manifestations that will facilitate the identification of the underlying cause of the illness. This information can assist in the development of an appropriate management plan.

The initial presentation of the patient determines the rapidity and direction of the interview. For a patient in acute distress, the history should be curtailed to a few questions about the patient's chief complaint and the precipitating events. For a patient in no obvious distress, the history should focus on current symptoms, the patient's medical history, and the family history. Specific items regarding each of these areas are outlined in Box 20.1.[1]

PRIORITY CLINICAL ASSESSMENT

The physical assessment helps establish baseline data about the physical dimensions of the patient's situation. The abdomen is divided into four quadrants (left upper, right upper, left lower, and right lower) with the umbilicus as the middle point, to specify the location of examination findings (Fig. 20.1 and Box 20.2).[2] The patient should empty his or her bladder before the examination, as a full bladder could distort the accuracy of the examination. The assessment should proceed when the patient is as comfortable as possible and in the supine position; however, the position may need readjustment if it elicits pain. To prevent stimulation of gastrointestinal (GI) activity, the order for the assessment should be changed to inspection, auscultation, percussion, and palpation.[3]

Inspection

Inspection of the patient focuses on three areas: (1) observation of the oral cavity, (2) assessment of the skin over the abdomen, and (3) evaluation of the shape of the abdomen. Inspection should be performed in a warm, well-lit environment, and the patient should be in a comfortable position, with the abdomen exposed.

Observation of the Oral Cavity

Although assessment of the GI system classically begins with inspection of the abdomen, the patient's oral cavity also must be inspected to determine any unusual findings. Abnormal findings of the mouth include temporomandibular joint tenderness, inflammation of gums, missing teeth, dental caries, ill-fitting dentures, and mouth odor.[4]

Assessment of the Skin Over the Abdomen

Observe the skin for pigmentation, lesions, striae, scars, petechiae, signs of dehydration, and venous pattern. Pigmentation may vary considerably and still be within normal limits because of race and ethnic background, although the abdomen usually is of a lighter color than other exposed areas of the skin. Abnormal findings include jaundice, skin lesions, and a tense and glistening appearance of the skin. A deviated umbilicus may be caused by a mass, hernia, fluid, or old scar tissue. An everted umbilicus is apparent with distention. Old striae (stretch marks) usually are silver, whereas pinkish purple striae may indicate Cushing syndrome.[5] Bluish discoloration of the umbilicus (Cullen sign) and of the flank (Grey Turner sign) indicates retroperitoneal bleeding.[2]

Evaluation of the Shape of the Abdomen

Observe the abdomen for contour, noting whether it is flat, slightly concave, or slightly round; observe for symmetry and for movement.[6] Marked distention is an abnormal finding. Ascites may cause generalized distention and bulging flanks. Asymmetric distention may indicate organ enlargement, large masses, hernia, or bowel obstruction.[5] Peristaltic waves should not be visible except in very thin patients. In the case of intestinal obstruction, hyperactive peristaltic waves may be observed. Pulsation in the epigastric area is often a normal finding, but increased pulsation may indicate an aortic aneurysm.[6] Symmetric movement of the abdomen with respirations is usually seen in men.[2]

Auscultation

Auscultation of the patient focuses on two areas: (1) evaluation of bowel sounds and (2) assessment of bruits. Auscultation of the abdomen provides clinical data regarding the status of bowel motility.

BOX 20.1 DATA COLLECTION

Gastrointestinal History

Common Gastrointestinal Symptoms
- Oral lesions
- Digestion or indigestion (heartburn)
- Dysphagia
- Nausea
- Vomiting
- Hematemesis
- Change in stool color or contents (e.g., clay-colored, tarry, fresh blood, mucus, undigested food)
- Constipation
- Diarrhea
- Abdominal pain
- Jaundice
- Anal discomfort
- Fecal incontinence

Patient Lifestyle
- Usual height and weight
- Dietary habits
- Usual number of meals or snacks per day
- Usual fluid intake per day
- Nutrient intake
- Types of food usually eaten at each meal or snack
- Food likes and dislikes
- Religious or medical food restrictions
- Food intolerances
- Patient's perceptions and concerns about adequacy of diet and appropriateness of weight
- Effects of lifestyle on food intake, weight gain, or loss
- Vitamins or nutritional supplements (e.g., type, amount, frequency)
- Bowel elimination
- Usual frequency of bowel movements
- Usual consistency and color of stool
- Ability to control elimination of gas and stool
- Any changes in bowel elimination patterns
- Use of enemas or laxatives (e.g., reason for use, frequency, type, response)
- Alcohol intake (e.g., frequency, usual amounts)
- Exercise patterns

Medical History
- Chronic illnesses
- Previous weight gain or loss
- Tooth extractions or orthodontic work
- GI disorders (e.g., peptic ulcer, inflammatory bowel disease, polyps, cholelithiasis, diverticular disease, pancreatitis, intestinal obstruction)
- Hepatitis or cirrhosis
- Abdominal surgery
- Abdominal trauma
- Cancer affecting GI system
- Spinal cord injury
- Women: episiotomy or fourth-degree laceration during delivery
- Exposure to infectious agents (e.g., foreign travel, water source)

Family History
- Investigate for history of following disorders, and document (+ or −) responses
- Hirschsprung disease
- Obesity
- Metabolic disorders
- Inflammatory disorders
- Malabsorption syndromes
- Familial Mediterranean fever
- Rectal polyps
- Polyposis syndromes
- Cancer of GI tract

Current Medication Use
- Laxatives
- Stool softeners
- Antiemetics
- Antidiarrheals
- Antacids
- Aspirin
- Acetaminophen
- Nonsteroidal antiinflammatory drugs
- Corticosteroids

GI, Gastrointestinal.

Initially, listen with the diaphragm of the stethoscope below and to the right of the umbilicus. The examination proceeds methodically through all four quadrants, lifting and then replacing the diaphragm of the stethoscope lightly against the abdomen (see Fig. 20.1).

Evaluation of Bowel Sounds

Normal bowel sounds include high-pitched, gurgling sounds that occur approximately every 5 to 10 seconds[5] or at a rate of 5 to 30 times per minute.[6] Colonic sounds are low-pitched sounds with a rumbling quality.

Abnormal findings include the absence of bowel sounds throughout a 5-minute period; extremely soft, widely separated sounds; and increased sounds with a high-pitched, loud rushing sound (peristaltic rush).[5] Hyperactive bowel sounds that are tinkling may indicate increased motility related to an early bowel obstruction, diarrhea, or gastroenteritis. Hypoactive bowel sounds may indicate

paralytic ileus after surgery, which is very common; peritoneal irritation; or bowel obstruction. Absent bowel sounds may result from inflammation; ileus; electrolyte disturbances; and ischemia, which requires immediate attention.[2]

Assessment of Bruits

Bruits are created by turbulent flow over a partially obstructed artery and are always considered an abnormal finding. The aorta, the right and left renal arteries, and the iliac arteries should be auscultated for the presence of bruits using the bell of the stethoscope (Fig. 20.2).[2,3]

Palpation

Palpation of the patient focuses on one area—detection of abdominal pathologic conditions. Light and deep palpation of each organ and quadrant should be completed. Light palpation, which has a palpation depth of approximately 1 cm, assesses to the depth of the skin and

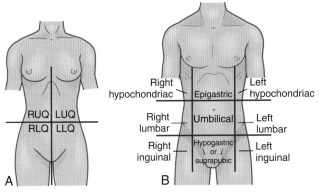

Fig. 20.1 Abdominal Quadrants and Regions. (A) Abdominal quadrants. (B) Abdominal regions. *LLQ,* Left lower quadrant; *LUQ,* left upper quadrant; *RLQ,* right lower quadrant; *RUQ,* right upper quadrant. (From Harding MM, ed. *Lewis's Medical-Surgical Nursing: Assessment and Management of Clinical Problems.* 11th ed. St. Louis: Elsevier; 2020.)

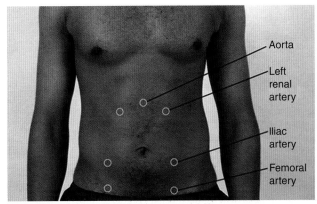

Fig. 20.2 Auscultation for Bruits. (From Jarvis C, ed. *Physical Examination and Health Assessment.* 8th ed. St. Louis: Elsevier; 2020.)

fascia. Deep palpation assesses the rectus abdominis muscle and is performed bimanually to a depth of 4 to 5 cm.[4] Deep palpation is most helpful in detecting abdominal masses.[3] Areas in which the patient complains of tenderness should be palpated last.

Detection of Abdominal Pathologic Conditions

Normal findings include no areas of tenderness or pain, no masses, and no hardened areas. Persistent involuntary guarding may indicate peritoneal inflammation, particularly if it continues after relaxation techniques are used. Rebound tenderness, in which pain increases with quick release of a palpated area, indicates an inflamed peritoneum.[3]

Percussion

Percussion of the patient focuses on one area: assessment of the deep organs. Percussion is used to elicit information about deep organs

such as the liver, spleen, and pancreas. Because the abdomen is a sensitive area, muscle tension may interfere with this part of the assessment. Percussion often helps relax tense muscles, and it is performed before palpation. Percussion in the absence of disease helps delineate the position and size of the liver and spleen, and it assists in the detection of fluid, gaseous distention, and masses in the abdomen.[6]

Assessment of Deep Organs

Percussion should proceed systematically and lightly in all four quadrants. Normal findings include tympany over the empty stomach, tympany or hyperresonance over the intestine, and dullness over the liver and spleen.[2] Abnormal areas of dullness may indicate an underlying mass. Tenderness over the liver may indicate inflammation or infection.[5] Solid masses, enlarged organs, and a distended bladder also produce areas of dullness. Dullness over both flanks may indicate ascites and necessitates further assessment.[3]

BOX 20.2 Anatomic Correlates of the Abdomen

Right Upper Quadrant
- Liver and gallbladder
- Pylorus
- Duodenum
- Head of pancreas
- Right adrenal gland
- Portion of right kidney
- Hepatic flexure of colon
- Portion of ascending and transverse colon

Right Lower Quadrant
- Lower pole of right kidney
- Cecum and appendix
- Portion of ascending colon
- Bladder (if distended)
- Ovary and salpinx
- Uterus (if enlarged)
- Right spermatic cord
- Right ureter

Left Upper Quadrant
- Left lobe of liver

- Spleen
- Stomach
- Body of pancreas
- Left adrenal gland
- Portion of left kidney
- Splenic flexure of colon
- Portions of transverse and descending colon

Left Lower Quadrant
- Lower pole of left kidney
- Sigmoid colon
- Portion of descending colon
- Bladder (if distended)
- Ovary and salpinx
- Uterus (if distended)
- Left spermatic cord
- Left ureter

Midline
- Aorta
- Uterus (if enlarged)
- Bladder (if distended)

LABORATORY STUDIES

The value of various laboratory studies used to diagnose and treat diseases of the GI system has been emphasized often. However, no single study provides an overall picture of the functional state of the various organs, and no single value is predictive by itself. Laboratory studies used in the assessment of GI function, liver function, and pancreatic function are presented in Tables 20.1 to 20.3.

DIAGNOSTIC PROCEDURES

To complete the assessment of a critically ill patient with GI dysfunction, the patient's diagnostic tests are reviewed. Although many procedures exist for diagnosing GI disease, their application in a critically ill patient is limited. Only procedures that are currently used in the critical care setting are presented here.

Endoscopy

Available in several forms, fiberoptic endoscopy is a diagnostic procedure for the direct visualization and evaluation of the GI tract. Endoscopy can provide information about lesions, mucosal changes, obstructions, and motility dysfunction, and a biopsy or removal of foreign objects may be performed during the procedure. The main difference between the various diagnostic forms is the length of the anatomic area that can be examined. Esophagogastroduodenoscopy permits viewing of the upper GI tract from the esophagus to the upper duodenum, and it is used to evaluate sources of upper GI bleeding. Colonoscopy permits viewing of the lower GI tract from the rectum to the distal ileum, and it is used to evaluate sources of lower GI bleeding. Enteroscopy permits viewing of the small bowel beyond the ligament of Treitz, and it is used to evaluate sources of GI bleeding that have not been identified previously with esophagogastroduodenoscopy or colonoscopy. Endoscopic retrograde cholangiopancreatography enables viewing of the biliary and pancreatic ducts, and it is used in the evaluation of pancreatitis. During this procedure, contrast medium is injected into the ducts through the endoscope, and radiographs are obtained.[7] Endoscopy also provides therapeutic benefits for various conditions, including GI bleeding.[8]

Angiography

Angiography is used as a diagnostic and a therapeutic procedure. Diagnostically, it is used to evaluate the status of the GI circulation.[7] Therapeutically, it is used to achieve transcatheter control of GI bleeding.[9] Angiography may be used for lower GI bleeding and as a way to isolate the bleeding source before surgery. Angiography is used in the diagnosis of upper GI bleeding only when endoscopy fails, and it is used to treat patients (approximately 15%) whose GI bleeding is not stopped with medical measures or endoscopic treatment.[9] Angiography also is used to evaluate cirrhosis, portal hypertension, intestinal ischemia, and other vascular abnormalities.[7]

During this procedure, a catheter is advanced over a guidewire into the vessel supplying the portion of the GI tract that is being studied.

TABLE 20.1 Selected Laboratory Studies of Gastrointestinal Function

Test	Normal Findings	Clinical Significance of Abnormal Findings
Stool studies	Resident microorganisms: clostridia, enterococci, *Pseudomonas*, a few yeasts	Detection of *Salmonella typhi* (typhoid fever), *Shigella* (dysentery), *Vibrio cholerae* (cholera), *Yersinia* (enterocolitis), *Escherichia coli* (gastroenteritis), *Staphylococcus aureus* (food poisoning), *Clostridium botulinum* (food poisoning), *Clostridium perfringens* (food poisoning), *Aeromonas* (gastroenteritis)
	Fat: 2–6 g/24 hr	Steatorrhea (increased values) resulting from intestinal malabsorption or pancreatic insufficiency
	Pus: none	Large amounts of pus associated with chronic ulcerative colitis, abscesses, and anorectal fistula
	Occult blood: none (ortho-toluidine or guaiac test)	Positive test results associated with bleeding
	Ova and parasites: none	Detection of *Entamoeba histolytica* (amebiasis), *Giardia lamblia* (giardiasis), and worms
d-Xylose absorption	5-hour urinary excretion: 4.5 g/L Peak blood level: >30 mg/dL	Differentiation of pancreatic steatorrhea (normal d-xylose absorption) from intestinal steatorrhea (impaired d-xylose absorption)
Gastric acid stimulation	11–20 mEq/hr after stimulation	Detection of duodenal ulcers, Zollinger-Ellison syndrome (increased values), gastric atrophy, gastric carcinoma (decreased values)
Manometry (use of water-filled catheters connected to pressure transducers passed into the esophagus, stomach, colon, or rectum to evaluate contractility)	Values vary at different levels of intestine	Inadequate swallowing, motility, sphincter function
Culture and sensitivity of duodenal contents	No pathogens	Detection of *S. typhi* (typhoid fever)
Breath Tests		
Glucose or d-xylose breath test	Negative for hydrogen or carbon dioxide	May indicate intestinal bacterial overgrowth
Urea breath test	Negative for isotopically labeled carbon dioxide	Presence of *Helicobacter pylori* infection
Lactose breath test	Negative for exhaled hydrogen	Lactose intolerance

From McCance KL, et al., eds. *Pathophysiology: The Biologic Basis for Disease in Adults and Children.* 8th ed. St. Louis: Elsevier; 2019.

TABLE 20.2 Common Laboratory Studies of Liver Function

Test	Normal Value	Interpretation
Serum Enzymes		
Alkaline phosphatase	35—150 units/L	Increases with biliary obstruction and cholestatic hepatitis
Gamma-glutamyl transpeptidase	Male, 12—38 units/L	Increases with biliary obstruction and cholestatic hepatitis
	Female, 9—31 units/L	
Aspartate aminotransferase (AST)[a]	Male 8—40 units/L	Increases with hepatocellular injury and injury in other tissues (e.g., skeletal and
	Female 6—34 units/L	cardiac muscle)
Alanine aminotransferase (ALT)[b]	Male 10—40 units/L	Increases with hepatocellular injury and necrosis
	Female 9—32 units/L	
Lactate dehydrogenase (LDH)	110—220 units/L	Isoenzyme lactate dehydrogenase (LD$_5$) is elevated with hypoxic and primary liver injury
5'-Nucleotidase	2—11 units/L	Increases with increase in alkaline phosphatase and cholestatic disorders
Bilirubin Metabolism		
Serum bilirubin		
Unconjugated (indirect)	0.1—1 mg/dL	Increases with hemolysis (lysis of red blood cells)
Conjugated (direct)	0.1—0.4 mg/dL	Increases with hepatocellular injury or obstruction
Total	<1 mg/dL	Increases with biliary obstruction
Urine bilirubin	0	Increases with biliary obstruction
Urine urobilinogen	0—4 mg/24 hr	Increases with hemolysis or shunting or portal blood flow
Serum Proteins		
Albumin	3.5—5.5 g/dL	Reduced with hepatocellular injury
Globulin	2—4 g/dL	Increases with hepatitis
Total	6—7 g/dL	
Albumin/Globulin (A/G) ratio	1.5—2.5:1	Ratio reverses with chronic hepatitis or other chronic liver disease
Transferrin	250—300 mcg/dL	Liver damage with decreased values, iron deficiency with increased values
Alpha-fetoprotein	6—20 ng/dL	Elevated values in primary hepatocellular carcinoma
Blood Clotting Functions		
Prothrombin time	10—13 seconds or 90%—100% of control	Increases with chronic liver disease (cirrhosis) or vitamin K deficiency
International normalized ratio (INR)	0.9—1.3	Increased values indicate high chance of bleeding; useful for monitoring effects of medications such as warfarin
Partial thromboplastin time (PTT)	22—37 seconds	Increases with severe liver disease or heparin therapy
Bromsulphthalein (BSP) excretion	<6% retention in 45 minutes	Increased retention with hepatocellular injury

From McCance KL, et al., eds. *Pathophysiology: The Biologic Basis for Disease in Adults and Children.* 8th ed. St. Louis: Elsevier; 2019.

After the catheter is in place, contrast medium is injected, and serial radiographs are obtained. If the procedure is undertaken to control bleeding, vasopressin (Pitressin Synthetic) or embolic material (Gelfoam) is injected after the site of the bleeding is located.[9]

Plain Abdominal Series

Although numerous radiologic studies are available to investigate GI dysfunction further, many of these studies are not performed on critically ill patients because of hemodynamic instability. The radiologic study that is performed most often is the plain abdominal series. An abdominal radiograph is useful in the diagnosis of bowel obstruction and perforation.[10]

Air in the bowel serves as a contrast medium to aid in the visualization of the bowel. Gas patterns (the presence of gas inside or outside the bowel lumen and the distribution of gas in dilated and nondilated bowel) are best revealed by plain radiographs. Common radiologic signs of free air in the abdomen include the presence of air on both sides of the bowel wall and the presence of air in the right upper quadrant anterior to the liver.[10] Free air in the abdomen suggests a perforated bowel, and the need for surgery is paramount. Table 20.4 lists common radiologic findings. Abdominal radiographs are used to verify nasogastric or feeding tube placement.

Abdominal Ultrasound

Abdominal ultrasound is useful in evaluating the status of the gallbladder and biliary system, the liver, the spleen, and the pancreas. It plays a key role in the diagnosis of many acute abdominal conditions such as acute cholecystitis and biliary obstructions, because it is sensitive in detecting obstructive lesions and ascites. Ultrasound is used to identify gallstones and hepatic abscesses, candidiasis, and hematomas. Intestinal gas, ascites, and extreme obesity can interfere with transmission of the sound waves and limit the usefulness of the procedure.[11]

The procedure uses sound waves to produce echoes that are converted into electrical energy and transferred to a screen for viewing. A transducer, which emits and receives sound waves, is moved slowly over the area of the abdomen being studied. Tissues with various densities produce different echoes, which translate into the different structures on the viewing screen.[11]

Computed Tomography of the Abdomen

Computed tomography (CT) is a radiographic examination that provides cross-sectional images of internal anatomy. It may be used to evaluate abdominal vasculature and identify focal points found on nuclear scans as solid, cystic, inflammatory, or vascular.[12] CT detects

TABLE 20.3   Common Laboratory Studies of Pancreatic Function

Test	Normal Value	Interpretation
Serum amylase	25–125 units/mL	Elevated levels with pancreatic inflammation
Serum lipase	20–240 units/mL	Elevated levels with pancreatic inflammation (may be elevated with other conditions; differentiates with amylase isoenzyme study)
Urine amylase	35–260 Somogyi units/hr	Elevated levels with pancreatic inflammation
Secretin test	Volume 1.8 mL/kg Bicarbonate concentration: >80 mEq/L Bicarbonate output: >10 mEq/L/30 sec	Decreased volume with pancreatic disease, because secretin stimulates pancreatic secretion
Stool fat	2–5 g/24 hr	Measures fatty acids: decreased pancreatic lipase increases stool fat
Fecal elastase	>200 mcg/g of stool	Decreased in pancreatic insufficiency

From McCance KL, et al., eds. *Pathophysiology: The Biologic Basis for Disease in Adults and Children.* 8th ed. St. Louis: Elsevier; 2019.

mass lesions greater than 2 cm in diameter and allows visualization and evaluation of many different aspects of GI disease. It is particularly useful in identifying pancreatic pseudocysts, abdominal abscesses, appendicitis, biliary obstructions, and various GI neoplastic lesions.[13]

The procedure involves taking the patient to the CT scanner, placing the patient on the table, and inserting the area to be studied into the opening of the scanner. Multiple scans are obtained at various angles, and a computer synthesizes images of the structures being studied. Intravenous or GI contrast medium may be used to facilitate imaging of the blood vessels or the GI tract, respectively.[12]

Hepatobiliary Scintigraphy

A hepatobiliary scan is a nuclear scan that is used to assess the status of the liver and the biliary system. It is valuable in detecting GI abnormalities such as acute and chronic cholecystitis, biliary obstruction, and bile leaks, and it yields additional information about organ size.[13]

The scan involves injecting an intravenous technetium-99m (^{99m}Tc)—labeled iminodiacetic agent (radiotracer), such as disofenin (^{99m}Tc DISIDA) or mebrofenin (^{99m}Tc TMBIDA). Serial images are obtained using a gamma (scintillation) camera. The liver cells take up 80% to 90% of the radiotracer, which is then secreted into the bile and

TABLE 20.4   Plain Film Findings

Finding	Appearance	Associations
Pneumoperitoneum	Air seen under diaphragm on upright chest or overlying right lobe of liver on left lateral decubitus films	Most commonly associated with bowel perforation, although other causes exist
Peritoneal fluid	Medial displacement of colon separated from flank stripes by fluid density on flat plate	Ascites or hemorrhage
Adynamic ileus	Dilation of entire intestinal tract, including stomach	Many causes, including trauma, infection (intra-abdominal and extra-abdominal), metabolic disease, and medications (e.g., opioids)
Sentinel loop	Single distended loop of small bowel containing air-fluid level	Represents localized ileus associated with localized inflammatory process such as cholecystitis, appendicitis, or pancreatitis
Small bowel obstruction	Dilated loops of small bowel (distinguished by valvulae conniventes, thin, transverse linear densities that extend completely across diameter of bowel) with air-fluid levels	Can be associated with other serious pathology such as incarcerated hernia, appendicitis, or mesenteric ischemia
Large bowel obstruction	Dilated loops, usually more peripheral in abdomen (distinguished by haustra—short, thick indentations that do not completely cross bowel and are less frequently spaced than valvulae conniventes)	Can be associated with diverticulitis and malignancy
Cecal volvulus	Usually found in middle or upper abdomen to the left; often kidney-shaped	
Sigmoid volvulus	Dilated loop of colon arising from left side of pelvis and projecting obliquely upward toward right side of abdomen	
Early ischemic bowel findings	May resemble mechanical obstruction with dilated loops and air-fluid levels	
Later ischemic bowel findings	May resemble adynamic ileus; thumbprinting (edema of bowel wall with convex indentations of lumen) and pneumatosis intestinalis (linear or mottled gas pattern in bowel wall)	
Gallbladder emergency findings	Ring of air outlining gallbladder Air in biliary tree combined with signs of small bowel obstruction, possibly with visible calculus in pelvis	Emphysematous cholecystitis Gallstone ileus
Abdominal aortic aneurysm (AAA)	Usually appears left of midline on supine film and anterior to spine in lateral projection; calcification in wall of aneurysm is variable	Ruptured or leaking AAA may reveal loss of psoas shadows or large soft tissue mass

From Hendrickson M, Naparst TR. Abdominal surgical emergencies in the elderly. *Emerg Med Clin North Am.* 2003;21(4):937–969.

transported throughout the biliary system, allowing visualization of the biliary tract, the gallbladder, and the duodenum.[14] Pooling of the iminodiacetic agent around the liver indicates poor uptake and hepatocellular dysfunction.[13]

Gastrointestinal Bleeding Scan

A GI bleeding scan is used to evaluate the presence of an active bleed, to identify the site of the bleed, and to assess the need for an arteriogram.[15] The GI bleeding scan is sensitive to low rates of bleeding (0.1 mL/min), but it is reliable only when the patient is actively bleeding and may need to be repeated in 1 to 2 days.[7,15]

The scan is usually performed with intravenous ^{99m}Tc-labeled sulfur colloid or ^{99m}Tc-labeled red blood cells (radiotracers). To tag the red blood cells, a blood sample is taken from the patient. The red blood cells are separated, tagged with ^{99m}Tc, and returned to the patient. Serial images are obtained using a gamma (scintillation) camera. Extravasation and accumulation or pooling of radiotracers in the bowel lumen indicates active bleeding is occurring and facilitates identification of the site.[7,15]

Magnetic Resonance Imaging

Magnetic resonance imaging (MRI) is used to identify tumors, abscesses, hemorrhages, and vascular abnormalities. Small tumors, whose tissue densities are different from those of the surrounding cells, can be identified before they would be visible on any other radiographic test.[7] Magnetic resonance angiography is a form of MRI that is used to assess blood vessels and blood flow.[12] Magnetic resonance cholangiopancreatography is a form of MRI used to evaluate the biliary and pancreatic ducts.[16]

During MRI, the patient is placed in a large magnetic field that stimulates the protons of the body. Introduction of radiofrequency waves causes resonance of these protons, which then emit an image that a computer can reconstruct for viewing. Intravenous administration of a non—iodine-based contrast medium enhances the image by influencing the magnetic environment and signal intensity.[12]

Percutaneous Liver Biopsy

Liver biopsy is a diagnostic procedure that is used to evaluate liver disease. Morphologic, biochemical, bacteriologic, and immunologic studies are performed on the tissue sample to diagnose liver disorders such as cirrhosis, hepatitis, infections, or cancer. A biopsy can also yield information about the progression of the patient's disease and response to therapy.[7,17]

Percutaneous liver biopsy can be performed at the bedside or in the imaging department and involves the use of an imaging-guided needle.[18] Before the test, the patient should maintain NPO status for 6 hours and have blood drawn for coagulation studies. The procedure is performed by anesthetizing the pericapsular tissue, inserting a coring or suction needle between the eighth and ninth intercostal space into the liver while the patient holds his or her breath on exhalation, withdrawing the needle with the sample, and applying pressure to stop the bleeding.[7] Puncturing of the gallbladder can cause leakage of bile into the abdominal cavity, resulting in peritonitis.[17]

Nursing Management

The nursing management of a patient undergoing a diagnostic procedure involves a variety of interventions. Nursing actions include preparing the patient psychologically and physically for the procedure, monitoring the patient's responses to the procedure, and assessing the patient after the procedure. Preparing the patient includes teaching the patient about the procedure, answering any questions, and transporting

and positioning the patient for the procedure. Monitoring the patient's responses to the procedure includes observing the patient for signs of pain, anxiety, or hemorrhage and monitoring vital signs. Assessing the patient after the procedure includes observing for complications of the procedure and medicating the patient for any postprocedural discomfort. Any evidence of GI bleeding should be immediately reported to the provider, and emergency measures to maintain circulation must be initiated.

ADDITIONAL RESOURCES

See Box 20.3 for Internet resources related to GI clinical assessment and diagnostic procedures.

BOX 20.3 Informatics   QSEN

Internet Resources: Gastrointestinal Clinical Assessment and Diagnostic Procedures

- American Gastroenterological Association: https://gastro.org/
- American College of Gastroenterology: https://gi.org/
- American Society for Gastrointestinal Endoscopy: https://www.asge.org/
- Society of Gastroenterology Nurses and Associates: https://www.sgna.org/
- World Gastroenterology Organisation: https://www.worldgastroenterology.org/

REFERENCES

1. Jarvis C, Eckhardt A. The interview. In: Jarvis C, ed. *Physical Examination and Health Assessment.* 8th ed. St. Louis: Elsevier; 2020.
2. Ball JW, Dains JE, Flynn JE, et al. Abdomen. In: Ball JW, Dains JE, Flynn JA, et al., eds. *Seidels's Guide to Physical Examination: An Interprofessional Approach.* 9th ed. St. Louis: Elsevier; 2018.
3. Bilal M, Voin V, Topale N, Iwanaga J, Loukas M, Tubbs RS. The clinical anatomy of the physical examination of the abdomen: a comprehensive review. *Clin Anat.* 2017;30(3):352—356.
4. Cox C, Steggall M. A step-by-step guide to performing a complete abdominal examination. *Gastrointest Nurs.* 2009;7(1):10—17.
5. Swartz MH. The abdomen. In: Swartz MH, ed. *Textbook of Physical Diagnosis: History and Examination.* 8th ed. Philadelphia: Elsevier; 2021.
6. Jarvis C. Abdomen. In: Jarvis C, ed. *Physical Examination and Health Assessment.* 8th ed. St. Louis: Elsevier; 2020.
7. Society of Gastroenterology Nurses and Associates. *Gastroenterology Nursing: A Core Curriculum.* 6th ed. St. Louis: Author; 2019.
8. Soetikno R, Ishii N, Kolb JM, Hammad H, Kaltenbach T. The role of endoscopic hemostasis therapy in acute lower gastrointestinal hemorrhage. *Gastrointest Endosc Clin N Am.* 2018;28(3):391—408.
9. Zurkiya O, Walker TG. Angiographic evaluation and management of nonvariceal gastrointestinal hemorrhage. *AJR Am J Roentgenol.* 2015;205(4):753—763.
10. Iaselli F, Mazzei MA, Firetto C, et al. Bowel and mesenteric injuries from blunt abdominal trauma: a review. *Radiol Med.* 2015;120(1):21—32.
11. Godfrey EM, Rushbrook SM, Carroll NR. Endoscopic ultrasound: a review of current diagnostic and therapeutic applications. *Postgrad Med J.* 2010;86(1016):346—353.
12. Cogbill TH, Ziegelbein KJ. Computed tomography, magnetic resonance and ultrasound imaging: basic principles, glossary of terms and patient safety. *Surg Clin North Am.* 2011;91(1):1—14.
13. McSweeney SE, O'Donoghue PM, Jhaveri K. Current and emerging techniques in gastrointestinal imaging. *J Postgrad Med.* 2010;56(2):109—116.
14. Ziessman HA. Hepatobiliary scintigraphy in 2014. *J Nucl Med.* 2014;55(6):967—975.

15. Mellinger JD, Bittner JG 4th, Edwards MA, Bates W, Williams HT. Imaging of gastrointestinal bleeding. *Surg Clin North Am.* 2011;91(1):93–108.

16. Wan J, Ouyang Y, Yu C, Yang X, Xia L, Lu N. Comparison of EUS with MRCP in idiopathic acute pancreatitis: a systematic review and meta-analysis. *Gastrointest Endosc.* 2018;87(5):1180–1188.

17. Sargent S, Farrington E. Percutaneous liver biopsy: an overview. *Gastrointest Nurs.* 2011;9(5):35–40.

18. Diehl DL. Endoscopic ultrasound-guided liver biopsy. *Gastrointest Endosc Clin N Am.* 2019;29(2):13–186.

21

Gastrointestinal Disorders and Therapeutic Management

Jacqueline Fitzgerald Close

ACUTE GASTROINTESTINAL HEMORRHAGE

Description and Etiology

Gastrointestinal (GI) hemorrhage is a potentially life-threatening emergency and a common complication of critical illness; it results in more than 300,000 hospital admissions yearly.[1] Despite advances in medical knowledge and nursing care, the mortality rate for patients with acute GI bleeding remains at 10% per annum in the United States.[1]

GI hemorrhage occurs from bleeding in the upper or lower GI tract. The ligament of Treitz is the anatomic division used to differentiate between the two areas. Bleeding proximal to the ligament is considered to be from the upper GI tract, and bleeding distal to the ligament is considered to be from the lower GI tract.[1-3] The various causes of acute GI hemorrhage are listed in Box 21.1.[4,5] The three main causes of GI hemorrhage commonly seen in the critical care unit are discussed further.

Peptic Ulcer Disease

Peptic ulcer disease (i.e., gastric and duodenal ulcers), which results from the breakdown of the gastromucosal lining, is the leading cause of upper GI hemorrhage, accounting for approximately 40% of cases.[6] Normally, protection of the gastric mucosa from the digestive effects of gastric secretions is accomplished in several ways. First, the gastro-duodenal mucosa is coated by a glycoprotein mucous barrier that protects the surface of the epithelium from hydrogen ions and other noxious substances present in the gut lumen.[6-8] Adequate gastric mucosal blood flow is necessary to maintain this mucosal barrier function. Second, gastroduodenal epithelial cells are protected structurally against damage from acid and pepsin because they are connected by tight junctions that help prevent acid penetration. Third, prostaglandins and nitric oxide protect the mucosal barrier by stimulating the secretion of mucus and bicarbonate and inhibiting the secretion of acid.[6-8]

Peptic ulceration occurs when these protective mechanisms cease to function, allowing gastroduodenal mucosal breakdown. After the mucosal lining is penetrated, gastric secretions autodigest the layers of the stomach or duodenum, leading to injury of the mucosal and submucosal layers. This results in damaged blood vessels and subsequent hemorrhage. The two main causes of disruption of gastroduodenal mucosal resistance are the bacterial action of *Helicobacter pylori* and nonsteroidal anti-inflammatory drugs.[4,9]

Stress-Related Mucosal Disease

Stress-related mucosal disease (SRMD) is an acute erosive gastritis that covers both types of mucosal lesions that are often found in critically ill patients: stress-related injury and discrete stress ulcers.[10-12] Additional terms used to describe this condition include *stress ulcers, stress erosions, stress gastritis, hemorrhagic gastritis,* and *erosive gastritis.* These abnormalities develop within hours of admission and range from superficial mucosal erosions to deep focal lesions and usually affect the upper GI tract.[11] SRMD occurs by means of the same pathophysiologic mechanisms as peptic ulcer disease, but the main cause of disruption of gastric mucosal resistance is increased acid production and decreased mucosal blood flow, resulting in ischemia and degeneration of the mucosal lining.[11] Patients at risk include patients in situations of high physiologic stress, as occurs with mechanical ventilation, extensive burns, severe trauma, major surgery, shock, sepsis, coagulopathy, or acute neurologic disease.[13] SRMD is decreasing in incidence because of advances in therapeutic techniques and prevention of hypoperfusion of the mucosa.[14]

Esophagogastric Varices

Esophagogastric varices are engorged and distended blood vessels of the esophagus and proximal stomach that develop as a result of portal hypertension caused by hepatic cirrhosis, a chronic disease of the liver that results in damage to the liver sinusoids (Fig. 21.1). Without adequate sinusoid function, resistance to portal blood flow is increased, and pressures within the liver are elevated. This leads to increased portal venous pressure (portal hypertension), causing collateral circulation to divert portal blood from areas of high pressure within the liver to adjacent areas of low pressure outside the liver, such as into the veins of the esophagus, spleen, intestines, and stomach. The tiny, thin-walled vessels of the esophagus and proximal stomach that receive this diverted blood lack sturdy mucosal protection. The vessels become engorged and dilated, forming esophagogastric varices that are vulnerable to damage from gastric secretions and that may result in subsequent rupture and massive hemorrhage.[15] The risk of variceal bleeding increases with disease severity and variceal size, but overall, bleeding occurs in 25% to 30% of patients within 2 years of diagnosis, with 20% to 30% mortality from each bleeding episode.[16,17]

Pathophysiology

GI hemorrhage is a life-threatening disorder that is characterized by acute, massive bleeding. Regardless of the cause, acute GI hemorrhage results in hypovolemic shock, initiation of the shock response, and development of multiple organ dysfunction syndrome if left untreated.[7] However, the most common cause of death in cases of GI hemorrhage is exacerbation of the underlying disease, not intractable hypovolemic shock.

BOX 21.1 Causes of Acute Gastrointestinal Hemorrhage

Upper Gastrointestinal Tract
- Peptic ulcer disease
- Stress-related erosive syndrome
- Esophagogastric varices
- Mallory-Weiss tear
- Esophagitis
- Neoplasm
- Aortoenteric fistula
- Angiodysplasia

Lower Gastrointestinal Tract
- Diverticulosis
- Angiodysplasia
- Neoplasm
- Inflammatory bowel disease
- Trauma
- Infectious colitis
- Radiation colitis
- Ischemia
- Aortoenteric fistula
- Hemorrhoids

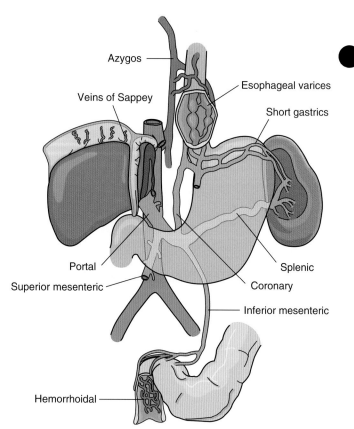

Fig. 21.1 Varices Related to Portal Hypertension. Portal vein, its major tributaries, and the most important shunts (collateral veins) between the portal and caval systems. (From Monahan FD, Neighbors M, Sands JK, et al., eds. *Phipps' Medical-Surgical Nursing: Concepts and Clinical Practice.* 8th ed. St. Louis: Mosby; 2007.)

Assessment and Diagnosis

The initial clinical presentation of a patient with acute GI hemorrhage is that of a patient in hypovolemic shock, and the clinical presentation depends on the amount of blood lost (Table 21.1). Hematemesis (bright red or brown, "coffee grounds" emesis), hematochezia (bright red stools), and melena (black, tarry, or dark red stools) are the hallmarks of GI hemorrhage.[2,18]

Hematemesis

A patient who is vomiting blood is usually bleeding from a source above the duodenojejunal junction; reverse peristalsis is seldom enough to cause hematemesis if the bleeding point is below this area. The hematemesis may be bright red or look like coffee grounds, depending on the amount of gastric contents at the time of bleeding and the length of time the blood has been in contact with gastric secretions. Gastric acid converts bright red hemoglobin to brown hematin, accounting for the "coffee grounds" appearance of the emesis. Bright red emesis results from profuse bleeding with little contact with gastric secretions.[19]

Hematochezia and Melena

The presence of blood in the GI tract results in increased peristalsis and diarrhea. Hematochezia occurs from massive lower GI hemorrhage and, if rapid enough, upper GI hemorrhage. Melena occurs from digestion of blood from an upper GI hemorrhage and may take several days to clear after the bleeding has stopped.

Laboratory Studies

Laboratory tests can help determine the extent of bleeding, although the patient's hemoglobin level and hematocrit are poor indicators of the severity of blood loss if the bleeding is acute. As whole blood is lost, plasma and red blood cells are lost in the same proportion; if the patient's hematocrit is 45% before a bleeding episode, it will be 45% several hours later.[7] It may take 24 to 72 hours for the redistribution of plasma from the extravascular space to the intravascular space to occur and cause the patient's hemoglobin level and hematocrit value to decrease.[19]

Diagnostic Procedures

To isolate and treat the source of bleeding, an urgent fiberoptic endoscopy is usually undertaken.[20] Before endoscopy, the patient must be hemodynamically stabilized.[21] Tagged red blood cell scanning, angiography, or both may be done to assist with localizing and treating a bleeding lesion in the GI tract when it is impossible to clearly view the GI tract because of continued active bleeding.[19]

Medical Management

Management of a patient at risk for GI hemorrhage may include prophylactic administration of pharmacologic agents for neutralization or suppression of gastric acids. These agents include histamine-2 (H_2) antagonists and proton-pump inhibitors (PPIs).[4,10,22] However, pharmacologic management to prevent stress ulcers is not without risks. Acid suppressive therapy is associated with increased bacterial colonization of the upper GI tract and increased risk of developing ventilator-associated pneumonia.[10] A meta-analysis suggested that patients who are receiving enteral feedings may not require stress ulcer prophylaxis.[10] Priorities in the medical management of a patient with GI hemorrhage include airway protection; fluid resuscitation to achieve hemodynamic stability; correction of comorbid conditions, if possible (e.g., coagulopathy); therapeutic procedures to control or stop

TABLE 21.1 Clinical Classification of Hemorrhage

Class	Blood Loss	Clinical Signs and Symptoms
1: Minimal blood loss	<15% <750 mL	Mental status: slightly anxious or apprehensive Heart rate: normal or mild increase Blood pressure: normal Capillary refill: brisk (<2 seconds) Skin: warm and pink Respiratory rate: normal Urine output: > 0.5 mL/kg/h (>30 mL/h)
2: Mild blood loss	15%–30% 750– 1500 mL	Mental status: irritable and confused Heart rate: increased ($\geq$100 beats/min) Blood pressure: normal Pulse pressure: decreased Peripheral pulses: diminished Capillary refill: delayed Skin: cool extremities, mottling Respiratory rate: mild increase Blood pressure: normal (supine) Urine output: mild oliguria (25–30 mL/h)
3: Moderate blood loss	30%–40% 2000 mL	Mental status: lethargic Heart rate: significantly increased ($\geq$120 beats/min) Blood pressure: hypotension Peripheral pulses: thready Capillary refill: prolonged Skin: cool extremities, pale Respiratory rate: moderate increase Urine output: oliguria (5–15 mL/h)
4: Severe blood loss	>40% >2000 mL	Mental status: lethargic, comatose Heart rate: severely increased ($\geq$140 beats/min) Blood pressure: severe hypotension Central pulses: thready Skin: cold extremities, pallor, cyanosis Respiratory rate: severe increase Urine output: anuria

bleeding; and diagnostic procedures to determine the exact cause of the bleeding.[4,21]

Stabilization

The initial treatment priority is the restoration of adequate circulating blood volume to treat or prevent shock. This is accomplished with the administration of intravenous infusions of crystalloids, blood, and blood products.[22] Hemodynamic monitoring can help guide fluid replacement therapy, particularly in patients at risk for heart failure. Supplemental oxygen therapy is initiated to increase oxygen delivery and improve tissue perfusion.[22] A large nasogastric tube may be inserted to confirm the diagnosis of active bleeding; facilitate gastric lavage; decrease the risk for aspiration; and prepare the esophagus, stomach, and proximal duodenum for endoscopic evaluation.[4]

Controlling Bleeding

Interventions to control bleeding are the second priority for a patient with GI hemorrhage after hemodynamic stability is achieved.

Peptic ulcer disease. In a patient with GI hemorrhage related to peptic ulcer disease, bleeding hemostasis may be accomplished by endoscopic injection therapy in conjunction with thermal or hemostatic clips.[20] Endoscopic thermal therapy uses heat to cauterize the bleeding vessel, and endoscopic injection therapy uses a variety of agents such as hypertonic saline, epinephrine, ethanol, and sclerosants to induce localized vasoconstriction of the bleeding vessel.[17] Intra-arterial infusion of vasopressin into the gastric artery or intra-arterial injection of an embolizing agent (e.g., Gelfoam pledgets, polyvinyl alcohol particles, coils) can be performed during arteriography to control bleeding after the site has been identified.[19]

Stress-related mucosal disease. In a patient with GI hemorrhage caused by SRMD, bleeding hemostasis may be accomplished by intra-arterial infusion of vasopressin and intra-arterial embolization. Endoscopic therapies provide minimal benefit because of the diffuse nature of the disease.[19]

Esophagogastric varices. In acute variceal hemorrhage, control of bleeding may be initially accomplished through the use of pharmacologic agents and endoscopic therapies.[23] Intravenous vasopressin, somatostatin, and octreotide can reduce portal venous pressure and slow variceal hemorrhaging by constricting the splanchnic arteriolar bed.[16] Two commonly used endoscopic therapies are endoscopic injection sclerotherapy and endoscopic variceal ligation (EVL).[4] Endoscopic injection sclerotherapy controls bleeding by injection of a sclerosing agent in or around the varices. This creates an inflammatory reaction that induces vasoconstriction and results in the formation of a venous thrombosis. During EVL, bands are placed around the varices to create an obstruction to stop the bleeding.[24]

If these initial therapies fail, transjugular intrahepatic portosystemic shunt (TIPS) may be necessary. In a TIPS procedure, a channel between the systemic and portal venous systems is created to redirect portal blood, reducing portal hypertension and decompressing the varices to control bleeding (Fig. 21.2).[23,24]

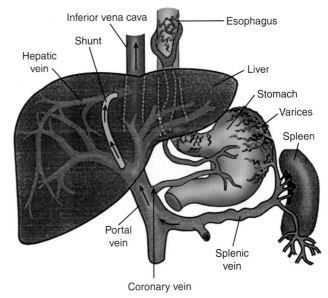

Fig. 21.2 Anatomic Location of Transjugular Intrahepatic Portosystemic Shunt (TIPS). (From Vargas HE, Gerber D, Abu-Elmagd K. Management of portal hypertension-related bleeding. *Surg Clin North Am.* 1999;79[1]:1–22.)

Surgical Intervention

A patient who remains hemodynamically unstable despite volume replacement may need urgent surgery.

Peptic ulcer disease. Surgical intervention is required to control bleeding in a few patients.[25] The operative procedure of choice to control bleeding from peptic ulcer disease is a vagotomy and pyloroplasty. During this procedure, the vagus nerve to the stomach is severed, eliminating the autonomic stimulus to the gastric cells and reducing hydrochloric acid production. Because the vagus nerve also stimulates motility, a pyloroplasty is performed to provide for gastric emptying.[26]

Stress-related mucosal disease. In the past, several operative procedures were used to control bleeding from SRMD. Because of the advent of stress ulcer prophylaxis, the incidence of hemorrhage from SRMD is markedly decreased.[22]

Esophagogastric varices. If medical treatment is unsuccessful and angiographic interventional TIPS procedure is not available, operative procedures to control bleeding gastroesophageal varices may be undertaken. Although rarely performed, operative interventions focus on some form of shunting (Fig. 21.3).[4] These shunt procedures are also referred to as *decompression procedures*, because they result in the diversion of portal blood flow away from the liver and decompression of the portal system. The portacaval shunt procedure has two variations: (1) an end-to-side portacaval shunt procedure, which involves the ligation of the hepatic end of the portal vein with subsequent anastomosis to the vena cava, and (2) a side-to-side portacaval shunt procedure, during which the side of the portal vein is anastomosed to the side of the vena cava. A mesocaval shunt procedure involves the insertion of a graft between the superior mesenteric artery and the vena cava. During a distal splenorenal shunt procedure, the splenic vein is detached from the portal vein and anastomosed to the left renal vein.[27]

Nursing Management

All critically ill patients should be considered at risk for stress ulcers and GI hemorrhage. Routine assessment of gastric fluid pH monitoring is controversial.[28] Maintaining the pH between 3.5 and 4.5 is a goal of prophylactic therapy. Gastric pH measurements made with litmus paper or direct nasogastric tube probes may be used to assess gastric fluid pH and the effectiveness of or need for prophylactic agents.[28] Patients at risk also should be assessed for the presence of bright red or coffee ground emesis; bloody nasogastric aspirate; and bright red, black, or dark red stools.[4] Any signs of bleeding should be promptly reported to the physician.

The patient care management plan for a patient experiencing acute GI hemorrhage incorporates a variety of patient problems (Box 21.2). The nurse plays a significant role in administering volume replacement, initiating gastric lavage, maintaining surveillance for complications, and educating the patient and family.

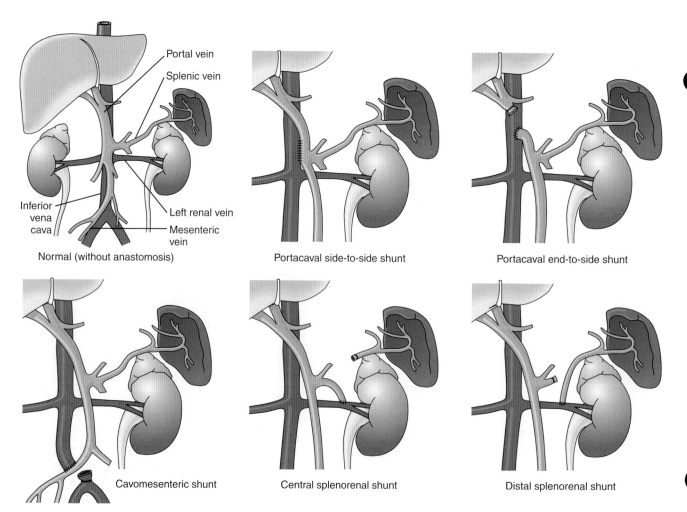

Fig. 21.3 Portosystemic Shunt Operative Procedures. (From Copstead LC, Banasik J, eds. *Pathophysiology.* 6th ed. St. Louis: Elsevier; 2019.)

BOX 21.2 PRIORITY PATIENT CARE MANAGEMENT

Acute Gastrointestinal Hemorrhage
- Hypovolemia due to absolute loss
- Impaired Cardiac Output due to alterations in preload
- Risk for Aspiration
- Impaired Nutritional Intake due to lack of exogenous nutrients and increased metabolic demand
- Powerlessness due to lack of control over current situation or disease progression
- Impaired Family Coping critically ill family member
- Lack of Knowledge of Treatment Regime due to lack of previous exposure to information (see Patient and Family Education Plan, Box 21.3)

Patient Care Management Plans are located in Appendix A.

Administer Volume Replacement

Measures to facilitate volume replacement include obtaining intravenous access and administering prescribed fluids and blood products. Two large-diameter peripheral intravenous catheters should be inserted to facilitate the rapid administration of prescribed fluids.[1]

Initiate Gastric Lavage

One measure to prepare the patient for endoscopy is the initiation of gastric lavage. It is used to evacuate blood from the stomach and improve visualization during endoscopy. Gastric lavage is performed by inserting a large-bore nasogastric tube into the stomach and irrigating it with normal saline until the returned solution is clear. It is important to keep accurate records of the amount of fluid instilled and aspirated to ascertain the true amount of bleeding.[1] However, this practice has been called into question as unnecessary and is no longer routinely recommended.[29]

Maintain Surveillance for Complications

The patient should be continuously observed for signs of gastric perforation. Although a rare complication, gastric perforation constitutes a surgical emergency. Signs and symptoms include sudden, severe, generalized abdominal pain with significant rebound tenderness and rigidity. Perforation should be suspected when fever, leukocytosis, and tachycardia persist despite adequate volume replacement.[30]

Educate the Patient and Family

Early in the hospital stay, the patient and family should be taught about acute GI hemorrhage and its causes and treatments. Closer to discharge, teaching should focus on the interventions necessary for preventing the recurrence of the precipitating disorder and steps to take if another bleed should occur. If the patient abuses alcohol, the patient should be encouraged to stop drinking and be referred to an alcohol cessation program (Box 21.3).

Interprofessional collaborative management of the patient with acute GI hemorrhage is outlined in Box 21.4.

Priority diagnostic assessments and priority nursing interventions for acute GI hemorrhage are displayed in Fig. 21.4.

ACUTE PANCREATITIS

Description and Etiology

Acute pancreatitis is an inflammation of the pancreas that produces exocrine and endocrine dysfunction that may also involve surrounding tissues, remote organ systems, or both. The clinical course can range from a mild, self-limiting disease to a systemic process characterized by

BOX 21.4 Teamwork and Collaboration
QSEN

Interprofessional Collaborative Practice: Acute Gastrointestinal Hemorrhage
- Initiate fluid resuscitation to achieve hemodynamic stability.
  - Crystalloids
  - Colloids
  - Blood and blood products
- Determine the cause of bleeding.
  - Gastric lavage
- Control bleeding.
  - Endoscopic interventions
  - Vasopressin, somatostatin, octreotide
  - Transjugular intrahepatic portosystemic shunt
  - Surgery (last resort)
- Provide comfort and emotional support.
- Maintain surveillance for complications.
  - Hypovolemic shock
  - Gastric perforation

BOX 21.3 PRIORITY PATIENT AND FAMILY EDUCATION

Gastrointestinal Disorders: Gastrointestinal Hemorrhage, Pancreatitis, and Liver Failure

Before discharge, the patient should be able to teach back the following topics:
- Specific cause of gastrointestinal hemorrhage, pancreatitis, or liver failure
- Precipitating factor modification
- Interventions to reduce further episodes
- Importance of taking medications
- Lifestyle changes
- Diet modifications
- Alcohol cessation
- Disorder specific modifications

- Stress management for patients with gastrointestinal hemorrhage and pancreatitis
- Smoking cessation for patients with gastrointestinal hemorrhage
- Diabetes management for patients with pancreatitis

Additional information for the patient can be found at the following websites:
- Alcoholics Anonymous: https://www.aa.org
- International Foundation for Functional Gastrointestinal Disorders (IFFGD): https://www.iffgd.org
- Office of Disease Prevention and Health Promotion (ODPHP): https://healthfinder.gov
- Web MD: https://www.webmd.com

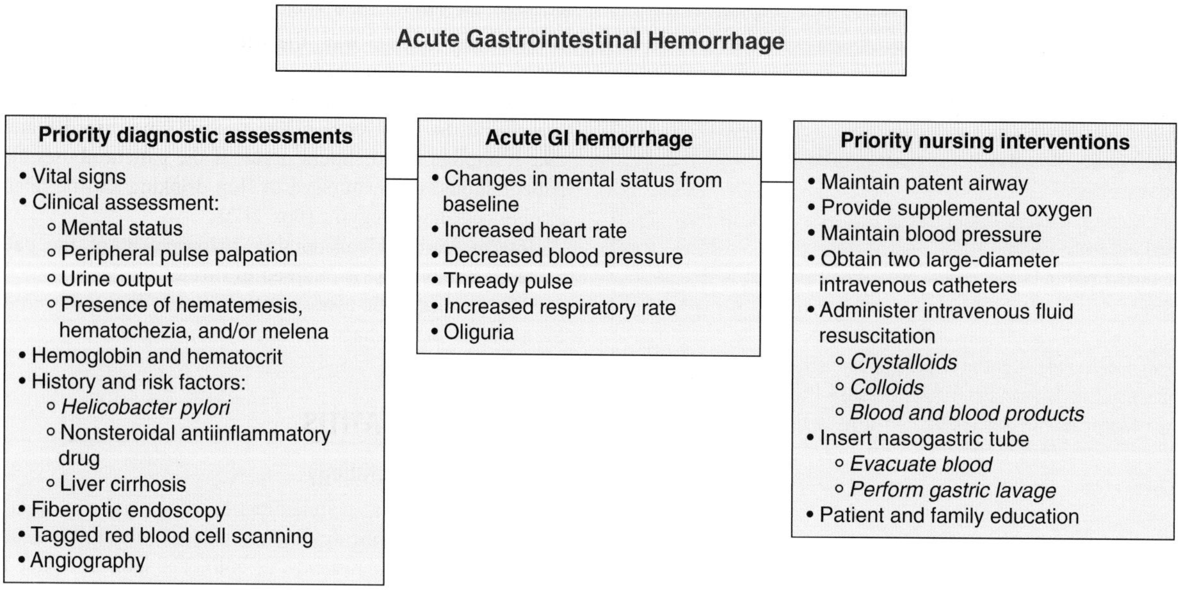

Acute Gastrointestinal Hemorrhage

Priority diagnostic assessments	Acute GI hemorrhage	Priority nursing interventions

• Vital signs
• Clinical assessment:
  ○ Mental status
  ○ Peripheral pulse palpation
  ○ Urine output
  ○ Presence of hematemesis,
    hematochezia, and/or melena
• Hemoglobin and hematocrit
• History and risk factors:
  ○ *Helicobacter pylori*
  ○ Nonsteroidal antiinflammatory
    drug
  ○ Liver cirrhosis
• Fiberoptic endoscopy
• Tagged red blood cell scanning
• Angiography
	• Changes in mental status from
	  baseline
	• Increased heart rate
	• Decreased blood pressure
	• Thready pulse
	• Increased respiratory rate
	• Oliguria
		• Maintain patent airway
		• Provide supplemental oxygen
		• Maintain blood pressure
		• Obtain two large-diameter
		  intravenous catheters
		• Administer intravenous fluid
		  resuscitation
		  ○ *Crystalloids*
		  ○ *Colloids*
		  ○ *Blood and blood products*
		• Insert nasogastric tube
		  ○ *Evacuate blood*
		  ○ *Perform gastric lavage*
		• Patient and family education

Fig. 21.4 Priority Diagnostic Assessments and Priority Nursing Interventions for Acute Gastrointestinal *(GI)* Hemorrhage.

organ failure, sepsis, and death. In approximately 80% to 90% of patients, it takes the milder form of interstitial edematous pancreatitis; the remaining 10% to 20% of patients develop severe necrotizing pancreatitis.[31] Acute pancreatitis can be further classified as mild, moderate, or severe based on associated complications. In mild acute pancreatitis there is an absence of local and systemic complications and organ failure. In moderate acute pancreatitis there are local or systemic complications without persistent organ failure or transient organ failure. In severe acute pancreatitis there is persistent failure of one or more organs.[32] Acute pancreatitis is one of the leading causes of hospital admissions, and treatment costs exceed $2.5 billion a year.[33] Reported mortality rates for severe acute pancreatitis are as high as 30%.[34]

Several prognostic scoring systems have been developed to predict the severity of acute pancreatitis.[35] One of the most commonly used is Ranson criteria (Box 21.5). If the patient has 0 to 2 factors present, the predicted mortality rate is 2%; with 3 to 4 factors, the rate is 15%; with 5 to 6 factors, the rate is 40%; and with 7 to 8 factors, the rate is 100%.[36]

The two most common causes of acute pancreatitis are gallstone migration and alcoholism. Together, they account for approximately 80% of cases. Less common causes are quite diverse and include hypertriglyceridemia, hypercalcemia, various toxins, ischemia, infections, and the use of certain medications (Box 21.6). In 20% of patients with acute pancreatitis, no etiologic factor can be determined.[37]

Pathophysiology

In acute pancreatitis, the normally inactive digestive enzymes become prematurely activated within the pancreas itself, leading to autodigestion of pancreatic tissue. The enzymes become activated through various mechanisms, including obstruction of or damage to the pancreatic duct system, alterations in the secretory processes of the acinar cells, infection, ischemia, and other unknown factors.[37]

Trypsin is the enzyme that becomes activated first. It initiates the autodigestion process by triggering the secretion of proteolytic enzymes, such as kallikrein, chymotrypsin and elastase, phospholipase A, and lipase. Release of kallikrein and chymotrypsin results in increased capillary membrane permeability, leading to leakage of fluid into the interstitium and the development of edema and relative hypovolemia.

BOX 21.5 Ranson Criteria

At Admission
- Age >55 years
- Hypotension
- Abnormal pulmonary findings
- Abdominal mass
- Hemorrhagic or discolored peritoneal fluid
- Increased serum LDH levels (>350 units/L)
- AST >250 units/L
- Leukocytosis (>16,000/mm^3)
- Hyperglycemia (>200 mg/dL; no diabetes history)
- Neurologic deficit (confusion, localizing signs)

During Initial 48 Hours of Hospitalization
- Fall in hematocrit >10% with hydration or hematocrit <30%
- Necessity for massive fluid and colloid replacement
- Hypocalcemia (<8 mg/dL)
- Arterial PO$_2$ <60 mm Hg with or without acute respiratory distress syndrome
- Hypoalbuminemia (<3.2 mg/dL)
- Base deficit >4 mEq/L
- Azotemia

AST, Aspartate aminotransferase; *LDH,* lactate dehydrogenase; *PO$_2$,* partial pressure of oxygen.
From Latifi R, McIntosh JK, Dudrick SJ. Nutritional management of acute and chronic pancreatitis. *Surg Clin North Am.* 1991;71(3):579–595.

Elastase is the most harmful enzyme in terms of direct cell damage. It dissolves the elastic fibers of blood vessels and ducts, leading to hemorrhage. Phospholipase A, in the presence of bile, destroys the phospholipids of cell membranes, causing severe pancreatic and adipose tissue necrosis. Lipase flows into the damaged tissue and is absorbed into the systemic circulation, resulting in fat necrosis of the pancreas and surrounding tissues.[7]

BOX 21.6 Causes of Acute Pancreatitis

- Alcohol
- Biliary disease (stones, sludge, common bile duct obstruction)
- Hypertriglyceridemia
- Toxins (ethyl alcohol, methyl alcohol, scorpion, venom, parathion)
- Medications (thiazides, immunosuppressive agents, anti-inflammatory drugs)
- Hypercalcemia (hyperparathyroidism)
- Tumors
- Infections (bacterial, viral, parasitic)
- Trauma (abdominal, surgical, endoscopic)
- Hypoperfusion
- Vasculitis
- Pregnancy
- Hypothermia
- Sphincter of Oddi dysfunction
- Autoimmune diseases
- Ampullary stenosis
- Idiopathic cause

BOX 21.7 Clinical Manifestations of Acute Pancreatitis

- Pain
- Location: left upper quadrant or midepigastrium radiating to the back
- Onset: sudden
- Quality: severe, deep, continuous
- Aggravating factors: food and alcohol
- Nausea and vomiting
- Flushing and diaphoresis
- Low-grade fever
- Abdominal distention
- Abdominal tenderness and guarding
- Abdominal tympany
- Hypoactive or absent bowel sounds
- Jaundice
- Palpable abdominal mass
- Ecchymoses or bluish discoloration of the flanks (Grey Turner sign) and/or the umbilical area (Cullen sign)
- Basilar crackles
- Tachypnea
- Tachycardia
- Hypotension

The extent of injury to the pancreatic cells determines the type of acute pancreatitis that develops. If injury to the pancreatic cells is mild and without necrosis, edematous pancreatitis develops. The acinar cells appear structurally intact, and blood flow is maintained through small capillaries and venules. This form of acute pancreatitis is self-limiting. If injury to the pancreatic cells is severe, acute necrotizing pancreatitis develops. Cellular destruction in pancreatic injury results in the release of toxic enzymes and inflammatory mediators into the systemic circulation and causes injury to vessels and other organs distant from the pancreas; this may result in systemic inflammatory response syndrome, multiorgan failure, and death. Local tissue injury results in infection, abscess and pseudocyst formation, disruption of the pancreatic duct, and severe hemorrhage and shock.[38]

Assessment and Diagnosis

The clinical manifestations of acute pancreatitis range from mild to severe and often mimic the manifestations of other disorders (Box 21.7). Acute onset of abdominal pain, nausea, and vomiting are hallmark symptoms.[39] Epigastric to periumbilical pain may vary from mild and tolerable to severe and incapacitating. Many patients report a twisting or knifelike sensation that radiates to the low dorsal region of the back. The patient may obtain some comfort by leaning forward or assuming a semifetal position.[40] Other clinical findings include fever, diaphoresis, weakness, tachypnea, hypotension, and tachycardia. Depending on the extent of fluid loss and hemorrhage, the patient may exhibit signs of hypovolemic shock.[37]

The diagnosis of acute pancreatitis requires two of these three features: (1) abdominal pain that is characteristic of acute pancreatitis; (2) serum lipase or serum amylase values that are at least three times the normal value; and (3) evidence of acute pancreatitis on contrast-enhanced computed tomography (CECT), magnetic resonance imaging (MRI), or ultrasonography.[32]

Physical Assessment

The results of a focused physical assessment usually reveal hypoactive bowel sounds and abdominal tenderness, guarding, distention, and tympany.[40] Findings that may indicate pancreatic hemorrhage include

Grey Turner sign (gray-blue discoloration of the flanks) and Cullen sign (discoloration of the umbilical region); however, these signs are rare and usually seen several days into the illness.[37] A palpable abdominal mass indicates the presence of a pseudocyst or abscess.

Laboratory Studies

Assessment of laboratory data usually demonstrates elevated levels of serum amylase and lipase. Serum lipase is more pancreas-specific than amylase and a more accurate marker for acute pancreatitis. Lipase remains elevated for 8 to 14 days. Amylase is present in other body tissues, and other disorders (e.g., intra-abdominal emergencies, renal insufficiency, salivary gland trauma, liver disease) may contribute to an elevated level. The serum amylase level may be elevated for only 2 to 4 days; if the patient delays seeking treatment, a normal level (false-negative result) may be detected.[40] A marker of severity may be determined with a serum cross-reactive (C-reactive) protein level. Additional laboratory tests include liver enzymes, blood urea nitrogen (BUN), creatinine, electrolytes, serum cholesterol and triglyceride, lactate, and complete blood count (CBC). Given the severity of the patient's condition, leukocytosis, hypocalcemia, hyperglycemia, hyperbilirubinemia, and hypoalbuminemia may also be present (Table 21.2).[41]

Diagnostic Procedures

An abdominal ultrasound scan is obtained as part of the diagnostic evaluation to determine the presence of biliary stones.[40] CECT is considered the gold standard for diagnosing pancreatitis and for ascertaining the overall degree of pancreatic inflammation and necrosis. An MRI may be performed in those patients who are at risk for contrast-related complications.[38] It is also more sensitive for identifying vascular and bile duct complications.[41]

Medical Management

Initial management of a patient with severe acute pancreatitis includes ensuring adequate pain management, fluid and electrolyte

TABLE 21.2 Laboratory Tests and Diagnostic Procedures for Acute Pancreatitis

Study	Finding in Pancreatitis
Laboratory Studies	
Serum amylase	Elevated
Urine amylase	Elevated
Serum lipase	Elevated
Serum triglycerides	Elevated
Cross-reactive protein	Elevated
Glucose	Elevated
Calcium	Decreased
Magnesium	Decreased
Potassium	Decreased
White blood cell count	Elevated
Bilirubin	May be elevated
Liver enzymes	May be elevated
Prothrombin time	Prolonged
Arterial blood gases	Hypoxemia, metabolic acidosis

replacement, providing nutrition support, and correcting metabolic alterations. Careful monitoring for systemic and local complications is critical. Current evidence-based guidelines for the management of a patient with acute pancreatitis are presented in Box 21.8.

Fluid Management

Because pancreatitis is often associated with massive fluid shifts, intravenous crystalloids are administered immediately to prevent hypovolemic shock and maintain hemodynamic stability. Electrolytes are monitored closely, and abnormalities such as hypocalcemia, hypokalemia, and hypomagnesemia are corrected. If hyperglycemia develops, exogenous insulin may be required.[42] Current guidelines do not recommend a specific type of fluid for resuscitation; however, there is evidence that Ringer's lactate solution may be superior to 0.9% sodium chloride solution due to the antiinflammatory effects of the lactate.[42,43] Fluids should be administered at 5 to 10 mL/kg/h. Aggressive fluid resuscitation should be avoided, because it has been shown to be associated with higher mortality rates.[44]

Nutrition Support

The philosophies regarding nutrition support have shifted over time. Previously, conventional nutrition management was to place the patient on a nothing by mouth (NPO) regimen and institute intravenous hydration. The rationale was to rest the inflamed pancreas and prevent enzyme release. This is no longer the standard of practice.[39] Current guidelines recommend starting oral feedings within 24 hours to protect the gut-mucosal barrier and reduce the incidence of bacterial translocation. Patients who are unable to take oral feedings should be started on enteral feedings, either via the nasogastric or nasoenteric (duodenal or jejunal) route. Enteral feeding is preferred over total parenteral nutrition.[42] Evidence has shown that enteral feeding is safe, cost-effective, and associated with fewer septic and metabolic complications than the parenteral route. Parenteral nutrition is only indicated if the patient is unable to tolerate enteral nutrition.[45] In the past, nasogastric suction was also recommended, but this intervention has not been shown to be beneficial and should be instituted only if the patient has persistent vomiting, obstruction, or gastric distention.

Systemic Complications

Acute pancreatitis can affect every organ system, and recognition and treatment of systemic complications are crucial to management of the patient (Box 21.9). The most serious complications are hypovolemic shock, acute respiratory distress syndrome (ARDS), acute kidney injury (AKI), and GI hemorrhage. Hypovolemic shock is the result of relative hypovolemia resulting from third spacing of intravascular volume and vasodilation caused by the release of inflammatory immune mediators. Fluid accumulates in the abdominal cavity, resulting in intra-abdominal hypertension and abdominal compartment syndrome. Inflammatory mediators also contribute to the development of ARDS and AKI. Other possible pulmonary complications include pleural effusions, atelectasis, and pneumonia.[7]

Local Complications

Local complications include the development of infected pancreatic necrosis and pancreatic pseudocyst. The necrotic areas of the pancreas can lead to development of a widespread pancreatic infection (infected pancreatic necrosis), which significantly increases the risk of death.[34]

Prophylactic antibiotics may not reduce mortality in patients suspected to have necrotizing pancreatitis. Intravenous antibiotics should not be used prophylactically,[42] but if sepsis, abscess, or biliary calculi are evident, they are indicated.[46] When the patient develops infected necrosis, surgical intervention is necessary. The procedure of choice is a minimally invasive necrosectomy, which entails careful débridement of the necrotic tissue in and around the pancreas.[34] A pancreatic pseudocyst is a collection of pancreatic fluid enclosed by a non-epithelialized wall. Cyst formation may result from liquefaction of a pancreatic fluid collection or from direct obstruction in the main pancreatic duct. A pancreatic pseudocyst may (1) resolve spontaneously; (2) rupture, resulting in peritonitis; (3) erode a major blood vessel, resulting in hemorrhage; (4) become infected, resulting in abscess; or (5) invade surrounding structures, resulting in obstruction. Treatment involves drainage of the pseudocyst surgically, endoscopically, or percutaneously.[44]

Nursing Management

The patient care management plan for a patient with pancreatitis incorporates a variety of patient problems (Box 21.10). The nurse plays a significant role in providing comfort and emotional support to the patient and the family, maintaining surveillance for complications, and educating the patient and family.

Provide Comfort and Emotional Support

Pain management is a major priority in acute pancreatitis. Administration of around-the-clock analgesics to achieve pain relief is essential. Morphine, fentanyl, and hydromorphone are the commonly used opioids for pain control. Relaxation techniques and the knee-chest position can also assist in pain control.

Maintain Surveillance for Complications

The patient is routinely monitored for signs of local or systemic complications (see Box 21.9). Intensive monitoring of each of the organ systems is imperative because organ failure is a major indicator of the severity of the disease. Intra-abdominal pressure monitoring is initiated if intra-abdominal hypertension is suspected. The patient is closely monitored for signs and symptoms of pancreatic infection, which include increased abdominal pain and tenderness, fever, and increased white blood cell count (Box 21.11).[19]

QSEN BOX 21.8 Evidence-Based Practice

Acute Pancreatitis Management Guidelines

A. Diagnosis of Acute Pancreatitis and Etiology

1. The definition of acute pancreatitis is based on the fulfillment of two out of three of the following criteria: clinical (upper abdominal pain), laboratory (serum amylase or lipase >3× upper limit of normal), or imaging (CT, MRI, ultrasonography) criteria. (GRADE 1B, strong agreement)
2. On admission, the etiology of acute pancreatitis should be determined using detailed personal (e.g., previous acute pancreatitis, known gallstone disease, alcohol intake, medication and drug intake, known hyperlipidemia, trauma, recent invasive procedures such as ERCP) and family history of pancreatic disease, physical examination, laboratory serum tests (e.g., liver enzymes, calcium, triglycerides), and imaging (e.g., right upper quadrant ultrasonography). (GRADE 1B, strong agreement)
3. In patients considered to have idiopathic acute pancreatitis, after negative routine work-up for biliary etiology, EUS is recommended as the first step to assess for occult microlithiasis, neoplasms, and chronic pancreatitis. If EUS is negative, (secretin-stimulated) MRCP is advised as a second step to identify rare morphologic abnormalities. CT of the abdomen should be performed. If etiology remains unidentified, especially after a second attack of idiopathic pancreatitis, genetic counseling (not necessarily genetic testing) should be considered. (GRADE 2C, weak agreement)

B. Prognostication/Prediction of Severity

4. Use of the SIRS criteria is advised to predict severe acute pancreatitis at admission, and the presence of persistent SIRS at 48 hours is an ongoing marker for severe acute pancreatitis. (GRADE 2B, weak agreement)
5. During admission, a three-dimensional approach is advised to predict outcome of acute pancreatitis combining host risk factors (e.g., age, co-morbidity, body mass index), clinical risk stratification (e.g., persistent SIRS), and monitoring response to initial therapy (e.g., persistent SIRS, blood urea nitrogen, creatinine). (GRADE 2B, strong agreement)

C. Imaging

6. The indication for initial CT assessment in acute pancreatitis can be (1) diagnostic uncertainty, (2) confirmation of severity based on clinical predictors of severe acute pancreatitis, or (3) failure to respond to conservative treatment or in the setting of clinical deterioration. Optimal timing for initial CT assessment is at least 72–96 hours after onset of symptoms. (GRADE 1C, strong agreement)
7. Follow-up CT or MRI in acute pancreatitis is indicated when there is a lack of clinical improvement, when there is clinical deterioration, or especially when invasive intervention is considered. (GRADE 1C, strong agreement)
8. It is recommended to perform multidetector CT with thin collimation and slice thickness (i.e., 5 mm or less), 100–150 mL of nonionic intravenous contrast material at a rate of 3 mL/s, during the pancreatic and/or portal venous phase (i.e., 50–70-second delay). During follow-up, only a portal venous phase (monophasic) is generally sufficient. For MRI, the recommendation is to perform axial fat-saturated T2 and fat-saturated T1 scanning before and after intravenous gadolinium contrast administration. (GRADE 1C, strong agreement)

D. Fluid Therapy

9. Ringer's lactate is recommended for initial fluid resuscitation in acute pancreatitis. (GRADE 1B, strong agreement)
10a. Goal-directed intravenous fluid therapy with 5–10 mL/kg/h should be used initially until resuscitation goals (see 10b) are reached. (GRADE 1B, weak agreement)
10b. The preferred approach to assessing the response to fluid resuscitation should be based on one or more of the following: (1) noninvasive clinical targets of heart rate <120 beats/min, mean arterial pressure 65–85 mm Hg (8.7–11.3 kPa), and urinary output >0.5–1 mL/kg/h; (2) invasive clinical targets of stroke volume variation and intrathoracic blood volume determination; and (3) biochemical targets of hematocrit 35%–44%. (GRADE 2B, weak agreement)

E. Intensive Care Management

11. Intensive care management is recommended for patients diagnosed with acute pancreatitis and one or more of the parameters identified at admission as defined by the guidelines of the Society of Critical Care Medicine. Furthermore, patients with severe acute pancreatitis as defined by the revised Atlanta Classification (i.e., persistent organ failure) should be treated in an intensive care setting. (GRADE 1C, strong agreement)
12. Management in, or referral to, a specialist center is necessary for patients with severe acute pancreatitis and for those who may need interventional radiologic, endoscopic, or surgical intervention. (GRADE 1C, strong agreement)
13. A specialist center in the management of acute pancreatitis is defined as a high-volume center with up-to-date intensive care facilities including options for organ replacement therapy and with daily (i.e., 7 days per week) access to interventional radiology, interventional endoscopy with EUS and ERCP assistance, and surgical expertise in managing necrotizing pancreatitis. Patients should be enrolled in prospective audits for quality control issues and into clinical trials whenever possible. (GRADE 2C, weak agreement)
14. Early fluid resuscitation within the first 24 hours of admission for acute pancreatitis is associated with decreased rates of persistent SIRS and organ failure. (GRADE 1C, strong agreement)
15. Abdominal compartment syndrome (ACS) is defined as a sustained intra-abdominal pressure >20 mm Hg that is associated with new-onset organ failure. (GRADE 2B, strong agreement)
16. Medical treatment of ACS should target (1) hollow viscera volume, (2) intravascular/extravascular fluid, and (3) abdominal wall expansion. Invasive treatment should be used only after multidisciplinary discussion in patients with a sustained intra-abdominal pressure >25 mm Hg with new-onset organ failure refractory to medical therapy and nasogastric/rectal decompression. Invasive treatment options include percutaneous catheter drainage of ascites, midline laparostomy, bilateral subcostal laparostomy, or subcutaneous linea alba fasciotomy. In case of surgical decompression, the retroperitoneal cavity and the omental bursa should be left intact to reduce the risk of infecting peripancreatic and pancreatic necrosis. (GRADE 2C, strong agreement)

F. Preventing Infectious Complications

17. Intravenous antibiotic prophylaxis is not recommended for the prevention of infectious complications in acute pancreatitis. (GRADE 1B, strong agreement)
18. Selective gut decontamination has shown some benefits in preventing infectious complications in acute pancreatitis, but further studies are needed. (GRADE 2B, weak agreement)
19. Probiotic prophylaxis is not recommended for the prevention of infectious complications in acute pancreatitis. (GRADE 1B, strong agreement)

G. Nutrition Support

20. Oral feeding in predicted mild pancreatitis can be restarted once abdominal pain is decreasing and inflammatory markers are improving. (GRADE 2B, strong agreement)
21. Enteral tube feeding should be the primary therapy in patients with predicted severe acute pancreatitis who require nutrition support. (GRADE 1B, strong agreement)
22. Either elemental or polymeric enteral nutrition formulations can be used in acute pancreatitis. (GRADE 2B, strong agreement)

Continued

QSEN BOX 21.8 **Evidence-Based Practice—cont'd**

23. Enteral nutrition in acute pancreatitis can be administered via either the nasojejunal or the nasogastric route. (GRADE 2A, strong agreement)
24. Parenteral nutrition can be administered in acute pancreatitis as second-line therapy if nasojejunal tube feeding is not tolerated and nutrition support is required. (GRADE 2C, strong agreement)

H. Biliary Tract Management

25. ERCP is not indicated in predicted mild biliary pancreatitis without cholangitis. (GRADE 1A, strong agreement) ERCP is probably not indicated in predicted severe biliary pancreatitis without cholangitis. (GRADE 1B, strong agreement) ERCP is probably indicated in biliary pancreatitis with common bile duct obstruction. (GRADE 1C, strong agreement) ERCP is indicated in patients with biliary pancreatitis and cholangitis. (GRADE 1B, strong agreement)
26. Urgent ERCP (<24 hours) is required in patients with acute cholangitis. Currently, there is no evidence regarding the optimal timing of ERCP in patients with biliary pancreatitis without cholangitis. (GRADE 2C, strong agreement)
27. MRCP and EUS may prevent a proportion of ERCPs that would otherwise be performed for suspected common bile duct stones in patients with biliary pancreatitis who do not have cholangitis, without influencing the clinical course. EUS is superior to MRCP in excluding the presence of small (<5 mm) gallstones. MRCP is less invasive, less operator-dependent, and probably more widely available than EUS. Therefore in clinical practice there is no clear superiority for either MRCP or EUS. (GRADE 2C, strong agreement)

I. Indications for Intervention in Necrotizing Pancreatitis

28. Common indications for intervention (radiologic, endoscopic, or surgical) in necrotizing pancreatitis are (1) clinical suspicion of or documented infected necrotizing pancreatitis with clinical deterioration, preferably when the necrosis has become "walled-off," and (2) in the absence of documented infected necrotizing pancreatitis, ongoing organ failure for several weeks after the onset of acute pancreatitis, preferably when the necrosis has become walled-off. (GRADE 1C, strong agreement)
29. Routine percutaneous FNA of peripancreatic collections to detect bacteria is not indicated, because clinical signs (i.e., persistent fever, increasing inflammatory markers) and imaging signs (i.e., gas in peripancreatic collections) are accurate predictors of infected necrosis in the majority of patients. Although the diagnosis of infection can be confirmed by FNA, there is a risk of false-negative results. (GRADE 1C, strong agreement)
30. Indications for intervention (radiologic, endoscopic, or surgical) in sterile necrotizing pancreatitis are (1) ongoing gastric outlet, intestinal, or biliary obstruction due to mass effect of walled-off necrosis (i.e., arbitrarily >4 —8 weeks after onset of acute pancreatitis); (2) persistent symptoms (e.g., pain, "persistent unwellness") in patients with walled-off necrosis without signs of infection (i.e., arbitrarily >8 weeks after onset of acute pancreatitis); and (3) disconnected duct syndrome (i.e., full transection of the pancreatic duct in the presence of pancreatic necrosis) with persisting

symptomatic (e.g., pain, obstruction) collections with necrosis without signs of infection (i.e., arbitrarily >8 weeks after onset of acute pancreatitis). (GRADE 2C, strong agreement)

J. Timing of Intervention in Necrotizing Pancreatitis

31. For patients with proven or suspected infected necrotizing pancreatitis, invasive intervention (i.e., percutaneous catheter drainage, endoscopic transluminal drainage/necrosectomy, minimally invasive or open necrosectomy) should be delayed where possible until at least 4 weeks after initial presentation to allow the collection to become walled-off. (GRADE 1C, strong agreement)
32. The best available evidence suggests that surgical necrosectomy should ideally be delayed until collections have become walled-off, typically 4 weeks after the onset of pancreatitis, in all patients with complications of necrosis. No subgroups have been identified that might benefit from earlier or delayed intervention. (GRADE 1C, strong agreement)

K. Intervention Strategies in Necrotizing Pancreatitis

33. The optimal interventional strategy for patients with suspected or confirmed infected necrotizing pancreatitis is initial image-guided percutaneous (retroperitoneal) catheter drainage or endoscopic transluminal drainage, followed, if necessary, by endoscopic or surgical necrosectomy. (GRADE 1A, strong agreement)
34. Percutaneous catheter or endoscopic transmural drainage should be the first step in the treatment of patients with suspected or confirmed (walled-off) infected necrotizing pancreatitis. (GRADE 1A, strong agreement)
35. There are insufficient data to define subgroups of patients with suspected or confirmed infected necrotizing pancreatitis who would benefit from a different treatment strategy. (GRADE 2C, strong agreement)

L. Timing of Cholecystectomy (or Endoscopic Sphincterotomy)

36. Cholecystectomy during index admission for mild biliary pancreatitis appears safe and is recommended. Interval cholecystectomy after mild biliary pancreatitis is associated with a substantial risk of readmission for recurrent biliary events, especially recurrent biliary pancreatitis. (GRADE 1C, strong agreement)
37. Cholecystectomy should be delayed in patients with peripancreatic collections until the collections either resolve or persist beyond 6 weeks, at which time cholecystectomy can be performed safely. (GRADE 2C, strong agreement)
38. In patients with biliary pancreatitis who have undergone sphincterotomy and are fit for surgery, cholecystectomy is advised, because ERCP and sphincterotomy prevent recurrence of biliary pancreatitis but not gallstone-related gallbladder disease (i.e., biliary colic and cholecystitis). (GRADE 2B, strong agreement)

CT, Computed tomography; *ERCP,* endoscopic retrograde cholangiopancreatography; *EUS,* endoscopic ultrasonography; *FNA,* fine-needle aspiration; *MRCP,* magnetic resonance cholangiopancreatography; *MRI,* magnetic resonance imaging; *SCCM,* Society of Critical Care Medicine; *SIRS,* systemic inflammatory response syndrome.
Modified from Working Group IAP/APA Acute Pancreatitis Guidelines. IAP/APA evidence-based guidelines for the management of acute pancreatitis. *Pancreatology.* 2013;13(4 suppl 2):e1—e15.

BOX 21.9   Complications of Acute Pancreatitis

Respiratory
- Early hypoxemia
- Pleural effusion
- Atelectasis
- Pulmonary infiltration
- Acute respiratory distress syndrome
- Mediastinal abscess

Cardiovascular
- Hypotension and shock
- Pericardial effusion
- ST-T changes

Renal
- Acute kidney injury
- Oliguria
- Renal artery or vein thrombosis

Hematologic
- Disseminated intravascular coagulation
- Thrombocytosis
- Hyperfibrinogenemia

Endocrine
- Hypocalcemia
- Hypertriglyceridemia
- Hyperglycemia

Neurologic
- Fat emboli

- Psychosis
- Encephalopathy and coma

Ophthalmic
- Purtscher retinopathy (sudden blindness)

Dermatologic
- Subcutaneous fat necrosis

Gastrointestinal or Hepatic
- Intra-abdominal hypertension/abdominal compartment syndrome
- Hepatic dysfunction
- Obstructive jaundice
- Stress ulceration
- Erosive gastritis
- Paralytic ileus
- Duodenal obstruction
- Pancreatic
- Pseudocyst
- Phlegmon
- Abscess
- Ascites
- Bowel infarction
- Massive intraperitoneal bleed
- Perforation
- Stomach
- Duodenum
- Small bowel
- Colon

Educate the Patient and Family

Early in the patient's hospital stay, the patient and family should be taught about acute pancreatitis and its causes and treatment. Closer to discharge, teaching should focus on the interventions necessary for preventing the recurrence of the precipitating disorder. If sustained, permanent damage to the pancreas has occurred, the patient will require teaching specific to diet modification and supplemental pancreatic enzymes. Diabetes education may also be necessary. If the patient abuses alcohol, the patient should be encouraged to stop drinking and be referred to an alcohol cessation program (see Box 21.11).

Interprofessional collaborative management of the patient with pancreatitis is outlined in Box 21.12.

BOX 21.10   PRIORITY PATIENT CARE MANAGEMENT

Acute Pancreatitis
- Acute Pain due to transmission and perception of cutaneous, visceral, muscular, or ischemia impulses
- Hypovolemia due to relative fluid loss
- Impaired Cardiac Output due to alterations in preload
- Impaired Breathing due to decreased lung expansion
- Impaired Nutritional Intake due to lack of exogenous nutrients or increased metabolic demand
- Anxiety due to threat to biologic, psychologic, or social integrity
- Impaired Family Coping due to critically ill family member
- Lack of Knowledge of Treatment Regime due to lack of previous exposure to information (see Patient and Family Education Plan, Box 21.3)

Patient Care Management Plans are located in Appendix A.

BOX 21.11   Signs and Symptoms of Pancreatic Infection

- Persistent abdominal pain
- Abdominal tenderness
- Prolonged fever
- Abdominal distention
- Palpable abdominal mass
- Nausea and vomiting
- Increased white blood cell count
- Persistent elevation of serum amylase
- Hyperbilirubinemia
- Elevated alkaline phosphatase level
- Positive culture and Gram stain

BOX 21.12   Teamwork and Collaboration

Interprofessional Collaborative Practice: Acute Pancreatitis
- Ensure adequate circulating volume.
- Provide nutrition support.
- Correct metabolic alterations.
- Minimize pancreatic stimulation.
- Provide comfort and emotional support.
- Maintain surveillance for complications.
  - Pancreatic pseudocyst
  - Infected pancreatic necrosis
  - Pancreatic abscess
  - Intra-abdominal compartment syndrome
  - Acute respiratory distress syndrome
  - Multiple organ dysfunction syndrome

ACUTE LIVER FAILURE

Description and Etiology

Acute liver failure (ALF) is a life-threatening condition characterized by severe and sudden liver cell dysfunction, coagulopathy, and hepatic encephalopathy.[47] Although uncommon, ALF is associated with a mortality rate of 40%, and it usually occurs in patients without pre-existing liver disease.[47] Because liver transplantation is one of the few definitive treatments, a patient with ALF should be transferred to a critical care unit and strongly considered for referral to a major medical center where transplantation services are available.[47]

The causes of ALF include infections, medications, toxins, hypoperfusion, metabolic disorders, and surgery (Box 21.13); however, viral hepatitis and medication-induced liver damage are the predominant causes in North America. Patients are usually healthy before the onset of symptoms, because ALF tends to occur in patients with no known liver history. A thorough medication and health history is imperative to determine a possible cause. The patient should be questioned about exposure to environmental toxins, hepatitis, intravenous drug use, sexual history, viral hepatitis, medication toxicity, and poisoning. Additional vascular causes such as thrombosis; ischemia; Budd-Chiari syndrome (blocked venous outflow from small hepatic veins to inferior vena cava from thrombosis); and metabolic disorders such as Reye syndrome (acute, often fatal liver disease), Wilson disease (disease of defective copper metabolism that damages liver and brain), galactosemia (rare disease in infants in which they cannot metabolize galactose, resulting in hepatocellular damage), and fructose intolerance should be considered.[47–51]

Pathophysiology

ALF is a result of massive necrosis of the hepatocytes. It results in numerous derangements, including impaired bilirubin conjugation, decreased production of clotting factors, depressed glucose synthesis, and decreased lactate clearance. This results in jaundice, coagulopathies, hypoglycemia, and metabolic acidosis. Other effects of ALF include increased risk of infection and altered carbohydrate, protein, and glucose metabolism. Hypoalbuminemia, fluid and electrolyte imbalances, and acute portal hypertension contribute to the development of ascites.[47] Hepatic encephalopathy is believed to result from failure of the liver to detoxify various substances in the bloodstream, and it may be worsened by metabolic and electrolyte imbalances.[7]

The patient may experience various other complications, including cerebral edema, cardiac dysrhythmias, acute lung failure, sepsis, and AKI. Cerebral edema and increased intracranial pressure (ICP) develop as a result of breakdown of the blood-brain barrier and astrocyte swelling. Circulatory failure that mimics sepsis is common in ALF and may exacerbate low cerebral perfusion pressure.[52] Hypoxemia, acidosis, electrolyte imbalances, and cerebral edema can precipitate the development of cardiac dysrhythmias. Acute lung failure progressing to ARDS, intrapulmonary shunting, ventilation-perfusion mismatch, sepsis, and aspiration may contribute to the universal arterial hypoxemia.[52]

BOX 21.13   Causes of Acute Liver Failure

Infections
- Hepatitis A, B, C, D, E, non-A, non-B, non-C
- Herpes simplex virus (types 1 and 2)
- Epstein-Barr virus
- Varicella zoster
- Dengue fever virus
- Rift Valley fever virus

Medications or Toxins
- Industrial substances (chlorinated hydrocarbons, phosphorus)
- *Amanita phalloides* (mushrooms)
- Aflatoxin (a toxic metabolite of fungus)
- Medications (isoniazid, rifampin, halothane, methyldopa, tetracycline, valproic acid, monoamine oxidase inhibitors, phenytoin, nicotinic acid, tricyclic antidepressants, isoflurane, ketoconazole, trimethoprim-sulfamethoxazole, sulfasalazine, pyrimethamine, octreotide)
- Acetaminophen toxicity
- Cocaine

Hypoperfusion
- Venous obstructions

- Budd-Chiari syndrome
- Veno-occlusive disease
- Ischemia

Metabolic Disorders
- Wilson disease
- Tyrosinemia
- Heat stroke
- Galactosemia

Surgery
- Jejunoileal bypass
- Partial hepatectomy
- Liver transplantation failure

Other Causes
- Reye syndrome
- Acute fatty liver of pregnancy
- Massive malignant infiltration
- Autoimmune hepatitis

Assessment and Diagnosis

Early recognition of ALF is essential. The diagnosis should include potentially reversible conditions (e.g., autoimmune hepatitis) and should differentiate ALF from decompensating chronic liver disease. Prognostic indicators such as coma grade, serum bilirubin, prothrombin time, coagulation factors, and pH should be assessed, and potential causes should be investigated.[47]

Signs and symptoms of ALF include headache, hyperventilation, jaundice, mental status changes, palmar erythema, spider nevi, bruises, and edema. The patient should be evaluated for the presence of asterixis, or "liver flap," which is best described as the inability to voluntarily sustain a fixed position of the extremities. Asterixis is best recognized by downward flapping of the hands when the patient extends the arms and dorsiflexes the wrists. Hepatic encephalopathy is assessed by using a grading system that stages the encephalopathy according to the patient's clinical manifestations (Box 21.14). Diagnostic findings include prolonged prothrombin times; elevated levels of serum bilirubin, aspartate aminotransferase, alkaline phosphatase, and serum ammonia; and decreased levels of serum albumin.[53] Arterial blood gases reveal respiratory alkalosis, metabolic acidosis, or both. Hypoglycemia, hypokalemia, and hyponatremia also may be present.[52,53]

Factors I (fibrinogen), II (prothrombin), V, VII, IX, and X are produced exclusively by the liver. Prothrombin time may be the most useful of these in the evaluation of acute ALF, because levels may be 40 to 80 seconds above control values. Test results show decreased levels of plasmin and plasminogen and increased levels of fibrin and fibrin-split products. Platelet counts may be less than 100,000/mm^3.[53]

Medical Management

Medical interventions are directed toward management of the various systems affected by ALF.

Ammonia Levels

Antibiotics such as neomycin, metronidazole, and rifaximin and lactulose, which is the gold standard, are administered to remove or decrease production of nitrogenous wastes in the large intestine. Antibiotics reduce bacterial flora of the colon; this aids in decreasing ammonia formation by decreasing bacterial action on the protein in feces. Side effects include renal toxicity and hearing impairment. Lactulose, a synthetic ketoanalogue of lactose split into lactic acid and acetic acid in the intestine, is given orally through a nasogastric tube or as a retention enema. The result is the creation of an acidic environment that results in ammonia being drawn out of the portal circulation. Lactulose has a laxative effect that promotes expulsion.[47,52]

Complications

Bleeding is best controlled through prevention. If an invasive procedure (e.g., central line placement, ICP monitor) will be performed or the patient develops active bleeding, vitamin K, fresh frozen plasma (to maintain a reasonable prothrombin time), and platelet transfusions are necessary.[53] Metabolic disturbances such as hypoglycemia, metabolic acidosis, hypokalemia, and hyponatremia should be monitored and treated appropriately. Prophylactic antibiotic administration may be initiated because the patient is at high risk for an infection.[53] The development of cerebral edema necessitates ICP monitoring. Treatment with mannitol has been shown to be beneficial in managing ICP in a patient with ALF, but it must be used with caution in patients with renal failure to avoid hyperosmolarity.[52] Other interventions to control ICP include elevating the head of the bed to 30 degrees, treating fever and hypertension, minimizing noxious stimulation, and correcting hypercapnia and hypoxemia.[47] AKI develops in 70% of patients with ALF; continuous renal replacement therapy provides renal support.[47] Hemodynamic instability is a common complication necessitating fluid administration and vasoactive medications to prevent prolonged episodes of hypotension. A pulmonary artery catheter may be used to guide clinical management.[47]

If ALF continues and the patient shows no immediate signs of improvement or reversal, the patient should be considered for a liver transplantation. Prompt referral to a transplantation center should be a high priority for patients experiencing ALF.[47]

Nursing Management

The patient management plan for a patient with ALF incorporates a variety of patient problems (Box 21.15). The nurse plays a significant role in protecting the patient from injury, maintaining surveillance for complications, and educating the patient and family.

Protect the Patient From Injury

Use of benzodiazepines and other sedatives is discouraged in a patient with ALF, because pertinent neurologic changes may be masked and hepatic encephalopathy may be exacerbated.[52] These patients are often very difficult to manage, because they may be extremely agitated and

---

BOX 21.14 Staging of Hepatic Encephalopathy

I. Euphoria or depression, mild confusion, slurred speech, disordered sleep rhythm; slight asterixis and normal EEG

II. Lethargy, moderate confusion; marked asterixis and abnormal EEG

III. Marked confusion, incoherent speech, sleeping but arousable; asterixis present and abnormal EEG

IV. Coma; initially responsive to noxious stimuli, later unresponsive; asterixis absent and abnormal EEG

EEG, Electroencephalogram.

◎ BOX 21.15 PRIORITY PATIENT CARE MANAGEMENT

Acute Liver Failure

- Impaired Breathing due to decreased lung expansion
- Impaired Gas Exchange due to ventilation-perfusion mismatching or intrapulmonary shunting
- Impaired Cardiac Output due to alterations in preload
- Impaired Cardiac Output due to alterations in heart rate or rhythm
- Decreased Intracranial Adaptive Capacity due to failure of normal compensatory mechanisms
- Risk for Infection
- Impaired Nutritional Intake due to lack of exogenous nutrients or increased metabolic demand
- Disturbed Body Image due to actual change in body structure, function, or appearance
- Impaired Family Coping due to critically ill family member
- Lack of Knowledge of Treatment Regime due to lack of previous exposure to information (see Patient and Family Education Plan, Box 21.3)
  Patient Care Management Plans are located in Appendix A.

combative. Physical restraint may be necessary to prevent injury to the patient; however, all other nursing interventions must be tried before restraints are considered.

Maintain Surveillance for Complications

As the neurologic condition worsens, respiratory depression and arrest can occur quickly. Continuous pulse oximetry monitoring and arterial blood gas analysis are helpful in assessing adequacy of respiratory efforts. A thorough neurologic assessment should be performed at least every hour, with changes reported immediately.

Educate the Patient and Family

Early in the patient's hospital stay, the patient and family should be taught about ALF and its causes and treatment. Closer to discharge, teaching should focus on the interventions necessary for preventing the recurrence of the precipitating cause. If the patient is considered a candidate for liver transplantation, the patient and family will need specific information regarding the procedure and care. Evaluation for liver transplantation may include screening for medical contraindications, human immunodeficiency virus serology, anticipated compliance, and assessment of the social support system. Psychiatric and other specialty team consultations are necessary for a thorough evaluation of the patient's suitability for a liver transplantation.

Interprofessional collaborative management of the patient with ALF is outlined in Box 21.16.

BOX 21.16   Teamwork and Collaboration

Interprofessional Collaborative Practice: Acute Liver Failure
- Decrease ammonia levels.
- Control bleeding.
- Correct metabolic alterations.
- Prevent infection.
- Prepare patient for liver transplantation, if necessary.
- Protect patient from injury.
- Provide comfort and emotional support.
- Maintain surveillance for complications:
  - Cerebral edema
  - Renal failure

GASTROINTESTINAL SURGERY

Types of Surgery

GI surgery refers to a wide variety of surgical procedures that involve the esophagus, stomach, intestine, liver, pancreas, or biliary tract. Indications for GI surgery are numerous and include bleeding or perforation from peptic ulcer disease, obstruction, trauma, inflammatory bowel disease, and malignancy. Patients may be admitted to the critical care unit for monitoring after GI surgery as a result of their underlying medical condition; however, this section focuses only on several surgical procedures that commonly require postoperative critical care.

Esophagectomy

Esophagectomy is usually performed for cancer of the distal esophagus and gastroesophageal junction. The technically difficult procedure involves the removal of part or all of the esophagus, part of the stomach, and lymph nodes in the surrounding area. The stomach is then pulled up into the chest and connected to the remaining part of the esophagus. If the entire esophagus and stomach must be removed, part of the bowel may be used to form the esophageal replacement (Figs. 21.5 and 21.6).[54]

Two approaches may be used for esophageal resection: transhiatal or transthoracic (see Figs. 21.5 and 21.6). In both approaches, the stomach is mobilized through an abdominal incision and then transposed into the chest. The anastomosis of the stomach to the esophagus is performed in the chest (transthoracic) or in the neck (transhiatal). The approach selected depends on the location of the tumor, the patient's overall health and pulmonary function, and the experience of the surgeon. After surgery, the patient has a nasogastric tube in place, and it should not be manipulated because of the potential to damage the anastomosis. Patients who undergo transthoracic esophagectomy have chest tubes.[54]

Pancreaticoduodenectomy

The standard operation for pancreatic cancer is a pancreaticoduodenectomy, also called the *Whipple procedure*. In the Whipple procedure, the pancreatic head, the duodenum, part of the jejunum, the common bile duct, the gallbladder, and part of the stomach are removed. The continuity of the GI tract is restored by anastomosing the remaining portion of the pancreas, the bile duct, and the stomach to the jejunum (Fig. 21.7).[54]

Bariatric Surgery

Bariatric surgery refers to surgical procedures of the GI tract that are performed to induce weight loss. Bariatric procedures are divided into three broad types: (1) restrictive, (2) malabsorptive, and (3) combined restrictive and malabsorptive.[55] Restrictive procedures such as vertical banded gastroplasty (Fig. 21.8A) and gastric banding (Fig. 21.8B) reduce the capacity of the stomach and limit the amount of food that can be consumed. Malabsorptive procedures such as biliopancreatic diversion (Fig. 21.8C) alter the GI tract to limit the digestion and absorption of food. The Roux-en-Y gastric bypass (Fig. 21.8D) combines both strategies by creating a small gastric pouch and anastomosing the jejunum to the pouch (Fig. 21.8E). Food then bypasses the lower stomach and duodenum, resulting in decreased absorption of digestive materials.[55]

Most bariatric procedures can be performed using an open or laparoscopic surgical technique. Although laparoscopic approaches are more technically difficult to perform, they have largely replaced open procedures because they are associated with decreased pulmonary complications, less postoperative pain, reduced length of hospital stay, fewer wound complications (e.g., infections, incisional hernia), and an earlier return to full activity.[54,55] Open procedures are performed on patients who have had prior upper abdominal surgery, who are morbidly obese, or who may be unable to tolerate the increased abdominal pressure associated with laparoscopic procedures.[54]

Preoperative Care

A thorough preoperative evaluation should be conducted to evaluate the patient's physical and mental status and identify risk factors that may affect the postoperative course. Because obesity is associated with a higher incidence of comorbidities such as cardiovascular disease, hypertension, diabetes, gastroesophageal reflux, obstructive sleep apnea, and heart failure, an extensive work-up may be required for the patient who will undergo bariatric surgery.[54,56]

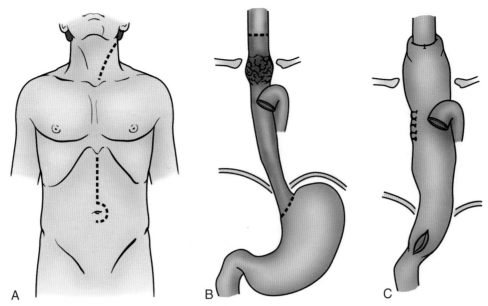

Fig. 21.5 Overview of Transhiatal Esophagectomy. (A) Transhiatal esophagectomy with (B) gastric mobilization and (C) gastric pull-up for cervical esophagogastric anastomosis. (Modified from Ellis FH. Esophagogastrectomy for carcinoma: technical considerations based on anatomic location of lesion. *Surg Clin North Am.* 1980;60[2]:265–279.)

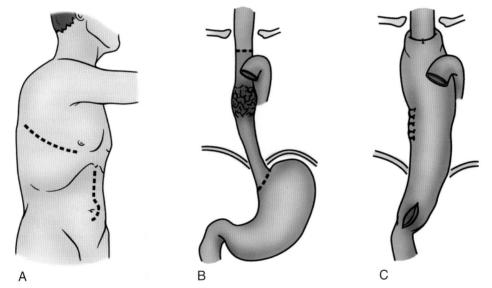

Fig. 21.6 Overview of Transthoracic Esophagectomy. Transthoracic esophagectomy with (A) esophageal resection, (B) gastric mobilization, and (C) intrathoracic anastomosis for a midesophageal tumor. (Modified from Ellis FH. Esophagogastrectomy for carcinoma: technical considerations based on anatomic location of lesion. *Surg Clin North Am.* 1980;60[2]:265–279.)

Complications and Medical Management

Several complications are associated with GI surgery, including respiratory failure, atelectasis, pneumonia, anastomotic leak, deep vein thrombosis, pulmonary embolus, and bleeding. Morbidly obese patients are at even greater risk for many postoperative complications.[55]

Pulmonary Complications

The risk for pulmonary complications is substantial after GI surgery, and adverse respiratory events such as atelectasis and pneumonia are twice as likely to occur in an obese patient.[56] Aggressive pulmonary exercise should be initiated in the immediate postoperative period. Early ambulation and adequate pain control assist in reducing the risk of developing atelectasis. Suctioning, chest physiotherapy, or bronchodilators may be needed to optimize pulmonary function. Patients should be closely monitored for the development of oxygenation problems. Treatment should be aimed at supporting adequate ventilation and gas exchange. Mechanical ventilation may be required in the event of respiratory failure.

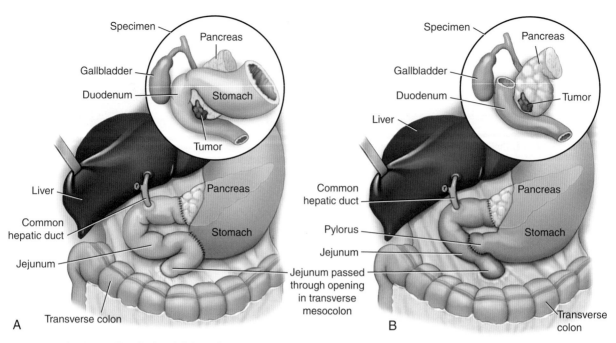

Fig. 21.7 Standard and Pylorus-Preserving Whipple Procedures. (A) The standard Whipple procedure involves resection of the gastric antrum, head of pancreas, distal bile duct, and entire duodenum with reconstruction as shown. (B) The pylorus-preserving Whipple procedure does not include resection of the distal stomach, pylorus, or proximal duodenum.

Anastomotic Leak

An anastomotic leak is a severe complication of GI surgery. It occurs when there is a breakdown of the suture line in a surgical anastomosis and results in leakage of gastric or intestinal contents into the abdomen or mediastinum (transthoracic esophagectomy).[56] The clinical signs and symptoms of a leak can be subtle and often go unrecognized. They include tachycardia, tachypnea, fever, abdominal pain, anxiety, and restlessness.[56] In a patient who had an esophagectomy, a leak of the esophageal anastomosis may manifest as subcutaneous emphysema in the chest and neck.[54] If undetected, a leak can result in sepsis, multiorgan failure, and death. Patients with progressive tachycardia and tachypnea should have a radiologic study (upper GI study with a contrast agent [Gastrografin] or CT scan with contrast medium) to rule out an anastomotic leak.[56] The type of treatment depends on the severity of the leak. If the leak is small and well contained, it may be managed conservatively by maintaining NPO status, administering antibiotics, and draining fluid percutaneously. If the patient is deteriorating rapidly, an urgent laparotomy is indicated to repair the defect.[54,56]

Deep Vein Thrombosis and Pulmonary Embolism

Pulmonary embolism is a very serious complication of any surgical procedure. Deep vein thrombosis prophylaxis should be initiated before surgery and continued until the patient is fully ambulatory to reduce the risk of clot development. Typically, a combination of sequential compression devices and subcutaneous unfractionated heparin or low-molecular-weight heparin is used. Patients determined to be at high risk for pulmonary embolism may benefit from prophylactic inferior vena cava filter placement.[54]

Bleeding

Upper GI bleeding is an uncommon but life-threatening complication of GI surgery. Early bleeding usually occurs at the site of the anastomosis and can usually be treated through endoscopic intervention. Surgical revision may be needed for persistent, uncontrolled bleeding. Late bleeding is usually a result of ulcer development. Medical therapy is aimed at the prevention of this complication through administration of H_2 antagonists or PPIs.[5]

Postoperative Nursing Management

The patient care management plan for a patient who has had GI surgery incorporates a variety of patient problems (Box 21.17). The nurse plays a significant role in optimizing pulmonary function and managing pain.

Pulmonary Management

Nursing interventions in the postoperative period are focused on promoting ventilation and adequate oxygenation and preventing complications such as atelectasis and pneumonia. After the patient is extubated, deep-breathing exercises and incentive spirometry should be initiated, and the patient should perform them regularly. Early ambulation is encouraged to promote maximal lung inflation, reducing the risk of pulmonary complications and the potential for pulmonary embolus.

Pain Management

It is imperative to manage the patient's pain appropriately after GI surgery. Adequate analgesia is necessary to promote the mobility of the patient and decrease pulmonary complications. Initial pain

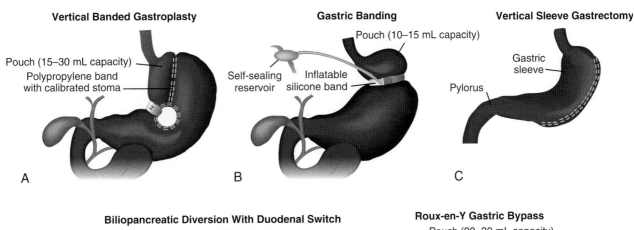

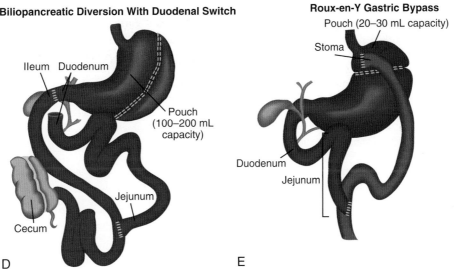

Fig. 21.8 Bariatric Surgical Procedures. (A) Vertical-banded gastroplasty involves creating a small gastric pouch. (B) Adjustable gastric banding uses a band to create a gastric pouch. (C) Vertical sleeve gastrectomy involves creating a sleeve-shaped stomach by removing approximately 80% of the stomach. (D) Biliopancreatic diversion with duodenal switch procedure creates an anastomosis between the stomach and intestine. (E) Roux-en-Y gastric bypass procedure involves constructing a gastric pouch whose outlet is a Y-shaped limb of small intestine. (From Harding MM, ed. *Lewis's Medical-Surgical Nursing: Assessment and Management of Clinical Problems.* 11th ed. St. Louis: Elsevier; 2020.)

◎ **BOX 21.17 PRIORITY PATIENT CARE MANAGEMENT**

Gastrointestinal Surgery
- Impaired Breathing due to decreased lung expansion
- Impaired Gas Exchange due to alveolar hypoventilation
- Impaired Cardiac Output due to alterations in preload
- Acute Pain due to transmission and perception of cutaneous, visceral, muscular, or ischemic impulses
- Anxiety due to threat to biologic, psychologic, or social integrity
- Disturbed Body Image due to actual change in body structure, function, or appearance
- Lack of Knowledge of Treatment Regime due to lack of previous exposure to information

Patient Care Management Plans are located in Appendix A.

---

management may be accomplished by intravenous opioid (morphine, hydromorphone) administration by means of a patient-controlled analgesia pump or through continuous epidural infusion of an opioid and local anesthetic (bupivacaine).[54] Oral pain medications can be started after an anastomotic leak is ruled out. Nonpharmacologic interventions such as positioning, application of heat or cold, and distraction may also be used. If the patient's pain is not being sufficiently relieved, the pain management service should be consulted.[54,56]

ENDOSCOPIC PROCEDURES

Gastrointestinal Intubation

Because GI intubation is used so often in critical care units, it is important for nurses to know the clinical indications and responsibilities inherent in tube use. The three categories of GI tubes are based on function: (1) nasogastric suction tubes, (2) long intestinal tubes, and (3) feeding tubes. Feeding tubes are discussed in Chapter 5.

Nasogastric Suction Tubes

Nasogastric tubes remove fluid regurgitated into the stomach, prevent accumulation of swallowed air, may partially decompress the bowel, and reduce the patient's risk for aspiration. Nasogastric tubes also can be used for collecting specimens, assessing the presence of blood, and administering tube feedings. The most common nasogastric tubes are the single-lumen Levin tube and the double-lumen Salem sump. The Salem sump has one lumen that is used for suction and drainage and another that allows air to enter the patient's stomach and prevents the tube from adhering to the gastric wall and damaging the mucosa. The tube is passed through the nose or mouth into the nasopharynx and then down through the pharynx into the esophagus and stomach. The length of time the nasogastric tube remains in place depends on its use. The tube is then placed to gravity, low intermittent suction, or low continuous suction, and in rare instances, it is clamped.

Patient care management focuses on preventing complications common to this therapy, such as ulceration and necrosis of the nares, esophageal reflux, esophagitis, esophageal erosion and stricture, gastric erosion, and dry mouth and parotitis from mouth breathing. Interference with ventilation and coughing, aspiration, and loss of fluid and electrolytes can be critical problems. Interventions include irrigating the tube every 4 hours with normal saline, ensuring the blue air vent of the Salem sump is patent and maintained above the level of the patient's stomach, and providing frequent mouth and nares care.

Long Intestinal Tubes

Miller-Abbott, Cantor, and Andersen tubes are examples of long, weighted-tip intestinal tubes that are placed preoperatively or intra-operatively. Their considerable length allows removal of the contents of the intestine to treat an obstruction that cannot be managed by a nasogastric tube. These tubes can decompress the small bowel and can splint the small bowel intraoperatively or postoperatively. Because progression of the tubes depends on bowel peristalsis, their use is contraindicated in patients with paralytic ileus and severe mechanical bowel obstructions.

Interventions used in the care of a patient with a long intestinal tube are similar to interventions used with a nasogastric tube. The patient should be observed for (1) gaseous distention of the balloon section, which makes removal difficult; (2) rupture of the balloon; (3) overinflation of the balloon, which can lead to intestinal rupture; and (4) reverse intussusception if the tube is removed rapidly. Intestinal tubes should be removed slowly; usually 6 inches of the tube is withdrawn every hour.

Endoscopic Injection Therapy

Endoscopic injection therapy is used to control bleeding of ulcers. It may be performed emergently, electively, or prophylactically. An endoscope is introduced through the patient's mouth, and endoscopy

of the esophagus and stomach is performed to identify the bleeding varices or ulcers. An injector with a retractable 23- to 25-gauge needle is introduced through the biopsy channel of the endoscope. The needle is then inserted in or around the varices or into the area around the ulcer, and a liquid agent is injected. The most commonly used agent is epinephrine, which results in localized vasoconstriction and enhanced platelet aggregation. Sclerosing agents such as ethanolamine, alcohol, and polidocanol also may be used. These agents cause an inflammatory reaction in the vessel that results in thrombosis and eventually produces a fibrous band. Repeated sclerotherapy results in the development of supportive scar tissue around the varices. Other embolic agents are used, including fibrinogen and thrombin, which when injected together react to form an active fibrin clot, and "glues" (N-butyl cyanoacrylate), which are used as a sealant to stop the bleeding.[57]

Endoscopic Variceal Ligation

EVL involves applying bands or metal clips around the circumference of the bleeding varices to induce venous obstruction and control bleeding. EVL has replaced endoscopic sclerotherapy of variceal hemorrhage. One or two days after the procedure, necrosis and scar formation promote band and tissue sloughing. Fibrinous deposits within the healing ulcer potentiate vessel obliteration. Band ligation is accomplished through endoscopy, with multiple bands placed per session.[16] The procedure may be repeated on an inpatient or outpatient basis every 1 or 2 weeks until all the varices are obliterated.[57] EVL controls bleeding in approximately 80% to 90% of cases.[57] The most common complication of EVL is the development of superficial mucosal ulcers. Varices may reoccur, as local banding does not affect portal pressure.[58]

Transjugular Intrahepatic Portosystemic Shunt

TIPS is an angiographic interventional procedure for decreasing portal hypertension. TIPS is advocated for (1) patients with portal hypertension who are also experiencing active bleeding or have poor liver reserve, (2) transplant recipients, and (3) patients with other operative risks.[58] The TIPS procedure is usually performed by a gastroenterologist, vascular surgeon, or interventional radiologist.

Portal hypertension is confirmed by direct measurement of the pressure in the portal vein (gradient greater than 10 mm Hg). Cannulation is achieved through the internal jugular vein, and an angiographic catheter is advanced into the middle or right hepatic vein. The midhepatic vein is then catheterized, and a new route is created by connecting the portal and hepatic veins using a needle and guidewire with a dilating balloon. A polytetrafluoroethylene-coated stent is then placed in the liver parenchyma to maintain that connection (Fig. 21.9). The increased resistance in the liver is bypassed.[59] TIPS may be performed in patients with bleeding varices, with refractory bleeding varices, or as a bridge to liver transplantation if the candidate becomes hemodynamically unstable. Postprocedural care should include observation for overt (cannulation site) or covert (intrahepatic site) bleeding, hepatic or portal vein laceration (resulting in rapid loss of blood volume), and inadvertent puncture of surrounding organs. Other complications include hepatic encephalopathy, liver failure, bacteremia, and stent stenosis.[59]

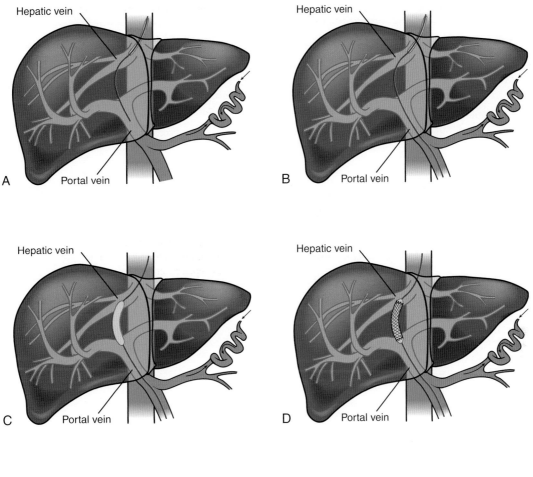

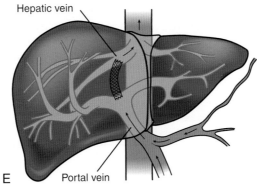

Fig. 21.9 Transjugular Intrahepatic Portosystemic Shunt (TIPS). (A) Needle directed through liver parenchyma to portal vein. (B) Needle and guidewire passed down to midportal vein. (C) Balloon dilation. (D) Deployment of stent. (E) Intrahepatic shunt from portal to hepatic vein. (From Urden LD, Stacy KM, Lough ME, eds. *Priorities in Critical Care Nursing.* 8th ed. St. Louis: Elsevier; 2020.)

GASTROINTESTINAL PHARMACOLOGY

Many pharmacologic agents are used in the care of patients with GI disorders. Table 21.3 reviews the various agents and any special considerations necessary for administering them.

ADDITIONAL RESOURCES

See Box 21.18 for Internet resources related to gastrointestinal disorders and therapeutic management.

TABLE 21.3 Pharmacologic Management Gastrointestinal Disorders.

Medication	Dosage	Actions	Special Considerations
Antacids	30–90 mL q1–2 h PO or NG; possibly titrated to NG pH	Used to buffer stomach acid and raise gastric pH	Can cause diarrhea or constipation and electrolyte disturbances Irrigate NG tube with water after administration because antacids can clog tube
Histamine-2 (H$_2$) Antagonists			
Cimetidine (Tagamet)	300 mg q6h IV or PO	Used to reduce volume and concentration of gastric secretions	Side effects include CNS toxicity (confusion or delirium) and thrombocytopenia
Ranitidine (Zantac)	150–300 mg q12h PO or 50 mg q8h IV		Separate administration of antacids and PO histamine blocking agents by 1 hour
Famotidine (Pepcid)	40 mg daily PO or 20 mg q12h IV		Dosage adjustments recommended for patients with moderate (creatinine clearance <50 mL/min) or severe (creatinine clearance <10 mL/min) renal insufficiency
Nizatidine (Axid)	150 mg q12h PO or 300 mg q24h		
Gastric Mucosal Agents			
Sucralfate (Carafate)	1 g q6h NG or PO, given 1 hour before meals and at bedtime	Forms an ulcer-adherent complex with proteinaceous exudates Covers ulcer and protects against acid, pepsin, and bile salts	Requires an acid medium for activation; do not administer within 30 minutes of antacid May cause severe constipation May cause decreased absorption of certain medications
Gastric Proton-Pump Inhibitors			
Omeprazole (Prilosec)	20–40 mg q12h PO	Inhibits gastric acid secretion by the gastric parietal cells	Capsules should be swallowed intact
Lansoprazole (Prevacid)	15–30 mg q24h PO 30 mg over 30 minutes q24h IV		May increase levels of phenytoin, diazepam, warfarin
Rabeprazole (AcipHex)	20–40 mg q24h PO		May be administered concomitantly with antacids
Esomeprazole (Nexium)	40 mg q12–24 h PO 20–40 mg q24h IV		Associated with higher incidence of *Clostridioides difficile* infection and ventilator-associated pneumonia
Pantoprazole (Protonix)	20–80 mg q24h PO 80 mg q8–12 h IV		
Vasopressin			
(Pitressin Synthetic)	Loading dose of 20 U over 20 minutes IV, followed by 0.2–0.4 units/min IV infusion Doses can be increased to 0.9 units/min, if necessary	Decreases splanchnic blood flow, reducing portal pressure	Side effects include coronary, mesenteric, and peripheral vasoconstriction May be administered concurrently with nitroglycerin to minimize side effects
Somatostatin			
Octreotide (Sandostatin)	Bolus dose of 25–50 mcg followed by IV infusion of 25–50 mcg/h for 48 hours	Decreases splanchnic blood flow, reducing portal pressure	May cause hyperglycemia or hypoglycemia when initiating drip and changing dosages

CNS, Central nervous system; *IV,* intravenous/intravenously; *NG,* nasogastric; *PO,* by mouth.
Data from *Clinical Key Drug Monographs.* https://www.clinicalkey.com. Accessed September 12, 2020.

QSEN   **BOX 21.18**   **Informatics**

Internet Resources: Gastrointestinal Disorders and Therapeutic Management

- National Digestive Diseases Information Clearinghouse (NDDIC): https://digestive.niddk.nih.gov
- International Foundation for Functional Gastrointestinal Disorders: https://www.iffgd.org
- American Pancreatic Association: https://www.american-pancreatic-association.org
- The National Pancreas Foundation (NPF): https://pancreasfoundation.org
- American Liver Foundation: https://www.liverfoundation.org
- American Association for the Study of Liver Diseases: https://www.aasld.org

REFERENCES

1. Khamaysi I, Gralnek IM. Acute upper gastrointestinal bleeding (UGIB)—initial evaluation and management. *Best Pract Res Clin Gastroenterol.* 2013; 27(5):633–638.
2. Nable JV, Graham AC. Gastrointestinal bleeding. *Emerg Med Clin North Am.* 2016;34(2):309–325.
3. Kim G, Sota JA, Morrison T. Radiologic assessment of gastrointestinal bleeding. *Gastroenterol Clin North Am.* 2018;47(3):501–514.
4. Feinman M, Haut ER. Upper gastrointestinal bleeding. *Surg Clin N Am.* 2014;94(1):43–53.
5. Feinman M, Haut ER. Lower gastrointestinal bleeding. *Surg Clin N Am.* 2014;94(1):55–63.
6. Schubert ML. Physiologic, pathophysiologic, and pharmacologic regulation of gastric acid secretion. *Curr Opin Gastroenterol.* 2017;33(6): 430–438.

7. Huether SE. Alterations of digestive function. In: McCance KL, Huether SE, eds. *Pathophysiology: The Biologic Basis for Disease in Adults and Children.* 8th ed. St. Louis: Elsevier; 2019.

8. Hunt RH, Camilleri M, Crowe SE, et al. The stomach in health and disease. *Gut.* 2015;64(10):1650–1668.

9. Lanas A, Chan FKL. Peptic ulcer disease. *Lancet.* 2017;390(10094):613–624.

10. Barbateskovic M, Marker S, Granholm A, et al. Stress ulcer prophylaxis with proton pump inhibitors or histamin-2 receptor antagonists in adult intensive care patients: a systematic review with meta-analysis and trial sequential analysis. *Intensive Care Med.* 2019;45(2):143–158.

11. Bardou M, Quenot JP, Barkun A. Stress-related mucosal disease in the critically ill patient. *Nat Rev Gastroenterol Hepatol.* 2015;12(5):98–107.

12. Toews I, George AT, Peter JV, et al. Interventions for preventing upper gastrointestinal bleeding in people admitted to intensive care units. *Cochrane Database Syst Rev.* 2018;6:CD008687.

13. Quenot JP, Dargent A, Barkun A. Prophylaxis for stress related gastrointestinal bleeding in the ICU: should we adjust to each patient's individual risk? *Anaesth Crit Care Pain Med.* 2019;38(2):99–101.

14. Tulassay Z, Herszenyi L. Gastric mucosal defense and cytoprotection. *Best Pract Res Clin Gastroenterol.* 2010;24(2):99–108.

15. Sartin JS. Liver diseases. In: Banasik JL, Copstead LC, eds. *Pathophysiology.* 6th ed. St. Louis: Elsevier; 2019.

16. Haq I, Tripathi D. Recent advances in the management of variceal bleeding. *Gastroenterol Rep (Oxf).* 2017;5(2):113–126.

17. Charif I, Saada K, Mellouki I, et al. Predictors of early rebleeding and mortality after acute variceal haemorrhage in patients with cirrhosis. *Open J Gastroenterol.* 2013;3(7):317–321.

18. Jessee MA. Stool studies: tried, true, and new. *Crit Care Nurs Clin Am.* 2010;22(1):129–145.

19. Kovacs TO, Jensen DM. Gastrointestinal hemorrhage. In: Goldman L, Schafer A, eds. *Goldman-Cecil Medicine.* 26th ed. Philadelphia, PA: Elsevier; 2020.

20. Nelms DW, Pelaez CA. The acute upper gastrointestinal bleed. *Surg Clin North Am.* 2018;98(5):1047–1057.

21. Wortman JR, Landman W, Fulwadhva UP, Viscomi SG, Sodickson AD. CT angiography for acute gastrointestinal bleeding: what the radiologist needs to know. *Br J Radiol.* 2017;90(1075):20170076.

22. Klein A, Gralnek IM. Acute, nonvariceal upper gastrointestinal bleeding. *Curr Opin Crit Care.* 2015;21(2):154–162.

23. Tripathi D, Stanley AJ, Hayes PC, et al. UK guidelines on the management of variceal haemorrhage in cirrhotic patients. *Gut.* 2015;64(11):1680–1704.

24. Opio CK, Garcia-Tsao G. Managing varices: drugs, bands, and shunts. *Gastroenterol Clin North Am.* 2011;40(3):561–579.

25. Chung KT, Shelat VG. Perforated peptic ulcer—an update. *World J Gastrointest Surg.* 2017;9(1):1–12.

26. Søreide K, Thorsen K, Harrison EM, et al. Perforated peptic ulcer. *Lancet.* 2015;386(10000):1288–1298.

27. Brand M, Prodehl L, Ede CJ. Surgical portosystemic shunts versus transjugular intrahepatic portosystemic shunt for variceal hemorrhage in people with cirrhosis. *Cochrane Database Syst Rev.* 2018;10:CD001023.

28. Miraglia C, Moccia F, Russo M, et al. Non-invasive method for the assessment of gastric acid secretion. *Acta Biomed.* 2018;89(8-S):53–57.

29. Cai JX, Saltzman JR. Initial assessment, risk stratification, and early management of acute nonvariceal upper gastrointestinal hemorrhage. *Gastrointest Endosc Clin N Am.* 2018;28(3):261–275.

30. Farrar FC. Management of acute gastrointestinal bleed. *Crit Care Clin North Am.* 2017;30(1):55–66.

31. Sarr MG, Banks PA, Bollen TL, et al. The new revised classification of acute pancreatitis 2012. *Surg Clin North Am.* 2013;93(3):549–562.

32. Banks PA, Bollen TL, Dervenis C, et al. Classification of acute pancreatitis—2012: revision of the Atlanta classification and definitions by international consensus. *Gut.* 2013;62(1):102–111.

33. Quinlan JD. Acute pancreatitis: international classification and nomenclature. *Clin Radiol.* 2016;71(2):121–133.

34. Trikudanathan G, Wolbrink DRJ, van Santvoort HC, Mallery S, Freeman M, Besselink MG. Current concepts in severe acute and necrotizing pancreatitis: an evidence-based approach. *Gastroenterology.* 2019;156(7):1994–2007.

35. Kuo DC, Rider AC, Estrada P, Kim D, Pillow MT. Acute pancreatitis: what's the score? *J Emerg Med.* 2015;48(6):762–770.

36. Ranson JH, Rifkind KM, Roses DF, Fink SD, Eng K, Spencer FC. Prognostic signs and the role of operative management in acute pancreatitis. *Surg Gynecol Obstet.* 1974;139(1):69–81.

37. Flood L, Nichol A. Acute pancreatitis: an intensive care perspective. *Anaesth Intensive Care Med.* 2017;19(3):119–124.

38. Chua TY, Walsh RM, Baker ME, Stevens T. Necrotizing pancreatitis: diagnose, treat, consult. *Cleve Clin J Med.* 2017;84(8):639–648.

39. Waller A, Long B, Koyfman A, Gottlieb M. Acute pancreatitis: updates for emergency clinicians. *J Emerg Med.* 2018;55(6):769–779.

40. Ney A, Pereira SP. Acute pancreatitis. *Med.* 2019;47(4):241–249.

41. Lankisch PG, Apte M, Banks PA. Acute pancreatitis. *Lancet.* 2015; 386(9988):85–96.

42. Hammad AY, Ditillo M, Castanon L. Pancreatitis. *Surg Clin N Am.* 2018;98(5):895–913.

43. Crockett SD, Wani S, Gardner TB, Falck-Ytter Y, Barkun AN, American Gastroenterological Association Institute Clinical Guidelines Committee. American Gastroenterological Association Institute guideline on initial management of acute pancreatitis. *Gastroenterology.* 2018;154(4): 1096–1101.

44. de-Madaria E, Herrera-Marante I, González-Camacho V, et al. Fluid resuscitation with lactated Ringer's solution vs normal saline in acute pancreatitis: a triple-bind, randomized, controlled trial. *United European Gastroenterol J.* 2018;6(1):63–71.

45. Goodchild G, Chouhan M, Johnson GJ. Practical guide to the management of acute pancreatitis. *Frontline Gastroenterol.* 2019;10(3):292–299.

46. Thomasset SC, Carter CR. Acute pancreatitis. *Surg (Oxford).* 2016;34(6): 292–300.

47. Grek A, Arasi L. Acute liver failure. *AACN Adv Crit Care.* 2016;27(4):420–429.

48. Grus T, Lambert L, Grusová G, Banerjee R, Burgetová A. Budd-Chiari syndrome. *Prague Med Rep.* 2017;119(2–3):69–80.

49. Lopez AM, Hendrickson RG. Toxin-induced hepatic injury. *Emerg Med Clin North Am.* 2014;32(1):103–125.

50. Roberts EA. Update on the diagnosis and management of Wilson disease. *Curr Gastroenterol Rep.* 2018;20(12):56.

51. Coelho AI, Rubio-Gozalbo ME, Vicente JB, Rivera I. Sweet and sour. An update on classic galactosemia. *J Inherit Metab Dis.* 2017;40(3):325–342.

52. Khan R, Koppe S. Modern management of acute liver failure. *Gastroenterol Clin North Am.* 2018;47(2):313–326.

53. Maher SZ, Schreibman IR. The clinical spectrum and manifestations of acute liver failure. *Clin Liver Dis.* 2018;22(2):361–374.

54. Devolder BE. Gastrointestinal surgery. In: Rothrock JC, McEwen DR, eds. *Alexander's Care of the Patient in Surgery.* 16th ed. St. Louis: Elsevier; 2019.

55. Caetano dos Santos J, Ferreira JDL, de Lima CLJ, et al. Nursing in the pre and postoperative of bariatric surgery. *Int Arch Med.* 2017;10(203):1–9.

56. Kreykes A, Choxi H, Rothberg A. Post-bariatric surgery patients: your role in their long-term care. *J Fam Pract.* 2017;66(6):356–363.

57. Kim JS, Park SM, Kim BW. Endoscopic management of peptic ulcer bleeding. *Clin Endosc.* 2015;48(2):106–111.

58. Sultanik P, Thabut D. Endoscopic therapy for variceal bleeding: from patient preparation to available techniques and rescue therapies. *Curr Hepatology Rep.* 2017;16(4):398–405.

59. Siramolpiwat S. Transjugular intrahepatic portosystemic shunts and portal hypertension-related complications. *World J Gastroenterol.* 2014; 20(45):16996–17010.

22

Endocrine Clinical Assessment and Diagnostic Procedures

Mary E. Lough

Assessment of a patient with endocrine dysfunction is a systematic process that incorporates history taking and physical examination. Most of the endocrine glands are deeply encased in the human body as shown in Fig. 22.1. This chapter describes clinical and diagnostic evaluation of the pancreas, the posterior pituitary, the thyroid gland, and the adrenal glands.

PANCREAS

Insulin, which is produced by the pancreas, is responsible for glucose metabolism. The clinical assessment provides information about pancreatic functioning. Clinical manifestations of abnormal glucose metabolism include hyperglycemia, which is the initial assessment priority for a patient with pancreatic dysfunction. Patients with hyperglycemia may be prediabetic, may be hyperglycemic in association with a severe critical illness, or may ultimately be diagnosed with type 1 or type 2 diabetes.[1] Each of these conditions has specific identifying features. Data collection questions to assist in the recognition of diabetes-related complications are outlined in Box 22.1.

Hyperglycemia
Focused Physical Assessment

Because severe hyperglycemia affects the entire body, all systems are assessed. The patient may complain of blurred vision, headache, weakness, fatigue, drowsiness, anorexia, nausea, and abdominal pain. On inspection, the patient has flushed skin, polyuria, polydipsia, vomiting, and evidence of dehydration. Progressive deterioration in the level of consciousness, from alert to lethargic or comatose, is observed as the hyperglycemia exacerbates. If ketoacidosis occurs, the patient's breathing becomes deep and rapid (Kussmaul respirations), and the breath may have a fruity odor. Auscultation of the abdomen may reveal hypoactive bowel sounds. Palpation elicits abdominal tenderness. Percussion may reveal diminished deep tendon reflexes. Hyperglycemia can lead to osmotic diuresis; therefore fluid volume status is assessed to evaluate hydration status. Signs of dehydration include tachycardia, orthostatic hypotension, and poor skin turgor.

Laboratory Studies: Pancreas

Pertinent laboratory tests for pancreatic function measure short-term and long-term blood glucose levels, which can identify and diagnose diabetes.

Blood Glucose

Fasting blood glucose. The fasting plasma glucose (FPG) level is assessed by a blood test when the patient has not eaten for 8 hours (Table 22.1).[1] A normal FPG level is between 70 and 100 mg/dL.[1] An FPG level between 100 and 125 mg/dL identifies prediabetes.[1] Individuals with prediabetes are at increased risk for complications of diabetes, such as coronary heart disease and stroke. An FPG level of 126 mg/dL (7 mmol/L) or higher is diagnostic of diabetes (see Table 22.1).[1]

Nonfasting blood glucose. After a meal, the concentration of glucose increases in the bloodstream. In the nonfasting state, normal postprandial blood glucose levels are expected to be less than 180 mg/dL (10 mmol/L) (see Table 22.1).[1]

Point-of-care blood glucose. All critically ill patients must have blood glucose levels monitored frequently while in the hospital. Clinical practice guidelines from the American Association of Clinical Endocrinologists and the American Diabetes Association recommend instituting insulin therapy when the blood glucose level is greater than 180 mg/dL in a critically ill patient.[2] A target blood glucose range of 140 to 180 mg/dL is recommended.[2] During administration of a continuous insulin infusion, point-of-care blood glucose testing is performed hourly or according to hospital protocol to achieve and maintain the blood glucose within the target range.[3,4]

HYPERglycemia. Multiple blood glucose levels about 180 mg/dL indicate hyperglycemia and may indicate that insulin administration is required with more intensive monitoring per hospital protocol.

HYPOglycemia. A blood glucose level less than 70 mg/dL (3.9 mmol/L) is defined as hypoglycemia.[1] A complication of intensive glucose control is that hypoglycemic episodes may occur more frequently both in the hospital and with self-management of glucose levels in diabetes.[2–4]

Before discharge to home, patients with diabetes are taught to monitor their blood glucose levels. This is because blood glucose levels

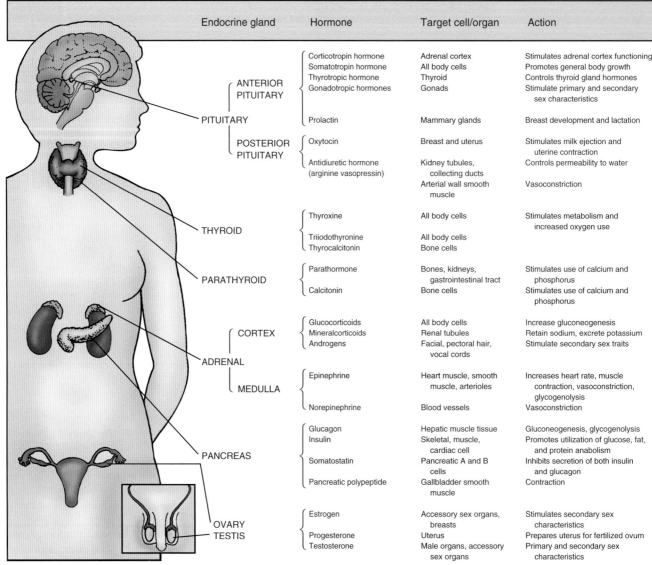

Endocrine gland	Hormone	Target cell/organ	Action
ANTERIOR PITUITARY	Corticotropin hormone	Adrenal cortex	Stimulates adrenal cortex functioning
	Somatotropin hormone	All body cells	Promotes general body growth
	Thyrotropic hormone	Thyroid	Controls thyroid gland hormones
	Gonadotropic hormones	Gonads	Stimulate primary and secondary sex characteristics
PITUITARY	Prolactin	Mammary glands	Breast development and lactation
POSTERIOR PITUITARY	Oxytocin	Breast and uterus	Stimulates milk ejection and uterine contraction
	Antidiuretic hormone (arginine vasopressin)	Kidney tubules, collecting ducts	Controls permeability to water
		Arterial wall smooth muscle	Vasoconstriction
THYROID	Thyroxine	All body cells	Stimulates metabolism and increased oxygen use
	Triiodothyronine	All body cells	
	Thyrocalcitonin	Bone cells	
PARATHYROID	Parathormone	Bones, kidneys, gastrointestinal tract	Stimulates use of calcium and phosphorus
	Calcitonin	Bone cells	Stimulates use of calcium and phosphorus
ADRENAL CORTEX	Glucocorticoids	All body cells	Increase gluconeogenesis
	Mineralcorticoids	Renal tubules	Retain sodium, excrete potassium
	Androgens	Facial, pectoral hair, vocal cords	Stimulate secondary sex traits
ADRENAL MEDULLA	Epinephrine	Heart muscle, smooth muscle, arterioles	Increases heart rate, muscle contraction, vasoconstriction, glycogenolysis
	Norepinephrine	Blood vessels	Vasoconstriction
PANCREAS	Glucagon	Hepatic muscle tissue	Gluconeogenesis, glycogenolysis
	Insulin	Skeletal, muscle, cardiac cell	Promotes utilization of glucose, fat, and protein anabolism
	Somatostatin	Pancreatic A and B cells	Inhibits secretion of both insulin and glucagon
	Pancreatic polypeptide	Gallbladder smooth muscle	Contraction
OVARY TESTIS	Estrogen	Accessory sex organs, breasts	Stimulates secondary sex characteristics
	Progesterone	Uterus	Prepares uterus for fertilized ovum
	Testosterone	Male organs, accessory sex organs	Primary and secondary sex characteristics

Fig. 22.1   Location of Endocrine Glands With the Hormones They Produce, Target Cells or Organs, and Hormonal Actions.

within the normal range are associated with fewer long-term diabetes-related complications.

Urine Glucose

Testing the urine for glucose is not recommended for patients with diabetes, because too much variation exists in the threshold for glucose when diabetes-related kidney damage has occurred. Urine glucose measurements are affected by variation in fluid intake; reflect an average glucose level, not a specific point in time; and are altered by some medications. Urine glucose testing also does not offer any help in the identification of hypoglycemia. For all these reasons, urine glucose testing should never be used.

Glycated Hemoglobin

A different blood test is used to achieve an objective measure of blood glucose over an extended period. The glycated hemoglobin (HbA$_{1c}$), or A$_{1c}$, provides information about the average amount of glucose that has been present in the patient's bloodstream over the previous

3 months.[5] During the 120-day life span of red blood cells (erythrocytes), the hemoglobin within each cell binds to the available blood glucose through a process known as *glycosylation*. Typically, 4% to 6% of hemoglobin contains the glucose group A$_{1c}$. The A$_{1c}$ is less than 5.7% in a person without diabetes.[6] The A$_{1c}$ value in a person with prediabetes is between 5.7% and 6.4%.[6] An acceptable target A$_{1c}$ less than 7% is appropriate for diabetic patients.[5] The A$_{1c}$ value correlates with specific blood glucose levels as shown in Table 22.2.[5] The American Diabetes Association recommends use of the A$_{1c}$ value both during initial assessment of diabetes mellitus and for follow-up to monitor treatment effectiveness.[5]

Blood Ketones

Ketone bodies are a by-product of rapid fat breakdown. Ketone blood levels rise in acute illness, in fasting states, and with sustained elevation of blood glucose in type 1 diabetes in the absence of insulin. In diabetic ketoacidosis, fat breakdown (*lipolysis*) occurs so rapidly that fat metabolism is incomplete, and the ketone bodies (acetone, beta-hydroxybutyric acid, and acetoacetic acid) accumulate in the blood (ketonemia) and are excreted in the urine (ketonuria). Elevated levels of ketones (ketonemia) may be detected by a fruity, sweet-smelling odor on the exhaled breath. This distinctive breath odor derives from the elimination of acetone as part of the compensatory response to maintain a normal pH.

It is recommended that all patients with diabetes perform self-testing or have their blood tested for the presence of ketones during any alteration in level of consciousness or acute illness accompanied by an elevated blood glucose level. Urine testing for ketones is no longer recommended.[7] Self-test meters to measure blood ketones from a fingerstick are now available.[8,9]

PITUITARY GLAND

The pituitary gland, recessed in the base of the cranium, is not accessible to physical assessment (Fig. 22.1). Therefore the critical care nurse must be aware of the systemic effects of a normally functioning pituitary to be able to identify dysfunction. One essential hormone formed in the hypothalamus but secreted through the posterior pituitary gland is antidiuretic hormone (ADH), also known as *arginine vasopressin* (AVP) or simply *vasopressin*.

Focused Physical Assessment

ADH controls the amount of fluid lost and retained within the body and is released from the posterior pituitary in response to hypovolemia, changes in plasma osmolality, hypoxia, and acidosis. ADH actions are both antidiuretic and vasoconstrictive.

Acute dysfunction of the posterior pituitary or the hypothalamus may result in insufficient or excessive ADH production. The clinical signs of posterior pituitary dysfunction often manifest as fluid volume deficit (insufficient ADH production) or fluid volume excess (excessive ADH production).

Hydration Status

A hydration assessment includes observations of skin integrity, skin turgor, and buccal membrane moisture. Moist, shiny buccal membranes indicate satisfactory fluid balance. Skin turgor that is resilient and returns to its original position in less than 3 seconds after being pinched or lifted indicates adequate skin elasticity. The skin over the forehead is the most reliable for testing tissue turgor, because this area of skin is less affected by aging.[9]

Other indicators that the patient's hydration status is adequate for metabolic demands include a balanced intake and output and absence of thirst. However, absence of thirst is an unreliable indicator of dehydration in critically ill patients. Other indicators of normal

---

TRENDING PRIORITIES IN HEALTHCARE

Zero Tolerance for Aggression Against Nurses by Patients and Families

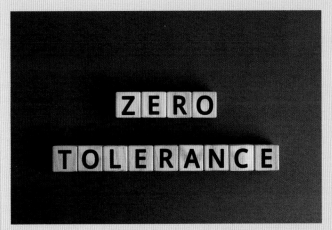

iStock.com/Roman Didkivskyi

Aggression toward nurses and other health care workers by patients, families, and visitors is a worrying trend that is increasing[1–4]:

- Physical assault by a patient or their family member is reported by 25% of nurses.[1]
- Verbal aggression by a patient or their family member is reported by 50% of nurses.[1]

According to the American Nurses Association (ANA) and the American Association of Critical Care Nurses (AACN), nurses often do not report verbal and physical abuse.[2–4]

Some reasons for nonreporting are:

- Concern over retaliation
- Unclear how to report the abuse
- Believe the incident was not serious enough to report
- Doubt that anything will be done about the violence

- Work in a health care culture that accepts aggression as routine against nurses

There has been a shift in attitudes about workplace violence. The emphasis is no longer on the individual nurse, but on the responsibility of health care organizations to provide a healthy workplace free of violence.[2–4] Some health care organizations now post signs to alert everyone that there will be zero tolerance for aggression and violence in health care by anyone.

The AACN and ANA position statements recommend that hospitals offer information to stop violence before it occurs by education about[2,3]:

- How to de-escalate a potentially violent situation?
- How to seek assistance when in a dangerous situation?

The AACN and ANA position statements recommend that hospitals[2,3]:

- Establish a clear and consistent reporting structure
- Encourage employees to press charges against an aggressor
- Evaluate staffing structures for safety
- Have security available to assist
- Schedule post-incident debriefings
- Collect data on the number of aggressive and violent incidents
- Support laws that will protect health care workers against violence

Health care organizations must take action to demonstrate *zero tolerance* for uncivil and aggressive behaviors targeting health care workers.

References

1. AL-Quadi MM. Workplace violence in nursing: a concept analysis. *J Occup Health.* 2021;63:e12226.
2. American Nurses Association (ANA). *Issue brief. Reporting incidents of workplace violence*; 2019. www.nursingworld.org/~4a4076/globalassets/practiceandpolicy/work-environment/endnurseabuse/endabuse-issue-brief-final.pdf.
3. American Association of Critical-Care Nurses (AACN). AACN position statement preventing violence against healthcare workers. *Am Assoc Crit Care Nurse*; 2019. www.aacn.org/policy-and-advocacy/aacn-position-statement-preventing-violence.
4. Jones M. Preventing workplace violence in healthcare. *Am Assoc Crit Care Nurse*; 2021. www.aacn.org/blog/preventing-workplace-violence-in-healthcare.

BOX 22.1 DATA COLLECTION

Complications of Diabetes

Current Health Status
- The body may be unable to adjust to increased insulin needs resulting from sudden physiologic changes such as infection, injury, or surgery. The nurse assesses whether the patient has a severe infection, surgical wound, or traumatic injury.
- Recent or current signs and symptoms:
  - Unexplained changes in weight, thirst, hunger
  - Headache, blurred vision
  - Long-standing, unhealed infection
  - Vaginitis, pruritus
  - Leg pain, numbness
- Unexplained change in urinary patterns (e.g., daytime and nighttime, frequency, volume)
- Energy or stamina changes
- Endurance level
- Weakness
- Unexplained, excessive fatigue
- Behavior or mental changes (also ask family member or significant other for input):
  - Memory loss
  - Orientation

Assessment of Current Illness: Onset, Characteristics, and Course
- Chronic illness: Physiologic or psychologic stress may increase endogenous glucose.
- Recent treatments that could be a source of exogenous glucose:
  - Hyperalimentation
  - Peritoneal dialysis
  - Hemodialysis
- Medications, including prescription and over-the-counter preparations: Pharmacologic agents may alter pancreatic function by increasing or decreasing the release of endocrine hormones. Medications also may interfere with hormonal action at the receptor site on the target cell.

Medical History: Questions
- Have you had prior pancreatic surgery?
- Have you ever been told that any of the following applied to you?
  - Too much sugar in the urine
  - Too much sugar in the blood
  - Will probably develop too much sugar later in life
- If you answered yes to any of these questions, what treatment, if any, was prescribed?
- Are you currently following such a treatment?

Family History: Questions
- Has a family member ever been diagnosed with diabetes or "sugar in the blood"?
- If so, how was the condition treated?

hydration include absence of edema, stable weight, and urine specific gravity within the normal range (1.005–1.030).

Vital Signs

Changes in heart rate, blood pressure, and central venous pressure (when available) are useful to determine fluid volume status.

Orthostatic hypotension, which occurs when intravascular fluid volume decreases, is identified by a drop in systolic blood pressure of 20 mm Hg or a drop in diastolic blood pressure of 10 mm Hg when the patient changes position from lying to standing.[10,11]

Weight Changes and Intake and Output

Daily weight changes coincide with fluid retention and fluid loss. Sudden changes in weight can result from a change in fluid balance; 1 L of fluid lost or retained is equal to approximately 2.2 lb, or 1 kg, of weight gained or lost. To use weight as a true determinant of fluid balance, all extraneous variables must be eliminated; this means the same scale is used at the same time each day. Precise measurement and notation of intake and output are used as criteria for fluid replacement therapy.

Laboratory Studies: Pituitary

No single diagnostic test identifies dysfunction of the posterior pituitary gland. A diagnosis usually is made through the patient's clinical presentation and history.

Serum Antidiuretic Hormone

Although serum measurement of ADH is available, it is rarely obtained in critically ill patients.

The normal serum ADH reference range is approximately 1 to 5 picograms/mL (pg/mL), although this range may vary according to the clinical laboratory doing the test. Before ADH measurement, all medications that may alter the release of ADH are withheld for a minimum of 8 hours. Common medications that affect ADH levels include morphine sulfate, lithium carbonate, chlorothiazide, carbamazepine, oxytocin, and selective serotonin reuptake inhibitors. Nicotine, alcohol, positive-pressure and negative-pressure ventilation, and emotional stress also influence ADH.

Serum ADH levels are compared with blood and urine osmolality to differentiate syndrome of inappropriate antidiuretic hormone (SIADH) from central diabetes insipidus (DI).[12] Increased ADH levels in the bloodstream compared with a low serum osmolality and elevated urine osmolality confirm the diagnosis of SIADH.[12] Reduced levels of serum ADH in a patient with high serum osmolality, hypernatremia, and reduced urine concentration indicate central DI. Typically, this diagnosis is based on urine output, serum sodium, and serum osmolality rather than serum ADH level.[12]

Serum and Urine Osmolality

Osmolality measurements determine the concentration of dissolved particles in a solution. The most accurate measures of the body's fluid balance are obtained when urine and blood samples are collected simultaneously.

Serum osmolality. Values for serum osmolality in the bloodstream range from 275 to 295 mOsm/kg H_2O; there are also variations in this range based on the clinical laboratory standard values. Increased serum osmolality stimulates the release of ADH, which reduces the amount of water lost through the kidney. Body fluid is retained at the kidney tubules and collecting ducts dilute the particle concentration in the bloodstream. According to one clinical guideline, the hypothalamic vasopressin (ADH) osmoreceptors are maximally inhibited at levels less than 280 mOsm/kg H_2O to eliminate water via the kidney.[12] In contrast, at levels greater than 290 mOsm/kg H_2O, the sensation of thirst and hypothalamic vasopressin (ADH) osmoreceptors are maximally stimulated to conserve water.[12] This is a narrow clinical range that is often disrupted in pituitary disease and critical illness.

TABLE 22.1 Blood Glucose Values and Clinical Significance

Clinical Significance	Fasting BG (mg/dL)	Fasting BG (mmol/L)
Hypoglycemia	<70	<3.9
Normal	70–100	>3.9–5.6
Prediabetes	100–125	5.6–6.9
Diabetes	≥126	≥7.0
	Nonfasting BG (mg/dL)	**Nonfasting BG (mg/dL)**
Diabetes (random blood test, nonfasting with symptoms)	≥200	≥11.1
PRE-prandial plasma glucose	80–130	4.4–7.2
POST-prandial plasma glucose	<180	10.0

BG, Blood glucose.
Data from American Diabetes Association. Classification and diagnosis of diabetes: Standards of Medical Care in Diabetes—2020. *Diabetes Care.* 2020;43(suppl 1):S14–S31 and S66–S76.

TABLE 22.2 Correlation Between Hemoglobin A₁c and Plasma Glucose Level

Hemoglobin A$_{1c}$ (%)	Mean Plasma Glucose Level (mg/dL)	Mean Plasma Glucose Level (mmol/L)
5	97 (76–120)	5.4 (4.2–6.7)
6	126 (100–152)	7.0 (5.5–8.5)
7	154 (123–185)	8.6 (6.8–10.3)
8	183 (147–217)	10.2 (8.1–12.1)
9	212 (170–249)	11.8 (9.4–13.9)
10	240 (193–282)	13.4 (10.7–15.7)
11	269 (217–314)	14.9 (12.0–17.5)
12	298 (240–347)	(13.3–19.3)

The numbers in parentheses represent the 95% confidence intervals (CI) for these values.
Hemoglobin A$_{1c}$, Glycosylated hemoglobin.
Data from American Diabetes Association. Glycemic targets: Standards of Medical Care in Diabetes—2020. *Diabetes Care.* 2020;43(suppl 1):S66–S76.

Decreased serum osmolality inhibits the release of ADH. The kidney tubules increase their permeability, and fluid is eliminated from the body in an attempt to regain normal concentration of particles in the bloodstream.

Urine osmolality. Urine osmolality in a person with normal kidneys depends on fluid intake. With high fluid intake, particle dilution is low, but it increases if fluids are restricted. This is the reason the expected range for urine osmolality is so wide, ranging from 50 to 1400 mOsm/kg.

Antidiuretic Hormone Test

The ADH test is used to differentiate central neurogenic DI from nephrogenic (kidney) DI. In central DI, the patient is producing large volumes of dilute urine and can quickly become dehydrated. The patient is challenged with 0.05 to 1.0 mL of intranasally administered ADH in the form of desmopressin (1-deamino-8-D-arginine vasopressin, commonly abbreviated as DDAVP). An intravenous line is inserted before ADH administration, and urine volume and osmolality are measured every 30 minutes for 2 hours before and after the ADH challenge:

- *Central DI.* In central DI (nonfunctional or poorly functional posterior pituitary), the kidney responds to the exogenous ADH by reabsorbing water at the kidney tubule, making the urine more concentrated.[13] This test is not done in critical care.
- *Nephrogenic DI.* In nephrogenic DI, the kidney does not respond to the exogenous ADH and urine osmolality remains unchanged (large volumes of dilute urine). This test is not performed in the

critical care unit because of the unstable hemodynamic and volume status of critically ill patients.

Copeptin

At the same time as ADH is released from the posterior pituitary, other biochemical biomarkers are also released. These biomarkers include *neurophysin 2* and the C-terminal part of the precursor pre-provasopressin (CTproAVP), more generally known as *copeptin.*[14–16] This has clinical benefits, because copeptin plasma levels reliably relate to ADH levels in both healthy persons and in critically ill patients.[14,15] Additionally, compared with ADH, copeptin is more stable in plasma, allowing reliable measurements.[14–16] For these reasons copeptin has the potential to be clinically useful in the diagnosis of both nephrogenic DI and partial central DI.[15]

Diagnostic Procedures: Pituitary

In addition to laboratory tests, radiographic examination, computed tomography (CT), and magnetic resonance imaging (MRI) are used to diagnose structural lesions such as cranial bone fractures, tumors, or blood clots in the region of the pituitary.[17,18] Although these procedures do not diagnose DI or SIADH, they are useful in uncovering the likely underlying cause.

Radiographic Examination

A basic radiographic examination of the inferior skull views the *sella turcica* and surrounding bone formation. Bone fractures or tissue swelling at the base of the brain, which are apparent on a radiograph, suggests interference with the vascular supply and nerve impulses to the hypothalamic-pituitary system. Dysfunction may occur if the hypothalamus, infundibular stalk, or pituitary gland is impaired.

Computed Tomography

CT of the base of the skull identifies pituitary tumors, blood clots, cysts, nodules, or other soft tissue masses. This rapid procedure causes no discomfort except that it requires the patient to lie perfectly still. CT studies can be performed with or without radiopaque contrast medium. The contrast dye is given intravenously to highlight the hypothalamus, infundibular stalk, and pituitary gland. This dye may cause allergic reactions in iodine-sensitive individuals, and the patient must be asked about iodine allergy before the test. The size and shape of the sella turcica and the position of the hypothalamus, infundibular stalk, and pituitary are identified.[11]

Magnetic Resonance Imaging

MRI enables the radiologist to visualize internal organs and cellular characteristics of specific tissues. MRI uses a magnetic field rather than radiation to produce high-resolution, cross-sectional images. The soft brain tissue and surrounding cerebrospinal fluid make the brain especially suited to assessment with MRI.[18]

THYROID GLAND

History

Information regarding the clinical manifestations of hypothyroidism or hyperthyroidism must be obtained from the patient, family, or others with knowledge of the health history. Sample questions pertinent to detection of thyroid disease are listed in Box 22.2.

Focused Physical Examination

The thyroid is palpated for tenderness, nodules, and enlargement and is auscultated for bruits. The normal-size thyroid gland usually is neither visible nor palpable in the anterior neck. Palpation may be done from an anterior or posterior approach. Auscultation of the thyroid is accomplished by use of the bell portion of the stethoscope to identify a bruit or blowing noise from the circulation through the thyroid gland. The presence of a bruit indicates enlargement of the thyroid, as evidenced by increased blood flow through the glandular tissue.

Laboratory Studies: Thyroid

Controversy exists about routine measurement of thyroid function in adults without clinical symptoms. The US Preventive Services Task Force 2015 review found the research evidence insufficient to recommend routine screening for thyroid disease in asymptomatic adults.[19] However, thyroid hormone blood test screening is recommended for adults 60 years old and older and for individuals with symptoms of thyroid dysfunction (hypofunction or hyperfunction).[19] There are no recommendations about thyroid hormone screening for critically ill patients.

Thyroid hormone blood tests measure the levels of circulating thyroid hormone and assess the integrity of the hormonal negative feedback response within the hypothalamic-pituitary-thyroid axis. Laboratory diagnosis is based on measurement of thyroid-stimulating hormone (TSH) or the simultaneous measurement of TSH and free thyroxine (FT_4).[20]

Normally, an inverse linear relationship exists between TSH and FT_4.[21] When the hypothalamic-pituitary-thyroid axis is normal, TSH production is inhibited by the presence of free thyroid hormone in the bloodstream (FT_4), and the TSH value is normal:

BOX 22.2 DATA COLLECTION

Hyperthyroidism and Hypothyroidism

The patient is the best source for the following information. If the patient is unable to respond, the following questions can be directed to family, friends, a significant other, or persons involved in admission of the patient to the critical care unit:

- Have you ever been diagnosed with overactive thyroid, increased metabolism, or hyperthyroidism? What about underactive thyroid, slowed metabolism, or hypothyroidism?
- Have you ever been treated for hyperthyroidism or hypothyroidism?
- Have you ever had an operation for thyroid disease?
- Have you ever received radioactive iodine for thyroid disease?
- Are you taking any medicine for thyroid disease? If so, what is the name of the medicine, and what is the prescribed dose and frequency?
- When did you first notice the constant restlessness or extreme fatigue?
- Has your weight been the same or changed over the past year?
- Has your appetite changed over the past 6 months?
- Have you lost weight even though your appetite has increased (may indicate hyperthyroidism)?
- Have you gained weight or stayed at the same weight even though you have not felt like eating over the past 6 months (may indicate hypothyroidism)?
- Do you always feel warm (may indicate hyperthyroidism)?
- Do you open windows in the house even in winter months?
- Do you wear lightweight clothing even when others are wearing layers of heavier clothing?
- Do you always feel cold (may indicate hypothyroidism)?
- Do you wear multiple layers of clothing despite warm weather or the use of a heater or furnace?
- Do you use several blankets and keep windows closed even in warm weather?
- Do you complain about never being able to "warm up"?
- Over the past 6 months to 1 year, have you developed any of the following?

HYPOthyroidism Indicators	HYPERthyroidism Indicators
Loss of coarse, dry scalp hair and outer edge of eyebrow	Hair thinning
Sleepiness, lethargy, depression	Swelling (face, eyes, legs)
Weight gain despite decreased appetite, severe constipation	Insomnia, nervousness, anxiety
Muscle and joint pain (hands, wrists, feet)	Weight loss despite increased appetite
Dry, itchy skin	Diarrhea
Increased sensitivity to cold	Muscle weakness or wasting
	Tremors
	Warm, moist skin
Bradycardia	Heat intolerance, sweating
Menstruation changes; impaired fertility	Tachycardia, atrial fibrillation
	Menstruation changes; impaired fertility

- Hypothyroidism: High TSH and low FT_4
- Hyperthyroidism: Low TSH, high FT_4, and an increased FT_3-to-FT_4 ratio

Thyroid-Stimulating Hormone

Clinical laboratory analysis of TSH has become more sensitive, allowing more accurate measurement of low levels of thyroid

TABLE 22.3 Thyroid Hormone Blood Tests

Name of Test	Abbreviation	Reference Value (SI)	Reference Value[a]
Thyroid-stimulating hormone (thyrotropin)	TSH	0.4—4.5 milliunits/L	
Total serum thyroxine	TT_4	581—154 nmol/L	4.0—12.0 mcg/dL
Free thyroxine	FT_4	9—23 pmol/L	0.7—1.8 ng/dL
Total serum triiodothyronine	TT_3	1.2—2.7 nmol/L	100—200 ng/dL
Free triiodothyronine	FT_3	3.2—9.2 pmol/L	208—596 pg/dL
Thyroglobulin[b]	Tg	3.0—40 mcg/L	

[a]Some tests are reported with more than one reference value, because clinical laboratories use various reference ranges depending on the specifics of the clinical test.

[b]Thyroglobulin (Tg) reference values should be determined locally, because serum Tg concentrations are influenced by local iodide intake.

SI, International Units.

Reference values from Demers LM. Thyroid disease: pathophysiology and diagnosis. *Clin Lab Med.* 2004;24(1):19.

hormone. Thyroid hormone reference ranges in adults are listed in Table 22.3.[22] Because serum values vary slightly between laboratory methods, it is imperative to know the normal reference values used by the hospital clinical laboratory.

The serum level of TSH increases as a person grows older, which may signal declining thyroid function, as greater stimulation of the thyroid gland by TSH is required.[20] In contrast, T_4 levels fall slightly with advanced age.[20] The average TSH level by age, from a study of 1200 persons (600 males, 600 females), is shown below[20]:

- TSH 0.4—4.3 mU/L between 20 to 59 years
- TSH 0.4—5.8 mU/L between 60 to 79 years
- TSH 0.4—6.7 mU/L older than 80 years

Thyroid Tests in Critically Ill Patients

The incidence of thyroid disease in hospitalized patients is low, estimated at 1% and 2% of all inpatients. In critically ill patients, TSH measurement is usually the first thyroid-related laboratory test that is obtained. Most experts recommend obtaining both TSH and FT_4 hormone levels.[23]

Medications and Thyroid Testing

Additional measurement difficulties involve concomitant use of certain medications that interfere with thyroid function and lower serum levels.[24]

TSH secretion is affected by several medications routinely administered in critical care units. Glucocorticoids in large doses may lower the serum level of FT_3 and inhibit TSH secretion.[22] Dopamine infusions at greater than 1 mcg/kg per minute directly block TSH release.[24] Amiodarone, an antidysrhythmic medication, is an iodine-rich compound that is structurally similar to T_3 and T_4.[25] At usual doses, amiodarone can increase the daily iodine amount by 50 to 100 times.[25]

Several medications increase the serum level of FT_4 by displacing protein-bound T_4.[24] Medications that displace protein-bound T_4 cause an increase in serum FT_4 levels.[24] Salicylates (aspirin), furosemide (Lasix), and unfractionated and low—molecular-weight heparins all raise FT_4 serum levels by this mechanism.[24] It is unclear whether it is necessary to adjust pharmacologic management of critically ill patients in response to these medication-laboratory interactions.

Diagnostic Procedures: Thyroid

Diagnostic tests often begin with ultrasonography to visualize a thyroid nodule or tumor.[26] To diagnose hypothyroidism, a nuclear medicine scan using an oral iodine radioactive isotope may be requested.[27] The thyroid-scanning procedure may also detect the presence of ectopic thyroid tissue, thyroid carcinomas, and the amount of viable thyroid glandular tissue after therapeutic irradiation.

ADRENAL GLAND

Primary Adrenal Disorders

Admission to the critical care unit with a primary adrenal disorder is rare. The term *primary* indicates that the principal problem lies within the adrenal gland. Secondary adrenal dysfunction is caused by dysfunction in another gland or by a clinical condition such as sepsis. The adrenal gland is actually two glands in one—defined by the cortex and the medulla—which make the history and presentation complex.

Adrenal Cortex

The adrenal cortex (outer layer) secretes two classes of hormones, and if deficient or released in excess, they may cause clinical symptoms:

- Cortisol. The glucocorticoid hormone cortisol is secreted in response to physiologic stress from infection, trauma, and hypoglycemia.
- Aldosterone. The mineralocorticoid hormone aldosterone is secreted in response to intravascular hypovolemia. Aldosterone release is the final step in the renin-angiotensin-aldosterone system (RAAS) pathway.

Adrenal Medulla

The adrenal medulla (inner layer) also secretes two hormones that are released in response to stress and that cause clinical symptoms if they are deficient or released in excess:

- Epinephrine also known as *adrenaline*
- Norepinephrine also known as *noradrenaline*

Clinical Assessment

History

A detailed history may help identify conditions or medications that may affect adrenal gland function. Primary endocrine disorders are rare, but a history of uncontrolled hypertension despite three or more oral medications may indicate whether endocrine-related hypertension should be investigated. The medication history may help determine whether the patient takes glucocorticoid tablets, and the patient or family should be asked about using steroid creams for dermatologic conditions and about using steroid-based inhalers for chronic obstructive lung disease.

Physical Examination

The signs and symptoms depend on the hormone involved, whether the problem is related to excess or deficiency and whether the dysfunction occurs within the adrenal cortex or the adrenal medulla. Consequently, a methodical approach to assessing all signs and symptoms is important, because adrenal disease is often missed or misdiagnosed.

Adrenal Cortex

Primary Cushing syndrome. Cushing syndrome is caused by excess release of the glucocorticoid hormone cortisol.[28–30] The excess cortisol results from a tumor of the pituitary gland or adrenal gland and produces the classic signs and symptoms listed in Box 22.3. Primary Cushing disease is rare, but if a patient is not taking exogenous steroids, it becomes a diagnosis of exclusion when the relevant constellation of signs and symptoms is present.[29,30] The first step is to obtain a serum adrenocorticotropic hormone (ACTH) level in a patient with overt signs of Cushing syndrome. A serum ACTH level less than 2.2 pmol/L (10 pg/mL) is considered diagnostic.[30] Imaging of the pituitary gland to search for a tumor or other injury is performed after the low

ACTH value has confirmed Cushing syndrome as the cause of the condition.[30]

Secondary Cushing syndrome. Symptoms identical to the symptoms of primary Cushing syndrome (Box 22.3) occur in patients with the secondary form who are on long-term glucocorticoid therapy. Pharmacologic glucocorticoid dosages are used to prevent solid-organ rejection after transplant, for patients with chronic obstructive lung disease, or patients with chronic inflammatory conditions. When patients are admitted to the critical care unit, it is important to ascertain whether they are steroid dependent to avoid the deleterious effects of abrupt steroid withdrawal.[30]

Primary Aldosteronism

In patients with primary aldosteronism, the adrenal cortex secretes excess mineralocorticoid (aldosterone) unrelated to the RAAS.[31] In other words, the aldosterone secretion is untethered from the normal RAAS feedback loop (see Fig. 11.16 in Chapter 11). Primary aldosteronism occurs in up to 10% of individuals with medication-resistant hypertension and in up to 20% in groups with hypertension and hypokalemia.[31] This rare condition may cause the patient to present emergently with severe hypertension and a critically low serum potassium (hypokalemia), which can be lethal if not identified and effectively treated.

Laboratory and diagnostic studies. The diagnostic laboratory test recommended for individuals at high risk is an aldosterone-to-renin ratio.[31] A CT scan of the adrenal-kidney structures is obtained to visualize tumors that may be secreting the excess aldosterone.[31,32] An invasive diagnostic test is adrenal venous sampling of cortisol and aldosterone levels, obtained by an interventional radiologist, to determine whether the condition affects one or both adrenal glands.[31,33] Surgical removal of an aldosterone-secreting tumor may be required.

Adrenal Insufficiency

Adrenal insufficiency is a rare disorder of the adrenal cortex that involves hyposecretion of glucocorticoids (cortisol), sometimes occurring with hyposecretion of mineralocorticoids (aldosterone). It is also known as *Addison disease* after Thomas Addison, who first described the condition.[34,35] Physiologically, adrenal insufficiency may be envisioned as the inverse of conditions with excess hormone secretion.

Laboratory studies. The laboratory diagnosis for adrenal disorders involves simultaneous measurements of the serum ACTH level with a cortisol serum level.[35] A low (or normal) serum cortisol in the presence of an elevated ACTH is diagnostic.[35] A serum cortisol value below 100 nmol/L in the early morning is also considered diagnostic.[35]

Adrenal Crisis

An adrenal crisis, also called an *Addisonian crisis*, is a life-threatening condition in which the adrenal gland is almost nonfunctional, usually because of destruction of adrenal tissue.[35] The patient presents acutely with critical hypotension, an elevated serum potassium level (hyperkalemia), a low serum sodium level (hyponatremia), and hypoglycemia.

Critical Illness—Related Corticosteroid Insufficiency

The adrenal gland is designed to respond to acute physiologic stress by increasing stress hormones via the hypothalamic-pituitary-adrenal axis. Early in critical illness, a rise in cortisol levels can be documented. However, over time, the adrenal glands are often unable to secrete adequate amounts of stress hormones, especially when critical illness is prolonged.[36] This is described as critical illness—related corticosteroid insufficiency (CIRCI).[36] Research into causes of CIRCI is ongoing.[36]

BOX 22.3   Causes of Cushing Syndrome

Cushing Syndrome

Cushing syndrome can result from several causes:

- Adrenocorticotropin-dependent Cushing Syndrome
- Adrenocorticotropin-independent Cushing Syndrome
- Secondary or Iatrogenic Cushing Syndrome

  Adrenocorticotropin is also known as *adrenocorticotropic hormone (ACTH)* or *corticotropin.*

ACTH-Dependent Cushing Syndrome

Most cases (80%) result from a pituitary adenoma that causes the pituitary gland to produce excess ACTH. Excess secretion of ACTH stimulates the adrenal cortex to release excess amounts of cortisol into the bloodstream, circumventing the normal inhibitory feedback loop.

  The other 20% of cases are caused by ectopic ACTH secretion from small cell cancers of the lung, metastases, and endocrine tumors.

ACTH-Independent Cushing Syndrome

Cases are usually caused by a unilateral adrenal tumor: adrenal adenoma (60%) or adrenal carcinoma (40%).

Secondary or Iatrogenic Cushing Syndrome

Occurs secondary to pharmacologic doses of glucocorticoids, which may be prescribed to prevent rejection after solid-organ transplantation or to treat chronic inflammatory conditions.

Clinical Signs and Symptoms of Cushing Syndrome

- Emotional lability (can range from depression to psychosis)
- Hyperglycemia and poorly controlled type 2 diabetes
- Obesity or weight gain in abdomen
- Rounded face
- Acne
- Thin skin, bruises easily, poor wound healing
- Hypertension
- Hirsutism (excess hair growth)
- Dorsocervical fat pad ("buffalo hump")
- Decreased libido
- Fatigue, weakness

BOX 22.4 Pheochromocytoma: Signs and Symptoms[a]

Signs	Symptoms
• Hypertension	• Headaches
• Tachycardia	• Dizziness or faintness
• Tachypnea	• Palpitations, chest pain
• Pallor or flushing	• Anxiety and nervousness
• Hyperglycemia or poorly controlled type 2 diabetes	• Excessive sweating
	• Weakness, fatigue
• Decreased gastrointestinal motility	• Weight loss
	• Constipation

[a]Not all patients have all signs and symptoms.

Adrenal Medulla

Pheochromocytoma. Pheochromocytomas are rare neuroendocrine tumors that arise from the catecholamine-producing chromaffin cells of the adrenal medulla.[37] Most produce norepinephrine, but some produce both norepinephrine and epinephrine. These tumors produce a far greater quantity of catecholamines than normal adrenal medullary tissue. The concentrations of catecholamines can be so high within the tumor that it has been likened to a volcano that is ready to erupt. When huge amounts of norepinephrine or epinephrine are released into the bloodstream, it creates a catecholamine storm and a hypertensive crisis that can be life-threatening. The body responds to the catecholamine surge as if to a severe fight-or-flight threat by hypertension, tachycardia, increased respiratory rate, and hyperglycemia. The patient may describe symptoms of headache, dizziness, palpitations, chest pain, anxiety, nervousness, and fatigue (Box 22.4).[37] Because the body perceives the catecholamine onslaught as a signal to be ready to escape a threatening situation, it slows down the gastrointestinal tract, and constipation is another symptom. Patients at greatest risk are patients who are admitted to a critical care unit or who undergo surgery and experience a hypertensive crisis during anesthesia.[37]

Laboratory studies. The recommended laboratory diagnosis of pheochromocytoma is by measurement of plasma and urine fractionated metanephrines.[37–39] Catecholamines are metabolized into *metanephrines.* Pheochromocytoma-secreted catecholamine levels fluctuate, making blood levels variable, but catecholamine metabolism into metanephrines is constant, which is the reason this test is preferred.[37] Before the metanephrine blood level is drawn, the patient should be supine and resting for 30 minutes.[37,38] A 24-hour urine collection of excreted catecholamines may be obtained.[37] Finally, genetic testing of the patient and immediate relatives may be requested.

Diagnostic Imaging Procedures: Adrenal

CT is the most widely used test to image the adrenal glands. Percutaneous adrenal biopsy is rarely performed and is unlikely to be performed in critically ill patients.

ADDITIONAL RESOURCES

See Box 22.5 for Internet resources pertaining to endocrine disorders and diagnosis.

REFERENCES

1. American Diabetes Association. Classification and diagnosis of diabetes: standards of medical care in diabetes—2020. *Diabetes Care.* 2020;43(suppl 1): S14–S31.
2. Moghissi ES, Korytkowski MT, DiNardo M, et al. American Association of Clinical Endocrinologists and American Diabetes Association consensus statement on inpatient glycemic control. *Diabetes Care.* 2009;32(6):1119.
3. Jacobi J, Bircher N, Krinsley J, et al. Guidelines for the use of an insulin infusion for the management of hyperglycemia in critically ill patients. *Crit Care Med.* 2012;40(12):3251.
4. Kitabchi AE, Umpierrez GE, Miles JM, Fisher JN. Hyperglycemic crises in adult patients with diabetes. *Diabetes Care.* 2009;32(7):1335.
5. American Diabetes Association. Glycemic targets: standards of medical care in diabetes—2020. *Diabetes Care.* 2020;43(suppl 1):S66–S76.
6. Centers for Disease Control (CDC). Diabetes tests. https://www.cdc.gov/diabetes/basics/getting-tested.html. Accessed April 15, 2022.
7. Brooke J, Stiell M, Ojo O. Evaluation of the accuracy of capillary hydroxybutyrate measurement compared with other measurements in the diagnosis of diabetic ketoacidosis: a systematic review. *Int J Environ Res Public Health.* 2016;13(9):837.
8. Guimont MC, Desjobert H, Fonfrède M, et al. Multicentric evaluation of eight glucose and four ketone blood meters. *Clin Biochem.* 2015;48(18): 1310–1316.
9. Morley JE. Dehydration, hypernatremia, and hyponatremia. *Clin Geriatr Med.* 2015;31:389.
10. Jones PK, Shaw BH, Satish RR. Orthostatic hypotension: managing a difficult problem. *Expert Rev Cardiovasc Ther.* 2015;13(11):1263.
11. Godbole BP, Aggarwal B. Review of management strategies for orthostatic hypotension in older people. *J Pharm Pract Res.* 2018;48:484–492.
12. Lamas C, del Pozo C, Villabona C, Neuroendocrinology Group of the SEEN. Clinical guidelines for management of diabetes insipidus and syndrome of inappropriate antidiuretic hormone secretion after pituitary surgery. *Endocrinol Nutr.* 2014;61(4):e15.
13. Refardt J. Diagnosis and differential diagnosis of diabetes insipidus: update. *Best Pract Res Clin Endocrinol Metab.* 2020;34(5):101398.
14. Koch A, Yagmur E, Hoss A, et al. Clinical relevance of copeptin plasma levels as a biomarker of disease severity and mortality in critically ill patients. *J Clin Lab Anal.* 2018;32:e22614.
15. Krychtiuk KA, Honeder MC, Lenz M, et al. Copeptin predicts mortality in critically ill patients. *PLoS One.* 2017;12(1):e0170436.

QSEN

BOX 22.5 Informatics

Internet Resources: Endocrine Disorders, Testing, and Diagnoses
- American Association of Clinical Endocrinology (AACE): https://www.aace.com/
- The Endocrine Society: https://www.endocrine.org/

Pancreas: Diabetes
- American Diabetes Association: https://www.diabetes.org/diabetes

Thyroid
- National Institutes of Health (NIH). Thyroid Tests: https://www.niddk.nih.gov/health-information/diagnostic-tests/thyroid

Pituitary and Adrenal
- Cushing's Support and Research Foundation: https://csrf.net/
- NIH, Cushing's Syndrome: https://www.ninds.nih.gov/disorders/all-disorders/cushings-syndrome-information-page
- National Cancer Institute (NCI), Rare Endocrine Tumors, Pheochromocytomas: https://www.cancer.gov/pediatric-adult-rare-tumor/rare-tumors/rare-endocrine-tumor/pheochromocytoma

16. Christ-Crain M, Fenske W. Copeptin in the diagnosis of vasopressin-dependent disorders of fluid homeostasis. *Nat Rev Endocrinol.* 2016;12(3):168–176.

17. Bresson D, Herman P, Polivka M, Froelich S. Sellar lesions/pathology. *Otolaryngol Clin North Am.* 2016;49:63.

18. Nunes RH, Abello AL, Zanation AM, Sasaki-Adams D, Huang BY. Imaging in endoscopic cranial skull base and pituitary surgery. *Otolaryngol Clin North Am.* 2016;49:33.

19. LeFevre ML, U.S. Preventive Services Task Force. Screening for thyroid dysfunction: U.S. Preventive Services Task Force recommendation statement. *Ann Intern Med.* 2015;162:641.

20. Fontes R, Coeli CR, Aguiar F, Vaisman M. Reference interval of thyroid stimulating hormone and free thyroxine in a reference population over 60 years old and in very old subjects (over 80 years): comparison to young subjects. *Thyroid Res.* 2013;6:13.

21. Razvi S, Bhana S, Mrabeti S. Challenges in interpreting thyroid stimulating hormone results in the diagnosis of thyroid dysfunction. *J Thyroid Res.* 2019;2019:4106816.

22. Demers LM. Thyroid disease: pathophysiology and diagnosis. *Clin Lab Med.* 2004;24(1):19.

23. Merchant NB, Mirza FS. Interpretation of thyroid function tests in hospitalized patients. *Hosp Clin Med.* 2015;4(2):243.

24. Kundra P, Burman KD. The effect of medications on thyroid function tests. *Med Clin North Am.* 2012;96(2):283.

25. Trohman RG, Sharma PS, McAninch EA, Bianco AC. Amiodarone and thyroid physiology, pathophysiology, diagnosis and management. *Trends Cardiovasc Med.* 2019;29(5):285–295.

26. Xie C, Cox P, Taylor N, LaPorte S. Ultrasonography of thyroid nodules: a pictorial review. *Insights Imaging.* 2016;7:77.

27. Hoang JK, Sosa JA, Nguyen XV, Galvin PL, Oldan JD. Imaging thyroid disease: updates, imaging approach, and management pearls. *Radiol Clin North Am.* 2015;53:145.

28. Nieman LK, Biller BM, Findling JW, et al. The diagnosis of Cushing's syndrome: an Endocrine Society Clinical Practice Guideline. *J Clin Endocrinol Metab.* 2008;93(5):1526.

29. Nieman LK, Biller BM, Findling JW, et al. The diagnosis of Cushing's syndrome: an Endocrine Society Clinical Practice Guideline. *J Clin Endocrinol Metab.* 2015;100(8):2807.

30. Lacroix A, Feelders RA, Stratakis CA, Nieman LK. Cushing's syndrome. *Lancet.* 2015;386:913.

31. Funder JW, Carey RM, Mantero F, et al. The management of primary aldosteronism: case detection, diagnosis, and treatment: an Endocrine Society Clinical Practice Guideline. *J Clin Endocrinol Metab.* 2016;101(5):1889–1916.

32. Allen BC, Francis IR. Adrenal imaging and intervention. *Radiol Clin North Am.* 2015;53(5):1021.

33. Rossi GP, Auchus RJ, Brown M, et al. An expert consensus statement on use of adrenal vein sampling for the subtyping of primary aldosteronism. *Hypertension.* 2014;63:151.

34. Bornstein SR, Allolio B, Arlt W, et al. Diagnosis and treatment of primary adrenal insufficiency: an Endocrine Society Clinical Practice Guideline. *J Clin Endocrinol Metab.* 2016;101(2):364.

35. Brooke AM, Monson JP. Addison's disease. *Medicine.* 2013;41(9):522.

36. Téblick A, Peeters B, Langouche L, Van den Berghe G. Adrenal function and dysfunction in critically ill patients. *Nat Rev Endocrinol.* 2019;15(7):417–427.

37. Thomas RM, Ruel E, Shantavasinkul PC, Corsino L. Endocrine hypertension: an overview on the current etiopathogenesis and management options. *World J Hypertens.* 2015;5(2):14.

38. Därr R, Kuhn M, Bode C, et al. Accuracy of recommended sampling and assay methods for the determination of plasma-free and urinary fractionated metanephrines in the diagnosis of pheochromocytoma and paraganglioma: a systematic review. *Endocrine.* 2017;56(3):495–503.

39. Lenders JW, Duh QY, Eisenhofer G, et al. Pheochromocytoma and paraganglioma: an Endocrine Society Clinical Practice Guideline. *J Clin Endocrinol Metab.* 2014;99(6):1915.

23

Endocrine Disorders and Therapeutic Management

Mary E. Lough

This chapter focuses on the neuroendocrine stress associated with critical illness and on disorders of three major endocrine glands: pancreas, posterior pituitary gland, and thyroid gland.

ACUTE NEUROENDOCRINE RESPONSE TO CRITICAL ILLNESS

Fight or Flight Response

Major neurologic and endocrine changes occur during physiologic stress caused by any critical illness, sepsis, trauma, major surgery, or underlying cardiovascular disease.[1] The normal "fight or flight" response that is initiated in times of physiologic or psychologic stress is exacerbated in critical illness through activation of the neuroendocrine system, specifically the hypothalamic-pituitary-adrenal (HPA) axis.[1,2] All endocrine organs are affected by acute critical illness, as shown in Table 23.1.

The fight or flight acute response to physiologic threat is a rapid discharge of the catecholamines *norepinephrine* and *epinephrine* into the bloodstream.[2] Norepinephrine is released from the nerve endings of the sympathetic nervous system. Epinephrine is released from the adrenal glands. These physiologic responses are initiated by the HPA axis.

Hypothalamus-Pituitary-Adrenal Pancreas in Critical Illness

The pituitary gland has two parts (anterior and posterior) that function under control of the hypothalamus.

Posterior Pituitary

The *posterior pituitary gland* releases antidiuretic hormone (ADH), also known as *vasopressin*, as a component of the physiologic stress response. This hormone is an antidiuretic with a powerful vasoconstrictive effect on blood vessels. The synergistic combination of vasopressin and epinephrine released from the adrenal glands quickly raises blood pressure (BP).

Anterior Pituitary

The *anterior pituitary gland* produces several hormones, including *corticotropin* (also called adrenocorticotropic hormone), which stimulates release of *cortisol* from the adrenal cortex. Cortisol release is an important protective response to stress. Increased cortisol levels alter carbohydrate, fat, and protein metabolism so that energy is immediately and selectively available to vital organs. This also contributes to the hyperglycemia observed in critical illness.

Adrenal Gland

The *adrenal gland* produces cortisol from the cortex and epinephrine from the medulla, contributing to the physiologic stress response. Initially, in response to critical illness, cortisol levels rise. However, when the illness is sustained, the adrenal glands may not be able to produce adequate amounts of stress hormones,[3] a condition known as *critical illness–related corticosteroid insufficiency* (CIRCI).[3]

Pancreas

In response to physiologic stress, *glucagon* is released by the pancreatic alpha cells and stimulates the liver to release glucose into the bloodstream. The physiologic purpose of glucagon is to prevent hypoglycemia by stimulating the liver to release additional glucose into the bloodstream. In critical illness, circulating glucagon can be increased five times the normal value, unrelated to insulin levels, causing hyperglycemia.[4]

Hyperglycemia Management in Critical Illness

Normal fasting blood glucose levels are between 70 and 100 mg/dL in a healthy person. Critically ill patients frequently have much higher blood glucose levels, and several retrospective analyses have reported that hyperglycemic patients have a higher mortality rate than patients with normal blood glucose values.[4] In 2001 a landmark prospective, randomized study showed a significant reduction in morbidity and mortality among critically ill surgical patients whose blood glucose concentration was maintained between 80 and 110 mg/dL with a continuous insulin infusion compared with patients whose blood glucose was treated only if it was greater than 180 mg/dL. These initial studies were greeted with tremendous enthusiasm, and many critical care units adopted stringent glucose control standards to reduce hyperglycemia-associated morbidity and mortality. However, reproducibility of such tight glucose control outside of a research trial was impossible, as shown by the results of follow-up clinical studies.[5-7] The most important trial was the NICE-SUGAR trial.[8] This was a prospective randomized trial of 6014 critically ill patients that compared continuous insulin infusion to achieve tight glucose control (target 81–108 mg/dL) with a conventional glucose control range (target below 180 mg/dL). In the tight glucose control group, 6.8% had episodes of severe hypoglycemia (less than 40 mg/dL); in the conventional control group, only 0.5% experienced severe hypoglycemia.[8] There was a 2.6% higher risk of death in the intensive glucose control group (27.5% died) compared with the conventional control group (24.9% died).[8]

TABLE 23.1   Endocrine Responses to Stress.

Gland or Organ	Hormone	Response or Physical Examination
Adrenal cortex	Cortisol	↑ Insulin resistance → ↑ glycogenolysis → ↑ glucose circulation
		↑ Hepatic gluconeogenesis → ↑ glucose available
		↑ Lipolysis
		↑ Protein catabolism
		↑ Sodium → ↑ water retention to maintain plasma osmolality by movement of extravascular fluid into the intravascular space
		↓ Connective tissue fibroblasts → poor wound healing
	Glucocorticoid	↓ Histamine release → suppression of immune system
		↓ Lymphocytes, monocytes, eosinophils, basophils
		↑ Polymorphonuclear leukocytes → ↑ infection risk
		↑ Glucose
		↓ Gastric acid secretion
	Mineralocorticoids	↑ Aldosterone → ↓ sodium excretion → ↓ water excretion → ↑ intravascular volume
		↑ Potassium excretion → hypokalemia
		↑ Hydrogen ion excretion → metabolic acidosis
Adrenal medulla	Epinephrine	↑ Endorphins → ↓ pain
	Norepinephrine, epinephrine	↑ Metabolic rate to accommodate stress response
		↑ Live glycogenolysis → ↑ glucose
		↑ Insulin (cells are insulin resistant)
		↑ Cardiac contractility
		↑ Cardiac output
		↑ Dilation of coronary arteries
		↑ Blood pressure
		↑ Heart rate
		↑ Bronchodilation → ↑ respirations
		↑ Perfusion to heart, brain, lungs, liver, and muscle
		↓ Perfusion to periphery of body
		↓ Peristalsis
	Norepinephrine	↑ Peripheral vasoconstriction
		↑ Blood pressure
		↑ Sodium retention
		↑ Potassium excretion
Pituitary	All hormones	↑ Endogenous opioids → ↓ pain
Anterior pituitary	Corticotropin	↑ Aldosterone → ↓ sodium excretion → ↓ water excretion → ↑ intravascular volume
		↑ Cortisol → ↑ blood volume
	Growth hormones	↑ Protein anabolism of amino acids to protein
		↑ Lipolysis → ↑ gluconeogenesis
Posterior pituitary	Antidiuretic hormone	↑ Vasoconstriction
		↑ Water retention → restoration of circulating blood volume
		↓ Urine output
		↑ Hypo-osmolality
Pancreas	Insulin	↑ Insulin resistance → hyperglycemia
	Glucagon	↑ Glycolysis (directly opposes action of insulin)
		↑ Glucose for fuel
		↑ Glycogenolysis
		↑ Gluconeogenesis
		↑ Lipolysis
Thyroid	Thyroxine	↓ Routine metabolic demands during stress
Gonads	Sex hormones	Energy and oxygen supply diverted to brain, heart, muscles, and liver

↑, Increased; →, causes; ↓, decreased.

Clinical Practice Guidelines for Blood Glucose Management in Critically Ill Patients

As a result of the studies just described, clinical practice guidelines were developed by the American Association of Clinical Endocrinologists and the American Diabetes Association (ADA) that recommend the use of continuous insulin infusions to maintain blood glucose in critical care patients between 140 and 180 mg/dL, with hourly monitoring of blood glucose.[9] The range of 140 to 180 mg/dL was selected to minimize the risk of hypoglycemia while avoiding extreme hyperglycemia. Other glucose control guidelines relevant to critical illness have also been published. The Society of Critical Care Medicine recommends initiating glycemic control when blood glucose rises above 150 mg/dL.[10] Insulin management must be initiated if the blood glucose level is greater than 180 mg/dL.[10] Stress hyperglycemia (greater than 180 mg/dL) occurs in almost one-third of critically ill patients.[4]

Point-of-care testing for blood glucose in critical illness. Monitoring the blood glucose with a point-of-care glucometer is the basis of targeted glucose control. As part of the comprehensive initial assessment, blood sugar is measured by a standard laboratory sample or by a fingerstick capillary blood sample. In many institutions, if blood sugar is greater than 180 mg/dL, the patient is started on a continuous intravenous (IV) insulin infusion.

Point-of-care testing with a handheld glucometer is frequently used to allow hourly rapid assessment of the blood glucose and titration of a continuous glucose infusion. The US Food and Drug Administration (FDA) requires that blood glucose testing devices used in the hospital meet standards specific to the inpatient setting.[11] For added safety, it is important to verify very high blood glucose values and low blood glucose values with a blood sample sent to the clinical laboratory for plasma glucose verification.

During hyperglycemia, blood sample measurements are usually obtained hourly to allow titration of the insulin drip to lower blood glucose.[10] After the blood glucose is stable, measurements can be spaced approximately every 2 hours based on individual hospital protocols.

Continuous Insulin Infusion

Many hospitals use insulin-infusion protocols for management of stress-induced hyperglycemia. These protocols are implemented and managed by the critical care nurse.[9,10] Effective glucose protocols gauge the insulin infusion rate based on two parameters: (1) the immediate blood glucose result and (2) the rate of change in the blood glucose level since the last hourly measurement. Protocols vary by hospital, but the underlying concepts are similar.

These three examples illustrate blood glucose management strategies that may be used:

- Patient A receives 3 units of continuous IV regular insulin per hour and has a blood glucose measurement of 110 mg/dL, but 1 hour ago it was 190 mg/dL. The insulin rate must be decreased to avoid sudden hypoglycemia.
- Patient B receives 3 units of continuous IV regular insulin per hour and has a blood glucose measurement of 110 mg/dL, but 1 hour ago it was 112 mg/dL. In this situation, no change is made in the insulin infusion rate.
- Patient C receives 3 units of continuous IV regular insulin per hour and has a blood glucose measurement of 190 mg/dL, and 1 hour ago it was 197 mg/dL. The insulin rate must be increased to move the patient's blood sugar more rapidly toward the targeted glucose range (i.e., 140–180 mg/dL, although this range varies by individual hospital protocol).

The important point to emphasize is that the *rate of change* of blood glucose is as important as the *most recent* blood glucose measurement. Each of the patients described in the examples may have the same insulin infusion rate, depending on their catabolic state, but individualization among patients with different diagnoses can be achieved safely if the rate of change is also considered.

A person's insulin requirement often fluctuates over the course of an illness. This fluctuation occurs in response to changes in the clinical condition such as development of an infection, caloric alterations caused by stopping or starting enteral or parenteral nutrition,

administration of therapeutic steroids, or because the person is less catabolic. A method to allow for corrective incremental changes (up or down) to adapt to the reality of clinical developments and maintain the glucose within the target range is essential. Some protocols alter only the infusion rate, whereas others incorporate bolus insulin doses if the glucose concentration is greater than a preestablished threshold (e.g., 180 mg/dL).

Transition From Continuous Insulin Infusion to Subcutaneous Insulin

The transition from a continuous insulin infusion to intermittent insulin coverage must be handled with care to avoid large fluctuations in blood glucose levels. Before the conversion, the regular insulin infusion should be at a stable and preferably low rate, and the patient's blood glucose level within the target range. The transition from IV to subcutaneous insulin administration depends on numerous factors, including whether the patient can eat a consistent amount of dietary carbohydrate. The number of units of insulin transitioned from IV to subcutaneous can range from 60% to 80% of the prior 24-hour total depending on individual patient needs.[9–11]

Clinicians use various methods to calculate the quantity of insulin to prescribe during the transition from IV to subcutaneous insulin to maintain stable blood glucose levels. Fig. 23.1 depicts hypothetical examples of how a combination of basal and bolus insulin regimens (prandial insulin) can work in clinical practice.

Many types of insulin are available for use. These include ultra–short-acting, short-acting, intermediate-acting, long-acting, and combination insulin replacement options. Some of these are listed in Table 23.2. After the transition to subcutaneous insulin is completed, blood glucose is monitored frequently to maintain blood glucose within the target range and detect hyperglycemia or hypoglycemia.

Corrective Insulin Coverage

A patient may be prescribed supplemental or corrective doses of insulin in addition to the basal/prandial insulin combination. The use of the trio of basal, prandial, and corrective insulin is designed to eliminate the use of the traditional sliding scale. Criticisms of the sliding scale method are that the dosages are rarely reevaluated or adjusted once established and that the scales treat hyperglycemia only after it has occurred; they are not proactive in the manner of the basal/bolus/corrective insulin method. The ADA does not recommend solo use of the sliding scale.[12,13]

Supplemental corrective insulin. A supplemental correction scale can be used to cover any episodes of hyperglycemia above the target range. The corrective insulin amount can be combined with scheduled blood glucose measurements and scheduled insulin administration.

After the transition to subcutaneous insulin, it is important to recheck the blood glucose level. The insulin dosage is adjusted based on the patient's *insulin sensitivity* or, stated another way, according to how much insulin is needed to metabolize each 15 g of carbohydrate intake. Patients who are *insulin resistant* require more insulin than patients who are *insulin sensitive*.

Hypoglycemia Management in Critical Illness

It is important to have a protocol for the management of hypoglycemia.[11] The major drawback to use of intensive insulin protocols is the potential for hypoglycemia. Whenever hypoglycemia is detected, it is important to *stop* any continuous infusion of insulin. An example of one protocol to reverse hypoglycemia follows:

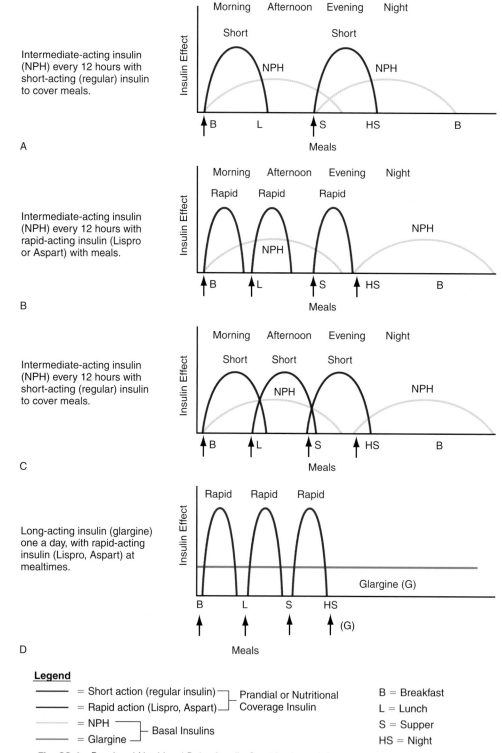

Fig. 23.1 Basal and Nutritional Bolus Insulin Combinations. *NPH,* Neutral protamine Hagedorn.

- Blood glucose level less than 40 mg/dL (severe hypoglycemia): Administer 50 mL of dextrose (25 g dextrose) in water ($D_{50}W$) as an IV bolus.
- Blood glucose level between 40 and 70 mg/dL (hypoglycemia): Administer 25 mL of $D_{50}W$ as an IV bolus.

The blood glucose concentration is monitored every 15 minutes until the blood glucose level has increased to greater than 70 mg/dL.

Collaborative Management

Standardized protocols designed to manage the complications of critical illness result in lower morbidity and mortality for patients.[10,14] Optimally, all disciplines concerned with the endocrine status of the patient will have participated in the hospital's guidelines related to targeted glucose control.[10,14] Evidence-based guidelines for blood glucose monitoring in critical illness are described in Box 23.1.

TABLE 23.2 Pharmacologic Management.

Insulin

Insulin	Route[b]	Action	Onset/Peak/Duration	Special Considerations
Ultra-Short-Acting Insulins				
Aspart (NovoLog)	Subcutaneous	Insulin replacement, rapid onset	5–15 minutes/30–90 minutes/ <5 hours	Insulin analog almost *immediately* absorbed; must be taken with food Insulin appearance should be clear Must be used in combination with intermediate-acting or long-acting basal insulin regimen; see Fig. 23.1
Lispro (Humalog)	Subcutaneous	Insulin replacement, rapid onset	5–15 minutes/30–90 minutes/ <5 hours	Insulin analog; almost *immediately* absorbed; must be taken with food Shorter duration of action than regular insulin; should be used with basal longer acting insulin; see Fig. 23.1
Glulisine (Apidra)	Subcutaneous	Insulin replacement, rapid onset	5–15 minutes/30–90 minutes/ <5 hours	Insulin analog
Short-Acting Insulin				
Regular	IV or Subcutaneous	Insulin replacement therapy	IV: <15 minutes Subcutaneous: 30–60 minutes/ 2–3 hours/5–8 hours	Only type of insulin suitable for IV continuous infusion or IV bolus administration
Intermediate-Acting Basal Insulin				
NPH	Subcutaneous	Insulin replacement, intermediate action	2–4 hours/4–10 hours/10–16 hours	NPH is not recommended for subcutaneous basal insulin because it has a peak with a less predictable time course than the long-acting insulin analogs.
Long-Acting Basal Insulins				
Glargine (Lantus)	Subcutaneous	Long-acting basal insulin analog	2–4 hours until steady state/no peak Concentration relatively constant over 20–24 hours	Synthetic insulin (analog); differs from human insulin by three amino acids, slow release over 24 hours; no peak Decrease dosage by 20% if switching from NPH to glargine Must not be diluted or mixed with other insulins; see Fig. 23.1
Detemir (Levemir)	Subcutaneous	Long-acting basal insulin analog	3–8 hours until steady state/no peak/5–23 hours	
Combination (Premixed) Insulins				
Various	Subcutaneous	Rapid plus intermediate or long-acting insulin combination	Varies according to combination used	Many combinations exist; examples (long-acting component/short-acting component) include 70/30 regular (70% NPH with 30% regular), NovoLog mix 70/30 (70% aspart-protamine suspension with 30% aspart), and Humalog mix 75/25 (75% lispro-protamine suspension with 25% lispro)

[a]Dosages are individualized according to patient's age and size.
[b]Only regular insulin is suitable for IV use.
IV, Intravenous; *NPH,* neutral protamine Hagedorn.

PANCREATIC DISORDERS

DIABETES MELLITUS

Diabetes mellitus is a progressive endocrinopathy with multiple manifestations that, without treatment, result in severe hyperglycemia.[15] Only type 1 and type 2 diabetes are discussed in this chapter:

- Type 1 diabetes describes a condition with an absolute loss of insulin that results from autoimmune destruction of the insulin-producing beta cells in the pancreas, so that exogenous insulin administration is required for life.[15]

- Type 2 diabetes describes an insulin deficiency caused by a progressive loss of insulin from the pancreatic beta cells.[15] There is also insulin resistance.[15] Type 2 diabetes can be managed by medications and alterations in lifestyle if the pancreas is producing some insulin.[16,17]

Diabetes Mellitus Diagnosis

Diabetes mellitus is diagnosed by measurement of the fasting plasma glucose (FPG) or by a *glycated hemoglobin* A_{1c} greater than 6.5%.[15] The blood glucose may also be called a fasting blood glucose. The benchmarks for a normal blood glucose value have been progressively

QSEN | BOX 23.1 Evidence-Based Practice

Hyperglycemia Management in Critical Illness

A summary is provided of evidence and evidence-based recommendations for controlling hyperglycemic symptoms related to physiologic stress of critical illness.

Strong Evidence to Support

- Initiate insulin therapy for persistent hyperglycemia greater than 180 mg/dL.
- Once a continuous insulin infusion is initiated, maintain target blood glucose level between 140 and 180 mg/dL.
- Perform frequent blood glucose monitoring to avoid hypoglycemia (hypoglycemia is defined as blood glucose level less than 70 mg/dL; severe hypoglycemia is less than 40 mg/dL).
- For patients who are eating, maintain preprandial blood glucose below 130 mg/dL; maintain 2-hour postprandial blood glucose below 180 mg/dL.
- A multidisciplinary team approach to implement institutional guidelines, protocols, and standardized order sets results in fewer hypoglycemic and hyperglycemic events.

References

American Diabetes Association. Classification and diagnosis of diabetes: standards of medical care in diabetes—2020. *Diabetes Care*. 2020;43(suppl 1):S14—S31.

Jacobi J, Bircher N, Krinsley J, et al. Guidelines for the use of an insulin infusion for the management of hyperglycemia in critically ill patients. *Crit Care Med*. 2012;40(12):3251.

Moghissi ES, Korytkowski MT, DiNardo M, et al. American Association of Clinical Endocrinologists and American Diabetes Association consensus statement on inpatient glycemic control. *Endocr Pract*. 2009;15(4):353—369.

lowered as more knowledge has been gained about the benefits of maintaining the plasma glucose level as close to normal as possible.

Blood glucose values endorsed by the ADA are as follows[15]:

- FPG level 70 to 100 mg/dL (5.6 mmol/L) is a normal fasting glucose.
- FPG level 100 to 125 mg/dL (5.6 and 6.9 mmol/L) denotes impaired fasting glucose.
- FPG level greater than 126 mg/dL (7 mmol/L) is diagnostic of diabetes (result is verified by testing more than once).

Glycated Hemoglobin A_{1c}

For individuals with diabetes, maintenance of blood glucose within a tight normal range is fundamental to avoid the development of microvascular and neuropathic secondary conditions. Although the plasma glucose value produces a snapshot of the blood glucose concentration at a single point in time, the *glycated hemoglobin* A_{1c} measures the percentage of glucose the red blood cells have absorbed from the plasma over the previous 3-month period. The optimal target for patients with diabetes is an A_{1c} less than 6.5%.[15]

Type 1 Diabetes

Type 1 diabetes mellitus accounts for 5% to 10% of all patients with diabetes.[15] It is an autoimmune disease that causes progressive destruction of the beta cells of the islets of Langerhans in the pancreas. Over time, the autoantibodies render the pancreatic beta cells incapable of secreting insulin and regulating intracellular glucose. In type 1 diabetes, the rate of beta cell destruction is highly variable. It occurs rapidly in some patients (mainly children) and more slowly in others (mainly adults). Children and adolescents often present emergently with ketoacidosis as the first manifestation of type1 diabetes.[15]

Management of Type 1 Diabetes

Patients with type 1 diabetes must receive IV or subcutaneous insulin therapy. Treatment with exogenous insulin replacement restores normal entry of glucose into the cells. The range of insulin replacements available is expanding, and it is essential that critical care nurses be knowledgeable about the different classes of insulin (see Table 23.2). Insulins can be long acting, intermediate acting, short acting, or rapid acting, or in many premixed combinations.[12,18] Without insulin, the rapid breakdown of noncarbohydrate substrate, particularly fat, leads to ketonemia, ketonuria, and diabetic ketoacidosis (DKA), a life-threatening complication associated with type 1 diabetes (see later discussion).

Type 2 Diabetes

Type 2 diabetes accounts for 90% to 95% of diabetes.[15] Type 2 diabetes is identified by decreased insulin secretion and insulin resistance, with a relative, versus absolute, insulin deficiency. Many patients with type 2 diabetes are obese, with excess adipose tissue concentrated in the abdominal area. The onset of hyperglycemia occurs gradually, and many people are unaware that they have diabetes. Initially, type 2 diabetes is managed by oral medications (noninsulin therapies) because the pancreatic beta cells remain functional. As progressive beta cell dysfunction occurs, a basal long-acting insulin is added to oral noninsulin medications.[12]

Insulin resistance describes a complex metabolic situation in which organ and tissue cells deny entry to insulin and glucose. This creates the clinical paradox in which elevated serum insulin levels and hyperglycemia are present at the same time. Insulin resistance has a strong association with obesity.

Lifestyle Management for Type 2 Diabetes

For most patients with type 2 diabetes, a program comprising weight reduction, increased physical exercise, and a change in diet pattern is the essential first step. The diet should contain less than 30% of calories from fat, with an increased quantity of whole grains, vegetables, and fruits. Crash diets are discouraged, and a gradual program of weight loss is recommended. The exercise program is tailored to the individual but might start with 30 minutes of brisk walking each day if the person was previously sedentary.[15,16,19]

Type 2 diabetes increases risk of contracting a wide range of cardiovascular and kidney complications that increase morbidity and mortality. In addition to taking medications to control blood glucose, some patients may need medications to lower their BP, lower cholesterol, and triglyceride levels, treat ischemic heart disease, or manage symptoms of heart failure.[19]

Pharmacologic Management of Type 2 Diabetes

If lifestyle changes are unsuccessful in reversing the pattern of type 2 diabetes, then noninsulin antihyperglycemic medications are prescribed as recommended by the ADA (Table 23.3 and Box 23.2). These medications are not oral forms of insulin and have many varied actions.

TABLE 23.3 Pharmacologic Management Type 2 Diabetes.

Medications for Type 2 Diabetes	Lower A$_{1c}$	Cardiovascular Disease	Cost	Route
Metformin	Yes		Low	Oral
Sulfonylureas	Yes		Low	Oral
Thiazolidinediones	Yes	Avoid in heart failure	Low	Oral
DPP-4 inhibitors	Yes	Avoid in heart failure	High	Oral
SGLT2 inhibitors	Yes	Added benefit	High	Oral
GLP-1 RA	Yes	Added benefit	High	Subcutaneous
Insulin	Yes		Low	Subcutaneous

Data from American Diabetes Association. Glycemic targets: standards of medical care in diabetes—2020. *Diabetes Care.* 2020;43 (suppl 1):S66—S76.

BOX 23.2 Antihyperglycemic Medications and Actions

Medications That Sensitize the Body to Insulin (Insulin Sensitizers)
- Biguanides
- Thiazolidinediones

Medications That Stimulate the Pancreas to Make More Insulin (Insulin Secretagogues)
- Sulfonylureas
- Glinides

Medications That Delay Carbohydrate Absorption From Small Intestine
- Alpha-glucosidase inhibitors

Medications That Augment Gut Incretin Hormone Effects
- Incretin mimetics
- Incretin enhancers

Medications That Increase Excretion of Glucose in the Urine
- Sodium-glucose cotransporter2 (SGLT2) inhibitors

Insulin in Type 2 Diabetes

In some situations, patients with type 2 diabetes will have insulin added to their medication regimen.[19] Patients with an A$_{1c}$ above 8.0% who are taking two oral antihyperglycemic medications, including metformin, may not benefit from adding a third oral antihyperglycemic medication.[19] One option is to add a long-acting basal insulin to the regimen. This requires more intensive blood glucose monitoring and increased education about insulin management.

Polypharmacy in Diabetes

The availability of varied pharmacologic approaches to reduce blood glucose and manage type 2 diabetes can reduce many long-term complications related to hyperglycemia. Often patients may be taking two or three medications for diabetes and taking additional medications for coexisting medical conditions.[19] One of the unintended consequences of having so many medications to manage type 2 diabetes is *polypharmacy* and risk of medication interactions and hypoglycemia; this is recognized as a particular problem for older adults.

HYPERGLYCEMIC EMERGENCIES

There are two hyperglycemic emergencies associated with diabetes: DKA and hyperglycemic hyperosmolar state (HHS).[20–24] In the United States, DKA and HHS account for 168,000 hospital admissions and 207,000 visits to the emergency department each year.[22] In both conditions, treatment focuses on administration of insulin, rehydration, and correction of electrolyte and acid–base imbalances.[20–22] Hyperglycemia emergencies include both DKA and HHS and a combined management algorithm is shown in Fig. 23.2. However, because there are significant differences between DKA and HHS, these conditions are discussed separately in this chapter.

Diabetic Ketoacidosis

DKA is a life-threatening complication of type 1 diabetes that occurs with new-onset type 1 diabetes or in a patient with established type 1 diabetes who is insulin dependent. DKA priority assessments and nursing interventions are listed in Fig. 23.3. The classic diagnostic criteria for DKA are[20]:
- Blood glucose greater than 250 mg/dL
- pH less than 7.3
- Serum bicarbonate less than 18 mEq/L
- Moderate or severe ketonemia or ketonuria

DKA is categorized as mild, moderate, or severe depending on the severity of the metabolic acidosis (assessed by blood pH, bicarbonate, ketones) and by the presence of altered mental status (Table 23.4).[20,23]

Plasma glucose levels for a patient with DKA typically are greater than 250 mg/dL.[21] However, elevated serum glucose levels alone do not define DKA; the other crucial determining factor is the presence of ketoacidosis as described in Table 23.4 and Fig. 23.3.[20] In addition to the low pH (less than 7.3), there is an increased anion gap (greater than 12), indicating metabolic acidosis.[21] Approximately 10% of patients present to the hospital with mild DKA with a plasma glucose less than 250 mg/dL.[20] This is known as *euglycemic DKA.*[21,23,24]

Precipitating Causes of DKA

Changes in the type of insulin, change in dosage, or increased metabolic demand can precipitate DKA in patients with type 1 diabetes.[20] Life cycle changes, such as growth spurts in an adolescent, require an increase in insulin intake, as do surgery, infection, and trauma. In young patients with diabetes, psychologic problems combined with eating disorders or depression are a contributing factor in up to 20% of cases of recurrent ketoacidosis.[20,21]

Ketoacidosis also occurs with acute pancreatitis. In addition to elevated glucose and acidosis, serum amylase and lipase are abnormally high, which helps to establish pancreatitis as a separate diagnosis

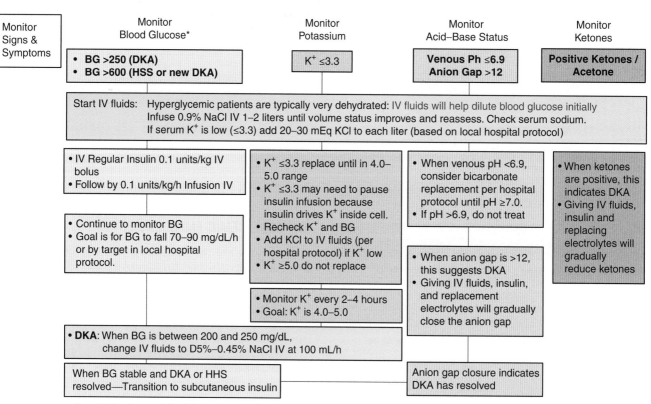

Fig. 23.2 Protocol for Management of Hyperglycemic Emergencies: Diabetic Ketoacidosis and Hyperglycemic Hyperosmolar State. *Different hospital protocols may use other BG target values to identify and resolve DKA and HHS. *BG,* Blood glucose; *DKA,* diabetic ketoacidosis; *HHS,* hyperglycemic hyperosmolar state; *IV,* intravenous; *K+,* potassium; *KCl,* potassium chloride; *NaCl,* sodium chloride; *pH,* a measure of the degree to which a solution is acidic or alkaline. (Data from Kitabchi AE, Umpierrez GE, Murphy MB, Kreisberg RA. Hyperglycemic crises in adult patients with diabetes: a consensus statement from the American Diabetes Association. *Diabetes Care.* 2006;29[12]:2739–2748; Umpierrez G, Korytkowski M. Diabetic emergencies—ketoacidosis, hyperglycaemic hyperosmolar state and hypoglycaemia. *Nat Rev Endocrinol.* 2016;12:222–232; Dhatariya KK, Vellanki P. Treatment of diabetic ketoacidosis [DKA]/hyperglycemic hyperosmolar state [HHS]: novel advances in the management of hyperglycemic crises [UK versus USA]. *Curr Diab Rep.* 2017;17[5]:33.)

from type 1 diabetes. Other nondiabetic causes of ketoacidosis are starvation ketosis and alcoholic ketoacidosis. These cases are distinguished from classic DKA by clinical history and usually by a plasma glucose less than 200 mg/dL.[20]

Pathophysiology

Insulin deficiency and DKA. Insulin is the metabolic key to the transfer of glucose from the bloodstream into the cell. Without insulin, glucose remains in the bloodstream, and cells are deprived of their energy source. A complex pathophysiologic chain of events follows. The release of glucagon from the liver is stimulated when insulin is ineffective in providing the cells with glucose for energy. Glucagon increases the amount of glucose in the bloodstream by breaking down stored glucose (glycogenolysis). Noncarbohydrates (fat and protein) are converted into glucose (gluconeogenesis).

Hyperglycemia and DKA. Hyperglycemia increases plasma osmolality, and the blood becomes hyperosmolar. Cellular dehydration occurs as the hyperosmolar extracellular fluid draws the more dilute intracellular and interstitial fluid into the vascular space. Cellular dehydration stimulates catecholamine production which stimulates glycogenolysis, lipolysis, and gluconeogenesis, pouring glucose into the bloodstream.

Without insulin to interrupt the cycle, this is an unstoppable process and death will ensue.

Fluid volume deficit and DKA. Excessive urine output (polyuria) and glucose in the urine (glucosuria) result from the excess glucose in the bloodstream that cannot be filtered by the kidney glomeruli. This causes volume loss in the urine as the glucose pulls water with it during urinary excretion (osmotic diuresis).

Electrolyte deficit and DKA. The presence of excess glucose in the bloodstream and other tissues causes movement of fluid and electrolytes from within the cell (intracellular space) to outside the cell (extracellular space). This results in an intracellular deficit of both fluid and electrolytes which predominantly affects potassium and magnesium, because these electrolytes are normally abundant within the cell. In addition, the osmotic diuresis allows excess excretion of potassium and magnesium. The result can be a total body electrolyte deficit.

Ketoacidosis and DKA. In a healthy individual, the presence of insulin in the bloodstream suppresses the manufacture of ketones. In insulin deficiency states, *ketoacidosis* occurs when free fatty acids are metabolized into ketones. The three ketones that are produced are: *beta-hydroxybutyrate, acetoacetate,* and *acetone.*

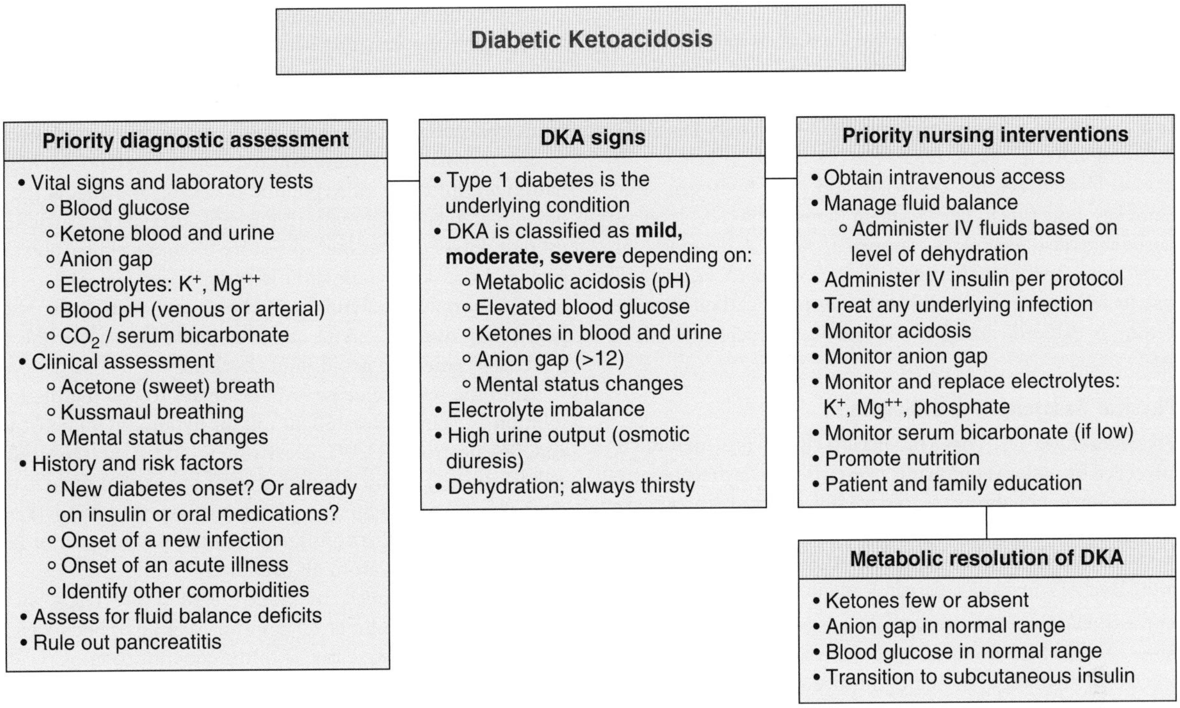

Diabetic Ketoacidosis

Priority diagnostic assessment

• Vital signs and laboratory tests
  ○ Blood glucose
  ○ Ketone blood and urine
  ○ Anion gap
  ○ Electrolytes: K^+, Mg^{++}
  ○ Blood pH (venous or arterial)
  ○ CO_2 / serum bicarbonate
• Clinical assessment
  ○ Acetone (sweet) breath
  ○ Kussmaul breathing
  ○ Mental status changes
• History and risk factors
  ○ New diabetes onset? Or already
    on insulin or oral medications?
  ○ Onset of a new infection
  ○ Onset of an acute illness
  ○ Identify other comorbidities
• Assess for fluid balance deficits
• Rule out pancreatitis

DKA signs

• Type 1 diabetes is the
  underlying condition
• DKA is classified as **mild,
  moderate, severe** depending on:
  ○ Metabolic acidosis (pH)
  ○ Elevated blood glucose
  ○ Ketones in blood and urine
  ○ Anion gap (>12)
  ○ Mental status changes
• Electrolyte imbalance
• High urine output (osmotic
  diuresis)
• Dehydration; always thirsty

Priority nursing interventions

• Obtain intravenous access
• Manage fluid balance
  ○ Administer IV fluids based on
    level of dehydration
• Administer IV insulin per protocol
• Treat any underlying infection
• Monitor acidosis
• Monitor anion gap
• Monitor and replace electrolytes:
  K^+, Mg^{++}, phosphate
• Monitor serum bicarbonate (if low)
• Promote nutrition
• Patient and family education

Metabolic resolution of DKA
• Ketones few or absent • Anion gap in normal range • Blood glucose in normal range • Transition to subcutaneous insulin

Fig. 23.3 Priority Diagnostic and Nursing Interventions for Diabetic Ketoacidosis. CO_2, Carbon dioxide; *DKA*, diabetic ketoacidosis; *IV*, intravenous; K^+, potassium; Mg^{++}, magnesium; *pH*, a measure of the degree to which a solution is acidic or alkaline.

TABLE 23.4 Diagnostic Criteria for Diabetic Ketoacidosis (DKA) and Hyperglycemic Hyperosmolar State (HHS).

	DKA			HHS
	Mild BG >250 mg/dL (13.9 mmol/L)	Moderate BG >250 mg/dL (13.9 mmol/L)	Severe BG >250 mg/dL (13.9 mmol/L)	Plasma Glucose >600 mg/dL
Arterial pH	7.25–7.30	7.00 to <7.24	<7.00	>7.30
Serum bicarbonate (mEq/L)	15–18	10 to <15	<10	>18
Urine ketone[a]	Positive	Positive	Positive	Negative, or small positive
Serum ketone[a]	Positive	Positive	Positive	Small
Urine or blood beta-hydroxybutyrate (mmol/L)	>3	>3	>3	<3
Effective serum osmolality[b]	Variable	Variable	Variable	>320 mOsm/kg
Anion gap[c]	>10	>12	>12	Variable
Mental status	Alert	Alert/drowsy	Stupor/coma	Stupor/coma

[a]Nitroprusside reaction method.
[b]Effective serum osmolality: 2[measured Na^+ (mEq/L)] + glucose (mg/dL)18.
[c]Anion gap: $(Na^+) - (Cl^- +)$ (mEq/L).
Data from Kitabchi AE, Umpierrez GE, Murphy MB, Kreisberg RA. Hyperglycemic crises in adult patients with diabetes: a consensus statement from the American Diabetes Association. *Diabetes Care.* 2009;32(7):1335–1343; Umpierrez G, Korytkowski M. Diabetic emergencies—ketoacidosis, hyperglycaemic hyperosmolar state and hypoglycaemia. *Nat Rev Endocrinol.* 2016;12:222–232; Dhatariya KK, Vellanki P. Treatment of diabetic ketoacidosis (DKA)/hyperglycemic hyperosmolar state (HHS): novel advances in the management of hyperglycemic crises (UK versus USA). *Curr Diab Rep.* 2017;17(5):33.

During normal metabolism, the ratio of beta-hydroxybutyrate to acetoacetate is 1:1, with acetone present in only small amounts. In DKA, because of lack of insulin, the quantities of all three ketones increase substantially, and the ratio of beta-hydroxybutyrate to acetoacetate can increase to 10:1. In DKA, the main ketone in the blood is beta-hydroxybutyrate, and the main ketone in the urine is its breakdown product, acetoacetate. Acetone does not cause acidosis and is safely excreted in the lungs, causing the characteristic fruity odor.

Ketones are measurable in the bloodstream (*ketonemia*). Blood tests that measure the quantity of beta-hydroxybutyric acid, the predominant ketone body in the blood, are the most useful.[20,23,24] Because ketones are excreted by the kidneys, they are also measurable in the urine (ketonuria). Ketone blood tests are preferred over urine tests for diagnosis and monitoring of DKA (see Table 23.4). When the blood and urine become clear of ketones, DKA is resolved.

Acid–base balance in DKA. The acid–base balance varies depending on the severity of DKA. A patient with mild DKA typically has a pH between 7.25 and 7.30. In severe DKA, the pH can drop below 7.00 (see Table 23.4).[20] Acid ketones dissociate and yield hydrogen ions, which accumulate and precipitate a fall in serum pH. The level of serum bicarbonate also decreases, consistent with a diagnosis of metabolic acidosis. Breathing becomes deep and rapid (Kussmaul respirations) to release carbonic acid in the form of carbon dioxide (CO_2). Acetone is exhaled, giving the breath its characteristic sweet fruity odor.

Focused Physical Assessment and Diagnosis

Clinical manifestations. DKA has a predictable clinical presentation. It is usually preceded by patient complaints of malaise, headache, polyuria (excessive urination), polydipsia (excessive thirst), and polyphagia (excessive hunger). Nausea, vomiting, extreme fatigue, dehydration, and weight loss follow. Central nervous system (CNS) depression, with changes in the level of consciousness, can lead quickly to coma.[20]

A patient with DKA may be stuporous or unresponsive, depending on the degree of fluid-balance disturbance. Physical examination reveals evidence of dehydration, including flushed dry skin, dry buccal membranes, and skin turgor that takes longer than 3 seconds to return to its original position after the skin has been lifted. Tachycardia and hypotension may signal profound fluid losses. Kussmaul respirations are present, and the fruity odor of acetone may be detected.

Laboratory studies. Considering the complexity and potential seriousness of DKA, the laboratory diagnosis is straightforward. When the patient has established type 1 diabetes and is insulin dependent, the presence of hyperglycemia, ketones, and acidosis on a venous blood gas provides rapid diagnostic confirmation of DKA[24] (see Table 23.4).

Other clues may be gleaned from the venous blood chemistry panel. CO_2, if measured, is low in the presence of uncompensated metabolic acidosis, and the anion gap is elevated. Serum sodium may be low because of the movement of water from the intracellular space into the extracellular (vascular) space.[20] The serum potassium level is often normal; a low serum potassium level in DKA suggests that a significant potassium deficiency may be present.[20]

Some patients may know their blood glucose and ketones are elevated because for self-management they have a ketone-test point-of-care meter and a blood glucose-test meter at home. However, if this is a new diagnosis, meaning the patient was not previously insulin dependent, the blood glucose can be very elevated, and the metabolic acidosis can be severe (see Table 23.4).

Medical Management

Diagnosis of DKA is based on the combination of presenting symptoms, patient history, medical history (type 1 diabetes), precipitating factors (if known), and results of serum glucose and urine ketone testing. After diagnosis, DKA requires aggressive clinical management to prevent progressive decompensation. The goals of treatment are to reverse dehydration, replace insulin, reverse ketoacidosis, and replenish electrolytes.

Reversing dehydration. A patient with DKA is dehydrated and may have lost 5% to 10% of body weight in fluids. Aggressive IV fluid replacement is provided to rehydrate the intracellular and extracellular compartments and prevent circulatory collapse (see Figs. 23.2 and 23.3).[20] Assessment of hydration is an important first step in the treatment of DKA.

IV isotonic normal saline (0.9% sodium chloride [NaCl]) is infused to replenish the vascular deficit and to reverse hypotension. For a severely dehydrated patient, 1 L of normal saline is infused immediately. Laboratory assessment of serum osmolality and the serum sodium concentration can help guide subsequent interventions. If the serum osmolality is elevated and serum sodium is high (hypernatremia), infusions of hypotonic NaCl (0.45%) follow the initial saline replacement. The replacement infusion typically includes 20 to 30 mEq of potassium per liter to restore the intracellular potassium debt, provided that kidney function is normal (see Fig. 23.2).[20] In patients without normally functioning kidneys and in patients with cardiopulmonary disease, careful attention must be paid to the volume of fluid replacement to avoid fluid overload.

After the serum glucose level decreases to 200 mg/dL, the infusing solution is changed to a 50/50 mix of hypotonic saline (0.45% NaCl) and 5% dextrose (D_5W). Dextrose is added to replenish depleted cellular glucose as the circulating serum glucose decreases to 200 mg/dL.[20] Dextrose infusion also prevents unexpected hypoglycemia when the insulin infusion is continued, but the patient cannot take in sufficient carbohydrate from an oral diet.

Insulin administration. In moderate to severe DKA, an initial IV bolus of regular insulin at 0.1 unit for each kg of body weight may be administered. Subsequently, a continuous infusion of regular insulin at 0.1 unit/kg/h is infused simultaneously with IV fluid replacement (see Fig. 23.2).[20,21] In a 70-kg adult, the infusion would be 7 units of insulin per hour. If the plasma glucose concentration does not fall by 50 to 70 mg/dL during the first hour of treatment, the glucose measurement should be rechecked. When the plasma glucose level is decreasing as expected, the insulin infusion is increased each hour until a steady blood glucose decline of between 50 and 70 mg/dL per hour is achieved.[20] It is important to emphasize that different hospitals' protocols may list other target requirements for decline of hourly blood glucose in DKA/HHS: for example, a decrease of 25 to 75 mg/dL per hour could also be the target reduction depending on the hospital protocol.[22]

Frequent assessment of the patient's blood glucose concentration is mandatory in moderate to severe DKA. Initially, blood glucose tests are performed hourly. The frequency decreases to every 2 to 4 hours as the patient's blood glucose level stabilizes and approaches normal. After the blood glucose level has decreased to between 200 and 250 mg/dL, the acidosis has been corrected, and rehydration has been achieved, the insulin infusion rate may be decreased by half to 0.05 unit/kg per hour.[21] This usually represents 3 to 6 units/h in an adult receiving a continuous IV insulin infusion. It is important to verify that the serum potassium concentration is not lower than 3.3 mEq/L and to replace potassium per local hospital protocol before administering the initial insulin bolus.[20]

Reversing ketoacidosis. Replacement of fluid volume and insulin interrupts the ketotic cycle and reverses the metabolic acidosis. In the presence of insulin, glucose enters the cells, and the body ceases to convert fats into glucose.

Adequate hydration and insulin replacement usually correct acidosis, and this treatment is sufficient for many patients with DKA. As shown in Fig. 23.2, replacement of bicarbonate is no longer routine except for a severely acidotic patient with a serum pH value lower than 7.0.[20] An indwelling arterial line provides access for hourly sampling of arterial blood gases to evaluate pH, bicarbonate, and other laboratory values in a patient with severe DKA.

Hyperglycemia usually resolves before ketoacidemia does.[20] Patients with type 1 diabetes and DKA may require 6 to 9 L of IV fluid replacement. Volume resuscitation occurs over 24 to 36 hours, with most IV crystalloid administered in the first 8 hours. Patients with a new diagnosis of type 1 diabetes take longer to clear urine ketones and require more insulin to achieve normal glycemic control. This is because the blood glucose is typically very elevated on the initial admission.

Replenishing electrolytes. Low serum potassium (hypokalemia) occurs as insulin promotes the return of potassium into the cell and metabolic acidosis is reversed. The potassium level must be 3.3 mEq or greater before administering insulin. The potassium level must be checked frequently, as insulin drives potassium into the cells and the serum potassium can drop precipitously. Potassium chloride is administered as soon as the serum potassium falls below normal. Frequent verification of the serum potassium concentration is required for a patient with DKA receiving fluid resuscitation and insulin therapy.

The serum phosphate level is sometimes low (hypophosphatemia) in DKA. Insulin treatment may make this more obvious as phosphate is returned to the interior of the cell. If the serum phosphate level is less than 1 mg/dL, phosphate replacement is recommended.[20]

Nursing Management

Nursing management of a patient with DKA incorporates a variety of patient diagnoses (Box 23.3). The nursing priorities are to administer prescribed fluids, insulin, and electrolytes; monitor response to therapy; and provide patient and family education.

Administering fluids, insulin, and electrolytes. Rapid IV fluid replacement requires the use of a volumetric pump. To ensure effective absorption, insulin is administered IV to patients who are severely dehydrated or have poor peripheral perfusion. Patients with DKA are kept on NPO status (nothing by mouth) until hyperglycemia is under control. The critical care nurse is responsible for monitoring the rate of plasma glucose decline in response to insulin. The goal is to achieve a fall in glucose levels of approximately 50 to 70 mg/dL each hour.[20] The coordination involved in monitoring blood glucose, potassium, and often blood gases on an hourly basis is considerable.

When the blood glucose level falls to, or below, 200 mg/dL, a D$_5$W with 0.45% NaCl solution is infused to prevent hypoglycemia.[20] At this time, it is likely that the insulin dose per hour will also be decreased. The infusion of regular insulin is not discontinued. The goal is to maintain the blood glucose level between 140 and 200 mg/dL until the ketoacidosis subsides, as identified by absence of ketones, until closure of the anion gap and return to a normal venous pH.[20,21]

◎ BOX 23.3 PRIORITY PATIENT CARE MANAGEMENT

Diabetic Ketoacidosis

- Risk for Infection
- Hypovolemia due to absolute loss
- Anxiety due to threat to biologic, psychologic, or social integrity
- Disturbed Body Image due to functional dependence on life-sustaining technology
- Powerlessness due to lack of control over current situation or disease progression
- Lack of Knowledge of Treatment Regime due to lack of previous exposure to information (see Box 23.5, Priority Patient and Family Education for Diabetic Ketoacidosis)

Patient Care Management plans are located in Appendix A.

Insulin is transitioned to the subcutaneous route after normalization of blood glucose levels, dehydration, hypotension, and acid–base balance, and the patient is sufficiently alert to eat an oral diet.

Monitoring response to therapy. Accurate intake and output (I&O) measurements must be maintained to monitor reversal of dehydration. Hourly urine output is an indicator of kidney function and provides information to prevent overhydration or insufficient hydration. Vital signs, especially heart rate (HR), hemodynamic values, and BP, are continuously monitored to assess response to fluid replacement. Evidence that fluid replacement is effective includes decreased HR, normal BP, and normalizing blood glucose levels. More invasive hemodynamic monitoring, such as a pulmonary artery catheter, is rarely needed. Further evidence of hydration improvement includes a change from a previously weak and rapid pulse to one that is strong and full and a change from hypotension to a gradual elevation of systolic BP. Respirations are assessed frequently for changes in rate, depth, and presence of the fruity acetone odor.

Blood glucose is measured each hour in the initial period. Sometimes potassium is measured just as frequently. The serum osmolality and serum sodium concentration are evaluated, and blood urea nitrogen (BUN) and creatinine levels are assessed for possible kidney impairment related to decreased organ perfusion. The purpose of these frequent assessments is to determine that the patient's clinical status is improving.

Transition to subcutaneous insulin. When the clinical laboratory indicators are stable and the patient is awake and alert, the transition to subcutaneous insulin and an oral diet can be made. Hyperglycemia is a risk if the subcutaneous insulin dosage is inadequate to maintain a normal blood glucose. In this situation, the anion gap may widen again. Hypoglycemia is also a risk during the transition period. For example, in anticipation of discontinuing the insulin and IV dextrose infusion, a patient receives a subcutaneous dose of insulin and is expected to eat a meal. However, if the patient is then unable to eat an adequate amount, hypoglycemia results from the administration of subcutaneous insulin without adequate carbohydrate.

Surveillance for complications. A patient with DKA can experience various complications, including fluid volume overload, hypoglycemia, hypokalemia or hyperkalemia, hyponatremia, cerebral edema, and infection.

Fluid volume overload. Fluid overload from rapid volume infusion is a serious complication that can occur in a patient with a compromised cardiopulmonary system or kidneys. Neck vein engorgement, dyspnea without exertion, and pulmonary crackles on auscultation signal circulatory overload. Reduction in the rate and volume of infusion, elevation of the head of the bed, and provision of oxygen may be required to manage increased intravascular volume. Hourly urine measurement is mandatory to assess kidney function and adequacy of fluid replacement.

Hypoglycemia. Hypoglycemia is defined as a serum glucose level lower than 70 mg/dL.[20] Most acute care hospitals have specific procedures for management of hypoglycemia (Box 23.4). For example, if hypoglycemia is detected by fingerstick point-of-care testing at the bedside, a blood sample is sent to the laboratory for verification; the physician is notified immediately; and replacement glucose is given IV or orally, depending on the patient's clinical condition, diagnosis, and level of consciousness.

Unexpected behavior changes or decreased level of consciousness, diaphoresis, and tremors are physical warning signs that the patient has become hypoglycemic. These symptoms are especially important to recognize if the frequency of blood glucose testing has lengthened to 2- to 4-hour intervals. Up to 30% of individuals who have type 1

BOX 23.4   Hypoglycemia Management

Hypoglycemia Prevention and Management
- Definition: Plasma blood glucose level below 70 mg/dL (3.9 mmol/L)
  - The American Diabetes Association recommends 70 mg/dL plasma blood glucose as the alert threshold for hypoglycemia. Most patients with diabetes do not have symptoms with this blood glucose, and this value provides some time to raise the blood glucose and avoid clinical symptoms.
  - Bedside POC glucometers results vary in accuracy. A POC blood glucose less than 70 mg/dL must be double-checked by sending a blood sample to the clinical laboratory *stat* to measure the plasma blood glucose.

Hypoglycemia Prevention
- Close monitoring of blood glucose for all hospitalized patients who receive insulin; use the laboratory threshold alert of 70 mg/dL, and do not wait for clinical symptoms.
- Approximately 10% of patients with diabetes admitted to critical care units experience at least one hypoglycemic episode (below 70 mg/dL).
- Blood glucose testing to detect hypoglycemia is vital, because many patients with diabetes do not experience symptoms. This is called *hypoglycemia unawareness.* In patients with diabetes who experience frequent episodes of hypoglycemia, the autonomic nervous system becomes less responsive. This is known as *hypoglycemia-associated autonomic failure.*
- Patient education before hospital discharge is essential to teach patients how blood glucose monitoring and dietary interventions are used to prevent hypoglycemia.

Clinical Signs and Symptoms of Acute Hypoglycemia
- Sedated and intubated patients may not have signs and symptoms
- Confusion
- Neurologic changes
- Seizures
- Death

Hypoglycemia Management
- Stop insulin infusion (if running).
- Administer 25 g of hypertonic dextrose (D_{50}) IV immediately.
- If blood glucose is dangerously low (below 40 mg/dL), some hospital protocols recommend 50 g D_{50} IV.
- Repeat blood glucose value in 15 minutes, and ongoing until blood glucose is greater than 70 mg/dL.
- Evaluate insulin regimen.
- Evaluate IV dextrose and carbohydrate nutrition regimen.
- If the patient can safely swallow, provide 25 g of carbohydrate orally and recheck blood glucose.
- Hold subcutaneous insulin. Recheck blood glucose level if subcutaneous insulin has been recently administered, and continue to check blood glucose level based on the duration of action of the subcutaneous insulin previously administered.

D50, 50% Dextrose; *IV,* intravenous; *POC,* point-of-care.
Data from Seaquist ER, Anderson J, Childs B, et al. Hypoglycemia and diabetes: a report of a workgroup of the American Diabetes Association and The Endocrine Society. *Diabetes Care.* 2013;36:1384–1395.

diabetes have impaired awareness of their low blood glucose, greatly increasing their risk of severe hypoglycemia.

Hypokalemia and hyperkalemia. Hypokalemia can occur within the first hours of rehydration and insulin treatment. Continuous cardiac monitoring is required because hypokalemia can cause ventricular dysrhythmias.

Hyperkalemia occurs with acidosis or with overaggressive administration of potassium replacement in patients with kidney disease. Severe hyperkalemia is demonstrated on the cardiac monitor by a large, peaked T wave; flattened P wave; and widened QRS complex (see Fig. 10.49 in Chapter 10). Ventricular fibrillation can follow.

Hyponatremia. Elimination of sodium from the body results from the osmotic diuresis and is compounded by the vomiting and diarrhea that can occur during DKA. Clinical manifestations of hyponatremia include abdominal cramping, postural hypotension, and unexpected behavioral changes. NaCl is infused as the initial IV solution. Maintenance of the saline infusion depends on clinical manifestations of sodium imbalance and serum laboratory values.

Level of consciousness. Cerebral edema occurs in 1% of children with DKA with a mortality rate between 20% and 40%[21]; this complication is rare in adults.[21] Changes in the patient's neurologic status may be insidious. Alterations in level of consciousness, pupil reaction, and motor function may be the result of fluctuating glucose levels and cerebral fluid shifts. Confusion and sudden complaints of headache are ominous signs that may signal cerebral edema. These observations require immediate action to prevent neurologic damage. Neurologic assessments are performed every hour or as needed during the acute phase of hyperglycemia and rehydration. Assessment of level of consciousness serves as the index of the patient's cerebral response to rehydration therapy.

Skin care. Skin care takes on new dimensions for patients with DKA. Dehydration, hypovolemia, and hypophosphatemia interfere with oxygen delivery at the cell site and contribute to inadequate perfusion and tissue breakdown. Patients must be repositioned frequently to relieve capillary pressure and promote adequate perfusion to body tissues. A typical patient with type 1 diabetes is of normal weight or underweight. Bony prominences must be assessed for tissue breakdown, and the patient's body weight must be repositioned every 1 to 2 hours. Irritation of skin from adhesive tape, shearing force, and detergents should be avoided. Maintenance of skin integrity prevents unwanted portals of entry for microorganisms.

Oral care. Care of the mouth, including toothbrushing and use of lip balm, helps keep lips supple and prevents cracking. Prepared sponge sticks or moist gauze pads can be used to moisten oral membranes of unconscious patients. Swabbing the mouth moistens the tissue and displaces the bacteria that collect when saliva, which has a bacteriostatic action, is curtailed by dehydration. Conscious patients must be provided the means to self-remove oral bacteria by toothbrushing and frequent oral rinsing.

Infection prevention. Strict sterile technique is used to maintain all IV systems. All venipuncture sites are checked every 4 hours for signs of inflammation, phlebitis, or infiltration. Strict surgical asepsis is used for all invasive procedures. Sterile technique is used if urinary catheterization is necessary to obtain urine samples for testing. Urinary catheter care is provided every 8 hours.

Patient and Family Education

It is important to be aware of the knowledge level and adherence history of patients with previously diagnosed diabetes to formulate an appropriate teaching plan (Box 23.5). Learning objectives include a discussion of target glucose levels, definition of hyperglycemia and its causes, harmful effects, symptoms, and how to manage insulin and diet when one is unwell and unable to eat. Additional objectives include a definition of DKA and its causes, symptoms, and harmful consequences. The patient and family are also expected to learn the principles of diabetes management. Universal precautions must be emphasized for all family caregivers. The patient and family must also

✵ BOX 23.5 PRIORITY PATIENT AND FAMILY EDUCATION

Diabetic Ketoacidosis

Acute Phase
- Explain rationale for critical care unit admission.
- Reduce anxiety associated with critical care unit.

Predischarge

Before discharge, the patient should be able to teach back the following topics:
- Target glucose levels
- Signs and symptoms of diabetic ketoacidosis
- Self-care monitoring of blood glucose level
- Self-care monitoring of blood ketones
- Insulin regimen
- Sick-day management
- Signs and symptoms to report to health care practitioner

learn the warning signs of DKA to report to a health care practitioner. Knowledge-based, independent self-management of blood glucose level and avoidance of diabetes-related complications are the ultimate goals of education of the patient, family, or other support persons using the teach-back method.

Hyperglycemic Hyperosmolar State

Epidemiology and Etiology. HHS is a potentially lethal complication of type 2 diabetes. The hallmarks of HHS are extremely high levels of plasma glucose with resultant elevation in serum osmolality causing osmotic diuresis. Ketosis is absent or mild. Inability to replace fluids lost through diuresis leads to profound dehydration and changes in level of consciousness. Hospitalizations for HHS account for only 1% of diabetes-related hospital admissions.[21] The HHS mortality rate is between 5% and 16%.[21] Because patients with HHS have type 2 diabetes as an underlying disorder, they are generally older adults with cardiovascular and other comorbidities as shown in the Priority Diagnostic Assessments and Nursing Interventions for HHS (Fig. 23.4).

The diagnostic criteria for HHS are as follows and as shown in Table 23.4[20]:
- Blood glucose greater than 600 mg/dL
- Arterial pH greater than 7.3
- Serum bicarbonate greater than 18 mEq/L
- Serum osmolality greater than 320 mOsm/kg H_2O (320 mmol/kg)
- Absent or mild ketonuria

Most patients with this level of metabolic disruption experience visual changes, mental status changes, and potentially hypovolemic shock.

HHS occurs when the pancreas produces an insufficient amount of insulin for the high levels of glucose that flood the bloodstream. Older adults with type 2 diabetes and cardiovascular conditions are at highest risk. Infection is the usual trigger for development of HHS; the most common infections are pneumonia and urinary tract infections.[21] Other precipitating causes of HHS include stroke, myocardial infarction, trauma, major surgery, and the physiologic stress of critical illness.

Differences Between Hyperglycemic Hyperosmolar State and Diabetic Ketoacidosis

Clinically, HHS is distinguished from DKA by the presence of extremely elevated serum glucose, more profound dehydration, and minimal or absent ketosis (see Tables 23.4 and 23.5). Another major difference is that protein and fats are not used to create new supplies of

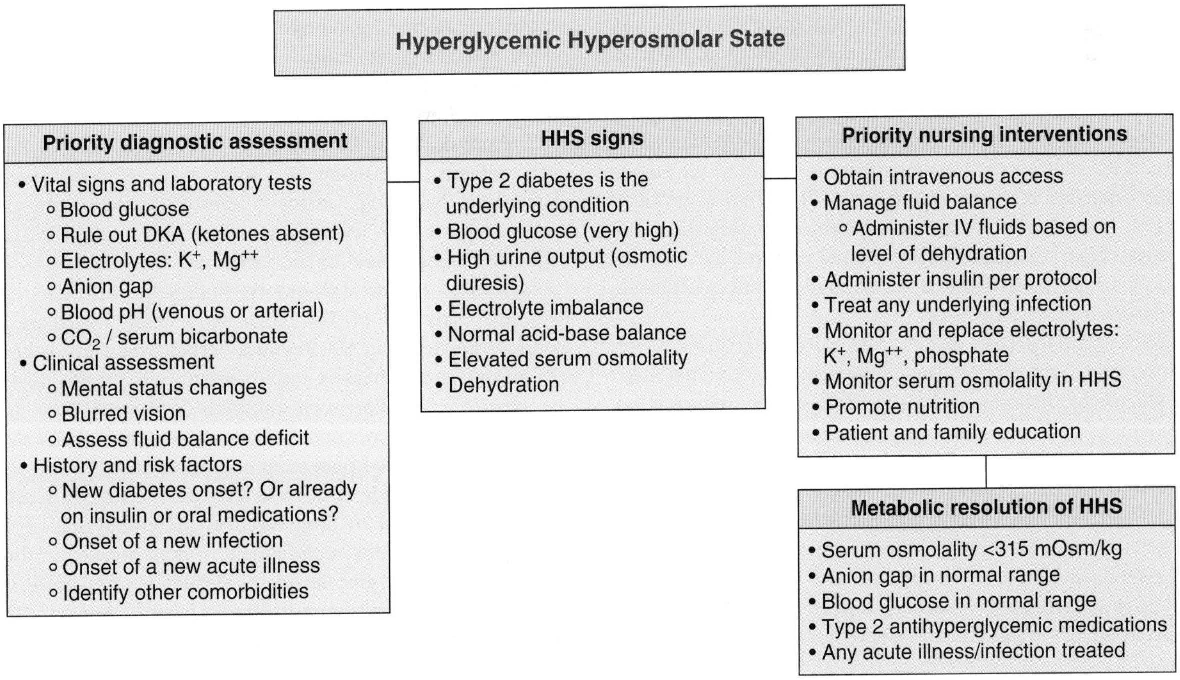

Hyperglycemic Hyperosmolar State

Priority diagnostic assessment	HHS signs	Priority nursing interventions

• Vital signs and laboratory tests
  ○ Blood glucose
  ○ Rule out DKA (ketones absent)
  ○ Electrolytes: K^+, Mg^{++}
  ○ Anion gap
  ○ Blood pH (venous or arterial)
  ○ CO_2 / serum bicarbonate
• Clinical assessment
  ○ Mental status changes
  ○ Blurred vision
  ○ Assess fluid balance deficit
• History and risk factors
  ○ New diabetes onset? Or already
    on insulin or oral medications?
  ○ Onset of a new infection
  ○ Onset of a new acute illness
  ○ Identify other comorbidities
	• Type 2 diabetes is the
	  underlying condition
	• Blood glucose (very high)
	• High urine output (osmotic
	  diuresis)
	• Electrolyte imbalance
	• Normal acid-base balance
	• Elevated serum osmolality
	• Dehydration
		• Obtain intravenous access
		• Manage fluid balance
		  ○ Administer IV fluids based on
		    level of dehydration
		• Administer insulin per protocol
		• Treat any underlying infection
		• Monitor and replace electrolytes:
		  K^+, Mg^{++}, phosphate
		• Monitor serum osmolality in HHS
		• Promote nutrition
		• Patient and family education

Metabolic resolution of HHS
- Serum osmolality <315 mOsm/kg
- Anion gap in normal range
- Blood glucose in normal range
- Type 2 antihyperglycemic medications
- Any acute illness/infection treated

Fig. 23.4 Priority Diagnostic and Nursing Interventions for Hyperglycemic Hyperosmolar State. *CO₂*, Carbon dioxide; *DKA*, diabetic ketoacidosis; *HHS*, hyperglycemic hyperosmolar state; *IV*, intravenous; *K⁺*, potassium; *Mg⁺⁺*, magnesium; *mOsmo/kg*, milliosmoles per kilogram of water; *pH*, a measure of the degree to which a solution is acidic or alkaline.

TABLE 23.5 Comparison of Diabetic Ketoacidosis and Hyperglycemic Hyperosmolar State.

Characteristics and Laboratory Tests	DKA	HHS
Characteristics		
Cause	Insufficient exogenous glucose for glucose needs	Insufficient exogenous/endogenous insulin for glucose needs
Onset	Sudden (hours)	Slow, insidious (days, weeks)
Precipitating factors	Noncompliance with type 1 diabetes therapy, illness, surgery, decreased activity	Recent acute illness in older patient; therapeutic procedures
Mortality (%)	9–14	10–50
Patients affected	Patients with type 1 diabetes	Patients with type 2 diabetes
Clinical manifestations	Dry mouth, polydipsia, polyuria, polyphagia, dehydration, dry skin, hypotension, weakness	Mental confusion, tachycardia, changes in level of consciousness
	Ketoacidosis, air hunger, acetone breath odor, respirations deep and rapid, nausea, vomiting	No ketosis, no breath odor, respirations rapid and shallow, usually mild nausea/vomiting
Laboratory Tests		
Glucose (mg/dL)	300–800	600–2000
Ketones	Strongly positive	Normal or mildly elevated
pH	<7.3	Normal[a]
Osmolality (mOsm/L)	<350	>350
Sodium	Normal or low	Normal or elevated
Potassium (K+)	Normal, low, or elevated (total body K+ depleted)	Low, normal, or elevated
Bicarbonate	<15 mEq/L	Normal
Phosphorus	Low, normal, or elevated (may decrease after insulin therapy)	Low, normal, or elevated (may decrease after insulin therapy)
Urine acetone	Strong	Absent or mild

[a]Exception: In severe HHS, lactic acidosis may develop as a result of dehydration and severe tissue hypoperfusion and ischemia.
DKA, Diabetic ketoacidosis; *HHS,* hyperglycemic hyperosmolar state.

glucose in HHS as they are in DKA; as a result, the ketotic cycle is never started or does not occur until the blood glucose level is extremely elevated.

Pathophysiology

HHS represents a deficit of insulin and an excess of glucagon. Reduced insulin levels prevent the movement of glucose into the cells, allowing glucose to accumulate in the plasma. The decreased insulin triggers glucagon release from the liver, and hepatic glucose is poured into the circulation. As the number of glucose particles increases in the blood, serum hyperosmolality increases. To decrease the serum osmolality, fluid is drawn from the intracellular compartment (inside the cells) into the extracellular vascular fluid. Profound intracellular volume depletion occurs if the patient's thirst sensation is absent or decreased. HHS may evolve over days or weeks.[20]

Hemoconcentration persists despite removal of large amounts of glucose in the urine (glycosuria). The glomerular filtration and elimination of glucose by the kidney tubules is ineffective in reducing the serum glucose level sufficiently to maintain normal glucose levels. The hyperosmolality and reduced blood volume stimulate release of ADH to increase the tubular resorption of water. However, ADH is powerless to overcome the osmotic pull exerted by the glucose load. Excessive fluid volume is lost at the kidney tubule, with simultaneous loss of potassium, sodium, and phosphate in the urine. This chain of events results in progressively worsening hypovolemia. Ketosis is absent or mild in HHS.[20] Kussmaul air hunger does not occur in HHS.

Focused Physical Assessment and Diagnosis

Clinical manifestations. HHS has a slow, subtle onset and develops over several days. Initially, the symptoms may be nonspecific and may be ignored or attributed to the patient's concurrent disease processes. History reveals malaise, blurred vision, polyuria, polydipsia (depending on the patient's thirst sensation), weight loss, and increasing weakness. Progressive dehydration follows and leads to mental confusion, convulsions, and eventually coma, especially in older patients.

The physical examination may reveal a profound fluid deficit. In older patients, assessment of clinical signs of dehydration can be challenging. Neurologic status is affected as the serum glucose increases, especially at levels greater than 1500 mg/dL. Without intervention, decreased level of conscious and coma occur.

Laboratory studies. Laboratory studies are used to establish a definitive diagnosis of HHS. Plasma glucose levels are strikingly elevated (greater than 600 mg/dL). Serum osmolality is greater than 320 mOsm/kg. Acidosis is absent (arterial pH greater than 7.3), and the serum bicarbonate concentration is greater than 18 mEq/L. Ketonuria is absent or mild.[20] The patient may have an elevated hematocrit and depleted potassium and phosphorus levels.

Point-of-care fingerstick or arterial line testing of glucose at the bedside is the usual method for frequent monitoring of the serum blood glucose. Insulin replacement is prescribed according to the blood glucose result. If point-of-care testing is unavailable, traditional serial laboratory tests keep the critical care team apprised of the fluctuating serum electrolyte levels and provide the basis for electrolyte replacement. Intracellular potassium and phosphate levels usually are depleted because of prior osmotic diuresis.[20] Metabolic acidosis usually is absent at lower glucose levels.

Medical Management

The goals of medical management are rapid rehydration, insulin replacement, and correction of electrolyte abnormalities, specifically potassium replacement. The underlying stimulus of HHS must be discovered and treated. The same basic principles used to treat DKA are used for patients with HHS.

Rapid rehydration. The primary intervention for HHS is rapid rehydration to restore the intravascular volume. The fluid deficit may be 150 mL/kg of body weight. The average 150-lb adult can lose more than 7 to 10 L of fluid. Physiologic saline solution (0.9%) is infused at 1 L/h, especially for a patient in hypovolemic shock if there is no cardiovascular contraindication. Several liters of volume replacement may be required to achieve a BP and central venous pressure (CVP) within normal range. Infusion volumes are adjusted according to the patient's hydration state and sodium level.[20]

Serum sodium concentration is the parameter that is monitored to determine whether to change from isotonic (0.9%) to hypotonic (0.45%) saline. For example, patients with sodium levels equal to or less than 140 mEq/L may be given 0.9% normal saline solution, whereas patients with levels greater than 140 mEq/L are given 0.45% saline solution (see Fig. 23.2).[20] It is difficult to assess the serum sodium level in the presence of hemoconcentration. Another recommendation is to calculate a *corrected sodium value.* This involves adding 1.6 mEq to the sodium laboratory value for each 100 mg/dL plasma glucose above normal.[20] Sodium input should not exceed the amount required to replace the losses. Careful monitoring of the serum sodium level is recommended to avoid a sodium-water imbalance and hemolysis as the hemoconcentration is reduced.

Insulin administration. Volume resuscitation lowers the serum glucose level and improves symptoms even without insulin administration. However, insulin replacement is recommended in the treatment of HHS because acidosis can develop if insulin is withheld, and insulin facilitates the cellular use of glucose.

Methods to lower the blood glucose level vary in HHS. One method is to administer an IV bolus of regular insulin (0.15 unit/kg of body weight) initially, followed by a continuous insulin drip. Regular insulin, infusing at an initial rate calculated as 0.1 unit/kg hourly (e.g., 7 units/h for a person weighing 70 kg) should lower the plasma glucose concentration by 50 to 70 mg/dL during the first hour of treatment. If the measured glucose level does not decrease by this amount, the insulin infusion rate may be doubled until the blood glucose is declining at a rate of 50 to 70 mg/dL each hour[20] or as listed in the local hospital protocol.

Insulin resistance. Type 2 diabetes is manifested not only by hyperglycemia but also by insulin resistance. HHS often develops secondary to an illness such as pneumonia or sepsis. In HHS, circulating counter-regulatory hormones, also known as *stress hormones* (cortisol, glucagon, epinephrine), increase blood glucose. Patients with HHS often require high doses of insulin initially to overcome the hyperglycemia and insulin resistance. Hourly serial monitoring of the blood glucose level permits safe glycemic management and avoids the most common complication, which is hypoglycemia caused by overzealous insulin administration.[20] After the patient has recovered from the hyperglycemic crisis and insulin has been discontinued, oral medications designed to decrease insulin resistance are individualized to the patient with type 2 diabetes (see Tables 23.2 and 23.3).

Electrolyte replacement. Increasing the circulating levels of insulin with therapeutic doses of IV insulin promotes the rapid return of potassium and phosphorus into the cell. Serial laboratory tests keep the clinician apprised of the serum electrolyte levels and provide the basis for electrolyte replacement. Potassium typically is added to the IV infusion (see Fig. 23.2). If the serum potassium concentration is lower than 3.3 mEq/L, it is essential to replenish the serum potassium before giving insulin.[20] Many hospitals have potassium replacement algorithms that are used to treat hypokalemia. Serum phosphate levels are carefully monitored, and phosphate is replaced if the level is lower than 1.0 mg/dL.[20]

Nursing Management

Nursing management of a patient with HHS incorporates a variety of patient diagnoses (Box 23.6). Priority nursing interventions are similar to the goals outlined for DKA. The critical care nurse administers prescribed fluids, insulin, and electrolytes; monitors the response to therapy; maintains surveillance for complications; and provides patient education.

Administering fluids, insulin, and electrolytes. Rigorous fluid replacement and continuous IV insulin replacement must be controlled with an electronic volumetric pump. Accurate I&O measurements are maintained to monitor fluid balance including the total of all fluids administered minus hourly losses, such as urine output and emesis. If the patient is alert, the fluid and electrolytes are replenished orally and via a peripheral IV line. If the patient manifests signs of hypovolemic shock, hemodynamic monitoring may include use of an arterial line and CVP measurements. Arterial line access is very helpful in monitoring serial blood glucose and electrolyte values. The use of a blood conservation system on the arterial line is essential to avoid iatrogenic exsanguination of the patient. Most critical care units have developed protocols or guidelines to ensure that patients in hyperglycemic crisis are managed safely (see Fig. 23.2). The major responsibility for delivery of insulin, hourly monitoring of blood glucose, and infusion of appropriate crystalloid solutions lies with the critical care nurse (Box 23.7). Many hospitals mandate a double-check procedure for medications such as insulin that have the potential to cause harm if wrongly administered.

Monitoring response to therapy. BP and HR are monitored to evaluate the degree of dehydration, the effectiveness of hydration therapy, and the patient's fluid tolerance. Because patients with HHS have underlying type 2 diabetes and, if older, are also likely to have preexisting illnesses such as heart failure and kidney failure, it is important to monitor for symptoms of circulatory overload. Symptoms to anticipate include tachycardia, bounding pulse, dyspnea, tachypnea,

---

◎ BOX 23.6 PRIORITY PATIENT CARE MANAGEMENT

Hyperglycemic Hyperosmolar State

- Risk for Infection
- Hypovolemia due to absolute loss
- Anxiety due to threat to biologic, psychologic, or social integrity
- Powerlessness due to lack of control over current situation or disease progression
- Lack of Knowledge of Treatment Regime due to previous lack of exposure to information (see Box 23.8, Priority Patient and Family Education for Hyperglycemic Hyperosmolar State)

Patient Care Management plans are located in Appendix A.

BOX 23.7 Hyperglycemia Prevention and Management

Hyperglycemia Definition: Plasma Blood Glucose Above 180 mg/dL

- Two serial blood glucose values above 180 mg/dL are evidence of hyperglycemia in critical care.
- Blood glucose target in critical care is between 150 and 180 mg/dL.

Hyperglycemia Prevention

- In a patient with hyperglycemia without a preexisting history of diabetes, the likely causes are hyperglycemia associated with critical illness or undiagnosed prediabetes.
- Type 1 diabetes: A preexisting diagnosis of type 1 diabetes means the patient can never be without insulin coverage. IV or subcutaneous insulin must always be provided and blood glucose checked frequently.
- Type 2 diabetes: A preexisting diagnosis of type 2 diabetes means the patient will have an elevated blood glucose when oral medications are stopped. Some patients with type 2 diabetes also have subcutaneous insulin. Hyperglycemia is prevented by use of subcutaneous or IV insulin.
- Use normal saline in IV infusions.
- Monitor blood glucose per hospital protocol.

Hyperglycemia: Clinical Signs and Symptoms

- Hyperglycemia with a history of type 1 diabetes is generally caused by lack of insulin leading to DKA. Symptoms associated with alteration in level of consciousness range from confusion to coma, with dehydration and ketoacidosis.
- Hyperglycemia with a history of type 2 diabetes is often associated with infection leading to HHS, which may take days to weeks to develop. HHS is associated with alteration in level of consciousness and extreme dehydration. Acidosis can develop in HHS when blood glucose levels are extremely high.

Hyperglycemia Management

- Identify the reason for the hyperglycemia (critical illness stress induced, DKA, HHS). Management varies according to the cause. It is essential to also treat the underlying medical/surgical cause of admission to critical care.
- Administer IV insulin according to hospital protocol, with hourly monitoring of blood glucose during the acute phase of hyperglycemia.
- Rehydrate according to hospital protocol and laboratory values.
- Replenish electrolytes according to hospital protocol and laboratory values.

DKA, Diabetic ketoacidosis; *HHS,* hyperglycemic, hyperosmolar syndrome; *IV,* intravenous.
Data from Jacobi J, Bircher N, Krinsley J, et al. Guidelines for the use of an insulin infusion for the management of hyperglycemia in critically ill patients. *Crit Care Med.* 2012;40(12):3251–3276; Kitabchi AE, Umpierrez GE, Miles JM, Fisher JN. Hyperglycemic crises in adult patients with diabetes. *Diabetes Care.* 2009;32(7):1335.

✳ BOX 23.8 PRIORITY PATIENT AND FAMILY EDUCATION

Hyperglycemic Hyperosmolar State

Acute Phase

- Explain rationale for critical care unit admission.

Predischarge

Before discharge, the patient should be able to teach back the following topics:
- Causes of hyperglycemic hyperosmotic state
- Self-care for type 2 diabetes, including medications
- Signs and symptoms to report to health care practitioner

Surveillance for complications. The potential complications of HHS are similar to the complications described for DKA and include hypoglycemia, hypokalemia or hyperkalemia, and infection. A patient with HHS is at risk for other complications specific to associated disease entities. A history of cardiovascular, pulmonary, or kidney disease, whether known or latent, places the patient with HHS at high risk for complications. Because HHS is an acute condition superimposed on the chronic health problem of type 2 diabetes, many health professionals work collaboratively to restore homeostasis.[25]

Patient and Family Education

As the patient's condition improves and the patient demonstrates readiness to learn, education about type 2 diabetes and avoiding a recurrence of HHS becomes a priority (Box 23.8). Most teaching occurs after the patient has left the critical care unit. Teaching topics include a description of type 2 diabetes and how it relates to HHS, dietary restrictions, exercise requirements, medication protocols, home testing of blood glucose, signs and symptoms of hyperglycemia and hypoglycemia, foot care, and lifestyle modifications.

PITUITARY GLAND DISORDERS

Two disorders of the pituitary gland are discussed in this chapter: diabetes insipidus (DI) and syndrome of inappropriate antidiuretic hormone (SIADH) secretion. Both are caused by disruptions in the release of ADH, also known as arginine vasopressin (AVP) or as vasopressin. DI and SIADH are clinical opposites. In DI, there is inadequate or no ADH released from the posterior pituitary. In SIADH, excess ADH is released from the pituitary or from another source (often malignancy-related) elsewhere in the body. These two conditions can be long-term chronic conditions or can occur in critical care as acute complications of other disorders. The focus in this chapter is on the acute presentation and management in critical care.

DIABETES INSIPIDUS

DI is recognized clinically by the vast quantities of very dilute urine that is produced in susceptible patients. In a critically ill patient, the extreme diuresis is most likely to be caused by a lack of ADH (vasopressin). This causes extreme dehydration due to extreme fluid loss. Any patient who has sustained a head trauma or had resection of a pituitary tumor has an increased risk of developing DI.

ADH is produced in the hypothalamus and stored in the posterior pituitary gland. Normally, ADH is released in response to even small

lung crackles, and engorged neck veins. The astute critical care nurse is aware of the clinical manifestations of fluid overload and observes for potential complications when rehydrating a patient with HHS and diseases involving the heart, lungs, or kidneys.

The serum glucose level should decrease by 50 to 70 mg/dL each hour with insulin administration.[20] This decrease is monitored by hourly blood glucose determinations. Based on the result, the critical care nurse can alter the infusion of insulin according to the local hospital protocol (see Fig. 23.2).

elevations in serum osmolality, and secondarily in reaction to hypovolemia or hypotension.

DI can occur if (1) the hypothalamus produces insufficient ADH, (2) the posterior pituitary fails to release ADH, or (3) the kidney nephron is resistant (unresponsive) to ADH.[26,27]

BOX 23.9 Causes of Diabetes Insipidus

Central Diabetes Insipidus

Primary Diabetes Insipidus (Rare in Critical Care)
- Antidiuretic hormone (ADH) deficiency caused by hypothalamic-hypophyseal malformation
- Congenital defect
- Idiopathic

Secondary Diabetes Insipidus (Most Common in Critical Care)
- ADH deficiency caused by damage to hypothalamic-hypophyseal system
- Trauma
- Infection
- Surgery
- Primary neoplasms
- Metastatic malignancies

Nephrogenic Diabetes Insipidus
- Inability of kidney tubules to respond to circulating ADH
- Decrease or absence of ADH receptors
- Cellular damage to nephron, especially loop of Henle
- Kidney damage (e.g., hydronephrosis, pyelonephritis, polycystic kidney)
- Untoward response to medication therapy (e.g., lithium carbonate, demeclocycline)

Dipsogenic Diabetes Insipidus
- Rare form of water intoxication
- Compulsive water drinking

Etiology

DI is divided into three types according to cause: central, nephrogenic, and dipsogenic (Box 23.9). Only central DI, also known as neurogenic DI because of its association with the brain, is encountered with any frequency in the critical care unit. The Priority Diagnostic Assessments and Nursing Interventions for Diabetes Insipidus are shown in Fig. 23.5.

Central Diabetes Insipidus

In central DI, an inadequate amount of ADH (AVP) results in inappropriately dilute urine.[26] In critical care, the most likely acute cause of central DI is neurosurgery, traumatic head injury, tumors, increased intracranial pressure (ICP), brain death, and infections such as encephalitis or meningitis. DI is seen with brain death 50% of the time,[26] and with traumatic brain injury in 20% to 30% of cases.[26]

Pathophysiology

The purpose of ADH is to maintain normal serum osmolality and circulating blood volume. Although there are several types of DI, this discussion focuses on neurogenic (central) DI, the condition encountered in the critical care unit after neurosurgery or head injury. In DI, the urine osmolality and specific gravity decrease (dilute urine). At the same time, in the bloodstream, the serum sodium concentration and serum osmolality increase. In a patient with decreased level of consciousness, the polyuria, if untreated, leads to severe hypernatremia, dehydration, decreased cerebral perfusion, seizures, loss of consciousness, and death.

Focused Physical Assessment and Diagnosis
Clinical Manifestations

The diagnosis is based on the increase in dilute urine output occurring in the absence of diuretics, a fluid challenge, or hyperglycemia. Central DI is anticipated in conditions in which the underlying disease process is likely to disrupt pituitary function.[26] Central DI that occurs because of increasing ICP is life-threatening, and it is imperative that the underlying condition causing ICP elevation be recognized and treated.

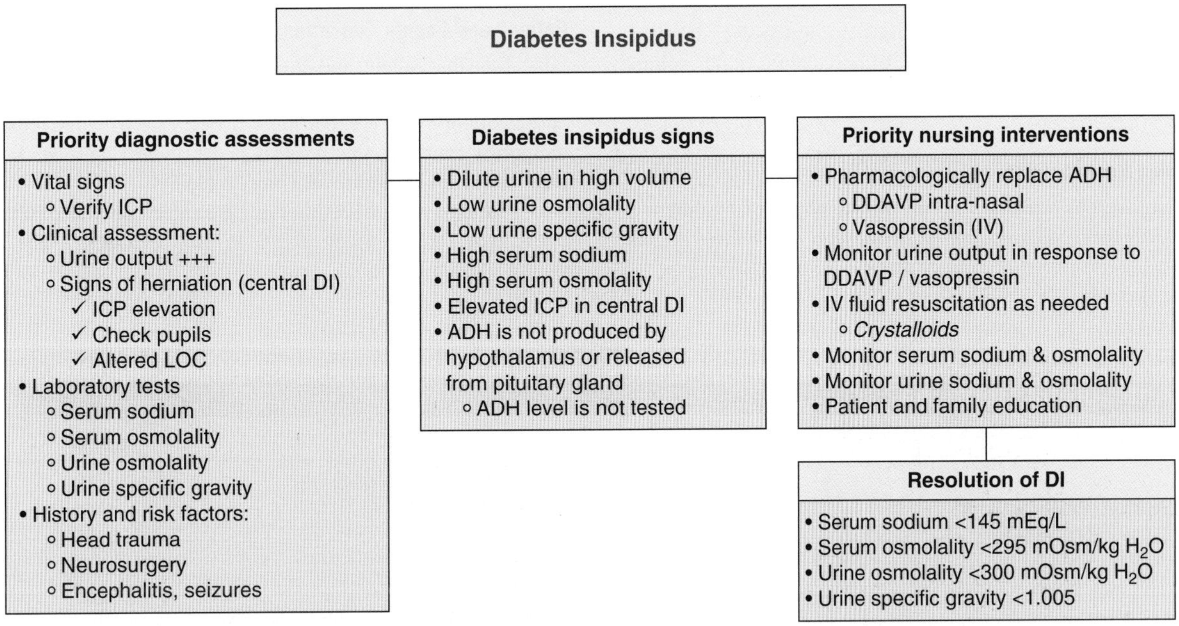

Diabetes Insipidus

Priority diagnostic assessments	Diabetes insipidus signs	Priority nursing interventions

• Vital signs
  ○ Verify ICP
• Clinical assessment:
  ○ Urine output +++
  ○ Signs of herniation (central DI)
    ✓ ICP elevation
    ✓ Check pupils
    ✓ Altered LOC
• Laboratory tests
  ○ Serum sodium
  ○ Serum osmolality
  ○ Urine osmolality
  ○ Urine specific gravity
• History and risk factors:
  ○ Head trauma
  ○ Neurosurgery
  ○ Encephalitis, seizures
	• Dilute urine in high volume
	• Low urine osmolality
	• Low urine specific gravity
	• High serum sodium
	• High serum osmolality
	• Elevated ICP in central DI
	• ADH is not produced by hypothalamus or released from pituitary gland
	  ○ ADH level is not tested
		• Pharmacologically replace ADH
		  ○ DDAVP intra-nasal
		  ○ Vasopressin (IV)
		• Monitor urine output in response to DDAVP / vasopressin
		• IV fluid resuscitation as needed
		  ○ *Crystalloids*
		• Monitor serum sodium & osmolality
		• Monitor urine sodium & osmolality
		• Patient and family education

Resolution of DI
• Serum sodium <145 mEq/L • Serum osmolality <295 mOsm/kg H$_2$O • Urine osmolality <300 mOsm/kg H$_2$O • Urine specific gravity <1.005

Fig. 23.5 Priority Diagnostic and Nursing Interventions for Diabetes Insipidus. *ADH,* Antidiuretic hormone; *DDAVP,* desmopressin acetate (synthetic analog of vasopressin); *DI,* diabetes insipidus; *ICP,* intracranial pressure; *IV,* intravenous; *LOC,* level of consciousness; *mEq/L,* milliequivalents per liter; *mOsmo/kg,* milliosmoles per kilogram of water.

Laboratory Studies

The diagnostic tests used to establish the presence of DI and evaluate the body's ability to balance fluid and electrolytes are not specific to the endocrine system. The specific tests are serum sodium, serum osmolality, and urine osmolality (Table 23.6). The combination of an obvious clinical picture of high volumes of hypotonic urine (greater than 3 L urine output/24 h) in the presence of these laboratory criteria, is sufficient to diagnose central DI[26,28]:

- Serum sodium level greater than 145 mEq/L
- Serum osmolality greater than 295 mOsm/kg H_2O (greater than 295 mmol/L)
- Urine osmolality less than 300 mOsm/kg H_2O (less than 300 mmol/L)
- Urine specific gravity less than 1.005

Serum sodium. The normal serum sodium concentration is 140 mEq/L (range, 135−145 mEq/L). In central DI, the serum sodium level can rise precipitously because of the loss of free water. Hypernatremia is usually associated with serum hyperosmolality.

Serum osmolality. Serum osmolality has a range of 275 to 295 mOsm/kg H_2O. Severe DI can increase serum osmolality to greater than 320 mOsm/kg H_2O. Normal values vary slightly between clinical laboratories (e.g., 280−295 mOsm/kg H_2O).[29,30]

Urine osmolality. Urine is dilute and urine osmolality is less than 300 mOsm/kg H_2O (300 mmol/L) in patients with central DI.[28] For accuracy, the urine sample should be collected and tested simultaneously with the blood sample. This test is rarely performed in the critical care unit.

Antidiuretic hormone measurement. Measurement of the baseline serum ADH level is an additional diagnostic step. This is not typically performed in critical care if the clinical circumstances (e.g., head injury with increased ICP) make further testing unnecessary.

Copeptin. Copeptin is co-released with ADH from the posterior pituitary gland. Unlike ADH, copeptin is stable in plasma, facilitating reliable measurements.[31] After pituitary surgery, copeptin levels below 2.5 pmol/L had a specificity of 97% for a diagnosis of DI.[26]

Medical Management

Immediate management of DI requires an aggressive approach. Treatment goals include restoration of circulating fluid volume, pharmacologic ADH replacement, and treatment of the underlying condition.[26]

Fluid Volume Restoration

Fluid replacement is provided in the initial phase of treatment to prevent circulatory collapse. For patients who are unable to take sufficient fluids orally, IV solutions are infused and carefully monitored to restore the hemodynamic balance.

Medications

The most prescribed medication for DI is the synthetic analog of ADH, *desmopressin* (DDAVP). DDAVP can be given intravenously, subcutaneously, or as a nasal spray with dosage titrated according to the patient's antidiuretic response. The urine output is recorded hourly to evaluate the response to the medication.

To avoid a medication error, it is important to be aware that DDAVP is also used to manage other conditions, including hemorrhage caused by platelet disorders, and that the dose ranges for these conditions are different. Medications to manage DI are listed in Table 23.7.

Nursing Management

Nursing management of a patient with DI incorporates a variety of patient diagnoses (Box 23.10). Priority nursing interventions are directed toward administration of prescribed fluids and medications, evaluation of response to therapy, surveillance for complications, and provision of patient and family education.

Administration of Fluids

Rapid IV fluid replacement requires the use of a volumetric pump. Initially, a hypotonic IV solution is used to replace fluids lost and reduce the serum hyperosmolality. With any signs of cardiovascular impairment, fluid intake is restricted until urine specific gravity is less than 1.015 and a normal urine output is resumed.

Critical assessment and management of fluid status are the most important initial concerns for patients with DI. Monitoring of HR, BP, and when available CVP, provides early indications of response to fluid volume replacement. I&O measurement, condition of buccal membranes, skin turgor, daily weight measurements, presence of thirst, and temperature provide a basic assessment list that is vital for the patient who is unable to regulate fluid needs and losses. Placement of a urinary catheter may be required to monitor the urinary output accurately.

Patient and Family Education

Educating the patient and the family about the disease process and how it affects thirst, urination, and fluid balance encourages patients to participate in their care. For most critical care patients, central DI is a temporary condition that resolves as the underlying medical condition (e.g., brain injury) improves (Box 23.11).

In patients who have undergone surgery on the pituitary gland, permanent DI can occur in 2% to 10% of cases.[28] The degree of

TABLE 23.6   Laboratory Values in Diabetes Insipidus and Syndrome of Inappropriate Antidiuretic Hormone.

Value	Normal	DI	SIADH
Serum ADH	1−5 pg/mL	Decreased in central DI	Elevated
Serum osmolality (mOsm/L)	275−295	>295	<270
Serum sodium (mEq/L)	135−145	>145	<120
Urine osmolality (mOsm/L)	300−1400	<300	Increased
Urine specific gravity	1.005−1.030	<1.005	>1.030
Urine output	1.0−1.5 L/day	1.0−1.5 L/h	Below normal

Use of diuretics negates the reliability of urine sodium and urine osmolality levels.
ADH, Antidiuretic hormone; *DI,* diabetes insipidus; *SIADH,* syndrome of inappropriate antidiuretic hormone.

TABLE 23.7 Pharmacologic Management Diabetes Insipidus.

Medication	Dosage	Actions	Special Considerations
Central Diabetes Insipidus			
DDAVP (available as IV injection, as nasal spray, rhinal tube)	Nasal: 10–40 mcg single dose or in divided doses Parenteral[a]: 2–4 mcg twice daily	Central DI Antidiuretic Increases water resorption in nephron Prevents and controls polydipsia, polyuria	Few side effects Observe for nasal congestion, upper respiratory infection, allergic rhinitis Monitor intake and output, urine osmolality, serum sodium level
Vasopressin (Pitressin)	IV, IM, subcutaneous Topical: nasal mucosa	Central DI antidiuretic Promotes resorption of water at kidney tubule Decreases urine output Increases urine osmolality Diagnostic aid Increases gastrointestinal peristalsis	Monitor fluid volume often, especially in older patients Assess cardiac status May precipitate angina, hypertension, or myocardial infarction if increased dosage is given to patient with cardiac history Parenteral extravasation can cause skin necrosis
Lypressin (Diapid)	Intranasal: 1–2 sprays (7–14 mcg) in each nostril four times daily	Central DI Synthetic ADH Increases resorption of sodium and water in nephron	Proper instillation is important for absorption and action Patient sits upright while holding bottle upright for administration Repeat sprays (>2–3) are ineffective and wasteful; if dosage is increased to two to three sprays, shorten time between dosing Cough, chest tightness, shortness of breath
Nephrogenic Diabetes Insipidus			
Thiazide diuretics	Varies according to diuretic chosen, patient's size, and age	Nephrogenic DI Leads to mild fluid depletion Increases resorption of water and sodium in proximal nephron; less fluid travels to distal nephron, excreting less water	Varies according to diuretic chosen
Dipsogenic Diabetes Insipidus			
Anticompulsive disorder medications, anxiolytics, psychopharmacologic agents	Dosage varies	Dipsogenic DI	Varies according to medication chosen

[a]IV or subcutaneous administration.
ADH, Antidiuretic hormone; *DDAVP*, desmopressin acetate; *DI*, diabetes insipidus; *IM*, intramuscular; *IV*, intravenous.

BOX 23.10 PRIORITY PATIENT CARE MANAGEMENT

Diabetes Insipidus

- Impaired Cardiac Output due to alterations in preload
- Hypovolemia due to absolute loss
- Lack of Knowledge of Treatment Regime due to lack of previous exposure to information (see Box 23.11, Priority Patient and Family Education for Diabetes Insipidus)

Patient Care Management plans are located in Appendix A.

hormone replacement required after surgery depends on the quantity of pituitary tissue that has been surgically or endoscopically removed.

Patients who are discharged with DI are taught, along with their families, the signs, and symptoms of dehydration and overhydration and procedures for accurate daily weight and urine specific gravity measurements. Printed information pertaining to medication actions, side effects, dosages, and timetable is provided along with an outline of factors to report to their clinical team.

Collaborative Management

Central DI is a life-threatening condition. The collaborative assessment and clinical skills of all health care professionals and use of a clear plan of care are essential to achieve optimal outcomes for each patient.

SYNDROME OF INAPPROPRIATE SECRETION OF ANTIDIURETIC HORMONE

The opposing syndrome to DI is SIADH, which manifests as a dilutional hyponatremia.[30] A patient with SIADH has an excess of ADH secreted into the bloodstream, much more than the amount needed to maintain normal blood volume and serum osmolality. Excessive water is reabsorbed at the kidney tubule, leading to dilutional hyponatremia.[30]

Etiology

SIADH can be precipitated by many conditions as described in Box 23.12. Specifically, CNS injury, tumors, and any diseases that interfere with the normal functioning of the hypothalamic-pituitary system can cause SIADH. An ectopic cause is malignant bronchogenic small cell carcinoma.[30] This type of malignant cell is capable of synthesizing and

✳ BOX 23.11 PRIORITY PATIENT AND FAMILY EDUCATION

Diabetes Insipidus

Acute Phase

- Explain rationale for critical care unit admission.

Predischarge

Before discharge, the patient should be able to teach back the following topics:

- Patient-specific cause of diabetes insipidus
- Measurement of fluid intake and output
- Urine specific gravity
- Causes of diabetes insipidus
- Disease process of diabetes insipidus
- Nutritional information to prevent constipation and diarrhea
- Medications: explain purpose, side effects, dosage, and how often to use
- Signs and symptoms to report to health care professional

releasing ADH regardless of the body's needs. The Priority Diagnostic and Nursing Interventions for SIADH are described in Fig. 23.6.

Pathophysiology

ADH regulates water and electrolyte balance in the body. In SIADH, profound fluid and electrolyte disturbances result from the continuous release of the ADH hormone into the bloodstream. Excessive ADH stimulates the kidney tubules to retain fluid regardless of need.

Excessive ADH and overhydration cause a severe dilutional hyponatremia and reduce the sodium concentration to critically low levels. Without ADH water is retained, urine output is diminished, and more sodium is excreted in the urine.

Focused Physical Assessment and Diagnosis
Clinical Manifestations

The clinical manifestations of SIADH relate to the excess circulating volume and the dilution of the circulating sodium. Edema usually is not present. Early clinical manifestations of dilutional hyponatremia include lethargy, anorexia, nausea, and vomiting. Symptoms of severe

BOX 23.12 Causes of Syndrome of Inappropriate Secretion of Antidiuretic Hormone

Malignant Disease Associated With Autonomous Production of Antidiuretic Hormone

- Bronchogenic small cell carcinoma
- Pancreatic adenocarcinoma
- Duodenal, bladder, ureter, and prostatic carcinomas
- Lymphosarcoma, Ewing sarcoma
- Acute leukemia, Hodgkin disease
- Cerebral neoplasm, thymoma

Central Nervous System Diseases That Interfere With Hypothalamic-Hypophyseal System and Increase Production or Release of Antidiuretic Hormone

- Head injury
- Brain abscess
- Hydrocephalus
- Pituitary adenoma
- Subdural hematoma
- Subarachnoid hemorrhage
- Cerebral atrophy
- Guillain-Barré syndrome

Neurogenic Stimuli Capable of Increasing Antidiuretic Hormone

- Decreased glomerular filtration rate
- Physical or emotional stress
- Pain
- Fear
- Trauma
- Surgery
- Myocardial infarction
- Acute infection
- Hypotension
- Hemorrhage
- Hypovolemia

Pulmonary Diseases Believed to Stimulate Baroreceptors and Increase Antidiuretic Hormone

- Pulmonary tuberculosis
- Viral and bacterial pneumonia
- Empyema
- Lung abscess

- Chronic obstructive lung disease
- Status asthmaticus
- Cystic fibrosis

Endocrine Disturbances That Hormonally Influence Antidiuretic Hormone

- Myxedema
- Hypothyroidism
- Hypopituitarism
- Adrenal insufficiency—Addison disease

Medications That Mimic, Increase Release of, or Potentiate Antidiuretic Hormone

- Hypoglycemics
  - Insulin
  - Tolbutamide
  - Chlorpropamide
- Potassium-depleting thiazide diuretics
- Tricyclic antidepressants
  - Imipramine
  - Amitriptyline
- Phenothiazine
  - Fluphenazine
  - Thioridazine
- Thioxanthenes
  - Thiothixene
  - Chlorprothixene
- Chemotherapeutic agents
  - Vincristine
  - Cyclophosphamide
- Opiates
- Carbamazepine
- Clofibrate
- Acetaminophen
- Nicotine
- Oxytocin
- Vasopressin
- Anesthetics

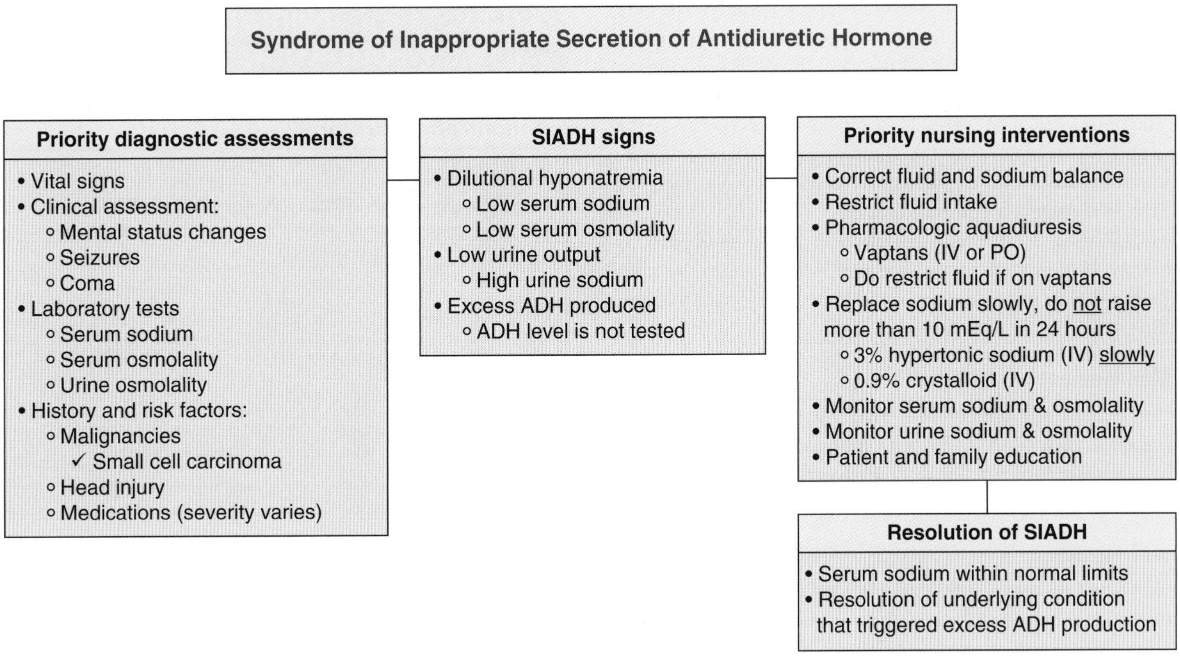

Syndrome of Inappropriate Secretion of Antidiuretic Hormone

Priority diagnostic assessments	SIADH signs	Priority nursing interventions

• Vital signs
• Clinical assessment:
  ○ Mental status changes
  ○ Seizures
  ○ Coma
• Laboratory tests
  ○ Serum sodium
  ○ Serum osmolality
  ○ Urine osmolality
• History and risk factors:
  ○ Malignancies
    ✓ Small cell carcinoma
  ○ Head injury
  ○ Medications (severity varies)
	• Dilutional hyponatremia
	  ○ Low serum sodium
	  ○ Low serum osmolality
	• Low urine output
	  ○ High urine sodium
	• Excess ADH produced
	  ○ ADH level is not tested
		• Correct fluid and sodium balance
		• Restrict fluid intake
		• Pharmacologic aquadiuresis
		  ○ Vaptans (IV or PO)
		  ○ Do restrict fluid if on vaptans
		• Replace sodium slowly, do <u>not</u> raise
		  more than 10 mEq/L in 24 hours
		  ○ 3% hypertonic sodium (IV) <u>slowly</u>
		  ○ 0.9% crystalloid (IV)
		• Monitor serum sodium & osmolality
		• Monitor urine sodium & osmolality
		• Patient and family education

Resolution of SIADH

- Serum sodium within normal limits
- Resolution of underlying condition that triggered excess ADH production

Fig. 23.6 Priority Diagnostic and Nursing Interventions for Syndrome of Inappropriate Secretion of Antidiuretic Hormone. *ADH*, Antidiuretic hormone; *IV*, intravenous; *SIADH*, syndrome of inappropriate secretion of antidiuretic hormone.

hyponatremia include inability to concentrate, mental confusion, apprehension, seizures, decreased level of consciousness, coma, and death. Severe neurologic symptoms usually do not develop until the serum sodium concentration is less than 120 mEq/L.

Laboratory Values

Patients with SIADH present with very dilute serum, hyponatremia, and concentrated urine. Laboratory values confirm this clinical picture. In SIADH, there is decreased plasma osmolality (less than 275 mOsm/kg H_2O)[32] with increased urine osmolality (greater than 100 mOsm/kg H_2O).[32] The low serum sodium (less than 125 mEq/L) is associated with increasingly severe neurologic symptoms. The urine sodium concentration is elevated (greater than 40 mEq/L), congruent with the concentrated urine output of SIADH.[32] Use of diuretics negates the reliability of the urine sodium and urine osmolality levels.[32] See Table 23.6 for the typical laboratory values associated with SIADH and with DI. Measurement of serum ADH levels is not recommended for the diagnosis of SIADH.[32]

Medical Management

In the critical care unit, SIADH often occurs as a secondary disease. If the patient is receiving any of the medications suspected to cause SIADH, stopping that medication may return ADH levels to normal. Some medications that alter ADH levels are listed in Box 23.12. The goals of medical management are to restore fluid and sodium balance. Yet research from the international Hyponatremia Registry[33] indicates that correction of serum sodium can be difficult to achieve and is not always successful.[33] Also, there are potentially many different causes of SIADH, and SIADH must be differentiated from other causes of hyponatremia.[34,35] Nonetheless, research demonstrates that patients had worse outcomes without treatment.[33]

Fluid Restriction

Fluid restriction is a cornerstone of the treatment plan for SIADH.[30,34] Fluids are generally restricted to 500 to 1000 mL/day.[30]

Sodium Replacement

Patients with severe hyponatremia (less than 125 mEq/L serum sodium) experience severe neurologic symptoms, including seizures. Too-rapid serum sodium correction must be avoided to reduce the risk of *osmotic demyelination*, which occurs in the white matter of the brain. Severe neurologic damage or death can result. The demyelination complication can be avoided by increasing the serum sodium slowly, conservatively by 8 mEq/L in 24 hours.[30] Serum sodium levels must be evaluated at least every 4 hours during the acute phase of sodium replacement. The serum sodium should not be increased more than 10 mEq/L in 24 hours.[30]

In SIADH in an emergency situation, a slow infusion of 3% saline (hypertonic saline) may be used to replenish the serum sodium without adding extra volume.[30] Hypertonic saline solution (3% or greater) can be dangerous if administered too quickly, causing demyelination as described earlier.

Calculation of the quantity of sodium that will be administered each hour and over 24 hours is advised. It is important to identify if the hyponatremia is transient, related to a medical condition such as pneumonia (vaptans not required), or caused by SIADH secondary to a small cell carcinoma in the lung that secretes ADH versus other SIADH subtypes.[35,36]

Medications

Medications are prescribed when water restriction is ineffective in correcting the SIADH. One pharmacologic option is to increase the action of ADH on the V_2 kidney tubule receptors so that more water is excreted.[30] Medications in this class (described subsequently) are known as vaptans.

Vasopressin receptor antagonists. *Vasopressin receptor antagonists* are used to treat euvolemic hyponatremia such as SIADH. Medications in this class are also called *vaptans*.

Conivaptan (Vaprisol) is approved for use only in hospitalized patients. These medications excrete water while conserving sodium, known as *aquadiuresis*. There is an initial 20-mg IV loading dose over 30 minutes, followed by a 20 mg/day continuous infusion for up to 4 days.[34] If the sodium correction is inadequate, the infusion dose can be increased to 40 mg/day.[34] Conivaptan is a nonselective vasopressin receptor antagonist, which means that it blocks V_1 receptors in the vasculature and V_2 receptors in the kidney. The patient must be observed carefully to avoid hypotension (caused by V_1 receptor blockade). Hypovolemia is a contraindication.

Tolvaptan (Samsca) is an oral medication in the same class. This medication may be initiated in the hospital, where serum sodium levels can be monitored to avoid a too-rapid increase in serum sodium after aquadiuresis.[34]

Nursing Management

Nursing management of a patient with SIADH addresses a variety of patient diagnoses (Box 23.13). Priority nursing interventions are directed toward restriction of fluids, surveillance for complications, and patient and family education.

Restriction of Fluids

Fluids are restricted to between 500 and 100 mL/day. Accurate measurement of I&O is required with serial measurements of urine output, serum sodium levels, and serum osmolality. Frequent mouth care (moistening of the buccal membrane) may give comfort during the period of fluid restriction. Daily weight may help track fluid retention or loss. Weight gain signifies continual fluid retention, whereas weight loss indicates loss of fluid.

Patient and Family Education

Rapidly occurring changes in the patient's neurologic status may worry visiting family members. Sensitivity to the family's fears can be shown by words that express empathy and by providing time for the patient and family to ask questions and express their concerns. Patient and family education about SIADH, its effect on water balance, and the reasons for fluid restrictions should be done using the teach-back method (Box 23.14).

Collaborative Management

SIADH is a complex condition that requires clinical judgment and a team approach to manage the fluid and electrolyte disruption.[32–36] Effective clinical management requires the skills of many health care professionals working as a team with goals that are clearly communicated to all team members.

THYROID GLAND DISORDERS

There are two emergency thyroid disorders. *Thyroid storm* is caused by an excess of thyroid hormone and is an exacerbation of

---

⊚ BOX 23.13 PRIORITY PATIENT CARE MANAGEMENT

Syndrome of Inappropriate Secretion of Antidiuretic Hormone

- Hypervolemia due to increased secretion of antidiuretic hormone
- Anxiety due to threat to biologic, psychologic, or social integrity
- Lack of Knowledge of Treatment Regime due to lack of previous exposure to information (see Box 23.11, Priority Patient and Family Education for Diabetes Insipidus)
   Patient Care Management plans are located in Appendix A.

✴ BOX 23.14 PRIORITY PATIENT AND FAMILY EDUCATION

Syndrome of Inappropriate Secretion of Antidiuretic Hormone

Acute Phase
- Explain reasons for admission to the critical care unit.
- Explain reasons for neurologic changes in inappropriate secretion of antidiuretic hormone (SIADH).

Predischarge
Before discharge, the patient should be able to teach back the following topics:
- Patient-specific cause of SIADH
- How to measure intake and output
- How to measure urine specific gravity (if indicated)
- Signs and symptoms to report to health care professional

---

hyperthyroidism. The clinical opposite is *myxedema coma*, which is caused by insufficient thyroid hormone and is an exacerbation of hypothyroidism.

Both hyperthyroidism and hypothyroidism are generally nonemergency conditions that are treated outside the hospital and are not discussed in this chapter. This section discusses recognition and management of the two thyroid emergency disorders that are rare but are occasionally seen in the critical care unit.

THYROID STORM

Description

Thyroid storm always occurs as a complication of preexisting hyperthyroidism.[37] Hyperthyroidism, also called *thyrotoxicosis*, occurs when the thyroid gland produces thyroid hormone in excess of the body's need.[37] The primary cause of hyperthyroidism is *Graves disease*, an autoimmune condition that affects 3% of women and 0.5% of men in the United States.[38] Graves disease is caused by circulating immunoglobulin G antibodies that attack the thyroid-stimulating hormone (TSH) receptor cells on the gland. The antidysrhythmic medication amiodarone causes a painless thyroiditis in 5% to 10% of patients.[37] Conditions associated with hyperthyroidism are described in Box 23.15.

Thyroid storm, also called *thyroid crisis*, is a rare and life-threatening exacerbation of hyperthyroidism. The pathophysiology underlying the transition from hyperthyroidism to thyroid storm is not fully understood, as thyroid hormone levels are not necessarily different from patients with hyperthyroidism. Activation of the sympathetic nervous system and enhanced sensitivity to the effects of thyroid hormone are apparent. Stopping antithyroid medications and major stressors such as infection, surgery, trauma, pregnancy, or critical illness can precipitate thyroid storm in any patient with preexisting hyperthyroidism. Mortality from thyroid storm is reported at 10%.[39]

Etiology

In thyroid storm, excessive endogenous thyroid hormone increases metabolic activity and stimulates the beta-adrenergic receptors, resulting in a heightened sympathetic nervous system response. There is hyperactivity of cardiac tissue, nervous tissue, and smooth muscle tissue, and tremendous heat production with a dangerously high

---

BOX 23.15 Conditions Associated With Hyperthyroidism

- Excessive pituitary production of thyroid-stimulating hormone
- Excessive ingestion of thyroid hormone
- Graves disease
- Toxic adenoma
- Toxic multinodular goiter
- Thyroiditis
- Painless thyroiditis, including amiodarone-induced, lymphocytic, and postpartum variations

---

temperature. The exact biochemical stimulus that precipitates the transition of hyperthyroidism into thyroid storm is unknown, although it is clear that an added external stressor such as surgery, pregnancy, or infection precipitates thyroid storm.[39] The Priority Diagnostic and Nursing Interventions for Thyroid Storm are described in Fig. 23.7.

Pathophysiology

Thyroid hormone increases cellular oxygen consumption in almost all metabolically active cells. Excess metabolism generates heat and critically high fever. Increased beta-adrenergic activity manifests as emotional lability, fine muscular tremors, agitation, delirium, hypertension, and dysrhythmias. Atrial fibrillation is a common dysrhythmia in patients with hyperthyroidism, and tachydysrhythmias should be anticipated in thyroid storm, especially in patients with underlying heart disease.[37,39]

Gastrointestinal peristalsis increases, resulting in diarrhea, nausea, and vomiting. These symptoms all lead to dehydration and compound malnutrition and weight loss. Metabolic acidosis is a potential complication. Clinical manifestations of thyroid storm are listed in Box 23.16.

Focused Physical Assessment and Diagnosis

The clinical presentation of thyroid storm is characterized by various organ systems:
1. **Thermoregulation**: fever
2. **Heart**: atrial fibrillation, supraventricular tachycardia, acute heart failure
3. **Neurologic**: agitation, restlessness, delirium
4. **Gastrointestinal**: nausea, vomiting, diarrhea

Early manifestations may be insidious or missed, creating a paradoxically abrupt presentation of apparently unrelated signs and symptoms. Use of a preestablished thyroid storm scoring system is one method to systematically diagnose thyroid storm (Table 23.8).[37] A score greater than 45 is indicative of thyroid storm.[37]

Laboratory Studies

Laboratory findings are used to confirm the suspicion raised by the clinical signs. The TSH value is extremely low, and thyroid hormones (triiodothyronine [T_3] and thyroxine [T_4]) are high compared with normal values. These results, in combination with the clinical picture, provide the diagnosis.

No laboratory test can differentiate thyroid storm from its predecessor, thyrotoxicosis, for which the laboratory values may be similar.[37,39] Thyroid storm is identified by a combination of the patient's medical history and exacerbation of clinical manifestations.

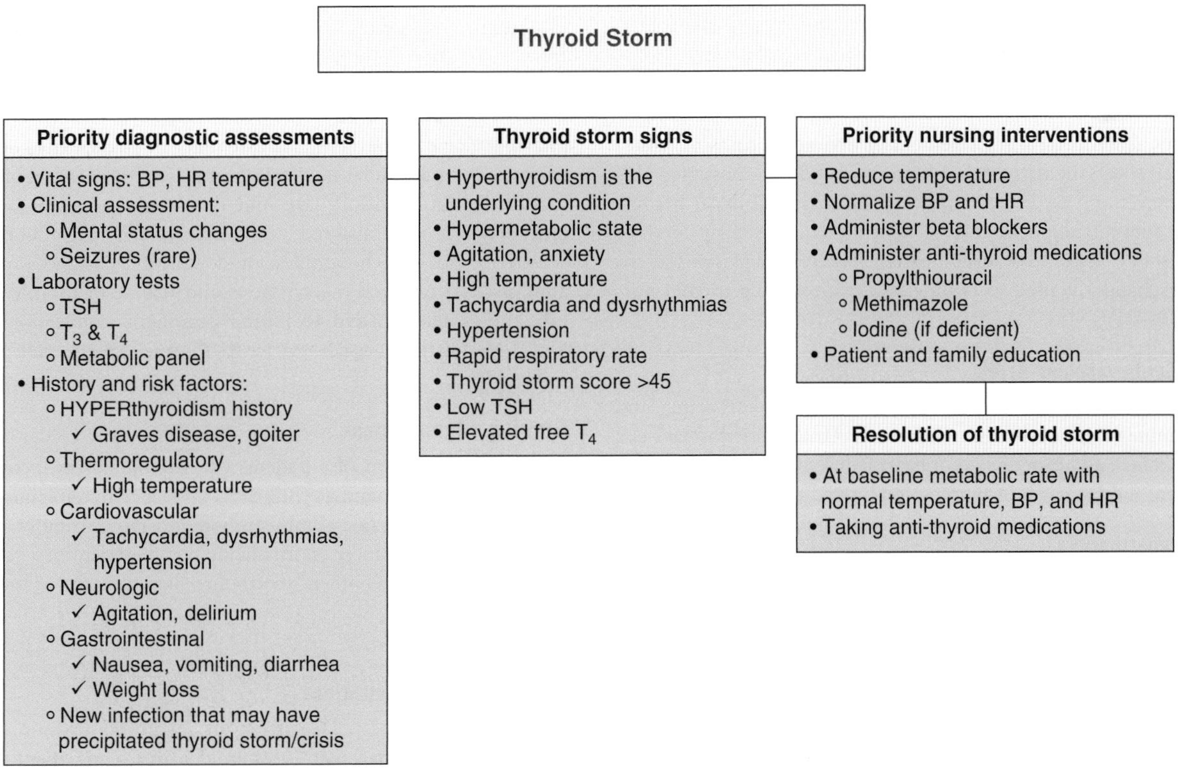

Fig. 23.7 Priority Diagnostic and Nursing Interventions for Thyroid Storm. *BP,* Blood pressure; *HR,* heart rate; *T₃,* triiodothyronine; *T₄,* thyroxine; *TSH,* thyroid-stimulating hormone.

BOX 23.16   Clinical Manifestations of Thyroid Storm

Cardiovascular System
Activation of Beta-Adrenergic (B_1) Receptors in Heart
- Tachycardia
- Systolic murmur
- Increased stroke volume
- Increased cardiac output
- Increased systolic blood pressure (BP)
- Decreased diastolic BP
- Extra systoles
- Paroxysmal atrial tachycardia
- Premature ventricular contraction
- Palpitations
- Chest pain
- Increased cardiac contractility
- Acute heart failure
- Pulmonary edema
- Cardiogenic shock

Central Nervous System
Resulting From Increased Catecholamine Response
- Hyperkinesis
- Nervousness
- Muscle weakness
- Confusion
- Convulsions
- Heat intolerance
- Fine tremor
- Emotional lability
- Frank psychosis
- Apathy

- Stupor
- Diaphoresis

Gastrointestinal System
- Nausea
- Vomiting
- Diarrhea
- Liver enlargement
- Abdominal pain
- Weight loss
- Increased appetite

Integumentary System
- Pruritus
- Hyperpigmentation of skin
- Fine, straight hair
- Alopecia

Thermoregulatory System
- Hyperthermia
- Heat dissipation
- Diaphoresis

Serum or Urine
- Hypercalcemia
- Hyperglycemia
- Hypoalbuminemia
- Hypoprothrombinemia
- Hypocholesterolemia
- Creatinuria

Medical Management

The goal of acute medical management of thyroid storm is to reduce the clinical effects of thyroid hormone as rapidly as possible. This includes preventing cardiac decompensation, reducing hyperthermia, and fluid administration to reverse dehydration caused by fever or gastrointestinal losses. In severe cases, *therapeutic plasmapheresis* (plasma exchange) is used to rapidly reduce circulating thyroid hormone levels.[37,39]

Prevent Cardiovascular Arrest

The body's heightened sensitivity to the increased adrenergic and catecholamine receptors must be suppressed. Atrial dysrhythmias need to be controlled, and progression of heart failure must be halted. Beta-blockers are the mainstay of therapy for cardiac protection.[37]

Reduce Hyperthermia

Reduction in body temperature is achieved by use of a cooling blanket and the antipyretic agent acetaminophen.[39] Salicylates (aspirin) are contraindicated, because they inhibit protein binding of T_3 to T_4, increasing the level of free, metabolically active thyroid hormone.[39]

Fluid Replacement

Vigorous fluid replacement must be instituted to treat or prevent dehydration. Antibiotic therapy may be warranted in the presence of systemic infection.

Pharmacologic Management

Pharmacologic treatment is essential in treatment of thyroid storm.[37] A multimodal medication approach is recommended, with monitoring in a critical care unit during the acute phase.[37] Beta-blockers are administered to decrease the peripheral cellular sensitivity to catecholamines, and antithyroid medications are administered to block the synthesis and release of thyroid hormone into the circulation and to inhibit peripheral conversion of T_4 to T_3.[37] Medications used to treat thyroid storm are listed in Table 23.9.

Nursing Management

Nursing management of a patient with thyroid storm incorporates a variety of patient diagnoses (Box 23.17). Priority nursing interventions are directed toward safe administration and monitoring of the effects of prescribed medications, normalizing body temperature, rehydration with correction of other metabolic derangements, and patient education.

Medication Administration

The timely and ordered sequence of medication administration is essential in the management of thyroid storm. The patient in thyroid storm is agitated, anxious, and will benefit from a calm environment. The effects of the antithyroid medications, iodides, and beta-

TABLE 23.8 Thyroid Storm Diagnostic Criteria.

Criteria	Points
Thermoregulatory Dysfunction	
Temperature (°F)	
99.0—99.9	5
100.0—100.9	10
101.0—101.9	15
102.0—102.9	20
103.0—103.9	25
≥104.0	30
Cardiovascular	
Tachycardia (beats/min)	
100—109	5
110—119	10
120—129	15
130—139	20
≥140	25
Atrial Fibrillation	
Absent	0
Present	10
Acute Heart Failure	
Absent	0
Mild	5
Moderate	10
Severe	20
Gastrointestinal-Hepatic Dysfunction	
Manifestation	
Absent	0
Moderate (diarrhea, abdominal pain, nausea/vomiting)	10
Severe (jaundice)	20
Central Nervous System Disturbance	
Manifestation	
Absent	0
Mild (agitation)	10
Moderate (delirium, psychosis, extreme lethargy)	20
Severe (seizure, coma)	30
Precipitant History	
Status	
Positive	0
Negative	10
Scores Totaled	
>45 Thyroid storm	
25—44 Impending storm	
<25 Storm unlikely	

Modified from Burch HB, Wartofsky L. Life-threatening thyrotoxicosis: thyroid storm. *Endocrinol Metal Clin North Am.* 1993;22:263; Bahn Chair RS, Burch HB, Cooper DS, et al. Hyperthyroidism and other causes of thyrotoxicosis: management guidelines of the American Thyroid Association and American Association of Clinical Endocrinologists. *Endocr Pract.* 2011;17(3):456.

adrenergic blocking agents gradually decrease the neurologic and cardiac symptoms related to catecholamine sensitivity.

Normalize Body Temperature

In thyroid storm, the patient has hyperthermia related to a hypermetabolic state, as evidenced by a critically high body temperature; diaphoresis; hot, flushed skin; intolerance to heat; tachycardia; and tachypnea. Temperature is assessed frequently until normal body temperature is attained. If antipyretic medications are required, acetaminophen is the agent of choice and salicylates are avoided.[39]

Rehydration and Correction of Metabolic Derangements

Hyperthermia, tachypnea, diaphoresis, vomiting, and diarrhea predispose the patient to a fluid volume deficit. Fluids and electrolytes are as vigorously replaced as possible. Glucose solutions are given to replace glycogen stores. Insulin is administered to treat hyperglycemia that results from mobilization of glucocorticoids. Hyponatremia from active vomiting is monitored by means of laboratory serum values. Hyponatremia is prevented or treated with isotonic IV fluid replacement.

Patient and Family Education

During the critical events surrounding the thyroid storm, the patient and family are given information to explain the causes of the high fever, anxiety, and cardiac dysrhythmias. The patient and family often are relieved to know that the agitation and nervousness result from circulating hormones that will be decreased by taking daily medications (Box 23.18).

For management of elevated temperature, patients are instructed to use acetaminophen rather than salicylates, because salicylates increase the amount of free thyroid hormone in circulation.

Collaborative Management

Management of patients with thyroid storm is derived from the guidelines issued by the *American Thyroid Association and American Association of Clinical Endocrinologists.*[37] A patient with thyroid storm requires interventions by many health care professionals, with clearly communicated goals to facilitate rapid recovery.

MYXEDEMA COMA

Description

A severe deficiency of thyroid hormone produces hypothyroidism.[40] Myxedema is differentiated from hypothyroidism by the extremely depressive effect on the CNS leading to altered level of conscious, stupor, or coma.[41]

Hypothyroidism affects all body cells and organs and slows the metabolic rate in every system. Hypothyroidism can be caused by damage to the thyroid gland (primary) or can be secondary to pituitary or hypothalamic dysfunction. There is a spectrum of hypothyroidism, as defined by laboratory tests and clinical symptoms, that ranges from mild to severe.

Mild hypothyroidism has subtle symptoms and is treated in the outpatient setting. *Myxedema coma* is an extreme exacerbation of hypothyroidism associated with respiratory depression, cardiogenic shock, hypothermia, coma, and death.[41,42] Mortality is reported to be 30% to 50%.[42]

Etiology

Myxedema coma is a rare condition, and a high index of suspicion is required to correctly recognize the signs and symptoms. A person may be admitted with myxedema coma after a prolonged period of unrecognized or poorly controlled hypothyroidism.[41,43,44] The precipitating event is generally a severe infection, trauma, acute illness, stroke, or acute myocardial infarction.[41,43,44] More women are affected than men.[44]

TABLE 23.9 Pharmacologic Management.

Thyroid Storm

Medication	Dosage	Actions	Special Considerations
Antithyroid Medications			
Propylthiouracil	Loading dose: 500–1000 mg Maintenance dosage: 250 mg every 4 hours	Blocks new thyroid hormone synthesis Blocks conversion of T_3 to T_4	May cause rash, nausea, vomiting, agranulocytosis, skin hyperpigmentation Administer with meals to reduce GI effects
Methimazole	60–80 mg/day	Blocks new thyroid hormone synthesis	Monitor signs listed for propylthiouracil. May cause rash, agranulocytosis
Iodine (saturated solution of potassium iodide)	Five drops (0.25 mL or 250 mg) orally every 6 hours	Blocks new hormone synthesis	Do not start until 1 hour after antithyroid medications have been administered
Hydrocortisone	Loading dose: 300 mg IV Maintenance dosage: 100 mg every 8 hours	May block conversion of T_4 to T_3	Prophylaxis against adrenal insufficiency Dexamethasone is an alternative medication
Beta-Blockers			
Propranolol	10–40 mg every 3–4 hours	Beta-adrenergic blockade	Monitor HR and BP response to beta-blockade
Atenolol	25–100 mg, every 12 hours or 1–2 times/day	Beta-adrenergic blockade	B_1 receptor selective
Metoprolol	25–50 mg every 8 hours or 2–3 times/day	Beta-adrenergic blockade	B_1 receptor selective
Esmolol	50–100 mcg/kg/min IV pump	Beta-adrenergic blockade	Monitor HR and BP response to beta-blockade in critical care unit

BP, Blood pressure; *GI*, gastrointestinal; *HR*, heart rate; *IV*, intravenous/intravenously; T_3, triiodothyronine; T_4, thyroxine.
Based on data from Ross DS, Burch HB, Cooper DS, et al. 2016 American Thyroid Association guidelines for diagnosis and management of hyperthyroidism and other causes of thyrotoxicosis. *Thyroid.* 2016;26(10):1343–1421.

BOX 23.17 PRIORITY PATIENT CARE MANAGEMENT

Thyroid Storm

- Hyperthermia due to increased metabolic rate
- Impaired Nutritional Intake due to lack of exogenous nutrients and increased metabolic demand
- Impaired Cardiac Output due to alterations in heart rate or rhythm
- Anxiety due to threat to biologic, psychologic, and social integrity
- Impaired Sleep due to fragmented sleep
- Lack of Knowledge of Treatment Regime due to lack of previous exposure to information (see Box 23.18, Priority Patient and Family Education: Thyroid Storm)

Patient Care Management plans are located in Appendix A.

BOX 23.18 PRIORITY PATIENT AND FAMILY EDUCATION

Thyroid Storm

Acute Phase
- Explain reasons for critical care unit admission.
- Explain reasons for extreme hypermetabolism.

Predischarge
Before discharge, the patient should be able to teach back the following topics:
- Patient-specific cause of thyroid storm
- Medications: purpose, dosage, how often to use, and side effects
- Signs and symptoms to report to health care professional

These features have been proposed as hallmarks of myxedema coma: precipitating illness, altered mental status, hypothermia, bradycardia, and abnormal thyroid blood levels, specifically, increased TSH and low free T_4.[41,42] See Table 22.3 in Chapter 22 for normal values of TSH, FT_3, and FT_4. The TSH level may be higher than 30 mU/L in myxedema coma.[42]

The diagnosis of myxedema coma is based on the clinical manifestations of end-stage hypothyroidism. Severe HYPERthyroidism (thyroid storm) and severe HYPOthyroidism (myxedema) are compared in Box 23.19. The Priority Diagnostic and Nursing Interventions for Myxedema Coma are described in Fig. 23.8.

Pathophysiology

The effects of hypothyroidism are widespread and varied. When the basal metabolic rate of oxygen consumption is reduced, cells are unable to maintain the processes necessary to sustain life. Hypothermia will occur. Metabolism of carbohydrate and fat is incomplete, and gluconeogenesis cannot supply additional sources of glucose. Lipolysis is ineffective, and cholesterol collects in the bloodstream.

Skin

The composition of the skin changes as deposits of *hyaluronic acid* (a gel-like substance capable of holding large amounts of fluid) accumulate in the interstitial spaces, giving rise to a fuller appearance of face, hands, and feet. The skin has an overall yellowish appearance resulting from increased carotene deposits from reduced carotene conversion to vitamin A.[44] The nails and hair are thin and brittle.

The hyaluronic acid deposits are evident in heart muscle; skeletal muscles; and muscles of the tongue, pharynx, and proximal esophagus.

BOX 23.19 Clinical Manifestations of Hyperthyroidism Compared With Hypothyroidism

HYPERthyroidism (Thyrotoxicosis, Thyroid Storm)	HYPOthyroidism (Myxedema, Myxedema Coma)
Elevated T_4, T_3	Decreased T_4, T_3
Decreased TSH	Elevated TSH
Hypercalcemia	Hyponatremia
Hyperglycemia	Hypoglycemia
Metabolic acidosis	Respiratory acidosis, metabolic acidosis
Tachycardia, palpitations, atrial fibrillation	Hypercholesterolemia
	Anemia
Angina	Bradycardia
ST segment wave changes	Peripheral vasoconstriction
Shortened Q-T interval	Flattened, inverted T waves
Hypertension	Prolonged Q-T and P-R intervals
AV block, acute heart failure	Decreased stroke volume, decreased
Hypovolemia	cardiac output
Shortness of breath, tachypnea	Enlarged heart, pericardial effusion
Hypermetabolism	Increased total body fluid with decreased
Polyphagia	effective arterial blood volume
Weight loss	Hypoventilation, possible CO_2 retention
Nausea, vomiting, increased peristalsis	Depressed metabolism
	Decreased lipolysis, increased cholesterol
Tremor	Weight gain
Extreme restlessness, insomnia, uneasiness, anxiety	Constipation
	Seizures
Emotional instability, despondency	Slowness, depression
	Impaired short-term memory
Diaphoresis	Slow, deliberate speech
Heat intolerance	Thickened tongue
Increased DTRs	Coarse, dry, scaly, edematous skin
Muscle weakness or muscle wasting	Hypothermia
	Delirium (myxedema madness)
Oligomenorrhea	Lethargy → stupor → coma (myxedema coma)
	Diminished DTRs
	Paresthesia of hands
	Menorrhagia

AV, Atrioventricular; *CO₂,* carbon dioxide; *DTRs,* deep tendon reflexes; *T₃,* triiodothyronine; *T₄,* thyroxine; *TSH,* thyroid-stimulating hormone.

These striated muscular changes of the tongue, pharynx, and esophagus contribute to the hoarse, husky voice. A lack of facial expression is notable in patients with hypothyroidism.[44] Absence of thyroid hormone also leads to decreased or absent sweat production.

Cardiopulmonary System

Interstitial edema impairs cardiac myocytes, resulting in bradycardia and low cardiac output. Serous fluid accumulation can accumulate in the pericardial sac causing cardiac tamponade. A decreased sensitivity to catecholamines is present, even though serum catecholamine levels are elevated. Resting HR and stroke volume are reduced, with a decreased BP. Electrocardiogram (ECG) typically reveals low-voltage QRS complexes and low-voltage, flattened, or inverted T waves and prolonged QT interval.

Pulmonary System

Hypoxic and hypercapnic ventilatory drives are severely impaired. Respiratory acidosis can occur. Pleural effusion, reduced vital capacity, and shallow respirations occur. Respiratory muscle weakness, sleep apnea, and upper airway obstruction may be present. Respiratory failure and a requirement for mechanical ventilation is typically the reason for admission to the critical care unit.

Kidneys and Fluid and Electrolyte Balance

Elimination of medications by the kidneys is severely slowed in hypothyroidism. Coexisting adrenal insufficiency should also be considered.[41]

Nutrition and Elimination

Decreased gastric motility or ileus is an expected complication for a patient with severe hypothyroidism. Intestinal hypomotility occurs, and serum cholesterol increases. Abdominal distention, slower intestinal peristalsis, and eventual paralytic ileus can lead to extreme constipation.

Thermoregulation

Heat production decreases due to insufficient energy to maintain the base metabolic rate within the cells and hypothermia occurs.[41]

Anemia

Anemia is present in many patients with hypothyroidism.[40] Erythropoiesis (red blood cell production) is impaired and coagulation abnormalities may coexist.[41,43,44]

Focused Physical Assessment and Diagnosis
Clinical Presentation

The diagnosis of end-stage hypothyroidism is based on the clinical presentation. Increasing signs of somnolence, depression, and diminished mental acuity occur. Organs become infiltrated with the mucoid-rich mucopolysaccharides, further compromising organ function. Patients present with cardiovascular collapse, hypothermia, decreased kidney function, fluid excess, weight gain, hypoventilation, and severe metabolic disorders.[41,43,44]

Hypothermia is a very distressing symptom. Most cases of myxedema are diagnosed in the winter months.[41] A myxedematous patient has hypotension, reduced total blood volume, decreased cardiac output, and bradycardia, all related to a decrease in beta-adrenergic stimulation.

Laboratory Studies

Thyroid hormone blood tests confirm the clinical picture of myxedema coma. TSH is the first test to order if hypothyroidism is suspected. Typically, patients with myxedema have primary hypothyroidism with a high TSH level and a low T_4 level.[41] If the TSH level is normal or low, other nonthyroidal causes of coma must be investigated.

Medical Management

The patient's primary admitting diagnosis may mask an underlying hypothyroidism. However, clinical manifestations can trigger the alert clinician to suspect a hypofunctioning thyroid. The primary disease condition and the myxedema coma must be treated immediately to improve the patient's chances for recovery. Myxedema coma often necessitates ventilator support, correction of fluid and electrolyte imbalance, correction of other multisystem abnormalities, corticosteroid supplementation, and thyroid hormone replacement.[41,43,44]

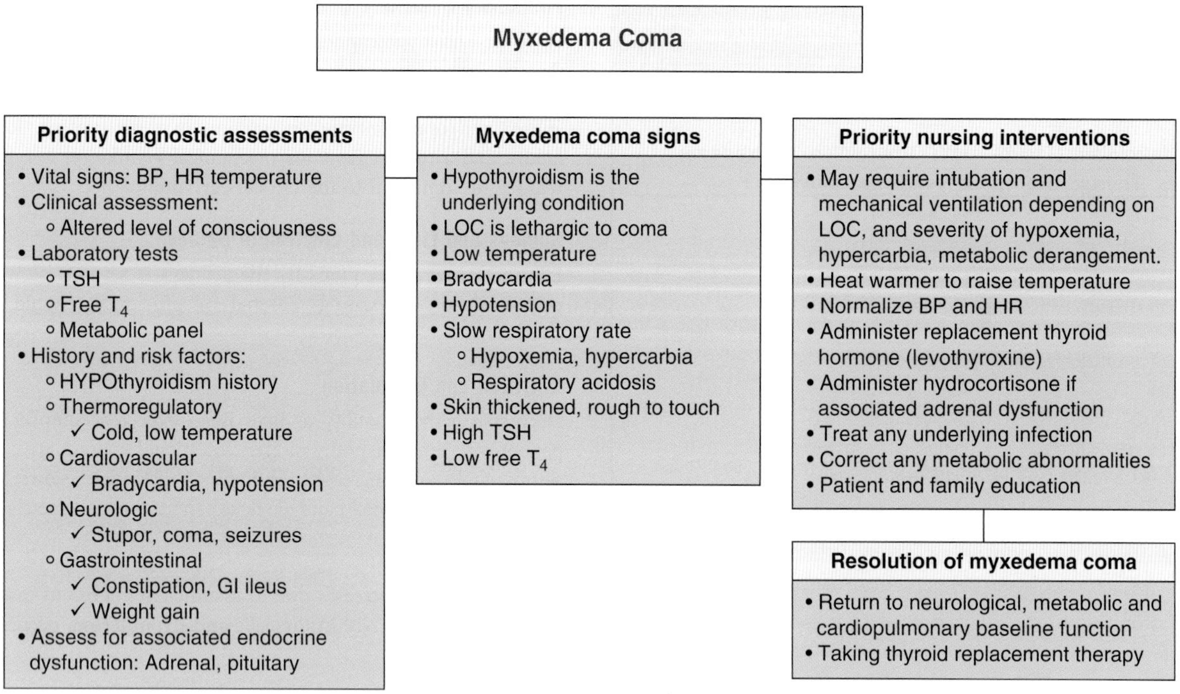

Myxedema Coma

Priority diagnostic assessments	Myxedema coma signs	Priority nursing interventions
• Vital signs: BP, HR temperature • Clinical assessment: 　○ Altered level of consciousness • Laboratory tests 　○ TSH 　○ Free T$_4$ 　○ Metabolic panel • History and risk factors: 　○ HYPOthyroidism history 　○ Thermoregulatory 　　✓ Cold, low temperature 　○ Cardiovascular 　　✓ Bradycardia, hypotension 　○ Neurologic 　　✓ Stupor, coma, seizures 　○ Gastrointestinal 　　✓ Constipation, GI ileus 　　✓ Weight gain • Assess for associated endocrine dysfunction: Adrenal, pituitary	• Hypothyroidism is the underlying condition • LOC is lethargic to coma • Low temperature • Bradycardia • Hypotension • Slow respiratory rate 　○ Hypoxemia, hypercarbia 　○ Respiratory acidosis • Skin thickened, rough to touch • High TSH • Low free T$_4$	• May require intubation and mechanical ventilation depending on LOC, and severity of hypoxemia, hypercarbia, metabolic derangement. • Heat warmer to raise temperature • Normalize BP and HR • Administer replacement thyroid hormone (levothyroxine) • Administer hydrocortisone if associated adrenal dysfunction • Treat any underlying infection • Correct any metabolic abnormalities • Patient and family education

Resolution of myxedema coma
• Return to neurological, metabolic and cardiopulmonary baseline function • Taking thyroid replacement therapy

Fig. 23.8 Priority Diagnostic and Nursing Interventions for Myxedema Coma. *BP,* Blood pressure; *HR,* heart rate; *LOC,* level of consciousness; *T$_4$,* thyroxine; *TSH,* thyroid-stimulating hormone.

◎ BOX 23.20 PRIORITY PATIENT CARE MANAGEMENT

Myxedema Coma

- Hypothermia due to decreased metabolic rate
- Impaired Breathing due to respiratory muscle fatigue or metabolic factors
- Activity Intolerance due to prolonged immobility or deconditioning
- Lack of Knowledge of Treatment Regime due to lack of previous exposure to information (see Box 23.21, Priority Patient and Family Education for Myxedema Coma)

　Patient Care Management plans are located in Appendix A.

✳ BOX 23.21 PRIORITY PATIENT AND FAMILY EDUCATION

Myxedema Coma

Acute Phase
- Explain reasons for critical care unit admission.
- Explain reasons for extreme hypometabolism.

Predischarge
Before discharge, the patient should be able to teach back the following topics:
- Patient-specific cause of hypothyroidism and myxedema coma
- Medications: purpose, dosage, how often to use, and side effects
- Signs and symptoms to report to health care professional

Pharmacologic Management

Thyroid hormone replacement including type and dosage to treat end-stage hypothyroidism (myxedema coma) is challenging, as dosages often are individualized for each patient. One method is to replete T$_4$ levels with an initial dose of levothyroxine (300–400 mcg administered IV) to saturate the previously empty T$_4$ binding sites, followed by daily administration of 50 to 100 mcg of levothyroxine.[45]

Nursing Management

Nursing management of a patient with myxedema coma involves management of a variety of patient problems (Box 23.20). Nursing actions are directed toward management of the precipitating disease and on the severe effect of hypothyroidism on multiple organ systems.

Pulmonary Care

A patient with myxedema coma who is admitted to the critical care unit may require intubation and mechanical ventilatory support. Arterial blood gas measurements are evaluated to monitor for CO$_2$ retention and respiratory acidosis.

Heart

Dysrhythmias are common in patients with myxedema and can quickly be identified by continuous ECG monitoring. Expected signs of myxedema, such as flattened or inverted T waves or prolonged QT and P-R intervals, resolve with thyroxine replacement therapy.

Thermoregulation

Hypothermia gradually improves as the patient is treated with thyroid hormone. Warm blankets and active warming devices are used. Continuous assessments are important to avoid too-rapid heating and vasodilation.

Thyroid Replacement Therapy

Improvements in the patient's cardiopulmonary and neurologic status, together with changes in T$_4$ and TSH laboratory values, are used to gauge the success of thyroid hormone replacement therapy.

QSEN

BOX 23.22 Informatics

Internet Resources: Endocrine Disorders, Testing, and Diagnoses
- American Association of Clinical Endocrinology (AACE): https://www.aace.com/
- The Endocrine Society: https://www.endocrine.org/

Pancreas: Diabetes
- American Diabetes Association: https://www.diabetes.org/diabetes

Thyroid
- American Thyroid Association Guidelines: https://www.thyroid.org/professionals/ata-professional-guidelines/

Pituitary and Adrenal
- Cushing's Support and Research Foundation: https://csrf.net/
- NIH Cushing's: https://www.ninds.nih.gov/disorders/all-disorders/cushings-syndrome-information-page
- National Cancer Institute (NCI), Neuroendocrine tumors, Pheochromocytomas: https://www.cancer.gov/pediatric-adult-rare-tumor/rare-tumors/rare-endocrine-tumor/pheochromocytoma

Skin Care

Patients with myxedema coma have rough, dry skin. Measures are taken to avoid skin breakdown related to decreased circulation and widespread edema. An emollient for skin hydration follows nonsoap baths. Frequent repositioning minimizes pressure over bony prominences.

Elimination

Constipation is managed to avoid impaction. Use of fiber-enriched enteral nutrition may be helpful. Increased fiber is preferable to use of enemas. Fluids are encouraged as the hypovolemia is corrected and BP stabilizes.

Patient and Family Education

Patients with myxedema coma have decreased comprehension and mental acuity.

All instructions given to the patient or family are given orally and in writing. The medication schedule and the frequency of the medication doses are explained. Side effects of each medication are described. All signs and symptoms to report to the health care provider are explained (Box 23.21).

Collaborative Management

There are no published guidelines that discuss acute collaborative care management of patients with hypothyroidism[40] and myxedema coma.[41,43,44] Collaborative management is required to decrease mortality in myxedema coma. Early recognition of symptoms and a willingness to request laboratory tests to confirm the diagnosis allow therapy to be instituted as early as possible.

ADDITIONAL RESOURCES

See Box 23.22 for Internet resources pertaining to endocrine disorders and therapeutic management.

REFERENCES

1. Russell G, Lightman S. The human stress response. *Nat Rev Endocrinol.* 2019;15:525–534.
2. Gibbison B, Angelini GD, Lightman SL. Dynamic output and control of the hypothalamic-pituitary-adrenal axis in critical illness and major surgery. *Br J Anaesth.* 2013;111(3):347.
3. Téblick A, Peeters B, Langouche L, Van den Berghe G. Adrenal function and dysfunction in critically ill patients. *Nat Rev Endocrinol.* 2019;15(7):417–427.
4. Harp JB, Yancopoulos GD, Gromada J. Glucagon orchestrates stress-induced hyperglycemia. *Diabetes Obes Metab.* 2016;18(7):648.
5. Van den Berghe G, Wouters P, Weekers F, et al. Intensive insulin therapy in critically ill patients. *N Engl J Med.* 2001;345:1359–1367.
6. Honiden S, Inzucchi SE. Metabolic management during critical illness: glycemic control in the ICU. *Semin Respir Crit Care Med.* 2015;36(6):859.
7. Clain J, Ramar K, Surani SR. Glucose control in critical care. *World J Diabetes.* 2015;6(9):1082.
8. NICE-SUGAR Study Investigators, Finfer S, Chittock DR, et al. Intensive versus conventional glucose control in critically ill patients. *N Engl J Med.* 2009;360(13):1283.
9. Moghissi ES, Korytkowski MT, DiNardo M, et al. American Association of Clinical Endocrinologists and American Diabetes Association consensus statement on inpatient glycemic control. *Diabetes Care.* 2009;32(6):1119.
10. Jacobi J, Bircher N, Krinsley J, et al. Guidelines for the use of an insulin infusion for the management of hyperglycemia in critically ill patients. *Crit Care Med.* 2012;40(12):3251.
11. American Diabetes Association. Diabetes care in the hospital. *Diabetes Care.* 2020;43(suppl 1):S193–S202.
12. American Diabetes Association. Pharmacologic approaches to glycemic treatment: standards of medical care in diabetes-2020. *Diabetes Care.* 2020;43(suppl 1):S98–S110.
13. Lambell KJ, Tatucu-Babet OA, Chapple LA, Gantner D, Ridley EJ. Nutrition therapy in critical illness: a review of the literature for clinicians. *Crit Care.* 2020;24:35.
14. Handelsman Y, Bloomgarden ZT, Grunberger G, et al. American Association of Clinical Endocrinologists and American College of Endocrinology - clinical practice guidelines for developing a diabetes mellitus comprehensive care plan—2015. *Endocr Pract.* 2015;21(suppl 1):1–87.
15. American Diabetes Association. Classification and diagnosis of diabetes: standards of medical care in diabetes—2020. *Diabetes Care.* 2020;43(suppl 1):S14–S31.
16. Fox CS, Golden SH, Anderson C, et al. Update on prevention of cardiovascular disease in adults with type 2 diabetes mellitus in light of recent evidence: a scientific statement from the American Heart Association and the American Diabetes Association. *Diabetes Care.* 2015;38(9):1777.
17. Arnett KK, Blumenthal RS, Albert MA, et al. 2019 ACC/AHA guideline on the primary prevention of cardiovascular disease: executive summary: a report of the American College of Cardiology/American Heart Association task force on clinical practice guidelines. *J Am Coll Cardiol.* 2019;74:1376–1414.
18. Davies MJ, D'Alessio DA, Fradkin J, et al. Management of hyperglycemia in type 2 diabetes, 2018. A consensus report by the American Diabetes Association (ADA) and the European Association for the Study of Diabetes (EASD). *Diabetes Care.* 2018;41(12):2669–2701.
19. Garber AJ, Handelsman Y, Grunberger G, et al. Consensus statement by the American Association of Clinical Endocrinologists and American College of Endocrinology on the comprehensive type 2 diabetes management algorithm—2020 executive summary. *Endocr Pract.* 2020;26(1):107–139.
20. Kitabchi AE, Umpierrez GE, Miles JM, Fisher JN. Hyperglycemic crises in adult patients with diabetes. *Diabetes Care.* 2009;32(7):1335.
21. Fayfman M, Pasquel FJ, Umpierrez GE. Management of hyperglycemic crises: diabetic ketoacidosis and hyperglycemic hyperosmolar state. *Med Clin North Am.* 2017;101(3):587–606.
22. Firestone RL, Parker PL, Pandya KA, Wilson MD, Duby JJ. Moderate-intensity insulin therapy is associated with reduced length of stay in

critically ill patients with diabetic ketoacidosis and hyperosmolar hyperglycemic state. *Crit Care Med.* 2019;47(5):700–705.

23. Umpierrez G, Korytkowski M. Diabetic emergencies—ketoacidosis, hyperglycaemic hyperosmolar state and hypoglycaemia. *Nat Rev Endocrinol.* 2016;12(4):222–232.

24. Dhatariya KK, Vellanki P. Treatment of diabetic ketoacidosis (DKA)/ hyperglycemic hyperosmolar state (HHS): novel advances in the management of hyperglycemic crises (UK versus USA). *Curr Diab Rep.* 2017;17(5):33.

25. Garber AJ, Abrahamson MJ, Barzilay JI, et al. Consensus statement by the American Association of Clinical Endocrinologists and American College of Endocrinology on the comprehensive type 2 diabetes management algorithm—2016 executive summary. *Endocr Pract.* 2016;22(1):84.

26. Harrois A, Anstey JR. Diabetes insipidus and syndrome of inappropriate antidiuretic hormone in critically ill patients. *Crit Care Clin.* 2019;35(2):187–200.

27. Baldweg SE, Ball S, Brooke A, et al. Society for Endocrinology clinical guidance: inpatient management of cranial diabetes insipidus. *Endocr Connect.* 2018;7(7):G8–G11.

28. Bockenhauer D, Bichet DG. Pathophysiology, diagnosis and management of nephrogenic diabetes insipidus. *Nat Rev Nephrol.* 2015;11(10):576.

29. Verbalis JG, Grossman A, Hoybye C, Runkle I. Review and analysis of differing regulatory indications and expert panel guidelines for the treatment of hyponatremia. *Curr Med Res Opin.* 2014;30(7):1201.

30. Verbalis JG. Disorders of water metabolism: diabetes insipidus and the syndrome of inappropriate antidiuretic hormone secretion. *Handb Clin Neurol.* 2014;124:37.

31. Christ-Crain M, Fenske W. Copeptin in the diagnosis of vasopressin-dependent disorders of fluid homeostasis. *Nat Rev Endocrinol.* 2016;12(3):168–176.

32. Spasovski G, Vanholder R, Allolio B, et al. Clinical practice guideline on diagnosis and treatment of hyponatraemia. *Intensive Care Med.* 2014;40(3):320–331.

33. Verbalis JG, Greenberg A, Burst V, et al. Diagnosing and treating the syndrome of inappropriate antidiuretic hormone secretion. *Am J Med.* 2016;129(5):537.e9–537.e20.

34. Verbalis JG, Goldsmith SR, Greenberg A, et al. Diagnosis, evaluation, and treatment of hyponatremia: expert panel recommendations. *Am J Med.* 2013;126(suppl 1):S1–S42.

35. Fenske W, Sandner B, Christ-Crain M. A copeptin-based classification of the osmoregulatory defects in the syndrome of inappropriate antidiuresis. *Best Pract Res Clin Endocrinol Metab.* 2016;30(2):219–233.

36. Hoorn EJ, Zietse R. Diagnosis and treatment of hyponatremia: compilation of the guidelines. *J Am Soc Nephrol.* 2017;28(5):1340–1349.

37. Ross DS, Burch HB, Cooper DS, et al. 2016 American Thyroid Association guidelines for diagnosis and management of hyperthyroidism and other causes of thyrotoxicosis. *Thyroid.* 2016;26(10):1343–1421.

38. Burch HB, Cooper DS. Management of Graves disease: a review. *J Am Med Assoc.* 2015;314(23):2544.

39. Chiha M, Samarasinghe S, Kabaker AS. Thyroid storm: an updated review. *J Intensive Care Med.* 2015;30(3):131–140.

40. Garber JR, Cobin RH, Gharib H, et al. Clinical practice guidelines for hypothyroidism in adults: cosponsored by the American Association of Clinical Endocrinologists and the American thyroid association. *Thyroid.* 2012;22(12):1200.

41. Torres MS, Emerson CH. Myxedema coma. In: Irwin RS, Rippe J, eds. *Irwin & Rippe's Intensive Care Medicine.* Philadelphia, PA: Wolters Kluwer Health, Lippincott Williams and Wilkins; 2018.

42. Chiong YV, Bammerlin E, Mariash CN. Development of an objective tool for the diagnosis of myxedema coma. *Transl Res.* 2015;166(3):233.

43. Popoveniuc G, Chandra T, Sud A, et al. A diagnostic scoring system for myxedema coma. *Endocr Pract.* 2014;20(8):808.

44. Pereira K. Hypothyroidism. In: Moini J, Pereira K, Samsam M, eds. *Epidemiology of Thyroid Disorders.* Elsevier Inc.; 2020.

45. Mathew V, Misgar RA, Ghosh S, et al. Myxedema coma: a new look into an old crisis. *J Thyroid Res.* 2011;2011:493, 462.

24

Trauma

Eugene E. Mondor

MECHANISM OF INJURY

Trauma occurs when an external force of energy impacts the body and causes structural or physiologic alterations, or *injury*. External forces can be radiation, electrical, thermal, chemical, or mechanical forms of energy. Trauma that occurs from high-velocity impact (mechanical energy) is most common. Mechanical energy can produce blunt or penetrating traumatic injuries. Understanding the mechanism of injury helps health care providers predict potential injuries and anticipate the associated care that may be required.

Blunt Trauma

Blunt trauma is seen most often with motor vehicle crashes (MVCs), falls, contact sports, or blunt-force injuries (e.g., trauma caused by a baseball bat). Blunt injury occurs because of the forces sustained during a rapid change in velocity (deceleration). To estimate the amount of force sustained in an MVC, multiply the person's weight by the miles per hour (speed) the vehicle was traveling. For example, a woman weighing 130 lb traveling in a vehicle 60 miles/h that hits a brick wall would sustain 7800 lb of force within milliseconds. As the body stops suddenly, tissues and internal organs continue to move forward. This sudden change in velocity can cause significant external and internal injury. Blunt injury may be difficult to diagnose, as injuries are not always obvious or readily apparent.

Penetrating Trauma

Penetrating injuries—those that puncture the body and result in damage to internal structures—occur with stabbings, firearms, or impalement. Damage is created along the path of penetration. Penetrating injuries can be misleading, because the appearance of the external wound may not accurately reflect the extent of internal injury. For instance, bullets can create internal cavitation several times larger than the diameter of the bullet itself. Several factors determine the extent of damage sustained as a result of penetrating trauma. For example, different weapons cause different types of injuries. The severity of a gunshot wound depends on the type of gun, ammunition used, and the distance and angle from which the gun was fired. Pellets from a shotgun blast expand on impact and cause multiple injuries to internal structures. Handgun bullets usually damage what is directly in the bullet's path. Inside the body, the bullet can ricochet off bone and create further damage.

With penetrating stab wounds, factors that determine the extent of injury include the type and length of object used and the angle of insertion. Stab wounds typically produce less serious injury (but not always), as most stabbings are typically low-velocity injuries.

Specific information that must be elicited pertaining to the mechanism of injury is summarized in Box 24.1.

PHASES OF TRAUMA CARE

Care of trauma victims during wartime has enhanced knowledge about trauma, triage, and the importance of rapid transport of injured individuals to medical facilities. Military experience has demonstrated that decreasing the time from injury to definitive care can save more lives. Care of critically injured individuals as a result of war has provided insight and knowledge that has helped improve civilian trauma care.

Historically, studies reported and statistics demonstrated that deaths as a result of trauma occurred in a trimodal distribution.[1] Development of the Advanced Trauma Life Support (ATLS) guidelines by the American College of Surgeons has enhanced assessment skills of prehospital care providers, expedited transport of critically injured patients, identified the importance of designated trauma care centers, created evidence-based protocols for injured patients, and focused on injury prevention, all which have affected the timing of death after trauma. At present, with improvements in trauma resuscitation described earlier, most deaths occur in a bimodal distribution (Fig. 24.1).[2]

The first peak of trauma deaths occurs within 48 hours after initial injury, and the second peak occurs days to weeks after injury. In the first peak, death often occurs on scene or very soon after admission to the hospital, usually as a result of severe traumatic brain injury (TBI) or hemorrhage. During the second peak, death frequently occurs in the critical care unit as a consequence of complications from the initial injury, such as infection or multiple-organ dysfunction syndrome (MODS). Trauma patients who develop MODS have increased mortality estimated to be as high as 30%.[3]

The *golden hour* of trauma resuscitation is often viewed as a critical time frame in which the injured patient will die unless definitive care is delivered. However, the golden hour should not be considered a time frame but rather a guideline for all trauma care providers. Components

BOX 24.1   History of Mechanism of Injury

Blunt Trauma
- Motor vehicle crash extrication time
- Ejection
- Steering wheel deformation
- Location in automobile (passenger, driver, front seat, back seat)
- Restraint status (lap belt, shoulder harness, or combination; unrestrained)
- Speed of automobiles, direction of impact
- Occupants (number and morbidity status)
- Height of fall

Penetrating Trauma
- Weapon used (handgun, shotgun, rifle, knife)
- Caliber of weapon
- Number of shots fired
- Position of victim and assailant when injury occurred

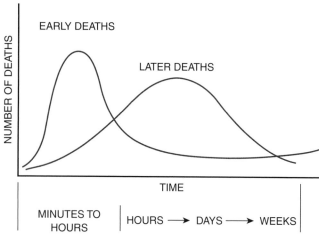

Fig. 24.1 Bimodal Distribution of Trauma Deaths.

of the golden hour incorporate activation of emergency medical services, stabilization and transport, triage, initial resuscitation, early surgical consultation, and provision of critical care. For a critically injured trauma patient, the primary goal is to minimize the time from injury to definitive care. There is no evidence to suggest that survival rates dramatically decrease in trauma patients after 60 minutes.

Major advances have been made in the management of patients with traumatic injuries in the prehospital, emergency department, and critical care settings. Nursing management of a patient with traumatic injury begins the moment a call for help is received and continues until the patient's death or return to the community. Patients with complex multisystem trauma are frequently admitted to critical care units, and these patients require complex nursing care. Care of a trauma patient is viewed on a continuum that includes multiple phases and locations: prehospital care, emergency department, damage control resuscitation, critical care, intermediate care, and rehabilitation.

Prehospital Care

The goal of prehospital care is immediate identification of life-threatening injuries and transport (ground or air) to the closest appropriate medical facility. Maintaining a patent airway, recognition

and control of external bleeding and shock, and immobilization of the patient are essential priorities. Initiation of a peripheral intravenous (IV) line, splinting of fractures, and pain management are also vital components. Prehospital personnel should communicate information needed for triage before arrival at the hospital. Advanced planning for multiple-injured patients by trauma teams is essential.

Emergency Department

The ATLS guidelines assist health care providers with the essential actions necessary for rapid assessment, immediate identification of life-threatening injuries, and initial resuscitation of trauma patients in the emergency department.[4] These guiding principles delineate a systematic approach to initial assessment and care of a trauma patient that includes a rapid primary survey, resuscitation of vital organ systems, a more detailed secondary survey, and initiation of the most appropriate care. Originally developed for physicians, these guidelines have been adopted worldwide by prehospital care providers and trauma teams, including emergency and critical care nurses, and provide the framework for the ABCDEs of trauma care.

Primary Survey

On arrival of the trauma patient in the emergency department, the primary survey is initiated. The purpose of this initial assessment is to identify and treat any life-threatening injuries that, if left untreated, could potentially cause the patient's death.

The five steps in the ATLS primary survey are commonly referred to as the *ABCDEs* of trauma resuscitation (Table 24.1):
- Airway maintenance with cervical spine protection
- Breathing and ventilation
- Circulation with hemorrhage control
- Disability: Neurologic status
- Exposure or environmental control

Although many trauma centers use this approach, there is ever-present awareness that many trauma patients die as a result of hemorrhage. Consequently, many trauma facilities have informally adopted the military's *C-ABCDE* approach, where the additional "C" stands for catastrophic hemorrhage.[5] This slight modification to the *ABCDE* approach of ATLS is intended to emphasize the importance of the immediate assessment, identification, and implementation of measures to control hemorrhage in a trauma patient without becoming overly preoccupied with other components of the primary survey.

Airway. The patient's airway is assessed for patency and possible airway obstruction. Trauma patients are at risk for ineffective airway clearance, especially in the presence of altered consciousness, effects of drugs and/or alcohol, and maxillofacial or thoracic injuries. Airway obstruction can be caused by foreign bodies, blood clots, or broken teeth. Airway patency is assessed by inspecting the oropharynx for foreign body obstruction and listening for air movement at the nose and mouth. If the patient can verbally communicate, it is likely that the airway is patent. Patients who have a Glasgow Coma Scale (GCS) score of 8 or less or are unable to protect their own airway often require placement of a definitive airway.[4] Airway placement must incorporate cervical spine immobilization. The patient's head and neck should not be rotated, hyperflexed, or hyperextended. The cervical spine must be immobilized at all times in all trauma patients until a cervical spinal cord injury (SCI) has been ruled out.

Breathing. The patient is assessed for signs of visible chest movement. An open, clear airway does not always ensure adequate ventilation and gas exchange. Assessment includes a visual inspection of chest wall integrity and respiratory rate, depth, and symmetry. Auscultation is performed to assess the presence or absence of breath

TABLE 24.1 Primary Survey of Trauma Patient.

Survey Component	Trauma Team Assessment	Immediate Care

A—Airway	Immediately assess patient's ability to speak
	Look
	  Are there obvious signs of airway trauma, tachypnea, accessory muscle use?
	Listen
	  Can you hear the patient breathing?
	Feel
	  For air exchange through the mouth
	  Palpate for tracheal deviation
		Immobilize spine
		Nondefinitive airway management
		  Oropharyngeal (unconscious patient)
		  Nasopharyngeal (conscious patient)
		When in doubt, secure the airway
		  Endotracheal intubation
		  Emergency cricothyrotomy

B—Breathing	Is the patient breathing?
	Look
	  Is the patient's chest rising and falling?
	  Respiratory rate, rhythm, symmetry
	  Is there any evidence of thoracic trauma?
	Listen
	  Quickly auscultate air entry
	  Is there air entry in all lobes?
	Palpate
	  Chest wall integrity
		Administer supplemental oxygen
		For life-threatening conditions (e.g., tension pneumothorax), immediate needle decompression or chest tube insertion
		Full-support mechanical ventilation (as required)

C—Circulation	Assess pulse quality and rate
	Assess for life-threatening conditions (e.g., uncontrolled bleeding, shock)
	Examine and feel patient's skin
	  Warm and dry
	  Cool, pale, and clammy
		Signs and symptoms of poor tissue perfusion
		  Initiate IV access
		  Administer 1 L of isotonic IV fluid, then reassess hemodynamic status
		If no pulse, begin CPR

D—Disability	Neurologic assessment
	  GCS score
	  Pupils: Size and reactivity?
	  Is patient moving all four limbs to command?
	  Any evidence of posturing?
		Consider early neurosurgical consultation
		  Consider early CT scan

E—Exposure	All clothing removed to inspect all body regions
	  Any lacerations, abrasions, bruises?
	  Stab wounds: Entrance?
	  Gunshot wounds: Entrance? Exit?
		Prevent hypothermia
		  Warm blankets
		  Warm IV fluids
		  Increase room temperature

CPR, Cardiopulmonary resuscitation; *CT,* computed tomography; *GCS,* Glasgow Coma Scale; *IV,* intravenous.

sounds. Decreased or absent breath sounds or alteration in chest wall integrity may necessitate chest tube placement. Supplemental oxygen is administered to some injured patients but may not be required in the spontaneously breathing trauma patient who is awake, alert, talking, and has an oxygen saturation with pulse oximetry (SpO₂) greater than 92%.[6] Endotracheal intubation may be required for patients who have compromised airways caused by mechanical factors, who are unconscious, or who have ventilatory problems. Needle or surgical cricothyroidotomy may be necessary when severe maxillofacial trauma exists and endotracheal intubation is not an option.[4]

Circulation. The next step is to assess for the presence of a palpable pulse, assess any evidence of external or internal hemorrhage, and, if possible, obtain a baseline measurement of the patient's vital signs. Rapid evaluation of circulatory status includes assessment of level of consciousness (LOC), skin color, and pulse.[7] The LOC provides data on cerebral perfusion. Facial color that is ashen or gray and extremities that are pale or slightly mottled may be ominous signs of hypovolemia and shock. Central pulses (femoral or carotid artery) are assessed bilaterally for rate, regularity, and quality. If a pulse is not present, cardiopulmonary resuscitation (CPR) must be initiated immediately.

All trauma patients are considered to be in shock. Trauma patients may or may not exhibit significant deterioration in hemodynamic stability. Trauma teams are aware that vital signs can initially remain stable even in the face of hemorrhage.[8] Measurement and trending of systolic and diastolic blood pressure, mean arterial pressure (MAP), and SpO₂ readings are more important than individual values. Hypotension in trauma should be attributed to hypovolemia until proven otherwise.[8] External exsanguination is identified and controlled by direct manual pressure on the wound. Internal hemorrhage in trauma requires urgent surgical consultation and transport to interventional radiology for diagnostic imaging or the operating room for immediate surgery.

Disability. A rapid neurologic assessment is performed. During this important step, the patient's baseline LOC and pupil size and reaction are assessed and documented. The *AVPU* method can be used to quickly describe the patient's LOC:
- **A:** Alert
- **V:** Responds to verbal stimuli
- **P:** Responds to painful stimuli
- **U:** Unresponsive

The GCS score can also be used (see Table 16.1).

Exposure. In the final step of the primary survey, all of the patient's clothing is removed to facilitate a thorough examination of all body surfaces for the presence of injury. The patient is turned (logrolled) while full spinal precautions are maintained. The spine is carefully palpated for obvious deformity. The occipital lobe, neck, back, buttocks, and extremities are quickly examined for wounds, impaled objects, and bleeding. After clothing is removed, the patient must be protected from hypothermia. This can be accomplished through warm blankets, increasing room temperature, and administering warm IV fluids.

Secondary Survey

The secondary survey begins when the primary survey is completed, potentially life-threatening injuries have been identified, and resuscitation initiated. In reality, both primary and secondary surveys may seem to occur almost simultaneously. However, the secondary survey is a more detailed, in-depth physical examination of the trauma patient. During the secondary survey, a head-to-toe approach is used to thoroughly examine each body region.

During the secondary survey, the nurse ensures the completion of all necessary procedures, such as an electrocardiogram, radiographic studies (chest, cervical spine, thorax, and pelvis), ultrasonography, and insertion of gastric and urinary catheters. Throughout this survey, the nurse continuously monitors the patient's vital signs (heart rate, blood pressure, MAP, and SpO_2) and response to resuscitation interventions. Emotional support to the patient and family also is imperative.

Patient history is also an important aspect of the secondary survey. The patient's pertinent past history can be assessed by use of the mnemonic *AMPLE*:
- **A:** Allergies
- **M:** Medications currently used
- **P:** Past medical illnesses/pregnancy
- **L:** Last meal
- **E:** Events/environment related to the injury

Head injury, shock, or the use of drugs and/or alcohol may preclude obtaining information from the patient. Prehospital care providers (paramedics, emergency medical technicians), family members, or sometimes bystanders can be excellent sources of information.

Volume resuscitation. Hypovolemic shock as a result of hemorrhage is the most common type of shock that occurs in trauma patients.[9] The traditional signs and symptoms of hemorrhagic hypovolemic shock may not appear until approximately 30% to 40% of circulating blood volume is lost.[4] Hemorrhage in trauma must be identified and treated rapidly. Two large-bore (14-gauge to 16-gauge) peripheral IV catheters, the intraosseous device, or central venous catheter is inserted. Initial blood samples to be drawn in trauma patients are identified in Box 24.2.

BOX 24.2 Recommended Initial Blood Samples in Trauma Patients

- Complete blood cell (CBC) count
- Electrolyte profile (Na^+, K^+, Cl^-, carbon dioxide, glucose, blood urea nitrogen, creatinine)
- Coagulation parameters: prothrombin time, partial thromboplastin time
- Type and screen (ABO compatibility)
- Amylase
- Toxicology screens
- Liver function studies
- Pregnancy test (for women of childbearing age)
- Lactate

The ideal IV fluid for trauma resuscitation has not been established. Current ATLS guidelines suggest an initial infusion of 1 L of 0.9% normal saline or lactated Ringer solution.[4] Both crystalloid solutions are physiologically isotonic, provide volume to the volume-depleted patient, and are often readily available.

When IV fluid is administered, trauma patients may be categorized as *responders, transient responders,* or *nonresponders.*[10] *Responders* are patients whose hemodynamics steadily improve with the administration of IV fluid. *Transient responders* may exhibit temporary stabilization of vital signs, followed by a decline in patient condition. *Nonresponders* are the most worrisome. These patients do not respond to IV fluid, which often indicates that internal bleeding may be present. Overaggressive volume resuscitation with IV fluids must be avoided to prevent unnecessary complications such as pulmonary edema or exacerbation of hemorrhage.

Damage control resuscitation. Damage control resuscitation is an evidence-based strategy employed in trauma centers worldwide to control and assist in stabilization of the trauma patient in hemorrhagic shock.[11,12] Components of damage control resuscitation include permissive hypotension, massive transfusion protocols (MTPs), and damage control surgery.[12] Damage control resuscitation begins in the field and continues through the emergency department, operating room, and critical care unit.

Permissive hypotension. Permissive hypotension is employed by most trauma providers. Permissive hypotension involves low-volume IV fluid resuscitation.[13] The goal is to maintain the blood pressure low enough to prevent worsening of hemorrhage but high enough to maintain perfusion of vital organs, including the brain. It is not, under any circumstances, to be considered as a substitute for surgical control of bleeding in the hemorrhaging trauma patient.

In adult trauma patients, some authors suggest targeting a systolic blood pressure (SBP) of 70 to 90 mm Hg and MAP of 50 mm Hg,[14] but these targets have not been universally adopted. Individualized assessment of each trauma patient is mandatory. Aggressively infusing IV fluid into a trauma patient may dilute clotting factors, disrupt any clots that have formed, and exacerbate hemorrhage.[15] Permissive hypotension is contraindicated in TBI.

Massive transfusion protocols. Given current emphasis on use of blood products over crystalloids and correction of trauma-induced coagulopathy, many trauma centers have developed *massive transfusion protocols* (MTP). Approximately 3% of all trauma patients require activation of the MTP.[16] Having a defined protocol serves as a system-based strategy to facilitate early, timely release of blood products in what can often be a chaotic situation. The MTP outlines the ratio of packed red blood cells, fresh frozen plasma, platelets, and cryoprecipitate to be administered. This is referred to as *hemostatic resuscitation,* where blood components are administered in a ratio that resembles whole blood.[17] The optimal ratio of blood components to be administered to bleeding trauma patients is a major focus in trauma research.

Tranexamic acid is an antifibrinolytic agent used to stop bleeding in trauma patients. It is given IV as a loading dose and subsequent IV infusion over 1 hour. *Thromboelastography,* or *TEG,* is a newer technique whereby real-time point-of-care testing of the coagulation profile can be done at the bedside of the trauma patient.[18] Based on the patient's coagulation profile, *TEG* helps identify the most important blood component required of the trauma patient at the time the sample is drawn and results obtained.

Damage control surgery. Trauma is sometimes referred to as a "surgical disease," because the nature and extent of injuries usually requires operative management. Damage control surgery is a well-established concept in trauma care. Damage control surgery is a strategy of providing essential surgical interventions to control hemorrhage and limit contamination.[19] The goal is to optimize physiology of the actively bleeding patient, not complete definitive repair. Permissive hypotension and massive transfusion protocols are often employed simultaneously during damage control surgery.[20] Reconstruction and formal closure of wounds are often not completed until after resuscitation and stabilization of the patient in the critical care unit have occurred.

Critical Care Phase

Critically injured trauma patients are frequently admitted to the critical care unit as direct transfers from the emergency department, diagnostic imaging, or operating room. It is essential that the critical care team be aware of all resuscitation strategies that have been initiated up until admission to the critical care unit. Information the critical care nurse must obtain from prehospital, emergency department, or operating room personnel can be summarized using the **SBAR** communication tool: Situation, Background, Assessment, and Recommendations (Box 24.3). This information is ideally obtained before the patient's admission to the critical care unit to ensure availability of needed personnel, equipment, and supplies, although this may not always be possible. Table 24.2 summarizes the effects of prehospital, emergency department, and operating room resuscitation measures that can affect initial management of the trauma patient in the critical care unit.

BOX 24.3 Nursing Report From Referring Area Using SBAR Method

S: Situation
- Age
- Sex
- Mechanism of injury/injuries sustained
- Admission diagnosis/chief complaint; any loss of consciousness and its duration with current Glasgow Coma Scale score
- Diagnostic tests and procedures completed
- Current issues, including derangements in any physical assessments requiring acute interventions

B: Background
- Significant medical and surgical history
- Home medications

A: Assessments
- Current assessment findings, including vital signs, level of consciousness, established airway, and mechanical ventilation settings
- Medications administered (opiates, sedatives, antibiotics, antifibrinolytics)
- Diagnostic test results (e.g., completed x-rays, angiography)
- Laboratory results (including implementation of massive transfusion protocol)
- Family members present and assessment of their current knowledge of nature and extent of injuries and treatment plan

R: Recommendations
- Identification of any immediate treatment required
- Description of resuscitation plan, including blood products, diagnostic imaging, possible surgery

---

Immediately after the patient's arrival in the critical care unit, the nurse repeats the primary and secondary surveys in accordance with ATLS guidelines. **Priority nursing care during the critical care phase includes (1) ongoing repeated physical assessments, (2) monitoring laboratory and diagnostic test results, and (3) observing trends in the patient's response to treatment.** The nurse is continually aware that the second peak of the bimodal distribution of trauma deaths occurs most often in the critical care setting as a result of complications including prolonged shock states, acute respiratory distress syndrome (ARDS), sepsis, and MODS. Ongoing nursing assessments are imperative for early detection and treatment of complications.

One of the most important nursing roles is ongoing assessment of the balance between oxygen delivery (supply) and oxygen demand (consumption). Oxygen delivery must be optimized to prevent further damage to bodily systems. The trauma patient is at high risk for impaired oxygenation as a result of various factors (Table 24.3). Risk factors must be promptly identified and treated to prevent life-threatening sequelae. Prevention and treatment of hypoxemia depend on accurate assessment of the adequacy of pulmonary gas exchange (arterial blood gas [ABG]), oxygen supply (fraction of inspired oxygen), and oxygen consumption (assessment of LOC, tissue perfusion, capillary refill, urinary output).

Acidosis (pH less than 7.2), hypothermia (temperature less than 35°C), and clinical coagulopathy are often present in trauma patients. This combination of factors is known as the *lethal triad of death*.[21] For example, hypothermia induced by an open visceral cavity in conjunction with massive blood transfusion can lead to coagulopathy and continued bleeding, which results in shock and metabolic acidosis. The triad of hypothermia, coagulopathy, and acidosis creates a self-propagating cycle that can eventually lead to an irreversible physiologic insult.[22]

One goal of the critical care nurse is to continue resuscitation and assist in correcting hypothermia, coagulopathy, and acidosis. For example, coagulation factors and platelets may be administered to correct coagulopathies and monitoring ABGs aids in determining acid–base balance. Rewarming techniques are described in Table 24.4.

End Points in Trauma Resuscitation

During resuscitation, all attempts are made to improve cellular oxygenation. Resuscitation is aimed at ensuring adequate perfusion of tissues with fluid, oxygen, and nutrients to support cellular function. No single resuscitation end point is sufficient. Resuscitation end points (variables or parameters) must be viewed across the continuum of trauma resuscitation.

During resuscitation from traumatic hemorrhagic shock, normalization of standard clinical parameters such as blood pressure, heart rate, and urine output is inadequate.[23] Resuscitation end points can be grouped into two major categories: hemodynamic variables and tissue perfusion variables.[23] Base deficit and lactic acid (lactate) values have been well studied to determine the adequacy of cellular oxygenation during trauma resuscitation.[24] Optimal resuscitation end points in different types of trauma are ongoing areas of research in trauma care.

Frequent and thorough assessments of all body systems are the cornerstone of medical and nursing management of critically injured trauma patients in critical care. The critical care nurse is able to detect subtle changes in patient condition and facilitate the implementation of timely therapeutic interventions to prevent complications often associated with trauma. The nurse must be knowledgeable about specific organ injuries and their associated sequelae. The focus of this chapter is nursing management of adult patients with traumatic injuries in the critical care setting.

TRENDING PRIORITIES IN HEALTHCARE

External Disaster Preparedness

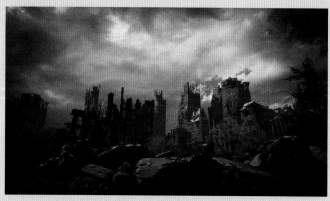

(From, iStock.com/Bulgac)

External disaster preparedness is needed to respond to events occurring outside of the hospital that may increase the demand on the hospital to treat immediate traumas as well as aftermath illnesses brought on by stress and pollutants days to months following the external disaster.[1] External disasters may be grouped into three categories: (1) natural disasters and weather conditions, (2) chemical, radiologic, nuclear, and explosive incidents, and (3) disease agents and toxins.[2]

Natural Disasters and Weather Conditions

Natural disasters and weather conditions are unexpected and unpredictable and may disrupt routine hospital operations, requiring focused efforts on disaster response or possible evacuation.[1] Some examples of natural disasters and weather conditions include earthquakes, volcanic eruptions, mass movements (e.g., rockfall, landslide, avalanche), floods, tornadoes, storms (e.g., hurricanes, typhoons, and cyclones), wildfires, and extreme temperatures (e.g., heat or cold waves).[1] It is important to become familiar with common natural disasters and weather conditions in the area where the hospital is located as some natural disasters and weather conditions produce likely injuries and illnesses for which the hospital may prepare.[1]

Chemical, Radiologic, Nuclear, and Explosive Incidents

Chemical reactivity hazards result from chemical exposures to other chemicals or particular physical conditions.[2] Radiation and nuclear emergencies result from accidental or intentional spills, transportation, misplacement, or misuse of radioactive or nuclear material.[2] These incidents can produce toxic fumes, fires, and explosions that negatively affect the health of populations and health care workers with the severity of illnesses being dependent on type, source, and dose of exposure and use of personal protective equipment.[2] In any of these chemical, radiologic, or nuclear incidents, it is recommended to stay away from known contamination sites, ensure building ventilation systems do not circulate contaminated air, and remove and seal contaminated materials.[2]

Disease Agents and Toxins

Biologic disease agents and toxins are microorganisms (e.g., bacteria, viruses, or fungi) and their associated toxins that result in mild to severe medical conditions.[2] These disease agents and toxins may spread directly or indirectly from person to person or through an insect vector.[2] Health care worker and hospital preparedness is specific to each disease agent and toxin.[2] More information on specific disease agents and toxins may be found on the Occupational Safety and Health Administration's website: www.osha.gov/biological-agents.

For additional information about preparing for external disasters, check out the following websites:

- Federal Emergency Management Agency—www.fema.gov/
- Office of the Assistant Secretary for Preparedness and Response—www. phe.gov/
- Robert T. Stafford Disaster Relief and Emergency Assistance Act—www. fema.gov/sites/default/files/2020-03/stafford-act_2019.pdf

References

1. Hidalgo J, Baez AA. Natural disasters. *Crit Care Clin.* 2019;35(4):591—607.
2. United States Department of Labor. Occupational Safety and Health Administration: Emergency preparedness and response. https://www.osha.gov/emergency-preparedness. Accessed October 17, 2021.

SPECIFIC TRAUMA INJURIES

Traumatic Brain Injuries

More than 69 million TBIs occur worldwide each year.[25] In the United States, it is estimated that 2.8 million TBIs occur annually. Of individuals who sustain TBI, approximately 56,000 Americans die and 288,000 are hospitalized.[26] More than 5.3 million Americans live with some form of long-term disability as a result of TBI.[26] TBI can be caused by both blunt and penetrating trauma. The leading causes of TBI include MVCs, violence (suicide and firearm injuries), and falls.[26] Adults 65 years old and older with a TBI that requires hospitalization have the highest percentage of TBI-related mortality.[4]

Pathophysiology

The pathophysiology of TBI can be divided into two main categories: primary brain injury and secondary brain injury. It is important that the nurse understands these two distinct phases of TBI, because critical care interventions are often directed at limiting the effects of and reducing morbidity and mortality from primary, but more importantly, secondary brain injury.

Primary injury. Primary TBI occurs at the moment of impact as a result of mechanical forces to the head. Primary injuries include those injuries that directly damage the brain parenchyma. Examples of primary TBIs include contusion, laceration, shearing injuries, and hemorrhage. Hemorrhage may significantly compress nearby structures. Primary injury may be mild, with little or no neurologic damage, or severe, with major brain and tissue damage. The extent of and recovery from injury are often related to whether the primary injury was localized (limited to a specific area) or diffuse (widespread) throughout the brain. Immediately after brain injury, a cascade of neural and vascular processes is activated.

Secondary injury. Secondary injury is the biochemical and cellular response to the initial trauma that can exacerbate the primary injury and cause additional damage and impairment in brain

TABLE 24.2 Effects of Trauma Resuscitation.

Aspect of Injury or Resuscitation	Effect on Critical Care Management
Prolonged extrication time	Loss of perfusion to vital organs
	Severity of shock state
Respiratory and/or cardiac arrest	Effects of loss of perfusion to brain (anoxic injury), kidneys, and other vital organs
Time on backboard	Potentiates risk of skin breakdown to occipital lobe, scapulae, sacrum, coccyx, and heels
Number of units of blood; whether any were not fully cross-matched; packed cells vs. whole blood used	Potentiates risk of ARDS, MODS
Prolonged transportation to definitive trauma facility	Worsening of patient condition during transport (e.g., hypotension, ongoing bleeding, acid–base imbalance, oxygenation, and/or ventilation issues)
	New-onset bleeding or rebleeding decreases perfusion to vital organs

ARDS, Acute respiratory distress syndrome; *MODS,* multiple-organ dysfunction syndrome.

TABLE 24.3 Factors Predisposing Trauma Patients to Impaired Oxygenation.

Factor	Impairment
Impaired ventilation	Injury to airway structures, loss of central nervous system regulation of breathing, impaired level of consciousness
Impaired pulmonary gas diffusion	Pneumothorax, hemothorax, aspiration of gastric contents
	Shifts to the left of oxyhemoglobin dissociation curve (can result from infusion of large volumes of banked blood, hypocarbia or alkalosis, or hypothermia)
Decreased oxygen supply	Reduced hemoglobin (from hemorrhage)
	Reduced cardiac output (cardiovascular injury, decreased preload from hemorrhage)

recovery. Secondary injury can be caused by ischemia, hypotension, hypercapnia, cerebral edema, seizures, or metabolic derangements.[27] Hypoxia and hypotension, the best-known culprits for secondary injury,[22] typically are the result of extracranial trauma. A self-perpetuating cycle develops that may cause worsening of the primary injury as a result of uncontrolled secondary factors.

Cerebral edema. Cerebral edema occurs as a result of the changes in the cellular environment caused by contusion, loss of autoregulation, and increased permeability of the blood-brain barrier. As pressure inside the cranial vault increases (in an attempt to perfuse the brain), cerebral perfusion decreases, which further compromises brain function. Cerebral edema can be localized around the area of contusion or diffuse as a result of hypotension or hypoxia. The combined effects of increasing pressure and decreasing perfusion precipitate a downward spiral of events. The extent of cerebral edema can sometimes be minimized by managing aspects of secondary injury, such as oxygenation, ventilation, and perfusion.

Hypotension. Significant hypotension will not adequately perfuse neural tissue. Hypotension is rarely observed in the patient with TBI on admission to the hospital unless terminal medullary failure has occurred. If a trauma patient is unconscious and hypotensive, a detailed assessment of the chest, abdomen, and pelvis must be performed to rule out internal injuries and hemorrhage.

However, hypertension in a trauma patient with severe TBI is common. With loss of autoregulation, an increase in blood pressure occurs, which results in increased intracranial blood volume and elevates intracranial pressure (ICP). Hypertension, observed most frequently after initial TBI, is the body's attempt to perfuse the brain when cerebral circulation is compromised.[28]

Ischemia. Tissue ischemia occurs in areas of poor cerebral perfusion as a result of primary injury, edema, hypotension, or hypoxia. The cells in ischemic areas become edematous. Extreme vasodilation of the cerebral vasculature occurs in TBI in an attempt to supply oxygen and nutrients to the cerebral tissue. This sudden increase in blood volume increases intracranial volume and raises ICP.

Hypercapnia. Hypercapnia is a powerful vasodilator of cerebral vessels. Most often caused by hypoventilation in an unconscious patient, hypercapnia results in cerebral vasodilation, increased cerebral

TABLE 24.4 Interventions for Rewarming Trauma Patients.

Intervention	External Rewarming Procedures	Internal Rewarming Procedures
Passive (protect patient from heat loss, patient will increase body temperature)	Remove all wet clothing and linen. Cover patient with blankets. Avoid bathing patient until normothermia achieved. Maintain a warm temperature in resuscitation room.	Administer warm, humidified oxygen. Administer warm IV fluids.
Active (delivery of heat to trauma patient, either externally or internally)	Use heating blankets or pads.	Perform thoracic or peritoneal lavage with warm solutions. Extracorporeal rewarming Intravascular catheters

IV, Intravenous.

blood flow (volume), and increased ICP. These three variables all contribute to worsening TBI.

Classification of Skull and Brain Injuries

Injuries of the skull and brain are described by the mechanism of injury, location of injury in the brain, and anatomic changes or losses that occur. Some of the most common abnormalities seen in neurologic trauma are described here.

Skull fracture. Skull fractures are common, but they do not by themselves cause neurologic deficits. Skull fractures can be classified as open (dura mater is torn) or closed (dura mater is not torn), or they can be classified as fractures of the vault or fractures of the base. Common vault fractures occur in the frontal and parietal regions. Basilar skull fractures are usually not visible on conventional skull x-rays; a computed tomography (CT) scan is typically required. Assessment findings may include cerebrospinal fluid (CSF) leakage—described as rhinorrhea (from nose) or otorrhea (from ear), Battle sign (ecchymosis overlying the mastoid process behind the ear), "raccoon eyes" (subconjunctival and periorbital ecchymosis), or palsy of the seventh cranial nerve.

The significance of a skull fracture is that it identifies a patient with a higher probability of having or developing an intracranial hematoma. A significant amount of force is required to fracture the skull. Open skull fractures require surgical intervention to remove bony fragments and close the dura mater. Major complications of basilar skull fractures are cranial nerve injury and CSF leakage. A CSF leak may result in a fistula, which increases the possibility of bacterial contamination and subsequent meningitis.

Concussion. A concussion is a brain injury accompanied by a brief loss of neurologic function, in particular, loss of consciousness. When loss of consciousness occurs, it may last for a few seconds to an hour. Neurologic dysfunctions include confusion, disorientation, and sometimes a period of anterograde or retrograde amnesia. Other clinical manifestations that occur after concussion are headache, dizziness, nausea, irritability, inability to concentrate, impaired memory, and fatigue. The diagnosis of concussion is based primarily on patient history.

Contusion. Contusion, or "bruising" of the brain, is frequently associated with acceleration-deceleration injuries, which result in hemorrhage into the superficial parenchyma. Frontal or temporal lobe contusions are most common and can be seen in a *coup-contrecoup mechanism of injury* (Fig. 24.2A). Coup injury affects the cerebral tissue directly under the point of impact. Contrecoup injury occurs in a line directly opposite the point of impact (Fig. 24.2B). The brain contusions caused by the coup and contrecoup impact are visible on a CT scan (Fig. 24.2C).

Clinical manifestations of a contusion are related to the location of the injury, the degree of contusion, and the presence of associated lesions. Contusions can be small, in which localized areas of dysfunction result in a focal neurologic deficit. Larger contusions can evolve over 2 to 3 days after injury as a result of further edema and hemorrhage. A large contusion can produce a mass effect that can cause a significant increase in ICP. Contusions may lead to the development of intracerebral hematomas.[4]

Contusions of the tips of the temporal lobe are a common occurrence and are of particular concern. Because the inner aspects of the temporal lobe surround the opening in the tentorium (where the midbrain enters the cerebrum), edema in this area can cause rapid deterioration in LOC and can lead to herniation. Because of the particular location of this injury, deterioration can occur with little or no warning.

Diagnosis of contusion is made by CT scan. If contusions are small, focal, or multiple, they are treated nonoperatively with serial neurologic assessments. Larger contusions that produce considerable mass effect may require surgical intervention to reduce edema and elevations in ICP. The nurse must pay specific attention to neurologic assessment findings and look for subtle changes in pupillary signs or vital signs, which may indicate potential worsening of the

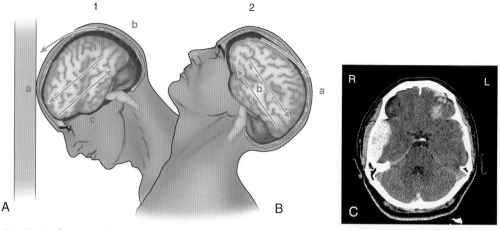

Fig. 24.2 Coup and Contrecoup Head Injury After Blunt Trauma. (A) Coup injury: impact against an object, showing the site of impact and *(a)* direct trauma to the brain, *(b)* shearing of subdural veins, and *(c)* trauma to the base of the brain. (B) Contrecoup injury: impact within the skull, showing *(a)* the site of impact from the brain hitting the opposite side of the skull and *(b)* shearing forces throughout the brain. These injuries occur in one continuous motion; the head strikes the wall (coup) and then rebounds (contrecoup). (C) Computed tomography (CT) scan of a coup and contrecoup head injury. The primary injury is located in the right parietal region, with the contrecoup injury in the left frontal/temporal area. Note that a CT scan is always shown as if the reader is looking in a mirror, so that right *(R)* and left *(L)* are reversed.

patient's condition. The outcome of cerebral contusion is highly variable.

Cerebral hematoma. Extravasation of blood creates a space-occupying lesion within the cranial vault that can lead to increased ICP. Three types of hematomas are discussed here and illustrated in Fig. 24.3. The first two, epidural hematoma (EDH) and subdural hematoma (SDH), are extraparenchymal (outside of brain tissue) and produce injury by pressure and displacement of intracranial contents. The third type is intraparenchymal, occurring within the brain tissue. Traumatic intracerebral hemorrhage (ICH) directly damages neural tissue and can produce further injury as a result of pressure and displacement of intracranial contents.

Epidural hematoma. Epidural hemorrhage or EDH is a collection of blood between the inner skull and the outermost layer of the dura mater (see Fig. 24.3A). EDH occurs as a result of trauma to the skull and meninges. EDHs are most often associated with skull fractures and middle meningeal artery lacerations (two-thirds of patients) or skull fractures with venous bleeding.[22] A blow to the head that causes a linear skull fracture on the lateral surface of the head may tear the middle meningeal artery. As the artery bleeds, it pulls the dura mater away from the skull, creating a pouch that expands into the intracranial space.

The incidence of EDH is relatively low. EDH can occur as a result of low-impact injuries (e.g., falls) or high-impact injuries such as MVCs.

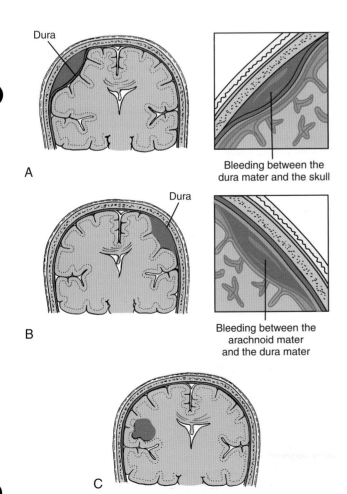

A   Bleeding between the dura mater and the skull

B   Bleeding between the arachnoid mater and the dura mater

C

Fig. 24.3 Intracranial Hematomas. (A) Epidural hematoma. (B) Subdural hematoma. (C) Intracerebral hematoma.

The classic clinical manifestations of EDH include brief loss of consciousness followed by a period of lucidity. Rapid deterioration in the LOC should be anticipated, because arterial bleeding into the epidural space can occur quickly. The patient may complain of a severe, localized headache and may be sleepy. A dilated and fixed pupil on the same side as the impact area is a hallmark of EDH.[22] Diagnosis is based on clinical symptoms and evidence of a collection of blood in the epidural space on CT scan. Treatment of EDH requires urgent surgical intervention to remove the blood and to cauterize the bleeding vessels.

Subdural hematoma. SDH, which is the accumulation of blood between the dura mater and underlying arachnoid membrane, is most often related to a rupture in the bridging veins between the cerebral cortex and the dura mater (see Fig. 24.3B). SDH accounts for approximately 30% of severe head injuries.[4] Acceleration-deceleration and rotational forces are major causes of SDH, which often is associated with cerebral contusions and ICH. Three types of SDH—acute, subacute, and chronic—are based on the time frame from injury and clinical symptoms.

Acute subdural hematoma. Acute SDHs are hematomas that occur after a severe blow to the head. The clinical presentation of acute SDH is determined by the severity of injury to the underlying brain tissue at the time of impact and the rate (speed) at which blood accumulates in the subdural space. The patient often presents with a decreased LOC; in other situations, the patient has a lucid period before deterioration. Careful observation for deterioration in the LOC or lateralizing signs such as inequality of pupils or motor movements is essential. Rapid surgical intervention, including craniectomy, craniotomy, or burr hole evacuation, can reduce mortality.

Subacute subdural hematoma. Subacute SDHs are hematomas that develop 4 days to 3 weeks after trauma.[29] An SDH occurs within the meninges in the subdural space. SDH is diagnosed by alteration in neurologic symptoms and by CT scan. In subacute subdural bleeding, expansion of the hematoma occurs at a rate slower than that observed in acute SDH and less than an epidural bleed. Clinical deterioration of a patient with a subacute SDH is also usually slower than deterioration with an acute SDH, but treatment by surgical intervention, when appropriate, is the same.

Chronic subdural hematoma. Chronic SDH is diagnosed when symptoms appear 21 days or more after injury. Most patients with chronic SDH are in late middle age or older. Individuals at risk for chronic SDH include patients with coordination or balance disturbances and patients receiving anticoagulation therapy. Clinical manifestations of chronic SDH are deceptive. The patient may report a variety of symptoms such as lethargy, absent-mindedness, headache, vomiting, stiff neck, and/or photophobia. They may also show signs of transient ischemic attack, seizures, pupillary changes, or hemiparesis. Because a history of trauma is often not significant enough to be recalled, chronic SDH seldom is seen as an initial diagnosis. CT evaluation confirms the diagnosis.

If surgical intervention is required, evacuation of chronic SDH may be accomplished by craniotomy, burr holes, or catheter drainage. Outcome after chronic SDH evacuation varies. Return of neurologic status often depends on the degree of neurologic dysfunction before intervention occurred. Because this condition is most common in older or debilitated patients, recovery may be slow.

Intracerebral hemorrhage and hematoma. ICH results when bleeding occurs deep within cerebral tissue. Traumatic causes of ICH include depressed skull fractures, penetrating injuries (bullet, knife), or sudden acceleration-deceleration motion. The ICH can act as a rapidly expanding space-occupying lesion; late ICH into the necrotic center of a contused area also is possible (see Fig. 24.3C). Sudden clinical deterioration of a patient 6 to 10 days after trauma may be the result of ICH.

Medical management of ICH may include nonsurgical or surgical approaches. Hemorrhages that are minimal or localized and do not cause significant neurologic or other problems are treated without surgery. Over time, the blood may be reabsorbed. If significant problems with neurologic status occur as a result of the ICH producing a mass effect, surgical intervention is required. The outcome of a patient with an ICH depends on the location of the hemorrhage. Size, mass effect, and displacement of other intracranial structures also affect the outcome.

Penetrating brain injury. Missile injuries are caused by objects that penetrate the skull to produce significant focal damage but little acceleration-deceleration or rotational injury. The injury may be depressed, penetrating, or perforating (Fig. 24.4). Depressed injuries are caused by fractures of the skull with penetration of bone into cerebral tissue. Penetrating injury is caused by a missile that enters the cranial cavity but does not exit. A low-velocity penetrating injury (knife) may involve only focal damage and no loss of consciousness. A high-velocity missile (bullet) can produce shock waves that are transmitted throughout the brain in addition to the injury caused by the bullet. Perforating injuries are missile injuries that enter and then exit the brain. Perforating injuries have much less ricochet effect but are still responsible for significant injury.

Risk of infection and cerebral abscess is a major concern in missile injuries. If fragments of the missile are embedded within the brain, surgery may be required. Careful consideration of the location and risk of increasing neurologic deficit is weighed against the risk of abscess, infection, or permanent disability. The outcome after missile injury is based on the degree of penetration, location of injury, and velocity of the missile.

Diffuse axonal injury. Diffuse axonal injury (DAI) is a term used to describe prolonged posttraumatic coma that is not caused by a mass lesion, although DAI with mass lesions has been reported. DAI covers a wide range of brain dysfunction typically caused by acceleration-deceleration and rotational forces. DAI occurs as a result of damage to the axons or disruption of axonal transmission of the neural impulses.

The pathophysiology of DAI is related to the stretching, shearing, and tearing of axons as a result of movement of the brain inside the cranium at the time of impact. The stretching and tearing of axons result in microscopic lesions throughout the brain, especially deep within cerebral tissue and the base of the cerebrum.[30] Disruption of axonal transmission of impulses results in loss of consciousness. DAI may not be visible on CT or magnetic resonance imaging (MRI) unless surrounding tissues areas are significantly injured, causing small hemorrhages.

DAI can be classified as mild, moderate, or severe based on the extent of lesions. A patient with mild DAI may be in a coma for 24 hours and exhibit periods of decorticate and decerebrate posturing. Patients with moderate DAI may be in a coma for longer than 24 hours and also have episodes of decorticate and decerebrate posturing. Severe DAI usually manifests as a prolonged, deep coma with periods of hypertension, hyperthermia, and excessive diaphoresis. Treatment of DAI includes support of vital functions. The outcome after severe DAI is often poor because of the extensive physiologic dysfunction of cerebral pathways.

Neurologic Assessment

Neurologic assessment is the most important tool for evaluating a patient with a severe TBI, because it can provide information about the severity of injury, offer prognostic information, and dictate the speed with which further evaluation and treatment must proceed.[31] The cornerstone of neurologic assessment is the GCS score, although assessment of the GCS score is not a complete neurologic examination. Pupillary and motor strength assessment must be incorporated into early and ongoing assessments. After specific injuries are identified, a more thorough, focused neurologic assessment, such as examination of the cranial nerves, is warranted. To assist with the initial assessment, TBIs are divided into three descriptive categories—mild, moderate, or severe—on the basis of the patient's GCS score and duration of the unconscious state.

Degree of traumatic brain injury

Mild brain injury. Mild TBI is described as a GCS score of 13 to 15 with a loss of consciousness that lasts up to 15 minutes. Patients with mild injury are seen in the emergency department and often discharged home with a family member who is instructed to evaluate

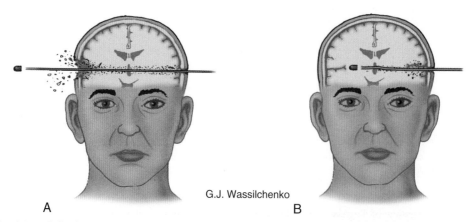

G.J. Wassilchenko

A   B

Fig. 24.4 Bullet Wounds of the Head. Bullet wounds or other penetrating missile injuries cause an open (compound) skull fracture and damage to brain tissue. Shock wave effects are transmitted throughout the brain. (A) Perforating injury. (B) Penetrating injury.

the patient routinely and to bring the patient back to the hospital if any further neurologic symptoms appear.

Moderate brain injury. Moderate TBI is described as a GCS score of 9 to 12 with a loss of consciousness for up to 6 hours. Patients with this type of TBI are usually hospitalized. They are at high risk for deterioration from increasing cerebral edema and ICP, and serial neurologic assessments are important. Hemodynamic and ICP monitoring and ventilatory support are usually not required for these patients unless other bodily injuries make them necessary. A CT scan is obtained on admission. Repeat CT scans are indicated if the patient's neurologic status deteriorates.

Severe brain injury. Patients with a GCS score of 8 or less after resuscitation or patients who deteriorate to that level within 48 hours of admission have a severe TBI.[32] Loss of consciousness may be 6 hours or longer. These patients are admitted to the critical care unit for continuous neurologic assessment, hemodynamic monitoring, mechanical ventilation, and management of complex care issues. Serial CT scans may be performed to rule out evidence of ongoing bleeding or mass lesions that can be surgically corrected.

Priority Clinical Assessment

As in all traumatic injuries, evaluation of a critically injured patient with TBI follows the *ABCDE* approach of ATLS. Immediate assessments of airway, breathing, and circulation (ABCs) are the first steps in patient assessment. Patients with moderate to severe TBI may require endotracheal intubation with mechanical ventilation to reduce the risk of hypoxia and hypercapnia. After stabilization of the ABCs, a thorough neurologic assessment is performed.

LOC, motor movements, pupillary response, respiratory function, and vital signs all are part of a complete neurologic assessment of a patient with TBI. LOC is a patient's degree of responsiveness and awareness.[7] Consciousness is assessed by obtaining the patient's response to verbal and painful stimuli. Determination of orientation to person, place, and time assesses mental alertness. Pupils are assessed for size, shape, equality, and reactivity. Asymmetry must be reported immediately. Pupils are also assessed for constriction to a light source (parasympathetic innervation) or dilation (sympathetic innervation). Because parasympathetic fibers are present in the brainstem, pupils that are slow to react to light may indicate a brainstem injury. A "blown" pupil is a term used to describe a fixed and dilated pupil that can be caused by compression of the third cranial nerve or transtentorial herniation (see Fig. 16.3). Bilateral fixed pupils can indicate midbrain involvement and are an indicator of poor neurologic outcome.

Neurologic assessments are continuous throughout the patient's stay in the critical care unit as part of ongoing assessments to detect subtle changes in the patient's condition. Serial assessments include changes in LOC, GCS score, pupils, and hemodynamic status. In these situations, careful clinical observation of trends in the patient's condition is essential. The use of analgesia, sedation, and muscle relaxants may mask neurologic signs in a patient with a severe head injury. When sedation of the patient is required, newer shorter-acting sedatives with a short half-life are used. For example, IV propofol can be turned off, and within minutes, a neurologic examination can be performed.

Diagnostic procedures. The cornerstone of diagnostic procedures for evaluation of TBI is the CT scan.[4,22] CT is a rapid, noninvasive procedure that can provide invaluable information about the presence of mass lesions (including hemorrhage) and cerebral edema. Serial CT scans may be obtained over a period of several days to assess areas of contusion and ischemia and to detect delayed hematomas. The critical

care nurse must always remain with a patient with a TBI during a CT scan and during transport to and from the scanner to provide continuous observation and monitoring. Transporting the patient, moving the patient from the bed to the CT table, and positioning the head flat during the CT scan all are stressful events and can cause severe increases in ICP and decreases in *cerebral perfusion pressure* (CPP).

Medical Management

Surgical management. If a lesion identified on CT scan is causing a shift of intracranial contents or increasing ICP, surgical intervention is necessary. A craniotomy is performed to remove the EDH, SDH, or large ICH. Patients may also undergo a *decompressive craniectomy* specifically for elevated ICP. This procedure involves removal of the overlying bone flap to allow the underlying brain tissue to expand and swell. This surgical strategy has demonstrated some benefits but remains controversial.[16,33]

Nonsurgical management. Nonsurgical management includes management of ICP, maintenance of adequate CPP, ensuring adequate oxygenation, and prevention and treatment of complications such as pneumonia or infection. The decision of when to initiate ICP monitoring is critical. ICP monitoring may be required for patients with a GCS score less than 8 and abnormal findings on a head CT scan.[34] Various methods to monitor brain tissue oxygenation may also be used.

Nursing Management

The patient care management plan for a patient with a TBI incorporates a variety of patient diagnoses (Box 24.4). **Nursing priorities focus on (1) recognition and reduction of increased ICP, (2) limiting or preventing secondary brain injury, and (3) stabilization of vital signs.** Ongoing neurologic assessments are the foundation of care for patients with TBI. Assessments are the primary mechanism for determining improvement or worsening of the patient's condition. If secondary injury is to be prevented, the critical care nurse (in collaboration with the physicians) must respond immediately to events that increase ICP, reduce MAP, and reduce CPP.

The initial management of severe TBI frequently occurs in the critical care unit. All aspects of care, including hemodynamic management, control of ICP, IV fluid therapy, pulmonary care, acid–base balance, maintenance of body temperature, and control of the environment, can affect outcome after TBI.[33,35]

In patients with TBI, changes in cardiovascular function and circulating catecholamines may contribute to hemodynamic instability. Heart rate and blood pressure are continually monitored. Although no specific hemodynamic parameters have been universally agreed upon, the Brain Trauma Foundation (BTF) TBI guidelines currently recommend SBP be maintained greater than 100 mm Hg for

---

⊚ BOX 24.4 PRIORITY PATIENT CARE MANAGEMENT

Traumatic Brain Injury
- Ineffective Tissue Perfusion due to decreased cerebral blood flow
- Decreased Intracranial Adaptive Capacity due to failure of normal intracranial compensatory mechanisms
- Impaired Verbal Communication due to cerebral speech center injury
- Impaired Breathing due to neuromuscular impairment
- Risk for Aspiration
- Powerlessness related to lack of control over current situation
Patient Care Management plans are located in Appendix A.

patients aged 50 to 69 years and greater than 110 mm Hg for patients 15 to 49 years and those over age 70.[36] Isotonic IV fluids (e.g., 0.9% normal saline) and vasopressors may be required if target SBP is not achieved. Arterial blood pressure should be continually monitored, because hypotension in a patient with TBI is rare and may indicate coexisting or undiagnosed injuries.

Ongoing monitoring of ICP may be necessary, and in some patients with TBI, insertion of an external ventricular drain may be required. When an external ventricular drain is in situ, best practice evidence suggests keeping ICP less than 20 mm Hg[16,37] (normal, 0–15 mm Hg) and maintaining CPP at between 60 and 70 mm Hg[36] to facilitate optimal patient outcomes. Aggressive attempts to maintain CPP greater than 70 mm Hg have not been supported in the literature and should be avoided secondary to increasing risk of cardiac or respiratory problems.[36]

When ICP is too high, the administration of IV mannitol or hypertonic saline may be necessary. Mannitol (an osmotic diuretic) and hypertonic saline (sterile salt solution) both pull fluid from brain parenchyma and decrease ICP. Mannitol and hypertonic saline are given as intermittent IV boluses. Whether mannitol or hypertonic saline is given to patients with TBI, careful monitoring of the patient's serum sodium and serum osmolality is required.

In severe TBI, the patient is often intubated, mechanically ventilated, and placed on a full support mode of mechanical ventilation. No clear consensus exists for mechanical ventilation in TBI, but best evidence suggests that low to normal lung ventilation volumes with the lowest amount of positive end-expiratory pressure (PEEP) that prevents hypoxemia, up to approximately 10 cm H_2O, appears safe.[4] Of utmost importance is ensuring that the TBI patient is not hypoxemic.

Capnography (monitoring of exhaled carbon dioxide levels) is suggested to monitor for hypercapnia. ABGs are frequently obtained, with particular attention to arterial partial pressure of carbon dioxide ($PaCO_2$). Most facilities caring for patients with TBI aim to keep the $PaCO_2$ level low normal at 35 to 40 mm Hg, as any increase in $PaCO_2$ would increase cerebral blood flow and worsen ICP. When $PaCO_2$ levels increase, the tidal volume or minute volume needs to be increased on the ventilator. Although pulmonary care must be instituted, endotracheal suctioning can elevate ICP. Techniques to counter elevation in ICP with suctioning are outlined in Box 24.5.

Cerebral oxygen consumption is increased during periods of increased body temperature. As a result, the goal is to achieve normothermia (36°C–37°C). Monitoring of the patient's temperature,

---

BOX 24.5 Recommendations for Suctioning Patients With Traumatic Brain Injury

- Hyperoxygenate the patient on 100% fraction of inspired oxygen (FiO_2) before passage of suction catheter.
- Intravenous lidocaine (blunts the increase in heart rate, mean arterial pressure, and intracranial pressure that can occur with suctioning).[a]
- Apply suction on removal of catheter for no longer than 10 seconds.
- Limit number of suction catheter passes, preferably to no more than two passes per suctioning episode.
- Minimize airway stimulation (e.g., stabilize endotracheal tube, avoid passing suction catheter all the way to carina).

[a]Singh S, Chouhan RS, Bindra A, Radhakrishna N. Comparison of effect of dexmedetomidine and lidocaine on intracranial and systemic hemodynamic response to chest physiotherapy and tracheal suctioning in patients with severe traumatic brain injury. *J Anesth.* 2018;32(4):518–523.

---

use of antipyretics, cooling blankets, and early identification and workup for infection are essential. A tremendous catecholamine surge after TBI has been associated with infectious complications and potentially preventable mortality.[33] The use of beta-blockers to suppress this catecholamine surge in patients with TBI has been shown to decrease mortality.[38]

In the early postinjury phase, the patient's environment must be controlled. Stimuli that produce pain, agitation, or discomfort can increase ICP. Nursing interventions should not be clustered, and care should be evenly distributed throughout the shift. Explanations can be provided to patients in a calm, soft-spoken manner. Families and significant others are informed about the importance of maintaining a quiet environment. Analgesics and sedatives should be administered as ordered by the physician and as required by the patient; they should not be routinely used as first-line agents when ICP increases. Patients should be provided several rest periods during hospitalization.

Newer pharmacologic agents have demonstrated some promise in the treatment of patients awakening from head trauma, but results have not been conclusive. One such medication is amantadine, a dopamine-receptor antagonist. Although its mechanism is only partially understood, it appears to enhance dopamine release at presynaptic neurons.[39] The latest research has identified amantadine to be of help in patients who experience feelings of aggressiveness after TBI.[40]

Spinal Cord Injuries

Approximately 17,700 new SCIs occur in the United States annually.[41] Since the 1970s, the median age at injury has increased from 28 years to the current median age of 43 years.[41] Over 70% of SCI patients are male. The most frequent cause of SCI is MVCs (38%), followed by falls (30%), violence (14.6%), and sporting activities (9%).[42] The diagnosis of SCI begins with a detailed history of events surrounding the incident, precise evaluation of sensory and motor function, and radiographic studies of the spine.

Pathophysiology

SCIs are the result of a mechanical force that disrupts neurologic tissue or its vascular supply or both. Similar to the pathophysiology of TBI, injury to the spinal cord occurs through both primary and secondary injury mechanisms (Box 24.6). Primary injury is the neurologic and vascular damage that occurs at the moment of impact, which may be caused by blunt or penetrating injury. Secondary injury, which occurs within minutes of injury, refers to the complex biochemical processes affecting cellular function that occur from inflammation, edema, hemorrhage, cytokine release, and vascular injury.[43]

This cascade of events that occurs immediately after SCI may lead to spinal cord ischemia and loss of neurologic function. Additionally, electrolyte and biochemical changes, the accumulation of glutamate (the most prevalent neurotransmitter in our brains), and disruption of the blood–spinal cord barrier promote cellular death.[44] Collectively, these secondary pathophysiologic events result in exacerbation of the injury, potentially extending the level of functional deficit and worsening long-term outcome. Knowledge of the pathophysiology of secondary processes has led to the development of newer therapies that aim to target cellular changes contributing to injury. Despite ongoing research efforts at repairing primary SCI, minimizing damage by reducing secondary injury has shown the most promise.

Mechanism of Injury

Hyperflexion, hyperextension, rotation, and axial loading are four distinct forces by which the spinal cord may be injured. The spinal cord may also be injured by penetrating trauma.

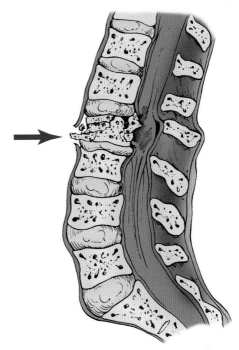

Fig. 24.5 Spinal Cord Compression Burst Fracture. Compression injuries cause burst fractures of the vertebral body that often send bony fragments into the spinal canal or directly into the spinal cord. Mechanisms of injury include hyperflexion, hyperextension, rotation, axial loading (vertical compression), and missile or penetrating injuries.

Hyperflexion. Hyperflexion injury is most often seen in the cervical area, especially at the level of C5 to C6, because this is the most mobile portion of the cervical spine. This type of injury most often is caused by sudden deceleration motion, as in head-on collisions. Injury occurs from compression of the cord as a result of fracture fragments or dislocation of the vertebral bodies. Instability of the spinal column occurs because of rupture or tearing of the posterior muscles and ligaments.

Hyperextension. Hyperextension injuries involve backward and downward motion of the head. With this injury, often seen in rear-end MVCs, the spinal cord is stretched and distorted. Neurologic deficits associated with this injury are often caused by contusion and ischemia of the cord without significant bony involvement. *Whiplash* is a mild form of hyperextension injury.

Rotation. Rotation injuries often occur in conjunction with a flexion or extension injury. This may occur in cervical, thoracic, or lumbar sections of the cord. Severe rotation of the neck or body results in tearing of the posterior ligaments and displacement (rotation) of the spinal column.

Axial loading. Axial loading, or compression injury, occurs from vertical force along the spinal cord. This is most commonly seen in a fall from a height in which the person lands on the feet or buttocks. Compression injuries may cause *burst fractures* of the vertebral body that often send bony fragments into the spinal canal or directly into the spinal cord (Fig. 24.5).

Penetrating injuries. Penetrating injury to the spinal cord can be caused by a bullet, knife, or any other object that penetrates the cord. These types of injuries often cause permanent damage by anatomically transecting the spinal cord.

Functional Injury of the Spinal Cord

Functional injury of the spinal cord refers to the degree of disruption of normal spinal cord function. This depends on what specific sensory and motor structures within the cord are damaged. SCIs are classified as complete or incomplete. The most frequent diagnosis at discharge has been incomplete tetraplegia (47.2%) followed by complete and incomplete paraplegia (20%).[41] SCI cannot be classified until spinal shock has resolved.

Complete injury. Complete SCI results in a total loss of sensory and motor function below the level of injury. Regardless of the mechanism of injury, the result is a complete dissection of the spinal cord and its neurochemical pathways, resulting in one of two conditions: tetraplegia or paraplegia.

Tetraplegia. With tetraplegia, the injury occurs between the C1 and T1 level. Residual muscle function depends on the specific cervical segments involved. The potential functional status resulting from different neurologic levels of injury is described in Table 24.5.

Paraplegia. With paraplegia, the injury occurs in the thoracolumbar region (T2—L1). Patients with injuries in this area may have full or limited use of the arms, and all require a wheelchair. In rare circumstances, a few patients may have limited ability to ambulate short distances with the assistance of crutches, braces, or other orthotic devices. Thoracic, L1, and L2 injuries produce paraplegia with variable innervation to intercostal and abdominal muscles.

Incomplete injury. Incomplete SCI results in a mixed loss of voluntary motor activity and sensation below the level of the lesion.

TABLE 24.5	Quadriplegia Functional Status.
Neurologic Level (Vertebrae) of Complete Injury	Functional Ability
C1—C4	Requires electric wheelchair with breath, head, or shoulder controls
C5	Needs electric wheelchair with hand control and/ or manual wheelchair with rim projections; may require adaptive devices to assist with ADLs
C6	Independent in manual wheelchair on level surface; may need hand controls; adaptive devices may be needed for ADLs
C7	Requires manual wheelchair on most surfaces
C8—T1	May need adaptive devices

ADL, Activities of daily living.

TABLE 24.6	Muscle Strength Scale.
5 =	Active movement against maximal resistance
4 =	Active movement through ROM against resistance
3 =	Active movement through ROM against gravity
2 =	Active movement through ROM with gravity eliminated
1 =	Flicker or trace of contraction
0 =	No contraction; total paralysis

ROM, Range of motion.

Incomplete SCI exists if any function remains below the level of injury. Incomplete injuries can result in a variety of syndromes, which are classified according to the degree of motor and sensory loss below the level of injury. Some of the more common incomplete injury syndromes are described here.

Brown-Séquard syndrome. Brown-Séquard syndrome is associated with damage to only one side of the cord as a result of penetrating trauma or crush injury. This produces loss of voluntary motor movement on the same side as the injury (hemiparaplegia), with coexisting loss of pain, temperature, and sensation on the opposite side (hemianesthesia).[45] Functionally, the side of the body with the best motor control has little or no sensation, whereas the side of the body with sensation has little or no motor control.

Central cord syndrome. Associated with cervical hyperextension-hyperflexion injury and damage to the central region of the spinal cord, central cord syndrome is the most common type of incomplete SCI. This injury produces motor deficits more pronounced in the upper extremities than in the lower extremities.[46] Various degrees of sensory impairment (pain, temperature) and bowel and bladder dysfunction may be present.

Anterior cord syndrome. Anterior cord syndrome occurs as a result of direct anterior spinal cord compression (occlusion) of the anterior spinal artery or hyperflexion of the cervical spine.[47] Injury occurs to the anterior gray horn cells (motor), spinothalamic tracts (pain), anterior spinothalamic tract (light touch), and corticospinal tracts (temperature). The result is a loss of motor function and loss of the sensations of pain and temperature below the level of injury. However, below the level of injury, position sense and sensations of pressure and vibration remain intact.

Posterior cord syndrome. Posterior cord syndrome is most often associated with blockage of the posterior spinal artery from a tumor. In trauma with cervical hyperextension injury, the posterior column may be damaged. This results in the loss of position sense, pressure, and vibration below the level of injury. Motor function and sensation of pain and temperature remain intact. These patients may be unable to ambulate because the loss of position sense impairs spontaneous movement. This type of SCI is extremely rare.

Neurotrauma assessment. Screening of the trauma patient for SCI is an integral part of the assessment for all trauma teams. However, the initial neurologic assessment may not be an accurate indication of eventual motor and sensory loss. The first assessment focuses on the rapid and accurate identification of present, absent, or impaired

functioning of the motor, sensory, and reflex systems that coordinate and regulate vital functions. Once the patient has been stabilized, a more detailed motor and sensory examination, which includes assessment of all 32 spinal nerves for evidence of dysfunction, can be performed.

Carefully mapped pathways for the sensory portion of the spinal nerves, called *dermatomes,* can assist in localizing the functional (sensory) level of injury. The American Spinal Injury Association (ASIA) suggests that motor function and strength may be graded on a six-point scale (Table 24.6). Initial evaluation must be performed correctly, and findings must be thoroughly documented in detail so that subsequent serial assessments can rapidly identify deterioration. ASIA has developed a form that outlines the necessary assessments for initial and ongoing classification of SCIs (Fig. 24.6). Ongoing spinal cord assessments must be documented during the critical care phase.

Nursing assessment. Attention to the ABCs of the ATLS approach is imperative in a patient with known or suspected SCI on admission to the critical care unit, similar to patients with TBI and all other trauma patients. Ensuring a patent airway is of primary concern. Assessment of breathing patterns and gas exchange is done after the airway has been secured. The level of SCI often dictates the degree of altered breathing patterns that exist (Table 24.7). Because injuries above the C3 level result in paralysis of the diaphragm, patients with these injuries require intubation and mechanical ventilation.

Stabilization of the spinal cord is mandatory to prevent further injury, and spinal precautions are maintained until otherwise ordered. This includes stabilization of the head and neck with manual (hand-held) traction during the initial assessment, including intubation and establishment of ventilatory support. Bed rest, a hard collar, and use of logrolling maneuvers are widely used across the country, although there is limited evidence to indicate true benefit.[48] However, until cervical and spinal x-rays have been completed, reviewed, and cleared, or definitive stabilization has been achieved, immobilization protocols are unlikely to produce any untoward consequences.

As discussed earlier, hypovolemic shock in trauma occurs in response to fluid volume deficit, often related to hemorrhage. *Spinal shock* is a condition that occurs shortly after traumatic injury to the spinal cord. Spinal shock is complete loss of all muscle tone and normal reflex activity below the level of injury,[4] including loss of rectal tone. In other words, spinal shock is a "concussion" of the spinal cord. Patients with spinal shock may appear completely without function below the area of injury, although not all of the area may be destroyed. It may occur 30 to 60 minutes after injury and on average last 4 to 12 weeks.[49]

Neurogenic shock results from injury to the descending sympathetic pathways in the spinal cord. This injury results in loss of vasomotor tone and sympathetic innervation to the heart. Patients with SCI at T6 or above may have profound neurogenic shock as a result of interruption of the sympathetic nervous system and loss of vasoconstrictor response below the level of the injury.[50] Hypotension, bradycardia,

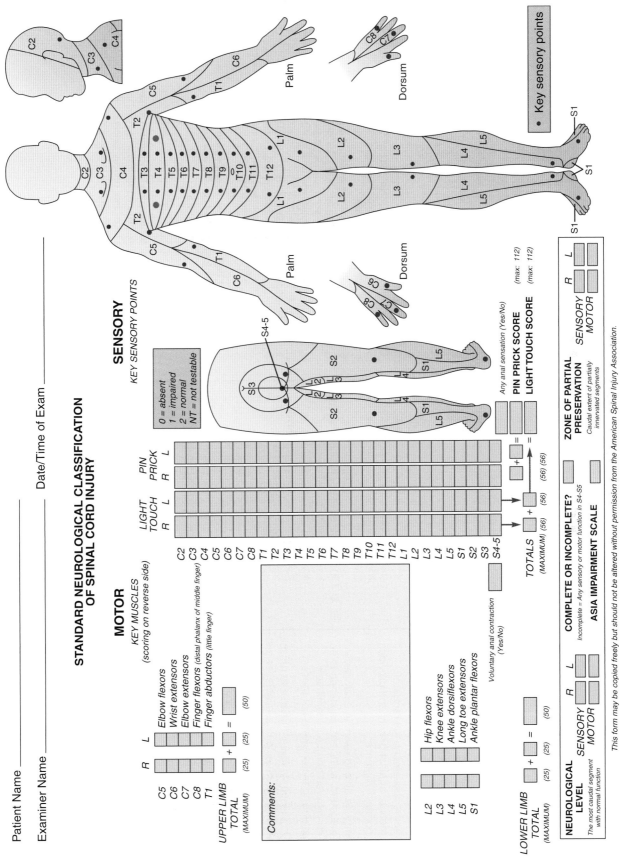

Fig. 24.6 American Spinal Injury Association Classification of Spinal Cord Injuries. ASIA, American Spinal Injury Association; SCI, cervical spinal cord injury.

MUSCLE GRADING

0   total paralysis

1   palpable or visible contraction

2   active movement, full range of motion, gravity eliminated

3   active movement, full range of motion, against gravity

4   active movement, full range of motion, against gravity and provides some resistance

5   active movement, full range of motion, against gravity and provides normal resistance

5* muscle able to exert, in examiner's judgment, sufficient resistance to be considered normal if identifiable inhibiting factors were not present

NT not testable. Patient unable to reliably exert effort or muscle unavailable for testing due to factors such as immobilization, pain on effort or contracture.

ASIA IMPAIRMENT SCALE

☐ **A = Complete**: No motor or sensory function is preserved in the sacral segments S4-S5.

☐ **B = Incomplete**: Sensory but not motor function is preserved below the neurological level and includes the sacral segments S4-S5.

☐ **C = Incomplete**: Motor function is preserved below the neurological level, and more than half of key muscles below the neurological level have a muscle grade less than 3.

☐ **D = Incomplete**: Motor function is preserved below the neurological level, and at least half of key muscles below the neurological level have a muscle grade of 3 or more.

☐ **E = Normal**: Motor and sensory function are normal.

CLINICAL SYNDROMES (OPTIONAL)

☐ Central Cord
☐ Brown-Sequard
☐ Anterior Cord
☐ Conus Medullaris
☐ Cauda Equina

STEPS IN CLASSIFICATION

The following order is recommended in determining the classification of individuals with SCI.

1. Determine sensory levels for right and left sides.

2. Determine motor levels for right and left sides.
   Note: in regions where there is no myotome to test, the motor level is presumed to be the same as the sensory level.

3. Determine the single neurological level.
   This is the lowest segment where motor and sensory function is normal on both sides, and is the most cephalad of the sensory and motor levels determined in steps 1 and 2.

4. Determine whether the injury is Complete or Incomplete.
   (sacral sparing).
   *If voluntary anal contraction = **No** AND all S4-5 sensory scores = **0** AND any anal sensation = **No**, then injury is COMPLETE. Otherwise injury is incomplete.*

5. Determine ASIA Impairment Scale (AIS) Grade:
   Is injury Complete?   If **YES**, AIS=A Record ZPP

   NO → (For ZPP record lowest dermatome or myotome on each side with some (non-zero score) preservation)

   Is injury motor incomplete? If **NO**, AIS=B

   YES → (Yes=voluntary anal contraction OR motor function more than three levels below the motor level on a given side.)

   Are at least half of the key muscles below the (single) neurological level graded 3 or better?

   NO → AIS=C   YES → AIS=D

   If sensation and motor function is normal in all segments, AIS=E
   Note: AIS E is used in follow up testing when an individual with a documented SCI has recovered normal function. If at initial testing no deficits are found, the individual is neurologically intact; the ASIA Impairment Scale does not apply.

Fig. 24.6 cont'd

TABLE 24.7 Effects of Spinal Cord Injury on Ventilatory Functions.

Neurologic Level (Vertebrae) of Complete Injury	Respiratory Function	Comment
C1–C2	Paralysis of diaphragm	Ventilator dependent
C3–C5	Various degrees of diaphragm paralysis	Some diaphragm control; may need ventilatory support; weaning depends on preinjury pulmonary status
C6–T11	Various degrees of impaired intercostal muscles and abdominal muscles	Compromised respiratory function; reduced inspiratory ability; paradoxical breathing patterns; ineffective cough, sneeze

and peripheral vasodilation are hallmark signs and symptoms of neurogenic shock. Blood pressure support may be required with the use of sympathomimetic medications. The duration of this shock state can persist for up to 1 month after injury.

The mechanism of injury often assists trauma teams in distinguishing between these three types of shock. In hypovolemic shock, the patient is often tachycardic. In neurogenic shock, the patient is generally bradycardic. In spinal shock, priapism may be present.

Diagnostic procedures. Radiographic evaluations can identify the severity of damage to the spinal cord. Initial evaluation on admission to the emergency department or critical care unit should include anteroposterior and lateral x-ray views of all areas of the spinal cord. In many medical centers, CT scan has replaced plain radiography as the principal modality for cervical spine assessment after trauma.[22] CT scans of all seven cervical vertebrae and the top of T1 must be obtained to rule out cervicothoracic injury. Flexion and extension views can identify subtle ligament injuries. MRI may also be used for definitive diagnosis of SCI.

The assessment and authorization to remove the cervical collar, known as *clearance of the cervical spine*, is challenging in a patient with SCI in the critical care unit. Clearance of the cervical spine is made difficult by alteration in mentation as a result of coexisting injury, analgesia, and sedation; intubation and mechanical ventilation; surgical procedures; and a focus on other more distracting injuries. The

Eastern Association of Surgeons in Trauma developed guidelines for clearance of the cervical spine (Table 24.8).

Medical Management

After initial assessment of the trauma patient has occurred and a diagnosis of SCI is confirmed, medical management begins. The primary goal is to preserve remaining neurologic function with either surgical or nonsurgical interventions.

Surgical management. Surgical intervention provides spinal column stability in the presence of an unstable injury. Unstable injuries include disrupted ligaments and tendons and a vertebral column that cannot maintain normal alignment. Identification and immobilization of unstable injuries are particularly important for a patient with incomplete neurologic deficit. Without adequate stabilization, movement and dislocation of the vertebral column may cause a complete neurologic deficit. Various surgical procedures may be performed to achieve decompression (relief of pressure on spinal nerves) and stabilization after SCI has occurred.

Laminectomy. In this procedure, the lamina (which forms the posterior portion of the spinal canal) is removed to allow decompression and removal of bony fragments or material from the canal.

Spinal fusion. This technique involves surgical fusion of two to six vertebral bodies to provide stability and to prevent motion. This may be

TABLE 24.8 EAST Guidelines for Cervical Spine Clearance.

Trauma Patient Population	Recommendation
Trauma patients who are awake, alert, not intoxicated, neurologically normal, no complaints of neck pain or tenderness with full range of motion of cervical spine	Neck is palpated in all directions for tenderness or pain. If physical examination is negative for pain or tenderness, CT of cervical spine is not required, and cervical collar may be removed.
All other trauma patients with suspected cervical injury must be radiologically evaluated, including patients with neck pain or tenderness, whether alert or with altered mental status/neurologic deficit, or distracting injury	Obtain axial CT from occiput to T1 with sagittal and coronal reconstructions. If CT is positive for injury, continue cervical collar, obtain spine consultation, and obtain MRI. In neurologically intact awake patient with neck pain, if CT is negative (no injury seen), MRI is negative, and adequate flexion/extension radiographs are negative, discontinue cervical collar.
Trauma patients who are obtunded with gross motor function of extremities	Obtain axial CT from occiput to T1 with sagittal and coronal reconstructions. If CT is negative (no injury seen), risk/benefit of additional MRI must be determined in each hospital. Options 1. Continue cervical collar until clinical examination can be performed. 2. Remove cervical collar on the basis of negative CT alone. 3. Obtain MRI. If MRI is negative, collar can be safely removed. Flexion/extension radiographs should not be performed.

CT, Computed tomography; *EAST,* Eastern Association of Surgeons in Trauma; *MRI,* magnetic resonance imaging.
Modified from Como JJ, Diaz JJ, Dunham CM, et al. Practice management guidelines for identification of cervical spine injuries following trauma: update from the Eastern Association for the Surgery of Trauma Practice Management Guidelines Committee. *J Trauma.* 2009;67(3):651.

accomplished by an anterior or posterior surgical approach. Fusion is accomplished through the use of bone chips taken from the iliac crest, bone bank, or artificial bone substitute, and by use of wires, pins, or rods.

Other spinal cord surgical options. Pedicle screw fixation has become one treatment option for thoracic and lumbar fracture fixation.[51] This procedure helps stabilize fractured thoracic and lumbar segments of the spinal column. Vertebral plates and bone grafting may also be used.

Nonsurgical management. If the injury to the spinal cord is stable, nonsurgical management is the treatment of choice. Nonsurgical management for cervical and thoracolumbar injuries is discussed in this section.

Cervical injury. Management of cervical injuries involves the immobilization of the fracture and realignment of any dislocation. This is accomplished through skeletal traction that involves the use of two-point tongs, which are inserted into the skull through shallow burr holes and are connected to weights. Several types of cervical tongs are used. Gardner-Wells and Crutchfield tongs are the most common. These tongs can be applied at the bedside by experienced personnel with the use of a local anesthetic. Weights are applied gradually, with frequent neurologic and radiographic evaluations, until the fracture is reduced (realigned).

After the procedure, the patient must be immobilized on a kinetic therapy bed or a regular bed. The kinetic therapy bed is advantageous for cervical immobilization because it maintains alignment of the spinal column while providing a constant turning motion to reduce pulmonary complications and incidence of skin breakdown.[52] Use of cervical skeletal traction on a regular bed is also acceptable, but it is more difficult to provide adequate care to the pulmonary and integumentary systems because of the extensive degree of immobility.

Halo traction braces may be used for some patients with a cervical spine injury. The halo vest consists of a metal ring secured to the skull with two occipital and two temporal screws. The metal ring is attached to steel bars that anchor to the plastic vest to provide cervical immobilization (Fig. 24.7). The halo traction brace immobilizes the cervical spine but allows the patient to ambulate and participate in self-care.

Thoracolumbar injury. Nonsurgical management of a patient with a thoracolumbar injury is undertaken in the absence of neurologic injury. Generally, this approach frequently involves immobilization. Immobilization is accomplished by bed rest (with the bed flat) or the use of a plastic or fiberglass jacket, a body cast, or a brace, which facilitates early mobility. There is no consensus on the optimal treatment.

Nursing Management

The patient care management plan for the patient with SCI incorporates a variety of patient diagnoses (Box 24.7). **Nursing priorities during the critical care phase focus on (1) optimizing hemodynamic stability and (2) preventing life-threatening complications while maximizing function of all organ systems.** Nursing interventions are aimed at preventing secondary damage to the spinal cord and managing the complications of the neurologic deficit. Because almost all body systems are affected by SCI, nursing management must include interventions that promote optimal functioning of each system. Moreover, patients with SCIs have complex psychosocial needs that require a great deal of emotional support from the critical care nurse.

Neurologic care. Assessment, monitoring, and trending of the patient's GCS score and sensory and motor function are important aspects of nursing the SCI patient in critical care. The use of methylprednisolone as a neuroprotective agent in SCI is controversial.[53] There is no clear

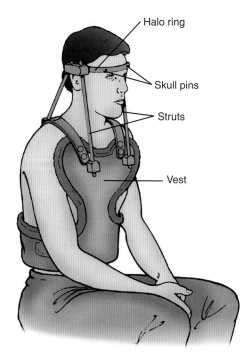

Fig. 24.7   Halo Vest. The halo traction device immobilizes the cervical spine, which allows the patient to ambulate and participate in self-care.

◎ BOX 24.7   PRIORITY PATIENT CARE MANAGEMENT

Spinal Cord Injury
- Impaired Gas Exchange due to alveolar hypoventilation
- Impaired Breathing due to musculoskeletal fatigue or neuromuscular impairment
- Impaired Cardiac Output due to sympathetic blockade
- Autonomic Dysreflexia due to excessive autonomic response to noxious stimuli
- Disturbed Body Image due to actual change in body structure, function, or appearance

Patient Care Management plans are located in Appendix A.

---

consensus on the efficacy of this medication or any other medication in enhancing recovery of cord function after injury. Current best practice guidelines suggest not administering corticosteroids in traumatic SCI.[54]

Cardiovascular care. Maintenance of hemodynamic stability and ensuring adequate tissue perfusion is a necessary prerequisite to promote recovery of injured spinal cord tissue. Hypotension (SBP less than 90 mm Hg) should be avoided or corrected as soon as possible after acute SCI. Alteration in tissue perfusion because of hypotension may require administration of IV fluids. After the fluid volume status has been optimized, inotropic or vasopressor support (or both) may be implemented if SBP or MAP remains low. Accurate assessment of fluid volume status is required because pulmonary edema is a threat to patients with SCI.

It is widely accepted as best practice to maintain the MAP greater than 85 to 90 mm Hg for the first 5 to 7 days post-SCI. This treatment helps facilitate optimal perfusion to the injured spinal cord[55] and helps facilitate functional recovery.

A patient with SCI is at high risk for, or may exhibit alterations in, cardiovascular stability, including dysrhythmias. The risk for cardiovascular instability is profound in patients with SCI at the C3 to C5 levels, although cardiovascular alterations occur with most injuries above T6. Symptomatic bradyarrhythmias may be treated with an inotropic medication such as isoproterenol or anticholinergic medication such as atropine. Both medications increase heart rate and also increase myocardial oxygen consumption. For persistent low heart rates that produce symptoms, another option may be a temporary transvenous pacemaker.

As with any immobilized patient, the risk for development of deep vein thrombosis (DVT) is high. However, detection of DVT is difficult because pain and tenderness are not applicable to a patient with SCI. Prevention of DVT is imperative and may include a combination of therapies such as low-dose heparin, low–molecular-weight heparin, sequential compression devices, and embolic hose.[53]

Pulmonary care.
Pulmonary complications are the most common cause of mortality in patients with SCI.[44] Initial and ongoing nursing assessments of respiratory status are vital for identifying actual or potential impairment in ventilation. Evaluations include assessment of respiratory rate and rhythm, observation of symmetry of chest expansion and use of accessory muscles, inspection of quantity and character of secretions, and auscultation of breath sounds. Serial ABG values provide information on the adequacy of gas exchange.

Intubation and mechanical ventilation are frequently required in acute SCI. The critical care nurse must be aware that the neuromuscular blocking agent *succinylcholine* (suxamethonium) should not be administered to patients with SCI. Use of this depolarizing agent in a patient with SCI not only may aggravate existing injury as a result of fasciculation during induction, but it also may produce hyperkalemic cardiac arrest.

Patients with lesions at C3 to C5 may eventually be able to be weaned from the ventilator. Some patients with C3 injuries may require mechanical ventilation only at night. Weaning can be a complex process because of the physiologic demands placed on the diaphragm and the psychologic effects of fear of the inability to breathe. Various weaning methods are available, and a well-coordinated approach by the nurse, physician, respiratory therapist, and patient is essential. Weaning difficulties are common, and reintubation, including insertion of a tracheostomy tube, is sometimes required.

Ineffective airway clearance and impaired gas exchange is a particular problem for a patient with SCI as a result of hypoventilation (paralysis of respiratory muscles), increased bronchial secretions, and atelectasis secondary to decreased cough. Nursing interventions are directed at improving and maintaining adequate gas exchange.

Frequent suctioning of the airway is required. Caution must be used with vigorous suctioning, because stimulation of the vagus nerve (which runs alongside the trachea) can cause profound bradycardia. Hyperoxygenation with 100% oxygen before suctioning is recommended.

Chest percussion and repositioning facilitate removal of secretions. Kinetic therapy beds, which can rotate up to 60 degrees on each side, may provide continual postural drainage and mobilization of secretions. To further aid in mobilizing secretions in the presence of an ineffective cough, a technique of cough assistance can be used. This procedure is similar to abdominal thrusts (formerly known as the Heimlich maneuver). Exact hand placement may vary, and it is important to assess which placement works best for the patient. Cough assist machines are also commercially available.

Gastrointestinal and genitourinary care.
Initially after SCI, bowel and bladder tone are flaccid. Abdominal distention, constipation, and fecal impaction are major problems encountered in care of patients with SCI. Innervation between the brain and defecation center in the sacral cord has been disrupted. A bowel program to prevent fecal impaction and encourage normal, regular bowel function may be initiated in the critical care phase. The patient should not go longer than 3 to 4 days without a bowel movement. Laxatives and stool softeners may be needed, especially if the patient is receiving opiates. Aspects of a successful bowel program include consistent timing of evacuation, proper positioning, physical activity, appropriate fluid intake, a high-fiber diet, and reflex stimulation for patients with upper motor neuron injuries.[56] Bowel retraining is a major focus of the intermediate care and rehabilitation phase of treatment.

The degree of bladder and urinary sphincter dysfunction depends on the location and completeness of the injury. A urinary drainage catheter is inserted on admission, but it should be removed 3 to 4 days later or as soon as possible, at which time the patient is placed on an intermittent catheterization schedule of every 4 to 6 hours. It is not unusual for male patients with an upper motor neuron injury to experience a reflexogenic erection when being catheterized. An overdistended bladder in a patient with an injury at T6 or above may trigger autonomic dysreflexia.

Autonomic dysreflexia is a life-threatening complication that occurs most commonly in the first year after SCI. This condition is caused by a massive sympathetic response to a noxious stimulus (e.g., full bladder, fecal impaction) that results in severe hypertension, bradycardia, facial flushing, and pounding headache.[54] Immediate intervention is needed to prevent cerebral hemorrhage and seizures. Treatment is aimed at alleviating the noxious stimuli. Suggestions for treatment of autonomic dysreflexia are provided in Box 24.8.

Integumentary and musculoskeletal care.
Patients with SCI are at extremely high risk for pressure injuries because of the lack of motor control and sensation. Prevention is the best treatment. Diligent assessments, meticulous skin care, and frequent position changes are required. Any evidence of skin breakdown or pressure injury development should be assessed, documented, and reported immediately to the most appropriate health care provider. Specialty surfaces or low-air-loss beds may be necessary for the prevention of pressure injury in patients with SCI.

Immobilized patients are at high risk for contractures. When a muscle is denervated, as in the case of SCI, muscle fibers shorten and produce a contracture. Irreversible contractures may result in skin breakdown, inability to perform activities of daily living, poor wheelchair posture, and inability to use adaptive devices. Physical therapy and occupational therapy personnel should be consulted early in the patient's hospitalization. Range-of-motion exercises are initiated as soon as the spine has been stabilized. Footdrop splints should be applied on admission to prevent contractures and prevent skin breakdown of the heels. Hand splints should be applied for individuals with quadriplegia. Hand and foot splints should be removed every 2 hours, and the extremities should be examined for evidence of skin breakdown.

Care management of a patient in skull traction or halo vest includes inspection of pins and traction for security, correct positioning, and maintenance of skin integrity. Traction bars of the halo vest must never be used to lift or reposition the patient, and the wrench that comes with the halo jacket must be immediately available at all times in case of cardiac arrest.

Another consequence of sympathetic nervous system dysfunction is loss of thermoregulation (poikilothermy), in which body temperature is regulated by the external environment. Use of heat or cold for therapeutic or comfort measures may be required but must be used cautiously. Profound changes in body temperature must be avoided. Before antipyretics are given for hyperthermia, a cooling blanket is typically used. Hypothermia can produce bradyarrhythmias and sinus arrest and may impair wound healing.

Maximizing psychosocial adaptation. Nursing management of the patient with SCI must include the provision of dedicated emotional support. In the critical care unit, the patient, family, and significant others often experience anxiety, grief, denial, anger, frustration, and hopelessness because of the nature of the injury, profound and immediate changes required in lifestyle, and the fact that long-term neurologic deficits may remain unknown.

Appropriate nursing interventions include promotion of support systems, which often involve family and friends, and use of coping mechanisms and adaptive skills. Simple, accurate, and consistent information may help alleviate some fear and anxiety. Feelings of powerlessness may be reduced by including the patient and family in patient care and decision making. Further psychosocial support can be provided by social workers, occupational therapists, psychologists, and members of the clergy.

Thoracic Injuries

Thoracic injuries involve trauma to the chest wall, lungs, heart, great vessels, and esophagus. Blunt thoracic trauma to the chest most often is caused by MVCs or falls. In penetrating thoracic injury, the object involved determines the degree of damage to underlying structures. Low-velocity weapons (e.g., .22-caliber gun, knife) usually damage only what is in the direct path of the weapon. Stab wounds that involve the anterior chest wall between the midclavicular lines, the angle of Louis, and the epigastric region are of particular concern, because of the proximity of the heart and great vessels. High-velocity weapons are capable of causing considerable thoracic injury because of greater kinetic energy.

Specific Thoracic Traumatic Injuries

Chest wall injuries

Rib fractures. Fractures of the ribs can be minimal and cause minor discomfort or be serious and life-threatening, particularly when

---

BOX 24.8 Autonomic Dysreflexia

- If patient is supine, immediately sit the patient up.
- Begin frequent vital sign monitoring, including blood pressure every 5 minutes.
- Loosen clothing and constrictive devices.
- Immediately begin assessment for underlying cause.
- If indwelling urinary catheter is not placed, catheterize the patient.
- If indwelling catheter is present, immediately:
  - Check system for kinks and obstructions to flow.
  - Use a bladder scanner to check if bladder is full.
  - Irrigate the bladder with small sterile amount of fluid, using strict aseptic technique.
  - If not draining, remove the catheter and replace using aseptic technique.
- If acute symptoms persist, suspect fecal impaction:
  - Perform digital examination to check for presence of stool; if present, gently remove.
  - If no stool is found and the abdomen is distended, consider administration of laxative.
- If systolic blood pressure is greater than 150 mm Hg, consider rapid-onset, short-duration antihypertensive agent.
- Do not hesitate to call for immediate medical assistance.

---

multiple ribs are fractured, when preexisting cardiopulmonary disease is present, or when the patient is an older adult. Fractures of the first and second ribs are frequently associated with intrathoracic vascular injuries of the brachial plexus, or great vessels. Because arteries and veins are protected by the scapula, clavicle, humerus, and muscles, vascular injury signifies a very high degree of force applied to the thorax. Fractures to the middle ribs may be associated with lung injury, including pulmonary contusion and pneumothorax. Fractures to the lower ribs (7th–12th) may be associated with abdominal trauma, such as spleen and liver injuries.

Localized pain that increases with respiration or that is elicited by rib compression may indicate rib fractures. The pain associated with rib fractures can be aggravated by chest wall movement. The patient often splints fractured ribs, takes shallow breaths, and may refuse to cough. This can result in atelectasis and pneumonia. Definitive diagnosis of rib fractures can be made with a chest x-ray.

Interventions include pain control to improve chest expansion and facilitate gas exchange, chest physiotherapy, and early mobilization. The primary goal of pain management in patients with rib fractures is patient comfort and prevention of pulmonary complications. Pain management interventions must be tailored to the individual patient and response to therapy. Nonsteroidal antiinflammatory drugs, intercostal nerve blocks, thoracic epidural analgesia, and opiates may be considered.[57] External splints are not recommended, because they may limit chest wall expansion and add to atelectasis. Surgical plating of fractured ribs has not yet gained widespread acceptance. This procedure is most often reserved for those patients with severe chest wall deformity, accompanied by pain and problems with oxygenation and ventilation, that without this newer surgical intervention would possibly require many months of hospitalization.[58]

Flail chest. Flail chest, caused by blunt trauma, disrupts the continuity of chest wall structures. Typically, a flail segment occurs when two or more ribs are fractured in two or more places and are no longer attached to the thoracic cage, producing a free-floating segment of the chest wall. A flail chest is a clinical diagnosis wherein the so-called flail segment (or floating segment) moves paradoxically compared with the rest of the chest wall (Fig. 24.8).

During inspiration, the intact portion of the chest wall expands while the injured part is sucked in. During expiration, the chest wall moves in, and the flail segment moves out. Although the flail segment increases the work of breathing, the main cause of hypoxemia is often underlying pulmonary contusions.[59] The physiologic effects of impaired chest wall motion of a flail chest include decreased tidal volume and vital capacity and impaired cough that lead to hypoventilation and atelectasis.

Inspection of the thorax reveals paradoxical chest movement. Palpation of the chest may indicate crepitus and tenderness near fractured ribs. With a flail chest, the chest x-ray reveals multiple rib fractures. Evidence of hypoxemia may be demonstrated by ABGs, but this does not aid in the diagnosis. Interventions focus on ensuring adequate oxygenation and analgesia to improve ventilation.[59] Intubation and mechanical ventilation may be required.

Lung injuries

Pulmonary contusion. A pulmonary contusion is a bruise of the lung. Pulmonary contusion is often associated with blunt trauma and other chest injuries, such as rib fractures and flail chest. Pulmonary contusions can occur unilaterally or bilaterally. A contusion manifests initially as a hemorrhage followed by alveolar and interstitial edema. The edema can remain localized in the contused part or can spread to other areas of the lung. Inflammation negatively affects gas exchange across the alveolar-capillary membrane. As inflammation and edema

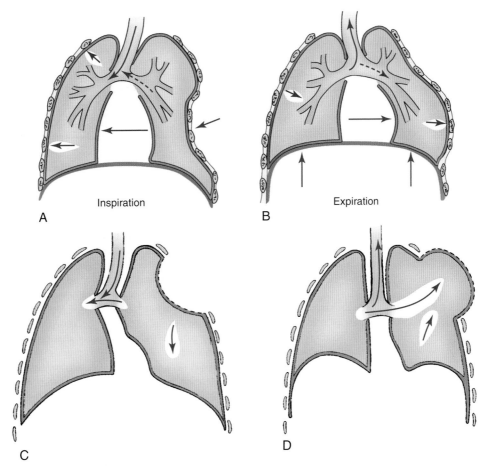

Fig. 24.8 Flail Chest. (A) Normal inspiration. (B) Normal expiration. (C) The area of the lung underlying the unstable chest wall sucks in on inspiration. (D) The same area balloons out on expiration. Notice the movement of the mediastinum toward the opposite lung on inspiration.

increase, a decrease in respiratory compliance, increased resistance, and decreased pulmonary blood flow may occur. These processes cause a ventilation-perfusion imbalance that results in progressive hypoxemia and poor ventilation.

Clinical manifestations of pulmonary contusion may take up to 24 hours after injury to develop.[60] Inspection of the chest wall may reveal ecchymosis at the site of impact. Diminished breath sounds and coarse crackles may be auscultated over the contused lung. The patient may have a cough and blood-tinged sputum. Abnormal lung function can manifest as arterial hypoxemia. Diagnosis is made primarily by imaging studies consistent with pulmonary infiltrates corresponding to the area of external chest impact that manifest within 12 to 24 hours of injury. Pulmonary contusions may worsen over 24 to 72 hours after injury and then slowly resolve unless complications from infection or ARDS occur.

Aggressive respiratory care is the cornerstone of care for nonintubated patients with pulmonary contusion. Interventions include deep-breathing exercises, incentive spirometry, early mobilization, or noninvasive positive-pressure ventilation.[60] Chest physiotherapy may not be tolerated if there are coexisting rib fractures. Adequate pain control is achieved with nonsteroidal antiinflammatory drugs, opiates, intercostal nerve blocks, or thoracic epidural analgesia. Removal of airway secretions is important to avoid infection and to improve ventilation. Patients with unilateral contusions are placed with the injured side up and uninjured side down ("good lung down"). This positioning helps correct the existing ventilation-perfusion mismatch.

Patients with severe pulmonary contusions may continue to exhibit signs of decompensation, such as respiratory acidosis and increased work of breathing, despite aggressive nursing management. Endotracheal intubation and mechanical ventilation with PEEP may be required. Complications resulting from pulmonary contusions include pneumonia, ARDS, lung abscesses, and pulmonary embolism.[61]

Pneumothoraces in trauma. Pleural damage is common in trauma. These conditions include *pneumothorax* (air in the pleural space), *hemothorax* (blood in the pleural space), or *hemopneumothorax* (air and blood in the pleural space). Pneumothoraces may be managed with chest tubes, analgesia, and surgical consultation, depending on the size of the pneumothorax, hemodynamic stability of the patient, and effects on oxygenation and ventilation. *Open pneumothorax, tension pneumothorax,* and *massive hemothorax,* three additional and potentially life-threatening respiratory problems in trauma, warrant special consideration.

Open pneumothorax. An open pneumothorax ("sucking chest wound") is caused by penetrating trauma. Large open thoracic wounds (greater than two-thirds the diameter of the trachea) allow communication between the atmosphere and intrathoracic cavity.[4] As air moves in and out of the hole in the chest, a sucking sound can be heard on inspiration. Respiratory mechanics become impaired. Dyspnea, tachycardia, and hypotension may be observed. *Subcutaneous emphysema* indicates that air is trapped in the tissues beneath the skin. This may be palpated around the wound as *crepitus,* a crackling sensation the examiner feels when lightly palpating the affected area.

Initial management of an open pneumothorax is accomplished by promptly inserting a chest tube. If a chest tube is not immediately available, covering the wound at end expiration with a sterile occlusive dressing taped securely on three sides and large enough to overlap the edges of the wound should be used.[4] As the patient breathes in, the dressing gets sucked in to occlude the wound and prevent air from entering the thoracic cavity. On expiration, the dressing moves outward, permitting the patient to exhale. Surgical intervention is often required to close the wound.

Tension pneumothorax. A tension pneumothorax is caused by an injury that perforates the chest wall or pleural space. During inspiration, air flows into the pleural space and becomes trapped. As pressure in the pleural space increases, the lung on the injured side collapses and causes the mediastinum to shift to the opposite side (Fig. 24.9). As pressure continues to build, the shift exerts pressure on the heart and thoracic aorta, which results in decreased venous return and decreased cardiac output. Tissue perfusion is affected because the collapsed lung does not participate in gas exchange.

Clinical manifestations of a tension pneumothorax include dyspnea, tachycardia, hypotension, and sudden chest pain extending to the back, neck, or shoulders. On the injured side, breath sounds may be decreased or absent. Percussion of the chest reveals a hyperresonant sound over the affected side. Tracheal deviation (a late sign in tension pneumothorax) can be observed as the trachea shifts away from the injured side. Diagnosis is made by immediate clinical assessment.

When a tension pneumothorax is suspected in any trauma patient, there is no time for a chest x-ray because this potentially lethal condition must be treated at once. Needle decompression, in which a large-bore (14-gauge) 5-cm needle is inserted over the second rib midclavicular line (on the affected side), is the immediate treatment of choice.[4] Alternative needle decompression sites include the fourth to fifth intercostal space anterior axillary or midaxillary line using a 5- or 8-cm needle.[62] This procedure allows release of air from the pleural space. A hissing sound is heard as the tension pneumothorax is converted to a simple pneumothorax. A chest tube is immediately inserted after needle decompression.

Massive hemothorax. Blunt or penetrating thoracic trauma can cause bleeding into the pleural space, resulting in a hemothorax (Fig. 24.10). A massive hemothorax results from the accumulation of

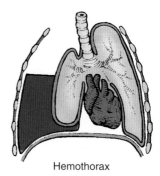

Hemothorax

Fig. 24.10 Blunt or penetrating thoracic trauma can cause bleeding into the pleural space to form a hemothorax.

more than 1500 mL of blood in the thoracic cavity.[16] The source of bleeding may be the intercostal or internal mammary arteries, lungs, heart, or great vessels. Lacerations to the lung parenchyma are low-pressure bleeds and typically stop bleeding spontaneously. Arterial bleeding from hilar vessels usually requires immediate surgical intervention. Increasing vascular blood loss into the pleural space causes decreased venous return and decreased cardiac output.

For patients with massive hemothorax, assessment findings reveal diminished or absent breath sounds over the affected lung and collapsed neck veins (hypovolemia) or distended neck veins (coexisting tension pneumothorax).[16] Massive hemothorax is diagnosed on the basis of hypotension associated with the absence of breath sounds or dullness to percussion on one side of the chest. Hypovolemic shock may be present.

This potentially life-threatening condition must be treated immediately. Resuscitation with IV fluids is initiated to treat hypovolemic shock. A chest tube is placed on the affected side to allow drainage of blood. Emergency thoracotomy may be necessary for patients who require persistent blood transfusions or who have significant bleeding (>20 mL/kg, or 200 mL/h for 2–4 hours, or more than 1500 mL on initial tube insertion) or when there are accompanying injuries to major cardiovascular structures.[63]

Heart and vascular injuries. Heart and vascular injuries can result from either blunt or penetrating trauma. The most common causes of blunt cardiac trauma include high-speed MVCs, direct blows to the chest, and falls. Because of its mobility and its location between the

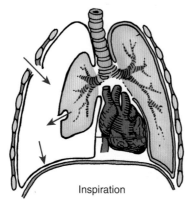

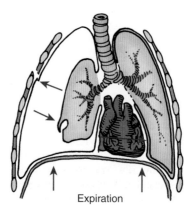

Inspiration   Expiration

Fig. 24.9 Tension Pneumothorax. Tension pneumothorax usually is caused by an injury that perforates the chest wall or pleural space. Air flows into the pleural space with inspiration and becomes trapped. As pressure in the pleural space increases, the lung on the injured side collapses and causes the mediastinum to shift to the opposite side. (From Marx J, Hockberger RS, Walls RM. *Rosen's Emergency Medicine: Concepts and Clinical Practice.* 5th ed. St. Louis: Mosby; 2002.)

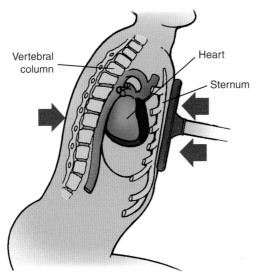

Fig. 24.11 Blunt Cardiac Trauma. Sudden acceleration (as from contact with the steering wheel) can cause the heart to be thrown against the sternum.

BOX 24.9 **EAST Guidelines for Screening of Blunt Cardiac Injury**

- Obtain an admission electrocardiogram (ECG) for all patients in whom there is suspected blunt cardiac injury (BCI).
- If ECG is abnormal, the patient should be admitted for continuous ECG monitoring for 24–48 hours.
- If the patient is hemodynamically unstable, an echocardiogram may be performed.
- Cardiac biomarkers such as cardiac troponin T values are not useful in predicting which patients will have complications related to BCI.

EAST, Eastern Association for the Surgery of Trauma.

sternum and thoracic vertebrae, the heart is particularly susceptible to blunt traumatic injury. Sudden acceleration (as from contact with a steering wheel) can cause the heart to be thrown against the sternum (Fig. 24.11). Sudden deceleration can also cause the heart to be thrown against the thoracic vertebrae by a direct impact to the chest, such as blows caused by a baseball, animal kick, or fall.

Penetrating cardiac trauma can occur from mechanical injuries as a result of bullets, knives, or impalements. The chest wall offers little protection to the heart from penetrating trauma. The most common site of injury is the right ventricle because of its anterior position in the mediastinum. Mortality rates from penetrating trauma to the heart are high. Prehospital mortality rates for penetrating cardiac injuries are significant, as most deaths occur within minutes after injury as a result of exsanguination or tamponade. Trauma teams need to be aware of three potentially lethal cardiac and vascular injuries, including blunt cardiac injury (BCI), cardiac tamponade, and blunt traumatic aortic injury (BTAI).

Blunt cardiac injury. BCI covers a wide spectrum of possible cardiac issues in trauma patients, including myocardial contusion, myocardial concussion, and rupture. The chambers most often injured are the right atrium and right ventricle because of their anterior position in the chest.

Few clinical signs and symptoms are specific for BCI. Evidence of external chest trauma, such as steering wheel imprint or sternal fractures, should raise suspicion for BCI. However, the presence of a sternal fracture does not predict the incidence of BCI. The patient may complain of chest pain that is similar to anginal pain, but the pain is not relieved with nitroglycerin. Chest discomfort is usually caused by associated injuries, including fractured ribs. Unexplained tachycardia or the presence of a new bundle branch block should increase awareness for BCI.[63]

Guidelines for screening of BCI from the Eastern Association of Surgeons in Trauma are listed in Box 24.9. The patient should be monitored for new onset of dysrhythmias. A 12-lead electrocardiogram may reveal dysrhythmias, ST segment changes, or bundle branch block. Cardiac biomarkers, such as troponin, are of little diagnostic help for BCI.[64] In symptomatic patients, echocardiography may reveal possible wall motion abnormalities, pericardial fluid, or valve tearing or rupture.[64]

Medical management is aimed at preventing and treating complications. This approach includes hemodynamic monitoring in a critical care unit and possible administration of antidysrhythmic medications. Surgical consultation may be required for ruptured valves and pericardial fluid accumulation.

Cardiac tamponade. Cardiac tamponade is the progressive accumulation of blood in the pericardial sac (Fig. 24.12). With cardiac tamponade, the accumulation of blood increases intracardiac pressure and compresses the atria and ventricles. The amount of blood needed to cause changes in patient hemodynamics depends on the amount of blood in the pericardial sac and the speed with which the fluid has accumulated.[65] As intracardiac pressure continues to increase, this leads to decreased venous return and decreased preload, which lead to decreased cardiac output. Myocardial hypoxia, heart failure, and cardiogenic shock may occur.

Classic assessment findings associated with cardiac tamponade include the presence of elevated central venous pressure (with neck vein distention), muffled heart sounds, and hypotension. This is known as *Beck's triad*. These signs are almost universally absent in traumatic cardiac tamponade.[16] Pulseless electrical activity in the absence of hypovolemia and tension pneumothorax strongly suggests cardiac tamponade.[16] Focused assessment with sonography for trauma (FAST) in the emergency department is rapid and extremely accurate, and it may be used to quickly identify cardiac tamponade in the trauma patient.[64,65] Immediate treatment is required to remove the accumulated fluid in the pericardial sac. Pericardiocentesis involves aspiration of fluid from the pericardium by use of a large-bore needle. The inherent risk in this procedure is potential laceration of the coronary artery. Longer-term definitive treatment may involve a pericardiotomy.[64]

Blunt traumatic aortic injury. BTAI is one of the most lethal thoracic injuries and the second most common cause of death in blunt trauma.[66] Of patients with BTAI, 80% die before reaching the hospital.[67] Associated injuries include a first or second rib fracture, high sternal fracture, left clavicular fracture at the level of the sternal margin, and massive hemothorax.

BTAI should be suspected in all trauma patients with a rapid deceleration or acceleration mechanism of injury. The thoracic aorta is relatively mobile and may tear at fixed anatomic points within the thorax. Approximately 75% of BTAI patients will rupture at the aortic isthmus (the most mobile portion of the aorta), followed by injury to the descending aorta (22%) and ascending aorta (4%).[68] A complete rupture of the aorta causes death by hemorrhage.

The critical care nurse must assess blood pressure in both arms, because a tear in the aortic arch may create a pressure gradient resulting in blood pressure changes between upper extremities.

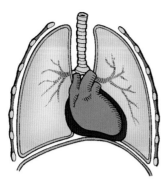

Fig. 24.12 Cardiac tamponade is the progressive accumulation of blood in the pericardial sac.

Additional clinical assessment findings include a pulse deficit at any site, unexplained hypotension, sternal pain, precordial systolic murmur, hoarseness, dyspnea, and lower extremity sensory deficits.

An initial chest x-ray is obtained in the upright position after spine x-rays have been completed and the spine is cleared. Radiographic findings suggesting aortic injury include widened mediastinum, obscured aortic knob, and deviation of the left main stem bronchus.[64] Although angiography and echocardiogram can also be used to help diagnose BTAI, computed tomographic angiogram is considered the gold standard.[66] The critical care nurse anticipates early surgical consultation and urgent endovascular repair.

During the resuscitation phase for a patient with blunt traumatic aortic injury, blood pressure management is the primary goal to minimize injury. Minimizing stress on the vessel is achieved by maintaining the heart rate less than 100 beats/min, ideally using a beta-blocker.[67] The aim is to keep SBP less than 100 mm Hg and MAP less than 80 mm Hg by using agents such as esmolol or labetalol.[66] If beta-blockers alone fail to achieve target goals, IV nitroglycerin or sodium nitroprusside[69] may be added.

Postoperative care is also directed toward blood pressure stabilization, with the goal of minimizing vessel stress while maintaining tissue perfusion, which typically is accomplished with the use of medications described earlier. Careful assessment for stroke and postoperative paraplegia is needed because of the degree of injury to the aorta. Paraplegia is closely related to the duration of aortic cross-clamping time intraoperatively. The critical care nurse monitors for bowel ischemia (e.g., tube feeding intolerance, lactic acidosis) and acute kidney injury, which may manifest by low urine output and rising serum creatinine, because blood flow to the mesentery and kidney may have been compromised as a result of the injury and/or surgery.

Abdominal Injuries

Abdominal injuries are frequently associated with multisystem trauma. Abdominal injuries are the third leading cause of death in trauma. Injuries to the abdomen may be the result of blunt or penetrating events.

Blunt abdominal injuries occur most often from MVCs, assaults, and falls. Blunt trauma to the abdomen can produce injuries to the liver, spleen, and diaphragm. Deceleration and direct forces can produce retroperitoneal hematomas. Penetrating abdominal trauma is primarily caused by knives, bullets, or other impalements. Commonly injured organs from stab wounds are the colon, liver, spleen, and diaphragm. Gunshot wounds to the abdomen usually are more serious than stab wounds. Inside the abdomen, a bullet can travel in erratic paths and ricochet off bone. Death from penetrating injuries depends on the injury to major vascular structures and resultant intra-abdominal hemorrhage.

Two major life-threatening conditions that can occur after abdominal trauma are hemorrhage and hollow viscus perforation with associated gastrointestinal bleeding and septic shock. The critical care nurse must pay particular attention to the abdomen after injury for immediate recognition of problems and prevention of complications.

Priority Clinical Assessment

Initial assessment of the trauma patient, whether in the emergency department or critical care unit, follows the primary and secondary survey techniques as outlined by ATLS guidelines.[4] The initial physical assessment of the abdomen may be nonspecific or unreliable, given possible coexisting influences of alcohol, illicit drugs, analgesics, or an altered LOC. The critical care nurse must be aware of specific assessment findings associated with abdominal trauma.

A distended abdomen may indicate the accumulation of blood, fluid, or gas resulting from a perforated organ or ruptured blood vessel. Purplish discoloration of the flanks or umbilicus (Cullen sign) may signify blood in the abdominal wall. Ecchymosis in the flank area (Grey-Turner sign) may indicate retroperitoneal bleeding or a pancreatic injury. A hematoma in the flank area suggests kidney injury. Auscultation may reveal normal or absent bowel sounds. The abdomen is assessed for rebound tenderness and rigidity, indicative of peritoneal inflammation. Referred pain to the left shoulder (Kehr sign) may indicate a ruptured spleen or irritation of the diaphragm from bile or other material in the peritoneum. The locations of entry and exit sites associated with penetrating trauma are identified and documented.

Diagnostic Procedures

Physical examination of the abdomen alone is unreliable in a patient suspected to have abdominal trauma. Insertion of a nasogastric tube serves as a useful diagnostic and therapeutic aid. A nasogastric tube can decompress the stomach, and drainage can be checked for blood.

Laboratory test results may be nonspecific for patients with abdominal trauma. Because of hemoconcentration, hemoglobin and hematocrit results may not reflect actual values. Serial measurements are helpful in diagnosing abdominal injuries. An increasing lactate level is highly suggestive of mesenteric hypoperfusion.[70]

Diagnostic imaging may occur during the ATLS secondary survey. The FAST scan, conventional chest and abdominal x-rays, and CT scan play important roles in evaluation of abdominal trauma. Diagnostic peritoneal lavage, an invasive technique in which a small catheter is inserted into the abdominal cavity and the abdomen is assessed for the presence of blood, is rarely performed. Bedside ultrasound and CT scan have largely replaced diagnostic peritoneal lavage as a superior diagnostic tool in abdominal trauma. FAST, a rapid bedside ultrasound test, is used widely for the detection of free fluid in the abdomen and hemoperitoneum after injury. FAST is an efficient means of rapid abdominal assessment, but success depends on the skill level of the operator.

The FAST test examines four areas of the abdomen for injury—the subxiphoid area (pericardial effusion and left lobe liver injury), the right upper quadrant (right liver, right kidney, Morrison pouch), the left upper quadrant (left kidney and spleen), and the suprapubic area (bladder and pouch of Douglas) (Fig. 24.13).[4] An extended FAST (e-FAST) examination may be completed in some centers to check for pneumothoraces. Although FAST has good sensitivity and specificity, it is not intended to replace the CT scan. Patients with abdominal obesity

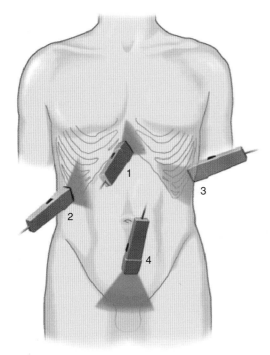

Fig. 24.13 Focused Assessment With Sonography for Trauma (FAST). Quadrants are examined for the presence of free fluid. (From Moore FA, Moore EE. Initial management of life-threatening trauma. In: Ashley SW, editorial chair. *ACS Surgery: Principles and Practice.* Hamilton, Ontario, Canada: Decker Publishing; 2012.)

TABLE 24.9 Liver Injury Scale.

Grade[a]	Injury	Criteria
I	Hematoma	Subcapsular, <10% surface area
	Laceration	Capsular tear, <1 cm parenchymal depth
II	Hematoma	Subcapsular, 10%—50% surface area; intraparenchymal <10 cm in diameter
	Laceration	1—3 cm parenchymal depth, <10 cm long
III	Hematoma	Subcapsular, >50% surface area or expanding; ruptured subcapsular or parenchymal hematoma; intraparenchymal hematoma >10 cm or expanding
	Laceration	>3 cm parenchymal depth
IV	Laceration	Parenchymal disruption involving 25%—75% of hepatic lobe
	Bleeding	Active bleeding beyond liver and into the peritoneum
V	Laceration	Parenchymal disruption involving >75% of hepatic lobe
	Vascular	Juxtahepatic venous injuries (retrohepatic vena cava, central major hepatic veins)

[a]Advance one grade for multiple injuries up to grade III.

and patients with ascites may have erroneous results, and further work-up for these patients is warranted. FAST is limited in its ability to diagnose diaphragmatic, intestinal, or pancreatic injuries. FAST is also unable to distinguish between blood and free intraperitoneal fluid.[71] Hemodynamically unstable patients with a positive FAST examination generally undergo damage control surgery to achieve hemostasis.

An initial negative FAST result does not preclude abdominal injury and may be followed by abdominal x-ray, CT scan, or MRI. CT is the mainstay of diagnostic evaluation in a hemodynamically stable patient with abdominal trauma. Abdominal CT provides information about specific organ injury, pelvic injury, and retroperitoneal hemorrhage.

Specific Abdominal Organ Injuries

Medical and nursing management vary according to specific organ injuries. Physical assessment findings and abdominal x-ray or CT scan aid in making the diagnosis of abdominal organ injury. Liver, spleen, and bowel injuries, which are seen most frequently in patients with multisystem trauma, are discussed here.

Liver injuries. The liver is a commonly injured abdominal organ in trauma and is a significant cause for hemorrhage after injury. Abdominal CT is considered to be the most reliable diagnostic tool to identify and assess the severity of injury to the liver.[4] The severity of liver injuries is graded to provide a mechanism for determining the amount of trauma sustained, the care needed, and possible outcomes (Table 24.9). Nonoperative management is considered the standard of care for hemodynamically stable patients with blunt liver injury.[72]

Patients with blunt or penetrating liver trauma who are hemodynamically unstable may require surgical intervention to achieve hemostasis. Resection of the devitalized tissue is required for massive injuries. Hemorrhage is common with liver injuries, and ligation of the hepatic arteries or veins may be required. Packing the liver in traumatic liver injury accompanied by hemorrhage is undertaken in damage control surgery.[64] Drains may be placed intraoperatively to prevent hematoma development.

Spleen injuries. The spleen is also a commonly injured organ in abdominal trauma and, like the liver, can be a source of life-threatening hemorrhage. Splenic injuries, similar to liver injuries, are graded for the purpose of determining the amount of trauma sustained, the care required, and possible outcomes (Table 24.10). Hemodynamically stable patients may be monitored in the critical care unit, trending serial hematocrit and hemoglobin values and vital signs. The current trend favors nonsurgical management.[64]

Embolization therapy is a possible option in all grades of spleen injury to help decrease blood loss from the spleen.[73] Patients with splenic injury who exhibit hemodynamic instability and progressive deterioration may require immediate surgical intervention with laparotomy.[73]

Hollow viscus injuries. The term *hollow viscus* refers to the hollow organs in the abdomen, such as the stomach, small intestine, and large intestine. Hollow viscus injuries can result from blunt or penetrating trauma. The diagnosis of a hollow viscus injury is challenging because these injuries may not be readily identifiable during the primary or secondary assessments or may not appear on initial CT scan or ultrasound. A delay in the time to diagnosis contributes to complications. Regardless of the mechanism of injury, intestinal contents (e.g., bile, stool, enzymes, bacteria) can leak into the peritoneum and cause numerous complications, including septic shock. Surgical resection and repair is almost always required.

Abdominal Compartment Syndrome

Abdominal compartment syndrome is defined as end-organ dysfunction caused by intraabdominal hypertension (IAH).[74] Increased pressure can be caused by bleeding, ileus, mesenteric edema, or a noncompliant abdominal wall. Increased pressure within the abdominal cavity can impinge on diaphragmatic excursion and can affect ventilation.

TABLE 24.10   Spleen Injury Scale.

Grade[a]	Injury	Criteria
I	Hematoma	Subcapsular, <10% surface area
	Laceration	Capsular tear <1 cm, parenchymal depth
II	Hematoma	Subcapsular 10%—50% surface area; intraparenchymal <5 cm in diameter
	Laceration	1—3 cm parenchymal depth
III	Hematoma	Subcapsular >50% surface area; ruptured subcapsular or intraparenchymal hematoma; intraparenchymal hematoma ≥5 cm or expanding
	Laceration	>3 cm parenchymal depth
IV	Bleeding	Any vascular injury in presence of injury to spleen or active bleeding *within* spleen capsule
	Laceration	Parenchymal laceration involving segmental or hilar vessels producing major devascularization (>25% of spleen)
V	Bleeding	Any vascular injury in presence of injury to spleen or active bleeding *beyond* spleen capsule into peritoneum Completely shattered spleen
	Vascular	Hilar vascular injury that devascularizes spleen

[a]Advance one grade for multiple injuries up to grade III.
Modified from AAST Patient Assessment Committee. Organ injury scaling 2018 update: spleen, liver, and kidney. *J Trauma Acute Care Surg.* 2018;85(6):1119—1122.

Clinical manifestations of abdominal compartment syndrome include decreased cardiac output, decreased tidal volume, increased peak pulmonary pressure, decreased urine output, and hypoxia.[74] IAP can be measured through various commercially available devices or a simple pressurized tubing setup. In both instances, the urinary bladder acts as a transducer to estimate the degree of IAP after the injection of 25 mL of sterile saline. IAH is defined as an IAP greater than or equal to 12 mm Hg (normal 5—7 mm Hg).[75] IAH may be graded as follows:

- IAH grade I (12—15 mm Hg)
- IAH grade II (16—20 mm Hg)
- IAH grade III (21—25 mm Hg)
- IAH grade IV (greater than 25 mm Hg)[75]

The abdominal perfusion pressure (APP) is calculated as MAP—IAP. APP should be maintained within 50 to 60 mm Hg to ensure adequate blood supply to the gut.

Surgical decompression of the abdomen may be required for abdominal pressures greater than 20 to 25 mm Hg accompanied by a taut, tense abdomen and signs of organ dysfunction such as deteriorating heart, lung, and kidney status. After surgical decompression is completed and the pressure is relieved, the patient may return to the critical care unit with an "open abdomen." For example, the abdomen may be temporarily closed with a sterile perforated plastic sheet, clips, vacuum-assisted device, or other option, and the skin and abdominal fascia are left open. The wound is closed permanently in the days or weeks following the surgery or, depending on its size, may be allowed to heal by secondary intention and eventual skin grafting.

Nursing Management

Vigilant assessment of the abdomen in a polytrauma patient warrants special consideration among critical care nurses. Signs and symptoms of abdominal trauma are often subtle and nonspecific, so synthesis of physical assessment findings, diagnostic imaging tests, and laboratory results are essential for early detection of abdominal complications. A fundamental nursing responsibility is to continually evaluate the patient's response to medical therapies.

Care of trauma patients with severe liver injuries can be challenging for critical care nurses. Serial serum hematocrit and hemoglobin levels and vital signs are monitored over several days. Hemodynamic instability can result from hemorrhage and hypovolemic shock, leading to fluid volume deficit, impaired cardiac output, and decreased tissue perfusion. Continued hemodynamic instability (e.g., hypotension, decreased cardiac output) despite aggressive medical intervention may indicate ongoing hemorrhage, in which case an exploratory laparotomy may be required to determine and correct the source of bleeding. A massive transfusion protocol may be implemented to restore blood volume and correct coagulopathies. The patient's postoperative course may be complicated by coagulopathy, acidosis, and hypothermia. Jaundice may occur as a sign of liver dysfunction, but it may also be caused by reabsorption of hematomas or the breakdown of transfused red blood cells.

Traditional postoperative care is provided after a splenectomy. The spleen plays a major role in preventing infection against different organisms, including *Streptococcus, Neisseria,* and *Haemophilus.*[76] Patients who have had a splenectomy are at risk for the development of postsplenectomy sepsis with streptococcal pneumonia. These patients require the polyvalent pneumococcal vaccine (Pneumovax) to help promote immunity against pneumococcal bacteria. Patients should also receive *Haemophilus influenzae* type B and meningococcal vaccines within 2 weeks of splenectomy.[77] Complications after splenic trauma include wound infection; sepsis; subdiaphragmatic abscess; and fistulas of the colon, pancreas, and stomach.

With hollow viscus injuries, the patient's postoperative course is usually affected by the spillage of intestinal contents and degree of septic shock. The critical care nurse will monitor vital signs, administer analgesia and antibiotics, trend hemoglobin and hematocrit values, and observe all fluid exiting from gastrointestinal tubes and drains. If frank blood is observed exiting from any tube or drain, the nurse will notify the most appropriate health care provider immediately. Enteral nutrition is generally not initiated until the bowel has had time to heal and only after consultation and approval by the surgeon. The patient is observed for signs of worsening hemodynamic instability and for abscess or fistula formation.

Genitourinary Injuries

Trauma to the genitourinary tract seldom occurs as an isolated injury. A genitourinary injury must be suspected in any patient with pelvic fracture; blunt trauma to the lower chest or flank; contusions, hematoma, or tenderness over the flank, lower abdomen, or perineum; genital swelling or discoloration; blood at the urethral meatus; hematuria after Foley catheter placement; or difficulty with micturition.[4] Similar to all other traumatic injuries, genitourinary injuries can result from blunt or penetrating trauma.

Priority Clinical Assessment

Evaluation of genitourinary trauma begins after the ATLS primary survey has been completed. Specific assessment findings may heighten suspicion for genitourinary trauma. A conscious patient may complain of flank pain or colic pain. Rebound tenderness can be elicited if intraperitoneal extravasation of urine has occurred. Inspection may reveal blood at the urethral meatus. Bluish discoloration of the flanks may indicate retroperitoneal bleeding, whereas perineal discoloration may indicate a pelvic fracture and possible bladder or urethral injury. Hematuria is common assessment finding with genitourinary trauma.[78] However, the absence of gross or microscopic hematuria does not exclude a urinary tract injury.

Diagnostic Procedures

The CT scan is considered the first-line diagnostic test to help evaluate the genitourinary system for evidence of blunt traumatic injury. Contrast-enhanced CT can be used to help identify the presence of upper and lower urinary tract for trauma. Penetrating kidney trauma may require a renal angiogram, which can also be used to embolize bleeding vessels. Sonography for testicular injury and MRI scan may also be used in genitourinary injury.

Specific Genitourinary Injuries

Kidney trauma. The kidney is another organ frequently injured in blunt abdominal trauma. Contusions or lacerations without urinary extravasation may occur. Injury to the kidney may be reflected by flank ecchymosis and fracture of inferior ribs or spinous processes. Gross or microscopic hematuria may be present; however, the degree of blood in the urine does not reflect the true extent of kidney damage. Gross hematuria can exist with minor injuries and sometimes clears within a few hours.

Kidney injury is graded I through V to assist trauma teams in determining the extent of injury. Grade I reflects small contusion and hematoma, and grade V identifies avulsion injury, devascularization, and active bleeding.[79] CT is the most accurate modality available for diagnosing kidney injury, because it can assess the extent of parenchymal laceration, urine extravasation, surrounding hemorrhage, and the presence of vascular injury.

Contusions and minor lacerations usually are treated with observation in hemodynamically stable patients. Operative interventions may be required in patients with kidney injuries who are hemodynamically unstable with a devascularized segment or are actively hemorrhaging. Angiographic embolization is used when possible. Postoperative and postinjury complications following kidney trauma include infection, hemorrhage, infarction, extravasation, calcification, and acute kidney injury.

Bladder trauma. A large percentage of bladder injuries result from blunt trauma,[78] although penetrating mechanisms can also induce injury. Physical findings may include lower abdominal bruising, distention, and pain. The patient may be unable to void. Bladder injuries are further subdivided as extraperitoneal ruptures (63%), intraperitoneal ruptures (32%), or combined injuries (4%).[78] Similarly, bladder injuries can be classified from grade I (mild injury with small hematoma) through grade V (lethal laceration that may extend into the neck of bladder). The type of injury depends on the location and strength of blunt force and volume of urine in the bladder at the time of injury. Extraperitoneal rupture of the bladder may be managed conservatively with catheterization and antibiotics for 7 to 10 days. Unresolved extravasation from intraperitoneal rupture requires surgical intervention.

Nursing Management

After admission to the critical care unit, assessment of the patient is done according to ATLS guidelines. Nursing priorities for the patient with genitourinary trauma include (1) assessing for hemorrhage, (2) maintaining fluid and electrolyte balance, and (3) maintaining patency of drains and tubes. Measurement of urinary output includes drainage from the urinary catheter, nephrostomy, or suprapubic tubes. Urinary output should be at least 0.5 mL/kg per hour.[4,22] Urine output is measured hourly until bloody drainage and clots have cleared. Gentle irrigation of drainage tubes may be required to clear clots and maintain patency. It is important to monitor the patient's hemoglobin, potassium, creatinine, and urea. Consultation with a urologist, if not already completed, may be necessary. The ideal treatment for bladder injury is unknown.

COMPLICATIONS OF TRAUMA

As a result of vast improvements in prehospital and emergency department care of trauma patients, many more patients are surviving their initial multisystem injuries, transport to hospital, and damage control operative procedures. Within the critical care unit, after resuscitation, stabilization, and damage control or definitive surgery, this is often a period of significant vulnerability for trauma patients. Ongoing nursing assessments are imperative for early detection of complications associated with traumatic injuries. Complications increase critical care and hospital length of stay, increase costs, and are associated with increased morbidity and mortality. Some of the most important complications in the care of critically injured patients in the critical care, intermediate care, and rehabilitation phases are identified in this section.

Central Nervous System Complications

Pain

Pain may come from many sources, including surgery, procedures, and the injuries themselves. Relief of pain is a major component in the care of trauma patients. Several different strategies of pain management may be used with the trauma patient, including continuous IV infusions, thoracic and lumbar epidural infusions, and intercostal nerve blocks. Pain relief measures are individualized for each patient based on injuries; contraindications; allergies; and patient, physician, and institutional preferences or protocols. Multimodal pain management approaches in the trauma patient may be required. See Chapter 7 for in-depth pain information.

Cardiovascular Complications

Compartment Syndrome

Compartment syndrome is a condition in which increased pressure within a limited space compromises circulation, resulting in ischemia and necrosis of tissues within that space. Among patients at high risk for the development of compartment syndrome are patients with upper and lower extremity trauma, including fractures, vascular ruptures, massive tissue injuries, or venous obstruction.

Clinical manifestations of compartment syndrome include obvious swelling and tightness of a limb, paresthesia, and extreme pain in the affected extremity.[16] Diminished pulses and decreased capillary refill do not reliably identify compartment syndrome because they may be intact until after irreversible damage has occurred. Elevated intracompartmental pressures confirm the diagnosis. Treatment can consist of simple interventions such as removing an occlusive dressing or bivalving (cutting) a cast or more complex interventions, including a surgical decompressive fasciotomy.

Venous Thromboembolism

Venous thromboembolism (VTE), which includes both DVT and pulmonary emboli, is an important cause of morbidity and mortality in a trauma patient with multiple injuries. Patients with major trauma are at very high risk for VTE. Factors that form the basis of VTE pathophysiology are exacerbated in trauma, including direct endothelial injury as a result of the trauma, hypercoagulopathy from trauma-induced coagulopathy, and blood stasis from immobility. VTE may develop into a life-threatening acute pulmonary embolism (see Acute Pulmonary Embolism in Chapter 14).

Trauma patients are at the greatest risk for developing VTE early in their hospitalization. Prevention is key. Routine thromboprophylaxis for a high-risk trauma patient includes use of low–molecular-weight heparin (starting as soon as it is considered safe to do so) and use of a mechanical method of prophylaxis, such as sequential compression devices.[64] Early mobilization, ensuring the comfort and safety of the patient and taking into consideration known injuries, can also help prevent development of VTE.

Pulmonary Complications

Acute Respiratory Distress Syndrome

Posttraumatic respiratory failure is often related to fractured ribs, pneumonia, or ARDS. ARDS can be caused by direct or indirect injury to the lungs (see Acute Respiratory Distress Syndrome in Chapter 14). Direct injuries in trauma patients, including aspiration, inhalation, and pulmonary contusion, or indirect injuries, including sepsis and massive transfusion, can all contribute to ARDS. When ARDS in trauma occurs, it generally develops 24 to 72 hours after the initial injury. Intubation, mechanical ventilation, low tidal-volume ventilation, and use of PEEP are the mainstays of ARDS treatment.[80] In severe cases of ARDS, and when spinal x-rays have been cleared and it is safe to do so, the trauma patient may need to be placed in the prone position.

Gastrointestinal and Genitourinary Complications

Hypermetabolism

Within 24 to 48 hours after traumatic injury, a predictable hypermetabolic response occurs. The metabolic response to injury mobilizes amino acids and accelerates protein synthesis to support wound healing and the immunologic response to invading organisms. Stress hypermetabolism also occurs after major injury and is characterized by increases in metabolic rate and oxygen consumption. Energy requirements increase to promote immune function and tissue repair. The goal of early nutrition is to maintain host defenses by supporting this hypermetabolism and to preserve lean body mass.

Nutrition support is an essential component in the care of critically ill trauma patients (see Chapter 5). Most nutrition experts advocate beginning enteral nutrition as early as possible. Current guidelines recommend enteral feedings be initiated, unless otherwise ordered, within 24 to 48 hours for all trauma patients.[81] Enteral feeding sites include the gastric route and any site beyond the pylorus of the stomach, including the duodenum and jejunum.

Prompt feeding tube placement by the critical care nurse is a priority. Diminished or absent bowel sounds are not a contraindication to initiation of tube feeds. Small bowel function and the ability to absorb nutrients remain intact despite the presence of gastroparesis and absent bowel sounds. Patients at risk for pulmonary aspiration as a result of gastric retention or gastroesophageal reflux should receive enteral feedings into the jejunum. If enteral feeding is unsuccessful, parenteral nutrition should be initiated.

Acute Kidney Injury

Assessment and ongoing monitoring of kidney function is critical to the survival of the trauma patient. The cause of posttraumatic acute kidney injury is complex and, besides the initial injury, may involve a variety of factors (Box 24.10).

BOX 24.10 Etiologic Factors in Posttraumatic Acute Kidney Injury

- Preexisting kidney disease
  - Hypertension
  - Heart failure
  - Diabetes
  - Chronic kidney disease
- Chronic liver disease
- Prolonged shock states
- Profound acidosis
- Systemic inflammatory response syndrome or reperfusion injury
- Abdominal compartment syndrome
- Muscle ischemia; myoglobinuria
- Microemboli
- Nephrotoxic medications
- Radiocontrast dye

Prevention of kidney failure is the best treatment, and it begins with ensuring sufficient IV fluid volume to provide adequate renal perfusion. Serial assessments of blood urea nitrogen and creatinine levels are commonly used to evaluate kidney function. Progressive deterioration in kidney function requires prompt diagnosis and treatment (see Acute Kidney Injury in Chapter 19).

Rhabdomyolysis and Myoglobinuria

Patients with muscle trauma and crush injuries are susceptible to the development of rhabdomyolysis and, if left untreated, can develop secondary kidney failure. Crush injuries can compromise blood flow. Decreased arterial blood flow results in insufficient oxygen transport and ischemia. This initiates a cascade of cellular events, including depletion of adenosine triphosphate (ATP) and failure of ATP pumps, which leads to the necrosis of skeletal muscle cells.[82]

As cells die, intracellular contents, particularly potassium and myoglobin, are released. Myoglobin, a muscular pigment, is a large molecule that gets lodged in the glomerulus, resulting in myoglobinuria (myoglobin in the urine). Circulating myoglobin can lead to the development of kidney failure by several mechanisms: volume depletion, decreased renal perfusion, cast formation with tubular obstruction, accumulation of iron, and direct toxic effects of myoglobin in the kidney tubules.[83]

Rhabdomyolysis should be suspected in all patients who experience crush injuries in which blood flow to the muscle is interrupted for a prolonged time. Dark tea–colored urine suggests myoglobinuria. Testing for myoglobin in the urine can be done but may take some time. The most rapid screening test is a serum creatine kinase level. Increased creatine kinase levels are associated with muscle damage and renal failure.[84] Urine output is monitored hourly, and trends in serial creatine kinase levels should be monitored frequently.

When rhabdomyolysis is diagnosed, treatment is aimed at prevention of subsequent kidney failure. Prevention of kidney dysfunction is paramount through the aggressive administration of IV fluids.[82] IV fluids increase renal blood flow and decrease the concentration of nephrotoxic pigments. Alkalinization of the urine and administration of diuretics have been studied, but their roles in the prevention or management of rhabdomyolysis are not firmly established. Nursing management is directed toward maintaining urinary output, achieving fluid and electrolyte balance, and optimizing hemodynamics to prevent deterioration in kidney function.

Integumentary and Musculoskeletal Complications
Fat Embolism Syndrome

Fat embolism syndrome can occur as a complication of orthopedic trauma. The clinical onset of fat embolism syndrome is normally up to 72 hours after initial injury but can occur as late as 2 weeks after injury.[85] Fat embolism syndrome appears to develop as a result of fat droplets that leak from fractured bone with embolization of the fat droplets to the lungs. These droplets are broken down into free fatty acids that are toxic to the pulmonary microvascular membranes. Pulmonary fat emboli alter pulmonary hemodynamics and pulmonary vascular permeability. The lung becomes highly edematous and hemorrhagic. This may lead to the development of ARDS.

Signs and symptoms may be subtle and nonspecific. The patient may become restless and slightly confused. Hypoxemia, neurologic impairment, and a petechial rash are classic signs and symptoms.[86] The patient may or may not exhibit tachypnea with some degree of respiratory distress. A chest x-ray may reveal patchy infiltrates; a CT scan is often performed to rule out pulmonary embolism. Diagnosis is clinical and based on patient history, which often involves orthopedic injury.[85] Nursing care is supportive.

Other Complications in Adult Trauma Patients
Infection

Infection is a major source of mortality and morbidity in critical care units. Trauma patients are at risk for infection because of contaminated wounds, intubation and mechanical ventilation, invasive catheters, host susceptibility (including preexisting medical conditions), adverse effects of trauma on the immune system, and the critical care environment. Nursing management must include interventions to decrease and eliminate the patient's risk of infection.

Wound contamination poses a major infection risk for trauma patients, especially with injuries resulting from deep or penetrating trauma. Exogenous bacteria (from the external environment) can enter through open wounds. Exogenous bacteria can be dirt, grass, or debris inoculated into the wound at the time of injury or microorganisms introduced by personnel during wound care. Endogenous bacteria (from the internal environment) can be released as a result of gastrointestinal or genitourinary perforation.

Meticulous wound care is essential. The goals of wound care include removing dead and devitalized tissue, allowing for wound drainage, and promoting wound epithelialization and contraction. Wound healing is accomplished through interventions that promote tissue perfusion, including administration of oxygen, IV fluids, and ensuring adequate nutritional support.

Standard interventions for the prevention of ventilator-associated pneumonia (VAP), catheter-associated urinary tract infection (CAUTI), and central line–associated bloodstream infection (CLABSI) apply to trauma patients. Strict aseptic technique is required for all invasive procedures, catheter care, and dressing changes. Prompt removal of unnecessary lines, tubes, and drains, and hand hygiene are paramount to supporting optimal patient outcomes.

Sepsis

A patient with multiple injuries is at risk for development of sepsis and septic shock, but it is not always clear who is most at risk for sepsis posttraumatic injury. In one study, the authors constructed a predictive scoring tool for the risk of sepsis among trauma patients admitted to critical care.[87] The study identified seven parameters, including injury severity score (ISS), GCS, temperature, heart rate, albumin level, international normalized ratio (INR), and C-reactive protein, to help predict risk of sepsis among injured patients. Although additional validation of the scale through more research is required, early results are encouraging.

Possible sources of sepsis in adult trauma patients are contaminated wounds, the presence of invasive catheters, and severe damage to internal organs and structures. The source of the septic nidus must be promptly investigated. Gram stain and cultures of blood, urine, sputum, invasive catheters, and wounds are obtained. Broad-spectrum antibiotic therapy is often initiated before receiving definitive positive culture results and is based on the patient's current condition, nature of traumatic injury, severity of hemodynamic stability, and probability of infection (see Sepsis and Septic Shock in Chapter 26).

Transfusion-Related Complications

A patient receiving multiple blood products, particularly red blood cells, must be monitored for *transfusion-related acute lung injury* (TRALI). Signs of TRALI are similar to signs of ARDS, although there is a time-based relationship between the new onset of respiratory distress and the transfusion of blood products.[88] TRALI may occur 6 hours after a transfusion, as evidenced by fever, hypoxemia, and hypotension. Bilateral infiltrates may appear on the chest x-ray, often described as a "white out" in clinical practice. Treatment is supportive, including lung-protective strategies (low tidal-volume ventilation and PEEP) and, if possible, avoidance of subsequent transfusions.

Missed Injury

Once the trauma patient's condition has stabilized, nursing assessment of a patient with multiple injuries may reveal missed injuries. Missed injuries have a reported incidence of approximately 0.6% to 39%.[89] Missed injuries, which are primarily orthopedic, may be a cause of morbidity and mortality. Several factors in critical care contribute to missed injury. Patient factors include patients with head injuries and a GCS score of 8 or less, patients who are intoxicated at time of admission, those with greater ISSs, and patients receiving analgesia and sedation.[89] Clinician factors may include lack of experience, error in radiologic interpretation, failure to engage other services, or responsibility for several trauma patients with competing demands.

In the critical care unit, a missed injury may be suspected if the patient fails to show appropriate response to medical or surgical intervention. Hypotension and a falling hematocrit level despite fluid administration may indicate new-onset or continued bleeding. Change in the character of drainage from wounds or catheters may represent biliary or duodenal injuries. The physician must be notified immediately, because potential complications of hemorrhage and infection may be life-threatening. In intermediate care units and rehabilitation facilities, small bone fractures and sprains may manifest as the patient begins to mobilize. Nurses and other health care team members play key roles in identifying missed injuries, particularly when patients regain consciousness and begin to increase their activity.

Multiple-Organ Dysfunction Syndrome

Trauma patients are at high risk for MODS, a clinical syndrome of progressive dysfunction of organ systems. It has been estimated that up to 30% of trauma patients in critical care will develop MODS.[90] MODS often appears after admission to the critical are unit and is still responsible for a significant number of patient deaths in the postinjury phase. Trauma patients may experience primary and secondary MODS. Primary (or early) MODS appears within a few days after critical care admission, often as a result of direct traumatic injury. Secondary (or prolonged) MODS may occur later in hospitalization and may be a continuum of primary MODS or identification of newer problems.[90] In both situations, the patient often remains in the critical care unit for prolonged periods. Treatment is supportive, and priorities include controlling or eliminating the source of inflammation, maintenance of oxygen delivery, minimizing oxygen consumption, and meeting nutrition and metabolic support for individual organs. See Chapter 26 for in-depth discussion of MODS.

SPECIAL CONSIDERATIONS IN TRAUMA

Intimate Partner Violence and Trauma

Intimate partner violence (IPV, previously known as domestic violence) constitutes a major public health issue in North America. It has been reported that approximately 1 in 4 women and 1 in 10 men (12 million people) endure some type of IPV (spouse, previous spouse, or partner) each year.[91] IPV takes many forms, including physical violence, sexual violence, and/or stalking. More than 43 million women and 38 million men have endured some form of psychological aggression by their partner at some point in their life.[91] IPV can occur in all age groups and cultures and in both heterosexual and same-sex relationships.

IPV is a leading cause of injury and death of women. Trauma care centers and emergency departments are seeing increased numbers of individuals affected by IPV.

In particular, women are more likely to present with serious injuries.[92] Injuries reported as a result of IPV include head injuries, lacerations, gastrointestinal bleeding, and sexually transmitted diseases. Posttraumatic stress disorder is also frequently observed in women who are the victims of IPV.

Many health care facilities and emergency departments routinely screen patients for IPV. Ensure that patients are provided privacy, ensure that they feel safe, and offer appropriate medical and social service assistance.[92] Key interventions for victims of IPV are listed in Box 24.11.

Alcohol and Substance Abuse and Trauma

Both alcohol and substance abuse have been implicated in traumatic injury. In 2016 more than 10,000 people died in alcohol-related MVCs, approximately 28% of all trauma deaths.[93] Alcohol can alter consciousness, affect behavior, and impair judgment and concentration. Alcohol screening is now included as a routine component of care in many trauma hospitals. A strong correlation exists between IPV, alcohol use, substance abuse, and violence-related injuries.[92]

Any substance is capable of being abused, including alcohol, prescription medications, and illegal drugs such as cocaine, heroin, and crystal methamphetamine. In 2016 legal and illegal drugs were involved in approximately 16% of MVCs.[93] Substance abuse embodies the potential to impair judgment and enhance impulsivity. Emergency and critical care teams screen trauma patients on admission for the presence of alcohol and illicit substances by obtaining blood and urine samples. The Alcohol Use Disorders Identification Test (Table 24.11) is an inexpensive, rapid test that has been validated in trauma centers and can be used to screen for problem drinking.

Trauma in Pregnancy

Physical trauma affects 1 in 12 pregnant women.[94] MVCs are the primary mechanism for most traumatic injury in pregnancy; penetrating trauma, falls, and IPV are also leading contributors. Placental

---

BOX 24.11 Key Interventions With Victims of Intimate Partner Violence

When intimate partner violence (IPV) is suspected or confirmed, health care providers can assist victims in many different ways:

Communication
- Discuss intimate partner violence with patients privately.
- Patients should be fully clothed.
- Respect confidentiality.
- Listen attentively, nonjudgmentally.
- Believe and validate the patient's experiences.

Assess the Patient
- Assess for possible injury and/or risk of immediate or future harm.

Provide Information
- Let the patient know that IPV is a common problem.
- Let the patient know that the IPV is not her/his fault.

Follow-Up
- Assist the patient with making a "safety" plan.
- Provide information/contact numbers on community resources.
- Offer information about local shelters to the patient in a way that it is safe for the patient to take with them. This could be a printed card for a purse or wallet or entering a shelter phone number into the patient's cell phone using a code name.
- The situation may need to involve social worker, social services.
- Notify law enforcement agencies when child abuse is suspected.
- Respect the patient's right to make decisions.

Adapted from Dicola D, Spaar E. Intimate partner violence. *Am Fam Physician.* 2016;94(8):646–651.

---

abruption is the most frequently observed complication for the pregnant patient with traumatic injury.[95] The admission of a pregnant trauma patient to the emergency department or critical care unit necessitates the ABC approach of the ATLS program, where the focus of trauma teams is on the health of both mother and fetus.

Trauma and the Older Adult

Older adults are predisposed to traumatic injuries because of the inevitable consequences of aging. The ability to react to or avoid environmental hazards is impaired because of age-related deterioration of the senses and changes in motor strength, postural stability, balance, and coordination.

Involvement of older adults in MVCs is a consequence of increasing age of the general population and the growing number of older drivers and occupants of motor vehicles. In 2015, 6800 older adults were killed and more than 260,000 older adult patients were triaged in emergency departments in the United States.[96] Factors that predispose older adults to MVCs are summarized in Box 24.12. Physiologic deterioration of cerebral and motor skills and alterations in visual and auditory acuity contribute to older drivers and pedestrians misjudging or being unable to avoid oncoming vehicles. Newly prescribed medication may interfere with one's ability to drive safely. Exacerbation of an acute or chronic medical condition while driving may have catastrophic consequences.

Older adults are most at risk for falls. Factors that predispose older people to falls are summarized in Box 24.13. Because falls are often caused by an underlying medical condition (syncope, dysrhythmias,

TABLE 24.11 AUDIT Alcohol Screening Questionnaire.

Question	Score[a]
How often do you have a drink containing alcohol?	Never
	Monthly or less
	2–4 times per month
	2–3 times per week
	4 or more times per week
How many standard drinks containing alcohol do you have on a typical day when drinking?	1 or 2
	3 or 4
	5 or 6
	7–9
	10 or more
How often do you have 6 or more drinks on one occasion?	Never
During the past year, how often have you found that you were not able to stop drinking once you had started?	Less than monthly
During the past year, how often have you failed to do what was normally expected of you because of drinking?	Monthly
During the past year, how often have you needed a drink in the morning to get yourself going after a heavy drinking session?	Weekly
During the past year, how often have you had a feeling of guilt or remorse after drinking?	Daily or almost daily
During the past year, have you been unable to remember what happened the night before because you had been drinking?	
Have you or someone else been injured as a result of your drinking?	No
Has a relative or friend or doctor or other health worker been concerned about your drinking or suggested you cut down?	Yes, but not in the past year
	Yes, during the past year

[a]Scores for each question range from 0 to 4, with the first response for each question (never) scoring 0, the second (less than monthly) scoring 1, the third (monthly) scoring 2, the fourth (weekly) scoring 3, and the fifth response (daily or almost daily) scoring 4. For the last two questions, which only have three responses, the scoring is 0, 2, and 4. A score of 8 or more is associated with harmful or hazardous drinking, and a score of 13 or more by women or 15 or more by men is likely to indicate alcohol dependence. See https://auditscreen.org for more information. *AUDIT*, Alcohol Use Disorders Identification Test.

BOX 24.12 Factors That Predispose Older Adults to Motor Vehicle Crashes

- Alterations in visual and auditory acuity
- Deterioration in strength and slower reaction times
- Diminution of cerebral skills
- Diminution of motor skills
- Exacerbation of acute or chronic medical conditions
- Medications that may interfere with safe driving

hypotension), management of an older adult who has experienced a fall must include an evaluation of events and conditions immediately preceding the traumatic injury.

The concept of *limited physiologic reserve* in an older adult trauma patient highlights the key difference between the average younger trauma patient with normal physiologic reserve and the older patient with underlying physiologic derangements.[97] Age-related changes that occur in virtually every organ system may not produce evidence of organ dysfunction in the resting state. At the same time, the ability of organs to augment function in response to traumatic stress may be greatly compromised. TBI; SCI; chest trauma; and fractures of the pelvis, hip, and extremities are frequently observed in the geriatric trauma population. Clinicians are increasingly recognizing that trauma protocols must be individualized for older trauma patients.[98] As an example, fluid resuscitation is an integral part of trauma resuscitation. Older adult patients on long-term diuretic therapy may require additional volume and enhanced potassium supplementation as a result of chronic volume and potassium depletion. At the same time, these patients may be less likely to tolerate aggressive fluid resuscitation because of preexisting cardiac or pulmonary issues. Similarly, many older adults take daily anticoagulants, antiplatelet medications, or both to prevent thrombotic or embolic complications from preexisting medical conditions. Traumatic injury in conjunction with a prolonged INR greatly increases the risk of major hemorrhage. When a head injury is suspected or confirmed, systemic anticoagulation must be corrected as soon as possible after admission, and a CT scan of the head is urgently obtained.

It is widely recognized that the best outcomes for this patient population are achieved through early, appropriate, aggressive trauma care, with admission to a trauma center with resources and protocols to provide excellent care to injured adults regardless of age. Trauma in older adults is associated with longer critical care stays, an increased number of life-threatening complications, and higher mortality rates, even when the injuries are less severe.[99] This is attributable to preexisting medical conditions, limited physiologic reserve, and decreased ability to compensate for severe injury.

Older patients who do survive traumatic injury are often faced with changes in functional status after injury. Relatively minor trauma can be the event that changes the lifestyle of an older person from one of relative independence to one that requires prolonged rehabilitation or skilled nursing care. Early advanced care planning in the critical care unit that involves both patient and family is of utmost importance.[99] Discharge planning and rehabilitation may also begin in the critical care or intermediate care unit. See Chapter 6 for in-depth discussion regarding the older adult.

Meeting Needs of Family Members and Significant Others

The effect of traumatic injury can be devastating for patients, family members, and significant others. Trauma can precipitate a crisis within the family. The family is often faced with an unexpected situation for

BOX 24.13   Risk Factors for Falls in Older Adults

Acute Illness
- Cerebrovascular accidents
- Dysrhythmias
- Syncope
- Diabetes

Cognitive Impairment
- Dementia

Neuromuscular Disorders
- Arthritis
- Lower extremity weakness
- Unstable gait

Medications
- Analgesics
- Antidepressants
- Benzodiazepines
- Diuretics
- Phenothiazines

BOX 24.14   Informatics

QSEN

Internet Resources: Trauma
- Centers for Disease Control and Prevention (CDC): Injury Prevention & Control: www.cdc.gov/injury/index.html
- Eastern Association for the Surgery of Trauma (EAST): www.east.org
- Emergency Nurses Association (ENA): www.ena.org
- ENA: Trauma Nursing Core Course (TNCC): www.ena.org/education/tncc
- Society of Trauma Nurses: www.traumanurses.org

which the members have had little time to prepare. Family members may exhibit physical and sociocultural reactions and a combination of emotional reactions including anger, fear, powerlessness, confusion, and mistrust. Recovery from traumatic injury can be long and frustrating for families. During this time, the family may exhaust social and financial support systems. Critical care nurses need to be able to assess, recognize, and address the effect of stressors on families of trauma patients.

A trend has evolved to move away from a paternalistic model of care to one that incorporates family into all aspects of trauma care. Although it is not uncommon for family members to be present during CPR, one question being asked is whether family members should be allowed to stay during trauma resuscitation.[100] Although many family members wish to remain close to their loved ones during hospitalization, should family be permitted to witness aggressive trauma interventions in a busy emergency department or critical care unit? Much more conversation is needed about this very important question.

Although it may be challenging, family members should be encouraged, to the extent that they are able and wish to do so, to participate in patient care while maintaining the comfort and safety of the patient. For example, bathing, brushing teeth, combing hair, and reading to the patient are excellent strategies to involve families in care of the injured patient.

Another valuable intervention is to bring families of trauma patients together in support groups. Trauma family support groups can offer sharing of experiences, expression of emotions, mutual support, sharing of coping strategies, and education about hospital and community resources and services.

ADDITIONAL RESOURCES

See Box 24.14 for additional resources for the management of the patient with trauma.

REFERENCES

1. Valdez C, Sarani B, Young H, Amdur R, Dunne J, Chawla LS. Timing of death after traumatic injury—a contemporary assessment of the temporal distribution of death. *J Surg Res.* 2016;200(2):604—609.
2. Bardes JM, Inaba K, Schellenberg M, et al. The contemporary timing of trauma deaths. *J Trauma Acute Care.* 2018;84(6):893—899.
3. Shepherd JM, Cole E, Brohi K. Contemporary patterns of multiple organ dysfunction syndrome in trauma. *Shock.* 2016;47(4):429—435.
4. American College of Surgeons. *Advanced Trauma Life Support.* 10th ed. Chicago: American College of Surgeons; 2018.
5. Ferrada P, Callcut RA, Skarupa DJ, et al. Circulation first—the time has come to question the sequencing of care in the ABCs of trauma; an American Association for the Surgery of Trauma multicenter trial. *World J Emerg Surg.* 2018;13:8. Available from: https://doi.org/10.1186/s13017-018-0168-3.
6. Eskesen TG, Baekgaard JS, Steinmetz J, Rasmussen LS. Initial use of supplementary oxygen for trauma patients: a systematic review. *BMJ Open.* 2018;8(7):e020880.
7. Smith D, Bowden T. Using the ABCDE approach to assess a deteriorating patient. *Nurs Stand.* 2017;32(14):51—63.
8. Tisherman SA, Stein DM. ICU management of trauma patients. *Crit Care Med.* 2018;46(12):1991—1997.
9. Buckman SA, Schuerer D. The multisystem trauma patient. In: Farcy DA, Chiu WC, Marshall JP, Osborn TM, eds. *Critical Care Emergency Medicine.* 2nd ed. New York: McGraw Hill; 2017.
10. Wise R, Faurie M, Malbrain MLNG, Hodgson E. Strategies for intravenous fluid resuscitation in trauma patients. *World J Surg.* 2017;41(5):1170—1183.
11. Cap AP, Pidcoke HF, Spinella P, et al. Damage control resuscitation. *Mil Med.* 2018;183(suppl 2):36—43.
12. Mizobata Y. Damage control resuscitation: a practical approach for severely hemorrhagic patients and its effects on trauma surgery. *J Intensive Care.* 2017;5:4.
13. Albreiki M, Voegeli D. Permissive hypotension resuscitation in adults with traumatic hemorrhagic shock: a systematic review. *Eur J Trauma Emerg Surg.* 2018;44(2):191—202.
14. Giamoudi M, Harwood P. Damage control resuscitation: lessons learned. *Eur J Trauma Emerg Surg.* 2016;42:273—282. Available from: https://doi.org/10.1007/s00068-015-0628-3.
15. Mizushima Y, Nakao S, Idoguchi K, Matsuoka T. Fluid resuscitation of trauma patients: how much fluid is enough to determine patient response? *Am J Emerg Med.* 2017;35(6):842—845.
16. American College of Surgeons. *ACS TQIP Massive Transfusion in Trauma Guidelines*; 2014. Available from: https://www.facs.org/-/media/files/quality-programs/trauma/tqip/transfusion_guildelines.ashx.
17. Phillips JB, Mohorn PL, Bookstaver RE, Ezekiel TO, Watson CM. Hemostatic management of trauma-induced coagulopathy. *Crit Care Nurse.* 2017;37(4):37—47.
18. Mohamed M, Majeske K, Sachwani GR, Kennedy K, Salib M, McCann M. The impact of early thromboelastography directed therapy in trauma resuscitation. *Scand J Trauma Resusc Emerg Med.* 2017;25(1):99.
19. Ball CG. Damage control surgery. *Curr Opin Crit Care.* 2015;21(6):538—543.

20. Bommiasamy AK, Schreiber MA. Damage control resuscitation: how to use blood products and manage major bleeding in trauma. *International Society of Blood Transfusion ISBT Science Series.* 2017.

21. Eick BG, Denke NJ. Resuscitative strategies in the trauma patient: the past, the present, and the future. *J Trauma Nurs.* 2018;25(4):254–263.

22. Emergency Nurses Association. *TNCC: Trauma Nursing Core Course.* 8th ed. Des Plaines, IL: Emergency Nurses Association. 2019. Available from: https://www.ena.org/enau/educational-offerings/tncc.

23. Cestero RF, Dent DL. Endpoints of resuscitation. *Surg Clin North Am.* 2015;95(2):319–336.

24. Davis JW, Dirks RC, Kaups KL, Tran P. Base deficit is superior to lactate in trauma. *Am J Surg.* 2018;215(4):682–685.

25. Dewan MC, Rattani A, Gupta S, et al. Estimating the global incidence of traumatic brain injury. *J Neurosurg.* 2018;130(4):1080–1097.

26. Centers for Disease Control and Prevention. *Traumatic Brain Injury and Concussion;* 2021. Available from: https://www.cdc.gov/traumaticbraininjury/index.html.

27. Pangilinan PH. Classification and complications of traumatic brain injury. *Medscape;* 2020. Available from: https://emedicine.medscape.com/article/326643-overview#a3.

28. Krishnamoorthy Y, Chaikittisilpa N, Kiatchai T, Vavilala M. Hypertension after severe traumatic brain injury: friend or foe? *J Neurosurg Anesthesiol.* 2018;29(4):382–387.

29. Meagher RJ. Subdural hematoma clinical presentation. *Medscape.* 2018. Available from: https://emedicine.medscape.com/article/1137207-clinical#b1.

30. March K. Head injury and dysfunction. In: Good VS, Kirkwood PL, eds. *Advanced Critical Care Nursing.* 2nd ed. St. Louis: Elsevier; 2018.

31. Royal College of Physicians and Surgeons of Glasgow. The Glasgow structured approach to assessment of the Glasgow Coma Scale. Available from: https://www.glasgowcomascale.org. Accessed September 25, 2021.

32. Marehbian J, Muehlschlegel S, Edlow BL, Hinson HE, Hwang DY. Medical management of the severe traumatic brain injury patient. *Neurocrit Care.* 2017;27(3):430–446.

33. Dash HH, Chavali S. Management of traumatic brain injury patients. *Korean J Anesthesiol.* 2018;71(1):12–21.

34. Marshall SA, Ling GSF. Critical care management of traumatic brain injury. In: Roberts PR, Todd SR, eds. *Comprehensive Critical Care: Adult.* 2nd ed. Mount Prospect, IL: Society of Critical Care Medicine; 2017.

35. Robba C, Citerio G. How I manage intracranial hypertension. *Crit Care.* 2019;23:243.

36. Carney N, Totten AM, O'Reilly C, et al. Guidelines for the management of severe traumatic brain injury. 4th ed. *Neurosurgery.* 2016;80(1):6–15.

37. Wittenberg CJ. Recognizing and managing traumatic brain injury. *Nursing 2018 Critical Care.* 2018;13(1):20–27.

38. Ley EJ, Leonard SD, Barmparas G, et al. Beta blockers in critically ill patients with traumatic brain injury: results from a multicentre, prospective, observational American Association for the Surgery of Trauma study. *J Trauma Acute Care Surg.* 2018;84(2):234–244.

39. Ghalaenovi H, Fattahi A, Koohpayehzadeh J, et al. The effects of amantadine on traumatic brain injury outcome: a double-blind, randomized, controlled, clinical trial. *Brain Inj.* 2018;32(8):1050–1055.

40. Hammond FM, Malec JF, Zafonte RD, et al. Potential impact of amantadine on aggression in chronic traumatic brain injury. *J Head Trauma Rehabil.* 2017;32(5):308.

41. National Spinal Cord Injury Statistical Center. *Spinal Cord Injury: Facts and Figures at a Glance;* 2021. Available from: https://www.nscisc.uab.edu/Public/Facts%20and%20Figures%202020.pdf.

42. Rabinstein AA. Traumatic spinal cord injury. *Continuum (Minneap Minn).* 2018;24(2, Spinal Cord Disorders):551–566.

43. Alizadeh A, Dyck SM, Karimi-Abdolrezaee S. Traumatic spinal cord injury: an overview of pathophysiology, models and acute injury mechanisms. *Front Neurol.* 2019;10:282. Available from: https://doi.org/10.3389/fneur.2019.00282.

44. Hachem LD, Ahuja CS, Fehlings MG. Assessment and management of acute spinal cord injury: from point of injury to rehabilitation. *J Spinal Cord Med.* 2017;40(6):665–675.

45. National Institute of Neurological Disorders and Stroke. Brown-Sequard information page; 2019. Available from: https://www.ninds.nih.gov/Disorders/All-Disorders/Brown-Sequard-Syndrome-Information-Page

46. National Institute of Neurological Disorders and Stroke. Central Cord Syndrome Information page; 2019. Available from: https://www.ninds.nih.gov/Disorders/All-Disorders/Central-Cord-Syndrome-Information-Page.

47. Syed SA. A boring guide to spinal cord syndromes. *Canadiem.* 2015. Available from: https://canadiem.org/a-boring-guide-to-spinal-cord-syndromes/.

48. McDonald NE, Curran-Sills G, Thomas RE. Outcomes and characteristics of non-immobilized, spine-injured trauma patients: a systematic review of prehospital selective immobilisation protocols. *Emerg Med J.* 2016;33:732–740. Available from: https://doi.org/10.1136/emermed-2015-204693.

49. Ko HY. Revisit spinal shock: pattern of reflex evolution during spinal shock. *Korean J Neurotrauma.* 2018;14(2):47–54.

50. Dave S, Cho JJ. *Neurogenic Shock.* [Updated 2021 Feb 19]. In: *StatPearls* [Internet]. Treasure Island (FL): StatPearls Publishing; 2021. Available from: https://www.ncbi.nlm.nih.gov/books/NBK459361/.

51. Mondal S, Dasgupta S, Naiya S, Ghosh A, Sarkar A. Unstable thoracolumbar spinal injuries treated by pedicle screw fixation: a short-term evaluation. *Saudi J Sports Med.* 2017;17(2):87–92.

52. Gosselink R, Clini E. Rehabilitation in intensive care. In: Clini E, Holland AE, Pitta F, Troosters T, eds. *Textbook of Pulmonary Rehabilitation.* New York: Springer International Publishing; 2018.

53. Fehlings MG, Tetreault LA, Wilson JR, et al. A clinical practice guideline for the management of acute spinal cord injury: introduction, rationale, and scope. *Global Spine J.* 2017;7(35):845–945.

54. Chin LS. Spinal cord injuries treatment and management. *Medscape.* 2018. Available from: https://emedicine.medscape.com/article/793582-treatment.

55. Sabolick EE, Menaker JA. Spinal cord injury. In: Farcy DA, Chiu WC, Marshall JP, Osborn TM, eds. *Critical Care Emergency Medicine.* 2nd ed. New York: McGraw Hill; 2017.

56. Wheeler TL, Bowel and Bladder Workshop Participants, de Groat W, et al. Translating promising strategies for bowel and bladder management in spinal cord injury. *Exp Neurol.* 2018;306:169–176. Available from: https://doi.org/10.1016/j.expneurol.2018.05.006.

57. Dennis BM, Bellister SA, Guillamondegui OD. Thoracic trauma. *Surg Clin North Am.* 2017;97(5):1047–1064.

58. Liu Y, Xu S, Yu Q, et al. Surgical versus conservative therapy for multiple rib fractures: a retrospective analysis. *Ann Transl Med.* 2018;6(22):439.

59. Jena RK, Agrawal A, Sandeep Y, Shrikhande NN. Understanding of flail chest injuries and concepts in management. *Int J Stud Res.* 2017;6(1):3–5.

60. Rendeki S, Molnar TF. Pulmonary contusion. *J Thorac Dis.* 2019;11(suppl 2):S141–S151.

61. Weiser TG. Pulmonary Contusion. *The Merck Manual.* 2020. Available from: https://www.merckmanuals.com/en-ca/professional/injuries-poisoning/thoracic-trauma/pulmonary-contusion.

62. Laan DV, Vu TD, Thiels CA, et al. Chest wall thickness and decompression failure: a systematic review and meta-analysis comparing anatomic locations in needle thoracostomy. *Injury.* 2016;47(4):797–804.

63. Legome E. Initial evaluation and management of blunt thoracic trauma in adults. In: Moreira ME, Khurana B, eds. *UpToDate.* UpToDate; 2021. Available from: https://www.uptodate.com/contents/initialevaluation-and-management-of-chest-wall-trauma-in-adults.

64. Sixta S, Kozar R. Management of the severely injured trauma patient. In: Roberts PR, Todd SR, eds. *Comprehensive Critical Care: Adult.* 2nd ed. Mount Prospect, IL: Society of Critical Care Medicine; 2017.

65. Yarlagadda C. Cardiac tamponade. *Medscape.* 2018. Available from: https://emedicine.medscape.com/article/152083-overview#a4.

66. Akhmerov A, DuBose J, Azizzadeh A. Blunt thoracic aortic injury: current therapies, outcomes and challenges. *Ann Vasc Dis.* 2019;12(1):1–5.

67. Fox N, Schwartz D, Salazar JH, et al. Evaluation and management of blunt traumatic aortic injury: a practice management guideline from the Eastern Association for the Surgery of Trauma. *J Trauma Acute Care Surg.* 2015;78(1):136–146.

68. Talaie T, Morrison JJ, O'Connor JV. Blunt thoracic aortic injury. *J Cardiothoracic Trauma.* 2018;3(1):11–18.

69. Neschis DG. Management of blunt thoracic aortic injury. In: Mills JL, Eidt JF, Bulger EM, eds. *UpToDate.* UpToDate; 2020. Available from: https://www.uptodate.com/contents/managementof-blunt-thoracic-aortic-injury.

70. Bellomy ML, Freundlich RE. Hyperglycemia and elevated lactate in trauma: where do we go from here? *Anesth Anal.* 2018;126(3):748–749.

71. Bloom BA, Gibbons RC. Focused assessment with sonography for trauma. *StatPearls;* 2019. Available from: https://www.ncbi.nlm.nih.gov/books/NBK470479/.

72. Taghavi S, Ashari R. Liver trauma. *StatPearls;* 2020. Available from: https://www.ncbi.nlm.nih.gov/books/NBK513236.

73. Coccolini F, Montori G, Catena F, et al. Splenic trauma: WSES classification and guidelines for adult and pediatric patients. *World J Emerg Surg.* 2017;12:40. Available from: https://doi.org/10.1186/s13017-017-0151-4.

74. Paula R. Abdominal compartment syndrome. *Medscape.* 2017. Available from: https://emedicine.medscape.com/article/829008-overview.

75. Fitzpatrick ER. The open abdomen in trauma and critical care. *Crit Care Nurse.* 2017;37(5):22–45.

76. Yuan VP. Splenic Injury. *The Merck Manual.* 2019. Available from: https://www.merckmanuals.com/en-ca/professional/injuries-poisoning/abdominal-trauma/splenic-injury.

77. Bonanni P, Grazzini M, Niccolai G, et al. Recommended vaccinations for asplenic and hyposplenic adult patients. *Hum Vaccin Immunother.* 2017;13(2):359–368.

78. Mahat Y, Leong JY, Chung PH. A contemporary review of adult bladder trauma. *Injury Violence.* 2019;11(2):101–106.

79. Kozar RA, Crandall M, Shanmuganathan K, et al. Organ injury scaling 2018 update: liver, spleen and kidney. *J Trauma Acute Care Surg.* 2018;85(6):1119–1122.

80. Howell MD, Davis AM. Management of ARDS in adults. *J Am Med Assoc.* 2018;319(7):711–712.

81. Miller KR, Smith JW, Harbrecht BG, Benns MV. Early enteral nutrition in trauma: is there still any doubt? *Current Trauma Reports.* 2016;2(2):73–78.

82. Torres PA, Helmstetter JA, Kaye AM, Kaye AD. Rhabdomyolysis: pathogenesis, diagnosis and treatment. *Ochsner J.* 2015;15(1):58–69.

83. Esposito P, Estienne L, Serpieri N, et al. Rhabdomyolysis-associated acute kidney injury. *Am J Kidney Dis.* 2018;71(6):A12–A14.

84. Cabral BMI, Edding SN, Portocarrero JP, Lerma EV. Rhabdomyolysis. *Dis Mon.* 2020;66(8):101015.

85. Singh S, Goyal R, Baghel PK, Sharma V. Fat embolism syndrome: a comprehensive review and update. *J Orthop Allied Sci.* 2018;6(2):56–63.

86. Aggarwal R, Banerjee A, Soni KD, Kumar A, Trikha A. Clinical characteristics and management of patients with fat embolism syndrome in level I apex trauma centre. *Chin J Traumatol.* 2019;22(3):172–176.

87. Lu H, Du J, Wen D, Sun J, Chen M. Development and validation of a novel predictive score for sepsis risk among trauma patients. *World J Emerg Surg.* 2019;14:11. Available from: https://doi.org/10.1186/s13017-019-0231-8.

88. Semple JW, Rebetz J, Kapur R. Transfusion-associated circulatory overload and transfusion-related acute lung injury. *Blood.* 2019;133(17):1840–1853.

89. Tammelin E, Handolin L, Soderlund T. Missed injuries in polytrauma patients after trauma tertiary survey in trauma intensive care unit. *Scand J Surg.* 2016;105(4):241–247.

90. Shepherd JM, Cole E, Brohi K. Contemporary patterns of multiple organ dysfunction in trauma. *Shock.* 2017;47(4):429–435.

91. Centers for Disease Control and Prevention. Violence prevention: intimate partner violence; 2020. Available from: https://www.cdc.gov/violenceprevention/intimatepartnerviolence/index.html.

92. Miller E, McCaw B. Intimate partner violence. *N Engl J Med.* 2019;380:850–857.

93. Centers for Disease Control and Prevention. Impaired driving: get the facts; *Centers for Disease Control and Prevention.* 2020. Available from: https://www.cdc.gov/transportationsafety/impaired_driving/impaired-drv_factsheet.html.

94. Jain V, Chari R, Maslovitz S, Farine D. Guidelines for the management of a pregnant trauma patient. *J Obstet Gynaecol Can.* 2015;37(6):553–571.

95. Huls CK, Detlefs C. Trauma in pregnancy. *Semin Perinatol.* 2018;42(1):13–20.

96. Greene WR, Smith R. Driving in the geriatric population. *Clin Geriatr Med.* 2019;35(1):127–131.

97. Llompart-Pou JA, Pérez-Bárcena J, Chico-Fernández M, Sánchez-Casado M, Raurich JM. Severe trauma in the geriatric population. *World J Crit Care Med.* 2017;6(2):99–106.

98. American College of Surgeons Committee on Trauma. *ACS TQIP Geriatric Trauma Management Guidelines.* American College of Surgeons; 2013. Available from: https://www.facs.org/-/media/files/quality-programs/trauma/tqip/geriatric_guidelines.ashx?la5en.

99. Verhoeff K, Glen P, Taheri A, et al. Implementation and adoption of advanced care planning in the elderly trauma patient. *World J Emerg Surg.* 2018;13:40. Available from: https://doi.org/10.1186/s13017-018-0201-6.

100. Traylor M. Should family be permitted in a trauma bay? *AMA J Ethics.* 2018;20(5):455–463.

25

Burns

Robyn Myers, Carrie M. Wilson, and Jennifer Seigel

ANATOMY AND FUNCTIONS OF THE SKIN

The skin is the largest organ of the human body, ranging from 0.2 m^2 in a newborn to more than 2 m^2 in an adult. The integumentary system consists of two major layers: (1) epidermis and (2) dermis (Fig. 25.1).

Epidermis

The outermost layer of the epidermis is 0.07 to 0.12 mm thick, with the deepest layer found on the soles of the feet and the palms of the hands. The epidermis is composed of dead, cornified cells that act as a tough protective barrier against the environment. It serves as a barrier to bacteria and moisture loss.[1]

From the surface inward, the five epidermal layers are: (1) stratum corneum, (2) stratum lucidum, (3) stratum granulosum, (4) stratum spinosum, and (5) stratum germinativum. The deepest layer of the epidermis contains fibronectin, which adheres the epidermis to the basement membrane. The epidermis regenerates every 2 to 3 weeks.

Dermis

The second, thicker layer, the dermis, is 1 to 2 mm thick and lies below the epidermis and regenerates continuously. The dermis is composed of two layers: (1) the more superficial, papillary layer next to the stratum germinativum and (2) the deeper, reticular layer. The dermis, composed primarily of connective tissue and collagenous fiber bundles made from fibroblasts, provides nutrition support to the epidermis.

The dermis contains blood vessels; sweat and sebaceous glands; hair follicles; nerves to the skin and capillaries that nourish the avascular epidermis; and sensory fibers that detect pain, touch, and temperature. Mast cells in the connective tissue perform the functions of secretion, phagocytosis, and production of fibroblasts.

ETIOLOGY AND PATHOPHYSIOLOGY OF BURN INJURY

Etiology

A burn injury results in tissue loss or damage. *Injury* to tissue can be caused by exposure to thermal, electrical, chemical, or radiation sources. The temperature or causticity of the burning agent and duration of tissue contact with the source determine the extent of tissue injury. Tissue damage can occur at various temperatures, usually between 40°C (104°F) and 44°C (111.2°F).

Pathophysiology

Tissue damage is caused by enzyme malfunction and denaturation of proteins. Prolonged exposure or higher temperatures can lead to cell necrosis and a process known as *protein coagulation*. The areas

extending outward from this central area of injury sustain various degrees of damage and are identified by zones of injury.[2,3]

Zones of Injury

Three concentric zones are present in burn injury: (1) zone of coagulation, (2) zone of stasis, and (3) zone of hyperemia (Fig. 25.2). The central zone, or *zone of coagulation*, is the site of most severe damage, and the peripheral zone is the site of least severe damage.

The central zone is usually the site of greatest heat transfer, leading to irreversible skin death. This area is surrounded by the *zone of stasis*, which is characterized by impaired circulation that can lead to cessation of blood flow caused by a pronounced inflammatory reaction. This area is potentially salvageable; however, local or systemic factors can convert it into a full-thickness injury.

The outermost area, the *zone of hyperemia*, has vasodilation and increased blood flow but minimal cell involvement. Early spontaneous recovery can occur in this area.[2,3]

CLASSIFICATION OF BURN INJURY

Burns are classified primarily according to the size and depth of injury. However, the type and location of the burn and the patient's age and medical history are also significant considerations. Recognition of the magnitude of burn injury, which is based on the previously mentioned factors, is crucial in the overall plan of care and in decisions concerning patient management and appropriate referral to a burn center[4] (Box 25.1).

The patient's age, burn size, and inhalation injury are the cardinal determinants of survival. A study of a large number of patients with burns found the biggest predictors of patient mortality to be age, percent total body surface area (TBSA) burned, and inhalation injury.

Size of Injury

Several different methods can be used to estimate the size of the burn area. A quick and easy method is the *rule of nines* (or *Berkow formula*), which often is used in the prehospital setting for initial triage of a patient with burns (Fig. 25.3). In this method, the adult body is divided into different surface areas of 9% per area, accounting for 7% of TBSA.

Designated burn centers have access to Berkow formula charts, but local hospitals may not have these charts. *Another method* uses the measure of the palmar surface of the victim's hand as a gauge for estimating burn area. The palmar surface (fingertip to wrist) represents 1% of the TBSA.[3]

In the hospital setting, the *Lund and Browder method* (Fig. 25.4) is the most accurate and accepted method for determining the percentage of

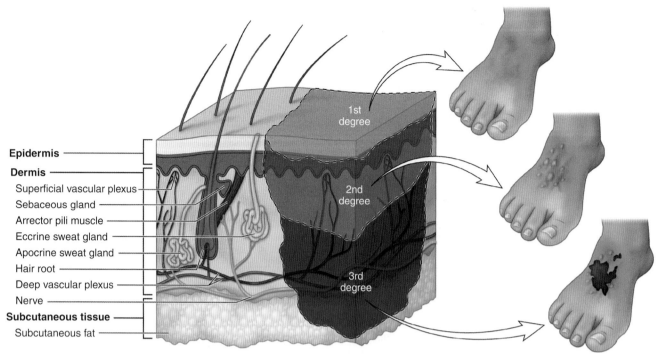

Fig. 25.1 Anatomy of the Skin. (From Dains JE. Integumentary system. In: Thompson JM, McFarland GK, Hirsch JE, et al., eds. *Mosby's Clinical Nursing.* 5th ed. St. Louis: Mosby; 2002.)

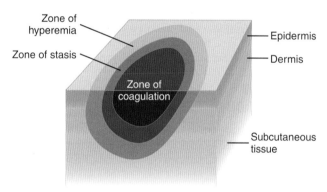

Fig. 25.2 Zones of Burn Injury.

burn. Surface area measurements are assigned to each body part in terms of the age of the patient.

This method is highly recommended for use with children younger than 10 years because it corrects for smaller surface areas of the lower extremities. It is also recommended for adult burn victims because of its accuracy.

Depth of Burn Injury

Traditionally, burn depth has been classified in degrees of injury based on the amount of injured epidermis, dermis, or both: first-degree, second-degree, third-degree, or fourth-degree burns. However, these terms are not descriptive of the burn surface. The depth of the burn is defined by how much of the skin's two layers are destroyed by the heat source.[3,5]

Burns are classified as superficial, partial-thickness, deep-dermal partial-thickness, or full-thickness burns. These descriptions are based on the surface appearance of the wound. *Superficial burns* include first-degree burns and are limited to the epidermis. *Partial-thickness burns*

BOX 25.1 Burn Center Referral

Patients with the following burn injuries are best treated in a certified burn center:

- Partial-thickness burns of 10% or more of total body surface area
- Full-thickness (third-degree) burns in any age group
- Burns of face, hands, feet, genitalia, perineum, or major joints that may result in cosmetic or functional disability
- Electrical burns, including lightning injury
- Inhalation injuries
- Chemical burns
- Burns in patients with preexisting medical disorders (e.g., diabetes mellitus, symptomatic cardiopulmonary disease) that could complicate management, prolong recovery, or affect mortality
- Burn injuries with concomitant trauma (e.g., fractures) in which the burn injury poses the greatest risk of morbidity or mortality may be stabilized initially in a trauma center before transfer to a burn center
- Burns in children in hospitals without qualified personnel or equipment for the care of children
- Burn injuries in patients who will require special social, emotional, or long-term rehabilitative intervention

include various stages of second-degree burns, and *full-thickness burns* include third-degree burns.[3,6] *Fourth-degree burns* extend through all skin layers and extend into muscle, tendon, and bone.

A *superficial (first-degree) burn* involves only the first two or three of the five layers of the epidermis. Erythema and mild discomfort characterize superficial partial-thickness wounds. Pain, the chief symptom, usually resolves in 48 to 72 hours.

Common examples of these burn injuries are sunburns and minor steam burns such as may occur while cooking. These wounds usually

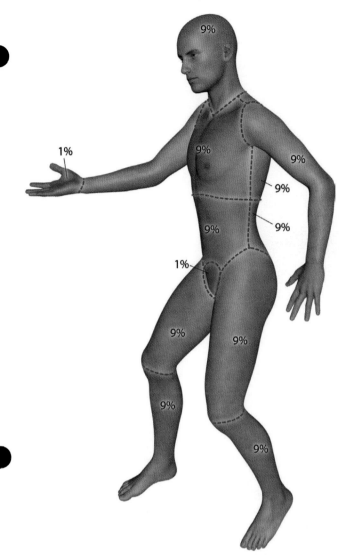

Fig. 25.3 Estimation of Adult Burn Injury. Rule of Nines. (From Singer AJ, Lee CC. Thermal burns. In: Walls R, Hockberger R, Gausche-Hill M, eds. *Rosen's Emergency Medicine Concepts and Clinical Practice*. 9th ed. St. Louis: Elsevier; 2018.)

heal in 2 to 7 days and do not require medical intervention aside from pain relief, management of pruritus (itching), and oral fluids. Swelling can be a common complication that may require intervention. Superficial burns are not included in the calculation of percent burn.

Partial-thickness (second-degree) burn involves all the epidermis and part of the underlying dermis.[3] These burns usually are caused by brief contact with flames, hot liquid, or exposure to dilute chemicals (Fig. 25.5). A light to bright red or mottled appearance characterizes superficial second-degree burns.

These wounds may appear wet and weeping, may contain bullae, and are extremely painful and sensitive to air currents. These burns blanch painfully.[3] The microvessels that perfuse this area are injured, and permeability is increased, resulting in leakage of large amounts of plasma into the interstitium.

This fluid lifts off the thin, damaged epidermis, causing blister formation. Despite the loss of the entire basal layer of the epidermis, a burn of this depth heals in 7 to 21 days. Minimal scarring can be expected. Mid-dermal partial-thickness wounds commonly take 4 to 6 weeks to heal.

Deep-dermal partial-thickness (second-degree) burns involve the entire epidermal layer and deeper layers of the dermis.[3] These burns often result from contact with hot liquids or solids or with intense radiant energy. A deep-dermal partial-thickness burn usually is not characterized by blister formation. Only a modest plasma surface leakage occurs because of severe impairment in blood supply.

The *wound surface* usually is red with patchy white areas that blanch with pressure. The appearance of the deep-dermal wound changes over time. Dermal necrosis and surface coagulated protein turn the wound from white to yellow (Fig. 25.6).

These wounds have a prolonged healing time. They can heal spontaneously as the epidermal elements germinate and migrate until the epidermal surface is restored, or they may require a skin substitute or surgical excision and grafting for wound closure. This process of healing by epithelialization can take up to 6 weeks.

Left untreated, these wounds can heal primarily with unstable epithelium, late hypertrophic scarring, and marked contracture formation.[3,6] Partial-thickness injuries can become full-thickness injuries if they become infected, if blood supply is diminished, or if further trauma occurs to the site. The treatment of choice is surgical excision and skin grafting.

A *full-thickness (third-degree) burn* involves destruction of all the layers of the skin down to and including the subcutaneous fat[3,6] (Fig. 25.7). The subcutaneous tissue is composed of adipose tissue, includes the hair follicles and sweat glands, and is poorly vascularized.

A full-thickness burn appears pale white or charred, red or brown, and leathery. The surface of the burn may be dry, and if the skin is broken, fat may be exposed. Full-thickness burns usually are *painless and insensitive to palpation*. Because all the epithelial elements are destroyed, the wound does not heal by reepithelialization.

Wound closure of small full-thickness burns (less than 4 cm² area) can be achieved with healing by contraction. All other full-thickness wounds require *skin grafting* for closure. Extensive full-thickness wounds leave the patient *extremely susceptible to* infections, fluid and electrolyte imbalances, alterations in thermoregulation, and metabolic disturbances.

The TBSA of the burn is calculated at the same time that assessment for wound depth occurs. This calculation provides the basis for determining the amount of fluid required for treatment. All burn wound surface area percentages except for superficial burns are used to calculate the patient's fluid requirements.

Types of Injury
Thermal Burns

The most common type of burn is a *thermal burn* caused by steam, scalds, contact with heat, or fire. Each year nearly 10,000 children experience severe disability as a result of thermal injury.[5] Toddlers are most often affected by scald burns, and mortality is highest in the 0- to 2-year age group because of their incompletely developed immune and organ systems.[5] Contact with hot foods (burns) is also common.[6]

The length of time the hot object is in contact with the skin determines the depth of injury. Children have thinner skin and will sustain a deeper burn at any temperature.[5] Non—food-related thermal burns can occur from fireworks, irons, curling irons, campfires, and fire pits in young children.

Burns associated with the use of lighters, lighter fluid, fire, firecrackers, and gasoline are seen in adolescents. Electrical burns are most likely to occur where there is exposure to live electrical wires from high-voltage lines, appliances, lightning, or faulty wiring.[6] Contact and flame burns tend to be deep-dermal or full-thickness injuries.

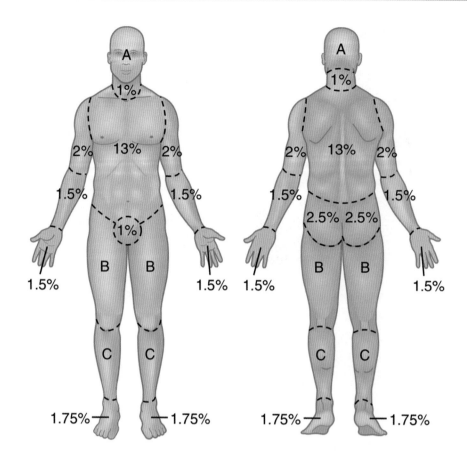

Relative percentages of areas affected by growth

Age	Half of head (A)	Half of one thigh (B)	Half of one leg (C)
Infant	9.5	2.75	2.5
1 yr	8.5	3.25	2.5
5 yr	6.5	4	2.75
10 yr	5.5	4.25	3
15 yr	4.5	4.25	3.25
Adult	3.5	4.75	3.5

Fig. 25.4 Lund and Browder Burn Estimate Chart and Diagram. (From Singer AJ, Lee CC. Thermal burns. In: Walls R, Hockberger R, Gausche-Hill M, eds. *Rosen's Emergency Medicine Concepts and Clinical Practice.* 9th ed. St. Louis: Elsevier; 2018.)

Electrical Burns

Electrical and lightning injuries result in 1000 deaths per year in the United States.[7] Electrical injuries account for 4% of patient admissions to burn centers.[4] Low-voltage (alternating) current (60–1000 V) or high-voltage (alternating or direct) current (greater than 1000 V) can cause electrical burns.[7]

Children have the highest incidence of electrical injury. These accidents occur as a result of insertion of an object into an outlet or by biting or sucking on an electrical cord. These burns can lead to tissue destruction and contracture formation.[6]

Electrical burns occur most often in the home for children; in adults, electrical injuries occur most often in the workplace.[7] Common situations that may increase the risk for electrical injuries include occupational exposure and accidents involving household current.

Chemical Burns

Acid and alkali agents cause chemical burns. Alkali burns commonly result in more severe injuries compared with acid burns. Acid and alkali agents are found in many household and industrial substances such as liquid concrete. Chemical burns most commonly occur in the domestic setting as a result of nonintentional exposure to household chemicals in children younger than 10 years of age and are preventable.[8]

Progression of injury from chemical burns to their complete depth may be delayed, and the full extent of the injury may not be apparent

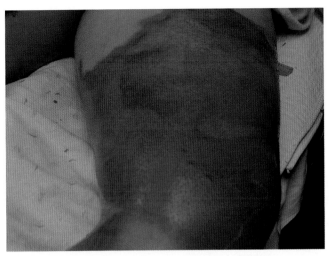

Fig. 25.5 Partial-Thickness Burn to Left Thigh.

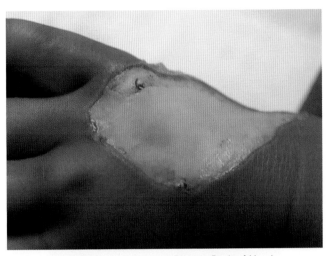

Fig. 25.7 Full-Thickness Burn to Back of Hand.

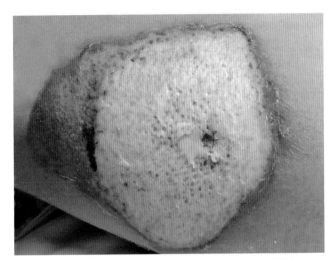

Fig. 25.6 Deep-Dermal Partial-Thickness Burn to Thigh.

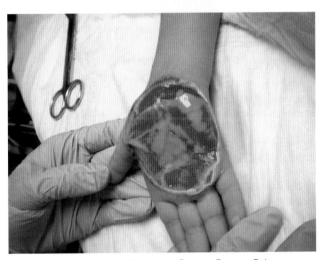

Fig. 25.8 Partial-Thickness Contact Burn to Palm.

until 48 hours after injury. Time must not be wasted in looking for a specific neutralizing agent, because the injury is related directly to the concentration of the chemical and the duration of the exposure, and the heat of neutralization can extend the injury.

Radiation Burns

Burns associated with radiation exposure are uncommon. *Radiation burns* usually are localized and indicate high radiation doses to the affected area. Radiation burns may appear identical to thermal burns.[9]

The major difference is the time between exposure and clinical manifestation; it can be days to weeks, depending on the level of the radiation dose. Radiation injury can occur with exposure to industrial equipment such as accelerators and cyclotrons and to equipment used for medical treatment.

Location of Injury

Location of injury can be a determining factor in differentiating the level of care required. According to triage criteria from the American College of Surgeons, burns on the face, hands, feet, genitalia, major joints, and perineum are best treated in a burn center. These burns involve functional areas of the body and often require specialized

intervention (Fig. 25.8). Injuries to these areas can result in significant long-term morbidity from impaired function and altered appearance.

Patient Age and History

Patient age and history are significant determinants of survival. Patients considered most at risk are children younger than 2 years and adults older than 60 years. Inhalation injury, electrical burns, and all burns complicated by trauma and fractures (considered major injuries) significantly increase the risk for death.

Obtaining the patient's medical history is important, especially a history related to cardiac, pulmonary, or kidney dysfunction; diabetes; and central nervous system (CNS) disorders. It is essential to obtain a thorough history, especially for nonverbal patients. Attention should be paid to the description of the burn event to rule out nonaccidental trauma (Fig. 25.9).

Social services such as child protective services and the police should be consulted if abuse or neglect is suspected. Education with caregivers, children, or older adults is key to burn injury prevention. Examples of prevention include having a fire safety plan, maintaining safe cooking, and ensuring proper water heater temperature. It is recommended to set water heater thermostats to 120°F or lower.[10]

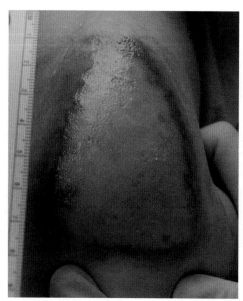

Fig. 25.9 Partial-Thickness Iron Burn to Right Buttock From Non-accidental Trauma.

Child Abuse

Burns account for approximately 5.8% to 8.8% of all abuse cases annually.[11] Most often, burns in children are accidental but are related to failure of the caregiver or parent to provide adequate supervision. However, the developmental age and size of the child are of key importance in ruling out accidental and nonaccidental burn injuries.

The *patterns of burns*—that is, inflicted burns consistent with immersion or dunking or contact—can be diagnostic of child abuse regardless of history.[11] A delay in seeking treatment or isolated scald or contact burns to the hands, feet, genitalia, or buttocks without a clearly defined mechanism should prompt further investigation for nonaccidental trauma.[6]

INITIAL EMERGENCY BURN MANAGEMENT

The *goals* of acute care of a patient with thermal injuries are to save life, minimize disability, and prepare the patient for definitive care. The burn injury may involve multiple organ systems, and the approach to the injured patient should be expeditious and methodical in identifying problems and establishing priorities of care.

The *resuscitation phase* begins immediately after the burn insult has occurred. Therefore the nurse is concerned with patient management at the scene until admission to an appropriate medical facility. As with any major trauma, the first hour after injury is crucial; however, the first 24 to 36 hours after injury also are important in management of patients with burns. Management during this period has a major effect on the patient's survival and ultimate rehabilitation (see Priority Patient Care Management, Box 25.2).

Obtaining a history regarding the nature of the injury is important in management of a patient with burns. A detailed patient history should include the mechanism of injury, patient's age, location and size of burn, type and amount of fluid already administered, known allergies, status of tetanus immunization, and significant medical history. All rings, watches, and jewelry are removed from injured limbs to avoid a tourniquet effect when edema occurs as a result of fluid shifts and fluid resuscitation.

Airway Management

The first priority of emergency burn care is to secure and protect the airway. If there is any possibility of underlying cervical instability, cervical precautions must be initiated. In patients with facial burns, exposure to fire in an enclosed space, or both, inhalation injury should be suspected.

Carbon monoxide poisoning is associated with high mortality rates. Carboxyhemoglobin (HbCO) levels are obtained, and oxygen therapy is initiated. Patients with HbCO level elevated greater than 10% and arterial partial pressure of oxygen (PaO_2)/fraction of inspired oxygen (FiO_2) ratio less than 200 have a high probability of needing respiratory support.[12]

All patients with major burns or suspected inhalation injury are initially administered 100% oxygen. Early intubation may be lifesaving in a patient who has an inhalation injury, because it may be impossible to perform this procedure later, when edema has obstructed the larynx. The need for frequent blood sampling and the benefit of continuous blood pressure monitoring may necessitate placement of an arterial line.

Respiratory Management

Circumferential, full-thickness burns to the chest wall can lead to restriction of chest wall expansion and decreased compliance. Decreased compliance requires higher ventilatory pressures to provide the patient with adequate tidal volumes. In a patient who has not undergone intubation, clinical manifestations of chest wall restriction include rapid, shallow respirations; poor chest wall excursion; and severe agitation.

Arterial blood gas analysis reveals a decrease in oxygen tension and an increasing arterial partial pressure of carbon dioxide ($PaCO_2$) level. Patients receiving mechanical ventilation have increasing peak airway pressure values.

Escharotomies (burn eschar incisions) may be needed immediately to increase compliance and for improved ventilation. These incisions usually are made bilaterally along the anterior axillary lines and are connected by a transverse incision at the costal margin (Fig. 25.10).

Circulatory Management

The extent and depth of the burn are assessed. The extent of TBSA of the burn is calculated for *estimation of fluid resuscitation requirements* (Table 25.1); the *Parkland formula* is the most widely used method of calculation.[1] Burn shock is caused by loss of fluid from the vascular compartment into the area of injury resulting in hypovolemia. The larger the percentage of burn area, the greater is the potential for development of shock. Lactated Ringer solution is infused through a large-bore cannula in a peripheral vein. Diuretics should not be given during the resuscitative phase of burn care.

According to the Parkland formula (see Table 25.1), 50% of the calculated amount of fluid is administered to the patient in the first 8 hours after injury, 25% is given in the second 8 hours, and 25% is given in the third 8 hours. Calculated fluid requirements are guidelines. Fluid resuscitation is a dynamic process. The rate of fluid administration is adjusted according to the individual's response, which is determined by monitoring urine output, heart rate, blood pressure, and level of consciousness.

Underresuscitation may result in inadequate cardiac output, leading to inadequate organ perfusion and the potential for wound conversion from a partial-thickness to full-thickness injury.

Overresuscitation may lead to moderate to severe pulmonary edema, to excessive wound edema causing a decrease in perfusion of unburned tissue in the distal portions of the extremities, or to edema inhibiting perfusion of the zone of stasis resulting in wound conversion. Fluid requirements may be much higher than estimated by using the Parkland formula.

Continuous monitoring with electrocardiograms (ECGs) should be used in patients with serious thermal burn injury and in the presence of electrical burns, inhalation injury, or associated traumatic injury. ECG lead placement may present a challenge with extensive burns, and nontraditional locations on nonburned skin should be selected instead.

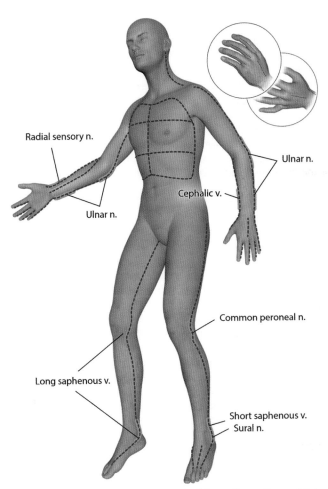

Fig. 25.10 Location of Escharotomy Incisions. (From Singer AJ, Lee CC. Thermal burns. In: Walls R, Hockberger R, Gausche-Hill M, eds. *Rosen's Emergency Medicine Concepts and Clinical Practice*. 9th ed. St. Louis: Elsevier; 2018.)

Kidney Management

If fluid resuscitation is inadequate, *acute kidney injury (AKI)* may occur. A urinary catheter may be necessary if the burn extends into the perineal area because of the presence or development of edema. Urinary catheters with temperature probes should be used whenever possible.

Gastrointestinal System Management

Patients with burns of greater than 20% of TBSA are prone to *gastric dilation* as a result of paralytic ileus. Nasogastric or orogastric tubes are placed in these patients to prevent abdominal distention, emesis, and potential aspiration. This decrease in gastrointestinal (GI) function is caused by the effects of hypovolemia and the neurologic and endocrine response to injury.

TABLE 25.1	Formulas for Fluid Replacement or Resuscitation in First 24 Hours.				
Fluid and Dose Rate	**ABA Consensus**	**Parkland**	**Modified Brooke**	**Brooke**	**Hypertonic**
Electrolyte solution	Ringer lactate	Ringer lactate	Ringer lactate	Ringer lactate	Hypertonic lactated saline (sodium, 250 mEq/L)
Dose: mL/kg/% burned[a]	2–4 50% of fluid over first 8 hours; 50% of fluid over next 16 hours	4	2	1.5	Rate based on urine output of 30–50 mL/h
Examples Using ABA Consensus Formula: An 85-kg Patient With 35% TBSA Burn					
2 mL × 85 kg × 35% = 5950 mL in first 24 hours 2975 mL in first 8 hours = 372 mL/h 2975 mL in next 16 hours = 186 mL/h		3 mL × 85 kg × 35% = 8925 mL in first 24 hours 4462 mL in first 8 hours = 558 mL/h 4462 mL in next 16 hours = 279 mL/h		4 mL × 85 kg × 35% = 11,900 mL in first 24 hours 5950 mL in first 8 hours = 744 mL/h 5950 mL in next 16 hours = 372 mL/h	

[a]Adjust these rates to maintain urine output >30 mL/h in adults or 1 mL/kg/h in children.
ABA, American Burn Association; *TBSA*, total body surface area.

GI activity usually returns in 24 to 48 hours. Prophylaxis with histamine blockers or sucralfate is initiated, because patients with burns are prone to *ileus*. These acute ulcerations of the duodenum are caused by sloughing of the gastric mucosa resulting from loss of plasma volume after severe burns.

Enteral nutrition has been shown to be protective of gastric mucosal integrity and to improve intestinal flow, gastric motility, and intestinal blood flow in patients with burns.[12] Enteral nutrition should be started as soon as possible. Patients with severe burns can be safely fed in the duodenum or jejunum within 6 hours of burn injury.[12] Enteral feeds should be promptly initiated for patients with burns via nasoduodenal or nasojejunal tube.

Extremity Pulse Assessment

Edema formation may cause *neurovascular compromise* to the extremities; frequent assessments are necessary to evaluate pulses, skin color, capillary refill, and sensation. Arterial circulation is at greatest risk with circumferential burns. If not corrected, reduced arterial flow causes ischemia and necrosis.

The *Doppler flow probe* is one of the best ways to evaluate arterial pulses. An *escharotomy* may be required to restore arterial circulation and to allow for further swelling. The escharotomy can be performed at the bedside with a sterile field and scalpel. Care must be taken to avoid major nerves, vessels, and tendons. The incision extends through the length of the eschar, over joints, and down to the subcutaneous fat. The incision is placed laterally or medially on the extremity.

If a single incision does not restore circulation, bilateral incisions are required (see Fig. 25.10). If escharotomy is required before the patient is transferred to a burn center, consultation with the receiving physician is advised.

Laboratory Assessment

Initial laboratory studies include complete blood count, electrolytes, blood urea nitrogen (BUN), creatinine, urinalysis, glucose, and blood screening. Special situations such as inhalation injury warrant arterial blood gas measurements, HbCO level determination, cultures, alcohol and drug screens, and cyanide levels.

Baseline assessment of nutrition status, including albumin and prealbumin, is helpful in monitoring future nutrition needs. Also, creatinine kinase, urinalysis, and urine myoglobin are good indicators of rhabdomyolysis seen in the setting of electrical burn injuries.[7] An ECG is obtained for all patients with electrical burns or preexisting heart disease. Serum lactate is also another good inflammatory marker indicating burn severity.[7]

Wound Care

After wounds have been assessed, topical antimicrobial therapy is *not a priority* during emergency care. However, the wounds must be covered with clean, dry dressings or sheets. Every attempt must be made to keep the patient warm because of the high risk of hypothermia. The administration of tetanus prophylaxis is recommended for all burns covering more than 10% of the TBSA and for patients with an unknown immunization history.

Burn Center Referral

After initial treatment and stabilization at an emergency department, referral to a burn center is considered (see Box 25.1). A burn center must be able to deliver all therapy required including rehabilitation and must perform personnel training and burn research. Patients meeting the criteria for referral need the expertise of a multidisciplinary team.

Referring hospitals must always contact the burn center in their region.[4]

Providers in the field should cover the burns with clean, dry cloths until arrival at the burn center. Early communication between the initial provider and the burn center is encouraged by the American Burn Association.[4]

SPECIAL MANAGEMENT CONSIDERATIONS

Inhalation Injury

Inhalation injury can occur in the presence or absence of cutaneous injury. Inhalation injuries are strongly associated with burns sustained in a closed or confined space, and they are associated with increased mortality.[13] Inhalation injury can occur in three basic forms, alone or in combination: carbon monoxide poisoning, direct heat injury, and chemical damage. The three types of inhalation injury are carbon monoxide poisoning, upper airway injury, and lower airway injury.

Carbon Monoxide Poisoning

Carbon monoxide poisoning is the leading cause of death in persons found dead at the scene of a fire who have few or no cutaneous thermal injuries. *Carbon monoxide* is a colorless, odorless, and tasteless gas. Inhalation of carbon monoxide, a by-product of the incomplete combustion of carbon, results in its bonding to available hemoglobin, producing *HbCO*, which effectively decreases oxygen saturation of hemoglobin.[14]

The affinity of hemoglobin molecules for carbon monoxide is approximately 200 to 250 times greater than that for oxygen.[12] HbCO binds poorly with oxygen, reducing the oxygen-carrying capacity of blood and causing hypoxemia. The shortage of oxygen at the tissue level is worsened by a shift to the left of the oxyhemoglobin dissociation curve, reflecting the fact that the oxygen in the hemoglobin is not readily given up to the cells.

Normal HbCO levels are less than 2%. HbCO levels of 40% to 60% often produce unresponsiveness; levels of 15% to 40% may result in various degrees of CNS dysfunction. Levels of 10% to 15%, which can be found in cigarette smokers, rarely produce serious symptoms but may cause a headache.

The major clinical manifestations of severe carbon monoxide poisoning are related to the CNS and the heart. Symptoms associated with carbon monoxide poisoning include headache, dizziness, nausea, vomiting, dyspnea, and confusion.[12] In severe cases, carbon monoxide poisoning may lead to myocardial ischemia, cardiac dysfunction, and CNS complications caused by reduced oxygen delivery and the already compromised circulatory system.

Early signs of carbon monoxide poisoning may include tachycardia, tachypnea, confusion, and lightheadedness. As the carbon monoxide level rises, patients exhibit a decreased level of responsiveness, which may progress to unresponsiveness and respiratory failure.

The treatment of choice for carbon monoxide poisoning is high-flow oxygen administered at 100% through a tight-fitting non-rebreathing mask or endotracheal intubation. Because of the rapid removal of carbon monoxide with the administration of 100% oxygen, the time required to transport a patient who has received oxygen in the field should always be considered to prevent possible underestimation of inhalation injury.

Upper Airway Injury

Burns of the upper respiratory tract include burns involving the pharynx, larynx, glottis, trachea, and larger bronchi. Injuries are caused by direct heat or by chemical inflammation and necrosis. Respiratory injury is most often confined to the upper airway. The heat exchange capability is so efficient that most heat absorption and damage occur in the pharynx and larynx above the vocal cords.

Heat damage may be severe enough to cause upper airway obstruction at any time, beginning from the moment of injury through the resuscitation period. Caution is needed for patients with severe hypovolemia, because supraglottic edema may be delayed until fluid resuscitation is underway and third spacing occurs.[13]

Patients must be monitored for hoarseness, stridor, audible airflow turbulence, and the production of carbonaceous sputum. Maximal edema occurs 24 hours after injury with upper airway injuries, and these patients should be observed in the critical care unit for a minimum of 24 hours.

Intubation is recommended whenever airway patency is questionable, rather than delaying intubation until airway obstruction is so severe that intubation becomes a challenge. After the airway is secure, priority is given to minimizing airway edema, maintaining pulmonary hygiene, and treating bronchospasm.

Elevating the head of the bed to 30 degrees or higher decreases airway edema. Fiberoptic bronchoscopy may be required to remove secretions in some patients. Mechanical ventilatory support is necessary when respiratory fatigue or failure occurs. Precautions to prevent ventilator-associated pneumonia should be implemented to avoid secondary infection.

Lower Airway Injury

Heated air rarely causes lower airway injury. If it does, it usually is associated with a higher mortality rate. Lower airway injuries are typically caused by chemical damage to mucosal surfaces. Tracheobronchitis with severe spasm and wheezing may occur in the first minutes to hours after injury. The onset of symptoms is unpredictable after smoke inhalation, and patients at risk must be closely monitored for at least 24 to 48 hours after injury.

Patients with inhalation injuries are at risk for developing pneumonia and acute respiratory distress syndrome (ARDS). Ventilator management strategies for hypoxia and ARDS in patients with burns can be challenging. Lung protective ventilation with low tidal volumes, higher levels of positive end-expiratory pressure, and permissive hypercarbia have shown optimal outcomes and minimized ventilator-induced lung injury.[13]

Treatment of lower airway injury is largely symptomatic. As with upper airway injury management, aggressive pulmonary hygiene, removal of secretions, ventilatory support, and careful fluid resuscitation so as to avoid exacerbating pulmonary edema and ARDS are indicated when caring for patients with burns and lower airway inhalation injuries.

Nonthermal Burns

Chemical Burns

Chemical burns can be caused by a variety of products. Acids, alkalis, and organic and inorganic compounds cause chemical burns. The acid or base quality determines the injurious nature of a product. The injury is caused by the pH of the product or by the concentration of the product.

Large amounts of water should be used to flush the area and clothing and shoes should be removed if they have been in contact with the chemical. Alkali burns of the eyes require continuous irrigation for many hours after the injury. Removal of contact lenses is necessary before irrigation. Litmus paper may be used to assess for neutrality or if further irrigation is needed.

Treatments for chemical burns vary. *Phenol burns* are first diluted, and then the skin is wiped quickly with polyethylene glycol or vegetable oil to decrease the severity of the burn.

Areas exposed to *hydrofluoric acid* must be copiously irrigated with water; the burned area then can be treated with 2.5% calcium gluconate gel.

The patient may need calcium gluconate supplements, because the fluoride ion precipitates serum calcium, causing hypocalcemia. White phosphorus can ignite if kept dry, and these wounds must be covered with a moist dressing.

After a *tar or asphalt injury*, the removal of tar or asphalt is best accomplished with the use of petroleum-containing distillates. One such product is Detachol Adhesive Remover (Ferndale Laboratories, Inc., Ferndale, MI). The solution can be placed directly on the wound and gently wiped off. Routine débridement of loose skin should be initiated after tar removal.

Electrical Burns

In electrical burns, consideration determining the amount of damage sustained is given to the:
1. type and voltage of the circuit,
2. resistance,
3. pathway of transmission through the body, and
4. duration of contact.

In these situations, *the rescuer* also may be injured if he or she becomes part of the electrical circuit. The rescuer must disconnect the electrical source to break the circuit or must know how to avoid becoming part of the circuit. The use of appropriately insulated equipment that diverts the circuit elsewhere is essential. Extreme caution must be used in the rescue of victims.

Electricity always travels toward the ground. The body conducts electrical current as a whole. Electrical burns are caused by the thermal conversion of electricity into heat within the tissues, which can cause the skin to only be minimally affected; however, there may be extensive damage to the underlying tissues.[15]

The electrical burn process can result in a profound alteration in acid—base balance and rhabdomyolysis, resulting in myoglobinuria, which poses a serious threat to kidney function. Myoglobin is a normal constituent of muscle. With extensive muscle destruction, it is released into the circulatory system and filtered by the kidneys. It can be highly toxic and can lead to AKI.

Fluid resuscitation for a patient with an electrical burn does not correlate with the Parkland formula, and the fluid is adjusted according to the patient's urine output. If myoglobin is present in the urine, a urine output of at least 1 mL/kg/h must be established until the urine is clear of all myoglobin pigment.[15]

If hemoglobinuria is identified, the clinician should assume that the patient has myoglobinuria and acidosis. Sodium bicarbonate may be administered to bring the pH level into the normal range, to correct a documented acidosis, or to alkalize urine to promote myoglobin excretion.

Diuretics such as mannitol also may be administered to increase renal blood flow and glomerular filtration rate to facilitate myoglobin clearance.[15] Sodium bicarbonate infusions and diuretic therapy are called *forced alkaline diuresis*.

BURN INJURY CLINICAL COURSE

Resuscitation Phase

Life-threatening airway and breathing problems, cardiopulmonary instability, and hypovolemia characterize the resuscitation phase, or shock phase. Burn injury affects the structure and function of almost every organ.[16] The magnitude of this pathophysiologic response is proportional to the extent of cutaneous injury. The goal of the resuscitation phase is to maintain vital organ function and perfusion. Emergent interventions for inhalation injury, airway management, and hypovolemia are concurrently addressed.

Oxygenation Alterations

Early diagnosis of inhalation injury is essential to minimize complications and to decrease the mortality rate. Three oxygenation complications are associated with smoke inhalation during the resuscitation phase: (1) *carbon monoxide poisoning*, (2) *upper airway obstruction*, and (3) *chemical pneumonitis*.

Impaired Gas Exchange

The most common pulmonary burn complication is carbon monoxide poisoning. High-flow oxygen should be administered at 100% through a nonrebreathing mask or endotracheal intubation until the HbCO level is less than 10% to 15%.

Chemical pneumonitis is caused by inhalation of the by-products of combustion of substances such as cotton, aldehydes, oxides of sulfur, and nitrogen. Burning polyvinyl chloride yields at least 75 potentially toxic compounds, including hydrochloric acid and carbon monoxide. Within days after a burn, ARDS commonly develops in patients with chemical pneumonitis.

Ineffective Airway Clearance

Laryngeal swelling and upper airway obstruction may occur at any time during the first 24 hours after a burn injury. Endotracheal intubation must be accomplished early, because this simple procedure can become extremely difficult in the presence of laryngeal edema.[12]

Extubation is done only when the patient can meet these criteria: level of consciousness assessed as awake, has intact cough and gag reflexes, and a respiratory effort greater than −25 cm H_2O in adults, vital capacity of 10 mL/kg, and decreased volume and tenacity of sputum.[13]

Fluid Resuscitation

Current resuscitation protocols emphasize fluid delivery rates based on the extent of burn injury and the patient's weight. The patient's weight measured in kilograms must be obtained on admission to the hospital. The extent of the burn is calculated by using one of the methods previously described. Several formulas are available to guide fluid resuscitation and should be used to assist in the management of fluid replacement (see Table 25.1).

Administration of crystalloid fluid (lactated Ringer solution) is given for the first 24 to 36 hours after the burn is the most common practice.[17] The addition of lactated Ringer solution with 5% dextrose should be considered as maintenance fluid, especially in the first 24 hours.

Colloid deficits can be considered for replacement in the next 24 hours with albumin. Colloid replacement can increase circulating volume and decrease fluid needs.[18]

In addition to colloid, maintenance fluids are given to replace evaporative losses, and the amount is adjusted according to the patient's serum electrolyte levels, urine output, weight, volume status, and clinical assessment.

Deficient fluid volume. In addition to the protein and electrolyte shift, an increased insensible water loss occurs. In a healthy adult, this loss is estimated to be 35 to 50 mL/h. Insensible water loss in a patient with burns may be 300 to 3000 mL/day. This increase may be related to temperature elevation, tracheostomy, and the size of the burn.

Burn shock is proportional to the extent and depth of injury. The loss of plasma begins almost immediately after the injury and reaches its peak within the first 48 hours. *Desired clinical responses to fluid resuscitation include*[19]:

1. Urinary output of 0.5 to 1 mL/kg per hour
2. Heart rate less than 120 beats/min
3. Blood pressure in the normal to high range
4. Mean arterial pressure (MAP) greater or equal to 65 mm Hg
5. Normal lactate
6. Clear lung sounds
7. Clear sensorium
8. Absence of intestinal events such as nausea and paralytic ileus

Heart rate, blood pressure, and central venous pressure (CVP) values are not always accurate or reliable predictors of successful fluid resuscitation. Electrolytes should be monitored frequently during resuscitation. *Hyperkalemia* can occur during this phase because of (1) the release of potassium from damaged cells; (2) metabolic acidosis; and (3) impaired kidney function caused by hemoglobinuria, myoglobinuria, or decreased renal perfusion.

Hypokalemia can occur during the resuscitation phase because of the massive loss of fluids and electrolytes through the burn wounds or because of hemodilution. During the acute phase, it may be related to hemodilution; inadequate replacement; loss associated with diuresis, diarrhea, vomiting, nasogastric drainage, and long hydrotherapy sessions; or the shift of potassium from the intravascular space to the cell after the acidosis has been corrected.

Hyponatremia is common during the *resuscitation phase* because of the loss of sodium through the burn wound, the shift of fluid into the interstitial space, vomiting, nasogastric drainage, diarrhea, and the use of hypotonic salt solutions during the early phase of resuscitation.

Hyponatremia also may occur during the *acute phase* because of hemodilution and loss through the wound, lengthy hydrotherapy sessions, and excessive diuresis resulting from the fluid shift back into the intravascular space.

Risk for Infection

The burn wound is the most common source of infection in the patient with burns. The loss of the protective mechanism of the skin and contamination from the patient's own bacterial flora can lead to bloodstream infections. Diagnosis of burn sepsis is based on evaluation of both clinical examination and laboratory findings.

Some centers advocate routine wound surveillance cultures and wound biopsy to identify infection early. Frequent wound inspection is needed to assess for changes in appearance such as an increase in exudate, odor, or color to minimize the risk of bacteremia. Patients should not be treated with antibiotics prophylactically; rather, treatment should be based on clinical examination and laboratory findings.[20]

Tissue Perfusion

Ineffective kidney tissue perfusion. Urinalysis to determine the myoglobin level may be performed soon after burn injury. Myoglobinuria can be detected grossly by the dark, port-wine color of the urine. Myoglobin is extremely toxic to the kidneys and can cause massive tubular destruction. It is best treated with rapid fluid administration and forced diuresis with diuretics such as mannitol, an osmotic diuretic.[15]

All other diuretics are avoided because they would deplete the already compromised intravascular volume. Sodium bicarbonate is sometimes given intravenously to alkalinize the urine and assist in the elimination of heme pigments.[15]

Maintaining and monitoring the renal system is vital in management of patients with burns. Impairment of the renal system may be related to hemoglobinuria, myoglobinuria, hypoperfusion, and hypovolemia. Urinary output must be monitored every hour for the first 48 to 72 hours, and specific gravity values can be used to determine the adequacy of hydration status and renal competency.

The urine glucose concentration is monitored, as are urine sodium, creatinine, and BUN levels. Oliguria may be associated with AKI but is usually related to inadequate fluid resuscitation in patients with burns. More commonly, AKI occurs early during resuscitation or late secondary to sepsis.[20] Other signs of kidney failure include increasing creatinine, BUN, phosphorus, and potassium levels; excessive fluid-weight gain; excessive edema; elevated blood pressure; lethargy; and confusion.

Ineffective cerebral tissue perfusion. The patient's neurologic status is assessed frequently during the first few days. Changes may be related to an associated head injury that occurred at the time of burn injury, hypoperfusion related to hypovolemia, hypoxemia associated with inadequate ventilation, carbon monoxide poisoning, or electrolyte imbalances.

Patients with *electrical burns or major thermal burns* may have peripheral neurologic injuries, which may not become evident for several days after the injury. The neurologic assessment includes use of the Glasgow Coma Scale.

It is not unusual for the patient to be agitated, restless, and extremely anxious during the resuscitation phase of burn injury as a result of hypovolemia, pain, and fear of disfigurement or death. Maintaining an adequate MAP is essential to ensure adequate cerebral perfusion pressure.

Ineffective peripheral tissue perfusion. Ineffective peripheral tissue perfusion results from *third spacing of* fluid during the resuscitation phase, which restricts blood flow to extremities.[18] As hypovolemia ensues, vasoconstriction increases, which can be potentiated by the loss of body temperature.

Monitoring the peripheral circulation is crucial in a patient with *circumferential, full-thickness* burns on the extremities. The resulting edema may severely compromise the venous system and then the arterial system. Neurovascular integrity of extremities with circumferential burns must be assessed every hour for the first 24 to 48 hours using the six Ps: *pulselessness, pallor, pain, paresthesia, paralysis,* and *poikilothermy.*

Numbness and paresthesia may occur only 30 minutes before loss of pulses. Irreversible nerve ischemia resulting in loss of function may begin after 12 to 24 hours. An *escharotomy* may become necessary to allow the underlying tissue to expand. In deeper wounds, a fasciotomy, which involves incision into the fascia, may be necessary.

Ineffective gastrointestinal tissue perfusion. Paralytic ileus is a common GI complication that can occur during resuscitation or when sepsis develops, because blood flow can decrease up to 60%.[20] If clinical manifestations of a paralytic ileus occur, oral intake is withheld, and a nasogastric tube may be inserted and placed on low suction.

Paralytic ileus can be related to hypokalemia, the sympathetic response to severe trauma, or decreased tissue perfusion related to hypovolemia. In large burns (>60% TBSA) or circumferential abdominal burns, the abdominal examination should include careful evaluation for abdominal compartment syndrome.

A *stress ulcer* may develop as a result of decreased tissue perfusion to the GI tract, a change in the quantity or quality of mucus (which has a pH of 1), or an increase in gastric acid secretion resulting from the stress response. Gastric acid should be maintained above a pH of 5 through the administration of antacids, histamine blockers, or proton-pump inhibitors to prevent the development of these ulcers.

Acute Care Phase

Immediately after injury, the body responds by initiating a series of physiologic changes to restore skin integrity. These physiologic changes include the inflammatory phase, proliferative phase, and maturation phase.

Inflammatory Phase

The *inflammatory phase* begins immediately after injury. A wound disrupts the blood vessels and results in bleeding, which induces the wound healing process. Vascular changes and cellular activity characterize this period. Changes in the severed vessels occur in an attempt to wall off the wound from the external environment.

Platelets, activated as a result of vessel wall injury, aggregate; blood coagulation is initiated; and in larger vessels, smooth muscle tissue contraction occurs, resulting in a reduction in the diameter of the vessel lumen.

These brief but important compensatory mechanisms protect the patient from excessive blood loss and increased exposure to bacterial contamination. As vasodilation occurs, blood supply to the wound site increases and is observed as erythema and exudates. Granulocytes invade the wound within 24 hours and initiate the phagocytosis of necrotic tissue and bacteria. Fibroblasts migrate to the wound and multiply, producing a bed of collagen.

Proliferative Phase

The *proliferative phase* of healing occurs approximately 4 to 20 days after injury. Formation of granulation tissue is key in this phase. The key cell in this phase of healing, the fibroblast, rapidly synthesizes collagen.

Collagen synthesis provides the needed strength for a healing wound. Epithelial cells migrate across the wound bed and multiply to a great extent. After these cells contact each other, the wound is covered. This process is known as *epithelialization*. The wound contraction process occurs when specialized fibroblasts known as *myofibroblasts* pull down the wound edges in an effort to close the wound.

Maturation Phase

The *maturation phase, or remodeling phase,* of healing occurs approximately 21 days after injury. During this period, the wound develops tensile strength, and the collagen becomes increasingly more organized. Both the quantity and quality of the new collagen determine the strength and integrity of the wound.

Scar remodeling may continue for 2 years after the injury. Regardless of how well collagen realigns itself, the tissue of the wound will never regain the degree of strength or intactness inherent in uninjured tissue.

Management of the Burn Wound

Management of the burn wound is the *top priority* after the resuscitation phase. The depth of the burn wound is the principal determinant of wound management. Expedient closure of the wounds decreases the potential for many complications such as fluid and electrolyte imbalances, loss of proteins and nitrogen, and infection. The major goal of burn wound care is wound closure.

Initial *débridement is* done by removal of blisters and loose skin. The assessment of wound depth by the clinician guides the treatment based on whether the wound will close in a reasonable time with dressings or will require surgical débridement. The assessment of wound depth can be a difficult challenge.

There are many alternative dressing regimens for wound closure that are temporary, semipermanent, or permanent. The following objectives must be met *for optimal wound closure*:

1. Control of infection through meticulous cleansing and débridement
2. Promotion of reepithelialization
3. Preparation of the wound for grafting and closure
4. Reduction of scarring and contracture formation
5. Providing patient comfort with appropriate psychologic support and pharmacologic intervention

Factors Affecting Healing of the Burn Wound

Because wound healing and clinical infection are inflammatory responses, it is essential to differentiate between normal wound inflammation in the presence of colonization of microorganisms and that of invading organisms. In diagnosing infection, the importance of microbiologic results must be evaluated in conjunction with clinical findings such as excessive erythema, edema, pain, and purulence.

Multidrug-resistant pathogens are increasing; therefore the appropriate diagnosis and choice of antimicrobial treatment should be guided by the intensity of colonization with these organisms as indicated by cultures from various sites. Clinical findings in conjunction with burn wound biopsy or culture results determine the diagnosis of wound infection.

A burn wound infection can delay healing and increase scarring, and invasive infection can result in death of the patient. Other *factors that affect wound healing* are:

- Tissue hypoxia from low blood flow to the burn wound
- Presence of *eschar* requiring débridement
- Exudate on the wound that can be harmful to the granulating wound or consume oxygen in the wound
- Trauma to the wound from daily dressing changes or lack of protection from the outside environment

Wound Cleansing

A variety of equally appropriate methods can be used to cleanse burn wounds (e.g., sterile normal saline at the bedside, tap water in a hydrotherapy room). At some centers, a mild antimicrobial cleansing agent may be used. Wounds are gently cleaned with a gauze dressing or washcloth and patted dry before application of topical agents. Hydrotherapy facilitates the removal of debris and loose eschar.

The prevalence of *immersion hydrotherapy* has been decreasing as more centers incorporate showering measures. Frequent cleansing and inspection of the wound and unburned skin are performed to assess for signs of healing and local infection.

Wound care exposure is limited as much as feasible to prevent hypothermia and decrease exposure to bacteria. Measures to reduce pain and hypothermia are used. Patients must receive adequate premedication with analgesics, opiates, and sedatives.

Wound Care

The most common regimen for burn wound care involves the application of a topical antimicrobial agent, followed by a primary nonstick dressing. An outer layer is applied to provide increased absorption, compression, and occlusion.

Another method is covering the wound with a thin layer of gauze or nonadherent dressing that can be impregnated with a petroleum product, with or without a topical antimicrobial. This method is useful for less severe wounds when the amount of drainage has decreased and

wound closure has almost been achieved. Lastly, a popular method for wound care is using silver-impregnated dressings. These dressings are more costly, but they reduce the dressing change frequency.

Topical antibiotic therapy. Effective antibacterial agents should control colonization so that specimens for wound biopsy reveal fewer than 10^5 microorganisms per gram of tissue. With more than 10^5 microorganisms per gram of tissue, control of wound sepsis with topical antibiotics is questionable, and oral or intravenous therapy may then be considered.

The *topical antibiotics* selected must meet several criteria: Side effects must be minimal, resistant strains must not develop with use, application must be easy and rapid, and use must be relatively economical.

The *most commonly used topical antibiotics* are silver sulfadiazine (SSD, Silvadene cream), mafenide acetate cream (Sulfamylon), bacitracin ointment, and silver impregnated into the primary dressing (Table 25.2). With multidrug-resistant pathogens increasing, deciding on the appropriate topical treatment is important.

SSD is a broad-spectrum antimicrobial agent with bactericidal action against many gram-negative and gram-positive bacteria associated with burn wound infection. SSD is indicated for use with partial-thickness and full-thickness wounds. It is a white cream that is applied once or twice daily to the burn wound.

Moisture provided by the wound exudate may give the SSD cream layer a yellow-gray pseudoeschar. A common side effect of SSD is leukopenia resulting from bone marrow suppression, which may develop 24 to 72 hours after application. Rebound to normal leukocyte levels follows onset within 2 to 3 days, and it is not necessary to discontinue SSD use.

Mafenide acetate cream penetrates through burn eschar and is bacteriostatic against many gram-negative and gram-positive organisms. Its use is limited because the application is uncomfortable for the patient, because it creates a burning sensation, and it is rapidly absorbed, requiring dressing changes two or three times daily. It is used routinely for coverage of small wounds involving anatomic areas that contain cartilage such as the ears and nose. Metabolic acidosis can result from the use of mafenide acetate. The patient must be observed closely for hyperventilation (see Table 25.2).

Bacitracin ointment is a topical agent applied to superficial burns and facial burns. Bacitracin is effective against gram-positive organisms such as *Staphylococcus aureus* and Streptococci.[21] Most gram-negative organisms and yeast are resistant. Bacitracin is applied to the wound one or two times daily and covered with a nonstick dressing. The ease of use, cost, and accessibility make it a common treatment in burn wounds. A yeast rash is commonly associated with repeated bacitracin usage.

Silver has long been used for the treatment of wounds because of its *broad-spectrum* bacteriostatic properties against gram-negative and gram-positive bacteria.[22] Silver has minimal side effects and minimal bacterial resistance. The wound moisture activates the silver and releases it into the wound.

An advantage of silver dressings is that the dressing does not need to be changed daily because of the sustained release of silver. Several silver-impregnated dressings are available from different manufacturers. These dressings are a popular choice by patients and providers because they decrease dressing change frequency.

Wound débridement. *Eschar* is the nonviable tissue that forms after a burn injury. This tissue has no blood supply, and polymorphonuclear leukocytes, antibodies, and systemic antibodies cannot reach these

TABLE 25.2 Pharmacologic Management: Topical Antimicrobial Agents.

Agent	Advantages	Disadvantages	Implications
SSD	Painless application Broad spectrum Easy application Rare sensitivities	May produce transient leukopenia by bone marrow suppression Minimal eschar penetration Some gram-negative resistance	Monitor WBC count Observe wounds for tunneling and subeschar infection Monitor culture reports
Mafenide acetate cream	Broad spectrum (especially *Pseudomonas* coverage) Easy application Penetrates eschar	Painful application Rare acid–base imbalance Frequent sensitivities	Provide adequate analgesia Monitor arterial blood gases Observe for hyperventilation Observe for rashes
Bacitracin	Painless application Nonirritating Transparent Nontoxic	No eschar penetration No gram-negative or fungal coverage	
Pure silver	Painless application Broad spectrum, including fungus and resistant organisms Rare sensitivity Less frequent dressing changes		Ensure knowledge of proper application

SSD, Silver sulfadiazine; *WBC*, white blood cell.

areas. Eschar provides an excellent medium for bacterial growth, and it is vital that loose eschar is débrided as necessary. *Débridement* facilitates wound healing by[23]:

1. Removing contaminated tissue of foreign bodies and bacteria
2. Controlling the inflammation
3. Removing the devitalized tissue, preparing the wound bed for grafting or biologic dressing application

The three types of débridement are mechanical, enzymatic, and surgical.

Mechanical débridement. *Mechanical débridement* includes rough débridement, wet-to-dry débridement, and sharp débridement with the use of scissors and forceps or curette (Fig. 25.11).[24] Wet-to-dry or wet-to-wet dressing to further débride the wound bed is less popular because of the related pain and tissue trauma.

Enzymatic débridement. *Enzymatic débridement* involves the topical application of proteolytic substances to the wound bed such as Santyl. These agents are useful in softening eschar and dissolving devitalized tissue while sparing healthy tissue. They promote the separation of eschar, which can lead to earlier wound closure.

Surgical débridement. *Surgical débridement*, which is performed by a surgeon,[23] is the gold standard. The goal here is to remove nonviable tissue down to bleeding viable tissue with an electric dermatome or surgical knife. Surgical excision is performed to mechanically remove necrotic tissue from the burn wound.

Skin Substitutes

To assist in wound closure, many temporary and permanent skin substitute dressings have gained popularity in the United States. A wide variety of products are available. Each dressing has specific indications for use. Temporary substitutes are designed for placement on partial-thickness or clean, excised wounds. Permanent substitutes provide a permanent skin replacement.

For application of skin substitutes, the wound must be clean and ideally should have a bacterial count of fewer than 10^5 microorganisms per gram of tissue. The burn wound must be free from eschar, and hemostasis must exist.

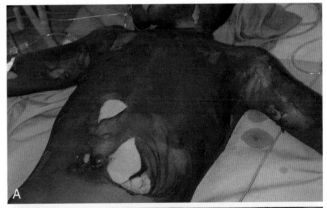
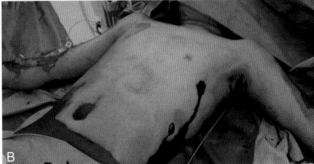

Fig. 25.11 Anterior Trunk and Bilateral Arm Burn. (A) Before mechanical débridement. (B) After mechanical débridement.

Definitive Burn Wound Closure

The primary goal of burn wound management is wound closure during the acute phase. Early excision and grafting of full-thickness (third-degree) burns is the standard in burn centers.[24] Some deep-dermal partial-thickness burns that have a prolonged healing time may also benefit from excision and grafting.

TABLE 25.3   Types of Grafts.

Graft	Use	Advantages	Disadvantages
Autograft	Provides permanent coverage of burn wounds Used in sheets or meshed form	Permanent coverage Nonantigenic Least expensive Meshing allows small amount of tissue to cover large area	Lack of available donor sites, which may delay wound coverage Donor sites are painful partial-thickness wounds Must be done in surgical suite
Homograft (allograft)	Temporary wound coverage	Can be placed at bedside or in operating room Allows for vascularization over deep wound Provides better control over bacterial growth than xenograft	Possibility of disease transmission Antigenic; body rejects in approximately 2 weeks Not readily available to all burn centers Expensive Requires rigorous quality controls

Early excision should be undertaken to improve functional and cosmetic results, decrease infection risk, decrease in-hospital time, and reduce the cost of burn care. Surgical débridement may begin 3 to 5 days after the burn insult, as soon as hemodynamic stability has been achieved. Some physicians operate within 24 hours of admission if the patient is hemodynamically stable.

To minimize contraction, burn wounds over joint surfaces should be excised and grafted as soon as possible. In patients with massive burns, excision procedures are commonly staged, requiring the patient to return to the operating room every 2 to 3 days until all wounds have been excised. Table 25.3 summarizes advantages and disadvantages of different graft types.

Autograft

An *autograft* is a skin graft harvested from a healthy, uninjured donor site on the patient with burns and then placed over the patient's burn wound to provide permanent coverage of the wound. Autografts are the only grafts that provide permanent wound coverage. Preferred sites for obtaining these grafts are the thighs, back, and abdomen; however, grafts can be harvested from almost anywhere on the body. Auto-grafting with the patient's own skin from a donor site is the preferred choice for wound closure.

With large TBSA burns, availability of donor sites can be prob-lematic. When an autograft is unavailable, many alternative methods are used to achieve this goal. Skin substitutes can be used until the patient's own skin is available for harvesting. Previously used and healed donor sites can be used again on later return visits to the operating room.

Sheets of the patient's epidermis and a partial layer of the dermis are harvested with use of a dermatome. These grafts are referred to as *split-thickness skin grafts* and can be applied to the wound bed as a sheet or in meshed form (Fig. 25.12). The size of the mesh is based on the areas requiring grafting and the availability of donor skin. This meshing prevents serum accumulation under the graft and permits coverage of a surface area larger than its original surface. Sheet grafts are placed on the face, neck, lower portions of the arms, and hands when possible. *Mesh grafts* can cover more area but may not produce the cosmetic appearance desired; therefore they are usually placed on areas covered by clothing.

Grafts can be secured with sutures, fibrin glue, or staples.[24] The choice of dressing that is placed over the graft varies widely based on physician and institution preference. One choice is fine mesh gauze impregnated with an emollient. It is placed over the graft, covered with a heavy gauze dressing, and secured to the patient with or without a splint, depending on the anatomic area of the graft.

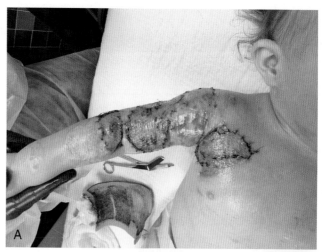

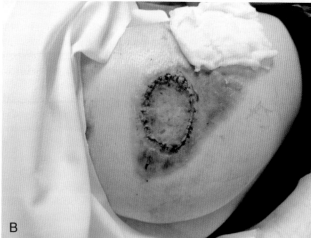

Fig. 25.12   (A) Split-thickness skin graft. (B) Sheet graft to left buttock.

A *vacuum-assisted closure* (VAC) device provides a safe and effective method for securing split-thickness skin grafts, and it is associated with improved graft survival.[24] VAC therapy can be used to secure the graft in place. The VAC is removed on postoperative day 3 to 5 for assessment of adherence and graft survival.

Great care must be taken not to disturb the graft. Care of the *donor site* is equally important, because it represents a wound similar to that of a partial-thickness injury. Donor sites can be covered with many different types of dressings depending on surgeon and institution preference.

Biosynthetic Skin Substitutes

Skin substitutes include homografts (allografts) and heterografts (xenografts). *Homograft* skin can be obtained from living donors or deceased donors (cadaver skin). With advances in cryopreservation, a homograft harvested from cadaver skin can be frozen and stored in a tissue bank. Because it is possible to transmit disease through the application of a homograft, tissue banks must adhere to strict guidelines.

Before application, homograft skin is tested for various transmissible diseases, including human immunodeficiency virus and hepatitis B surface antigens. Homograft skin can be applied as a *biological dressing* for débridement at the bedside or as *temporary wound coverage* on excised burn wounds. Vascular ingrowth occurs, and the homograft seals the wound and protects it from bacterial invasion; however, it is rejected approximately 2 weeks after its application.

Disadvantages include the homograft antigenicity, lack of accessibility, difficulties with storage and quality control, expense of procurement, and possibility of disease transmission from the donor.

Homografts are harvested during the first 4 hours after death, and they are taken from the abdomen, thighs, and back. Homografts usually are available only in centers in which the rigorous processing procedure can be achieved. These centers usually have skin and tissue bank facilities. Procurement of the allograft is much the same as for any other donated organ.

A *xenograft (heterograft)* is a graft transferred between two different species to provide temporary wound coverage. The most common and widely accepted xenograft is *pigskin* (porcine skin). Pigskin is available in frozen and shelf forms.

It can be *meshed or nonmeshed* and can be used for temporary coverage of burn wounds and donor sites. After the pigskin is in place, it may be dressed with antibacterial-impregnated dressings or other forms of dressings. Pigskin usually is removed or dissolves because of lack of blood supply in 5 to 7 days (see Table 25.3).

Synthetic Skin

The lack of available donor sites for major burn injury often delays wound closure. In an effort to minimize infection and to promote healing, many attempts have been made to develop skin substitutes that seal the wound in a functional and cosmetically acceptable fashion.

Integra has become a very popular dermal substitute, with its ultrathin layer of epidermal autograft used successfully. Integra is intended to be placed on freshly excised, full-thickness burns, and the outer silicone membrane is replaced with an ultrathin epithelial autograft 2 to 3 weeks later.

A technique that involves the growth and subsequent graft placement of *cultured epithelial autograft (CEA)* has also become an adjunct to the treatment of burn wounds. A complex process that allows for separation of keratinocytes is performed. The CEA is grown over 2 to 3 weeks to achieve a graft size of 25 cm^2. This represents an expansion of 50 to 70 times the original specimen. These confluent sheets of cultured epithelial cells are attached to a gauze backing and placed on the wound.

Even when grafts take initially, graft loss can occur later. Compared with other methods, the CEA also is more fragile, and the technique is costly. This therapy is being recommended as an adjunct for traditional split-thickness skin grafts, and it continues to be investigated and combined with newer dermal skin substitutes.

Nutrition Management
Imbalanced Nutrition: Less Than Body Requirements

The basal metabolic rate of a patient with burns may be elevated 40% to 100% above the normal rate, depending on the amount of TBSA involved. The metabolic rate is influenced by the amount of protein and albumin lost through the wounds; the catabolic response associated with stress, injuries, fluid loss, fever, infection, and immobility; sex; and height and weight of the patient before the injury. Without proper nutrition, healing may be slower and can decrease the immune system.[25]

A 10% loss of total body mass leads to immune dysfunction; 20% leads to decreased wound healing; 30% leads to severe infections; a 40% loss leads to death. Severely burned, catabolic patients can lose 25% of total body mass after acute severe burn injury.

The goal in nutrition management of a patient with burns is to provide adequate calories to enhance wound healing. To achieve this goal, nutrition support and a reduction of energy demand are imperative.

Because of the increased nutrition needs of patients with large-surface-area burns, oral feedings are usually inadequate, and supplemental enteral feedings are necessary. After burn injury, intestinal mucosal damage and increased bacterial translocation occur, resulting in decreased absorption of nutrients.

Nutritional support should ideally be initiated within 24 hours of injury via an enteral route.[26] Enteral feedings may be gastric or postpyloric; both are widely used. Caloric requirements are calculated on the basis of the size of the burn; the age, height, and weight of the patient; and stress factors. The daily protein requirement may increase to two to four times the normal 0.8 g/kg of body weight.

Carbohydrates and fat are used for energy and to spare proteins required for wound healing. Daily caloric intake can be 2 to 20 times higher than normal. Vitamins and minerals are usually given in doses higher than normal. Serum albumin, prealbumin, iron, zinc, calcium, phosphate, and potassium values are monitored, and supplements are given as needed.

Pain Management

Burn injuries are very painful. Pain management must be addressed early and frequently reassessed. Pain is an individualized and subjective phenomenon, and it has physiologic and psychologic components. Pain results from the acute burn injury and occurs throughout the phases of healing.

Initially after burn injury, opioids are administered intravenously in small doses and titrated to effect. The constant background pain may be addressed with the use of a patient-controlled analgesia (PCA) device. After hemodynamic stability has occurred and GI function has returned, oral opioids can be useful. Intramuscular or subcutaneous injections must not be administered, because absorption by these routes is unpredictable.

Additional premedication and analgesics are necessary during therapeutic procedures. Acetaminophen and nonsteroidal antiinflammatory drugs can be useful in patients who are not at risk for bleeding. Anxiolytics and antidepressants also should be considered and used appropriately. Nonpharmacologic techniques such as imagery, hypnosis, virtual reality, and distraction can be effective in reducing anxiety and the pain experience.[27] Treatment strategies need to be individualized. See Chapter 7 for more information on pain and pain management.

Rehabilitation Phase

The rehabilitation phase is one of recuperation and healing physically and emotionally. This phase can last several years. Psychologic rehabilitation is equal in importance to physical rehabilitation in patients with burns. The patient may require extensive reconstructive surgery.

Psychologically, the patient focuses on attaining specific personal goals related to achieving as much preburn function as possible. A person's preburn level of physical and emotional functioning can greatly affect the course of recovery. Minor and major accomplishments must be praised. This phase is characterized by scar management techniques and by physical and occupational therapies.

The burn team and the patient prepare for the transition to the outside world. Group therapy is a valuable tool used at many burn centers. Patients, family members, and health care providers express ideas and feelings. Patients with burns often establish priorities and make realistic decisions about their lives. Staff intervention during this phase is primarily of a supportive nature.

Impaired Physical Mobility

Tremendous advances have been made in the physical care of patients with burns. As more patients with larger and deeper burns survive, the challenge to maintain their optimal mobility and cosmetic appearance has been met with increased success. Despite advances in other areas of burn care, contractures still develop after a burn injury.

A *contracture is* the shortening of a scar over a joint surface and is the primary cause of functional deficits in patients with burns[28] (Fig. 25.13). Contractures develop as a result of various factors including the extent, depth, location, and configuration of the burn; the position of comfort the patient most frequently assumes; the relative underlying muscle strength; and the patient's motivation and compliance. The affected body parts should be positioned to prevent long-term deformity.

Splints can be used to prevent or correct contracture or to immobilize joints after grafting. If splints are used, they must be checked daily for proper fit and effectiveness. Splints that are used to immobilize body parts after grafting must be left on at all times except to assess the graft site for pressure points during every shift. Splints to correct severe contracture may be off for 2 hours per shift to allow burn care and range-of-motion exercises.

Active exercise is encouraged and is preferred, although active-assisted or gentle-passive exercises also may be an important part of the rehabilitation program. Before range-of-motion exercises and activities of daily living are performed, the need for pain medication must be assessed.

Scar Management

A person's skin response to a burn injury can be barely noticeable, such as slight color change, or can lead to cosmetic disfigurement and dysfunction. The goal of scar management is to minimize scarring, making the skin flat, elastic, and close to the original color.

It is important to inform the patient that the tissue may not return to the preburn texture or appearance. The highest risk for scar tissue development is associated with deep partial-thickness and full-thickness burns because of their depth and increased risk of infection.

Areas of the skin that required skin grafting also have a visible scar (Fig. 25.14). Scar maturation occurs 6 months to 2 years from the time of the injury. One method to reduce scar formation is timely application of uniform pressure. Custom-made *elastic pressure garments* are worn for 6 months to 1 year, if needed. These garments reduce scar blood flow and may provide force that helps developing collagen to organize.

Additional approaches to reduce scarring are scar massage, high-SPF sun protection, silicone gel sheeting, laser therapy, and steroid treatment. *Scar massage* works by stretching the scar and providing moisture and is most helpful in preventing contractures. *Sun protection* over the healed burn may decrease the long-term pigment change to the injured area.

Silicone gel sheets are used alone over the scar or in conjunction with compression to soften the scar by maintaining scar hydration and tension reduction. *Injectable steroids* are used for treatment of hypertrophic scars; however, they have some side effects that may make them undesirable.

Corticosteroid injections inhibit fibroblast growth and enhance collagen breakdown, leading to a flatter and softer scar. If less-invasive techniques have been unsuccessful for troublesome scars that cause pain or inhibit full range of motion, surgical excision may be recommended.

Itching

Pruritus is common in the maturing burn wound and commonly replaces burn pain. Itching can be extremely uncomfortable for the patient and should be continually assessed. Research has shown that burn pruritus can continue for years after the healed burn injury and has negative long-term effects for the patient.[29]

A mild, *non—alcohol-based skin cream or lotion* is applied every 4 hours and as needed to healed areas to lubricate the skin until natural lubrication occurs. Patients can be relieved of discomfort by the administration of an antipruritic agent such as *diphenhydramine* and by the application of *moisturizing creams*.

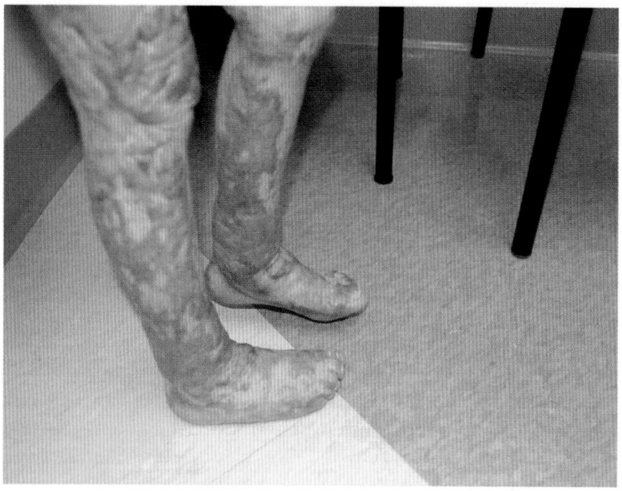

Fig. 25.13 Severe Contracture to Bilateral Lower Extremities.

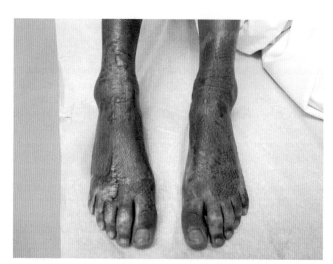

Fig. 25.14 Healed Split-Thickness Skin Graft to Bilateral Feet.

BOX 25.3 Informatics

Internet Resources: Burns
- American Burn Association: http://www.ameriburn.org
- https://www.uptodate.com/contents/skin-autografting
- https://www.acf.hhs.gov/cb/resource/child-maltreatment-2017
- https://www.urmc.rochester.edu/burn-trauma/burn-center/nutrition
- https://msktc.org
- https://www.cdc.gov/safechild/burns
- https://www.phoenix-society.org
- https://www.cdc.gov/niosh/topics/co-comp/

Multidisciplinary Collaborative Care

A multidisciplinary collaborative approach to burn treatment is an integral part of providing quality care. This approach involves considering all aspects of the patient's care when treatment decisions are made.

The burn team works together to address all needs of the patient and the family, and meets frequently to review patient care and maximize patient and family support. The multidisciplinary team includes, but is not limited to, physicians and nurses and individuals from social work, nutrition, physical and occupational therapy, respiratory therapy, pharmacy, psychology, pain service, child life services, and utilization review.

Support of the Patient With Burns

Burn injuries are physically and psychologically traumatic and life altering for the patient. The family of the patient with burns is also affected, and their needs should be remembered during the healing process. *Guilt i*s often associated with burn injuries, especially when the victim is a child. It is important for care providers to support the patient with burns physically and psychologically. Health care providers heal and support the patient throughout the hospital stay but often forget that the patient's biggest challenges may still lie ahead after hospitalization.

Many *resources* are available to help patients with burns cope after they are home, and these resources should be provided by the hospital team during the inpatient stay. Research has shown that many patients have difficulty returning to work and desire a coordinator during the rehabilitation process to assess work capacity. Programs are available to help with issues including social and school reentry, support for sexual considerations, and dealing with scars.[30]

STRESSORS OF BURN NURSING

Burn units can be stimulating workplaces in that they offer the fast-paced, high-technology atmosphere of any critical care setting; the complexity of advanced nursing management; and the dynamics of an interdisciplinary, collaborative model of practice. However, all these elements combined contribute to a potentially stressful work environment for the staff.

The physical environment can be a difficult one for a variety of reasons. The amount of equipment necessary to maintain the patient can be overwhelming and can limit the workspace dramatically. The temperature of the room usually is kept at approximately 85°F and can become much warmer, depending on the amount of equipment in the room.

The various odors in the room may be very unpleasant. Noise levels within a unit also are distressing. Research has shown that although nurses are emotionally supportive to patients and families, the emotional support available to staff is lacking. Self-care and care of other nurses and staff are issues just as important as the care of the patient and the family.[31] The decision to specialize in burn nursing requires careful consideration.

ADDITIONAL RESOURCES

Internet resources related to this chapter are located in Box 25.3.

REFERENCES

1. Haines E, Fairbrother H. Optimizing emergency management to reduce morbidity and mortality in pediatric burn patients. *Pediatr Emerg Med Pract*. 2015;12(5):1–24.
2. Kaddoura I, Abu-Sittah G, Ibrahim A, Karamanoukian R, Papazian N. Burn injury: review of pathophysiology and therapeutic modalities in major burns. *Ann Burns Fire Disasters*. 2017;30(2):95–102.
3. Douglas HE, Dunne JA, Rawlins J. Management of burns. *Surgery*. 2017;35(9):511–518.
4. American Burn Association. *Burn incidence and treatment in United States fact sheet*; 2016. http://www.ameriburn.org. Accessed October 27, 2021.
5. Palmieri TL. Pediatric burn resuscitation. *Crit Care Clin*. 2016;32(4):547–559.
6. Shah AR, Liao LF. Pediatric burn care: unique considerations in management. *Clin Plast Surg*. 2017;44:603–610.
7. Zemaitis MR, Foris LA, Lopez RA, Huecker MR. Electrical injuries. In: *StatPearls*. Treasure Island (FL): StatPearls Publishing; 2019.
8. D'Cruz R, Pang TC, Harvey JG, Holland AJ. Chemical burns in children: aetiology and prevention. *Burns*. 2015;41:764–769.
9. Hundeshagen G, Milner SM. Radiation injuries and vesicant burns. In: Herndon DN, ed. *Total Burn Care*. Elsevier; 2017.
10. Centers for Disease Control and Prevention. Injuries among children and teens. https://www.cdc.gov/safechild/burns. Accessed October 27, 2021.
11. Hodgman EI, Pastorek RA, Saeman MR, et al. The Parkland Burn Center experience with 297 cases of child abuse from 1974 to 2010. *Burns*. 2016;42:1121–1127.
12. Rose JJ, Wang L, Xu Q, et al. Carbon monoxide poisoning: pathogenesis, management, and future directions of therapy. *Am J Respir Crit Care Med*. 2017;195(5):596–606.
13. Sheridan RL. Fire-related inhalation injury. *N Engl J Med*. 2016;375(5):464–469.
14. Centers for Disease Control and Prevention. Carbon monoxide. https://www.cdc.gov/niosh/topics/co-comp/. Accessed October 28, 2021.
15. Gibran N. Electrical injuries. In: Greenghalgh DG, ed. *Burn Care for General Surgeons and General Practitioners*. Springer International Publishing; 2016:193–200.
16. Kraft R, Herndon DN, Finnerty CC, Shahrokhi S, Jeschke MG. Occurrence of multiorgan dysfunction in pediatric burn patients—incidence and clinical outcome. *Ann Surg*. 2014;259:381–387.
17. Guilabert G, Usúa G, Martín N, Abarca L, Barret JP, Colomina MJ. Fluid resuscitation management in patients with burns: update. *Br J Anaesth*. 2016;117(3):284–296.
18. Gillenwater J, Garner W. Acute fluid management of large burns: pathophysiology, monitoring, and resuscitation. *Clin Plast Surg*. 2017;44(3):495–503.
19. Nunez Lopez O, Cambiaso-Daniel J, Branski LK, Norbury WB, Herndon DN. Predicting and managing sepsis in burn patients: current perspectives. *Ther Clin Risk Manag*. 2017;13:1107–1117.
20. Nielson CB, Duethman NC, Howard JM, Moncure M, Wood JG. Burns: pathophysiology of systemic complications and current management. *J Burn Care Res*. 2017;38(1):469–481.
21. Cambiaso-Daniel J, Boukovalas S, Bitz GH, Branski LK, Herndon DN, Culnan DM. Topical antimicrobials in burn care. *Ann Plast Surg*. 2018. https://doi.org/10.1097/SAP.000000000001297.

22. Nherera LM, Trueman P, Roberts CD, Berg L. A systematic review and meta-analysis of clinical outcomes associated with nanocrystalline silver use compared to alternative silver delivery systems in the management of superficial and deep partial thickness burns. *Burns*. 2017;43(5):939—948.

23. Block L, King TW, Gosain A. Debridement techniques in pediatric trauma and burn-related wounds. *Adv Wound Care (New Rochelle)*. 2015;4(10):596—606.

24. Leon-Villapalos J, Dziewulski P. *Skin Autografting*. UpToDate; 2020. https://www.uptodate.com/contents/skin-autografting.

25. University of Rochester Medical Center. Nutrition: Burn recovery diet. https://www.urmc.rochester.edu/burn-trauma/burn-center/nutrition. Accessed October 27, 2021.

26. Clark A, Imran J, Madni T, Wolf SE. Nutrition and metabolism in burn patients. *Burns Trauma*. 2017;5(1):11.

27. James DL, Jowza M. Principles of burn pain management. *Clin Plast Surg*. 2017;44(4):737—747.

28. Goverman J, Mathews K, Goldstein R, et al. Adult contractures in burn injury: A burn model system national database study. *J Burn Care Res*. 2017; 38(1):e328—e336.

29. Nedelec B, Carrougher GJ. Pain and pruritus postburn injury. *J Burn Care Res*. 2017;38(3):142—145.

30. Model Systems Knowledge Translation Center. https://msktc.org. Accessed April 24, 2022.

31. Phoenix Society for Burn Survivors. Supporting the burn community. https://www.phoenix-society.org. Accessed April 24, 2022.

Shock, Sepsis, and Multiple Organ Dysfunction Syndrome

Julie-Kathryn Graham

SHOCK SYNDROME

Description and Etiology

Shock is an acute, widespread process of impaired tissue perfusion that results in cellular, metabolic, and hemodynamic alterations. Ineffective tissue perfusion occurs when an imbalance develops between cellular oxygen supply and cellular oxygen demand. This imbalance can occur for a variety of reasons and eventually results in cellular dysfunction and death. All types of shock involve ineffective tissue perfusion and acute circulatory failure. The shock syndrome is a pathway involving a variety of pathologic processes that may be categorized in four stages: initial, compensatory, progressive, and refractory. Progression through each stage varies with the patient's prior condition, duration of initiating event, response to therapy, and correction of the underlying cause (Fig. 26.1).

Shock can be classified as hypovolemic, cardiogenic, or distributive, depending on the pathophysiologic cause and hemodynamic profile. Hypovolemic shock results from a loss of circulating or intravascular volume. Cardiogenic shock results from the impaired ability of the heart to pump. Distributive shock results from maldistribution of circulating blood volume and can be further classified as septic, anaphylactic, or neurogenic. Septic shock is the result of the host's dysregulated response to microorganisms entering the body. Anaphylactic shock is the result of a severe antibody-antigen reaction. Neurogenic shock is the result of the loss of sympathetic tone.[1]

Pathophysiology

During the initial stage, cardiac output (CO) is decreased, and tissue perfusion is threatened. Almost immediately, the compensatory stage begins as the body's homeostatic mechanisms attempt to maintain CO, blood pressure, and tissue perfusion. The compensatory mechanisms are mediated by the sympathetic nervous system (SNS) and consist of neural, hormonal, and chemical responses. The neural response includes an increase in heart rate and contractility, arterial and venous vasoconstriction, and shunting of blood to the vital organs. Hormonal compensation includes activation of the renin response and stimulation of the anterior pituitary and adrenal medulla. Activation of the renin response results in the production of angiotensin II, which causes vasoconstriction and the release of aldosterone and antidiuretic hormone, leading to sodium and water retention. Stimulation of the anterior pituitary results in the secretion of adrenocorticotropic hormone (ACTH), which stimulates the adrenal cortex to produce glucocorticoids, causing an increase in blood glucose levels. Stimulation of

the adrenal medulla causes the release of epinephrine and norepinephrine, which further enhance the compensatory mechanisms.[2–4]

During the progressive stage, the compensatory mechanisms begin failing to meet tissue metabolic needs, and the shock cycle is perpetuated. As tissue perfusion becomes ineffective, the cells switch from aerobic to anaerobic metabolism to produce energy. Anaerobic metabolism produces small amounts of energy but large amounts of lactic acid, producing lactic acidemia. Vasodilation and increased vascular permeability from endothelial and epithelial hypoxia and inflammatory mediators result in intravascular hypovolemia, tissue edema, and further decline in tissue perfusion. A systemic release of inflammatory mediators in response to tissue hypoxia, especially in gut tissue, produces microcirculatory impairment and derangement of cellular metabolism, facilitating progression of the shock cycle.[5] Some cells die as a result of apoptosis, an injury-activated, preprogrammed cellular suicide. Others die as the sodium-potassium pump in the cell membrane fails, causing the cell and its organelles to swell. Cellular energy production comes to a complete halt as the mitochondria swell and rupture. At this point, the problem becomes one of oxygen use instead of oxygen delivery. Even if the cell were to receive more oxygen, it would be unable to use it because of damage to the mitochondria. The cell's digestive organelles swell and leak destructive enzymes into the cell, accelerating cell death.[2–4]

Every system in the body is affected by this process (Box 26.1). Cardiac dysfunction develops as a result of the release of myocardial depressant cytokines. Ventricular failure eventually occurs, further perpetuating the entire process. Central nervous system dysfunction develops as a result of cerebral hypoperfusion, leading to failure of the SNS, cardiac and respiratory depression, and thermoregulatory failure. Endothelial injury from hypoxia and inflammatory cytokines and impaired blood flow result in microvascular thrombosis. Hematologic dysfunction occurs from impaired blood product production secondary to bone marrow, liver and kidney failure, release of inflammatory cytokines, and dilutional thrombocytopenia. As a result, disseminated intravascular coagulation (DIC) eventually may develop. Pulmonary dysfunction occurs as a result of increased pulmonary capillary membrane permeability, pulmonary microemboli, and pulmonary vasoconstriction. Ventilatory failure and acute respiratory distress syndrome (ARDS) develop. Renal dysfunction develops secondary to renal vasoconstriction and renal hypoperfusion, leading to acute kidney injury (AKI). Gastrointestinal (GI) dysfunction occurs as a result of splanchnic vasoconstriction and hypoperfusion and leads to failure of the gut organs. Disruption of the intestinal mucosal barrier

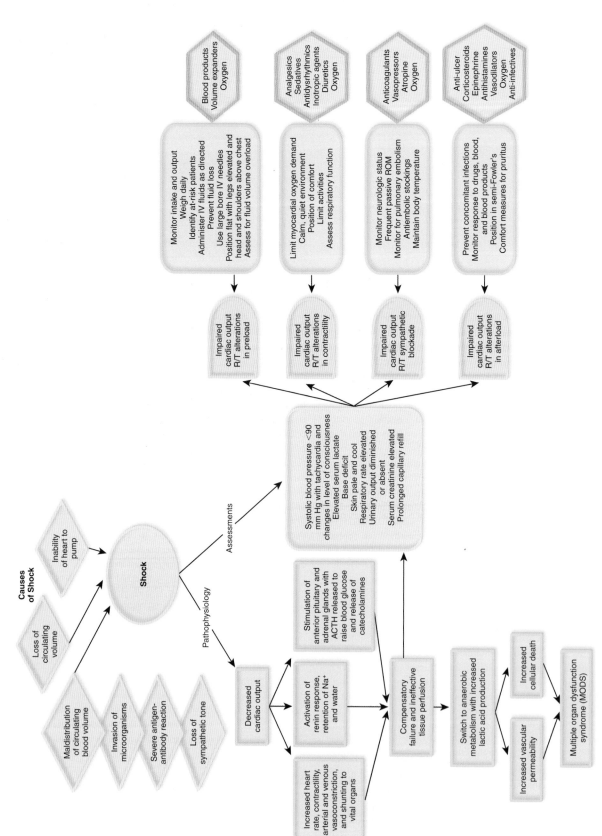

Fig. 26.1 Overview of Shock. *ACTH,* Adrenocorticotropic hormone. (Modified from Urden LD, Stacy KM, Lough ME, eds. *Critical Care Nursing: Diagnosis and Management.* 6th ed. St. Louis: Mosby; 2010.)

BOX 26.1 Consequences of Shock

Cardiovascular
- Ventricular failure
- Microvascular thrombosis

Neurologic
- Sympathetic nervous system dysfunction
- Cardiac and respiratory depression
- Thermoregulatory failure
- Coma

Pulmonary
- Acute lung failure
- Acute respiratory distress syndrome

Renal
- Acute kidney injury

Hematologic
- Disseminated intravascular coagulation

Gastrointestinal
- Gastrointestinal tract failure
- Liver failure
- Pancreatic failure

releases proinflammatory substances into the systemic circulation that further perpetuate the entire shock syndrome.[2-4]

During the refractory stage, shock becomes unresponsive to therapy and is considered irreversible. As the individual organ systems die, multiple organ dysfunction syndrome (MODS)—defined as failure of two or more body systems—occurs. Death is the final outcome. Regardless of the etiologic factors, death occurs from ineffective cellular consumption of oxygen from either a perfusion deficit or an inability of the cell to downregulate oxygen into useable energy (adenosine triphosphate; ATP).[2-4]

Assessment and Diagnosis

A patient with a mean arterial blood pressure (MAP) of less than 60 mm Hg or with evidence of global tissue hypoperfusion is considered to be in a shock state.[3] Because shock is a dynamic physiologic phenomenon, hypotension may occur late in the process or may normalize even when tissue perfusion is still inadequate.[6] Clinical manifestations vary according to the underlying cause of shock, the stage of the shock, and the patient's response to shock.[7]

Compensatory mechanisms may produce normal hemodynamic values even when tissue perfusion is compromised. Global indicators of systemic perfusion include serum lactate, arterial base deficit, serum bicarbonate, and mixed venous oxygen saturation levels.[8,9] Inadequate cellular oxygenation results in anaerobic metabolism, and increased metabolic lactate production increases the serum lactate level.[6] The level and duration of this hyperlactatemia are predictive of morbidity and mortality, and management guided by lactate levels has been effective in improving outcomes. The base deficit derived from arterial blood gas (ABG) values also reflects global tissue acidosis and is useful to assess the severity of shock. Serum bicarbonate is a measure of metabolic acidosis and has been found to correlate well with arterial base deficit.[8] The sections on different types of shock discuss clinical assessment and diagnosis of the patient in shock.

Medical Management

The major focus of treatment of shock is the improvement and preservation of tissue perfusion. Adequate tissue perfusion depends on an adequate supply of oxygen being transported to the tissues and the cell's ability to use it. Oxygen transport is influenced by pulmonary gas exchange, CO, and hemoglobin level. Oxygen use is influenced by the internal metabolic environment and mitochondrial function. Management of a patient in shock focuses on supporting oxygen delivery.[2,3]

Adequate pulmonary gas exchange is critical to oxygen transport. Establishing and maintaining an adequate airway are the first steps in ensuring adequate oxygenation. After the airway is patent, emphasis is placed on improving ventilation and oxygenation. Therapies include administration of supplemental oxygen and mechanical ventilatory support.

An adequate CO and hemoglobin level are crucial to oxygen transport. CO depends on heart rate, preload, afterload, and contractility. Various fluids and medications are used to manipulate these parameters. The types of fluids used include crystalloids and colloids. The categories of medications used include vasoconstrictors, vasodilators, positive inotropes, and antidysrhythmics.

Fluid administration is indicated for decreased preload related to intravascular volume depletion, and it can be accomplished by use of a crystalloid or colloid solution, or both depending on the situation.[10] Examples of crystalloid solutions used in shock situations are normal saline and lactated Ringer solution. Balanced crystalloid solutions (e.g., lactated Ringer's, Plasma-Lyte) are increasingly being used as an alternative to normal saline as they have a sodium, potassium, and chloride content closer to that of extracellular fluid and have fewer adverse effects on acid–base balance.[11] Colloids are protein-containing or starch-containing solutions. Examples of colloid solutions are blood and blood components, such as albumin, and pharmaceutical plasma expanders, such as dextran and mannitol.

The quantity and type of fluid are a subject of debate and depend on the situation.[10-13] Excessive volume expansion, more than what increases preload and stroke volume (SV), worsens organ function and may produce coagulopathy, cytokine activation, and abdominal compartment syndrome.[14] Methods to measure preload responsiveness include respiratory or positional variations in pulse pressure, systolic pressure, and SV and are more accurate than central venous pressure (CVP).[7,14] One method for assessing fluid response is passive leg raising, which involves placing the patient in a supine position and raising the patient's legs to 45 degrees. If the patient needs fluid, the systemic pressure will increase, and this will in turn increase venous return and CO. If the patient does not respond, then the patient should not be given additional volume.[7] Noninvasive ultrasound is also used to evaluate hemodynamic response to fluid augmentation, although it requires physician interpretation. Fluid resuscitation with normal saline or with albumin produces similar outcomes regardless of baseline serum albumin level.[12] Crystalloid solutions are inexpensive and effective. Advantages of colloids include faster restoration of intravascular volume and use of smaller amounts. Colloids are believed to stay in the intravascular space, in contrast to crystalloids, which readily leak into the extravascular space. Disadvantages include expense, allergic reactions, and difficulties in typing and cross-matching blood. Colloids also can leak out of damaged capillaries and cause a variety of additional problems, particularly in the lungs. Hypertonic or hyperoncotic fluids offer no additional benefit over isotonic crystalloids and are not recommended.[10,13,14]

Blood may be considered to augment oxygen transport if the patient's hemoglobin level is critically low, although what threshold value should be used for a patient in shock or with acute cardiac disease is still undetermined.[14,15] Transfusion of stored red blood cells (RBCs) does not substantially increase oxygen consumption and has been associated with immunosuppression, infection, impairment of microcirculatory flow, increased pulmonary vascular resistance, coagulopathy, and increased mortality. Restrictive transfusion practice has demonstrated lower mortality in a wide variety of patients, including critically ill patients.[16] Transfusion-related acute lung injury (TRALI) resulting from immune and nonimmune neutrophil activation has become the leading cause of transfusion-related death and may occur with transfusion of any plasma-containing blood or blood product.[17]

Vasoconstrictor agents are used to increase afterload by increasing the systemic vascular resistance (SVR) and improving the patient's blood pressure level. Vasodilator agents are used to decrease preload or afterload, or both, by decreasing venous return and SVR. Positive inotropic agents are used to increase contractility. Antidysrhythmic agents are used to influence heart rate. Box 26.2 lists examples of each of these agents.

Sodium bicarbonate is not recommended in the treatment of shock-related lactic acidosis.[18] No overall benefit has been found, and the risks associated with its use are significant. These risks include shifting of the oxyhemoglobin dissociation curve to the left, rebound increase in lactic acid production, development of hyperosmolar state, fluid overload resulting from excessive sodium, and rapid cellular electrolyte shifts.[18]

A critically ill patient should be started on enteral nutrition support therapy within 24 to 48 hours.[19] The type of nutrition supplementation initiated varies according to the cause of shock, and it should be tailored to the individual patient's needs, as indicated by the underlying condition, laboratory data, and treatment. When enteral feeding is contraindicated, parenteral nutrition should be considered, although a delay of 7 days is recommended for better outcomes. Supplementation of enteral feeding with parenteral nutrition to increase caloric intake is a subject of debate but has not been shown to improve patient outcomes.[20] A delay of 1 week is recommended before consideration of this strategy.[19]

Glucose control to a target level of 140 to 180 mg/dL is recommended for all critically ill patients.[21] Benefits of glucose control in critically ill patients include lower incidences of infection, renal failure, sepsis, and death.[21]

Nursing Management

The patient care management for the patient in shock is a complex and challenging responsibility. It requires an in-depth understanding of the pathophysiology of the disease and the anticipated effects of each intervention, as well as a solid understanding of the nursing process. Later sections discuss specific interventions for patients in shock.

The psychosocial needs of the patient and family dealing with shock are extremely important. These needs are based on situational, familial, and patient-centered variables. Nursing priorities for managing the psychosocial stress of critical illness include (1) providing information on patient status, (2) explaining procedures and routines, (3) supporting the family, (4) encouraging the expression of feelings, (5) facilitating problem solving and shared decision making, (6) individualizing visitation schedules, (7) involving the family in the patient's care, and (8) establishing contacts with necessary resources. The consensus of all relevant professional organizations is that patients and families should be given the option of family presence during invasive procedures and resuscitation.[22–25] Interprofessional collaborative management of a patient with shock is outlined in Box 26.3.

HYPOVOLEMIC SHOCK

Description and Etiology

Hypovolemic shock occurs from inadequate fluid volume in the intravascular space. The lack of adequate circulating volume leads to decreased tissue perfusion and initiation of the general shock response. Hypovolemic shock is the most commonly occurring form of shock (Fig. 26.2).

Hypovolemic shock can result from absolute or relative hypovolemia. Absolute hypovolemia occurs when there is a loss of fluid from the intravascular space. This can result from an external loss of fluid from the body or from internal shifting of fluid from the intravascular space to the extravascular space. Fluid shifts can be due to a loss of intravascular integrity, increased capillary membrane permeability, or decreased colloidal osmotic pressure. Relative hypovolemia occurs when vasodilation produces an increase in vascular capacitance relative to circulating volume (Box 26.4).

Pathophysiology

Hypovolemia results in a loss of circulating fluid volume. A decrease in circulating volume leads to a decrease in venous return, which results in a decrease in end-diastolic volume or preload. Preload is a major determinant of SV and CO. A decrease in preload results in a decrease in SV and CO. The decrease in CO leads to inadequate cellular oxygen supply and ineffective tissue perfusion.

BOX 26.2 Agents Used in the Treatment of Shock

Vasoconstrictors
- Epinephrine (Adrenalin)
- Norepinephrine (Levophed)
- Alpha-range dopamine (Intropin)
- Phenylephrine (Neo-Synephrine)
- Vasopressin (Pitressin)

Vasodilators
- Nitroprusside (Nipride, Nitropress)
- Nitroglycerin (Nitrol, Tridil)
- Hydralazine (Apresoline)
- Labetalol (Normodyne, Trandate)

Inotropes
- Beta-range dopamine (Intropin)
- Dobutamine (Dobutrex)
- Epinephrine (Adrenalin)
- Norepinephrine (Levophed)
- Milrinone (Primacor)

Antidysrhythmics
- Amiodarone (Cordarone)
- Adenosine (Adenocard)
- Procainamide (Pronestyl)
- Labetalol (Normodyne, Trandate)
- Verapamil (Calan, Isoptin)
- Esmolol (Brevibloc)
- Diltiazem (Cardizem)
- Lidocaine (Xylocaine)

BOX 26.3 Collaborative Management of Shock

- Support oxygen transport.
  - Establish a patent airway.
  - Initiate mechanical ventilation.
  - Administer oxygen.
  - Administer fluids (crystalloids, colloids, blood, and other blood products).
  - Administer vasoactive medications.
  - Administer positive inotropic medications.
  - Ensure sufficient hemoglobin and hematocrit.
- Support oxygen use.
  - Identify and correct cause of lactic acidosis.
  - Ensure adequate organ and extremity perfusion.
  - Initiate nutrition support therapy.
- Identify underlying cause of shock and treat accordingly.
- Provide comfort and emotional support.
- Institute evidence-based practice protocols to prevent complications.
- Assess response to therapy.
- Prevent and maintain surveillance for complications.

Assessment and Diagnosis

The clinical manifestations of hypovolemic shock depend on the severity of fluid loss and the patient's ability to compensate for it. A clinical classification developed by the American College of Surgeons to describe the levels of severity of hypovolemic shock in the trauma setting has been widely accepted, but a test of the validity of this classification suggests that modifications are necessary.[26]

A simpler approach of classifying hypovolemic shock as mild, moderate, or severe is also commonly used. Class I, or mild shock, indicates a fluid volume loss up to 15% to 20% or an actual volume loss up to approximately 750 mL. Compensatory mechanisms maintain CO, and the patient appears free of symptoms other than possibly slight anxiety. As volume loss worsens, the patient may develop cool extremities and increased capillary refill time in response to peripheral vasoconstriction.[3]

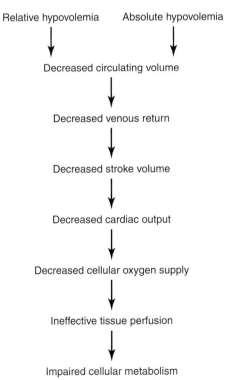

Fig. 26.2 Pathophysiology of Hypovolemic Shock. (From Urden LD, Stacy KM, Lough ME, eds. *Critical Care Nursing: Diagnosis and Management.* 6th ed. St. Louis: Mosby; 2010.)

Class II and class III hypovolemia is consistent with moderate shock. Class II hypovolemia occurs with a fluid volume loss of approximately 15% to 30% or an actual volume loss of 750 to 1500 mL. Falling CO activates more intense compensatory responses. Anxiety increases. The heart rate may increase to more than 100 beats/min in response to increased SNS stimulation unless blocked by preexisting beta-blocker therapy. The pulse pressure narrows as the diastolic blood pressure increases because of vasoconstriction. Postural hypotension develops. The respiratory rate increases as blood loss worsens, and ABG specimens drawn during this phase may reveal respiratory alkalosis, as evidenced by a low partial pressure of carbon dioxide ($PaCO_2$). Urine output starts to decline to 20 to 30 mL/h as renal perfusion decreases. The urine sodium level decreases, whereas urinary osmolality and specific gravity increase as the kidneys start to conserve sodium and water. The patient's skin becomes pale and cool with delayed capillary refill because of peripheral vasoconstriction. Jugular veins appear flat as a result of decreased venous return.[3]

Class III hypovolemic shock occurs with a fluid volume loss of 30% to 40% or an actual volume loss of 1500 to 2000 mL. This level of severity may produce the progressive stage of shock as compensatory mechanisms become overwhelmed and ineffective tissue perfusion develops. Blood pressure decreases but often after tissue hypoperfusion is already significant. The heart rate may increase to more than 120 beats/min, and dysrhythmias may develop as myocardial ischemia ensues. During this phase, serum lactate levels increase, and ABG values reveal metabolic acidosis, as evidenced by a low bicarbonate (HCO_3^-) and elevated base deficit. Decreased renal perfusion results in the development of oliguria. Blood urea nitrogen and serum creatinine levels start to rise as the kidneys begin to fail. The patient's skin becomes ashen, cold, and clammy, with marked delayed capillary refill. The patient may appear confused as cerebral perfusion decreases.[3]

Class IV hypovolemic shock is severe shock and usually refractory in nature. It occurs with a fluid volume loss of greater than 40% or an actual volume loss of greater than 2000 mL. As the compensatory mechanisms of the body become insufficient, tachycardia and hemodynamic instability worsen, and hypotension ensues. Severe lactic acidosis is present. Peripheral pulses and capillary refill become absent because of marked peripheral vasoconstriction. The skin may appear cyanotic, mottled, and extremely diaphoretic. Organ failure occurs. Urine output ceases. The patient may be confused and agitated, eventually becoming unresponsive. Various clinical manifestations associated with failure of the different body systems develop.[3]

Assessment of the hemodynamic parameters of a patient in hypovolemic shock varies by stage but commonly reveals a decreased CO and cardiac index (CI). Loss of circulating volume leads to a decrease in venous return to the heart, which results in a decrease in the preload of

BOX 26.4 Etiologic Factors in Hypovolemic Shock

Absolute Factors
- Loss of whole blood
  - Trauma or surgery
  - Gastrointestinal bleeding
- Loss of plasma
  - Thermal injuries
  - Large lesions
- Loss of other body fluids
  - Severe vomiting or diarrhea
  - Massive diuresis
  - Loss of intravascular integrity
  - Ruptured spleen
  - Long bone or pelvic fractures
  - Hemorrhagic pancreatitis
  - Hemothorax or hemoperitoneum
  - Arterial dissection or rupture

Relative Factors
- Vasodilation
  - Sepsis
  - Anaphylaxis
  - Loss of sympathetic stimulation
- Increased capillary membrane permeability
  - Sepsis
  - Anaphylaxis
  - Thermal injuries
- Decreased colloidal osmotic pressure
  - Severe sodium depletion
  - Hypopituitarism
  - Cirrhosis
  - Intestinal obstruction

the right and left ventricles. This is evidenced by a decline in the CVP or right atrial pressure (RAP) and pulmonary artery occlusion pressure (PAOP). Vasoconstriction of the arterial system results in an increase in the afterload of the heart, as evidenced by an increase in the SVR. This vasoconstriction may produce inaccurate systolic and diastolic blood pressure values when measured by arterial catheter or noninvasive oscillometry. MAP is more accurate in this low-flow state.[27]

Medical Management

The major goals of therapy for a patient in hypovolemic shock are to correct the cause of the hypovolemia, restore tissue perfusion, and prevent complications. This approach includes identifying and stopping the source of fluid loss, administering fluid to replace circulating volume, and administering vasopressor therapy to maintain tissue perfusion until volume is restored. Fluid administration can be accomplished with use of a crystalloid solution, a colloid solution, blood products, or a combination of fluids. The type of solution used depends on the type of fluid lost, the degree of hypovolemia, the severity of hypoperfusion, and the cause of hypovolemia.

Aggressive fluid resuscitation in trauma and surgical patients is a subject of great debate. Limited or hypotensive (systolic blood pressure 60–80 mm Hg or MAP 40–60 mm Hg) volume resuscitation in patients with uncontrolled hemorrhage has been shown to lessen bleeding and improve survival.[10,28–30] The type and amount of solutions used for fluid resuscitation and the rate of administration influence immune function; inflammatory mediator release; coagulation; and the incidence of cardiac, pulmonary, renal, and GI complications.[10,13,14] Consensus on the optimal resuscitative strategy for hypovolemic shock is lacking and is likely situation specific, especially in the case of traumatic hemorrhage.[14,28,30]

Nursing Management

Prevention of hypovolemic shock is one of the primary responsibilities of the nurse in the critical care unit. Preventive measures include the identification of patients at risk and frequent assessment of the patient's fluid balance. Accurate monitoring of intake and output and daily weights are essential components of preventive nursing care. Early identification and treatment result in decreased mortality.

The patient care management plan for a patient in hypovolemic shock may include numerous patient problems, depending on the

progression of the process (Box 26.5). A patient in hypovolemic shock requires continuous evaluation of intravascular volume, tissue perfusion, and response to therapy. Nursing priorities are directed toward (1) minimizing fluid loss, (2) administering volume replacement and vasopressor agents (if needed), (3) assessing response to therapy, (4) providing comfort and emotional support, and (5) preventing and maintaining surveillance for complications.

Measures to minimize fluid loss include limiting blood sampling, observing lines for accidental disconnection, and applying direct pressure to bleeding sites. Measures to facilitate the administration of volume replacement include insertion of large-bore peripheral intravenous (IV) catheters and rapid administration of prescribed fluids. Monitoring the patient for adequate tissue perfusion and for clinical manifestations of fluid overload or complications related to fluid and blood product administration is essential for preventing further problems. It is also essential to monitor the patient for organ failure, which may occur for up to several days after resuscitation.

CARDIOGENIC SHOCK

Description and Etiology

Cardiogenic shock is a result of failure of the heart to effectively pump blood forward. It can occur with dysfunction of the right or the left ventricle, or both. The lack of adequate pumping function leads to decreased tissue perfusion and circulatory failure (Fig. 26.3). It occurs in approximately 5% to 8% of the patients with an ST segment myocardial infarction (MI), and it is the leading cause of death of

⊚ BOX 26.5 PRIORITY PATIENT CARE MANAGEMENT

Hypovolemic Shock
- Hypovolemia due to absolute loss
- Hypovolemia due to relative loss
- Impaired Cardiac Output due to alterations in preload
- Anxiety due to threat to biologic, psychologic, or social integrity

Patient Care Management plans are located in Appendix A.

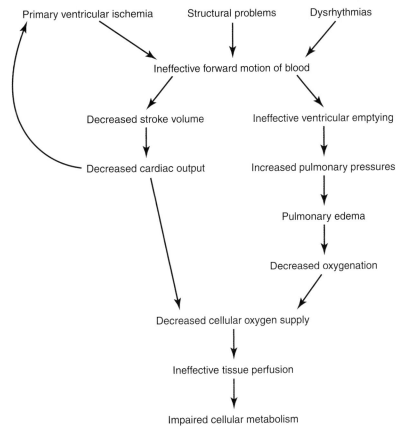

Fig. 26.3 Pathophysiology of Cardiogenic Shock. (From Urden LD, Stacy KM, Lough ME, eds. *Critical Care Nursing: Diagnosis and Management.* 6th ed. St. Louis: Mosby; 2010.)

patients hospitalized with MI.[31] The mortality rate for cardiogenic shock has decreased with the advent of early revascularization therapy and is currently approximately 40% to 65%.[31–33]

Cardiogenic shock can result from problems affecting the muscular function or the mechanical function of the heart or the cardiac rhythm. The most common cause is acute MI resulting in the loss of 40% or more of the functional myocardium. It can occur with ST segment elevation or non–ST segment elevation MI.[31] The damage to the myocardium may occur after one massive MI (usually of the anterior wall), or it may be cumulative as a result of several smaller MIs or a small MI in a patient with preexisting ventricular dysfunction.[31] Cardiomyopathy may cause cardiogenic shock as left ventricular function becomes unable to maintain adequate CO. Examples of problems affecting the mechanical function of the heart to fill and eject adequately include severe valvular disease; acute papillary muscle, chordal, or septal rupture; cardiac tamponade; and massive pulmonary embolus (Box 26.6).[33]

Pathophysiology

Cardiogenic shock results from the impaired ability of the ventricle to pump blood forward, which leads to a decrease in SV and an increase in the blood left in the ventricle at the end of systole. The decrease in SV results in a decrease in CO, which leads to decreased cellular oxygen supply and ineffective tissue perfusion. Typically, myocardial performance spirals downward as compensatory vasoconstriction increases myocardial afterload and low blood pressure worsens myocardial ischemia. As left ventricular contractility declines and ventricular compliance decreases, an increase in end-systolic volume

results in blood backing up into the pulmonary system and the subsequent development of pulmonary edema. Pulmonary edema causes impaired gas exchange and decreased oxygenation of the arterial blood, which further impair tissue perfusion.[34] In a substantial number of patients, the pathophysiology may follow a different course secondary to activation of inflammatory cytokines. An inflammatory response results with systemic vasodilation and, possibly, normalization of the CO. Whether this process contributes to the genesis or the outcome of cardiogenic shock is uncertain, but it is thought to be activated by acute MI and to facilitate development of sepsis.[35] Death caused by cardiogenic shock results from cardiopulmonary collapse or multiple organ failure.[34]

Assessment and Diagnosis

Various clinical manifestations occur in patients in cardiogenic shock depending on etiologic factors, the patient's underlying medical status, and the severity of the shock state. Although some clinical manifestations are caused by failure of the heart as a pump, many are related to the overall shock response (Box 26.7).

Initially, clinical manifestations reflect the decline in CO. These signs and symptoms include systolic blood pressure less than 90 mm Hg, MAP less than 65 mm Hg, or an acute drop in systolic or mean blood pressure of 30 mm Hg or more; decreased sensorium; cool, pale, moist skin; and urine output of less than 30 mL/h. The patient also may complain of chest pain. Tachycardia develops to compensate for the decrease in CO. A weak, thready pulse develops, and diminished S_1 and S_2 heart sounds may occur as a result of the decreased contractility. The respiratory rate increases to improve oxygenation. ABG

BOX 26.6 Etiologic Factors in Cardiogenic Shock

Muscular
- Ischemic injury
  - Acute myocardial infarction
  - Cardiopulmonary arrest
- Acute decompensated heart failure
- Cardiomyopathy
- Acute myocarditis
- Myocardial contusion
- Prolonged cardiopulmonary bypass
- Septic shock
- Hemorrhagic shock
- Medications (beta-adrenergic blockers, calcium channel antagonists, cytotoxic agents)

Mechanical
- Valvular dysfunction

- Papillary muscle dysfunction or rupture
- Septal wall rupture
- Free wall rupture
- Ventricular aneurysm
- Obstructive hypertrophic cardiomyopathy
- Intracardiac tumor
- Pulmonary embolus
- Atrial thrombus
- Cardiac tamponade
- Massive pulmonary embolus
- Constrictive pericarditis

Rhythmic
- Bradydysrhythmias
- Tachydysrhythmias

BOX 26.7 Clinical Manifestations of Cardiogenic Shock

- Systolic blood pressure <90 mm Hg
- Acute drop in blood pressure >30 mm Hg
- Heart rate >100 beats/min
- Weak, thready pulse
- Diminished heart sounds
- Change in sensorium
- Cool, pale, moist skin
- Urine output <30 mL/h
- Chest pain

- Dysrhythmias
- Tachypnea
- Crackles
- Decreased cardiac output
- Cardiac index <2.2 L/min/m^2
- Increased pulmonary artery occlusion pressure
- Increased right atrial pressure
- Variable systemic vascular resistance

values at this point indicate respiratory alkalosis, as evidenced by a decrease in PaCO$_2$. Urinalysis findings demonstrate a decrease in urine sodium level and an increase in urine osmolality and specific gravity as the kidneys start to conserve sodium and water. Serum B-type natriuretic peptide levels are likely to be elevated.[31,33,34]

As the left ventricle fails, auscultation of the lungs may disclose crackles and rhonchi, indicating the development of pulmonary edema. Hypoxemia occurs, as evidenced by a fall in PaO$_2$ and SaO$_2$ as measured by ABG values. S$_3$ and S$_4$ heart sounds may occur. Jugular venous distention is evident with right-sided failure. The patient also may experience dysrhythmias in response to tissue hypoxia, the underlying problem, and medication therapy.[31]

Assessment of the hemodynamic parameters of a patient in cardiogenic shock reveals decreased CO with CI less than 2.2 L/min/m^2 in the presence of an elevated PAOP.[32] A proportional pulse pressure (systolic blood pressure/pulse pressure) less than 25% is indicative of left ventricular failure and CI less than 2.2 L/min/m^2 and may be useful when direct measurement of CI is unavailable.[36] Increased filling pressures are necessary to rule out hypovolemia as the cause of circulatory failure. The increase in PAOP reflects an increase in the left ventricular end-diastolic pressure and left ventricular end-diastolic volume resulting from decreased SV. With right ventricular failure, the RAP also increases. Compensatory vasoconstriction typically results in an increase in the afterload of the heart, as evidenced by an increase in the SVR, unless inflammation produces vasodilation

and a normal or decreased SVR. Echocardiography confirms the diagnosis of cardiogenic shock, provides noninvasive estimates of PAOP and ejection fraction, and often clarifies etiologic factors.[32,37]

As compensatory mechanisms fail and ineffective tissue perfusion develops, other clinical manifestations appear. Myocardial ischemia progresses, as evidenced by continued increases in heart rate, dysrhythmias, and chest pain. Pulmonary function deteriorates, which leads to respiratory distress. ABG values during this phase reveal respiratory and metabolic acidosis and hypoxemia, as indicated by a high PaCO$_2$, low HCO$_3^-$, and low PaO$_2$. Renal failure occurs, as exhibited by the development of anuria and increases in blood urea nitrogen and serum creatinine levels. Cerebral hypoperfusion manifests as a decreasing level of consciousness.[37]

Medical Management

Treatment of a patient in cardiogenic shock requires an aggressive approach. The major goals of therapy are to treat the underlying cause, enhance the effectiveness of the pump, and improve tissue perfusion. This approach includes identifying and treating the etiologic factors of heart failure and administering pharmacologic agents or using mechanical devices to enhance CO. Inotropic agents are used to increase contractility and maintain adequate blood pressure and tissue perfusion.[37] A vasopressor, preferably norepinephrine, may be necessary to maintain blood pressure when hypotension is severe.[32] Because both of these therapies increase myocardial oxygen demand, the lowest possible doses should be used.[32] Diuretics may be used for preload reduction. Vasodilating agents are used for preload and afterload reduction only in specific situations in conjunction with an inotrope or when the patient is no longer in shock. Antidysrhythmic agents should be used to suppress or control dysrhythmias that can affect CO. Intubation and mechanical ventilation are usually necessary to support oxygenation.[37]

The cause of pump failure should be identified as quickly as possible so that measures can be taken to correct the problem if possible. In the setting of acute MI, emergent revascularization by percutaneous coronary intervention or coronary artery bypass graft surgery provides significant survival benefit and is recommended by national guidelines.[32] Fibrinolytic agents may be used in select patients. Procedural or surgical intervention may be necessary to remedy mechanical etiology.[37]

Mechanical circulatory assist devices are used if adequate tissue perfusion cannot be immediately restored. Options include an intra-aortic balloon pump (IABP), percutaneous ventricular assist device (VAD), or extracorporeal membrane oxygenator. The IABP is used to decrease myocardial workload by improving myocardial supply and decreasing myocardial demand. It achieves this goal by improving coronary artery perfusion and reducing left ventricular afterload. However, IABP therapy is no longer recommended for cardiogenic shock associated with acute MI, because results of several more recent studies have confirmed a lack of short-term and long-term survival benefit in these patients.[32,37,38] The other mechanical assist devices provide a means to sustain effective organ perfusion, allowing time for effective intervention, healing, permanent placement of a VAD, or cardiac transplantation. Chapter 12 provides more information about these therapies.[37]

Nursing Management

Prevention of cardiogenic shock is one of the primary responsibilities of the nurse in the critical care unit. Preventive measures include the identification of patients at risk, facilitation of early reperfusion therapy for acute MI, and frequent assessment and management of the patient's cardiopulmonary status.

The patient care management plan for a patient in cardiogenic shock may include numerous patient problems, depending on the progression of the process (Box 26.8). Nursing priorities are directed toward (1) limiting myocardial oxygen demand, (2) enhancing myocardial oxygen supply, (3) maintaining adequate tissue perfusion, (4) providing comfort and emotional support, and (5) preventing and maintaining surveillance for complications. Measures to limit myocardial oxygen demand include administering analgesics, sedatives, and agents to control afterload and dysrhythmias; positioning the patient for comfort; limiting activities; providing a calm and quiet

---

BOX 26.8 PRIORITY PATIENT CARE MANAGEMENT

Cardiogenic Shock
- Impaired Cardiac Output due to alterations in contractility
- Impaired Cardiac Output due to alterations in heart rate or rhythm
- Impaired Nutritional Intake due to lack of exogenous nutrients and increased metabolic demand
- Risk for Infection
- Impaired Family Coping due to a critically ill family member

Patient Care Management plans are located in Appendix A.

---

environment and offering support to reduce anxiety; and teaching the patient about the condition. Measures to enhance myocardial oxygen supply include administering supplemental oxygen, monitoring the patient's respiratory status, administering prescribed medications, and managing device therapy.

Effective nursing management of cardiogenic shock requires precise monitoring and management of heart rate, preload, afterload, and contractility. This is accomplished through accurate measurement of hemodynamic variables and controlled administration of fluids and inotropic and vasoactive agents. Close assessment and management of respiratory function is also essential to maintain adequate oxygenation. Dysrhythmias are common and require immediate recognition and treatment.

Patients who require mechanical device therapy (IABP, VAD, or extracorporeal membrane oxygenator) need to be observed frequently for complications. Complications of mechanical circulatory assist devices include infection, bleeding, thrombocytopenia, hemolysis, embolus, stroke, device malfunction, circulatory compromise of a cannulated extremity, and sepsis.

ANAPHYLACTIC SHOCK

Description and Etiology

Anaphylactic shock, a type of distributive shock, is the result of an immediate hypersensitivity reaction. It is a life-threatening event that requires prompt intervention. The severe and systemic response leads to decreased tissue perfusion and initiation of the general shock response (Fig. 26.4).

Anaphylaxis is a systemic reaction caused by an immunologic antibody-antigen response or nonimmunologic activation of mast cells and basophils. Numerous triggers have been identified that, when introduced by injection or ingestion or through the skin or respiratory tract, can cause a reaction. This list includes foods, food additives, diagnostic agents, biologic agents, environmental agents, medications, and venoms (Box 26.9). Anaphylaxis can also be triggered by physical factors and can be idiopathic in nature with no known trigger.[39] In the hospital environment, latex was once an extremely problematic antigen for patients and health care providers, but efforts to minimize and prevent exposure have been highly successful.[40]

Pathophysiology

Both immunologic and nonimmunologic activation of the mast cells and basophils results in the release of biochemical mediators. These mediators include histamine; tryptase; chymase; carboxypeptidase A3; platelet-activating factor (PAF); heparin; leukotrienes; prostaglandins; and cytokines such as interleukin (IL)-6, IL-33, and tumor necrosis factor (TNF)-alpha, among others. The activation of the biochemical mediators causes vasodilation; increased capillary permeability; laryngeal edema; bronchoconstriction; excessive mucus secretion; coronary vasoconstriction; inflammation; cutaneous reactions; and constriction of the smooth muscle in the intestinal wall, bladder, and uterus. Coronary vasoconstriction causes severe myocardial depression. Cutaneous reactions cause stimulation of nerve endings, followed by itching and pain.[41,42]

Peripheral vasodilation results in relative hypovolemia and decreased venous return. Increased capillary membrane permeability results in the loss of intravascular volume into the interstitial space, as much as 35% within 10 minutes, worsening the hypovolemic state. Decreased venous return results in decreased end-diastolic volume and SV. The decline in SV leads to decreased CO and ineffective tissue

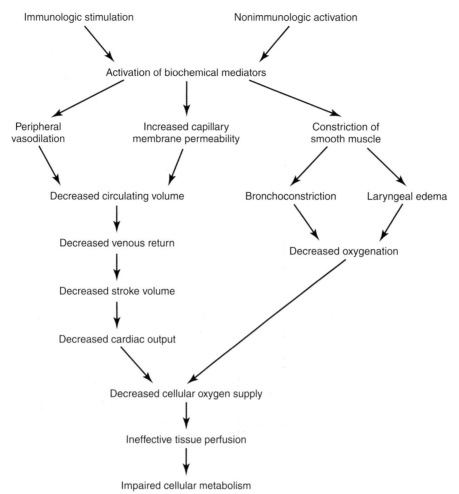

Fig. 26.4 Pathophysiology of Anaphylactic Shock. (From Urden LD, Stacy KM, Lough ME, eds. *Critical Care Nursing: Diagnosis and Management*. 6th ed. St. Louis: Mosby; 2010.)

perfusion. Death may result from airway obstruction or cardiovascular collapse, or both.[39]

Assessment and Diagnosis

Anaphylactic shock is a severe systemic reaction that can affect multiple organ systems. Various clinical manifestations occur in a patient in anaphylactic shock, depending on the extent of multisystem involvement. The symptoms usually start to appear within minutes of exposure to the antigen, but they may not occur for hours (Box 26.10).[39] Symptoms may also reappear after a 1- to 72-hour window of resolution in what is termed a *biphasic reaction*. These late-phase reactions may be similar to the initial anaphylactic response, milder, or more severe. In protracted anaphylaxis, symptoms may last 32 hours.[43]

The cutaneous effects may appear first and include pruritus, generalized erythema, urticaria, and angioedema. Commonly seen on the face and in the oral cavity and lower pharynx, angioedema develops as a result of fluid leaking into the interstitial space. The patient may appear restless, uneasy, apprehensive, and anxious and may complain of being warm. Respiratory effects include the development of laryngeal edema, bronchoconstriction, and mucous plugs. Clinical manifestations of laryngeal edema include inspiratory stridor, hoarseness, a sensation of fullness or a lump in the throat, and dysphagia. Bronchoconstriction causes dyspnea, wheezing, and chest

tightness. GI and genitourinary (GU) manifestations, which may develop as a result of smooth muscle contraction, include vomiting, diarrhea, cramping, and abdominal pain.[39,42,43]

Hypotension and reflex tachycardia may develop quickly in response to massive vasodilation and rapid loss of circulating volume. Jugular veins appear flat as right ventricular end-diastolic volume is decreased. The eventual outcome is circulatory failure and ineffective tissue perfusion.[39] The patient's level of consciousness may deteriorate to unresponsiveness.

Assessment of the hemodynamic parameters of a patient in anaphylactic shock reveals a decreased CO and CI. Venous vasodilation and massive volume loss lead to a decrease in preload, which results in a decline in the RAP and PAOP. Vasodilation of the arterial system results in a decrease in the afterload of the heart, as evidenced by a decrease in the SVR. Box 26.11 outlines the clinical criteria for diagnosing anaphylaxis.

Medical Management

Treatment of anaphylactic shock requires an immediate and direct approach to prevent death. The goals of therapy are to remove the offending antigen, reverse the effects of the biochemical mediators, and promote adequate tissue perfusion. When the hypersensitivity reaction occurs as a result of administration of medications, dye, blood, or blood products, the infusion should be immediately

BOX 26.9   Etiologic Factors in Anaphylactic Shock

Common Foods and Food Additives
- Eggs and milk
- Fish and shellfish
- Nuts and seeds
- Legumes and cereals
- Soy
- Wheat
- Strawberries
- Avocados
- Food coloring
- Preservatives

Diagnostic Agents
- Radiocontrast media
- Dehydrocholic acid (Decholin)
- Iopanoic acid (Telepaque)

Biologic Agents
- Blood and blood components
- Insulin and other hormones
- Gammaglobulin
- Seminal fluid
- Vaccines and antitoxins

Environmental Agents
- Pollens, molds, and spores

- Sunlight
- Cold or heat
- Animal dander
- Latex

Medications
- Antibiotics
- Aspirin
- Nonsteroidal antiinflammatory drugs
- Opioids
- Dextran
- Vitamins
- Muscle relaxants
- Neuromuscular blocking agents
- Barbiturates
- Nonbarbiturate hypnotics
- Protamine
- Infliximab (Remicade)
- Ethanol

Venoms
- Bees, hornets, yellow jackets, and wasps
- Snakes, jellyfish
- Deer flies
- Fire ants

BOX 26.10   Clinical Manifestations of Anaphylactic Shock

Cardiovascular
- Hypotension
- Tachycardia
- Bradycardia
- Chest pain

Respiratory
- Lump in throat
- Cough
- Dyspnea
- Dysphagia
- Hoarseness
- Stridor
- Wheezing
- Rhinitis
- Chest tightness

Cutaneous
- Pruritus
- Erythema
- Urticaria
- Angioedema
- Sense of warmth

Neurologic
- Restlessness

- Uneasiness
- Apprehension
- Anxiety
- Dizziness
- Headache
- Sense of impending doom
- Confusion
- Syncope or near syncope

Gastrointestinal
- Nausea
- Vomiting
- Diarrhea
- Cramping abdominal pain

Genitourinary
- Incontinence

Hemodynamic Parameters
- Decreased cardiac output
- Decreased cardiac index
- Decreased right atrial pressure
- Decreased pulmonary occlusion pressure
- Decreased systemic vascular resistance

BOX 26.11 Clinical Criteria for Diagnosing Anaphylaxis

Anaphylaxis is highly likely when one of the following three criteria is fulfilled:

1. Acute onset of an illness (minutes to several hours) with involvement of the skin or mucosal tissue or both (e.g., generalized hives; pruritus or flushing; swollen lips, tongue, and uvula) *and at least one of the following:*
   a. Respiratory compromise (e.g., dyspnea, wheeze [bronchospasm], stridor, reduced peak expiratory flow, hypoxemia)
   b. Reduced blood pressure or associated symptoms of end-organ dysfunction (e.g., collapse, syncope, incontinence)

2. Two or more of the following that occur rapidly after exposure *to a likely allergen for that patient* (minutes to several hours):
   a. Involvement of the skin and mucosal tissue (e.g., generalized hives; pruritus or flushing; swollen lips, tongue, and uvula)
   b. Respiratory compromise (e.g., dyspnea, wheeze [bronchospasm], stridor, reduced peak expiratory flow, hypoxemia)
   c. Reduced blood pressure or associated symptoms of end-organ dysfunction (e.g., collapse, syncope, incontinence)
   d. Persistent gastrointestinal symptoms (e.g., crampy abdominal pain, vomiting, diarrhea)

3. Reduced blood pressure after exposure *to known allergen for that patient* (minutes to several hours):
   a. Infants and children: Low systolic blood pressure (age-specific) or >30% decrease in systolic blood pressure[a]
   b. Adults: Systolic blood pressure of <90 mm Hg or >30% decrease for the person's baseline

From Sampson HA, Muñoz-Furlong, Campbell RL, et al. Second symposium on the definition and management of anaphylaxis: summary report—Second National Institute of Allergy and Infectious Disease/Food Allergy and Anaphylaxis Network symposium. *J Allergy Clin Immunol.* 2006;117(2):391–397.

[a]Low systolic blood pressure is defined as <70 mm Hg for children aged 1 month to 1 year, less than (70 mm Hg + [2 × age]) for children aged 1 to 10 years, and <90 mm Hg for children aged 11–17 years.

discontinued. It is often impossible to remove the antigen because it is unknown or has already entered the patient's system.

Reversal of the effects of the biochemical mediators involves the preservation and support of the patient's airway, ventilation, and circulation. This is accomplished through oxygen therapy, intubation, mechanical ventilation, and administration of medications and fluids.[41]

Epinephrine is the first-line treatment of choice for anaphylaxis and should be administered when initial signs and symptoms occur.[41,44–46] It promotes bronchodilation, vasoconstriction, and increased myocardial contractility and inhibits further release of biochemical mediators. In mild cases of anaphylaxis, 0.2 to 0.5 mg (0.3–0.5 mL) of a 1:1000 dilution of epinephrine is administered by intramuscular injection into the anterolateral thigh and repeated every 5 to 15 minutes until anaphylaxis is resolved.[42,45] Subcutaneous injection is no longer recommended.[46] For anaphylactic shock with hypotension, epinephrine is administered intravenously. The IV dose is 0.05 to 0.1 mg (1 mL) of a 1:10,000 dilution administered over 5 minutes.[46] If hypotension persists, a continuous infusion of epinephrine is recommended, administered at 1 to 4 mcg/min with titration up to 10 mcg/min as needed.[46] Patients receiving beta-blockers may have a limited response to epinephrine. IV glucagon administered as a 20- to 30-mcg/kg bolus over 5 minutes followed by continuous infusion at 5 to 15 mcg/min is recommended to treat bronchospasm and hypotension in these patients.[46]

Rapid volume replacement with crystalloid or colloid solutions is also used for patients with hypotension. Administration of up to 1 L in 5 to 10 minutes is suggested if needed to restore perfusion. Vasopressors may be necessary to reverse the vasodilation and increase blood pressure.[39,41]

Several medications are used as second-line or third-line adjunctive therapy but are not to be used as substitutes for epinephrine. Inhaled beta-adrenergic agents are used to treat bronchospasm unresponsive to epinephrine.[42,46] Diphenhydramine (Benadryl), 1 to 2 mg/kg (25–50 mg) given by a slow IV push, is used to block histamine response.[44,45] Ranitidine or cimetidine given in conjunction with diphenhydramine has been found helpful to control cutaneous reactions.[46] Corticosteroids are not effective in the immediate treatment of acute anaphylaxis but may be given with the goal of preventing a prolonged or delayed reaction.[47]

Nursing Management

Prevention of anaphylactic shock is one of the primary responsibilities of the nurse in the critical care unit. Preventive measures include the identification of patients at risk and cautious assessment of the patient's response to the administration of medications, blood, and blood products. A complete and accurate history of the patient's allergies is an essential component of preventive nursing care. In addition to a list of the allergies, a detailed description of the type of response for each allergy should be obtained.

The patient care management plan for a patient in anaphylactic shock may include numerous patient problems, depending on the progression of the process (Box 26.12). Nursing priorities are directed toward (1) administering epinephrine, (2) facilitating ventilation, (3) administering volume replacement, (4) providing comfort and emotional support, (5) maintaining surveillance for recurrent reactions, and (6) preventing and maintaining surveillance for complications.

Measures to facilitate ventilation include positioning the patient to assist with breathing and instructing the patient to breathe slowly and deeply. Airway protection through prompt administration of prescribed medications is essential. Measures to facilitate the administration of volume replacement include inserting large-bore peripheral IV catheters and rapidly administering prescribed fluids. Measures to promote comfort include administering medications to relieve itching and applying warm soaks to skin. Observing the patient for clinical manifestations of a delayed or recurrent reaction is critical. Patient

◎ BOX 26.12 PRIORITY PATIENT CARE MANAGEMENT

Anaphylactic Shock

- Hypovolemia due to relative loss
- Impaired Cardiac Output due to alterations in afterload
- Impaired Breathing due to decreased lung expansion
- Impaired Gas Exchange due to ventilation-perfusion mismatching or intrapulmonary shunting
- Impaired Family Coping due to a critically ill family member

Patient Care Management plans are located in Appendix A.

education about how to avoid the precipitating allergen is essential for preventing future episodes of anaphylaxis. Education about how to recognize and respond to a future episode including self-administration of epinephrine is essential to prevent a future life-threatening event.

NEUROGENIC SHOCK

Description and Etiology

Neurogenic shock, another type of distributive shock, is the result of the loss or suppression of sympathetic tone. The lack of sympathetic tone leads to decreased tissue perfusion and initiation of the general shock response (Fig. 26.5). Neurogenic shock is the most uncommon form of shock.

Neurogenic shock can be caused by anything that disrupts the SNS. The problem can occur as the result of interrupted impulse transmission or blockage of sympathetic outflow from the vasomotor center in the brain. The most common cause is spinal cord injury (SCI). Neurogenic shock may mistakenly be referred to as *spinal shock*. The latter condition refers to loss of neurologic activity below the level of SCI, but it does not necessarily involve ineffective tissue perfusion.[48]

Pathophysiology

Loss of sympathetic tone results in massive peripheral vasodilation, inhibition of the baroreceptor response, and impaired thermoregulation. Arterial vasodilation leads to a decrease in SVR and a fall in

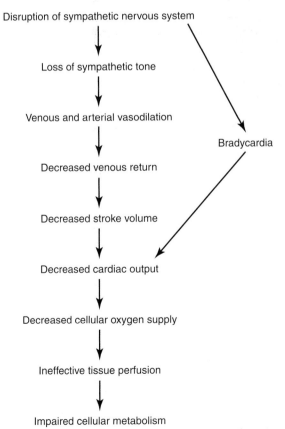

Fig. 26.5 Pathophysiology of Neurogenic Shock. (From Urden LD, Stacy KM, Lough ME, eds. *Critical Care Nursing: Diagnosis and Management.* 6th ed. St. Louis: Mosby; 2010.)

blood pressure. Venous vasodilation leads to relative hypovolemia and pooling of blood in the venous circuit. The decreased venous return results in a decrease in end-diastolic volume or preload, causing a decrease in SV and CO. The fall in blood pressure and CO leads to inadequate or ineffective tissue perfusion. Loss of sympathetic tone and inhibition of the baroreceptor response result in bradycardia.[48,49] The slow heart rate worsens CO, which further compromises tissue perfusion. Impaired thermoregulation occurs because of loss of vasomotor tone in the cutaneous blood vessels that dilate and constrict to maintain body temperature. The patient becomes poikilothermic, or dependent on the environment for temperature regulation.[49]

Assessment and Diagnosis

A patient in neurogenic shock characteristically presents with hypotension, bradycardia, and warm, dry skin. The decreased blood pressure results from massive peripheral vasodilation. The decreased heart rate is caused by inhibition of the baroreceptor response and unopposed parasympathetic control of the heart. Consensus on the specific blood pressure and heart rate thresholds for the diagnosis of neurogenic shock has not been established. Hypothermia develops from uncontrolled peripheral heat loss. The warm, dry skin occurs as a consequence of pooling of blood in the extremities and loss of vasomotor control in surface vessels of the skin that control heat loss.[48]

Assessment of the hemodynamic parameters of a patient in neurogenic shock reveals a decreased CO and CI. Venous vasodilation leads to a decrease in preload, which results in a decline in RAP and PAOP. Vasodilation of the arterial system causes a decrease in the afterload of the heart, as evidenced by a decrease in the SVR.

Medical Management

Treatment of neurogenic shock requires a careful approach. The goals of therapy are to treat or remove the cause, prevent cardiovascular instability, and promote optimal tissue perfusion. Cardiovascular instability can result from hypovolemia, bradycardia, and hypothermia. Specific treatments are aimed at preventing or correcting these problems as they occur.

Hypovolemia is treated with careful fluid resuscitation. The minimal amount of fluid is administered to ensure adequate tissue perfusion. Volume replacement is initiated for systolic blood pressure less than 90 mm Hg or evidence of inadequate tissue perfusion.[50,51] Base deficit or lactate levels are recommended to guide fluid resuscitation in patients with SCI.[52] The patient is carefully observed for evidence of fluid overload. Vasopressors are used as necessary to maintain blood pressure and organ perfusion. Higher than typical MAPs are commonly needed for patients with acute SCI to prevent cord ischemia, but optimal pressures have not been determined.[51] Bradycardia associated with neurogenic shock rarely requires specific treatment, but atropine, IV infusion of a beta-adrenergic agent, or electrical pacing can be used when necessary.[53] Hypothermia is treated with warming measures and environmental temperature regulation.

Nursing Management

Prevention of neurogenic shock is one of the primary responsibilities of the nurse in the critical care unit. This includes the identification of patients at risk and constant assessment of the neurologic status. Vigilant immobilization of SCIs and slight elevation of the head of the patient's bed after spinal anesthesia are essential components of preventive nursing care. Early identification allows for early treatment and decreased mortality.

The patient care management plan for a patient in neurogenic shock may include numerous patient problems, depending on the

⊚ BOX 26.13 PRIORITY PATIENT CARE MANAGEMENT

Neurogenic Shock
- Hypovolemia due to relative loss
- Impaired Cardiac Output due to sympathetic blockade
- Hypothermia due to exposure to cold environment, trauma, or damage to the hypothalamus
- Anxiety due to threat to biologic, psychologic, or social integrity
- Impaired Family Coping due to a critically ill family member

Patient Care Management plans are located in Appendix A.

progression of the process (Box 26.13). Nursing priorities are directed toward (1) treating hypovolemia and maintaining tissue perfusion, (2) maintaining normothermia, (3) monitoring for and treating dysrhythmias, (4) providing comfort and emotional support, and (5) preventing and maintaining surveillance for complications.

Venous pooling in the lower extremities promotes the formation of deep vein thrombosis (DVT), which can result in a pulmonary embolism. All patients at risk for DVT should be started on prophylaxis therapy. Prophylactic measures include monitoring of passive range-of-motion exercises, application of sequential pneumatic stockings, and administration of prescribed anticoagulation therapy.

SEPSIS AND SEPTIC SHOCK

Description and Etiology

Sepsis is a life-threatening clinical syndrome caused by an infection and dysregulated physiologic systemic response. The host response results in perfusion abnormalities with organ dysfunction (sepsis) and eventually circulatory, cellular, and metabolic abnormalities (septic shock) (Table 26.1). Septic shock differs from sepsis in that the complications are more severe, and the risk of patient mortality is greater.[54]

The primary mechanisms of this type of shock are maldistribution of blood flow to the tissues, hypovolemia, and myocardial dysfunction (Fig. 26.6).[55] Sepsis is estimated to result in more than 1.7 million hospitalizations annually in the United States, with an estimated in-hospital mortality rate of 15.6%.[56] It is the leading cause of in-hospital death and the 12th leading cause of all deaths in the United States.[56,57]

Sepsis is caused by a wide variety of microorganisms, including gram-negative and gram-positive aerobes, anaerobes, fungi, and viruses. Common sources of infection include the respiratory, GU, and GI systems; the skin; and the soft tissues.[58] Sepsis and septic shock are associated with a wide variety of intrinsic and extrinsic precipitating factors (Box 26.14). All these factors interfere directly or indirectly with the body's anatomic and physiologic defense mechanisms. Several of the intrinsic factors are not modifiable or are very difficult to control. Several of the extrinsic factors may be required for diagnosis and management.[59] Therefore all critically ill patients are at risk for septic shock.

Pathophysiology

The syndrome encompassing sepsis and septic shock is a complex systemic response that is initiated when a microorganism enters the body and stimulates the inflammatory/immune system. In a host-pathogen interaction, both the invading organism and the injured tissue release intracellular proteins activating neutrophils, monocytes, lymphocytes, macrophages, mast cells, and platelets, as well as numerous plasma enzyme cascades (complement, kinin/kallikrein, coagulation, and fibrinolytic factors). When this reaction is localized, infection is contained and eradicated. However, when the magnitude of the infectious insult is great or the patient is physiologically unable to generate an effective host response, containment fails. The result is a systemic release of the pathogen, activated cells, and mediators, including cytokines, which initiate a chain of complex interactions leading to an uncontrolled, dysregulated response.[60]

With systemic activation, various physiologic and pathophysiologic events occur that affect clotting, the distribution of blood flow to the tissues and organs, capillary membrane permeability, and the metabolic state of the body. Subsequently, a systemic imbalance between cellular oxygen supply, demand, and consumption develops that results in cellular hypoxia, damage, hibernation, and death.[55]

Hallmarks of sepsis are endothelial damage and coagulation dysfunction.[61] Tissue factor is released from endothelial cells and monocytes in response to stimulation by inflammatory cytokines.[60] Release of tissue factor initiates the coagulation cascade, producing widespread microvascular thrombosis and further stimulation of the systemic inflammatory pathways. Diffuse endothelial damage impairs endogenous anticlotting mechanisms. Mediator-induced suppression of fibrinolysis slows clot breakdown. The result can be DIC with eventual consumption of coagulation factors, bleeding, and hemorrhage.[62]

Significant alterations in cardiovascular hemodynamics are caused by the activation of inflammatory cytokines and endothelial damage. Ventricular contractility is impaired.[63] Massive peripheral vasodilation results in the development of relative hypovolemia. Increased capillary permeability produces a loss of intravascular volume to the interstitium, which accentuates the reduction in preload and CO. These changes in global hemodynamics coupled with complex microvascular alterations and thrombosis produce maldistribution of circulating blood volume, decreased tissue perfusion, and inadequate oxygen delivery to the cells. Microcirculatory failure is a key feature of this distributive shock. Even if global hemodynamics are restored, occult hypoperfusion secondary to microcirculatory impairment may persist.[55,64]

Activation of the central nervous system and endocrine system also occurs as part of the response to invading microorganisms. This activation leads to stimulation of the SNS and the release of ACTH. These events trigger the release of epinephrine, norepinephrine, glucocorticoids, aldosterone, glucagon, renin, and growth hormone, contributing to vasoconstriction of the renal, pulmonary, and splanchnic beds.[65] Selective vasoconstriction in the splanchnic bed may contribute to hypoperfusion of the GI mucosal barrier, an area particularly vulnerable to the effects of inflammatory cytokines. The resulting gut injury propagates the inflammatory response.[66]

Several metabolic alterations occur as a result of central nervous system, endocrine system, and cytokine activation. Lactic acid is produced as a result of increased metabolic lactate production and hypoxic anaerobic metabolism.[67] Glucocorticoids, ACTH, epinephrine, glucagon, and growth hormone all are catabolic hormones that are released as part of this response. In conjunction with the inflammatory cytokines, these hormones stimulate catabolism of protein stores in the visceral organs and skeletal muscles to fuel glucose production in the liver, hyperglycemia, and insulin resistance. The cytokines also stimulate the use of fats for energy production (lipolysis).[68]

TABLE 26.1 Definitions of Sepsis and Septic Shock.

Term	Basic Definition	Comments
Infection	A pathologic process that results from an invasion of a normal part of the body by pathogenic or potentially pathogenic microorganisms	Suspicion of infection necessitates immediate identification of possible pathogens, bacteria, fungi, or viruses with blood culture(s). Without benefit of microbiologic confirmation, clinical judgment should be used to identify signs, symptoms, and risk stratification of potential infection to promote early identification.
Bacteremia	Presence of viable bacteria in the blood	Insufficient to make a diagnosis of sepsis, especially in the absence of organ dysfunction.
Sepsis	Life-threatening organ dysfunction caused by a dysregulated host response to infection	Common organ systems showing dysfunction are the respiratory, hematologic, cardiac, renal, hepatic, and central nervous systems. Additional clinical signs, symptoms, biomarkers, and variables that may be used to identify inflammation, inadequate tissue perfusion, and organ dysfunction: 1 General variables a. Fever >38°C (100.4°F) or hypothermia <36°C (96.8°F) b. Tachycardia, heart rate >90 beats/min c. Tachypnea d. Progressive deterioration of mental status e. Altered mental status f. Significant edema or positive fluid balance (>20 mL/kg over 24 hours) g. Hyperglycemia (blood glucose >140 mg/dL) in the absence of diabetes 2 Inflammatory variables a. Leukocytosis or leukopenia (WBC >12,000/mm^3, <4000/mm^3, or >10% bands) b. CRP >2 SD above the normal value c. PCT >2 SD above the normal value 3 Hemodynamic variables a. Arterial hypotension (SBP <90 mm Hg; MAP <70 mm Hg, or an SBP decrease >40 mm Hg) b. SvO$_2$ >70% c. Cardiac index > 3.5 L/min 4 Organ dysfunction variables a. Arterial hypoxemia (PaO$_2$/FiO$_2$ <300 mm Hg) b. Acute oliguria (urine output <0.5 mL/kg/h or 45 mL for at least 2 hours) c. Creatinine increase >0.5 mg/dL d. Coagulation abnormalities (INR >1.5 or PTT >60 seconds) e. Ileus f. Thrombocytopenia (platelet count <100,000/m^3) g. Hyperbilirubinemia (plasma total bilirubin >4 mg/dL or 70 mmol/L) 5 Tissue perfusion variables a. Hyperlactatemia (>1 mmol/L) b. Decreased capillary refill or mottling
Septic shock	A subset of sepsis in which particularly profound circulatory, cellular, and metabolic abnormalities are associated with a greater risk of mortality than with sepsis alone	Clinically identified by a vasopressor requirement to maintain a mean arterial pressure of 65 mm Hg or greater and serum lactate level greater than 2 mmol/L (>18 mg/dL) in the absence of hypovolemia.

CRP, Plasma C-reactive protein; *INR*, international normalized ratio; *MAP*, mean arterial pressure; *PaO$_2$/FiO$_2$*, partial pressure of oxygen in arterial blood/fraction of inspired oxygen; *PCT*, plasma procalcitonin; *PTT*, partial thromboplastin time; *SBP*, systolic blood pressure; *SD*, standard deviation; *SvO$_2$*, mixed venous oxygen saturation; *Temp*, core temperature; *WBC*, white blood cell(s).

Data from Dellinger RP, et al. Surviving sepsis campaign: international guidelines for management of severe sepsis and septic shock: 2012. *Crit Care Med.* 2013;41(2):580–637; Levy MM, et al. 2001 SCCM/ESICM/ACCP/ATS/SIS International Sepsis Definitions Conference. *Crit Care Med.* 2003;312:1250; Opal SM. Severe sepsis and septic shock: defining the clinical problem. *Scand J Infect Dis.* 2003;35:529; Seymour CW, et al. Assessment of clinical criteria for sepsis: for the Third International Consensus Definitions for Sepsis and Septic Shock (Sepsis-3). *JAMA.* 2016:315(8);762–774; Shankar-Hari M, et al. Developing a new definition and assessing new clinical criteria for septic shock: for the Third International Consensus Definitions for Sepsis and Septic Shock (Sepsis-3). *JAMA.* 2016;315(8):775–787; Singer M, et al. The Third International Consensus Definitions for Sepsis and Septic Shock (Sepsis-3). *JAMA.* 2016;315(8):801–810.

Modified from McCance KL, Huether SE, eds. *Pathophysiology: The Biological Basis for Disease in Adults and Children.* 8th ed. Elsevier: St. Louis; 2019.

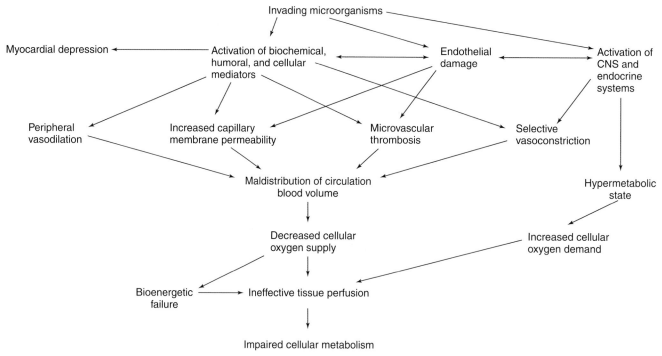

Fig. 26.6 Pathophysiology of Septic Shock. *CNS,* Central nervous system. (From Urden LD, Stacy KM, Lough ME, eds. *Critical Care Nursing: Diagnosis and Management.* 6th ed. St. Louis: Mosby; 2010.)

BOX 26.14　Risk Factors Associated With Septic Shock

Intrinsic Factors
- Extreme of age
- Male sex
- Coexisting diseases
- Malignancies
- Burns
- Immunosuppressive disorders
- Diabetes
- Substance abuse
- Dysfunction of one or more of the major body systems
- Malnutrition

Extrinsic Factors
- Invasive devices
- Medication therapy
- Fluid therapy
- Surgical and traumatic wounds
- Surgical and invasive diagnostic procedures
- Immunosuppressive therapy

Metabolic derangements in sepsis and septic shock include an inability of the cells to use oxygen even if blood flow is adequate. Mitochondrial dysfunction plays an important role in the development of tissue ischemia and multiple organ dysfunction. These complex and interrelated pathophysiologic changes produce a pathologic imbalance between cellular oxygen demand and cellular oxygen supply and consumption.[55,69]

The dysregulated systemic inflammatory response associated with sepsis and septic shock results in cell death via both ischemic necrosis and, to a large degree, apoptosis. Apoptosis is a programmed cell death or cellular suicide mediated by caspase-3, a cysteine protease, and affecting endothelial, GI epithelial, and immune cells. Apoptosis of immune cells results in immunosuppression and secondary infection, as well as release of immune cell toxins.[70] The potentially host-toxic effects of cytokines and immune cell toxins are discussed later in the chapter. Ischemic necrosis and apoptosis stimulate further inflammation, propagating an ongoing cycle of infection, tissue injury, and inflammation. If unabated, this situation ultimately results in MODS and death.[55]

Assessment and Diagnosis

Effective treatment of sepsis and septic shock depends on timely recognition.[71] Earlier guidelines advocated the use of the Sequential (Sepsis-related) Organ Failure Assessment (SOFA) score or the quick SOFA (qSOFA) score to facilitate early identification of patients.[54] The SOFA score is a mortality prediction tool that is based on the degree of dysfunction of six different organ systems (respiratory, cardiovascular, hepatic, coagulation, renal, and neurologic).[54] However, the latest guidelines no longer recommend using the SOFA or qSOFA score for early identification, as the instrument was developed as a mortality prediction tool and not a sepsis screening tool.[71]

The two most common organs to demonstrate dysfunction in sepsis are the cardiovascular system and the lungs. A patient with persistent hypotension requiring vasopressor therapy despite adequate volume resuscitation is demonstrating cardiovascular dysfunction.[63] Pulmonary dysfunction is manifested by a PaO_2/fraction of inspired oxygen (FiO_2) ratio of less than 300, indicating ARDS.[72] Signs indicating septic shock are hypotension despite adequate fluid resuscitation and the presence of perfusion abnormalities such as lactic acidosis, oliguria, or acute change in mentation. Signs of individual organ dysfunction are discussed later in the chapter.

A patient in sepsis or septic shock may present with a variety of clinical manifestations that may change dynamically as the condition progresses (Box 26.15). During the initial stage, massive vasodilation occurs in the venous and arterial beds. Dilation of the venous system leads to a decrease in venous return to the heart, which results in a decrease in the preload of the right and left ventricles. This is evidenced by a decline in RAP and PAOP. Dilation of the arterial system results in a decrease in the afterload of the heart, as evidenced by a decrease in the SVR. The patient's skin becomes pink, warm, and flushed as a result of the massive vasodilation. Myocardial contractility is decreased, as evidenced by a decline in the left ventricular SV index and ejection fraction.

The heart rate increases in response to increased SNS, metabolic, and adrenal gland stimulation. If circulating volume and preload are adequate, this results in a normal-to-high CO and CI despite impaired contractility. The pulse pressure widens as the diastolic blood pressure decreases because of the vasodilation, and the systolic blood pressure increases because of the elevated CO. A full, bounding pulse develops. The net result of these changes is a relatively normal blood pressure in sepsis. However, as the reduction in preload and afterload becomes overwhelming and contractility fails, hypotension ensues, resulting in septic shock.

In the lungs, ventilation-perfusion mismatching develops because of pulmonary vasoconstriction and the formation of pulmonary microemboli. Hypoxemia occurs, and the respiratory rate increases to compensate for the lack of oxygen. Crackles develop as increased pulmonary capillary membrane permeability leads to pulmonary edema.[72]

The level of consciousness starts to change as a result of decreased cerebral perfusion, immune mediator activation, hyperthermia, and lactic acidosis. This septic encephalopathy is demonstrated by acute onset of impaired cognitive functioning, or delirium, which may fluctuate during its course.[73] The patient may appear disoriented, confused, combative, or lethargic.

ABG values initially reveal hypocarbia, hypoxemia, and metabolic acidosis. This is demonstrated by low PaO_2 (hypoxemia), low $PaCO_2$ (hypocarbia), and low HCO_3^- (metabolic acidosis) levels. The respiratory alkalosis is caused by the patient's increased respiratory rate. As pathologic pulmonary changes progress and the patient becomes fatigued, the effectiveness of respirations decreases, and $PaCO_2$ increases, resulting in respiratory acidosis. The metabolic acidosis is the result of a lack of oxygen to the cells and the development of lactic acidemia. Serum lactate levels increase above 2 mmol/L because of anaerobic metabolism.[74] The white blood cell (WBC) count is elevated as part of the immune response to the invading microorganisms. The WBC differential count reveals an increase in immature neutrophils (shift to the left). This increase occurs because the body has to mobilize increasing numbers of WBCs to fight the infection. An elevated procalcitonin level is a valuable biomarker of significant bacterial infection, and procalcitonin levels have been used in clinical trials to guide antibiotic therapy with positive outcomes.[74] Serum glucose levels increase as part of the response and the development of insulin resistance.[68] The patient's temperature is elevated in response to pyrogens released from the invading microorganisms, immune mediator activation, and increased metabolic activity. Urine output decreases because of decreased perfusion of the kidneys. As impaired tissue perfusion develops, other clinical manifestations appear that indicate the development of MODS.

Medical Management

Treatment of a patient in sepsis or septic shock requires a multifaceted approach. The goals of treatment are to control the infection, reverse the pathophysiologic responses, and promote metabolic support. This approach includes identifying and treating the infection, supporting the cardiovascular system and enhancing tissue perfusion, limiting the systemic inflammatory response, restoring metabolic balance, and initiating nutrition therapy. Dysfunction of the individual organ systems must be prevented. Early treatment reduces mortality.[75] Guidelines for the management of sepsis and septic shock have been developed and updated under the auspices of the Surviving Sepsis Campaign (SSC), an international effort of more than 11 organizations to improve patient outcomes.[71] From these guidelines, a group ("bundle") of selected interventions were identified as having the greatest effect on patient outcomes (Box 26.16). Early recognition and treatment of sepsis and septic shock is critical for optimal patient outcomes. The Hour-1 Bundle lists interventions that should be implemented within the first hour after recognition.[76]

BOX 26.15 Clinical Manifestations of Septic Shock

- Increased heart rate
- Decreased blood pressure
- Wide pulse pressure
- Full, bounding pulse
- Pink, warm, flushed skin
- Increased respiratory rate (early) or decreased respiratory rate (late)
- Crackles
- Change in sensorium
- Decreased urine output
- Increased temperature
- Increased cardiac output and cardiac index
- Decreased systemic vascular resistance
- Decreased right atrial pressure
- Decreased pulmonary artery occlusion pressure
- Decreased left ventricular stroke work index
- Decreased PaO_2
- Decreased $PaCO_2$ (early) or increased $PaCO_2$ (late)
- Decreased HCO_3^-

HCO_3^-, Bicarbonate; $PaCO_2$, partial pressure of carbon dioxide; PaO_2, partial pressure of oxygen.

BOX 26.16 Evidence-Based Practice QSEN

Surviving Sepsis Campaign 1-Hour Bundle
- Measure lactate level
- Remeasure lactate if initial lactate is elevated (>2 mmol/L)
- Obtain blood cultures before administering antibiotics
- Administer broad-spectrum antibiotics
- Begin rapid administration of 30 mL/kg crystalloid for hypotension or lactate level ≥4 mmol/L
- Apply vasopressors if hypotensive during or after fluid resuscitation to maintain mean arterial blood pressure (MAP) ≥65 mm Hg

Modified from Surviving Sepsis Campaign 2021 Adult Guidelines. *Society of Critical Care Medicine.* 2019. https://www.sccm.org/SurvivingSepsisCampaign/Guidelines/Adult-Patients.

A patient in sepsis or septic shock requires immediate resuscitation of the hypoperfused state. Specific interventions have been aimed at increasing cellular oxygen supply and decreasing cellular oxygen demand. These treatments include administration of fluids, vasopressors, and possibly positive inotropic agents. This therapy includes aggressive fluid resuscitation to augment intravascular volume in the fluid-responsive patient. Balanced crystalloids are the initial fluid of choice as opposed to normal saline.[71] Initial resuscitation of at least 30 mL/kg of IV balanced crystalloids should be given within the first 3 hours. The guidelines suggest using capillary refill time (in addition to other measures of perfusion) to guide resuscitative efforts.[71] Albumin may also be used in patients who have received large volumes of crystalloids.[71] The guidelines recommend against using starches or gelatin.[71]

Vasopressors should be administered as necessary to maintain a MAP of at least 65 mm Hg.[71] These agents reverse the massive peripheral vasodilation and increase SVR. Norepinephrine is recommended as the first-choice agent because of evidence of its superiority in reducing mortality rates and a higher risk of dysrhythmias when dopamine is used.[71] When indicated, norepinephrine should be initiated quickly, because delay in starting this therapy has been found to significantly worsen survival.[77] Vasopressin is recommended as an alternative agent if response to norepinephrine is poor.[71] If MAP remains low despite norepinephrine and vasopressin, epinephrine should be started.[71] Invasive arterial blood pressure monitoring should be initiated as soon as possible to facilitate accurate and reliable data measurement.[71] A central line is also recommended for any patient requiring vasopressor therapy; however, rather than delay initiation of the medication, it should be started via peripheral venous access until central venous access is secured.[71] Serum lactate values are used to evaluate the effectiveness of these interventions to restore adequate tissue oxygenation.[71] In the past, CVP, ScVO$_2$, or SVO$_2$ monitoring were recommended to guide therapy, but this recommendation is no longer part of the newest guidelines and has been refuted by the results of three major trials and a meta-analysis.[71,78-81]

Intubation and mechanical ventilatory support are usually required to optimize oxygenation and ventilation for a patient in sepsis or septic shock. Ventilation with lower than traditional tidal volumes (6 mL/kg vs. 12 mL/kg) in patients with ARDS decreases mortality.[82] Current guidelines recommend the goals of 6 mL/kg of predicted body weight and plateau pressures no more than 30 cm H$_2$O for patients with sepsis-inducted ARDS.[71] Higher levels of positive end-expiratory pressure (PEEP) should be used for patients with moderate to severe sepsis-induced ARDS. In addition, prone positioning should be employed for greater than 12 hours a day.[71] If neuromuscular blocking agents are needed, current guideline suggest using intermittent IV boluses versus a continuous IV infusion to prevent prolonged blockade after discontinuation.[71]

A key measure in the treatment of septic shock is the early initiation of appropriate antibiotic therapy to eradicate the cause of the infection. If it can be accomplished without delaying antibiotic administration, at least two blood cultures plus urine, sputum, and wound cultures should be obtained to find the location of the infection before such therapy is initiated.[71] Antimicrobial therapy should be started within 1 hour of recognition of septic shock (or high suspicion of sepsis) without delay for cultures.[71] Each hour of delay in initial antibiotic administration is associated with a substantial decrease in the survival rate.[76] If the patient has a medium likelihood of sepsis, antimicrobial therapy should start within 3 hours, thus giving some additional time to identify the source.[71] If the microorganism is unknown, antimicrobial therapy with one or more agents known to be effective against likely pathogens should be initiated, with daily reassessment of the regimen.[71] Surgical intervention to débride infected or necrotic tissue or to drain abscesses may be necessary to facilitate removal of the septic source. Intravascular devices that may be the source of the infection should be removed after establishment of alternative vascular access.[71]

The administration of IV corticosteroids should be considered for the patient in septic shock who remains hypotensive despite adequate fluid resuscitation and vasopressor therapy.[71] Steroid therapy is to be weaned when vasopressors are no longer required. In a meta-analysis, no support for the use of steroids at any dose was found.[83] Continuous infusion of IV insulin is recommended by current guidelines when blood glucose level exceeds 180 mg/dL with a goal blood glucose level between 140 and 180 mg/dL.[71] Glucose levels should be monitored every 1 to 2 hours until stable and then every 4 hours. Low glucose levels measured by capillary testing may be inaccurate in this population. RBC transfusions are recommended when the hemoglobin level is less than 7 g/dL to obtain a target value of 7 to 9 g/dL.[71] Stress ulcer prophylaxis using H$_2$-receptor antagonists or proton-pump inhibitors is recommended for patients who have risk factors for GI bleeding.[71] DVT prophylaxis is recommended for all patients with sepsis or septic shock.[71] The use of sodium bicarbonate therapy for the treatment of lactic acidemia is not recommended unless the pH is less than 7.20 and the patient is experiencing AKI.[71]

The initiation of nutrition therapy is critical in the management of a patient in sepsis or septic shock. The goal is to improve the patient's overall nutrition status, enhance immune function, and promote wound healing. A daily caloric intake of 20 to 30 kcal/kg of usual body weight is recommended for critically ill patients. The enteral route is strongly preferred. Compared with enteral nutrition, parenteral nutrition or a combination of both methods has been associated with higher risk for secondary infection and higher mortality in patients with sepsis or septic shock.[19] Sufficient protein needs to be provided because of the metabolic derangements that develop in the hypermetabolic state. A range of 1.5 to 2.0 g/kg actual body weight per day is recommended for patients with a body mass index less than 30, with progressively larger amounts for patients with a higher body mass index.[68] Enteral nutrition should be initiated within 72 hours.[71]

Nursing Management

Patient care management of the patient with sepsis focuses on infection prevention and transmission, early recognition and treatment of sepsis and septic shock, and supportive nursing care. Prevention of sepsis and septic shock is one of the primary responsibilities of the nurse in the critical care unit. These measures include identification of patients at risk and reduction of their risk factors, including exposure to invading microorganisms. Handwashing, aseptic technique, and an understanding of evidence-based practice to reduce nosocomial infection in critically ill patients are essential components of preventive nursing care. Early identification allows for early treatment and decreases mortality. There are a number of screening tools that are used by different organizations to identify patients with sepsis. Continual observation to detect subtle changes that indicate the progression of the septic process is vitally important, as is evidence-based practice to prevent further infection. Immunosuppression is common as sepsis progresses,[55] and more recent research has found that a resurgence in opportunistic infection in patients with sepsis and septic shock occurs in the later stages, more than 2 weeks after initial diagnosis and treatment.[84] Evidence-based practice to prevent complications of critical illness and prolonged bed rest are essential to prevent further compromise and negative short-term and long-term

BOX 26.17 PRIORITY PATIENT CARE MANAGEMENT

Septic Shock
- Hypovolemia due to relative loss
- Impaired Cardiac Output due to alterations in contractility
- Impaired Gas Exchange due to ventilation-perfusion mismatching or intrapulmonary shunting
- Impaired Nutritional Intake due to lack of exogenous nutrients and increased metabolic demand
- Impaired Family Coping due to a critically ill family member

Patient Care Management plans are located in Appendix A.

BOX 26.18 Evidence-Based Practice

Sepsis and Septic Shock Management Guidelines
The current guidelines for the management of sepsis and septic shock can be found at the Surviving Sepsis Campaign website at
https://www.sccm.org/Clinical-Resources/Guidelines/Guidelines/Surviving-Sepsis-Guidelines-2021

outcomes. For survivors of sepsis, ongoing mortality and impaired quality of life persist in the months and years after hospital discharge.[85]

The nursing management plan for a patient in septic shock may include numerous patient problems, depending on the progression of the process (Box 26.17). Nursing priorities are directed toward (1) early identification of sepsis and septic shock; (2) administering prescribed fluids, medications, and nutrition; (3) providing comfort and emotional support; and (4) preventing and maintaining surveillance for complications. Current guidelines for management of a patient with sepsis or septic shock are outlined in Box 26.18.

MULTIPLE ORGAN DYSFUNCTION SYNDROME

Description and Etiology

MODS results from progressive physiologic failure of two or more separate organ systems in an acutely ill patient such that homeostasis cannot be maintained without intervention.[7] MODS is the major cause of death in patients in critical care units. Mortality is closely linked to the number of organ systems involved. Dysfunction or failure of two or more organ systems is associated with an estimated mortality rate of 54%, which increases to 100% when five organ systems fail.[86] Survivors of MODS may develop generalized polyneuropathy and a chronic form of pulmonary disease from ARDS, complicating recovery. These patients often require prolonged, expensive rehabilitation.[87]

Trauma patients are particularly vulnerable to developing MODS, because they often experience ischemia-reperfusion events resulting from hemorrhage, blunt trauma, or SNS-induced vasoconstriction.[88] Other high-risk patients include patients who have experienced infection, a shock episode, various ischemia-reperfusion events, acute pancreatitis, sepsis, burns, aspiration, multiple blood transfusions, or surgical complications.[86] Patients 65 years old or older are at increased risk because of their decreased organ reserve and comorbidities.[54]

Organ dysfunction may be the direct consequence of an initial insult (primary MODS) or can manifest latently and involve organs not directly affected in the initial insult (secondary MODS). Patients can experience both primary and secondary MODS (Fig. 26.7).

Primary MODS results from a well-defined insult in which organ dysfunction occurs early and is directly attributed to the insult itself. Direct insults initially cause localized inflammatory responses. Primary MODS accounts for only a small percentage of MODS cases. Examples of primary MODS include the immediate consequences of posttraumatic pulmonary failure, thermal injuries, AKI, or invasive infections.[88] These cellular or microcirculatory insults may lead to a loss of critical organ function induced by failure of delivery of oxygen and substrates, coupled with the inability to remove end products of metabolism. The inflammatory response in primary MODS has a less apparent presentation and may resolve without long-term implications. However, primary MODS may "prime" physiologic systems for a more sustained exaggerated inflammatory response that leads to secondary MODS.[86]

Secondary MODS is a consequence of widespread sustained systemic inflammation that results in dysfunction of organs not involved in the initial insult. Secondary MODS develops latently after an initial insult.[88] The early impairment of organs normally involved in immunoregulatory function, such as the liver and the GI tract, intensifies the host response to the insult.[89] The initial insult may prime the inflammatory system in such a way that even a mild second insult (hit) may perpetuate a sustained hyperinflammatory response. This "two-hit hypothesis" has been increasingly recognized as an important contributor to morbidity and mortality in patients with secondary MODS.[90]

Sepsis is a common initiating event in the development of secondary MODS. When inflammation is not contained locally, consequences occur systemically that lead to organ dysfunction, including intense, uncontrolled activation of inflammatory cells; direct damage of vascular endothelium; disruption of immune cell function; persistent hypermetabolism; and maldistribution of circulatory volume to organ systems. Inflammation becomes a systemic, self-perpetuating process that is inadequately controlled and results in organ dysfunction.[90]

During hypermetabolism, changes occur in cellular anabolic and catabolic function, resulting in autocatabolism. Autocatabolism manifests as a severe decrease in lean body mass, severe weight loss, anergy, and increased CO and oxygen consumption (VO_2) resulting from profound alterations in carbohydrate, protein, and fat metabolism.[86] Concurrently, GI, hepatic, and immunologic dysfunction may occur, which intensifies systemic inflammation. Clinical consequences may affect gut function, wound healing, muscle wasting, host response, respiratory function, and continued promotion of the hypermetabolic response.

Pathophysiology

Secondary MODS results from altered regulation of the patient's acute immune and inflammatory responses. Dysregulation, or failure to control the host inflammatory response, leads to the excessive production of inflammatory cells and biochemical mediators that cause widespread damage to vascular endothelium and organ damage.[60,90]

Certain cellular and biochemical activity evokes the inflammatory and immune responses implicated in MODS. The mediators associated with MODS can be classified as inflammatory cells, biochemical mediators, or plasma protein systems (Box 26.19). Activation of one mediator often leads to activation of another.[60] The biologic activity of inflammatory cells, biochemical mediators, and plasma protein

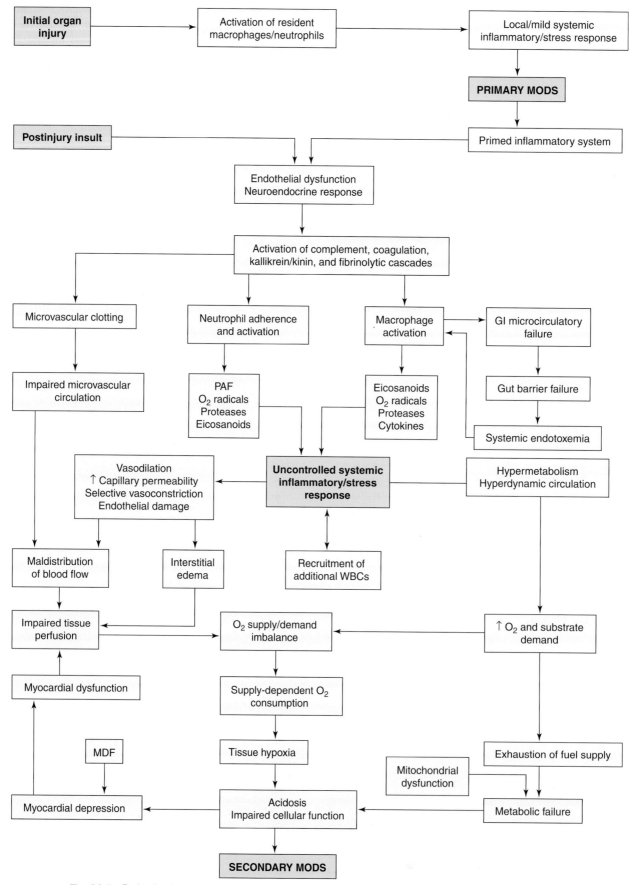

Fig. 26.7 Pathophysiology of Multiple Organ Dysfunction Syndrome. *GI,* Gastrointestinal; *MDF,* myocardial depressant factor; *MODS,* multiple organ dysfunction syndrome; O_2, oxygen; *PAF,* platelet-activating factor; *WBCs,* white blood cells. (From McCance KL, Huether SE, eds. *Pathophysiology: The Biological Basis for Disease in Adults and Children.* 8th ed. St. Louis: Elsevier; 2019.)

BOX 26.19 Inflammatory Mediators Associated With Multiple Organ Dysfunction Syndrome

Inflammatory Cells
- Neutrophils
- Macrophages or monocytes
- Mast lymphocytes
- Endothelial

Plasma Protein Systems
- Complement
- Kinin
- Coagulation

Biochemical Mediators
- Reactive oxygen species
  - Superoxide radical

- Hydroxyl radical
- Hydrogen peroxide
- Tumor necrosis factor
- Interleukins
- Platelet-activating factor
- Arachidonic acid metabolites
  - Prostaglandins
  - Leukotrienes
  - Thromboxanes
- Proteases

---

systems and how they work in concert to cause MODS have not been totally determined.

Assessment and Diagnosis

Secondary MODS is a systemic disease with organ-specific manifestations. Organ dysfunction is influenced by numerous factors, including organ host defense function, response time to the injury, metabolic requirements, organ vasculature response to vasoactive medications, organ sensitivity to damage, and physiologic reserve. The responses of the GI, hepatobiliary, cardiovascular, pulmonary, renal, and hematologic systems are discussed in the following paragraphs. Clinical manifestations of organ dysfunction are outlined in Box 26.20.

Gastrointestinal Dysfunction

The GI tract plays an important role in MODS. GI organs normally have immunoregulatory functions, and the GI tract contains approximately 70% to 80% of the immunologic tissue of the entire body. A normally functioning GI tract prevents bacteria from entering the systemic circulation. Normal gut flora and gut environment are altered in patients with severe inflammation. Healthy probiotics are decreased in an inflammatory state, and pathogenic organisms proliferate.[66]

With microcirculatory failure to the GI tract, the gut's barrier function may be lost, which leads to bacterial translocation, sustained inflammation, endogenous endotoxemia, and MODS.[90–93] Hypoperfusion and shock-like states damage the normal GI mucosa barrier by decreasing mesenteric blood flow, leading to hypoperfusion of the villi, mucosal edema, ischemic necrosis, sloughing of the mucosa, and malabsorption. The GI tract is extremely vulnerable to oxygen metabolite–induced reperfusion injury. Endothelial injury and GI lesions occur in response to mediator-induced tissue damage. Ischemic events and the absence of feedings can disrupt the normal metabolism of the gastric or intestinal lumen and the normal protective function of the gut barrier.[66]

The translocation of GI bacteria through a "leaky gut" into the systemic circulation initiates and perpetuates an inflammatory focus in a critically ill patient.[90,91] The GI tract harbors organisms that present an inflammatory focus when carried from the gut via the intestinal lymphatics. After hemorrhagic shock, trauma, or a major burn injury, gut-released proinflammatory and tissue injurious factors may lead to ARDS, bone marrow failure, myocardial dysfunction, neutrophil activation, RBC injury, and endothelial cell activation and injury. These factors, released from the gut and carried in the mesenteric lymphatics, are capable of causing a septic state and secondary MODS.

The "gut-lymph hypothesis" proposes that gut ischemia-reperfusion injury leads to loss of a gut protective barrier, bacterial translocation, and a gut inflammatory response. Gut-derived inflammatory factors are carried in the mesenteric lymph, leading to a septic state and distant organ failure and MODS.[91]

Last, the oropharynx of a critically ill patient also becomes colonized with potentially pathogenic organisms from the GI tract. Pulmonary aspiration of colonized secretions presents an inflammatory focus that can contribute to concomitant pulmonary dysfunction.

Hepatobiliary Dysfunction

The liver plays a vital role in host homeostasis related to the acute inflammatory response. The liver responds to sustained inflammation by selectively altering carbohydrate, fat, and protein metabolism. Consequently, hepatic dysfunction threatens the patient's survival. The liver normally controls the inflammatory response by several mechanisms. Kupffer cells, which are hepatic macrophages, detoxify substances that may normally induce systemic inflammation and vasoactive substances that cause hemodynamic instability. Failure to detoxify gram-negative bacteria causes endotoxemia, perpetuates inflammation, and may lead to MODS. The liver also produces proteins and antiproteases to control the inflammatory response; however, hepatic dysfunction limits this response.[90]

Common causes of liver failure in critically ill patients are infection-related cholestasis and hepatocellular injury in response to toxins and toxins themselves. In infection-related cholestasis, bacterial toxins and released cytokines affect the uptake and excretion of bilirubin leading to jaundice. In hepatocellular injury, endotoxins and bacteria are phagocytized by Kupffer cells that release hepatotoxic substances that cause cellular damage. Hepatic dysfunction may also occur with organ hypoperfusion, hemolysis, and hepatotoxic medications. Measurements of liver enzymes, bilirubin, ammonia, and liver-produced proteins should be carefully monitored.[86]

The liver and gallbladder are extremely vulnerable to ischemic injury from organ hypoperfusion. Ischemic hepatitis occurs after a prolonged period of physiologic shock and is associated with centrilobular hepatocellular necrosis. The degree of hepatic damage is related directly to the severity and duration of the shock episode. Anoxic and reperfusion injuries damage hepatocytes and the vascular endothelium. Patients at high risk for ischemic hepatitis after a hypotensive event include patients with a history of heart failure or cardiac dysrhythmias. Clinical manifestations of hepatic insufficiency are evident 1 to 2 days after the insult. Jaundice and transient

BOX 26.20   Clinical Manifestations of Organ Dysfunction

Pulmonary
- Acute respiratory distress syndrome (ARDS) pattern of respiratory failure (dyspnea, patchy infiltrates, refractory hypoxemia, respiratory acidosis, abnormal O_2 indices)
- Pulmonary hypertension

Gastrointestinal
- Abdominal distention and ascites
- Intolerance to enteral feedings
- Paralytic ileus
- Upper or lower gastrointestinal bleeding
- Diarrhea
- Ischemic colitis
- Mucosal ulceration
- Decreased bowel sounds
- Bacterial overgrowth in stool

Liver
- Jaundice
- Hepatomegaly
- Increased serum bilirubin (hyperbilirubinemia)
- Increased liver enzymes
- Increased serum ammonia
- Decreased serum transferrin

Gallbladder
- Right upper quadrant tenderness or pain
- Abdominal distention
- Unexplained fever
- Decreased bowel sounds

Metabolic and Nutrition
- Decreased lean body mass
- Muscle wasting
- Severe weight loss
- Negative nitrogen balance
- Hyperglycemia
- Hypertriglyceridemia
- Increased serum lactate

- Decreased serum albumin, serum transferrin, prealbumin, and retinol-binding protein

Kidney
- Increased serum creatinine and blood urea nitrogen
- Oliguria, anuria, or polyuria consistent with prerenal azotemia or acute kidney injury
- Urinary indices consistent with prerenal azotemia or acute kidney injury

Cardiovascular
Hyperdynamic
- Decreased pulmonary artery occlusion pressure
- Decreased systemic vascular resistance
- Decreased right atrial pressure
- Decreased left ventricular stroke work index
- Increased oxygen consumption
- Increased cardiac output, cardiac index, and heart rate

Hypodynamic
- Increased systemic vascular resistance
- Increased right atrial pressure
- Increased left ventricular stroke work index
- Decreased oxygen delivery and consumption
- Decreased cardiac output and cardiac index

Central Nervous System
- Lethargy
- Altered level of consciousness
- Fever
- Hepatic encephalopathy

Coagulation or Hematologic
- Thrombocytopenia
- Disseminated intravascular coagulation

Immune
- Infection
- Decreased lymphocyte count
- Anergy

---

elevations in serum transaminase and bilirubin levels occur. Hyperbilirubinemia results from hepatocyte anoxic injury and an increased production of bilirubin from hemoglobin catabolism. Ischemic hepatitis may resolve spontaneously or progress to acute liver failure. Although ischemic hepatitis is not a life-threatening complication, it can contribute to morbidity and mortality as a component of MODS.[92] Acute liver failure is discussed further in Chapter 21.

Acalculous cholecystitis manifests 3 to 4 weeks after an insult. Its pathogenesis is unclear, but it may be related to ischemic reperfusion injury, PEEP greater than 5 cm H_2O, volume depletion, total parenteral nutrition, opioids, and cystic duct obstruction as a result of hyperviscous bile. Visceral hypotension and vasoactive medication use may decrease perfusion of the gallbladder mucosa contributing to ischemia. Bacterial invasion may stimulate activation of factor XII and initiate the coagulation pathway. Clinical manifestations of acalculous cholecystitis may mimic acute cholecystitis with gallstones. However, patients may demonstrate vague symptoms, including right upper quadrant pain and tenderness. Critical to the detection of acalculous cholecystitis is the recognition of abdominal distention, unexplained fever, loss of bowel sounds, and sudden deterioration in the patient's condition. Approximately 50% of patients with acalculous cholecystitis have gallbladder gangrene, and 10% have gallbladder perforation requiring a cholecystectomy.[93]

Pulmonary Dysfunction

The lungs are common and early target organs for mediator-induced injury and are usually the first organs affected. ARDS is the pulmonary manifestation of MODS. Patients who develop MODS usually have pulmonary symptoms; however, not all patients with ARDS develop secondary MODS. Patients with ARDS who develop sepsis concurrently with acute lung failure are at the greatest risk for MODS.[90]

ARDS associated with MODS usually occurs 24 to 72 hours after the initial insult. Patients initially exhibit a low-grade fever, tachycardia, dyspnea, and mental confusion. With progression of ARDS dyspnea, hypoxemia, and the work of breathing increase, requiring intubation and mechanical ventilation. ARDS results in refractory hypoxemia caused by intrapulmonary shunting, decreased pulmonary compliance, and altered airway mechanics; there usually is radiographic evidence of noncardiogenic pulmonary edema.[94]

Mediators associated with ARDS include inflammatory cells such as polymorphonuclear cells, macrophages, monocytes, endothelial cells, and mast cells and biochemical mediators such as arachidonic acid (AA) metabolites, toxic oxygen metabolites, proteases, TNF, PAF, and interleukins. Intense mediator activity damages the pulmonary vascular endothelium and the alveolar epithelium, resulting in surfactant deficiency, mild pulmonary hypertension, and increased pulmonary capillary permeability leading to increased lung water (noncardiogenic pulmonary edema).[72] ARDS is discussed further in Chapter 14.

Kidney Dysfunction

AKI is a common manifestation of MODS. The kidney is highly vulnerable to hypoperfusion and reperfusion injury. Consequently, kidney ischemia-reperfusion injury may be a major cause of kidney dysfunction in MODS. A patient with AKI may demonstrate oliguria or anuria resulting from decreased renal perfusion and relative hypovolemia. Early oliguria is likely caused by decreases in renal perfusion related to shock-like states; late oliguria is typically a sign of evolving kidney injury and ischemia. Renal function may become refractory to diuretics, fluid challenges, and vasoactive medications. Prerenal azotemia from impaired renal blood flow may progress to AKI, necessitating continuous renal replacement therapies. Frequent use of nephrotoxic medications also intensifies the risk of AKI.[95]

Early recognition of AKI is imperative. However, the lack of early and reliable biomarkers for AKI leads to a delay in initiating treatment. The instability of kidney function in a critically ill patient decreases the validity of measures that are based on creatinine assessment. An elevated serum creatinine level is usually a late sign, but it is typically accepted as the index for renal dysfunction. However, serum creatinine concentrations can vary for reasons other than renal function in patients with organ failure and are rarely at a steady state. It may be preferable to use 8-, 12-, or 24-hour urinary creatinine clearance values to estimate glomerular filtration rate in critically ill patients, especially when determining medication dosages.[95] Additional signs of kidney impairment include decreased erythropoietin-induced anemia, vitamin D malabsorption, and altered fluid and electrolyte balance. AKI is discussed further in Chapter 19.

Cardiovascular and Hematologic System Dysfunction

The initial cardiovascular response in sepsis is myocardial depression; decreased RAP and SVR; and increased venous capacitance, CO, and heart rate. Despite an increased CO, myocardial depression occurs and is accompanied by decreased SVR, increased heart rate, and ventricular dilation. These compensatory mechanisms help maintain CO during the early phase of sepsis. An inability to increase CO in response to a low SVR may indicate myocardial failure or inadequate fluid resuscitation, and it is associated with increased mortality. VO_2 may be twice the normal value and may be flow dependent.[63]

As MODS progresses, heart failure develops. Cardiac dysfunction is characterized by ventricular dilation, decreased diastolic compliance, and decreased systolic contractile function. Cardiovascular function becomes vasopressor dependent. Heart failure may be caused by immune mediators, TNF-alpha, acidosis, or myocardial depressant factor, a substance secreted by the pancreas. Myocardial depression is exacerbated by myocardial hypoperfusion from a low CO state and

persistent lactic acidosis. Cardiogenic shock and biventricular failure occur and lead to death.[63] Heart failure is discussed further in Chapter 11, and more information on cardiogenic shock can be found earlier in this chapter.

The most common manifestations of hematologic dysfunction in sepsis or MODS are thrombocytopenia, coagulation abnormalities, and anemia. The most severe is coagulation system dysfunction manifesting as DIC. DIC is a complex, consumptive coagulopathy that occurs in patients with a variety of disorders, including sepsis, tissue injury, and shock; it is overstimulation of the normal coagulation process. DIC results simultaneously in microvascular clotting and hemorrhage in organ systems, leading to thrombosis and fibrinolysis in life-threatening proportions. Clotting factor derangement leads to further inflammation and further thrombosis. Microvascular damage leads to further organ injury. Cell injury and damage to the endothelium activate the intrinsic or extrinsic coagulation pathways. Low platelet counts and elevated D-dimer concentrations and fibrinogen degradation products are clinical indicators of DIC.[62] DIC is discussed further in Chapter 27.

Medical Management

A patient with MODS requires multidisciplinary collaboration in clinical management. The focus of management includes fluid resuscitation and hemodynamic support, prevention and treatment of infection, maintenance of tissue oxygenation, nutrition and metabolic support, comfort and emotional support, and preservation of individual organs. The use of investigational therapies may be part of the patient's clinical management.

Identification and Treatment of Infection

Identification and treatment of the underlying source of inflammation or infection are important ways to reduce mortality. Medical and surgical intervention to remove sources of infection or contamination may limit the inflammatory response and improve chances of recovery. Surgical procedures such as early fracture stabilization, removal of infected organs or tissue, and burn excision are helpful. Appropriate antibiotics are needed if the cause cannot be removed by surgical débridement or incision and draining.[58]

Maintenance of Tissue Oxygenation

Normally under steady-state conditions, VO_2 is relatively constant and independent of oxygen delivery (DO_2) unless delivery becomes severely impaired. The relationship is called *supply-independent oxygen consumption*. Consequently, a percentage of oxygen is not used (physiologic reserve). Patients with MODS often develop supply-dependent oxygen consumption, in which VO_2 becomes dependent on DO_2, rather than demand, at a normal or high DO_2. When VO_2 does not equal demand, a tissue oxygen debt develops, subjecting organs to failure.[86]

Hypoperfusion and resultant organ hypoxemia often occur in patients at high risk for MODS, subjecting essential organs to failure. Effective fluid resuscitation and early recognition of flow-dependent VO_2 is essential, and patients at risk for MODS require hemodynamic monitoring, frequent measurements or surrogate measurements of DO_2 and VO_2, and serum lactate levels to guide therapy. Serum lactate levels provide information regarding the severity of impaired perfusion and the presence of lactic acidosis and differ significantly in survivors of MODS and nonsurvivors. Failure to maintain adequate oxygenation to vital organs results in organ dysfunction. Despite adequate DO_2, VO_2 may not meet the needs of the body during MODS.

⊚ BOX 26.21   **PRIORITY PATIENT CARE MANAGEMENT**

Multiple Organ Dysfunction Syndrome
- Impaired Cardiac Output due to alterations in contractility
- Impaired Gas Exchange due to ventilation-perfusion mismatching or intrapulmonary shunting
- Imbalanced Nutrition: Less Than Body Requirements due to lack of exogenous nutrients and increased metabolic demand
- Anxiety due to threat to biologic, psychologic, or social integrity
- Compromised Family Coping due to a critically ill family member

Patient Care Management plans are located in Appendix A.

Patients with MODS commonly manifest supply-dependent oxygen consumption and are unable to use oxygen appropriately despite normal delivery. Interventions that decrease oxygen demand and increase oxygen delivery are essential. Sedation, mechanical ventilation, rest, and temperature and pain control may be able to decrease oxygen demand. Oxygen delivery may be increased by maintaining normal hematocrit and PaO_2 levels, using PEEP, increasing preload or myocardial contractility to enhance CO, or reducing afterload to increase CO. Various methods of kinetic or prone therapies are available and may enhance alveolar recruitment, improve oxygenation delivery, and decrease other potential complications.

Nutrition and Metabolic Support

Hypermetabolism in MODS results in profound weight loss, cachexia, and loss of organ function.[65] The goal of nutrition support is the preservation of organ structure and function. Although nutrition support may not definitely alter the course of organ dysfunction, it prevents generalized nutrition deficiencies and preserves gut integrity. Enteral nutrition may exert a physiologic effect that downregulates the systemic immune response and reduces oxidative stress.[89] The enteral route is preferable to parenteral support. Enteral feedings are given distal to the pylorus to reduce the risk of pulmonary aspiration.[19] Enteral feedings may limit bacterial translocation.[89] In addition to early nutrition support, the pharmacologic properties of enteral feeding formulas may limit inflammation for selected critical care populations. Nutrition support is discussed further in Chapter 5.

Nursing Management

Preventive measures include a multitude of assessment strategies to detect early organ manifestations of this syndrome. Patients who continue to experience sites of inflammation, septic foci, and inadequate tissue perfusion may be at higher risk. Handwashing, aseptic technique, and an understanding of how microorganisms can invade the body are essential components of preventive nursing care.

The patient care management plan for a patient with MODS incorporates a variety of patient problems (Box 26.21). Nursing priorities are directed toward (1) preventing development of infection, (2) facilitating oxygen delivery and limiting tissue oxygen demand, (3) facilitating nutrition support, (4) providing comfort and emotional support, and (5) preventing and maintaining surveillance for complications.

Patients are assessed closely for inflammation and infection. Subtle expressions of infection warrant investigation. Nursing measures include strict adherence to standards of practice to prevent infection. Practices related to infection control with invasive hemodynamic monitoring, urinary catheters, endotracheal tubes, intracranial pressure monitoring devices, total parenteral nutrition, and wound care must be stringent to prevent further infection.

Measures to limit tissue oxygen consumption include administering analgesics and sedatives, positioning the patient for comfort, limiting activities, offering support to reduce anxiety, providing a calm and quiet environment, and educating the patient and family about the condition. Measures to enhance tissue oxygen supply include administering supplemental oxygen, monitoring the patient's respiratory status, and administering prescribed fluids and medications. Interprofessional collaborative management of a patient with MODS is outlined in Box 26.22.

ADDITIONAL RESOURCES

Additional resources about sepsis, septic shock, and MODS can be found in Box 26.23.

BOX 26.22   **Collaborative Management of Multiple Organ Dysfunction Syndrome**

- Support oxygen transport:
  - Establish a patent airway.
  - Initiate mechanical ventilation.
  - Administer oxygen.
  - Administer fluids (crystalloids, colloids, blood, and other blood products).
  - Administer vasoactive medications.
  - Administer positive inotropic medications.
  - Administer antidysrhythmic medications.
  - Ensure sufficient hemoglobin and hematocrit.
- Support oxygen use:
  - Identify and correct cause of lactic acidosis.
  - Ensure adequate organ and extremity perfusion.
- Decrease oxygen demand:
  - Administer sedation or paralytics.
  - Administer antipyretics and external cooling measures.
- Administer pain medications.
- Identify underlying cause of inflammation and treat accordingly:
  - Remove infected organs or tissue.
  - Administer antibiotics.
  - Initiate nutrition support.
- Treat individual organ dysfunction:
  - Gastrointestinal
  - Hepatobiliary
  - Pulmonary
  - Renal
  - Cardiovascular
  - Coagulation system
- Prevent and maintain surveillance for complications, particularly infection.
- Provide comfort and emotional support.

QSEN

BOX 26.23 Informatics

Internet Resources: Shock, Sepsis, and Multiple Organ Dysfunction Syndrome

- American Association of Critical-Care Nurses (AACN): www.aacn.org
- American College of Surgeons (ACS): www.facs.org
- American Medical Association (AMA): www.ama-assn.org
- American Society for Parenteral and Enteral Nutrition (ASPEN): www.nutritioncare.org
- Anaphylaxis Campaign (AC): www.anaphylaxis.org.uk

- College of Physicians (ACP): www.acponline.org
- European Society of Intensive Care Medicine: www.esicm.org
- International Sepsis Forum (ISF): www.internationalsepsisforum.com
- Sepsis Alliance (SA): www.sepsis.org
- Society of Critical Care Medicine (SCCM): www.sccm.org
- Surviving Sepsis Campaign: www.sccm.org/SurvivingSepsisCampaign/Home
- The Food Allergy & Anaphylaxis Network (FARE): www.foodallergy.org
- National Institutes for Health: www.nih.gov

REFERENCES

1. Wacker DA, Winters ME. Shock. *Emerg Med Clin North Am.* 2014;32(4):747−758. Available from: https://doi.org/10.1016/j.emc.2014.07.003.
2. Kumar A, Tremblay V, Vazquez-Grande G, et al. Shock: classification, pathophysiology, and approach to management. In: Parrillo JE, Dellinger RP, eds. *Critical Care Medicine: Principles of Diagnosis and Management in the Adult.* 5th ed. Philadelphia: Elsevier; 2019.
3. Pugh AM. Shock. In: Sutton JM, Beckwith MA, Johnson BL, et al., eds. *The Mont Reid Surgical Handbook.* Philadelphia: Elsevier; 2018.
4. Astiz ME. Pathophysiology and classification of shock states. In: Vincent JL, Abraham E, Moore FA, et al., eds. *Textbook of Critical Care.* 7th ed. Philadelphia: Elsevier; 2017.
5. Otani S, Coopersmith CM. Gut integrity in critical illness. *J Intensive Care.* 2019;7:17. Available from: https://doi.org/10.1186/s40560-019-0372-6.
6. Hallsey SD, Greenwood JC. Beyond mean arterial pressure and lactate: perfusion end points for managing the shocked patient. *Emerg Med Clin North Am.* 2019;37(3):395−408.
7. Simmon J, Ventetuolo CE. Cardiopulmonary monitoring of shock. *Curr Opin Crit Care.* 2017;23(3):223−231.
8. Surbatovic M, Radakovic S, Jevtic M, et al. Predictive value of sodium bicarbonate, arterial base deficit/excess and SAPS III score in critically ill patients. *Gen Physiol Biophys.* 2009;28(Spec No):271−276.
9. Hatog C, Bloos F. Venous oxygen saturation. *Best Pract Res Clin Anaesthesiol.* 2014;28(4):419−428.
10. Martin GS, Bassett P. Crystalloids vs. colloids for fluid resuscitation in the intensive care unit: a systematic review and meta-analysis. *J Crit Care.* 2019;50:144−154. Available from: https://doi.org/10.1016/j.jcrc.2018.11.031.
11. Semler MW, Kellum JA. Balanced crystalloid solutions. *Am J Respir Crit Care Med.* 2019;199(8):952−960.
12. Lewis SR, Pritchard MW, Evans DJ, et al. Colloids versus crystalloids for fluid resuscitation in critically ill patients. *Cochrane Database Syst Rev.* 2018;2018(8):CD000567.
13. Vincent JL. Fluid management in the critically ill. *Kidney Int.* 2019;96(1):52−57.
14. Pieracci FM, Biffl WL, Moore EE. Current concepts in resuscitation. *J Intensive Care Med.* 2012;27(2):79−96.
15. Carson JL, Stanworth SJ, Roubinian N, et al. Transfusion thresholds and other strategies for guiding allogenic red blood cell transfusion. *Cochrane Database Syst Rev.* 2016;2016(10):CD002042.
16. Cable CA, Razavi SA, Roback JD, Murphy DJ. RBC transfusion strategies in the ICU: a concise review. *Crit Care Med.* 2019;47(11):1637−1644.
17. Jongerius I, Porcelijn L, van Beek AE, et al. The role of complement in transfusion-related acute lung injury. *Transfus Med Rev.* 2019;33(4):236−242.
18. Kimmoun A, Novy E, Auchet T, Ducrocq N, Levy B. Hemodynamic consequences of severe lactic acidosis in shock states: from bench to bedside. *Crit Care.* 2015;19:175. Available from: https://doi.org/10.1186/s13054-015-0896-7.
19. Taylor BE, McClave SA, Martindale RG, et al, Society of Critical Care Medicine; American Society of Parenteral and Enteral Nutrition. Guidelines for the provision and assessment of nutrition support therapy in the adult critically ill patient: Society of Critical Care Medicine (SCCM) and American Society for Parenteral and Enteral Nutrition (ASPEN). *Crit Care Med.* 2016;44(2):390−438.
20. Fuentes Padilla P, Martínez G, Vernooij RW, et al. Early enteral nutrition (within 48 hours) versus delayed enteral nutrition (after 48 hours) with or without supplemental parenteral nutrition in critically ill adults. *Cochrane Database Syst Rev.* 2019;2019(10):CD012340.
21. American Diabetes Association. Diabetes care in the hospital: standards of medical care in diabetes—2021. *Diabetes Care.* 2021;44(suppl 1):S211−S220.
22. American Association of Critical-Care Nurses: AACN Practice Alert. Family presence during resuscitation and invasive procedures. *Crit Care Nurse.* 2016;36(1):e11−e14.
23. Davidson JE, Aslakson RA, Long AC, et al. Guideline for family centered care in the neonatal, pediatric, and adult ICU. *Crit Care Med.* 2017;45(1):103−128.
24. 2017 ENA Clinical Practice Guideline Committee. Clinical practice guideline: family presence. *J Emerg Nurs.* 2019;45(1):76.e1−76.e29.
25. Mancini ME, Diekema DS, Hoadley TA, et al. Part 3: ethical issues: 2015 American Heart Association guidelines for cardiopulmonary resuscitation and emergency cardiovascular care. *Circulation.* 2015;132(18 suppl 2):S383−S396.
26. Parks J, Vasileiou G, Parreco J, et al. Validating the ATLS Shock Classification for predicting death, transfusion, or urgent intervention. *J Surg Res.* 2020;245:163−167. Available from: https://doi.org/10.1016/j.jss.2019.07.041.
27. Dries DJ. Hypovolemia and traumatic shock: nonsurgical management. In: Parrillo JE, Dellinger RP, eds. *Critical Care Medicine: Principles of Diagnosis and Management in the Adult.* 5th ed. Philadelphia: Elsevier; 2019.
28. Kwan I, Bunn F, Chinnock P, Roberts I. Timing and volume of fluid administration for patients with bleeding. *Cochrane Database Syst Rev.* 2014;2014(3):CD002245.
29. Duan C, Li T, Liu L. Efficacy of limited fluid resuscitation in patients with hemorrhagic shock: a meta-analysis. *Int J Clin Exp Med.* 2015;8(7):11645−11656.
30. Cap AP, Pidcoke HF, Spinella P, et al. Damage control resuscitation. *Mil Med.* 2018;183(suppl 2):36−43.
31. Tewelde SZ, Liu SS, Winters ME. Cardiogenic shock. *Cardiol Clin.* 2018;36(1):53−61.
32. Levy B, Bastien O, Karim B, et al. Experts' recommendations for the management of adult patients with cardiogenic shock. *Ann Intensive Care.* 2015;5(1):52.
33. Wilcox SR. Nonischemic causes of cardiogenic shock. *Emer Med Clin North Am.* 2019;37(3):493−509.
34. Hollenberg SM, Parrillo JE. Cardiogenic shock: nonsurgical management. In: Parrillo JE, Dellinger RP, eds. *Critical Care Medicine: Principles of Diagnosis and Management in the Adult.* 5th ed. Philadelphia: Elsevier; 2019.
35. Muller-Werdan U, Prondzinsky R, Wedan K. Effect of inflammatory mediators on cardiovascular function. *Curr Opin Crit Care.* 2016;22(5):453−463.
36. Petrie CJ, Ponikowski P, Metra M, et al. Proportional pulse pressure relates to cardiac index in stabilized acute heart failure patients. *Clin Exp Hypertens.* 2018;40(7):637−643.

37. van Diepen S, Katz JN, Albert NM, et al. Contemporary management of cardiogenic shock: a scientific statement from the American Heart Association. *Circulation*. 2017;136(16):e232—e268.

38. Cui K, Lyu S, Liu H, et al. Timing of initiation of intra-aortic balloon pump in patients with acute myocardial infarction complicated by cardiogenic shock: a meta-analysis. *Clin Cardiol*. 2019;42(11):1126—1134.

39. De Backer D. Anaphylaxis and anaphylactic shock. In: Parrillo JE, Dellinger RP, eds. *Critical Care Medicine: Principles of Diagnosis and Management in the Adult*. 5th ed. Philadelphia: Elsevier; 2019.

40. Raulf M. Current state of occupational latex allergy. *Curr Opin Allergy Clin Immunol*. 2020;20(2):112—116.

41. Lieberman P, Nicklas RA, Randolph C, et al. Anaphylaxis-a practice parameter update. *Ann Allergy Asthma Immunol*. 2015;115(5):341—384.

42. Reber LL, Hernandez JD, Galli SJ. The pathophysiology of anaphylaxis. *J Allergy Clin Immunol*. 2017;140(2):335—348.

43. Rance K, Goldberg P. Anaphylaxis overview: addressing unmet patient needs. *J Nurse Pract*. 2015;11(3):352—359.

44. Fineman SM. Optimal treatment of anaphylaxis: antihistamine versus epinephrine. *Postgrad Med*. 2014;126(4):73—81.

45. Shaker MS, Wallace DV, Golden DBK, et al. Anaphylaxis-a 2020 practice parameter update, systematic review, and Grading of Recommendations, Assessment, Development and Evaluation (GRADE) analysis. *J Allergy Clin Immunol*. 2020;145(4):1082—1123.

46. Pflipsen MC, Vega Colon KM. Anaphylaxis: recognition and management. *Am Fam Physician*. 2020;102(6):355—362.

47. Choo KJ, Simons FE, Sheikh A. Glucocorticoids for the treatment of anaphylaxis. *Cochrane Database Syst Rev*. 2012;2012(4):CD007596.

48. Eckert MJ, Martin MJ. Trauma: spinal cord injury. *Surg Clin North Am*. 2017;97(5):1031—1045.

49. Galeiras Vázquez R, Ferreiro Velasco ME, Mourelo Fariña M, Montoto Marqués A, Salvador de la Barrera S. Update on traumatic acute spinal cord injury. Part 1. *Med Intensiva*. 2017;41(4):237—247.

50. Wang S, Singh JM, Fehlings MG. Medical management of spinal cord injury. In: Winn HR, ed. *Youmans and Winn Neurological Surgery*. 7th ed. Philadelphia: Elsevier; 2017.

51. Casha S, Christie S. A systematic review of intensive cardiopulmonary management after spinal cord injury. *J Neurotrauma*. 2011;28(8):1479—1495.

52. Consortium for Spinal Cord Medicine. Early acute management in adults with spinal cord injury: a clinical practice guideline for health-care professionals. *J Spinal Cord Med*. 2008;31(4):403—479.

53. Panchal AR, Bartos JA, Cabañas JG, et al. Part 3: adult basic and advanced life support: 2020 American Heart Association guidelines for cardiopulmonary resuscitation and emergency cardiovascular care. *Circulation*. 2020;142(16 suppl 2):S366—S468.

54. Singer M, Deutschman CS, Seymour CW, et al. The third international consensus definitions for sepsis and septic shock. *J Am Med Assoc*. 2016;315(8):801—810.

55. Dellinger RP, Roy A, Parrillo JE. Severe sepsis and septic shock. In: Parrillo JE, Dellinger RP, eds. *Critical Care Medicine: Principles of Diagnosis and Management in the Adult*. 5th ed. Philadelphia: Elsevier; 2019.

56. Rhee C, Dantes R, Epstein L, et al. Incidence and trends of sepsis in US hospitals using clinical vs claims data, 2009-2014. *J Am Med Assoc*. 2017;318(13):1241—1249.

57. Murphy SL, Xu J, Kochanek KD, Arias E, Tejada-Vera B. *Deaths: Final Data for 2018*; 2021. Available from: https://www.cdc.gov/nchs/data/nvsr/nvsr69/nvsr69-13-508.pdf.

58. Oliver ZP, Perkins J. Source identification and source control. *Emerg Med Clin North Am*. 2017;35(1):43—58.

59. Fathi M, Markazi-Moghaddam N, Ramezankhani A. A systematic review on risk factors associated with sepsis in patients admitted to intensive care units. *Aust Crit Care*. 2019;32(2):155—164.

60. Qiu Y, Tu GW, Ju MJ, Yang C, Luo Z. The immune system regulation in sepsis: from innate to adaptive. *Curr Protein Pept Sci*. 2019;20(8):799—816.

61. Ait-Oufella H, Bourcier S, Lehoux S, Guidet B. Microcirculatory disorders during septic shock. *Curr Opin Crit Care*. 2015;21(4):271—275.

62. Semeraro N, Ammollo CT, Semeraro F, et al. Coagulation of acute sepsis. *Semin Thromb Hemost*. 2015;41(6):650—658.

63. Tartavoulle T, Fowler L. Cardiogenic shock in the septic patient: early identification and evidence-based management. *Crit Care Nurs Clin North Am*. 2018;30(3):379—387.

64. Russell JA, Rush B, Boyd J. Pathophysiology of septic shock. *Crit Care Clin*. 2018;34(1):43—61.

65. Ingels C, Gunst J, Van den Berghe G. Endocrine and metabolic alterations in sepsis and implications for treatment. *Crit Care Clin*. 2018;34(1):81—96.

66. Fay KT, Ford ML, Coopersmith CM. The intestinal microenvironment in sepsis. *Biochim Biophys Acta (BBA)—Mol Basis Dis*. 2017;1863(10 Pt B):2574—2583.

67. Dries DJ. Sepsis: 2018 update. *Air Med J*. 2018;37(5):277—281.

68. Wischmeyer PE. Nutrition therapy in sepsis. *Crit Care Clin*. 2018;34(1):107—125.

69. Nagar H, Piao S, Kim CS. Role of mitochondrial oxidative stress in sepsis. *Acute Crit Care*. 2018;33(2):65—72.

70. Cao C, Yu M, Chai Y. Pathological alteration and therapeutic implications of sepsis-induced immune cell apoptosis. *Cell Death Dis*. 2019;10(10):782.

71. Evans L, Rhodes A, Alhazzani W, et al. Surviving Sepsis Campaign: international guidelines for management of sepsis and septic shock 2021. *Crit Care Med*. 2021;49(11):e1063—e1143.

72. Perl M, Lomas-Neira J, Venet F, Chung CS, Ayala A. Pathogenesis of indirect (secondary) acute lung injury. *Expert Rev Respir Med*. 2011;5(1):115—126.

73. Jacob A, Brorson JR, Alexander JJ. Septic encephalopathy: inflammation in man and mouse. *Neurochem Int*. 2011;58(4):472—476.

74. Rello J, Valenzuela-Sánchez F, Ruiz-Rodriguez M, Moyano S. Sepsis: a review of advances in management. *Adv Ther*. 2017;34(11):2393—2411.

75. Simpson N, Lamontagne F, Shankar-Hari M. Septic shock resuscitation in the first hour. *Curr Opin Crit Care*. 2017;23(6):561—566.

76. Levy MM, Evans LE, Rhodes A. The surviving sepsis campaign bundle: 2018 update. *Intensive Care Med*. 2018;44(6):925—928.

77. Dalimonte MA, DeGrado JR, Anger KE. Vasoactive agents for adult septic shock: an update and review. *J Pharm Pract*. 2020;33(4):523—532.

78. Angus DC, Barnato AE, Bell D, et al. A systematic review and meta-analysis of early goal-directed therapy for septic shock: the ARISE, ProCESS and ProMISE investigators. *Intensive Care Med*. 2015;41(9):1549—1560.

79. ProMISEe Trial Investigators. Trial of early goal-directed resuscitation for septic shock. *N Engl J Med*. 2015;372(14):1301—1311.

80. ARISE Investigators. Goal-directed resuscitation for patients with early septic shock. *N Engl J Med*. 2014;371(16):1496—1506.

81. ProCESSS Investigators. A randomized trial of protocol-based care for early septic shock. *N Engl J Med*. 2014;370(18):1683—1693.

82. Brower RB, Matthay MA, Morris A, et al. The Acute Respiratory Distress System Network. Ventilation with lower tidal volumes as compared with traditional tidal volumes for acute lung injury and the acute respiratory distress syndrome. *N Engl J Med*. 2000;342(18):1301—1308.

83. Volbeda M, Wetterslev J, Gluud C, Zijlstra JG, van der Horst IC, Keus F. Glucocorticosteroids for sepsis: systematic review with meta-analysis and trial sequential analysis. *Intensive Care Med*. 2015;41(7):1220—1234.

84. Otto GP, Sossdorf M, Claus RA, et al. The late phase of sepsis is characterized by an increased microbiological burden and death rate. *Crit Care*. 2011;15(4):R183.

85. Martin JB, Badeaux JE. Beyond the intensive care unit: posttraumatic stress disorder in critical ill patients. *Crit Care Nurs Clin North Am*. 2018;30(3):333—342.

86. Martin LL, Cheek DJ, Morris SD. Shock, multiple organ dysfunction syndrome, and burns in adults. In: McCance KL, Heuther SE, eds. *Pathophysiology: The Biologic Basis for Disease in Adults and Children*. 8th ed. St Louis: Elsevier; 2019.

87. Hermans G, Van den Berghe G. Clinical review: intensive care unit acquired weakness. *Crit Care*. 2015;19:274. Available from: https://doi.org/10.1186/s13054-015-0993-7.

88. Sauaia A, Moore FA, Moore EE. Postinjury inflammation and organ dysfunction. *Crit Care Clin*. 2017;33(1):167—191.

89. Meng M, Klingensmith NJ, Coopersmith CM. New insights into the gut as the driver of critical illness and organ failure. *Curr Opin Crit Care.* 2017;23(2):143—148.

90. Osterbur K, Mann FA, Kuroki K, DeClue A. Multiple organ dysfunction syndrome in humans and animals. *J Vet Intern Med.* 2014;28(4):1141—1151.

91. Assimakopoulos SF, Triantos C, Thomopoulos K, et al. Gut-origin sepsis in the critically ill patient: pathophysiology and treatment. *Infection.* 2018; 46(6):751—760.

92. Woźnica EA, Inglot M, Woźnica RK, Łysenko L. Liver dysfunction in sepsis. *Adv Clin Exp Med.* 2018;27(4):547—551.

93. Barie PS, Eachempati SR. Acute acalculous cholecystitis. *Gastroenterol Clin North Am.* 2010;39(2):343—357.

94. Matthay MA, Zemans RL, Zimmerman GA, et al. Acute respiratory distress syndrome. *Nat Rev Dis Primers.* 2019;5(1):18.

95. Doi K. Role of kidney injury in sepsis. *J Intensive Care.* 2016;4:17. Available from: https://doi.org/10.1186/s40560-016-0146-3.

Hematologic and Oncologic Emergencies

Carol Ann Suarez

DISSEMINATED INTRAVASCULAR COAGULATION

Description and Etiology

Disseminated intravascular coagulation (DIC) is a condition characterized by systemic activation of coagulation, potentially leading to thrombotic obstruction of small and midsize vessels, thereby contributing to organ dysfunction.[1] An understanding of the etiologic and pathophysiologic mechanisms of DIC can assist in anticipating occurrence of the syndrome, recognizing its signs and symptoms, and prompting intervention. Also known as *consumptive coagulopathy*, DIC is characterized by bleeding and thrombosis, both of which result from depletion of clotting factors, platelets, and red blood cells (RBCs). If not treated quickly, DIC will progress to multiple organ failure and death.[2]

Many clinical events can prompt the development of DIC in a critically ill patient, but the exact underlying trigger may not be identifiable (Box 27.1). DIC is always secondary to an underlying condition, such as severe infection, solid or hematologic malignancies, trauma, or obstetric calamities.[1]

Sepsis, particularly sepsis resulting from gram-negative organisms, can be identified as the cause of DIC in 20% of cases, making it the most common cause of DIC. Endotoxins serve as a trigger for activation of tissue factor and the extrinsic coagulation pathway. Metabolic acidosis and hypoperfusion associated with shock syndromes can result in increased formation of free radicals and damage to tissues. Tissue factor is activated, resulting in DIC. Massive trauma or burns are frequently associated with DIC. Direct tissue damage activates the extrinsic coagulation pathway, and damage to endothelial surfaces activates the intrinsic pathway.[3] Obstetric emergencies, such as abruptio placentae, retained placenta, or incomplete abortion, are also associated with the development of DIC. Tissue factor is concentrated in the placenta, and damage or disruption of this structure can activate coagulation pathways, resulting in coagulopathy.[4]

Pathophysiology

Regardless of the cause, the common thread in the development of DIC is damage to the endothelium that results in activation of the coagulation mechanism (Fig. 27.1).[1] The extrinsic coagulation pathway plays a major role in the development of DIC. Direct damage to the endothelium results in the release of tissue factor and activation of this pathway. The secondary surge of thrombin formation as a result of activation of the intrinsic coagulation pathway leads to the massive disruption of the delicate balance that is hemostasis. Excessive thrombin formation results in rapid consumption of coagulation factors and depletion of regulatory substances—protein C, protein S, and antithrombin.[5] With no checks and balances, thrombi continue to form

along damaged epithelial walls, resulting in occlusion of the vessels. As occlusion reaches a critical level, tissue ischemia ensues, leading to further tissue damage and perpetuating the process. Eventually, end-organ function is affected by the ischemia, and failure is evident.[5]

In response to the formation of clots, the fibrinolytic system is activated. As plasmin breaks down the fibrin clots, fibrin split products are released, and they act as anticoagulants.[2,3] Coupled with depletion of circulating clotting factors, activation of fibrinolysis results in excessive bleeding. The end result is shock and further tissue ischemia that aggravate end-organ dysfunction and failure. Death is imminent if this destructive cycle is not interrupted.[4]

Assessment and Diagnosis

Favorable outcomes for patients with DIC depend on accurate and timely diagnosis of the condition. Realization of the role underlying pathology plays, recognition of clinical manifestations, and assessment of appropriate laboratory values are key steps in this process.

Clinical Manifestations

Clinical manifestations are related to the two primary pathophysiologic mechanisms of DIC: the formation of thrombi and bleeding. Thrombi in peripheral capillaries can lead to cyanosis, particularly in the fingers, toes, ears, and nose. In severe, untreated cases, this peripheral ischemia may progress to gangrene.[2,3] As the condition progresses, ischemia worsens and end organs are affected. The result of this more central ischemia can be respiratory insufficiency and failure, acute kidney injury, bowel infarction, and ischemic stroke. The tissue damage that results perpetuates the anomalies of DIC.[3]

As coagulation factors are depleted, bleeding from intravenous and other puncture sites is observed. Ecchymoses may result from routine interventions such as the use of a manual blood pressure cuff, bathing, or turning. Bloody drainage may also occur from surgical sites, drains, and urinary catheters. With the progression of DIC, the patient is at risk for severe gastrointestinal or subarachnoid hemorrhage.[2,6] Table 27.1 lists common signs and symptoms of DIC.

Laboratory Findings

Laboratory tests used to diagnose DIC essentially assess the four basic characteristics of this syndrome: (1) increased coagulant activity, (2) increased fibrinolytic activity, (3) impaired regulatory function, and (4) end-organ failure.[2,3]

Continuous activation of the coagulation pathways results in the consumption of coagulation factors. Because of this, prothrombin time, activated partial thromboplastin time, and international normalized ratio values are elevated. Although the platelet count may be within normal ranges, serial examination reveals a declining trend

BOX 27.1 Causes of Disseminated Intravascular Coagulation

Obstetric Complications
- Abruptio placentae
- Placenta previa
- Retained dead fetus
- Septic abortion
- Amniotic fluid embolism
- Toxemia of pregnancy

Infections
- Gram-negative sepsis
- Gram-positive sepsis
- Meningococcemia
- Rocky Mountain spotted fever
- Histoplasmosis
- Aspergillosis
- Malaria

Neoplasms
- Carcinomas of pancreas, prostate, lung, and stomach
- Acute promyelocytic leukemia
- Tumor lysis syndrome
- Chemotherapy

Massive Tissue Injury
- Trauma
- Crush injuries
- Burns
- Extensive surgery
- Heat stroke
- Acute transplant rejection

Miscellaneous
- Acute intravascular hemolysis
- Snakebite
- Giant hemangioma
- Shock
- Heat stroke
- Vasculitis
- Aortic aneurysm
- Liver disease
- Cardiac arrest

in values. An unexpected drop of at least 50% in the platelet count, particularly in the presence of known contributing factors and associated signs and symptoms, strongly indicates DIC.[5] Fibrinogen levels drop as more and more clots are formed. Thrombus formation in small vessels narrows the vessel lumen, forcing RBCs to squeeze through. The resulting damage and fragmentation of these cells can be seen on microscopic examination of blood samples. Damaged, fragmented RBCs are called *schistocytes*.[2,3]

In response to the excess clotting activity, the fibrinolytic process accelerates, and levels of by-products increase. This is reflected in markedly elevated levels of fibrin degradation products. Another key laboratory test used to evaluate the degree of clot dissolution and the severity of the coagulopathy is the D-dimer level.[1] D-dimers exclusively indicate clot degradation because, in contrast to fibrin degradation products, which also result from the breakdown of free circulating fibrin, D-dimers result only from dissolution of clots.[3] With progression of the

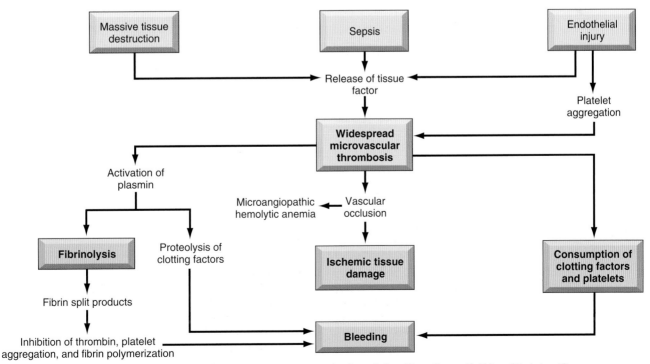

Fig. 27.1 Pathophysiology of Disseminated Intravascular Coagulation. (From Kumar V, Abbas AK, Aster JC, eds. *Robbins and Cotran Pathologic Basis of Disease*. 10th ed. Philadelphia: Elsevier; 2021.)

TABLE 27.1 Signs and Symptoms of Disseminated Intravascular Coagulation.

System	Signs Related to Hemorrhage	Signs Related to Thrombi
Integumentary	Bleeding from gums, venipunctures, and old surgical sites; epistaxis; ecchymoses	Peripheral cyanosis, gangrene
Cardiopulmonary	Hemoptysis	Dysrhythmias, chest pain, acute myocardial infarction, pulmonary embolus, respiratory failure
Renal	Hematuria	Oliguria, acute kidney injury
Gastrointestinal	Abdominal distention, hemorrhage	Diarrhea, constipation, bowel infarct
Neurologic	Subarachnoid hemorrhage	Altered level of consciousness, ischemic stroke

coagulopathy, normal regulatory mechanisms are disrupted, as reflected in decreasing levels of inhibitory factors such as protein C, factor V, and antithrombin III.[2,3,6]

Unchecked DIC resulting in occlusion of vessels and tissue ischemia leads to end-organ dysfunction. Common findings in advanced DIC include respiratory failure, indicated by abnormal arterial blood gas (ABG) levels; liver failure, indicated by increasing liver enzymes; and renal impairment, indicated by increasing blood urea nitrogen (BUN) and creatinine levels.[6]

No single laboratory study can confirm the diagnosis of DIC, but several key results are strong indicators of the condition (Table 27.2). The International Society on Thrombosis and Hemostasis emphasizes early detection of DIC through observation of abnormal trends in laboratory values.[7]

Medical Management

The primary intervention in DIC is prevention. Being aware of the conditions that commonly contribute to the development of DIC and treating them vigorously and without delay provide the best defense against this devastating condition.[2,3,6] After DIC is identified, maintaining organ perfusion and slowing consumption of coagulation factors are paramount to achieving a favorable outcome.[3,5]

Multiple-organ dysfunction syndrome (MODS) frequently results from DIC and exacerbates the underlying pathology.[4] It is essential to prevent end-organ ischemia and damage by supporting blood pressure and circulating volume. Administration of intravenous fluids and inotropic agents and, if overt hemorrhaging is evident, infusion of packed RBCs are appropriate interventions to replace blood volume and essential oxygen-carrying RBCs.

In the presence of severe platelet depletion (less than 50,000/mm³) and severe hemorrhage, platelet transfusions are often indicated.[2,6] However, caution must be used when administering platelets, because antiplatelet antibodies may be formed. These antibodies may become activated during future platelet transfusions and elicit DIC.[3]

Replacement of clotting factors in a patient with DIC is thought by some authorities to perpetuate the coagulopathy; however, there is little scientific evidence to support this theory.[5] Fibrinogen levels less than 100 mg/dL indicate the appropriateness of administering cryoprecipitate. A prolonged prothrombin time indicates the need for fresh frozen plasma.[2,3,6]

Slowing consumption of coagulation factors by inhibiting the processes involved in clot formation is another strategy used to treat DIC. The use of heparin, particularly low–molecular-weight heparin, to prevent formation of future clots is controversial.[2] It is contraindicated in patients with DIC associated with recent surgery or with gastrointestinal or central nervous system bleeding. However, heparin has been beneficial in obstetric emergencies such as retained placenta or incomplete abortion, severe arterial occlusions, or MODS caused by microemboli.[2,3] Inhibitors such as aminocaproic acid may be used in conjunction with heparin.[2,3]

Thrombin production in DIC surpasses production of antithrombins and other regulatory factors that would normally be present to inactivate thrombin and its subsequent actions. The use of antithrombin III has been approved in the United States. Ongoing research is yielding mixed results in the treatment of DIC.[3]

Nursing Management

The patient care management plan for a patient with DIC incorporates a variety of patient problems (Box 27.2). Assessment and monitoring are the primary weapons in the arsenal against DIC. Knowing the diseases and conditions that are most often associated with DIC and understanding the pathophysiologic mechanisms involved enable appropriate monitoring and intervention should the situation arise. Nursing actions are driven by the specific cause of the DIC, although some common interventions are appropriate for all patients with DIC. Priority patient care interventions include supporting the patient's vital functions, initiating bleeding precautions, providing comfort and emotional support, and maintaining surveillance for complications.

TABLE 27.2 Laboratory Studies in Disseminated Intravascular Coagulation.

Test	Value
Prothrombin time (PT)	>12.5 seconds
Platelets	<50,000/mm³ or at least 50% drop from baseline
Activated partial thromboplastin time (aPTT)	>40 seconds
D-dimer	>250 ng/mL
Fibrin degradation products (FDP)	>40 mg/mL
Fibrinogen	<100 mg/dL

◎ BOX 27.2 PRIORITY PATIENT CARE MANAGEMENT

Disseminated Intravascular Coagulation
- Hypovolemia due to absolute loss
- Impaired Cardiac Output due to alterations in preload
- Risk for infection
- Anxiety due to threat to biological, psychological, or social integrity
- Impaired Family Coping due to a critically ill family member

Patient Care Management plans are located in Appendix A.

Supporting the Patient's Vital Functions

Supporting the patient's vital physiologic functions is critical to the outcome of the patient. The administration of intravenous fluids, blood products, and medications is essential to providing adequate hemodynamic support and ensuring adequate tissue oxygenation to combat DIC and prevent end-organ damage. Blood products may include packed RBCs, fresh frozen plasma, platelet concentrates, and cryoprecipitates. The patient should be closely monitored for any adverse reaction to blood products. Medications may include heparin, antibiotics for infection (depending on the underlying cause), vasoactive agents for hemodynamic support, and analgesics for pain.

Close monitoring of vital signs, hemodynamic parameters, intake and output, and appropriate laboratory values assists in the administration and titration of appropriate agents. Frequent assessments of the patient's neurologic status, kidney function, cardiopulmonary function, and integumentary condition facilitate the early identification of impaired tissue or organ perfusion. Particular parameters to include are mental status and level of consciousness; BUN and creatinine levels; prothrombin time, activated partial thromboplastin time, and international normalized ratio values; urine output; vital signs and hemodynamic values including cardiac rhythm and oxygen saturation; and skin integrity.

Initiating Bleeding Precautions

Awareness of the patient's bleeding potential necessitates adjustments to normal nursing interventions (Box 27.3). Unnecessary venipunctures or arterial punctures that may result in bleeding, bruising, or hematomas are avoided. Blood is drawn from existing arterial or venous lines. The use of manual or automatic blood pressure cuffs is avoided whenever possible. If tracheal or oral suctioning is necessary, the use of low-level suction is recommended. Meticulous skin care is advised, keeping the skin moist and using specialty mattresses and

beds as appropriate to prevent breakdown. Gentle care is used when bathing or turning the patient to prevent bruising or hematoma formation. The patient is continually assessed for signs of bleeding, petechiae, and ecchymosis.

Providing Comfort and Emotional Support

The development of DIC in an already critically ill patient can be stressful for the patient and his or her family members. It is imperative to provide psychosocial support throughout this crisis. Calm reassurance and uncomplicated explanations of the care the patient is receiving can help allay much of the anxiety experienced. All treatments and interventions are explained before carrying them out, and questions should be answered at a level understandable to the patient and family. The use of an interpreter when English is not the primary language can enhance understanding and help avoid misconceptions. Providing spiritual support as requested may also be of assistance.

Interprofessional collaborative management of the patient with DIC is outlined in Box 27.4.

HEPARIN-INDUCED THROMBOCYTOPENIA

Description and Etiology

One form of thrombocytopenia seen in critical care patients is heparin-induced thrombocytopenia (HIT). There are two distinct types of HIT. The most common form is non–immune-mediated HIT, formally known as *type 1 HIT*.[8] Seen in 30% of patients receiving heparin therapy, this non–autoimmune condition manifests within a few days of initiation of therapy. Platelet depletion is moderate, counts are usually less than 100,000/mm^3, and the condition is transient, often resolving spontaneously. Discontinuation of heparin is not required. The second form is *type 2 HIT*, or *immune-mediated HIT*,[8] which is less commonly encountered but is more severe.[8,9] This discussion is limited to immune-mediated HIT.

Immune-mediated HIT is a response to the administration of heparin therapy. It has been observed in 0.5% to 5% of patients

BOX 27.3 Safety

Bleeding Precautions and Injury Prevention
- Handle the patient gently.
  - Use a draw sheet when repositioning the patient in bed.
  - Instruct the patient to notify the nurse immediately if bleeding or bruising is noted.
- Protect the patient from trauma.
  - Avoid rectal temperatures, enemas, and suppositories.
  - If suppositories are prescribed, lubricate liberally and administer with caution.
  - Initiate fall precautions.
  - Instruct the patient to notify the nurse immediately if any trauma occurs.
- Avoid IM injections and venipunctures.
  - If necessary, use a small-gauge needle or IV cannula.
- Apply firm pressure to any puncture sites for at least 10 minutes or until site no longer oozes blood.
- Apply ice to areas of trauma.
- Avoid the use of manual or automatic blood pressure cuff.
  - If necessary, remove cuff immediately after using it.
  - Do not leave cuff on the patient.
- Observe IV sites every few hours for bleeding.
- Shave the patient with an electric shaver only.
- Use a soft-bristled toothbrush when providing mouth care.
- Test urine and stool for occult blood as ordered.

IM, Intramuscular; *IV*, intravenous.

BOX 27.4 Summary of Management of Disseminated Intravascular Coagulation

- Identify and eliminate underlying cause.
- Provide hemodynamic support to prevent end-organ ischemia.
  - Intravenous fluids
  - Positive inotropic agents
- Administer blood and blood components.
  - Fresh frozen plasma
  - Platelets
  - Cryoprecipitate
  - Antithrombin III
- Administer medications.
  - Heparin
  - Aminocaproic acid
- Initiate bleeding precautions.
- Maintain surveillance for complications.
  - Hypovolemic shock
  - Peripheral ischemia
  - Central ischemia
  - Multiple-organ dysfunction syndrome
- Provide comfort and emotional support.

treated with unfractionated heparin and has occurred after exposure to low–molecular-weight heparin, although to a lesser degree.[8] The disorder is characterized by severe thrombocytopenia during heparin therapy. Diagnostically, it is identified by a platelet count less than 50,000/mm^3 or at least a 50% decrease from the baseline platelet count from the initiation of therapy. Onset usually occurs 5 to 10 days from the first exposure to heparin, but the onset can occur within hours of a reexposure to heparin.[8,9] The risk of developing HIT is higher in women, surgical patients, and patients with major trauma.[8] High-risk surgical procedures include cardiac surgery and orthopedic surgery.[8]

Pathophysiology

The thrombocytopenia that occurs with immune-mediated HIT is related to the formation of heparin-antibody complexes. These complexes release a substance known as *platelet factor 4*. Platelet factor 4 attracts heparin molecules, forming immunogenic complexes that adhere to platelet and endothelial surfaces (Fig. 27.2). Activation of platelets stimulates the release of thrombin and the subsequent formation of platelet clumps.[8,9]

Patients with immune-mediated HIT are at greater risk for thrombosis than bleeding. Thrombotic complications develop in 20% to 50% of patients and can occur in both the venous and the arterial system.[8] Vessel occlusion can result in the need for limb amputation, stroke, acute myocardial infarction, and death.[8–10] The resultant formation of fibrin- and platelet-rich thrombi is the primary characteristic of HIT that distinguishes it from other forms of thrombocytopenia and gives rise to its more descriptive name: white clot syndrome.[9]

Assessment and Diagnosis

HIT can be associated with severe consequences. Rapid recognition of risk factors and subsequent development of signs and symptoms are essential in treating this condition.

Clinical Manifestations

Common signs and symptoms are listed in Table 27.3. The clinical manifestations of HIT are related to the formation of thrombi and subsequent vessel occlusion.[8] Most thrombotic events are venous, although venous and arterial thrombosis can occur. Thrombotic events typically include deep vein thrombosis, pulmonary embolism, limb ischemia thrombosis, thrombotic stroke, and myocardial infarction.[8,11] The presence of blanching and the loss of peripheral pulses, sensation, or motor function in a limb indicate peripheral vascular thrombi. Neurologic signs and symptoms such as confusion, headache, and impaired speech can signal the onset of cerebral artery occlusion and stroke. Acute myocardial infarction may be heralded by dyspnea, chest pain, pallor, and alterations in blood pressure. Thrombi in the pulmonary vasculature may be evidenced by pleuritic pain, rales, and dyspnea.

Laboratory Findings

The key indicator for identifying HIT is the platelet count. General consensus in the literature considers a platelet count of less than 100,000/mm^3 or a sudden drop of 50% from the patient's baseline after initiation of heparin therapy to strongly indicate HIT.[8–11]

Two types of assays are available to assist in confirming the diagnosis of HIT: activation assays, based on platelet aggregation or the release of granular contents such as serotonin, and assays that identify the HIT

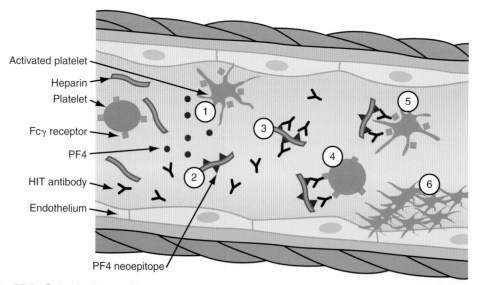

Activated platelet
Heparin
Platelet
Fcγ receptor
PF4
HIT antibody
Endothelium
PF4 neoepitope

Fig. 27.2 Pathophysiology of Heparin-Induced Thrombocytopenia (HIT). (1) Activated platelets release procoagulant proteins from α-granules, including platelet factor 4 (PF4). Administered heparin binds PF4 (2), which undergoes a conformation change and expresses a new antigen (neoepitope). Individuals with HIT produce an immunoglobulin G (IgG) antibody that specifically reacts (3) with multiple identical neoepitopes on the heparin-PF4 complex. The reaction forms heparin-PF4-IgG immune complexes. Platelets express FcγRIIa receptors (Fcγ receptor) that react (4) with the Fc portion of IgG in immune complexes. Cross-linking of Fc receptors (5) results in FcγRIIa-dependent platelet activation. The activated platelets mediate a series of events that lead to further activation of the coagulation cascade, resulting in thrombin generation. Further release of PF4 from newly activated platelets leads to a cycle of continuing platelet activation and (6) formation of a primary clot. The reaction can be enhanced by the release of platelet-derived microparticles that are rich in surface phosphatidylserine and increase activation of coagulation and by the binding of heparin-PF4 complexes and HIT-IgG to the vascular endothelium (not shown). (From McCance KL, Huether SE, eds. *Pathophysiology: The Biologic Basis for Disease in Adults and Children.* 8th ed. St. Louis: Elsevier; 2019.)

TABLE 27.3 Diagnostic Data for Heparin-Induced Thrombocytopenia.

System or Study	Signs and Symptoms
Cardiac	Chest pain, diaphoresis, pallor, alterations in blood pressure, dysrhythmias
Vascular	Arterial: pain, pallor, pulselessness, paresthesia, paralysis
	Venous: pain, tenderness, unilateral leg swelling, warmth, erythema, palpable cord, pain on passive dorsiflexion of foot, spontaneous maintenance of relaxed foot in abnormal plantar flexion (Homans sign)
Pulmonary	Dyspnea, pleuritic pain, rales, chest pain, chest wall tenderness, back pain, shoulder pain, upper abdominal pain, syncope, hemoptysis, shortness of breath, wheezing
Renal	Thirst, decreased urine output, dizziness, orthostatic hypotension
Gastrointestinal	Abdominal pain, vomiting, bloody diarrhea, abnormal bowel sounds
Neurologic	Confusion, headache, impaired speech patterns, hemiparesis or hemiplegia, vision disturbances, dysarthria, aphasia, ataxia, vertigo, nystagmus, sudden decrease in consciousness
Laboratory	Platelets <50,000/mm^3 or sudden drop of 30%—50% from baseline; positive results for HIPA, SRA, ELISA

ELISA, Enzyme-linked immunosorbent assay; *HIPA*, heparin-induced platelet aggregation; *SRA*, serotonin release assay.

antigen. Activation assays are highly sensitive in detecting the presence of HIT. The most common assay used is heparin-induced platelet aggregation. Serotonin release assay is used by a few institutions. The enzyme-linked immunosorbent assay identifies the presence of the HIT antigen.[9,10]

Medical Management

Early identification is critical to managing the effects of immune-mediated HIT. Current guidelines suggest that platelet count monitoring be performed every 2 or 3 days from day 4 to day 14 for high-risk patients.[12] When a decrease in the platelet count is detected, heparin therapy is discontinued immediately, and the patient is tested for the presence of heparin antibodies.[8–12] If the original indication for heparin still exists or new thromboses occur, an alternative form of anticoagulation is usually necessary.[12]

Direct Thrombin Inhibitors

Direct thrombin inhibitors (DTIs) are being used with increasing frequency to treat HIT. DTIs bind directly to the thrombin molecule, inhibiting its action.[11] Argatroban is the only medication approved for use in the United States at the present time. Warfarin, although commonly used to treat deep vein thrombosis, is not indicated as a sole agent in treating HIT because of its prolonged onset of action. Studies have shown that the use of warfarin without concomitant use of DTIs can significantly increase the incidence of thrombosis in patients with HIT.[11]

Nursing Management

The patient care management plan for a patient with HIT incorporates a variety of patient problems (Box 27.5). Priority patient care interventions

include decreasing the incidence of heparin exposure, maintaining surveillance for complications, providing comfort and emotional support, and educating the patient and family. Prevention of HIT is a major nursing focus, because most critically ill patients receive heparin as part of their plan of care and thus are at risk for this disorder. Initial assessment is crucial to identifying patients at risk for HIT. A medical history that includes previous heparin therapy, deep vein thrombosis, or cardiovascular surgery that involved the use of cardiopulmonary bypass can signal potential problems.

Decreasing the Incidence of Heparin Exposure

Ensuring that all heparin has been removed from the patient's hemodynamic pressure monitoring system, avoiding the use of heparin-coated catheters and discontinuing heparin flushes to maintain the patency of other intravenous lines are essential elements of nursing management.

Maintaining Surveillance for Complications

Patients with HIT remain at high risk for thrombotic complications for several days or weeks after cessation of heparin. Key nursing actions include vigilant monitoring, early recognition of signs and symptoms, and strategies to prevent deep vein thrombosis. Prompt notification of the physician of any complications that occur is critical to patient outcome.

Educating the Patient and Family

Early in the patient's hospital stay, the patient and family are taught about HIT, its etiologies, and its treatment (Box 27.6). Education of the patient and family is part of prevention of subsequent episodes in patients sensitized to heparin. Closer to discharge, the patient's education plan focuses on the interventions necessary for preventing the reoccurrence of HIT, including measures to avoid future exposure to heparin. The use of medical alert bracelets and listing heparin allergies in the medical record are necessary to avoid this serious complication in the future.

Interprofessional collaborative management of the patient with HIT is outlined in Box 27.7.

SICKLE CELL ANEMIA

Description and Etiology

Sickle cell anemia (SCA) is a hereditary disease in which RBCs form an abnormal sickle or crescent shape. RBCs carry oxygen to the body and are normally shaped like a disk.[13,14] The sickle-shaped cells have a shortened life span; are unable to carry adequate oxygen to tissues and become trapped in the vasculature because of their shape; and can cause severe pain, increased risk of infection, and life-threatening complications.[13,14]

SCA is an autosomal recessive genetic disorder. An individual with normal hemoglobin has two copies of hemoglobin A (HbA) gene. An individual with SCA has two copies of hemoglobin S (HbS) gene. Individuals who have one gene for HbS and one gene for HbA are known as *carriers* of the sickle cell trait (HbAS). When two carriers have a child, there is a 25% chance that the child will have SCA (HbSS), a 50% chance that the child will have sickle cell trait (HbAS), and a 25% chance that the child will have entirely normal hemoglobin (HbAA).[15] This genetic trait is found in people of African, Caribbean, Central American, South American, Saudi Arabian, Indian, and Mediterranean descent.[14] Most patients in the United States are African American.[14] The disease is not prevalent in persons of Asian or Pacific Islander descent.

◎ BOX 27.5   PRIORITY PATIENT CARE MANAGEMENT

Heparin-Induced Thrombocytopenia
- Impaired Peripheral Tissue Perfusion due to decreased blood flow
- Ineffective Tissue Perfusion due to decreased myocardial blood flow
- Ineffective Tissue Perfusion due to decreased kidney blood flow
- Ineffective Tissue Perfusion due to decreased gastrointestinal blood flow
- Ineffective Tissue Perfusion due to decreased cerebral blood flow
- Powerlessness due to lack of control over current situation or disease progression
- Lack of Knowledge of Treatment Regime due to lack of previous exposure to information (see Box 27.6, Priority Patient and Family Education for Heparin-Induced Thrombocytopenia)

Patient Care Management plans are located in Appendix A.

✳ BOX 27.6   PRIORITY PATIENT AND FAMILY EDUCATION

Heparin-Induced Thrombocytopenia
Before discharge, the patient should be able to teach back the following topics:
- Pathophysiology of disease
- Purpose of heparin
- Measures to avoid future exposure to heparin
- Identify different types of heparin (unfractionated and low-molecular-weight forms)
- Encourage the purchase of a medical alert bracelet or similar type of warning device
- Tell any new health care provider about the heparin allergy and previous reaction

Additional information for the patient can be found at these websites:
- My Healthfinder: https://health.gov/myhealthfinder
- WebMD: https://www.webmd.com/

BOX 27.7   Summary of Management of Heparin-Induced Thrombocytopenia

- Stop all heparin exposure.
  - Unfractionated and low—molecular-weight heparin by any route
  - Heparin flushes
  - Heparin-coated vascular access devices
- Begin therapy with an alternative anticoagulant.
  - Argatroban
- Maintain surveillance for complications.
  - Deep vein thrombosis
  - Pulmonary emboli
  - Acute limb ischemia
  - Ischemic stroke
  - Acute myocardial infarction
- Administer antifibrinolytic therapy (as indicated) if thrombosis occurs.
- Prepare patient for surgical embolectomy (as indicated) if thrombosis occurs.
- Provide comfort and emotional support.

SCA is usually diagnosed during the first few years of life secondary to manifestation of initial symptoms. Prenatal screening that consists of DNA analysis from fetal cells is now available for at-risk couples.[15] This screening should be offered as part of their prenatal counseling. More than 40 states offer universal neonatal screening for hemoglobinopathies.[15]

Pathophysiology

Sickle cell disease (SCD) is a chronic inflammatory condition that is characterized by hemolysis and vasoocclusion. The cause of SCA is a mutation in the genetic sequence in the beta chain gene of the hemoglobin. This results in a sequence of the replacement of valine with glutamic acid at the N-terminal amino acid position 6 of the protein chain.[13] This substitution leads to the production of HbS.[14]

Normal RBCs contain hemoglobin that are flexible, biconcave disks. When deoxygenated, RBCs containing predominantly HbS distort into a crescent or sickle shape. In this form, the hemoglobin becomes rigid and friable, causing vasoocclusion in the small vessels of the circulatory system.[13] This tends to occur during times of physiologic stress, such as physical overexertion, muscle tissue ischemia, dehydration, infection, or extreme temperatures.[14] Although these conditions have a tendency to exacerbate the condition, most of the sickling events have no identifying cause.[14]

The RBCs become lodged in the vasculature and the microcirculation causing stasis and obstruction of blood flow and damage to the surrounding organs, tissue ischemia, infarction, and, if not corrected, eventually necrosis (Fig. 27.3). In addition, hemolysis of the RBCs occurs, resulting in anemia.[13]

Assessment and Diagnosis

SCA can be associated with severe consequences. Rapid recognition of signs and symptoms is essential in treating this condition.

Clinical Manifestations

Various clinical manifestations are associated with SCA (Fig. 27.4). The patient may present with a low-grade fever, bone or joint pain, pinpoint pupils, inability to follow commands, photophobia, tachycardia, tachypnea, decreased respiratory excursion, hepatomegaly, nonpalpable spleen, and pretibial ulcers.[16]

Laboratory Studies

Initial laboratory studies include a complete blood count, a peripheral blood smear, and a quantitative hemoglobin electrophoresis. Sickle cells constitute 5% to 10% of the blood smear. The elevated reticulocyte count (greater than 10%) is characteristically accompanied by the presence of Howell-Jolly bodies. Howell-Jolly bodies are small remnants of nuclear material from hemolyzed erythrocytes reflective of hyposplenia or autoinfarction and target cells (an erythrocyte with a deeply stained core surrounded by a lighter stained margin that resembles a target with a bull's eye). Typically, an elevated white blood cell (WBC) count occurs during and after a crisis. Other tests might include an indirect bilirubin level, which will be elevated following hemolysis. The haptoglobin level will be low or absent because it cannot be replaced quickly enough after severe hemolysis. Haptoglobin, a glycoprotein, exists to bind free hemoglobin that is released from hemolyzed erythrocytes.

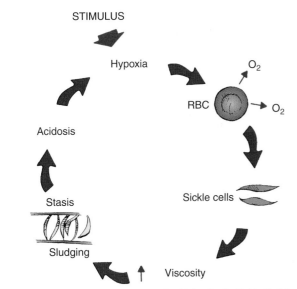

STIMULUS

Hypoxia

O_2

RBC

O_2

Acidosis

Stasis

Sickle cells

Sludging

↑ Viscosity

Fig. 27.3 Cycle Causing Vasoocclusive Episodes in Sickle Cell Anemia. *RBC,* Red blood cell. (From Hockenberry M, Coody D. *Pediatric Oncology and Hematology: Perspectives on Care.* St. Louis: Mosby; 1986.)

Medical Management

SCA is an incurable disease; however, treatment options are available for management of symptoms and complications. Bone marrow transplant offers a cure in a limited number of cases.[13] Medical interventions are aimed at preventing infections, managing pain, transfusing RBCs, and administering hydroxyurea. Patients with chronic disease are more effectively managed through a multidisciplinary approach.[13] It is also important to look at other issues that may exacerbate the patient disease process, such as diet, poor housing, inadequate housing, lack of education, poor access to services, and poor lifestyle choices.

Prevent Infection

Both children and adults with SCA are more prone to infection and have a more difficult time fighting off infection.[16] SCA can result in damage to the spleen from constant sickling of the RBCs, and damage to the spleen can prevent the destruction of bacteria in the blood. Prophylactic administration of oral antibiotics starting at age 2 months can decrease the chances of a pneumococcal infection and early death. Vaccinations against pneumococcal infections, meningitis, hepatitis, and influenza are important to prevent future infections.[16]

Pain Management

Pain associated with SCA can be acute or chronic in nature. The most common type of pain associated with SCA is vasoocclusive pain. It is commonly treated with antiinflammatory and opioid or nonopioid analgesics.[16,17] The pain associated with SCA can vary enormously; therefore numerous different approaches may be required. The medication of choice is influenced by the patient's history of analgesia use. Some patients may have extremely intricate medication regimens.[16] Paracetamol and nonsteroidal antiinflammatory drugs are used for mild to moderate pain relief. If this approach is ineffective, oral or parenteral opiates may be an alternative.[16,17]

For patients who wish to try nonpharmacologic pain control, approaches include psychologic support, massage, acupuncture, and transcutaneous electrical nerve stimulation. Distraction can be another valuable tool to use. Television, video games, repeating inspirational phrases, and mental calculations can also be a form of distraction. Studies suggested that cognitive behavioral therapy can help teach patients coping strategies for acute and chronic pain.[16]

Transfusion Therapy

RBC transfusion therapy in SCD is an important lifesaving treatment option but should be performed only after careful consideration. Transfusion therapy is primarily used for treatment of patients who are experiencing complications secondary to SCD or as an emergency measure.[17] Transfusion therapy is used with extreme caution because of risks such as iron overload; exposure to hepatitis, human immunodeficiency virus, and other infectious agents; alloimmunization; induction of hyperviscosity; and limitations on resources. The indications for having a blood transfusion or exchange are recurrent painful vasoocclusive crises with long hospital admissions, acute chest syndrome, stroke, priapism, and leg ulcers. Blood transfusions or exchange can also be performed before major operations, such as hip replacement because of avascular necrosis of the hip bone.[16]

Administration of Hydroxyurea

Hydroxyurea is an oral agent that is a safe and effective treatment for children and adults with SCA. It works by increasing the level of fetal hemoglobin in the RBCs, reducing the concentration of sickle hemoglobin and sickling itself.[16] The patient is usually started at a dosage of 15 mg/kg orally once a day. The dosage is increased by 5 mg/kg every 12 weeks until 35 mg/kg is reached, provided that the patient's blood count remains within an acceptable range. Research shows that patients receiving hydroxyurea had fewer episodes of pain and acute chest syndrome and had a decreased need for blood transfusion and hospitalizations compared with patients who received no treatment. Research showed that hydroxyurea can be used as an alternative to regular blood transfusions.[17]

Nursing Management

The patient care management plan for a patient with SCA incorporates a variety of patient problems (Box 27.8). Priority patient care interventions include supporting the patient's vital functions, providing comfort and emotional support, maintaining surveillance for complications, and educating the patient and family.

Supporting the Patient's Vital Functions

The nurse must recognize and support the patient's vital physiologic functions. Administration of intravenous fluids, blood products, and inotropic agents to provide adequate hemodynamic support and tissue oxygenation is essential in preventing or combating end-organ damage. Close monitoring of vital signs, hemodynamic parameters, intake and output, and appropriate laboratory values assists the critical care nurse in administering and titrating appropriate agents.[17] Frequent assessments include parameters for neurologic status, kidney function, cardiopulmonary function, and skin integrity that indicate impaired tissue or organ perfusion. Particular parameters to include are mental status, BUN and creatinine levels, urine output, vital signs, hemodynamic values, cardiac rhythm, ABG and pulse oximetry values, skin breakdown, ecchymoses, or hematomas.[17]

Maintaining Surveillance for Complications

The nurse needs to be vigilant for signs of life-threatening complications such as septicemia, acute myocardial infarction, priapism,

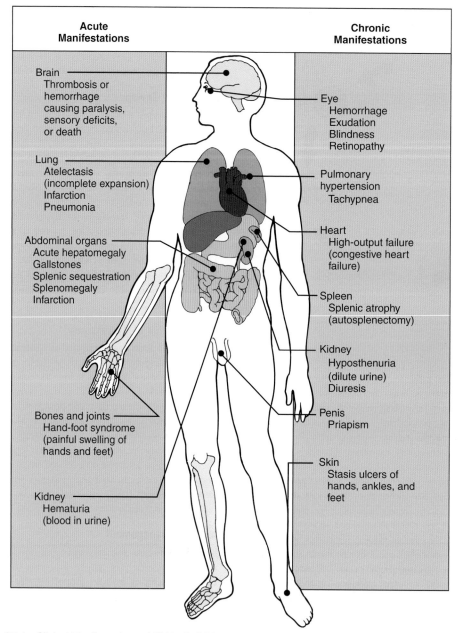

Acute Manifestations	**Chronic Manifestations**

Brain
Thrombosis or hemorrhage causing paralysis, sensory deficits, or death

Lung
Atelectasis (incomplete expansion)
Infarction
Pneumonia

Abdominal organs
Acute hepatomegaly
Gallstones
Splenic sequestration
Splenomegaly
Infarction

Bones and joints
Hand-foot syndrome (painful swelling of hands and feet)

Kidney
Hematuria (blood in urine)

Eye
Hemorrhage
Exudation
Blindness
Retinopathy

Pulmonary hypertension
Tachypnea

Heart
High-output failure (congestive heart failure)

Spleen
Splenic atrophy (autosplenectomy)

Kidney
Hyposthenuria (dilute urine)
Diuresis

Penis
Priapism

Skin
Stasis ulcers of hands, ankles, and feet

Fig. 27.4 Clinical Manifestations of Sickle Cell Disease. (From McCance KL, Huether SE, eds. *Pathophysiology: The Biologic Basis for Disease in Adults and Children.* 8th ed. St. Louis: 2019; Elsevier.)

ischemic stroke, and shock.[13] If there are any significant concerns, these must be reported immediately. Other issues that may arise are dehydration, hypoxia, infection, skin and tissue viability, and decreased hemoglobin levels.

Educating the Patient and Family

Although there is no cure for SCA, the focus of care is prevention. Early in the patient's hospital stay, the patient and family are taught about SCA, its etiologies, and its treatment (Box 27.9). The patient and family education plan focuses on measures to help prevent recurrence of painful episodes. If the patient smokes, he or she is encouraged to stop smoking and is referred to a *smoking cessation program.* In addition, the importance of continuous medical follow-up is stressed. While research continues to try to find a cure, nurses must continue to

be sensitive to the effects of the disease on the patient and the family and the need to be culturally sensitive.[13]

Interprofessional collaborative management of the patient with SCA is outlined in Box 27.10.

TUMOR LYSIS SYNDROME

Description and Etiology

Tumor lysis syndrome (TLS) refers to a variety of metabolic disturbances that may be seen with the treatment of cancer. A potentially lethal complication of various forms of cancer treatment, TLS occurs when large numbers of neoplastic cells are rapidly killed, resulting in the release of large amounts of potassium, phosphate, and uric acid

⊚ BOX 27.8 PRIORITY PATIENT CARE MANAGEMENT

Sickle Cell Anemia
- Acute Pain due to transmission and perception of cutaneous, visceral, muscular, or ischemic impulses
- Impaired Peripheral Tissue Perfusion due to decreased blood flow
- Ineffective Tissue Perfusion due to decreased kidney blood flow
- Ineffective Tissue Perfusion due to decreased gastrointestinal blood flow
- Ineffective Tissue Perfusion due to decreased cerebral blood flow
- Powerlessness due to lack of control over current situation or disease progression
- Lack of Knowledge of Treatment Regime due to lack of previous exposure to information (see Box 27.9, Priority Patient and Family Education for Sickle Cell Anemia)

Patient Care Management plans are located in Appendix A.

BOX 27.10 Summary of Management of Sickle Cell Anemia

- Prevent infection.
  - Prophylactic antibiotics
  - Vaccinations
- Manage pain.
  - Pharmacologic management
  - Nonpharmacologic management
- Administer blood.
- Administer hydroxyurea.
- Maintain surveillance for complications.
  - Septicemia
  - Acute kidney injury
  - Acute myocardial infarction
  - Acute limb ischemia
  - Ischemic stroke
  - Anemia
- Provide comfort and emotional support.

into the systemic circulation. It is most commonly seen in patients with lymphoma, leukemia, large bulky tumors, or multiple metastatic conditions who are receiving cytotoxic chemotherapy.[18,19]

Although most often associated with the use of chemotherapeutic medications, TLS has also been associated with immunotherapy, monoclonal antibody therapy, radiation therapy, and hormone therapy.[18–20] In rare instances, TLS can occur spontaneously.[18] Certain preexisting conditions can place the patient at higher risk for developing TLS, including dehydration, hypotension, elevated uric acid, splenomegaly, and chronic renal insufficiency.[18,20]

Pathophysiology

The primary mechanism involved in the development of TLS is the destruction of massive numbers of malignant cells by chemotherapy or radiation therapy (Fig. 27.5). Massive destruction of cells releases large amounts of potassium, phosphorus, and nucleic acids, leading to severe metabolic disturbances such as hyperuricemia, hyperkalemia, hyperphosphatemia, and hypocalcemia (Table 27.4). Vomiting, diarrhea, and other insensible fluid losses from fever or tachypnea also contribute to these electrolyte disturbances.[18] Death of patients with TLS is most often caused by complications of acute kidney injury or cardiac arrest.[18–20]

Hyperuricemia

Hyperuricemia occurs 48 to 72 hours after the initiation of anticancer therapy.[18] Tumor cells undergo rapid growth and development, and large amounts of nucleic acids are present within them. When therapy is initiated, tumor cell destruction releases nucleic acids, which are metabolized into uric acid. Metabolic acidosis ensues, resulting in crystallization of the uric acid in the distal tubules of the kidney and leading to obstruction of urine flow. Glomerular filtration rates decrease as the kidneys are unable to clear the increasing amounts of uric acid. Consequently, acute kidney injury eventually occurs.[21] Acute kidney injury is discussed further in Chapter 19.

Hyperuricemia associated with TLS can be potentiated by several other factors, including elevated uric acid levels before the initiation of therapy. Other causes of increased uric acid production are elevated WBC counts; destruction of WBCs; and enlargement of the lymph nodes, spleen, or liver.[18]

Hyperkalemia

Hyperkalemia occurs within 6 to 72 hours after the initiation of chemotherapy. This is the most deleterious of all the manifestations of TLS.[18] In addition to the release of nucleic acids, tumor cell destruction also results in the release of potassium. Renal insufficiency related to hyperuricemia prevents adequate excretion of potassium, and levels rise. The resultant hyperkalemia may have a profound effect on intracellular and extracellular fluid levels.[22] Left

✴ BOX 27.9 PRIORITY PATIENT AND FAMILY EDUCATION

Sickle Cell Anemia
Before discharge, the patient should be able to teach back the following topics:
- Pathophysiology of disease
- Precipitating factor modification
- Importance of taking medications
- Maintenance of adequate hydration (especially during febrile periods and hot weather)
- Use of pharmacologic and nonpharmacologic methods of pain management
- Avoidance of situations that can precipitate condition such as extreme cold
- Smoking cessation and avoidance of secondhand smoke

- Importance of plenty of rest and relaxation and avoiding exhaustive exercise
- Genetic screening
- Encourage the purchase of a medical alert bracelet or similar type of warning device

Additional information for the patient can be found at these websites:
- Sickle Cell Disease Association of America: https://www.sicklecelldisease.org/
- Smokefree.gov: https://smokefree.gov/
- My Healthfinder: https://health.gov/myhealthfinder
- WebMD: https://www.webmd.com/

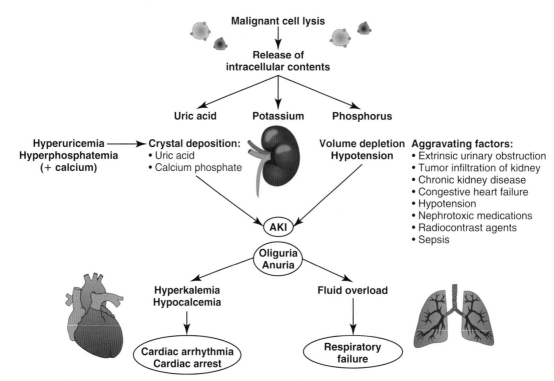

Fig. 27.5 Tumor Lysis Syndrome. Metabolic abnormalities in tumor lysis syndrome and clinical consequences. *AKI*, Acute kidney injury. (From Abu-Alfa AK, Younes A. Tumor lysis syndrome and acute kidney injury: evaluation, prevention and management. *Am J Kidney Dis.* 2010;55[5 Suppl 3]:S1–S13.)

untreated, hyperkalemia can have devastating consequences, including cardiac arrest and death.[18]

Hyperphosphatemia and Hypocalcemia

Hyperphosphatemia and hypocalcemia occur 24 to 48 hours after the initiation of therapy.[18] Phosphorus levels also rise as a consequence of tumor cell destruction. Calcium ions then bind with the excess phosphorus, creating calcium phosphate salts and bringing about hypocalcemia. These salts precipitate in the kidney tubules, worsening renal insufficiency. Hypocalcemia causes tetany and cardiac dysrhythmias, which can result in cardiac arrest and death.[21,22]

Assessment and Diagnosis

Detection and recognition of TLS is accomplished through assessment of clinical manifestations, evaluation of laboratory findings, and other diagnostic tests. Table 27.5 summarizes common findings in TLS.[18,20]

Clinical Manifestations

Clinical manifestations are related to the metabolic disturbances associated with TLS.[20] The patient's history reveals an unexplained weight gain after initiation of chemotherapy or radiation therapy. The weight gain is associated with fluid retention secondary to electrolyte disturbances. Other early signs heralding the onset of TLS include

TABLE 27.4 Electrolyte Abnormalities in Tumor Lysis Syndrome.

Electrolyte	Pathophysiology	Clinical Consequence	Treatment Options
Potassium	Rapid expulsion of intracellular K$^+$ into circulation due to cell lysis	Adverse skeletal and cardiac manifestations (e.g., ventricular dysrhythmias, weakness, paresthesias)	Insulin/glucose, sodium bicarbonate, inhaled beta-agonist, K$^+$-binding resins, dialysis, calcium gluconate
Phosphate	Release of intracellular PO$_4^-$ due to cell lysis May be compounded by renal dysfunction	Muscle cramps, tetany, dysrhythmias, seizures	Dialysis, phosphate binders
Calcium	Precipitation of calcium phosphate complex because of rapid increase in phosphorus concentration	Muscle cramps, tetany, dysrhythmias, seizures, acute kidney injury (acute nephrocalcinosis)	Calcium gluconate (treatment should be reserved for patients with neuromuscular irritability)
Uric acid	Cell lysis leads to increased levels of purine nucleic acids into circulation that are metabolized to uric acid	Renal failure (uric acid nephropathy)	Hydration, dialysis, xanthine oxidase inhibitors, alkalization of urine, urate oxidase

From Davidson MB, Thakkar S, Hix JK, Bhandarkar ND, Wong A, Schreiber MJ. Pathophysiology, clinical consequences, and treatment of tumor lysis syndrome. *Am J Med.* 2004;116(8):546–554.

TABLE 27.5 Diagnostic Data for Tumor Lysis Syndrome.

Diagnostic Parameter	Findings
Clinical	Weight gain, edema, diarrhea, lethargy, muscle cramps, nausea and vomiting, paresthesia, weakness, oliguria, uremia, seizures
Laboratory	↑ Potassium, phosphorus, uric acid, BUN, Cr ↓ Calcium, Cr clearance, pH, bicarbonate, PaCO$_2$
Diagnostic	Positive Chvostek and Trousseau signs, hyperactive deep tendon reflexes, dysrhythmias, ECG changes

BUN, Blood urea nitrogen; *Cr*, creatinine; *ECG*, electrocardiogram; *PaCO$_2$*, arterial partial pressure of carbon dioxide; ↑, increased; ↓, decreased.

diarrhea, lethargy, muscle cramps, nausea, vomiting, paresthesias, and weakness.[19]

Laboratory Findings

Laboratory findings demonstrate electrolyte disturbances such as elevated potassium and phosphorus levels and a decreased calcium level. Uric acid levels are increased. Elevated levels of BUN and creatinine and decreased creatinine clearance also indicate TLS. Metabolic acidosis is confirmed by the presence of decreased pH, bicarbonate levels, and arterial partial pressure of carbon dioxide (PaCO$_2$) on ABG measurements.[19]

Other Diagnostic Tests

Physical examination reveals positive Chvostek and Trousseau signs related to hypocalcemia. Hyperactive deep tendon reflexes indicate hyperkalemia and hypocalcemia.[20] Potassium and calcium disturbances result in changes that can be seen on the electrocardiogram, such as peaked or inverted T waves, altered QT intervals, widened QRS complexes, and dysrhythmias.[18]

Medical Management

Medical interventions are aimed at maintaining adequate hydration, treating metabolic imbalances, and preventing life-threatening complications (see Table 27.4).[19,22]

Adequate Hydration

Administration of intravenous fluids may be necessary early in the course of treatment if inadequate hydration exists. The administration of isotonic saline (0.9% normal saline) reduces serum concentrations of uric acid, phosphate, and potassium.[20] The use of nonthiazide diuretics to maintain adequate urine output may be required. If acute kidney injury occurs, hemodialysis is considered.[20]

Metabolic Imbalances

Electrolytes and ABGs are closely monitored. Dietary restrictions of potassium and phosphorus may be necessary. The goals in treating hyperuricemia are to inhibit uric acid formation and to increase renal clearance.[22] This can be accomplished through the administration of sodium bicarbonate to increase the pH of the urine to greater than 7.0, which increases the solubility of uric acid, preventing subsequent crystallization. Allopurinol administration can also inhibit uric acid formation.[20]

Life-Threatening Complications

If potassium levels rise dangerously, sodium polystyrene sulfonate (Kayexalate) may be given orally, or if the patient is unable to tolerate oral medications because of nausea and vomiting, rectal instillation may be used. If the patient is oliguric, glucose and insulin infusions may be given to facilitate lowering the potassium levels. A 10% solution of calcium gluconate may be administered to stabilize cardiac tissue membranes to prevent life-threatening dysrhythmias.[23] Phosphorus-binding antacids can be used for treating hyperphosphatemia. Stool softeners may be necessary to treat the constipation often associated with the administration of these antacids. Calcium gluconate may be required to replace calcium, but it should be used judiciously.[18]

Nursing Management

The patient care management plan for a patient with TLS incorporates a variety of patient problems (Box 27.11). Priority patient care interventions include monitoring fluid and electrolytes, providing comfort and emotional support, maintaining surveillance for complications, and education of the patient and family.

Monitoring Fluid and Electrolytes

Assessment and continued monitoring of the patient is an important role of the critical care nurse when caring for a patient with TLS. Recognizing critical laboratory changes or development of symptoms and notifying the physician in a timely manner are essential. Insertion of a urinary catheter and maintenance of the intravenous line site are necessary to ensure adequate intake and output. Vital signs are monitored frequently and the patient's weight is monitored daily.

Maintaining Surveillance for Complications

Nursing interventions are aimed at preventing complications. Seizure precautions are instituted, especially if calcium levels are disrupted. Insertion of a nasogastric tube is appropriate if nausea or vomiting occurs. Dietary adjustments are necessary, such as potassium and phosphorus restrictions in the presence of elevated serum levels and providing additional fiber to combat the constipation associated with the administration of antacids.[23]

Educating the Patient and Family

Early in the patient's hospital stay, the patient and family are taught about TLS, its etiologies, and its treatment. All treatments and interventions are explained before carrying them out, and questions should be answered at a level understandable to the patient and family. Before discharge, potential risk factors and identification of early signs and symptoms are reviewed.

Interprofessional collaborative management of the patient with TLS is outlined in Box 27.12.

BOX 27.11 PRIORITY PATIENT CARE MANAGEMENT

Tumor Lysis Syndrome
- Hypervolemia due to renal dysfunction
- Impaired Cardiac Output due to alterations in contractility
- Anxiety due to threat to biologic, psychologic, or social integrity
- Impaired Adaptation due to a situational crisis and personal vulnerability

Patient Care Management plans are located in Appendix A.

BOX 27.12 Summary of Management of Tumor Lysis Syndrome

- Facilitate adequate kidney function.
  - Volume hydration with 0.9% normal saline
  - Nonthiazide diuretics
- Treat hyperkalemia.
  - Kayexalate
  - Glucose and insulin
- Treat hyperuricemia.
  - Sodium bicarbonate
  - Allopurinol
- Treat hyperphosphatemia.
  - Dietary restrictions
  - Phosphorus-binding antacids
- Treat hypocalcemia.
  - Calcium gluconate
- Maintain surveillance for complications.
  - Acute kidney injury
  - Cardiac dysrhythmias
- Provide comfort and emotional support.

QSEN

BOX 27.13 Informatics

Internet Resources: Hematologic and Oncologic Emergencies
- American Association of Critical-Care Nurses (AACN): https://www.aacn.org/
- American College of Physicians (ACP): https://www.acponline.org/
- American College of Surgeons: https://www.facs.org/
- American Medical Association (AMA): https://www.ama-assn.org/
- American Society of Clinical Oncology (ASCO): https://www.asco.org/
- American Society of Hematology: https://www.hematology.org/
- British Society for Haematology: https://b-s-h.org.uk/
- Cancer Network: https://www.cancernetwork.com/
- National Heart, Lung, and Blood Institute: https://www.nhlbi.nih.gov/
- Society of Critical Care Medicine (SCCM): https://www.sccm.org/Home

ADDITIONAL RESOURCES

See Box 27.13 for Internet resources pertaining to hematologic disorders and oncologic emergencies.

REFERENCES

1. Levi M, Scully M. How I treat disseminated intravascular coagulation. *Blood.* 2018;131(8):845–854.
2. Iba T, Levi M, Levy JH. Sepsis-induced coagulopathy and disseminated intravascular coagulation. *Semin Thromb Hemost.* 2019;116(1):89–95.
3. Levi M. Pathogenesis and diagnosis of disseminated intravascular coagulation. *Int J Lab Hematol.* 2018;40(suppl 1):15–20.
4. Erez O, Mastrolia SA, Thachil J. Disseminated intravascular coagulation in pregnancy: insights in pathophysiology, diagnosis and management. *Am J Obstet Gynecol.* 2015;213(4):452–463.
5. Huether KL, Rote NS, McCance KL. Structure and function of the hematologic system. In: McCance KL, Huether SE, eds. *Pathophysiology: The Biologic Basis for Disease in Adults and Children.* 8th ed. St. Louis: Elsevier; 2019.
6. Levi M, Sivapalaratnam S. Disseminated intravascular coagulation: an update on pathogenesis and diagnosis. *Expert Rev Hematol.* 2018;11(8):663–672.
7. Levi M, van der Poll T. A short contemporary history of disseminated intravascular coagulation. *Semin Thromb Hemost.* 2014;40(8):874–880.
8. Hogan M, Berger JS. Heparin-induced thrombocytopenia (HIT): review of incidence, diagnosis, and management. *Vasc Med.* 2020;25(2):160–173.
9. Warkentin TE, Greinacher A. Management of heparin-induced thrombocytopenia. *Curr Opin Hematol.* 2016;23(5):462–470.
10. Arepally GM, Cines DB. Pathogenesis of heparin-induced thrombocytopenia. *Transl Res.* 2020;225:131–140. http://doi.org/10.1016/j.trsl.2020.04.014.
11. Frazer CA. Heparin-induced thrombocytopenia. *J Infus Nurs.* 2017;40(2):98–100.
12. Cuker A, Arepally GM, Chong BH, et al. American Society of Hematology 2018 guidelines for management of heparin-induced thrombocytopenia. *Blood Adv.* 2018;2(22):3360–3392.
13. Ware RE, de Montalembert M, Tshilolo L, Abboud MR. Sickle cell disease. *Lancet.* 2017;390(10091):311–323.
14. Strouse J. Sickle cell disease. *Handb Clin Neurol.* 2016;138:311–324. https://doi.org/10.1016/B978-0-12-802973-2.00018-5.
15. Jorde LB. Genes and genetic diseases. In: McCance KL, Huether SE, eds. *Pathophysiology: The Biologic Basis for Disease in Adults and Children.* 8th ed. St. Louis: Elsevier; 2019.
16. Lovett PB, Sule HP, Lopez BL. Sickle cell disease in the emergency department. *Hematol Oncol Clin North Am.* 2017;31(6):1061–1079.
17. Azar S, Wong TE. Sickle cell disease: a brief update. *Med Clin North Am.* 2017;101(2):375–393.
18. Strauss PZ, Hamlin SK, Dang J. Tumor lysis syndrome: a unique solute disturbance. *Nurs Clin North Am.* 2017;52(2):309–320.
19. Delaney E, Nilolai C, Coe K. Metabolic emergencies. In: Brant JM, ed. *Core Curriculum for Oncology Nursing.* 6th ed. St. Louis: Elsevier; 2020.
20. Wagner J, Arora S. Oncologic metabolic emergencies. *Hematol Oncol Clin North Am.* 2017;31(6):941–957.
21. Dubbs SB. Rapid fire: tumor lysis syndrome. *Emerg Med Clin North Am.* 2018;36(3):517–525.
22. Criscuolo M, Fianchi L, Dragonetti G, Pagano L. Tumor lysis syndrome: review of pathogenesis, risk factors and management of a medical emergency. *Expert Rev Hematol.* 2016;9(2):197–208.
23. Williams SM, Killeen AA. Tumor lysis syndrome. *Arch Pathol Lab Med.* 2019;143(3):386–393.

Patient Care Management Plans

Kathleen M. Stacy

◎ PATIENT CARE MANAGEMENT PLAN

Activity Intolerance

Activity Intolerance Due to Cardiopulmonary Dysfunction

Signs and Symptoms

- Chest pain with activity
- Electrocardiogram (ECG) changes with activity
- Heart rate is >15 beats/min above baseline with activity for patients on beta-blockers or calcium channel blockers
- Heart rate remains elevated above baseline 5 minutes after activity
- Breathlessness with activity
- SpO_2 <92% with activity
- Postural hypotension when moving from supine to upright position
- Patient reports fatigue with activity

Outcomes

- Heart rate is <20 beats/min above baseline with activity and is <10 beats/min above baseline with activity for patients on beta-blockers or calcium channel blockers.
- Heart rate returns to baseline 5 minutes after activity.
- Chest pain with activity is absent.
- Patient reports tolerance to activity.

Interventions and Rationale

1. Encourage active or passive range-of-motion exercises while the patient is in bed **to keep joints flexible and muscles stretched.**
2. Teach the patient to refrain from holding breath while performing exercises and **to avoid Valsalva maneuver.**
3. Encourage performance of muscle-toning exercises at least three times daily because a toned muscle uses less oxygen when performing work than an untoned muscle.
4. Progress ambulation to increase tolerance to activity.
5. Teach the patient to take pulse **to determine activity tolerance:** Take pulse for a full minute before exercise and then for 10 seconds and multiply by 6 at exercise peak.
6. Collaborate with the practitioner regarding administration of fluids to ensure that the patient is hydrated to 24-hour fluid requirements per body surface area **to increase preload and increase stroke volume and cardiac output.**

Activity Intolerance Due to Prolonged Immobility or Deconditioning

Signs and Symptoms

- Decrease in systolic blood pressure is >20 mm Hg.
- Increase in heart rate is >20 beats/min with postural change.
- Syncope occurs with postural change.
- Patient reports lightheadedness with postural change.

Outcomes

- Decrease in systolic blood pressure is <10 mm Hg.
- Increase in heart rate is <10 beats/min with postural change.
- Syncope or lightheadedness is absent with postural change.
- Hypoxemia is absent.
- Patient reports tolerance to activity.

Interventions and Rationale

1. Collaborate with the practitioner regarding the patient's activity level and the need for physical therapy **to ensure the patient's safety.**
2. Collaborate with the physical therapist to develop a progressive activity plan for the patient **to return to prior level of function.**

   For Patient on Bed Rest
1. Instruct the patient how to perform straight-leg raises, dorsiflexion or plantar flexion, and quadriceps-setting and gluteal-setting exercises **to increase muscular and vascular tone.**
2. Reposition the patient incrementally **to avoid syncope:**
   a. Head of bed to 45 degrees and hold until symptom-free
   b. Head of bed to 90 degrees and hold until symptom-free
   c. Dangle until symptom-free
   d. Stand until symptom-free and ambulate

   For Patient on Mechanical Ventilation
1. Collaborate with the practitioner, respiratory care practitioner, and physical therapist regarding the patient's eligibility for early progressive mobility **to ensure patient is ready and able to participate.**
2. Initiate early progressive mobility program when the patient is ready **to limit the effects of prolonged immobility.**
   a. Elevate the head of the bed.
   b. Turn patient every 2 hours.
   c. Perform passive range of motion at least three times a day.
   d. Progress patient to active range of motion when ready.
   e. Place bed in chair position to position patient in upright/leg-down position.
   f. Initiate bed mobility activities such as sitting on the edge of the bed (dangling).
   g. Initiate transfer training.
   h. Implement pregait activities such as standing at the side of the bed and marching in place.
   i. Progress patient to ambulation.
3. Monitor the patient's response to activity and discontinue activity if patient shows signs of intolerance **to ensure patient safety:**
   a. Hypoxemia
   b. Hypotension
   c. Dysrhythmias or ECG changes

◎ PATIENT CARE MANAGEMENT PLAN

Acute Pain
Acute Pain Due to Transmission and Perception of Cutaneous, Visceral, Muscular, or Ischemic Impulses
Signs and Symptoms
Subjective
- Patient verbalizes presence of pain
- Patient rates pain on a scale of 1—10 using a visual analog scale

Objective
- Increase in blood pressure, heart rate, and respiratory rate
- Pupillary dilation
- Diaphoresis, pallor
- Skeletal muscle reactions (e.g., grimacing, clenching fists, writhing, pacing, guarding, or splinting of affected part)
- Apprehension, fearful appearance
- May not exhibit any physiologic change

Outcomes
- Patient verbalizes that pain is reduced to a tolerable level or is totally relieved.
- Patient's pain rating is lower on a scale of 1—10.
- Blood pressure, heart rate, and respiratory rate return to baseline 5 minutes after intravenous (IV) administration of an opioid analgesic or 20 minutes after intramuscular administration of an opioid analgesic.

Interventions and Rationale
1. Modify variables that heighten the patient's experience of pain.
   a. Explain to the patient that frequent, detailed, and seemingly repetitive assessments will be conducted to allow the nurse to better understand the patient's pain experience, not because the existence of pain is in question.
   b. Explain the factors responsible for pain production in the individual. Estimate the expected duration of the pain if possible.
   c. Explain diagnostic and therapeutic procedures to the patient in relation to sensations the patient should expect to feel.
   d. Reduce the patient's fear of addiction by explaining the difference between drug tolerance and drug dependence. **Drug tolerance is a physiologic phenomenon in which a medication begins to lose effectiveness after repeated doses; drug dependence is a psychological phenomenon in which opioids are used regularly for emotional, not medical, reasons.**
   e. Instruct the patient to ask for pain medication when pain is beginning and not to wait until it is intolerable.
   f. Explain that the practitioner will be consulted if pain relief is inadequate with the present medication.
   g. Instruct the patient in the importance of adequate rest, especially when it reduces pain **to maintain strength and coping abilities and to reduce stress.**
2. Collaborate with the practitioner regarding pharmacologic interventions.
   a. For postoperative or posttraumatic cutaneous, muscular, or visceral pain, perform the following:
      (1) Medicate with an opioid analgesic to break the pain cycles as long as level of consciousness and vital signs are stable.
      (2) Check the patient's previous response to similar dosage and opioids.
      (3) Establish optimal analgesic dose that brings optimal pain relief.
      (4) Offer pain medication at prescribed regular intervals rather than making the patient ask for it **to maintain more steady blood levels.**
      (5) Consider waking the patient to avoid loss of opiate blood levels during sleep.

(6) If administering medication on as-needed (PRN) basis, give it when the patient's pain is just beginning, rather than at its peak.
   (a) Advise the patient to intercept pain, not endure it, or several hours and higher doses of opioid analgesics may be necessary to relieve pain, leading to a cycle of undermedication and pain alternating with overmedication and drug toxicity.
(7) Perform rehabilitation exercises (turn, deep breathe, leg exercises, ambulate) shortly before peak of drug effect **because this will be the optimal time for the patient to increase activity with the least risk of increasing pain.**
(8) When making the transition from one drug to another or from intramuscular or IV to oral medication, use an equianalgesic chart. **Equianalgesic means approximately the same pain relief. The patient's response should be closely monitored to determine whether the right analgesic choice was made.**
(9) To assess effectiveness of pain medication, do the following:
   (a) Reevaluate pain 15—30 minutes after IV and 30—60 minutes after oral medication administration; observe the patient's behavior, and ask the patient to rate pain on a scale of 1—10.
   (b) Collaborate with the practitioner to add or delete other medications that potentiate the action of analgesics, such as antiemetics, hypnotics, sedatives, or muscle relaxants.
   (c) Observe for indicators of undertreatment: report of pain not relieved; observed restlessness, sleeplessness, irritability, and anorexia; decreased activity level.
   (d) Observe for indicators of overtreatment: hypotension or bradycardia; respiratory rate <10/min; excessive sedation.
(10) Evaluate the patient's level of sedation and respiratory rate at regular intervals **to avoid oversedation.**
   (a) Respirations should be counted for a full minute and qualified according to rhythm and depth of chest excursion.
   (b) Consider the use of capnography (end-tidal carbon dioxide monitoring) as an early indicator of hypoventilation and oversedation.
(11) If patient-controlled analgesia (PCA) is used, perform the following:
   (a) Instruct the patient on what the drug is, the dose, and how often it can be self-administered by pushing the button to activate the PCA machine. For example, "When you have pain, instead of asking the nurse to bring medication, push the button that activates the machine and a small dose of the pain medicine will be injected into your IV line. You can keep your pain under control by administering additional medicine as soon as your pain begins to return or increases. Push the button before undertaking a painful activity, such as ambulation. Try to balance your pain relief against sleepiness, and don't activate the machine if you start to feel sleepy. If your pain medicine seems to stop working despite pushing the button several times, call the nurse to check your IV. If you are not receiving adequate pain relief, the nurse will call your doctor."
   (b) Monitor vital signs, especially blood pressure and respiratory rate, every hour for the first 4 hours, and assess postural heart rate and blood pressure before initial ambulation.
   (c) Monitor respiratory rate every 2 hours while the patient is on PCA.
   (d) If the patient's respiratory rate decreases to <10 breaths/min or if patient is overly sedated, anticipate administration of naloxone.

◉ PATIENT CARE MANAGEMENT PLAN—Cont'd

(12) If epidural opioid analgesia is used, do the following:

(a) Keep the patient's head elevated 30—45 degrees after injection **to prevent respiratory depressant effects.**

(b) Observe closely for respiratory depression for 24 hours after injection. Monitor respiratory rate every 15 minutes for 1 hour, every 30 minutes for 7 hours, and every hour for the remaining 16 hours.

(c) Assess for adequate cough reflex.

(d) Avoid use of other central nervous system depressants, such as sedatives.

(e) Observe for reports of pruritus, nausea, and vomiting.

(f) Anticipate administration of naloxone for respiratory depression (and smaller doses of naloxone for pruritus).

(g) Assess for and treat urinary retention.

(h) Assess epidural catheter site for local infection. Keep the catheter taped securely **to prevent catheter migration**.

b. For peripheral vascular ischemic pain (hypothetic vascular occlusion of leg), do the following:

(1) Correctly identify and differentiate ischemic pain from other types of pain. **(NOTE: Ischemic pain is usually a burning, aching pain made worse by exercise and lessened or relieved by rest. Eventually, the pain occurs at rest. Coldness and pallor of the extremity may be noted, especially if the limb is elevated above the heart level. Rubor and mottling of the skin may be evident from prolonged tissue anoxia and inability of damaged vessels to constrict. Eventually, cyanosis and gangrenous tissue will be evident. Chronic ischemia leads to visible changes in the limb, such as flaking skin, brittle nails and hair, leg ulcers, and cellulitis.)**

(2) Administer pain medications, and evaluate their effectiveness as previously described. **The pain of ischemia is chronic and continuous and can make the patient irritable and depressed.**

(3) Treat the cause of the ischemic pain, and institute measures **to increase circulation to the affected part**.

3. Initiate nonpharmacologic interventions.

a. Treat contributing factors.

b. Apply comfort measures.

(1) Use relaxation techniques, such as back rubs, massage, warm baths, music, and aromatherapy.

(a) Use blankets and pillows to support the painful part and reduce muscle tension.

(b) Encourage slow, rhythmic breathing.

(2) Encourage progressive muscle relaxation techniques.

(a) Instruct the patient to inhale and tense (tighten) specific muscle groups and then relax the muscles as exhalation occurs.

(b) Suggest an order for performing the tension and relaxation cycle (e.g., start with facial muscles and move down body, ending with toes).

(3) Encourage guided imagery.

(a) Ask the patient to recall an experienced image that is very pleasurable and relaxing and involves at least two senses.

(b) Have the patient begin with rhythmic breathing and progressive relaxation and then travel mentally to the scene.

(c) Have the patient slowly experience the scene (e.g., how it looks, sounds, smells, feels).

(d) Ask the patient to practice this imagery in private.

(e) Instruct the patient to end the imagery by counting to three and saying, "Now I'm relaxed." If the person does not end the imagery and falls asleep, the purpose of the technique is defeated.

◉ PATIENT CARE MANAGEMENT PLAN

Anxiety
Anxiety Due to Threat to Biologic, Psychological, or Social Integrity
Signs and Symptoms
Subjective

- Verbalizes increased muscle tension
- Expresses frequent sensation of tingling in hands and feet
- Relates continuous feeling of apprehension
- Expresses preoccupation with a sense of impending doom
- Reports difficulty falling asleep
- Repeatedly expresses concerns about changes in health status and outcome of illness

Objective

- Psychomotor agitation (fidgeting, jitteriness, restlessness)
- Tightened, wrinkled brow
- Strained (worried) facial expression
- Hypervigilance (scans environment)
- Startles easily
- Distractibility
- Sweaty palms
- Fragmented sleep patterns
- Tachycardia
- Tachypnea

Outcomes

- Patient effectively uses learned relaxation strategies.
- Patient demonstrates significant decrease in psychomotor agitation.
- Patient verbalizes reduction in tingling sensations in hands and feet.
- Patient is able to focus on the tasks at hand.
- Patient expresses positive, future-based plans to family and staff.
- Patient's heart rate and rhythm remain within limits commensurate with physiologic status.

Interventions and Rationale

1. Instruct the patient in the following simple, effective relaxation strategies:

a. If not contraindicated for cardiovascular reasons, tense and relax all muscles progressively from toes to head. **Progressive toe-to-head relaxation releases the muscular tension that may be a stress-related effect resulting from the threat or change in the patient's health status and outcome of illness.**

b. Perform slow deep-breathing exercises. **Deep-breathing exercises provide slow, rhythmic, controlled breathing patterns that relax the patient and distract him or her from the effects of his or her illness and hospitalization.**

c. Focus on a single object or person in the environment. **Focusing on a single object or person helps the patient dismiss myriad disorienting stimuli from his or her visual-perceptual field, which can have a dizzying, distorted effect. A**

Continued

◎ PATIENT CARE MANAGEMENT PLAN—Cont'd

clear sensorium allows him or her to feel more in control of his or her environment.

d. Listen to soothing music or relaxation tapes with eyes closed. **Music or words expressed in soft, low tones tend to produce soothing, relaxing effects that counteract or inhibit escalating anxiety and provide respites from the patient's situational crisis. Closed eyes eliminate distracting visual stimuli and promote a more restful environment.**

2. Actively listen to and accept the patient's concerns regarding the threats from his or her illness, outcome, and hospitalization. **Active listening and unconditional acceptance validate the patient as a worthwhile individual and assure him or her that his or her concerns, no matter how great, will be addressed. Knowledge that he or she has an avenue for ventilation will assuage anxiety.**

3. Help the patient distinguish between realistic concerns and exaggerated fears through clear, simple explanations. *Sample statements:* "Your lab results show that you're doing okay right now." "The shortness of breath you're experiencing is not unusual." "The pain you described is expected, and this medication will relieve it." **A patient who is informed about his or her progress and is reassured about expected symptoms and management of care will be better equipped to maintain a more realistic perspective of his or her illness and its outcome. Anxiety emanating from imagined or exaggerated fears will likely be assuaged or averted.**

4. Provide simple clarification of environmental events and stimuli that are not related to the patient's illness and care. *Sample statements:* "That loud noise is coming from a machine that is helping another patient." "The visitor behind the curtain is crying because she's had an upsetting day." "That gurney is here to take another patient to x-ray." **Clarification of events and stimuli that are unrelated to the patient helps to disengage him or her from the extant anxiety-provoking situations surrounding him or her, avoiding further anxiety and apprehension.**

5. Assist the patient in focusing on building on prior coping strategies to deal with the effects of his or her illness and care. *Sample statements:* "What methods have helped you get through difficult times in the past?" "How can we help you use those methods now?" (See the patient management plan for Impaired Adaptation for interventions that assist patients to use coping strategies effectively.) **Use of previously successful coping strategies in conjunction with newly learned techniques arms the patient with an arsenal of weapons against anxiety, providing him or her with greater control over the situational crisis and decreased feelings of doom and despair.**

6. Give the patient permission to deny or suppress the effects of his or her illness and hospitalization with which he or she cannot cope or control. *Sample statements:* "It's perfectly okay to ignore things you can't handle right now." "How can we help ease your mind during this time?" "What are some things or tasks that may help distract you?" **Adaptive denial can be helpful in reducing feelings of anxiety in patients with a life-threatening illness.**

◎ PATIENT CARE MANAGEMENT PLAN

Autonomic Dysreflexia
Autonomic Dysreflexia Due to Excessive Autonomic Response to Noxious Stimuli
Signs and Symptoms

- Paroxysmal hypertension (sudden increase in both systolic and diastolic blood pressure [BP] >20 mm Hg above patient's normal BP); for many patients with spinal cord injury, normal BP may be 90/60 mm Hg
- Pounding headache
- Bradycardia (may be a relative slowing, so the heart rate may still appear within the normal range)
- Profuse sweating (above the level of the injury) especially in the face, neck, and shoulders
- Pilomotor erection (goose bumps) above the level of the injury
- Cardiac dysrhythmias (atrial fibrillation, premature ventricular contractions, and atrioventricular conduction abnormalities)
- Flushing of the skin (above the level of the injury) especially in the face, neck, and shoulders
- Blurred vision
- Appearance of spots in the visual fields
- Nasal congestion
- Feelings of apprehension or anxiety

Outcomes

- BP returns to patient's baseline level.
- Heart rate and rhythm returns to patient's baseline level.
- Headache is absent.
- Sweating, flushing, and piloerection above level of injury are absent.
- Visual disturbances and nasal congestion are absent.
- Feelings of apprehension or anxiety are absent.

Interventions and Rationale

1. Place the patient on a cardiac monitor, and assess for bradycardia or other dysrhythmias. Disturbances of cardiac rate and rhythm can occur because of autonomic dysfunction associated with dysreflexia.
2. Check the patient's BP every 3—5 minutes, as BP may fluctuate very quickly.
3. Sit the patient upright and lower his or her legs, if possible, to decrease venous return and BP.
4. Loosen any clothing or constrictive devices to decrease venous return and BP.
5. Investigate for and remove the instigating cause of dysreflexia:
   a. Bladder
      (1) If an indwelling catheter is not in place, catheterize the patient immediately.
         (a) Before inserting the catheter, instill 2% lidocaine jelly into the urethra and wait 2 minutes, if possible.
         (b) Drain 500 mL of urine and recheck BP.
         (c) If BP is still elevated, drain another 500 mL of urine.
         (d) If BP declines after the bladder is empty, serial BPs must be monitored closely because the bladder can go into severe contractions, causing hypertension to recur.
      (2) If an indwelling catheter is in place, check the catheter and tubing for kinks, folds, constrictions, or obstructions and for correct placement. If a problem is found, correct it immediately.
      (3) If the catheter is plugged, irrigate it gently with no more than 10—15 mL of sterile normal saline solution at body temperature.
      (4) If unable to irrigate the catheter, remove it and prepare to reinsert a new catheter. Proceed with its lubrication, drainage, and observation as outlined above.
      (5) Avoid manually compressing or tapping on the bladder.
   b. Bowel: If systolic BP is >150 mm Hg, proceed to Step 6 before checking for a fecal impaction.

◎ PATIENT CARE MANAGEMENT PLAN—Cont'd

(1) With a gloved hand, instill a topical anesthetic agent (2% lidocaine jelly) generously into the rectum **to decrease flow of impulses from bowel**.

(2) Wait 2 minutes, if possible, **for sensation in area to decrease.**

(3) With a gloved hand, insert a lubricated finger into the rectum and check for the presence of stool.

(4) If stool is felt, gently remove, if possible.

c. Skin

(1) Loosen clothing or bed linens as indicated.

(2) Inspect skin for pimples, boils, pressure ulcers, and ingrown toenails, and treat as indicated.

6. If symptoms of dysreflexia do not subside, collaborate with the practitioner regarding the administration of antihypertensive medications (e.g., nifedipine [immediate-release form], nitrates [sodium nitroprusside, isosorbide dinitrate, or nitroglycerin ointment], hydralazine, mecamylamine, diazoxide, phenoxybenzamine, captopril, prazosin).

a. Administer medications and monitor their effectiveness.

b. Assess BP and heart rate.

7. Instruct the patient about causes, symptoms, treatment, and prevention of dysreflexia.

8. Encourage the patient to carry a medical bracelet or informational card to present to medical personnel in the event dysreflexia may be developing.

◎ PATIENT CARE MANAGEMENT PLAN

Decreased Intracranial Adaptive Capacity

Decreased Intracranial Adaptive Capacity Due to Failure of Normal Intracranial Compensatory Mechanisms

Signs and Symptoms

- Intracranial pressure (ICP) >15 mm Hg, sustained for 15–30 minutes
- Headache
- Vomiting, with or without nausea
- Seizures
- Decrease in Glasgow Coma Scale score of 2 or more points from baseline
- Alteration in level of consciousness, ranging from restlessness to coma
- Change in orientation: disoriented to time, place, or person, or all three
- Difficulty or inability to follow simple commands
- Increasing systolic blood pressure of more than 20 mm Hg with widening pulse pressure
- Bradycardia
- Irregular respiratory pattern (e.g., Cheyne-Stokes, central neurogenic hyperventilation, ataxic, apneustic)
- Change in response to painful stimuli (e.g., purposeful to inappropriate or absent response)
- Signs of impending brain herniation:
  - Hemiparesis or hemiplegia
  - Hemisensory changes
  - Unequal pupil size (1 mm or more difference)
  - Failure of pupil to react to light
  - Disconjugate gaze and inability to move one eye beyond midline if third, fourth, or sixth cranial nerves involved
  - Loss of oculocephalic or oculovestibular reflexes
  - Possible decorticate or decerebrate posturing

Outcomes

- ICP is <15 mm Hg.
- Cerebral perfusion pressure is >60 mm Hg.
- Clinical signs of increased ICP are absent.

Interventions and Rationale

1. Maintain adequate cerebral perfusion pressure.

   a. Collaborate with the practitioner regarding administration of volume expanders, vasopressors, or antihypertensives **to maintain the patient's blood pressure within normal range**.

   b. Implement measures to reduce ICP.

   (1) Elevate head of bed 30–45 degrees **to facilitate venous return**.

   (2) Maintain head and neck in neutral (avoid flexion, extension, or lateral rotation) **to enhance venous drainage from the head.**

   (3) Avoid extreme hip flexion.

   (4) Collaborate with the practitioner regarding administration of steroids, osmotic agents, and diuretics and need for drainage of cerebrospinal fluid if a ventriculostomy is in place.

   (5) Assist the patient to turn and move self in bed (instruct the patient to exhale while turning or pushing up in bed) **to avoid isometric contractions and Valsalva maneuver.**

2. Maintain patent airway and adequate ventilation, and supply oxygen **to prevent hypoxemia and hypercarbia.**

3. Monitor arterial blood gas values and maintain arterial partial pressure of oxygen (PaO_2) >80 mm Hg, arterial partial pressure of carbon dioxide ($PaCO_2$) >35 mm Hg, and pH at 7.35–7.45 **to prevent cerebral vasodilation.**

4. Avoid suctioning beyond 10 seconds at a time; hyperoxygenate and hyperventilate before and after suctioning **to avoid hypoxemia.**

5. Plan patient care activities and interventions around the patient's ICP response. Avoid unnecessary additional disturbances, and allow the patient up to 1 hour of rest between activities as frequently as possible. **Studies have shown the direct correlation between patient care activities and increases in ICP.**

6. Maintain normothermia with external cooling or heating measures as necessary. Wrap hands, feet, and male genitalia in soft towels before cooling measures **to prevent shivering and frostbite.**

7. Collaborate with the practitioner to control seizures with prophylactic and PRN anticonvulsants. **Seizures can greatly increase the cerebral metabolic rate.**

8. Collaborate with the practitioner regarding administration of sedatives, barbiturates, or paralyzing agents **to reduce cerebral metabolic rate.**

9. Counsel family members to maintain a calm atmosphere and avoid disturbing topics of conversation (e.g., patient condition, pain, prognosis, family crisis, financial difficulties).

10. If signs of impending brain herniation are present, implement the following:

    a. Notify the practitioner at once.

    b. Ensure that head of bed is elevated 45 degrees and that the patient's head is in a neutral plane.

    c. Administer a mainline intravenous infusion slowly to the keep-open rate.

    d. Drain cerebrospinal fluid as ordered if a ventriculostomy is in place.

    e. Prepare to administer osmotic agents and/or diuretics.

    f. Prepare the patient for an emergency computed tomography head scan and/or emergency surgery.

PATIENT CARE MANAGEMENT PLAN

Delirium
Delirium Due to Sensory Overload, Sensory Deprivation, and Sleep Pattern Disturbance
Signs and Symptoms
Early Symptoms
- Sudden onset of global cognitive function impairment (hours to days)
- Restlessness, agitation, and combative behavior
- Drowsiness (can lead to loss of consciousness)
- Slurring of speech, inappropriate statements or "word salad," mumbling, or inappropriate gestures
- Short attention span (needs questions repeated); inability to learn new material
- Disordered sleep/wake cycle
- Disorientation to person, time, place, and situation
- Difficulty in separating dreams from reality (may experience bizarre dreams or nightmares)
- Anger at staff for continued questions about his or her orientation

Later Symptoms
- Symptoms that tend to fluctuate throughout the day and night
- Continuations of early symptoms, which may be more frequent or of longer duration
- Illusions
- Hallucinations
- Extreme agitation (e.g., attempts to climb out of bed, pull out catheters, rip off dressings)
- Calling out in loud voice, swearing, or attempting to bite or hit people who approach patient

Outcomes
- Absence of or diminished confusion.
- Absence of or diminished sensory overload.
- Absence of or diminished sensory deprivation.
- Absence of or diminished sleep pattern disturbance.

Interventions and Rationale
1. Determine and document the patient's dominant spoken language, his or her literacy, and the languages in which he or she is literate. **Sometimes people are not literate in their spoken language, or, less commonly, they are literate only in their second language.**
2. Determine and document the patient's premorbid degree of orientation, cognitive capabilities, and any sensory/perceptual deficits.

For Sensory Overload
1. Initiate each nurse-patient encounter by calling the patient by name and identifying yourself by name. This fosters reality orientation and assists the patient in filtering irrelevant or impersonal conversation.
2. Assess the patient's immediate physical environment from his or her viewpoint, and explain equipment, its sounds, and its therapeutic purpose. Demonstrate audible and visual alarms, and explain possible alarm conditions. This decreases alienation of the patient from the technologic environment and reduces the inherent sense of fear and urgency accompanying alarm conditions.
3. Provide preparatory sensory information by explaining procedures in relation to the sensations the patient will experience, including duration of sensations. Preparatory sensory information enhances learning and lessens anticipatory anxiety.
4. Limit noise levels. Audible alarms cannot and must not be silenced, and many critical but noisy activities must take place in the critical care unit. However, it has been shown that noise levels produced by clinical personnel exceed levels designated as acceptable and are often greater than levels generated by technologic devices.
   a. Keep staff conversations soft enough that they are inaudible to the patient whenever possible.
   b. Assume that everything said at or around a patient's bedside is intended for that patient's awareness and that it will be interpreted as pertaining to him or her. **As in the discussion that follows, conversations about the patient but not to him or her foster depersonalization and delusions of reference.**
   c. Enforce nighttime noise limits.
5. Readjust alarm limits on physiologic monitoring devices as the patient's condition changes (improves or deteriorates) **to lessen unnecessary alarm states.**
6. Consider use of headphones and digital music player with the patient's favorite music and/or subliminal or classical music. This can effectively filter out assaultive noise of the critical care environment and supplant it with familiar, soothing sounds and rhythms.
7. Modify lighting. Day and night cycles need to be simulated with environmental lighting.
   a. Never turn on overhead fluorescent lights abruptly without warning the patient, assisting him or her out of the supine position, and shielding his or her eyes with gauze or a face cloth. **Continuous bright lighting sustains anxiety and promotes circadian rhythm desynchronization.**
8. Shield patients from viewing urgent and emergent events in the critical care unit. Resuscitation efforts, albeit difficult to conceal, engender fear in the patient and a sense of instability and vulnerability (e.g., "I'm next").
   a. When such an event occurs, elicit the patient's cognitive and emotional reaction; thoughts, impressions, and feelings need to be shared, and misconceptions need to be clarified.
9. Ensure patients' privacy, modesty, and dignity. Physical exposure and nudity, although they seemingly pale in importance compared with priorities such as physiologic assessment and stabilization, are primal indignities for all individuals.
   a. Keep the patient minimally exposed. When it becomes necessary to expose the patient, verbally apologize for this necessity. **To be naked is to feel vulnerable; to be vulnerable is to feel fearful.**

For Sensory Deprivation
1. Provide reality orientation in four spheres (personal, place, time, and situation) at more frequent intervals than when testing.
   a. Convey this information in the context of routine conversation. *Sample statements:* "Mr. Clark, this is Tuesday morning and you're in University Hospital. Your heart surgery was yesterday morning, and you're doing well. My name is Joe, and I'm your nurse today." **The patient is made to feel patronized by repetitions such as, "Do you know where you are?" Given the effects of general anesthesia, opioid analgesics, sedatives, and sleep, it is expected that some degree of disorientation will exist normally.**
2. Ensure the patient's visual access to a calendar.
3. Apprise the patient of daily news events and the weather.
4. Touch patients for the express purpose of communicating caring. Hold their hands, stroke their brows, and rub the skin on an aspect of the arms. **Touch is the universal language of caring. In the setting of critical care, in which there is considerable physical body manipulation, it is useful and important to contrast assaultive touch with comforting touch. Touch can be used as a technique for distraction from painful stimuli when used in conjunction with uncomfortable procedures.** (See later discussion of the use of touch in management of the patient experiencing hallucinations.)

PATIENT CARE MANAGEMENT PLAN—Cont'd

5. Foster liberal visitation by family members and significant others. Encourage significant others to touch the patient as consistent with their individual comfort level and cultural norms.

6. Structure and identify opportunities for the patient to exercise decision-making skills, however small. **Although not so designated, patients with sensory alterations also experience a type of cognitive deprivation.**

7. Assist patients to find meaning in their experiences. Patients need to find meaning and to identify their roles in the experience of critical illness and critical care.

   a. Explain the therapeutic purpose of all they are asked to do for themselves and all that is done with them and for them.

   b. Avoid statements such as, "Will you turn to that side for me?" or "I need you to swallow this medication." **These statements implicitly convey that the maneuver has some value for the nurses instead of the patients.**

   c. Similarly, use "thank you" judiciously. This simple salutation, when used indiscriminately, suggests something was done to benefit the nurses, not the patients.

For Hallucinations

1. Approach the patient with a calm, matter-of-fact demeanor. The goal of this interaction is for the nurse to demonstrate external control. This helps decrease the anxiety and fear that generally accompany hallucinations and allows the patient to feel safe. Anxiety is transferable.

2. Address the patient by name. This is a useful presentation of reality because self-identity is the last sphere of orientation to vanish.

3. In responding to the patient's description of the hallucination, do not deny, argue, or attempt to disprove the existence of the perceived event. Statements such as, "There are no voices coming from that air vent," or "Look, I'm brushing my hand across the wall, and there are no bugs," confuse the patient further because the hallucination, although frightening, is his or her perceived reality.

4. Express to the patient that your experiences are dissimilar and acknowledge how frightening his or hers must be. *Sample statements:* "I don't hear (or see) what you do, but I know how frightening such an experience must be to you. I'm Joe, your nurse, and I'm going to stay with you until the voices (or visions) go away." Validating the patient's feelings demonstrates acceptance and sensitivity to the experience and promotes trust.

5. Remain with any patient who is experiencing a hallucination. Feelings of fear and anxiety often accelerate when a patient is left alone. He or she needs someone to represent a nonthreatening reality.

6. Do not explore the content of the hallucination with the patient by asking about its nature or character. The nurse is the patient's link with reality. Pursuit of a detailed description of a hallucination may signify to the patient that the nurse accepts his or her sensory distortion as factual. This may further confuse the patient and distance him or her more from reality.

   a. Ascertain that the voices are not telling the patient to harm himself or herself by asking simply and concretely, "What are the voices saying?" **The nurse can help bridge the gap between the patient's misperception and reality by addressing the feelings (e.g., fear, anxiety) and/or meanings (e.g., danger, death) engendered by the hallucination.**

   b. Determine how the misperception affects the patient emotionally, acknowledge those feelings, and use a calm, controlled, matter-of-fact approach to provide the trust and comfort the patient needs to tolerate this frightening experience. **In other words, the nurse should deal with the intent more than the content of the hallucination. The resultant decrease in anxiety will enable the patient to focus more accurately on his or her immediate environment.**

7. Talk concretely with the patient about things that are really happening. *Sample statements:* "How does your chest incision feel this afternoon, Mr. Clark?" "Your sister Kate was here to see you, but you were sleeping. She went down to the cafeteria and will be back." "Your secretions are a little easier for you to cough up today." **Interpretation of reality-based stimuli by the nurse encourages the patient to focus on actual circumstances and discourages a preoccupation with sensory misperceptions.**

8. Distract the patient by changing the topic. This tactic is useful in situations of escalating anxiety and confusion or when all else fails. Topics need to consist of basic themes that are universally understood and culturally congruent such as music, food, or weather, or topics of special interest to the patient such as hobbies, crafts, or sports.

   a. Avoid topics that evoke strong emotions such as politics, religion, or sexuality. This is especially true in regard to a patient with reality distortions; sometimes hallucinations and delusions are expressions of repressed conflicts associated with religious, sexual, or aggressive issues. Pursuit of such subjects could increase confusion and anxiety.

9. Avoid the use of touch as an intervention strategy for any patient who demonstrates escalating anxiety or paranoid, suspicious, or mistrustful thoughts. **Although touch can be useful in the management of patients with sensory alterations, for patients experiencing hallucinations (as well as delusions and illusions), touch can be readily misinterpreted as aggression or pain, and it can provide the basis for a tactile illusion.**

10. For auditory hallucinations:

   a. *Patient behaviors:* Head cocked as if listening to an unseen presence; lips moving.

   b. *Therapeutic nurse responses:* "Mr. Clark, you appear to be listening to something." If the patient acknowledges voices: "I don't hear any voices, but I know this is troubling you. The voices will go away. Nothing is going to harm you. I'm Joe, your nurse, and I'll be here with you."

   c. *Nontherapeutic nurse responses:* "Tell me about your conversations with these voices." "To whom do these voices belong—anyone you know?"

11. For visual hallucinations:

   a. *Patient behaviors:* Staring into space as if focused on an unseen object; startled movements and anxious facial expression.

   b. *Therapeutic nurse responses:* "Mr. Clark, something seems to be troubling you. Tell me what it is." If the patient states he visualizes people, images, or the devil in his environment and implies a sense of danger, respond, "There are only nurses and doctors here, Mr. Clark. I know this must be upsetting, but these images will go away. We're here with you in the hospital. Nothing will happen to you."

   c. *Nontherapeutic nurse responses:* "Describe the people you see. What are they wearing?" "What does the devil mean in your life? What about God?"

For Delusions

1. Explain all unseen noises, voices, and activity simply and clearly. **They readily feed a delusional system.** Sample statements: "That is Dr. Smith. He's come to see you and other patients here in the hospital." "The voices and activity you hear are from the bedside of the patient behind this curtain. He's being helped by one of the nurses."

2. Avoid the "negative challenge" of the patient's delusions (e.g., "Nobody here stole your belongings" or "Doctors and nurses do not harm people"). Similarly, avoid defending the referents of the patient's belief: "Nurses are good," or "Doctors mean well." **A delusion is a belief, albeit false, that cannot be changed with logic. To attempt this change is to**

Continued

PATIENT CARE MANAGEMENT PLAN—Cont'd

challenge the patient's belief system and escalate his or her anxiety, further blurring the boundaries between reality and the patient's internally based "logic."

3. For a patient with persecutory delusions who refuses food, fluids, or medications because of a belief that he or she has been poisoned or the medications are tainted, permit the refusal unless it is a life-threatening event. Try again in 20 minutes; allow the patient to choose an alternative selection of food or to read the label on the unit's medication. **Coercion, show of force, or engagement in complicated, logical justifications will heighten the patient's suspiciousness and possibly reinforce the delusional belief. When the patient feels more in control, he or she need not rely on the "paradoxical" quality of the delusion to equip him or her with a false sense of power. His or her power instead is derived from making reality-based decisions.**

4. Staff members should be particularly careful not to engage in unnecessary laughter or whispering within view of a delusional patient. **The delusional patient is hypervigilant, scanning the environment for evidence to corroborate or confirm his or her belief that staff members are colluding against him or her; laughter and whispers easily suggest this belief, this delusion of reference. This rationale also pertains to the patient experiencing hallucinations and/or illusions.**

5. Observe the principles detailed in the third intervention in the "For Hallucinations" section.

For Illusions

1. Interpret a reality-based stimulus for the patient in a calm, matter-of-fact manner. Seen and unseen noises, voices, activity, and people can provide the stimulus for a sensory misinterpretation, an illusion.

2. Minimize stimulation in the patient's immediate environment. Interventions detailed previously under "For Sensory Overload" are especially relevant here.

3. Address the feeling and meaning associated with the experience, not the content of the sensory misinterpretation.

   a. *Patient behaviors:* Eyes darting, startled movements, frightened facial expression. "I know who you are. You're the devil come to take me to hell."

   b. *Therapeutic nurse responses:* "I'm Joe, your nurse. I know this experience is troubling for you. You're in the hospital, and no one here will harm you."

   c. Nontherapeutic nurse responses: "There are no such things as devils and angels." "Do you think the devil would be dressed in white?" **The first nontherapeutic nurse response carries a parental tone (e.g., "You know better than that."), infantilizing the patient and adding to his or her feelings of powerlessness over the environment. The second nontherapeutic response reflects obvious logic, which is not in the patient's sensory domain; it cannot be processed and only adds to his or her confused state.**

4. Observe the principles detailed in the fifth intervention of the "For Hallucinations" section.

PATIENT CARE MANAGEMENT PLAN

Disturbed Body Image
Disturbed Body Image Due to Actual Change in Body Structure, Function, or Appearance
Signs and Symptoms

- Actual change in appearance, structure, or function
- Avoidance of looking at body part
- Avoidance of touching body part
- Hiding or overexposing body part (intentional or unintentional)
- Trauma to nonfunctioning part
- Change in ability to estimate spatial relationship of body to environment
- Verbalization of the following:
  - Fear of rejection or reaction by others
  - Negative feeling about body
  - Preoccupation with change or loss
  - Refusal to participate in or to accept responsibility for self-care of altered body part
  - Personalization of part or loss with a name
  - Depersonalization of part or loss by use of impersonal pronouns
  - Refusal to verify actual change

Outcomes

- Patient verbalizes the specific meaning of the change to him or her.
- Patient requests appropriate information about self-care.
- Patient completes personal hygiene and grooming daily with or without help.
- Patient interacts freely with family or other visitors.
- Patient participates in the discussions and conferences related to planning his or her medical and patient management in the critical care unit and transfer from the unit.

- Patient talks with trained visitors (support group representatives) at least twice about his or her loss.

Interventions and Rationale

1. Evaluate the patient's mental, physical, and emotional state; recognize assets, strengths, response to illness, coping mechanisms, past experience with stress, and support system.

2. Apprise the response of the family and significant others. Body image is derived from the "reflected appraisals" of family and significant others.

3. Determine the patient's goals and readiness for learning.

4. Provide the necessary information to help the patient and family adapt to the change. Clarify misconceptions about future limitations.

5. Permit and encourage the patient to express the significance of the loss or change; note nonverbal behavior responses.

6. Allow and encourage the patient's expression of anxiety. Anxiety is the most predominant emotional response to a body image disturbance.

7. Recognize and accept the use of denial as an adaptive defense mechanism when used early and temporarily.

8. Recognize maladaptive denial as that which interferes with the patient's progress and/or alienates support systems. Use confrontation.

9. Provide an opportunity for the patient to discuss sexual concerns.

10. Touch the affected body part to provide the patient with sensory information about altered body structure and/or function.

11. Encourage and provide movement of the altered body part to establish kinesthetic feedback. This enables the patient to know his or her body as it now exists.

12. Prepare the patient to look at the body part. Call the body part by its anatomic name (e.g., stump, stoma, limb) as opposed to "it." **The use of**

PATIENT CARE MANAGEMENT PLAN—Cont'd

impersonal pronouns increases a sense of fantasy and depersonalization of the body part.

13. Allow the patient to experience excellence in some aspect of physical functioning—walking, turning, deep breathing, healing, self-care—and point out progress and accomplishment. **This helps to balance the patient's sense of dysfunction with function.**

14. Avoid false reassurance. Acknowledge the difficulty of incorporating the altered body part or function into one's body image. **This evidences the nurse's sensitivity and promotes trust.**

15. Talk with the patient about his or her life, generativity, and accomplishments. Patients with disturbances in body image frequently see themselves in a distortedly "narrow" sense. Encouraging a wider focus of themselves and their life reduces this distortion.

16. Help the patient explore realistic alternatives.

17. Recognize that incorporating a body change into one's body image takes time. Avoid setting unrealistic expectations and **inadvertently reinforcing a low self-esteem.**

18. Suggest the use of additional resources such as trained visitors who have mastered situations similar to those of the patient.
    a. Refer the patient to a psychiatric nurse, psychologist, or psychiatrist if needed.

Disturbed Body Image Due to Functional Dependence on Life-Sustaining Technology
Signs and Symptoms
- Actual change in function requiring permanent or temporary replacement
- Refusal to verify actual loss
- Verbalization of the following: feelings of helplessness, hopelessness, powerlessness, fear of failure to wean from technology

Outcomes
- Patient verifies actual change in function.
- Patient does not refuse or fight technologic intervention.
- Patient verbalizes acceptance of expected change in lifestyle.

Interventions and Rationale
1. Evaluate the patient's response to the technologic intervention.
2. Assess responses of the family and significant others. **Body image is derived from the "reflected appraisals" of family and significant others.**
3. Provide information needed by the patient and family.
4. Promote trust, security, comfort, and privacy.
5. Recognize anxiety. Allow and encourage its expression. **Anxiety is the most predominant emotion accompanying body image alterations.** Implement a patient management plan for Anxiety Due to Threat to Biologic, Psychological, or Social Integrity.
6. Assist the patient to recognize his or her own functioning and performance in the face of technology. For example, assist the patient to distinguish spontaneous breaths from mechanically delivered breaths. **The activity will assist in weaning the patient from the ventilator when feasible. To establish realistic, accurate body boundaries, a patient needs to help separate himself or herself from the technology that is supporting his or her functioning. Any participation or function on the part of the patient during periods of dependency is helpful in preventing and/or resolving an alteration in body image.**
7. Plan for discontinuation of the treatment (e.g., weaning from a ventilator). Explain the procedure that will be followed and be present during its initiation.
8. Plan for transfer from the critical care environment.
9. Document care, ensuring an up-to-date management plan is available to all involved caregivers.

PATIENT CARE MANAGEMENT PLAN

Hyperthermia
Hyperthermia Due to Increased Metabolic Rate
Signs and Symptoms
- Increased body temperature above normal range
- Seizures
- Flushed skin
- Increased respiratory rate
- Tachycardia
- Skin warm to touch
- Diaphoresis

Outcomes
- Temperature is within normal range.
- Respiratory rate and heart rate are within patient's baseline range.
- Skin is warm and dry.

Interventions and Rationale
1. Monitor temperature every 15 minutes to 1 hour until within normal range and stable, then every 4 hours to maintain close **surveillance for temperature fluctuations and evaluate effectiveness of interventions.**
    a. Use temperature taken from the pulmonary artery catheter or bladder catheter if available **because these methods closely reflect core body temperature**.
    b. Use tympanic membrane temperature if core body temperature devices are unavailable.
    c. Use rectal temperature if none of the aforementioned methods are available.
2. Collaborate with the practitioner regarding administration of antithyroid medications **to block the synthesis and release of thyroid hormone.**
3. Collaborate with the practitioner regarding the use of a cooling blanket **to facilitate heat loss by conduction**.
    a. Wrap hands, feet, and male genitalia to protect them from maceration during cooling and decrease chance of shivering.
    b. Avoid rapidly cooling the patient and overcooling the patient because this initiates the heat-conserving response (i.e., shivering).
4. Place ice packs in patient's groin and axilla **to facilitate heat loss by conduction.**
5. Maintain the patient on bed rest to decrease the effects of activity on the patient's metabolic rate.
6. Provide tepid sponge baths to facilitate heat loss by evaporation.

Continued

PATIENT CARE MANAGEMENT PLAN—Cont'd

7. Decrease the patient's room temperature to facilitate radiant heat loss.
8. Place a fan near the patient to circulate cool air to facilitate heat loss by convection.
9. Provide the patient with a nonrestrictive gown and lightweight bed coverings to allow heat to escape from the patient's trunk.
10. Collaborate with the practitioner and the respiratory care practitioner regarding administration of oxygen to maintain oxygen saturation >90%

because the patient has increased oxygen consumption resulting from an increased metabolic rate.
11. Collaborate with the practitioner regarding use of antipyretic medications **to facilitate patient comfort.**
12. Collaborate with the practitioner regarding the use of intravenous (IV) and oral fluids **to maintain adequate hydration of the patient.**

PATIENT CARE MANAGEMENT PLAN

Hypervolemia

Hypervolemia Due to Increased Secretion of Antidiuretic Hormone (ADH)

Signs and Symptoms

- Headache
- Decreased sensorium
- Weight gain over short period
- Intake greater than output
- Increased pulmonary artery occlusion pressure
- Increased right atrial pressure
- Urine output is <30 mL/h
- Serum sodium is <120 mEq/L
- Serum osmolality is <275 mOsm/kg
- Urine osmolality greater than serum osmolality
- Urine sodium is >200 mEq/L
- Urine specific gravity is >1.03

Outcomes

- Weight returns to baseline.
- Urine output is >30 mL/h.
- Serum sodium is 135–145 mEq/L.
- Urine specific gravity is 1.005–1.030.

Interventions and Rationale

1. Monitor cardiac rhythm continuously for dysrhythmias **caused by electrolyte imbalance.**
2. Restrict the patient's fluids to 500 mL less than output per day **to decrease fluid retention.**
3. Provide the patient chilled beverages high in sodium content such as tomato juice or broth **to increase sodium intake.**
4. Collaborate with the practitioner regarding administration of demeclocycline, lithium, or opioid agonists **to inhibit renal response to ADH.**
5. Collaborate with the practitioner regarding administration of hypertonic saline and furosemide **for rapid correction of severe sodium deficit and diuresis of free water**.
   a. Administer hypertonic saline at a rate of 1 to 2 mL/kg/h until the patient's serum sodium is increased no greater than 1 to 2 mEq/L/h.
6. Weigh the patient daily (at same time, in same amount of clothing, and preferably with same scale) **to ensure accuracy of readings.**
7. Provide frequent mouth care to prevent breakdown of oral mucous membranes.
8. Initiate seizure precautions because the patient is at high risk as a result of hyponatremia.
   a. Pad the side rails of the bed to protect the patient from injury.
   b. Remove any objects from the immediate environment that could injure the patient in the event of a seizure.

c. Keep an appropriate-size oral airway at bedside to assist with airway management after the seizure.
9. Collaborate with the practitioner regarding the administration of medications to prevent constipation **caused by decreased fluid intake and immobility.**
10. Maintain surveillance for symptoms of hyponatremia (e.g., headache, abdominal cramps, weakness) and congestive heart failure (e.g., dyspnea, rales, increased central venous pressure, and pulmonary artery occlusion pressure).

Hypervolemia Due to Renal Dysfunction

Signs and Symptoms

- Weight gain that occurs during a 24- to 48-hour period
- Dependent pitting edema
- Ascites in severe cases
- Fluid crackles on lung auscultation
- Exertional dyspnea
- Oliguria or anuria
- Hypertension
- Engorged neck veins
- Decrease in urinary osmolality as renal failure progresses
- Right atrial pressure is >8 mm Hg
- Pulmonary artery occlusion pressure is >12 mm Hg

Outcomes

- Weight returns to baseline.
- Edema or ascites is absent or reduced to baseline.
- Lungs are clear to auscultation.
- Exertional dyspnea is absent.
- Blood pressure returns to baseline.
- Heart rate returns to baseline.
- Neck veins are flat.
- Mucous membranes are moist.

Interventions and Rationale

1. Promote skin integrity of edematous areas by frequent repositioning and elevation of areas where possible. Avoid massaging pressure points or reddened areas of skin **because this results in further tissue trauma.**
2. Plan patient care to provide rest periods **so as not to heighten exertional dyspnea.**
3. Weigh the patient daily at same time, in same amount of clothing, and preferably with same scale.
4. Instruct the patient about the correlation between fluid intake and weight gain, using commonly understood fluid measurements; for example, ingesting four cups (1000 mL) of fluid results in an approximate 2-lb weight gain in the anuric patient.

PATIENT CARE MANAGEMENT PLAN

Hypothermia
Hypothermia Due to Decreased Metabolic Rate
Signs and Symptoms
- Reduction in body temperature below normal range
- Shivering
- Pallor
- Piloerection
- Hypertension
- Skin cool to touch
- Tachycardia
- Decreased capillary refill

Outcomes
- Temperature is within normal range.
- Heart rate is within patient's baseline range.
- Skin is warm and dry.
- Capillary refill is normal.

Interventions and Rationale
1. Monitor temperature every 15 minutes to 1 hour until within normal range and stable and then every 4 hours **to maintain close surveillance for temperature fluctuations and to evaluate effectiveness of interventions**.
   a. Use temperature taken from pulmonary artery catheter or bladder catheter if available **because these methods closely reflect core body temperature**.
   b. Use tympanic membrane temperature if core body temperature devices are unavailable.
   c. Use rectal temperature if none of the aforementioned methods are available.
2. Collaborate with the practitioner regarding administration of thyroid medications **to replace lacking thyroid hormone.**
3. Collaborate with the practitioner regarding the use of a fluid-filled heating blanket **to facilitate rewarming by conduction.**
4. Initiate forced air–warming therapy **to facilitate convective heat gain.**
5. Provide the patient with warm blankets **to facilitate heat transfer to the patient.**
6. Increase the patient's room temperature **to decrease radiant heat loss.**
7. Replace wet patient gown and bed linen promptly **to decrease evaporative heat loss.**
8. Warm intravenous fluids and blood products **to facilitate rewarming by conduction.**

Hypothermia Due to Exposure to Cold Environment, Trauma, or Damage to the Hypothalamus
Signs and Symptoms
- Core body temperature <35°C (95°F)
- Skin cold to touch
- Slurred speech, incoordination
- At temperature <33°C (91.4°F):
  - Cardiac dysrhythmias (atrial fibrillation, bradycardia)
  - Cyanosis
  - Respiratory alkalosis
- At temperatures <32°C (89.6°F):
  - Shivering replaced by muscle rigidity

- Hypotension
- Dilated pupils
- At temperatures <28°C to 29°C (82.4°F to 84.2°F):
  - Absent deep tendon reflexes
  - Three to four breaths/min to apnea
  - Ventricular fibrillation possible
- At temperatures <26°C to 27°C (78.8°F to 80.6°F):
  - Coma
  - Flaccid muscles
  - Fixed, dilated pupils
  - Ventricular fibrillation to cardiac standstill
  - Apnea

Outcomes
- Core body temperature is >35°C (95°F).
- Patient is alert and oriented.
- Cardiac dysrhythmias are absent.
- Acid–base balance is normal.
- Pupils are normoreactive.

Interventions and Rationale
1. Monitor the patient's core body temperature continuously.
2. Collaborate with the practitioner regarding the need for intubation and mechanical ventilation.
   a. Heated air or oxygen can be added **to help rewarm the body core**.
   b. Do not hyperventilate a patient with hypothermia because carbon dioxide production is low, and this action may induce severe alkalosis and precipitate ventricular fibrillation.
3. Maintain cardiopulmonary resuscitation and advanced cardiac life support until core body temperature is at least 29.5°C (85.1°F) before determining that the patient cannot be resuscitated. **Electrical defibrillation is usually successful in terminating ventricular fibrillation if the temperature is >28°C (82.4°F).**
4. Administer cardiac resuscitation drugs sparingly because as the body warms, peripheral vasodilation occurs. Drugs that remain in the periphery are suddenly released, leading to a bolus effect that may cause fatal dysrhythmias.
5. Monitor arterial blood gas values to direct further therapy and ensure that pH, arterial partial pressure of oxygen (PaO_2), and arterial partial pressure of carbon dioxide ($PaCO_2$) are corrected for temperature.
6. Rewarm the patient rapidly because the pathophysiologic changes associated with chronic hypothermia have not had time to evolve.
   a. Institute rapid, active rewarming by immersion in warm water (38°C to 43°C) (100.4°F to 109.4°F).
   b. Apply thermal blanket at 36.6°C to 37.7°C (97.9°F to 99.9°F). Some researchers suggest rewarming only the torso or trunk first, leaving the extremities exposed to room temperature. **This is done to prevent early peripheral vasodilation with abrupt redistribution of intravascular volume. This also prevents colder blood trapped in the extremities from returning to the body core before the heart is rewarmed.**
   c. Perform rapid core rewarming with heated (37° to 43°C [98.6° to 109.4°F]) intravenous infusion, hemodialysis, peritoneal dialysis, and colonic or gastric irrigation fluids.
7. Monitor peripheral circulation because gangrene of the fingers and toes is a common complication of accidental hypothermia.

◎ PATIENT CARE MANAGEMENT PLAN

Hypovolemia
Hypovolemia Due to Absolute Loss
Signs and Symptoms
- Cardiac output is <4 L/min
- Cardiac index is <2.2 L/min
- Pulmonary artery occlusion pressure is <6 mm Hg
- Right atrial pressure is <2 mm Hg
- Tachycardia
- Narrowed pulse pressure
- Systolic blood pressure is <100 mm Hg
- Urinary output is <30 mL/h
- Pale, cool, moist skin
- Apprehensiveness

Outcomes
- Cardiac output is >4 L/min, and cardiac index is >2.2 L/min.
- Pulmonary artery occlusion pressure is >6 mm Hg or returns to baseline level.
- Right atrial pressure is >2 mm Hg or returns to baseline level.
- Heart rate is normal or returns to baseline level.
- Systolic blood pressure is >90 mm Hg.
- Urinary output is >30 mL/h.

Interventions and Rationale
1. Secure the airway and administer oxygen to maintain oxygen saturation >92%.
2. Place the patient in the supine position with the legs elevated **to increase preload.** For the patient with a head injury, consider using the low-Fowler position with legs elevated.
3. For fluid repletion, use the 3:1 rule, replacing three parts of fluid for every unit of blood lost.
4. Administer crystalloid solutions using the fluid challenge technique: Infuse precise boluses of fluid (usually 5–20 mL/min) over 10-minute periods; monitor hemodynamic pressures serially **to determine successful challenging.** If the pulmonary artery occlusion pressure elevates >7 mm Hg above the beginning level, the infusion should be stopped. If the pulmonary artery occlusion pressure rises only to 3 mm Hg above baseline or falls, another fluid challenge should be administered.
5. Replete fluids first before considering use of vasopressors because vasopressors increase myocardial oxygen consumption out of proportion to the reestablishment of coronary perfusion in the early phases of treatment.
6. When blood replacement is indicated, replace it with fresh-packed red blood cells and fresh-frozen plasma **to keep clotting factors intact.**
7. Move or reposition the patient minimally *to decrease or limit tissue oxygen demands.*
8. Evaluate the patient's anxiety level, and intervene through patient education or sedation **to decrease tissue oxygen demands.**
9. Maintain surveillance for signs and symptoms of fluid overload.

Hypovolemia Due to Decreased Secretion of Antidiuretic Hormone (ADH)
Signs and Symptoms
- Confusion and lethargy
- Decreased skin turgor
- Thirst
- Weight loss over short period
- Decreased pulmonary artery occlusion pressure
- Decreased right atrial pressure
- Urinary output is >6 L/day
- Serum sodium is >148 mEq/L
- Serum osmolality is >295 mOsm/kg
- Urine osmolality is <100 mOsm/kg
- Urine specific gravity is <1.005

Outcomes
- Weight returns to baseline.
- Urinary output is >30 mL/h and <200 mL/h.
- Serum osmolality is 280–295 mOsm/kg.
- Urine specific gravity is 1.010–1.030.

Interventions and Rationale
1. Record intake and output every hour, noting color and clarity of urine **because color and clarity are an indication of urine concentration.**
2. Monitor cardiac rhythm continuously for dysrhythmias **caused by electrolyte imbalance.**
3. Collaborate with the practitioner regarding administration of vasopressin or desmopressin **to replace ADH.**
   a. Monitor the patient for adverse effects of medications (e.g., headache, chest pain, abdominal pain) **caused by vasoconstriction.**
   b. Report adverse effects to the practitioner immediately.
4. Collaborate with the practitioner regarding intravenous fluid and electrolyte replacement therapy **to restore fluid balance, correct dehydration, and maintain electrolyte balance.**
   a. Administer hypotonic saline **to replace free water deficit.**
5. Provide oral fluids low in sodium such as water, coffee, tea, or orange juice **to decrease sodium intake.**
6. Weigh the patient daily at same time, in same amount of clothing, and preferably with same scale **to ensure accuracy of readings.**
7. Reposition the patient every 2 hours to prevent skin integrity issues caused by dehydration.
8. Provide mouth care every 4 hours to prevent breakdown of oral mucous membranes.
9. Collaborate with the practitioner regarding administration of medications to prevent constipation **caused by dehydration.**
10. Maintain surveillance for symptoms of hypernatremia (muscle twitching, irritability, seizures), hypovolemic shock (hypotension, tachycardia, decreased central venous pressure and pulmonary artery occlusion pressure), and deep vein thrombosis (calf pain, tenderness, swelling).

Hypovolemia Due to Relative Loss
Signs and Symptoms
- Pulmonary artery occlusion pressure <6 mm Hg
- Right atrial pressure <2 mm Hg
- Tachycardia
- Narrowed pulse pressure
- Systolic blood pressure <100 mm Hg
- Urinary output <30 mL/h.
- Increased hematocrit level

Outcomes
- Pulmonary artery occlusion pressure is >6 mm Hg or returns to baseline level.
- Right atrial pressure is >2 mm Hg or returns to baseline level.
- Systolic blood pressure is >90 mm Hg.
- Urinary output is >30 mL/h.
- Hematocrit level is normal.

Interventions and Rationale
1. Collaborate with the practitioner regarding administration of intravenous fluid replacements (usually normal saline solution or lactated Ringer solution) at a rate sufficient to maintain urinary output >30 mL/h. Colloid solutions are avoided in the initial phases (but can be used later) because of the possibility of increased edema formation **as a result of increased capillary permeability.**

PATIENT CARE MANAGEMENT PLAN

Impaired Adaptation

Impaired Adaptation Due to Situational Crisis and Personal Vulnerability

Signs and Symptoms

- Verbalization of inability to cope. *Sample statements:* "I can't take this anymore." "I don't know how to deal with this."
- Ineffective problem solving (problem lumping). *Sample statements:* "I have to eliminate salt from my diet. They tell me I can no longer mow the lawn. This hospitalization is costing a mint. What about my kids' future? Who's going to change the oil in the car? This is an incredible amount of time away from work."
- Ineffective use of coping mechanisms
- Projection: blames others for illness or pain
- Displacement: directs anger and/or aggression toward family. *Sample statements:* "Get out of here. Leave me alone."
- Cursing, shouting, or demanding attention; striking out or throwing objects
- Denial: of severity of illness and need for treatment
- Noncompliance. *Examples:* activity restriction; refusal to allow treatment or to take medications
- Suicidal thoughts (verbalizes desire to end life)
- Self-directed aggression. *Examples:* disconnects or attempts to disconnect life-sustaining equipment; deliberately tries to harm self
- Failure to progress from dependent to more independent state (refusal or resistance to care for self)

Outcomes

- Patient verbalizes beginning ability to cope with illness, pain, and hospitalization. *Sample statements:* "I'm trying to do the best I can." "I want to help myself get better."
- Patient demonstrates effective problem solving (lists and prioritizes problems from most to least urgent).
- Patient uses effective behavioral strategies to manage the stress of illness and care.
- Patient demonstrates interest or involvement in illness or environment. *Examples:* Patient does the following:
  - Requests medications when anticipating pain
  - Questions course of treatment, progress, and prognosis
  - Asks for clarification of environmental stimuli and events
  - Seeks out supportive individuals in his or her environment
  - Uses coping mechanisms and strategies more effectively to manage situational crisis
  - Demonstrates significant reduction in impulsive, angry, or aggressive outbursts (projection, shouting, cursing) directed toward family
  - Verbalizes future-based plans with cessation of self-directed aggressive acts and suicidal thoughts
  - Willingly complies with treatment regimen
  - Begins to participate in self-care

Interventions and Rationale

1. Actively listen and respond to the patient's verbal and behavioral expressions. Active listening signifies unconditional respect and acceptance for the patient as a worthwhile individual. It builds trust and rapport, guides the nurse toward problem areas, encourages the patient to express concerns, and promotes compliance.
2. Offer effective coping strategies to help the patient better tolerate the stressors related to his or her illness and care. Give permission to vent feelings in a safe setting. Sample statements: "I don't blame you for feeling angry or frustrated." "Others who are ill like you have expressed similar feelings." "I will listen to anything you want to share with me." "We don't have to talk; I'd like to sit here with you." "It's perfectly okay to cry."

Individuals who are provided with opportunities to express their feelings will be better able to release pent-up emotions and derive a greater sense of relief and comfort. They are less likely to resort to overly impulsive, aggressive acts, which may harm self or others.

3. Inform the family of the patient's need to displace anger occasionally but that you will be working with the patient to help him or her release his or her feelings in a more constructive, effective way. Family members who are well informed are better equipped to cope with their loved one's emotional anguish and outbursts. They are less likely to waste energy on feelings of guilt, fear, anger, or despair and can use their strength to help the patient in more constructive ways. The knowledge that their loved one is being cared for emotionally as well as physically provides family members with a greater sense of comfort and understanding. They will feel nurtured and respected by the nurse's attempt to include them in the process.

4. With the patient, list and number problems from the most to least urgent. Assist the patient in finding immediate solutions for the most urgent problems, postpone finding solutions for problems that can wait, delegate some problems to family members, and help the patient to acknowledge problems that are beyond his or her control. Listing and numbering problems in an organized fashion helps to break them down into more manageable "pieces" so that the patient is better able to identify solutions for problems that are solvable and to suppress problems that are less relevant or not amenable to interventions.

5. Identify individuals in the patient's environment who best help him or her to cope, and identify those who do not. Validate your observations with the patient. Sample statements: "I notice you seemed more relaxed during your daughter's visit." "After the chaplain left, you were able to sleep a bit longer than usual; would you like to see him more often?" "Your grandson was a bit upset today; I'll be glad to talk to him if you like." Supportive persons can invoke a calming effect on the patient's physiologic and psychological states. Conversely, well-meaning but nonsupportive individuals can have a deleterious effect on the patient's ability to cope and must be carefully screened and counseled by the nurse.

6. Teach the patient effective cognitive strategies to help him or her better manage the stress of critical illness and care. Help the patient construct pleasant thoughts, situations, or images that can simultaneously inhibit unpleasant realities. Examples: a day at the beach, a walk in the park, drinking a glass of wine, or being with a loved one. Pleasant thoughts and images constructed during critical illness and care tend to inhibit or reduce the intensity of the unpleasant, stressful effects of the experience.

7. Assist the patient in using coping mechanisms more effectively so that the patient can better manage his or her situational crisis.
   a. Suppression of problems beyond his or her control
   b. Compensation for illness and its effects; focusing on his or her strengths, interests, family, and spiritual beliefs
   c. Adaptive displacement of anger, fear, or frustration through healthy, verbal expressions to staff. Effective use of coping mechanisms helps to assuage the patient's painful feelings in a safe setting. The patient is strengthened and need not resort to the use of more ineffective defenses to eliminate anxiety.

8. Initiate a suicidal assessment if the patient verbalizes the desire to die, states that life is not worth living, or exhibits self-directed aggression.

Continued

PATIENT CARE MANAGEMENT PLAN—Cont'd

Sample statement: "We know that this is a bad time for you. You're saying repeatedly that you want to die. Are you planning to harm yourself?" If the response is "yes," remain with the patient, alert staff members, and provide for psychiatric consultation as soon as possible. Continue to express concern to the patient and protect him or her from harm. **Suicidal thoughts as a result of ineffective coping or exhaustion of coping devices are a common occurrence in critically ill patients. If the mood state is distressing enough, a patient may seek relief by attempting a self-destructive act. Although the patient may not imminently have the energy to succeed in his or her attempt, voicing a specific plan signifies a depressed mood state and depletion of coping strategies. Immediate intervention is needed because the attempt may be successful when the patient's energy is restored.**

9. Encourage the patient to participate in self-care activities and treatment regimens in accordance with his or her level of progress. Offer praise for his or her efforts toward self-care. **Patients who take an active role in their own treatment and progress are less apt to feel like helpless or powerless victims. This greater sense of control over their illness and environment will guide them more swiftly toward becoming as independent as possible.**

PATIENT CARE MANAGEMENT PLAN

Impaired Airway Clearance
Impaired Airway Clearance Due to Excessive Secretions or Abnormal Viscosity of Mucus
Signs and Symptoms

- Abnormal breath sounds (displaced normal sounds, adventitious sounds, diminished or absent sounds)
- Ineffective cough with or without sputum
- Tachypnea, dyspnea
- Verbal reports of inability to clear airway

Outcomes

- Cough produces thin mucus.
- Lungs are clear to auscultation.
- Respiratory rate, depth, and rhythm return to baseline.

Interventions and Rationale

1. Assess sputum for color, consistency, and amount.
2. Assess for clinical manifestations of pneumonia.
3. Provide for maximal thoracic expansion by repositioning, deep breathing, splinting, and pain management **to avoid hypoventilation and atelectasis.** If hypoventilation is present, implement the patient management plan for Impaired Breathing Due to Decreased Lung Expansion.
4. Maintain adequate hydration by administering oral and intravenous fluids (as ordered) **to thin secretions and facilitate airway clearance.**
5. Provide humidification to airways by an oxygen delivery device or artificial airway **to thin secretions and facilitate airway clearance.**
6. Administer bland aerosol every 4 hours **to facilitate expectoration of sputum.**
7. Collaborate with the practitioner regarding administration of the following:
   a. Bronchodilators to treat or prevent bronchospasms and facilitate expectoration of mucus.
   b. Mucolytics and expectorants to enhance mobilization and removal of secretions.
   c. Antibiotics to treat infection.
8. Assist with directed coughing exercises **to facilitate expectoration of secretions**. If the patient is unable to perform cascade cough, consider using huff cough (patients with hyperactive airways), end-expiratory cough (patient with secretions in the distal airway), or augmented cough (patient with weakened abdominal muscles).
   a. Cascade cough—instruct the patient to do the following:
      (1) Take a deep breath, and hold it for 1–3 seconds.
      (2) Cough out forcefully several times until all air is exhaled.
      (3) Inhale slowly through the nose.
      (4) Repeat once.
      (5) Rest, and then repeat as necessary.
   b. Huff cough—instruct the patient to do the following:
      (1) Take a deep breath, and hold it for 1–3 seconds.
      (2) Say the word "huff" while coughing out several times until air is exhaled.
      (3) Inhale slowly through the nose.
      (4) Repeat as necessary.
   c. End-expiratory cough—instruct the patient to do the following:
      (1) Take a deep breath, and hold it for 1–3 seconds.
      (2) Exhale slowly.
      (3) At the end of exhalation, cough once.
      (4) Inhale slowly through the nose.
      (5) Repeat as necessary, or follow with cascade cough.
   d. Augmented cough—instruct the patient to do the following:
      (1) Take a deep breath, and hold it for 1–3 seconds.
      (2) Perform one or more of the following maneuvers to increase intraabdominal pressure:
         (a) Tighten knees and buttocks.
         (b) Bend forward at the waist.
         (c) Place a hand flat on the upper abdomen just under the xiphoid process and press in and up abruptly during coughing.
         (d) Keep hands on the chest wall and press inward with each cough.
      (3) Inhale slowly through the nose.
      (4) Rest and repeat as necessary.
9. Suction the patient as necessary **to assist with secretion removal.**
10. Reposition the patient at least every 2 hours or use kinetic therapy **to mobilize and prevent stasis of secretions.**
11. Allow rest periods between coughing sessions, suctioning, or any other demanding activities **to promote energy conservation.**

◎ PATIENT CARE MANAGEMENT PLAN

Impaired Breathing

Impaired Breathing Due to Decreased Lung Expansion

Signs and Symptoms

- Abnormal respiratory patterns (hypoventilation, hyperventilation, tachypnea, bradypnea, obstructive breathing)
- Arterial blood gas (ABG) values (increased arterial partial pressure of carbon dioxide [$PaCO_2$], decreased pH)
- Unequal chest movement
- Shortness of breath, dyspnea

Outcomes

- Respiratory rate, rhythm, and depth return to baseline.
- Minimal or absent use of accessory muscles
- Chest expands symmetrically.
- ABG values return to baseline.

Interventions and Rationale

1. Treat pain, if present, **to prevent hypoventilation and atelectasis.** Implement the patient management plan for Acute Pain Due to Transmission and Perception of Cutaneous, Visceral, Muscular, or Ischemic Impulses.
2. Position the patient in high-Fowler or semi-Fowler position **to promote diaphragmatic descent and maximal inhalation.**
3. Assist with deep-breathing exercises and incentive spirometry with sustained maximal inspiration 5–10 times/h **to help reinflate collapsed portions of the lung.**
   a. Deep breathing—instruct the patient to do the following:
   (1) Sit up straight or lean forward slightly while sitting on edge of bed or chair (if possible).
   (2) Take in a slow, deep breath.
   (3) Pause slightly or hold breath for at least 3 seconds.
   (4) Exhale slowly.
   (5) Rest, and repeat.
   b. Incentive spirometry—instruct the patient to do the following:
   (1) Exhale normally.
   (2) Place lips around the mouthpiece and close mouth tightly around it.
   (3) Inhale slowly and as deeply as possible, noting the maximal volume of air inspired.
   (4) Hold maximal inhalation for 3 seconds.
   (5) Take the mouthpiece out of mouth and slowly exhale.
   (6) Rest and repeat.
4. Assist the practitioner with intubation and initiation of mechanical ventilation as indicated.

Impaired Breathing Due to Musculoskeletal Fatigue or Neuromuscular Impairment

Signs and Symptoms

- Unequal chest movement
- Shortness of breath, dyspnea
- Use of accessory muscles
- Tachypnea
- Thoracoabdominal asynchrony
- Abnormal ABG values (increased $PaCO_2$, decreased pH)
- Nasal flaring
- Assumption of three-point position

Outcomes

- Respiratory rate, rhythm, and depth return to baseline.
- Use of accessory muscles is minimal or absent.
- Chest expands symmetrically.
- ABG values return to baseline.

Interventions and Rationale

1. Prevent unnecessary exertion to limit drain on the patient's ventilatory reserve.
2. Instruct the patient in energy-saving techniques **to conserve the patient's ventilatory reserve.**
3. Assist with pursed-lip and diaphragmatic breathing techniques **to facilitate diaphragmatic descent and improved ventilation.**
   a. Diaphragmatic breathing—instruct the patient to do the following:
   (1) Sit in the upright position.
   (2) Place one hand on the abdomen just above the waist and the other on the upper chest.
   (3) Breathe in through the nose and feel the lower hand push out; the upper hand should not move.
   (4) Breathe out through pursed lips, and feel the lower hand move in.
4. Position the patient in the high-Fowler or semi-Fowler position **to promote diaphragmatic descent and maximal inhalation.**
5. Assist the practitioner with intubation and initiation of mechanical ventilation as indicated.

Impaired Breathing Due to Respiratory Muscle Fatigue or Metabolic Factors

Signs and Symptoms

- Dyspnea and apprehension
- Increased metabolic rate
- Increased restlessness
- Increased use of accessory muscles
- Decreased tidal volume
- Increased heart rate
- Abnormal ABG values (decreased arterial partial pressure of oxygen [PaO_2], increased arterial partial pressure of carbon dioxide [$PaCO_2$], decreased pH, decreased arterial oxygen saturation [SaO_2])
- Decreased cooperation

Outcomes

- Metabolic rate and heart rate are within the patient's baseline.
- Patient experiences eupnea.
- ABG values are within the patient's baseline.

Interventions and Rationale

1. Collaborate with the practitioner regarding application of pressure support to the ventilator to assist the patient in overcoming the work of breathing imposed by the ventilator and endotracheal tube.
2. Carefully snip excess length from the proximal end of the endotracheal tube **to decrease dead space and decrease the work of breathing.**
3. Collaborate with the practitioner and dietitian to ensure that at least 50% of the diet's nonprotein caloric source is in the form of fat rather than carbohydrates **to prevent excess carbon dioxide production.**
4. Collaborate with the practitioner and respiratory care practitioner regarding the best method of weaning for individual patients **because each situation is different, and various weaning options are available.**
   a. Consider initiating a daily spontaneous awakening trial ("sedation vacation") and spontaneous breathing trial.
   b. Monitor the patient for signs of weaning intolerance.
5. Collaborate with the practitioner and physical therapist regarding a progressive ambulation and conditioning plan **to promote overall muscle conditioning and respiratory muscle functioning.** Implement the patient management plan for Activity Intolerance Due to Prolonged Immobility or Deconditioning.

Continued

PATIENT CARE MANAGEMENT PLAN—Cont'd

6. Determine the most effective means of communication for the patient **to promote independence and reduce anxiety.**

7. Develop a daily schedule and post it in the patient's room to coordinate care and facilitate the patient's involvement in the plan.

8. Treat pain, if present, **to prevent respiratory splinting and hypoventilation.** Implement the patient management plan for Acute Pain Due to Transmission and Perception of Cutaneous, Visceral, Muscular, or Ischemic Impulses.

9. Ensure that the patient receives at least 2- to 4-hour intervals of uninterrupted sleep in a quiet, dark room. Collaborate with the practitioner and respiratory care practitioner regarding use of full ventilatory support at night **to provide respiratory muscle rest.**

10. Place the patient in the semi-Fowler position or in a chair at the bedside **for best use of ventilatory muscles and to facilitate diaphragmatic descent.**

11. Explain the weaning procedure to the patient before the trial so that the patient will understand what to expect and how to participate.

12. Monitor the patient during the weaning trial for evidence of respiratory muscle fatigue **to avoid overtiring the patient.**

13. Collaborate with the practitioner and occupational therapist to provide diversional activities during the weaning trial **to reduce the patient's anxiety.**

14. Collaborate with the practitioner and respiratory care practitioner regarding removal of the ventilator and artificial airway **after the patient has been successfully weaned.**

PATIENT CARE MANAGEMENT PLAN

Impaired Cardiac Output
Impaired Cardiac Output Due to Alterations in Preload
Signs and Symptoms
- Cardiac output is <4.0 L/min
- Cardiac index is <2.5 $L/min/m^2$
- Heart rate is >100 beats/min
- Urine output is <30 mL/h or 0.5 mL/kg/h
- Decreased mentation, restlessness, agitation, confusion
- Diminished peripheral pulses
- Blue, gray, or dark purple tint to tongue and sublingual area
- Systolic blood pressure <90 mm Hg
- Subjective complaints of fatigue

Reduced Preload
- Right atrial pressure is <2 mm Hg
- Pulmonary artery occlusion pressure is <6 mm Hg

Excessive Preload
- Right atrial pressure is >8 mm Hg
- Pulmonary artery occlusion pressure is >12 mm Hg

Outcomes
- Cardiac output is 4–8 L/min.
- Cardiac index is 2.5–4 $L/min/m^2$.
- Right atrial pressure is 2–8 mm Hg.
- Pulmonary artery occlusion pressure is 6–12 mm Hg.

Interventions and Rationale
1. Collaborate with the practitioner regarding administration of oxygen to maintain peripheral oxygen saturation (SpO_2) >92% **to prevent tissue hypoxia.**

2. Maintain surveillance for signs of decreased tissue perfusion and acidosis **to facilitate early identification and treatment of complications.**

3. Monitor fluid balance and daily weights to facilitate regulation of the patient's fluid balance.

For Reduced Preload Resulting From Volume Loss

1. Collaborate with the practitioner regarding administration of crystalloids, colloids, blood, and blood products **to increase circulating volume.**

2. Limit blood sampling, observe intravenous lines for accidental disconnection, apply direct pressure to bleeding sites, and maintain normal body temperature **to minimize fluid loss.**

3. Position the patient with legs elevated, trunk flat, and head and shoulders above the chest **to enhance venous return.**

4. Encourage oral fluids (as appropriate), administer free water with tube feedings, and replace fluids that are lost through wound or tube drainage **to promote adequate fluid intake.**

5. Maintain surveillance for signs of fluid volume excess and adverse effects of blood and blood product administration **to facilitate early identification and treatment of complications.**

For Reduced Preload Resulting From Venous Dilation

1. Collaborate with the practitioner regarding administration of vasoconstrictors **to increase venous return.**

2. Maintain surveillance for adverse effects of vasoconstrictor therapy **to facilitate early identification and treatment of complications.**

3. If the patient is hyperthermic, administer tepid bath, hypothermia blanket, or ice bags to the axilla and groin **to decrease temperature and promote vasoconstriction.**

For Excessive Preload Resulting From Volume Overload

1. Collaborate with the practitioner regarding administration of the following:
   a. Diuretics to remove excessive fluid
   b. Vasodilators to decrease venous return
   c. Inotropes to increase myocardial contractility

2. Restrict fluid intake and double-concentrate intravenous drips **to minimize fluid intake.**

3. Position the patient in the semi-Fowler or high-Fowler position **to reduce venous return.**

4. Maintain surveillance for signs of fluid volume deficit and adverse effects of diuretic, vasodilator, and inotropic therapies **to facilitate early identification and treatment of complications.**

For Excessive Preload Resulting From Venous Constriction

1. Collaborate with the practitioner regarding administration of vasodilators **to promote venous dilation.**

2. Maintain surveillance for adverse effects of vasodilator therapy **to facilitate early identification and treatment of complications.**

3. If the patient is hypothermic, wrap him or her in warm blankets or administer a hyperthermia blanket **to increase temperature and promote vasodilation.**

Impaired Cardiac Output Due to Alterations in Afterload
Signs and Symptoms
- Cardiac output is <4 L/min
- Cardiac index is <2.5 $L/min/m^2$
- Heart rate is >100 beats/min
- Urine output is <30 mL/h
- Decreased mentation, restlessness, agitation, confusion

◎ PATIENT CARE MANAGEMENT PLAN—Cont'd

- Diminished peripheral pulses
- Blue, gray, or dark purple tint to tongue and sublingual area
- Systolic blood pressure is <90 mm Hg
- Subjective complaints of fatigue

Reduced Afterload
- Pulmonary vascular resistance is <100 dyn • sec • cm^{-5}
- Systemic vascular resistance is <800 dyn • sec • cm^{-5}

Excessive Afterload
- Pulmonary vascular resistance is >250 dyn • sec • cm^{-5}
- Systemic vascular resistance is >1200 dyn • sec • cm^{-5}

Outcomes
- Cardiac output is 4—8 L/min.
- Cardiac index is 2.5—4 L/min/m^2.
- Pulmonary vascular resistance is 80—250 dyn • sec • cm^{-5}.
- Systemic vascular resistance is 800—1200 dyn • sec • cm^{-5}.

Interventions and Rationale
1. Collaborate with the practitioner regarding administration of oxygen to maintain SpO$_2$ >92% **to prevent tissue hypoxia.**
2. Maintain surveillance for signs of decreased tissue perfusion and acidosis **to facilitate early identification and treatment of complications.**

For Reduced Afterload
1. Collaborate with the practitioner regarding administration of vasoconstrictors **to promote arterial vasoconstriction and prevent relative hypovolemia.** If decreased preload is present, implement patient management plan for Impaired Cardiac Output Due to Alterations in Preload.
2. Maintain surveillance for adverse effects of vasoconstrictor therapy **to facilitate early identification and treatment of complications.**
3. If the patient is hyperthermic, administer a tepid bath, hypothermia blanket, or ice bags to the axilla and groin **to decrease temperature and promote vasoconstriction.**

For Excessive Afterload
1. Collaborate with the practitioner regarding administration of vasodilators **to promote arterial vasodilation.**
2. Collaborate with the practitioner regarding initiation of an intraaortic balloon pump **to facilitate afterload reduction.**
3. Promote rest and relaxation and decrease environmental stimulation **to minimize sympathetic stimulation.**
4. Maintain surveillance for adverse effects of vasodilator therapy **to facilitate early identification and treatment of complications.**
5. If the patient is hypothermic, wrap the patient in warm blankets or administer hyperthermia blanket **to increase temperature and promote vasodilation.**
6. If the patient is in pain, treat pain **to reduce sympathetic stimulation.** Implement patient management plan for Acute Pain Due to Transmission and Perception of Cutaneous, Visceral, Muscular, or Ischemic Impulses.

Impaired Cardiac Output Due to Alterations in Contractility
Signs and Symptoms
- Cardiac output is <4 L/min
- Cardiac index is <2.5 L/min/m^2
- Heart rate is >100 beats/min
- Urine output is <30 mL/h
- Decreased mentation, restlessness, agitation, confusion
- Diminished peripheral pulses
- Blue, gray, or dark purple tint to tongue and sublingual area
- Systolic blood pressure is <90 mm Hg
- Subjective complaints of fatigue

- Right ventricular stroke work index is <7 g/m^2/beat
- Left ventricular stroke work index is <35 g/m^2/beat

Outcomes
- Cardiac output is 4—8 L/min.
- Cardiac index is 2.5—4 L/min/m^2.
- Right ventricular stroke work index is 7—12 g/m^2/beat.
- Left ventricular stroke work index is 35—85 g/m^2/beat.

Interventions and Rationale
1. Collaborate with the practitioner regarding administration of oxygen to maintain SpO$_2$ >92% **to prevent tissue hypoxia.**
2. Maintain surveillance for signs of decreased tissue perfusion and acidosis **to facilitate early identification and treatment of complications.**
3. Ensure preload is optimized. If preload is reduced or excessive, implement the patient management plan for Impaired Cardiac Output Due to Alterations in Preload.
4. Ensure afterload is optimized. If afterload is reduced or excessive, implement the patient management plan for Impaired Cardiac Output Due to Alterations in Afterload.
5. Ensure electrolytes are optimized. Collaborate with the practitioner regarding administration of electrolyte replacement therapy **to enhance the cellular ionic environment.**
6. Collaborate with the practitioner regarding administration of inotropes **to enhance myocardial contractility.**
7. Monitor the ST segment continuously **to determine changes in myocardial tissue perfusion.** If myocardial ischemia is present, implement the patient management plan for Ineffective Tissue Perfusion Due to Decreased Myocardial Blood Flow.

Impaired Cardiac Output Due to Alterations in Heart Rate or Rhythm
Signs and Symptoms
- Cardiac output is <4 L/min
- Cardiac index is <2.5 L/min/m^2
- Heart rate is >100 beats/min or <60 beats/min
- Urine output is <30 mL/h or 0.5 mL/kg/h
- Decreased mentation, restlessness, agitation, confusion
- Diminished peripheral pulses
- Blue, gray, or dark purple tint to tongue and sublingual area
- Systolic blood pressure is <90 mm Hg
- Subjective complaints of fatigue
- Dysrhythmias

Outcomes
- Cardiac output is 4—8 L/min.
- Cardiac index is 2.5—4 L/min/m^2.
- Dysrhythmias are absent or return to baseline.
- Heart rate is >60 beats/min or <100 beats/min.

Interventions and Rationale
1. Collaborate with the practitioner regarding administration of oxygen to maintain SpO$_2$ >92% **to prevent tissue hypoxia.**
2. Ensure electrolytes are optimized. Collaborate with the practitioner regarding administration of electrolyte therapy **to enhance cellular ionic environment and avoid precipitation of dysrhythmias.**
3. Collaborate with the practitioner and pharmacist regarding the patient's current medications and their effect on heart rate and rhythm **to identify any prodysrhythmic or bradycardic side effects.**

Continued

PATIENT CARE MANAGEMENT PLAN—Cont'd

4. Maintain surveillance for signs of decreased tissue perfusion and acidosis **to facilitate early identification and treatment of complications.**
5. Monitor ST segment continuously **to determine changes in myocardial tissue perfusion.** If myocardial ischemia is present, implement the patient management plan for Ineffective Tissue Perfusion Due to Decreased Myocardial Blood Flow.

For Lethal Dysrhythmias or Asystole
1. Initiate advanced cardiac life support interventions, and notify the practitioner immediately.

For Nonlethal Dysrhythmias
1. Collaborate with the practitioner regarding administration of antidysrhythmic therapy, synchronized cardioversion, or overdrive pacing **to control dysrhythmias.**
2. Maintain surveillance for adverse effects of antidysrhythmic therapy **to facilitate early identification and treatment of complications.**

For Heart Rate <60 Beats/Min
1. Collaborate with the practitioner regarding initiation of temporary pacing **to increase heart rate.**

Impaired Cardiac Output Due to Sympathetic Blockade
Signs and Symptoms
- Decreased cardiac output and cardiac index
- Systolic blood pressure <90 mm Hg or below patient's baseline
- Decreased right atrial pressure and pulmonary artery occlusion pressure
- Decreased systemic vascular resistance
- Bradycardia
- Cardiac dysrhythmias
- Postural hypotension

Outcomes
- Cardiac output and cardiac index are within normal limits.

- Systolic blood pressure is >90 mm Hg or returns to baseline.
- Right atrial pressure and pulmonary artery occlusion pressure are within normal limits.
- Systemic vascular resistance is within normal limits.
- Sinus rhythm is present.
- Dysrhythmias are absent.
- Fainting or dizziness with position change is absent.

Interventions and Rationale
1. Implement measures to prevent episodes of postural hypertension:
   a. Change the patient's position slowly to allow the cardiovascular system time to compensate.
   b. Apply pneumatic compression stockings to promote venous return.
   c. Perform range-of-motion exercises every 2 hours to prevent venous pooling.
   d. Collaborate with the practitioner and physical therapist regarding the use of a tilt table to progress the patient from supine to upright position.
2. Collaborate with the practitioner regarding administration of the following:
   a. Crystalloids and/or colloids to increase the patient's circulating volume, **which increases stroke volume and subsequently cardiac output**
   b. Vasopressors if fluids are ineffective to constrict the patient's vascular system, **which increases resistance and subsequently blood pressure**
3. Monitor cardiac rhythm for bradycardia and/or dysrhythmias, **which can further decrease cardiac output.**
4. Avoid any activity that can stimulate the vagal response **because bradycardia can result.**
5. Treat symptomatic bradycardia and symptomatic dysrhythmias according to unit's emergency protocol or advanced cardiac life support guidelines.

PATIENT CARE MANAGEMENT PLAN

Impaired Family Coping
Impaired Family Coping Due to Critically Ill Family Member
Signs and Symptoms
- Disruption of usual family functions and roles
- Inability to accept or deal with crisis situation; use of defense mechanisms (e.g., denial, anger); unrealistic expectations of patient's outcome and care provided; judgmental toward health care practitioners
- Nonrecognition that family is in state of crisis
- Inappropriate emotional outbursts; arguments among family and with others; inability to respond to each other's feelings or support each other
- Misinterpretation of information; short attention span with repeated questions about information already provided; members not sharing information with each other
- Inability to make decisions regarding changes in family structure or about course of care for ill member; noncooperation among family members
- Expressions of grief, hopelessness, powerlessness, and isolation; do not seek or respond to support services
- Hesitancy to spend time with ill person in the critical care unit or inappropriate behavior when visiting (may upset patient)
- Neglect of own personal health; fatigue, apathy; refusal of offers for respite time

Outcomes
- The family will express an understanding of course and prognosis of illness, therapies, and alternative measures.
- The family will diminish or resolve conflicts and cooperate in decision making.
- The family will develop trust and mutual support for each member and form a cohesive unit.
- The family will support the ill person in making decisions (if capable) or respect prior wishes regarding provision of health care.
- Family efforts will be directed toward a purpose and readjust to changes in life patterns and role function. Members will accept responsibility for changes.
- The family will identify and use effective coping strategies.
- The family will identify and use available resources as needed to facilitate resolution of the crisis.
- The family will have a sense of control and confidence in meeting personal and collective needs.

Interventions and Rationale
1. Identify family's perception of the crisis situation. All initial interventions should be directed toward resolving the crisis situation. Understanding and

PATIENT CARE MANAGEMENT PLAN—Cont'd

using family theory principles will facilitate this process and individualize care.

a. Determine family structure; developmental phase of roles; and ethnic, cultural, and belief factors that may affect communication with family and the plan of care.

b. Identify strengths of the family.

2. Provide honest and accurate information in language persons can understand. Give updated information as appropriate. Listen. **This facilitates open communication among family and health care practitioners, projects a caring attitude and concern for them and the patient, and assists the family in making decisions and being involved with the plan and goals of care.**

3. Encourage liberal visitation with the patient.

a. Before the visit, prepare family members for what they will observe in a technical environment. **This prevents a strong emotional reaction to an unfamiliar and frightening situation.**

(1) Inform them about the patient's appearance and behaviors that may be distressing to them.

(2) Explain the cause of the patient's responses to stimuli (e.g., pain, trauma, surgery, medication), and explain that these behaviors are being monitored and are usually temporary.

b. Encourage them to touch the patient and let the patient know of their presence.

4. Identify and support effective coping behaviors. This aids in the family's sense of control and resolution of helplessness/powerlessness.

5. Observe for signs of fatigue and the need for emotional/spiritual support and respite from hospital waiting routine. This provides support and comfort, facilitates hope, resolves sense of isolation, gives sense of security, and diminishes guilt feeling for attending to personal needs.

a. Encourage family to verbalize feelings.

b. Provide information on available resources.

c. Alert interdisciplinary team members (social, psychological, spiritual) to family needs.

d. Provide pager device (if available) or obtain phone numbers when family leaves the hospital premises.

6. Instruct family in simple caregiving techniques, and encourage participation in the patient's care. This facilitates giving a sense of normalcy to the experience, self-confidence, and assurance that good care is being provided.

7. Serve as an advocate for the patient and family. Teach the family how to negotiate with the health care delivery system, and include them in health care team conferences when appropriate. **This facilitates informed decision making, promotes control and satisfaction, and permits mutual goal setting.**

8. Consider nonbiologic or nonlegal family relationships. Encourage contact with the patient and participation in care. **This facilitates holistic care and support of emotional ties and demonstrates respect for the family unit and relationships.**

9. Provide emotional support and compassion when the patient's condition worsens or deteriorates. **The use of touch and expression of concern for the patient and family convey comfort and trust in the health care practitioner and respect and assurance that the family's loved one will receive appropriate care and attention.**

PATIENT CARE MANAGEMENT PLAN

Impaired Gas Exchange
Impaired Gas Exchange Due to Alveolar Hypoventilation
Signs and Symptoms

- Abnormal arterial blood gas (ABG) values (decreased arterial partial pressure of oxygen [PaO_2], increased arterial partial pressure of carbon dioxide [$PaCO_2$], decreased pH, decreased arterial oxygen saturation [SaO_2])
- Somnolence
- Neurobehavioral changes (e.g., restlessness, irritability, confusion)
- Tachycardia or dysrhythmias
- Central cyanosis

Outcomes
- ABG values are within patient's baseline.
- Central cyanosis is absent.

Interventions and Rationale
1. Initiate continuous pulse oximetry or monitor peripheral oxygen saturation (SpO_2) every hour.
2. Collaborate with the practitioner and respiratory care practitioner regarding administration of oxygen to maintain SpO_2 >90%.

a. Administer supplemental oxygen by an appropriate oxygen delivery device **to increase driving pressure of oxygen in the alveoli.**

b. If supplemental oxygen alone is ineffective, administer high-flow oxygen via high-flow nasal cannula, bilevel positive airway pressure (BiPAP) via noninvasive ventilation (NIV), or positive end-expiratory pressure (PEEP) via invasive mechanical ventilation **to open collapsed alveoli and increase the surface area for gas exchange.**

3. Prevent hypoventilation.

a. Position the patient in high-Fowler or semi-Fowler position **to promote diaphragmatic descent and maximal inhalation.**

b. Assist with deep-breathing exercises and/or incentive spirometry with sustained maximal inspiration 5–10 times/h **to help reinflate collapsed portions of the lung.** See the patient management plan for Impaired Breathing Due to Decreased Lung Expansion for further instructions.

c. Treat pain, if present, **to prevent hypoventilation and atelectasis.** Implement the patient management plan for Acute Pain Due to Transmission and Perception of Cutaneous, Visceral, Muscular, or Ischemic Impulses.

4. Assist the practitioner with intubation and initiation of mechanical ventilation as indicated.

Impaired Gas Exchange Due to Ventilation-Perfusion Mismatching or Intrapulmonary Shunting
Signs and Symptoms
- Abnormal ABG values (decreased PaO_2, decreased SaO_2)
- Somnolence
- Neurobehavioral changes (restlessness, irritability, confusion)
- Central cyanosis

Outcomes
- ABG values are within patient's baseline.
- Central cyanosis is absent.

Interventions and Rationale
1. Initiate continuous pulse oximetry, or monitor SpO_2 every hour.

Continued

PATIENT CARE MANAGEMENT PLAN—Cont'd

2. Collaborate with the practitioner and respiratory care practitioner regarding administration of oxygen to maintain an SpO_2 >90%.
   a. Administer supplemental oxygen by an appropriate oxygen delivery device **to increase driving pressure of oxygen in the alveoli**.
   b. If supplemental oxygen alone is ineffective, administer high-flow oxygen via high-flow nasal cannula, BiPAP via NIV, or positive end-expiratory pressure (PEEP) via invasive mechanical ventilation **to open collapsed alveoli and increase the surface area for gas exchange.**
3. Position the patient to optimize ventilation-perfusion matching.
   a. For a patient with unilateral lung disease, position with the good lung down because gravity will improve perfusion to this area, and this will best match ventilation with perfusion.
   b. For a patient with bilateral lung disease, position with the right lung down because this lung is larger than the left and affords a greater area for ventilation and perfusion, or change position every 2 hours, favoring positions that improve oxygenation.

c. For a patient with diffuse bilateral disease, collaborate with the practitioner regarding the use of prone positioning **to encourage perfusion to the anterior region of the lungs, which are usually less damaged than the posterior region.**
   d. Avoid any position that seriously compromises oxygenation status.
4. Perform procedures only as needed, and provide adequate rest and recovery time in between **to prevent desaturation.**
5. Collaborate with the practitioner regarding administration of the following:
   a. Sedatives to decrease ventilator asynchrony and facilitate the patient's sense of control.
   b. Neuromuscular blocking agents to prevent ventilator asynchrony and decrease oxygen demand.
   c. Analgesics **to treat pain if present.** Implement the patient management plan for Acute Pain Due to Transmission and Perception of Cutaneous, Visceral, Muscular, or Ischemic Impulses.
6. Evaluate the patient for the presence of secretions. If secretions are present, implement the patient management plan for Impaired Airway Clearance Due to Excessive Secretions or Abnormal Viscosity of Mucus.

PATIENT CARE MANAGEMENT PLAN

Impaired Health Maintenance
Impaired Health Maintenance Due to Cognitive or Perceptual Learning Limitations
Signs and Symptoms
- Verbalized statement of inadequate knowledge of skills
- Verbalization of inadequate recall of information
- Verbalization of inadequate understanding of information
- Evidence of inaccurate follow-through of instructions
- Inadequate demonstration of a skill
- Lack of compliance with prescribed behavior

Outcomes
- Patient participates actively in necessary and prescribed health behaviors.
- Patient verbalizes adequate knowledge or demonstrates adequate skills.

Interventions and Rationale
1. Determine the specific cause of the patient's cognitive or perceptual limitation.
2. Provide an uninterrupted rest period before the teaching session to decrease fatigue and encourage the optimal state for learning and retention.
3. Manipulate the environment as much as possible to provide quiet and uninterrupted learning sessions.
   a. Ensure that lights are bright enough to see teaching aids but not too bright.
   b. Schedule care and medications to allow uninterrupted teaching periods.
   c. Move the patient to a quiet, private room for teaching if possible.

4. Adapt teaching sessions and materials to the level of education and ability to understand the patient and family.
   a. Provide printed material appropriate to reading level.
   b. Use terminology understood by the patient.
   c. Provide printed materials in the patient's primary language if possible.
   d. Use interpreters during teaching sessions *when necessary*.
5. Teach only present-tense focus during periods of sensory overload.
6. Determine potential effects of medications on ability to retain or recall information. Avoid teaching critical content while the patient is taking sedatives, analgesics, or other medications that affect memory.
7. Reinforce new skills and information in several teaching sessions. Use several senses when possible in a teaching session (e.g., see a film, hear a discussion, read printed information, demonstrate skills related to self-injection of insulin).
8. Reduce the patient's anxiety.
   a. Listen attentively and encourage verbalization of feelings.
   b. Answer questions as they arise in a clear and succinct manner.
   c. Elicit the patient's concerns, and address those issues first.
   d. Give only correct and relevant information.
   e. Continually assess response to teaching session, and discontinue if anxiety increases or physical condition becomes unstable.
   f. Provide nonthreatening information before more anxiety-producing information is presented.
   g. Plan for several teaching sessions so that information can be divided into small, manageable packages.

PATIENT CARE MANAGEMENT PLAN

Impaired Nutritional Intake

Impaired Nutritional Intake Due to Lack of Exogenous Nutrients and Increased Metabolic Demand

Signs and Symptoms

- Unplanned weight loss of 20% of body weight within past 6 months
- Serum albumin <3.5 g/dL
- Total lymphocytes <1500/mm^3
- Anergy
- Negative nitrogen balance
- Fatigue; lack of energy and endurance
- Nonhealing wounds
- Daily caloric intake less than estimated nutrition requirements
- Presence of factors known to increase nutrition requirements (e.g., sepsis, trauma, multiple-organ dysfunction syndrome)
- Maintenance of nothing by mouth (NPO) status for >10 days
- Long-term use of intravenous 5% dextrose
- Documentation of suboptimal calorie counts
- Drug or nutrient interaction that might decrease oral intake (e.g., chronic use of bronchodilators, laxatives, anticonvulsives, diuretics, antacids, opioids)
- Physical problems with chewing, swallowing, choking, and salivation and presence of altered taste, anorexia, nausea, vomiting, diarrhea, or constipation

Outcomes

- Patient exhibits stabilization of weight loss or weight gain of 0.5 lb daily.
- Serum albumin is >3.5 g/dL.
- Total lymphocytes are <1500/mm^3.
- Patient has positive response to cutaneous skin antigen testing.
- Patient is in positive nitrogen balance.
- Wound healing is evident.
- Daily caloric intake equals estimated nutrition requirements.
- Increased ambulation and endurance are evident.

Interventions and Rationale

1. Inquire whether the patient has any food allergies and food preferences **to ensure the food provided to the patient is not contraindicated.**
2. Monitor the patient's caloric intake and weight daily **to ensure adequacy of nutrition interventions.**
3. Collaborate with the dietitian regarding the patient's nutrition and caloric needs **to determine the appropriateness of the patient's diet to meet those needs.**
4. Monitor the patient for signs of nutrition deficiencies **to facilitate evaluation of the extent of nutrition deficit.**
5. Provide the patient with oral care before eating **to ensure optimal consumption of diet.**
6. Assist the patient to eat as appropriate **to ensure optimal consumption of diet.**
7. Collaborate with the practitioner and dietitian regarding administration of parenteral and enteral nutrition as needed.

PATIENT CARE MANAGEMENT PLAN

Impaired Peripheral Tissue Perfusion

Impaired Peripheral Tissue Perfusion Due to Decreased Blood Flow

Sign and Symptoms

- Weak and/or unequal peripheral pulses
- Delayed capillary refill
- Ischemic pain from extremity
- Cool skin on extremity
- Pale extremity
- Paresthesias from extremity

Outcomes

- Peripheral pulses are full and equal bilaterally.
- Capillary refill is equal bilaterally.
- Ischemic pain is absent.
- Skin temperature is equal in both extremities.
- Skin is pink and warm in both extremities.
- Paresthesias are absent.

Interventions and Rationale

1. Collaborate with the practitioner regarding administration of antiplatelet, anticoagulant, or fibrinolytic therapy.
2. Collaborate with the practitioner regarding pain management. Implement the patient management plan for Acute Pain Due to Transmission and Perception of Cutaneous, Visceral, Muscular, or Ischemic Impulses.
3. Ensure the patient is adequately hydrated **to decrease blood viscosity.**
4. Maintain the affected extremity in dependent position, if possible, **to enhance blood flow.**
5. Keep the affected extremity warm and protect it from injury. Do not apply heat directly to the affected extremity because this can result in injury.
6. Maintain surveillance for pain, pallor, pulselessness, paresthesia, paralysis, and poikilothermia **as indicators of abrupt change in blood flow.**
7. Maintain surveillance for tissue breakdown and arterial ulcers **as indicators of injury.**
8. Prepare the patient for possible surgery or interventional procedure to restore blood flow.

PATIENT CARE MANAGEMENT PLAN

Impaired Sleep

Impaired Sleep Due to Fragmented Sleep

Signs and Symptoms

- Decreased sleep during one block of sleep time
- Daytime sleepiness
- Decreased sleep
- Less than one-half of normal total sleep time
- Decreased slow-wave or rapid-eye-movement (REM) sleep
- Anxiety
- Fatigue
- Restlessness
- Disorientation and hallucinations
- Combativeness
- Frequent awakenings

Outcomes

- Patient's total sleep time approximates patient's normal sleep time.
- Patient can complete sleep cycles of 90 minutes without interruption.
- Patient has no delusions or hallucinations.
- Patient has reality-based thought content.

Interventions and Rationale

1. Assess the normal sleep pattern on admission and any history of sleep disturbance or chronic illness that may affect sleep or sedative/hypnotic use.
   a. Promote normal sleep activity while the patient is in the critical care unit.
   b. Assess sleep effectiveness by asking the patient how his or her sleep in the hospital compares with sleep at home.
2. Promote comfort, relaxation, and a sense of well-being.
   a. Treat pain; change, smooth, or refresh bed linens at bedtime; and provide oral hygiene.
   b. Eliminate stressful situations before bedtime.
   c. Use relaxation techniques, imagery, music, massage, or warm blankets.

   d. Have a close family member sit beside the bed and provide the patient with his or her own garments or coverings.
   e. Provide quiet or background noise of the television or music (patient preference) **to best promote sleep.**
   f. Provide a comfortable room temperature.
3. Minimize noise, particularly noise generated by the staff and equipment.
   a. Reduce the level of environmental stimuli.
   b. Dim the lights at night.
4. Foods containing tryptophan (e.g., milk, turkey) may be appropriate **because these promote sleep.**
5. Plan nap times to assist in approximating the patient's normal 24-hour sleep time.
6. Minimize awakenings to allow for at least 90-minute sleep cycles.
   a. Continually assess the need to awaken the patient, particularly at night. Distinguish between essential and nonessential patient care tasks.
   b. Organize patient management to allow for maximal amount of uninterrupted sleep while ensuring close monitoring of the patient's condition. Whenever possible, monitor physiologic parameters without waking the patient.
   c. Coordinate awakenings with other departments, such as laboratory and radiography, **to minimize sleep interruptions.**
7. Be aware of the effects of commonly used medications on sleep. **Many sedative/hypnotic medications decrease REM sleep**.
   a. Use sedative and analgesic medications that minimally disrupt sleep to complement comfort measures, with dosages reduced gradually as the medication is no longer necessary.
   b. Do not abruptly withdraw REM-suppressing medications **because this can result in REM rebound.**
8. Document the amount of uninterrupted sleep per shift, especially sleep episodes lasting longer than 2 hours. Sleep pattern disturbance is diagnosed, treated, and resolved more efficiently when formally documented in this manner.

PATIENT CARE MANAGEMENT PLAN

Impaired Spiritual Status

Impaired Spiritual Status Due to Change in Health Status That Alters Ability to Experience Meaning in Life Through Self-Expression

Signs and Symptoms

- Anxiety
- Crying
- Fear
- Expression of hopelessness
- Expression of loss of connectedness
- Insomnia
- Anger
- Questioning previously held sources of meaning
- Withdrawal from significant others
- Increased dependence on health care personnel
- Refusal to participate in care
- Avoidance of spiritual advisors
- Avoidance of previously pursued activities

Outcomes

- Patient expresses feelings, fears, and concerns.
- Patient expresses sense of hope in the future.
- Patient expresses feelings of connectedness and meaning in life.

Interventions and Rationale

1. Assess for signs and symptoms in patients with acute or chronic health problems. Changes in health status can bring about spiritual confusion in patients who are experiencing unfamiliar life circumstances. Early intervention can prevent serious spiritual problems.
2. Assess patient's mental/emotional status using active listening. Active listening can help identify central points of concern for the patient.
3. Assist the patient to identify spiritual beliefs and practices and express acceptance of those beliefs and practices. Verbalizing beliefs can help the patient regain connectedness to their familiar sources of support. An accepting atmosphere from the nurse will promote the supportive relationship.
4. Encourage the patient to engage in preferred spiritual expression. Spiritual expression is a positive method of coping and can promote a sense of well-being.

PATIENT CARE MANAGEMENT PLAN—Cont'd

5. Assist patient to identify sources of gratitude and hope. Focusing on familiar and reliable sources of strength can provide avenues for spiritual relief.

6. Include family as appropriate in discussion and support. Significant others are a primary source of support for patients, and they will be most familiar with the beliefs, strengths, and limitations of the patient in trying circumstances.

7. Offer or suggest a consultation with a spiritual advisor. **Spiritual care can promote connectedness and spiritual relief.**

8. Consider complementary therapies: meditation, guided imagery, journaling, art, or music as a means to promote relaxation and decrease anxiety. **Complementary therapies provide distraction and provide avenues of self-expression.**

PATIENT CARE MANAGEMENT PLAN

Impaired Swallowing

Impaired Swallowing Due to Neuromuscular Impairment, Fatigue, and Limited Awareness

Signs and Symptoms

- Evidence of difficulty swallowing:
  - Drooling
  - Difficulty handling oral secretions
  - Absence of gag, cough, or swallow reflex
  - Moist, wet, gurgling voice quality
  - Decreased tongue and mouth movements
  - Presence of dysarthria
- Difficulty handling solid foods:
  - Uncoordinated chewing or swallowing
  - Stasis of food in oral cavity
  - Wet-sounding voice or change in voice quality
  - Sneezing, coughing, or choking with eating
  - Delay in swallowing of more than 5 seconds
  - Change in respiratory patterns
- Difficulty handling liquids:
  - Momentary loss of voice or change in voice quality
  - Nasal regurgitation of liquids
  - Coughing with drinking
- Evidence of aspiration:
  - Hypoxemia
  - Productive cough
  - Frothy sputum
  - Wheezing, crackles, or rhonchi
  - Temperature elevation

Outcomes

- Evidence of swallowing difficulties is absent.
- Evidence of aspiration is absent.

Interventions and Rationale

1. Collaborate with the practitioner and speech therapist regarding the swallowing evaluation and rehabilitation program **to decrease the incidence of aspiration.**

2. Collaborate with the practitioner and dietitian regarding a nutrition assessment and nutrition plan **to ensure that the patient is receiving adequate nutrition.**

3. Place the patient in an upright position with the head midline and the chin slightly down **to keep food in the anterior portion of the mouth and to prevent it from falling over the base of the tongue into the open airway.**

4. Provide the patient with single-textured soft foods (e.g., cream cereals) that maintain their shape **because these foods require minimal oral manipulation.**

5. Avoid particulate foods (e.g., hamburger) and foods containing more than one texture (e.g., stew) **because these foods require more chewing and oral manipulation.**

6. Avoid dry foods (e.g., popcorn, rice, crackers) and sticky foods (e.g., peanut butter, bananas) **because these foods are difficult to manipulate orally.**

7. Provide the patient with thick liquids (e.g., fruit nectar, yogurt) **because thick liquids are more easily controlled in the mouth.**

8. Thicken thin liquids (e.g., water, juice) with a thickening preparation or avoid them **because thin liquids are easily aspirated.**

9. Place foods in the uninvolved side of the mouth because oral sensitivity and function are greatest in this area.

10. Avoid the use of straws because they can deposit the liquid too far back in the mouth for the patient to handle.

11. Serve foods and liquids at room temperature because the patient may be overly sensitive to heat or cold.

12. Offer solids and liquids at different times to avoid swallowing solids before being properly chewed.

13. Provide oral hygiene after meals to clear food particles from the mouth that could be aspirated.

14. Collaborate with the practitioner and pharmacist regarding oral medication administration to adjust the medication regimen to prevent aspiration and choking and to ensure all prescribed medications are swallowed.

15. Crush tablets (if appropriate) and mix with food that is easily formed into a bolus, use thickened liquid medications (if available), or embed small capsules into food **to facilitate oral medication administration.**

16. Inspect the mouth for residue after all medication administration **to ensure medication has been swallowed.**

17. Educate the patient and family on the swallowing problem, rehabilitation program, and emergency measures for choking.

PATIENT CARE MANAGEMENT PLAN

Impaired Ventilatory Weaning
Impaired Ventilatory Weaning Due to Physical, Psychosocial, or Situational Factors
Signs and Symptoms
Mild Impairment

- Responds to lowered levels of mechanical ventilator support with:
  - Restlessness
  - Slightly increased respiratory rate from baseline
  - Expressed feelings of increased need for oxygen, breathing discomfort, fatigue, warmth
  - Queries about possible machine malfunction
  - Increased concentration on breathing

Moderate Impairment

- Responds to lowered levels of mechanical ventilator support with:
  - Slight baseline increase in blood pressure <20 mm Hg
  - Slight baseline increase in heart rate <20 beats/min
  - Baseline increase in respiratory rate <5 breaths/min
  - Hypervigilance to activities
  - Inability to respond to coaching
  - Inability to cooperate
  - Apprehension
  - Diaphoresis
  - Eye widening ("wide-eyed look")
  - Decreased air entry on auscultation
  - Color changes: pale, slight cyanosis
  - Slight respiratory accessory muscle use

Severe Impairment

- Responds to lowered levels of mechanical ventilator support with:
  - Agitation
  - Deterioration in arterial blood gases from current baseline
  - Baseline increase in blood pressure >20 mm Hg
  - Baseline increase in heart rate >20 beats/min
  - Respiratory rate increased significantly from baseline
  - Profuse diaphoresis
  - Full respiratory accessory muscle use
  - Shallow, gasping breaths
  - Paradoxical abdominal breathing
  - Discoordinated breathing with the ventilator
  - Decreased level of consciousness
  - Adventitious breath sounds, audible airway secretions
  - Cyanosis

Outcomes

- Airway is clear.
- Underlying disorder is resolving.
- Patient is rested, and pain is controlled.
- Nutrition status is adequate.
- Patient has feelings of perceived control, situational security, and trust in the nurses.
- Patient is able to adapt to selected levels of ventilator support without undue fatigue.

Interventions and Rationale

1. Communicate interest and concern for the patient's well-being, and demonstrate confidence in ability to manage weaning process **to instill trust in the patient.**

2. Use normalizing strategies (e.g., grooming, dressing, mobilizing, social conversation) **to reinforce the patient's self-esteem and feeling of identity.**

3. Identify parameters of the patient's usual functioning before the weaning process begins **to facilitate early identification of problems.**

4. Identify the patient's strengths and resources that can be mobilized **to enhance the patient's coping and maximize weaning effort.**

5. Note concerns that adversely affect the patient's comfort and confidence, and manage them discreetly **to facilitate the patient's ease.**

6. Praise successful activities, encourage a positive outlook, and review the patient's positive progress **to increase the patient's perceived self-efficacy.**

7. Inform the patient of his or her situation and weaning progress **to permit the patient as much control as possible.**

8. Teach the patient about the weaning process and how he or she can participate in the process.

9. Negotiate daily weaning goals with the patient **to gain cooperation.**

10. Position the patient with the head of the bed elevated **to optimize respiratory efforts.**

11. Coach the patient in breath control by regular demonstrations of slow, deep, rhythmic patterns of breathing **to assist with dyspnea.**

12. Remain visible in the room and reassure the patient that help is immediately available if needed **to reduce the patient's anxiety and fearfulness.**

13. Encourage the patient to view weaning trials as a form of training, regardless of whether the weaning goal is achieved, **to avoid discouragement.**

14. Encourage the patient to maintain emotional calmness by reassuring, being present, comforting, talking down if emotionally aroused, and reinforcing the idea that he or she can and will succeed.

15. Monitor the patient's status frequently **to avoid undue fatigue and anxiety.**

16. Provide regular periods of rest by reducing activities, maintaining or increasing ventilator support, and providing oxygen as needed before fatigue advances.

17. Provide distraction (e.g., visitors, radio, television, conversation) when the patient's concentration starts to create tension and increases anxiety.

18. Ensure adequate nutrition support, sufficient rest and sleep time, and sedation or pain control **to promote the patient's optimal physical and emotional comfort.**

19. Start weaning early in the day **when the patient is most rested.**

20. Restrict unnecessary activities and visitors who do not cooperate with weaning strategies **to minimize energy demands on the patient during the weaning process.**

21. Coordinate necessary activities to promote adequate time for rest and relaxation. Implement the patient management plan for Activity Intolerance Due to Prolonged Immobility or Deconditioning.

22. Monitor the patient's underlying disease process **to ensure it is stabilized and under control.**

23. Advocate for additional resources (e.g., sedation, analgesia, rest) needed by the patient **to maximize comfort status.**

24. Develop and adhere to an individualized plan of care **to promote the patient's feelings of control.**

PATIENT CARE MANAGEMENT PLAN

Impaired Verbal Communication
Impaired Verbal Communication Due to Cerebral Speech Center Injury

Signs and Symptoms
- Inappropriate or absent speech or responses to questions
- Inability to speak spontaneously
- Inability to understand spoken words
- Inability to follow commands appropriately through gestures
- Difficulty or inability to understand written language
- Difficulty or inability to express ideas in writing
- Difficulty or inability to name objects

Outcome
- Patient is able to make basic needs known.

Interventions and Rationale
1. Collaborate with the practitioner and speech pathologist to determine the extent of the patient's communication deficit (e.g., whether fluent, nonfluent, or global aphasia is involved).
2. Have the speech therapist post a list of appropriate ways to communicate with the patient in the patient's room so that all health care personnel can be consistent in their efforts.
3. Assess the patient's ability to comprehend, speak, read, and write.
    a. Ask questions that can be answered with "yes" or "no." If a patient answers "yes" to a question, ask the opposite (e.g., "Are you hot?" "Yes." "Are you cold?" "Yes."). **This may help determine whether the patient understands what is being said**.
    b. Ask simple, short questions, and use gestures, pantomime, and facial expressions to give the patient additional clues.
    c. Stand in the patient's line of vision, giving a good view of your face and hands.
    d. Have the patient try to write with a pad and pencil. Offer pictures and alphabet letters at which to point.
    e. Make flash cards with pictures or words depicting frequently used phrases (e.g., glass of water, bedpan).
4. Maintain an uncluttered environment, and decrease external distractions **to enhance communication.**
5. Maintain a relaxed and calm manner, and explain all diagnostic, therapeutic, and comfort measures before initiating them.
6. Do not shout or speak in a loud voice. Hearing loss is not a factor in aphasia, and shouting will not help.
7. Have only one person talk at a time. It is more difficult for the patient to follow a multisided conversation.
8. Use direct eye contact, and speak directly to the patient in unhurried, short phrases.
9. Give one-step commands and directions, and provide cues through pictures and gestures.
10. Try to ask questions that can be answered with a "yes" or a "no," and avoid topics that are controversial, emotional, abstract, or lengthy.
11. Listen to the patient in an unhurried manner, and wait for his or her attempt to communicate.
    a. Expect a time lag from when you ask the patient something until the patient responds.
    b. Accept the patient's statement of essential words without expecting complete sentences.
    c. Avoid finishing the sentence for the patient if possible.
    d. Wait approximately 30 seconds before providing the word the patient may be attempting to find (except when the patient is very frustrated and needs something quickly, such as a bedpan).
    e. Rephrase the patient's message aloud **to validate it.**
    f. Do not pretend to understand the patient's message if you do not.
12. Encourage the patient to speak slowly in short phrases and to say each word clearly.
13. Ask the patient to write the message, if able, or draw pictures if only verbal communication is affected.
14. Observe the patient's nonverbal clues for validation (e.g., answers "yes" but shakes head "no").
15. When handing an object to the patient, state what it is **because hearing language spoken is necessary to stimulate language development.**
16. Explain what has happened to the patient, and offer reassurance about the plan of care.
17. Verbally address the problem of frustration over the inability to communicate, and explain that both the nurse and the patient need patience.
18. Maintain a calm, positive manner, and offer reassurance (e.g., "I know this is very hard for you, but it will get better if we work on it together").
19. Talk to the patient as an adult. Be respectful, and avoid talking down to the patient.
20. Do not discuss the patient's condition or hold conversations in the patient's presence without including him or her in the discussion. **This may be the reason some aphasic patients develop paranoid thoughts.**
21. Do not exhibit disapproval of emotional utterances or spontaneous use of profanity; instead, offer calm, quiet reassurance.
22. If the patient makes an error in speech, do not reprimand or scold, but try to compliment the patient by saying, "That was a good try."
23. Delay conversation if the patient is tired. The symptoms of aphasia worsen if the patient is fatigued, anxious, or upset.
24. Be prepared for emotional outbursts and tears from patients who have more difficulty in expressing themselves than with understanding. **The patient may become depressed, refuse treatment and food, ignore relatives, and push objects away.** Comfort the patient with statements such as, "I know it's frustrating and you feel sad, but you are not alone. Other people who have had strokes have felt the way you do. We will be here to help you get through this."

⊚ PATIENT CARE MANAGEMENT PLAN

Ineffective Tissue Perfusion
Ineffective Tissue Perfusion Due to Decreased Cerebral Blood Flow
Signs and Symptoms
- Decreased level of consciousness
- Hemiparesis or hemiplegia
- Visual changes
- Aphasia
- Dysphagia
- Facial droop
- Cognitive deficits
- Ataxia

Outcomes
- Patient is oriented to time, place, person, and situation.
- Pupils are equal and normoreactive.
- Blood pressure is within baseline or ordered parameters.
- Motor function is bilaterally equal.
- Headache, nausea, and vomiting are absent.
- Patient verbalizes importance of and displays compliance with reduced activity.
- Neurologic deficits are absent.

Interventions and Rationale
For Ischemia
1. Collaborate with the practitioner regarding administration of fibrinolytic therapy **to facilitate lysis of the clot and restoration of blood flow to the affected area.**
2. Monitor the patient for alterations in blood pressure, oxygenation, temperature, rhythm, and glucose levels.
3. Collaborate with the practitioner regarding administration of vasodilators for hypertension **to maintain the patient's blood pressure within the desired range.** Use caution in lowering blood pressure, **as hypotension decreases cerebral blood flow.**
    a. Patients receiving fibrinolytic therapy: keep systolic blood pressure <185 mm Hg and diastolic blood pressure <110 mm Hg.
    b. Patients not receiving fibrinolytic therapy: keep systolic blood pressure <220 mm Hg and diastolic blood pressure <120 mm Hg.
4. Collaborate with the practitioner regarding administration of intravenous fluids and vasoconstrictors for hypotension, **as hypotension decreases cerebral blood flow.**
5. Collaborate with the practitioner regarding administration of oxygen to maintain oxygen saturation measured >95% **to prevent hypoxemia and potential worsening of the neurologic injury.**
6. Collaborate with the practitioner regarding administration of acetaminophen for elevated temperature **because hyperthermia is associated with increased morbidity in patients with stroke.**
7. Collaborate with the practitioner regarding the treatment of dysrhythmias **resulting from increased sympathetic nervous system stimulation.**
8. Collaborate with the practitioner regarding administration of insulin for hyperglycemia, **as elevated blood glucose has been linked to an increase in the area of infarct.**
9. Collaborate with the speech therapist regarding the patient's ability to swallow before initiating oral feedings **to ensure the patient is not at risk for aspiration.**
10. Collaborate with the physical therapist to assess the patient's ability to ambulate safely **to ensure the patient is not at risk for falling** and ability to perform activities of daily living **to facilitate discharge home.**

11. Maintain surveillance for complications such as increased intracranial pressure, seizures, and acute lung failure.
12. Collaborate with the practitioner and rehabilitation specialist regarding the patient's need for rehabilitation **to maximize the patient's independence.**

For Hemorrhage
1. Assess for indicators of increased intracranial pressure and brain herniation (see the patient management plan for Decreased Intracranial Adaptive Capacity Due to Failure of Normal Intracranial Compensatory Mechanism).
2. Collaborate with the practitioner regarding administration of anticonvulsant medications **to prevent the onset of seizures or to control seizures.**
3. Collaborate with the practitioner regarding administration of vasodilators for hypertension **to avoid further bleeding.** Use caution in lowering blood pressure, **as hypotension decreases cerebral blood flow.**
    a. If systolic blood pressure is >200 mm Hg or mean arterial pressure (MAP) is >150 mm Hg, aggressive reduction in blood pressure is indicated.
    b. If systolic blood pressure is >180 mm Hg or MAP is >130 mm Hg in the presence of increased intracranial pressure, cautious reduction in pressure is indicated, maintaining cerebral perfusion pressure >60–80 mm Hg.
    c. If systolic blood pressure is >180 mm Hg or MAP is >130 mm Hg in the absence of elevated intracranial pressure, reduction in blood pressure is indicated, with a target of 160/90 mm Hg.
4. Collaborate with the practitioner regarding administration of insulin for hyperglycemia, **as elevated blood glucose has been linked to an increase in the area of infarct.**
5. Collaborate with the practitioner regarding administration of acetaminophen for elevated temperature **because hyperthermia is associated with increased morbidity in patients with stroke.**
6. Initiate precautions **to prevent rebleeding.**
    a. Ensure bed rest in a quiet environment **to lessen external stimuli.**
    b. Maintain a darkened room to lessen symptoms of photophobia.
    c. Restrict visitors, and instruct them to keep conversation as nonstressful as possible.
    d. Administer sedatives as prescribed **to reduce anxiety to promote rest.**
    e. Administer analgesics as prescribed **to relieve or lessen headache.**
    f. Provide a soft, high-fiber diet and stool softeners to prevent constipation, which can lead to straining and increased risk of rebleeding.
    g. Assist with activities of daily living (feeding, bathing, dressing, toileting).
    h. Avoid any activity that could lead to increased intracranial pressure; ensure that the patient does not flex hips beyond 90 degrees and avoids neck hyperflexion, hyperextension, or lateral hyper-rotation **that could impede jugular venous return.**
7. Collaborate with the physical therapist to assess the patient's ability to ambulate safely **to ensure the patient is not at risk for falling** and ability to perform activities of daily living **to facilitate discharge home.**
8. Collaborate with the practitioner and rehabilitation specialist regarding the patient's need for rehabilitation **to maximize the patient's independence.**

Ineffective Tissue Perfusion Due to Decreased Gastrointestinal Blood Flow
Signs and Symptoms
- Abdominal pain
- Melena
- Abdominal distention

PATIENT CARE MANAGEMENT PLAN—Cont'd

- Hyperactive to absent bowel sounds range from hyperactive to absent
- Guarding
- Fever
- Hypotension
- Tachycardia
- Altered mental status
- Urine output is <30 mL/h

Outcomes
- Normal bowel sounds are present.
- Abdominal pain, distention, and guarding are absent.
- Vital signs are at baseline.
- Urine output is >30 mL/h.

Interventions and Rationales
1. Collaborate with the practitioner regarding administration of crystalloids, colloids, blood, and blood products **to maintain adequate circulating volume.** Implement the patient management plan for Hypovolemia Due to Absolute Loss.
2. Collaborate with the practitioner regarding pain management. Implement the patient management plan for Acute Pain Due to Transmission and Perception of Cutaneous, Visceral, Muscular, or Ischemic Impulses.
3. Collaborate with the practitioner regarding administration of oxygen to maintain oxygen saturation >92% **to prevent hypoxemia and potential worsening of the gastrointestinal injury.**
4. Collaborate with the practitioner regarding administration of electrolyte replacement therapy **to maintain adequate electrolyte balance.**
5. Collaborate with the dietitian regarding administration of nutrition **because the patient will be unable to eat.** Implement the patient management plan for Impaired Nutritional Intake.
6. Maintain surveillance for complications such as gastrointestinal hemorrhage, hypovolemic shock, and septic shock.
7. Collaborate with the practitioner regarding preparation for surgery **to remove infarcted bowel.**

Ineffective Tissue Perfusion Due to Decreased Kidney Blood Flow
Signs and Symptoms
- Anuria or oliguria
- Decreased urinary creatinine clearance
- Increased serum creatinine
- Increased blood urea nitrogen (BUN)
- Electrolyte abnormalities: sodium and potassium
- Increased MAP, pulmonary artery occlusion pressure (PAOP), pulmonary artery diastolic (PAD) pressure, central venous pressure (CVP) secondary to fluid overload
- Sinus tachycardia
- Metabolic acidosis
- Crackles on lung auscultation
- Engorged neck veins
- Fluid weight gain
- Pitting edema
- Mental status changes
- Anemia

Outcomes
- Electrolytes are within normal range.
- Serum creatinine and blood urea nitrogen are within normal range.
- Normal acid–base balance is present.
- Urinary output is within normal limits, or patient is stable on dialysis.
- Hemoglobin and hematocrit values are stable.

Interventions and Rationale
1. Monitor intake and output, urine output, and the patient's weight.
2. Collaborate with the practitioner regarding administration of crystalloids, colloids, blood, and blood products **to increase circulating volume and maintain mean arterial pressure >70 mm Hg.**
3. Collaborate with the practitioner regarding administration of inotropes **to enhance myocardial contractility and increase cardiac index to >2.5 L/min.**
4. Collaborate with the practitioner regarding administration of diuretics to oliguric patient **to flush out cellular debris and increase urine output.**
5. Minimize the patient's exposure to nephrotoxic medications **to decrease damage to kidneys.**
6. Monitor blood levels of drugs cleared by kidneys **to avoid accumulation.**
7. Monitor the patient for signs of electrolyte imbalance **as a result of impaired electrolyte regulation.**
8. Maintain surveillance for signs and symptoms of fluid overload.
9. Monitor the patient's clinical status and response to dialysis therapy **to ensure the patient is receiving safe and effective dialytic therapy.**

Ineffective Tissue Perfusion Due to Decreased Myocardial Blood Flow
Signs and Symptoms
- Angina for more than 30 minutes
- ST-segment elevation on 12-lead electrocardiogram (ECG)
- Elevated biomarkers
- Apprehension
- Shortness of breath

Outcomes
- Systolic blood pressure is >90 mm Hg.
- Mean arterial pressure is >60 mm Hg.
- Heart rate is <100 beats/min.
- Pulmonary artery pressures are within normal limits or back to baseline.
- Cardiac index is >2.2 L/min/m^2.
- Urine output is >0.5 mL/kg/h or >30 mL/h.
- The 12-lead ECG is normalized without new Q waves.
- Chest pain is absent.
- CK-MB enzymes, troponin I, and myoglobin levels are within normal range.

Interventions and Rationale
1. Collaborate with the practitioner regarding administration of fibrinolytic therapy or the preparation of the patient for percutaneous coronary intervention **to restore myocardial blood flow.**
2. Collaborate with the practitioner regarding administration of oxygen at 2 L/min to achieve oxygen saturation measured >90% **to maximize myocardial oxygen supply.**
3. Collaborate with the practitioner regarding administration of sublingual nitroglycerin and/or intravenous nitroglycerin infusion **to augment coronary blood flow and reduce cardiac work by decreasing preload and afterload**.
   a. Do not administer nitrates to patients who have taken phosphodiesterase inhibitors for erectile dysfunction within the last 24 or 48 hours (depending on the medication), **as severe hypotension may occur**.
4. Collaborate with the practitioner regarding administration of morphine **to control pain.**

Continued

◎ PATIENT CARE MANAGEMENT PLAN—Cont'd

5. Collaborate with the practitioner regarding administration of aspirin, antiplatelet therapy, and heparin **to prevent recurrent thrombosis and inhibit platelet function.**
6. Collaborate with the practitioner regarding administration of beta-blockers **to decrease myocardial oxygen demand and prevent recurrent ischemia.**
7. Collaborate with the practitioner regarding administration of angiotensin-converting enzyme inhibitors **to block the conversion of angiotensin I to angiotensin II, a potent vasoconstrictor.**
8. Maintain the patient on bed rest with bedside commode privileges **to minimize myocardial oxygen demand.**
9. Monitor the patient's hemodynamic and cardiac rhythm status:
   a. Select cardiac monitoring leads based on infarct location and rhythm to obtain the best rhythm for monitoring.
   b. Evaluate cardiac rhythm for the presence of dysrhythmias, which are common complications of myocardial ischemia.
   c. Collaborate with the practitioner regarding administration of anti-dysrhythmic medications.
   d. Assess serum electrolytes (potassium and magnesium) and arterial blood gases.
   e. Collaborate with the practitioner regarding administration of electrolytes to correct any imbalances.
   f. Monitor the ST segment continuously to determine changes in myocardial tissue perfusion.
   g. Monitor the patient's blood pressure at least every hour, as many conditions (e.g., drugs, dysrhythmias, myocardial ischemia) may cause hypotension (systolic blood pressure <90 mm Hg).
   h. Treat symptomatic dysrhythmias according to the unit's emergency protocol or advanced cardiac life support guidelines.
10. Instruct the patient to avoid the Valsalva maneuver, as forced expiration against a closed glottis causes sudden and intense changes in systolic blood pressure and heart rate.

◎ PATIENT CARE MANAGEMENT PLAN

Lack of Knowledge of Treatment Regime
Lack of Knowledge of Treatment Regime Due to Lack of Previous Exposure to Information
Signs and Symptoms
- Verbalized statement of inadequate knowledge or skills
- New diagnosis or health problem requiring self-management or care
- Lack of prior formal or informal education about the specific health problem
- Demonstration of inappropriate behaviors related to management of the health problem

Outcomes
- Patient verbalizes adequate knowledge about or performs skills related to disease process, its causes, factors related to onset of symptoms, and self-management of disease or health problem.
- Patient actively participates in health behaviors required for performance of a procedure or in behaviors enhancing recovery from illness and preventing recurrence or complications.

Interventions and Rationale
1. Determine the existing level of knowledge or skill.
2. Assess factors that affect the knowledge deficit:
   a. Learning needs, including the patient's priorities and the necessary knowledge and skills for safety
   b. Learning ability of the patient, including language skills, level of education, ability to read, and preferred learning style
   c. Physical ability to perform prescribed skills or procedures; consider effect of limitations imposed by treatment such as bed rest, restriction of movement by intravenous or other equipment, or effect of sedatives or analgesics
   d. Psychological effect of stage of adaptation to disease
   e. Activity tolerance and ability to concentrate
   f. Motivation to learn new skills or gain new knowledge
3. Reduce or limit barriers to learning:
   a. Provide consistent nurse-patient contact to encourage development of a trusting and therapeutic relationship.
   b. Structure the environment to enhance learning and control unnecessary noise or interruptions.
   c. Individualize the teaching plan to fit the patient's current physical and psychological status.
   d. Delay teaching until the patient is ready to learn.
   e. Conduct teaching sessions during a time of day when the patient is most alert and receptive.
   f. Meet the patient's immediate learning needs as they arise (e.g., give a brief explanation of procedures when they are performed).
4. Promote active participation in the teaching plan by the patient and family:
   a. Solicit input during the development of the plan.
   b. Develop mutually acceptable goals and outcomes.
   c. Solicit expression of feelings and emotions related to new responsibilities.
   d. Encourage questions.
5. Conduct teaching sessions, using the most appropriate teaching methods.
6. Use the "teach-back" method to confirm that you have explained to the patient what they need to know in a manner that the patient understands.
   a. Use simple lay language, explain the concept, or demonstrate the process to the patient/caregiver.
      (1) Avoid technical terms to avoid misunderstandings.
      (2) If the patient/caregiver has limited English proficiency, use a professional translator to reduce miscommunication.
   b. Ask the patient/caregiver to repeat in his or her own words how he or she understands the concept explained. If a process was demonstrated to the patient, ask the patient/caregiver to demonstrate it independent of assistance.
   c. Identify and correct misunderstandings of or incorrect procedures by the patient/caregiver.
   d. Ask the patient/caregiver to demonstrate his or her understanding or procedural ability again **to ensure the aforementioned misunderstandings are now corrected.**
   e. Repeat steps until convinced the patient/caregiver comprehends the concept or possesses the ability to perform the procedure accurately and safely.
7. Provide written materials that enhance health literacy:
   a. Limit content to one or two key objectives. Do not provide too much information or try to cover everything at once.
   b. Limit content to what patients really need to know. Avoid information overload.
   c. Use only words that are well known to individuals without medical training.

◎ PATIENT CARE MANAGEMENT PLAN—Cont'd

d. Ensure that content is appropriate for the age and culture of the target audience.

e. Write at or below the sixth-grade level.

f. Use words of one or two syllables.

g. Use short paragraphs.

h. Use active voice.

i. Avoid all but the simplest tables and graphs. Clear explanations (legends) should be placed adjacent to the table or graph as well as in the text.

j. Use large font (minimum 12 point) with serifs. (Serif text has the little horizontal lines that you see at the bottoms of letters such as "f," "x," "n," and others.)

k. Do not use more than two or three font styles on a page. **Consistency in appearance is important.**

l. Use uppercase and lowercase text. ALL-UPPERCASE TEXT IS HARD TO READ.

m. Ensure a good amount of empty space on the page. Do not clutter the page with text or pictures.

n. Use headings and subheadings to separate blocks of text.

o. Bulleted lists are preferable to blocks of text in paragraphs.

p. Illustrations are useful if they depict common, easy-to-recognize objects. Images of people, places, and things should be age and culturally appropriate to the target audience. Avoid complex anatomic diagrams.

8. Initiate referrals for follow-up if necessary:

a. Health educators

b. Home health care

c. Rehabilitation programs

d. Social services

9. Evaluate effectiveness of teaching plan based on the patient's ability to meet preset goals and objectives **to determine need for further teaching.**

◎ PATIENT CARE MANAGEMENT PLAN

Powerlessness
Powerlessness Due to Lack of Control Over Current Situation or Disease Progression
Signs and Symptoms
Severe

- Verbal expressions of having no control or influence over situation
- Verbal expressions of having no control or influence over outcome
- Verbal expressions of having no control over self-care
- Depression over physical deterioration that occurs despite patient's compliance with regimens
- Apathy

Moderate

- Nonparticipation in care or decision making when opportunities are provided
- Expressions of dissatisfaction and frustration about inability to perform previous tasks and/or activities
- Lack of progress monitoring
- Expressions of doubt about role performance
- Reluctance to express true feelings, fearing alienation from caregivers
- Passivity
- Inability to seek information about care
- Dependence on others that may result in irritability, resentment, anger, and guilt
- No defense of self-care practices when challenged

Low

- Passivity

Outcomes

- Patient verbalizes increased control over situation by wanting to do things his or her way.
- Patient actively participates in planning care.
- Patient requests needed information.
- Patient chooses to participate in self-care activities.
- Patient monitors progress.

Interventions and Rationale

1. Evaluate the patient's feelings and perception of the reasons for lack of power and sense of helplessness.

2. Determine as far as possible the patient's usual response to limited-control situations. Determine through ongoing assessment the patient's usual locus of control (i.e., believes that influence over his or her life is exerted by luck, fate, or powerful persons [external locus of control] or that influence is exerted through personal choices, self-effort, self-determination [internal locus of control]).

3. Support the patient's physical control of the environment by involving him or her in care activities; knock before entering room if appropriate; ask permission before moving personal belongings. Inform the patient that although an activity may not be to his or her liking, it is necessary. **This gives the patient permission to express dissatisfaction with the environment and the regimen.**

4. Personalize the patient's care using his or her preferred name. **This supports the patient's psychological control.**

5. Provide a therapeutic rationale for all the patient is asked to do for himself or herself and for all that is being done for and with him or her. Reinforce the practitioner's explanations; clarify misconceptions about the illness situation and treatment plans. **This supports the patient's cognitive control.**

6. Include the patient in care planning by encouraging participation and allowing choices wherever possible (e.g., timing of personal care activities; deciding when pain medicines are needed). Point out situations in which no choices exist.

7. Provide opportunities for the patient to exert influence over himself or herself and his or her body, affecting an outcome. For example, share with the patient the nurse's assessment of his or her breath sounds and explain that they can be improved by self-initiated deep-breathing exercises. **Feedback that the patient has been successful in helping clear his or her lungs reinforces the influence he or she does retain.**

8. Encourage the family to permit the patient to do as much independently as possible **to foster perception of personal power.**

9. Assist the patient to establish realistic short-term and long-term goals. Setting unrealistic or unattainable goals inadvertently reinforces the patient's perception of powerlessness.

10. Document care to provide for continuity so that the patient can maintain appropriate control over the environment.

Continued

◎ PATIENT CARE MANAGEMENT PLAN—Cont'd

11. Assist the patient to regain strength and activity tolerance as appropriate, **increasing a sense of control and self-reliance.**
12. Increase the sensitivity of the health team members and significant others to the patient's sense of powerlessness. Use power over the patient carefully. Use the words *must, should,* and *have to* with caution

because they communicate coercive powers and imply that the objects of "musts" and "shoulds" are of benefit to the nurse instead of the patient.
13. Plan with the patient for transfer from the critical care unit to the intermediate unit and eventually to home.

◎ PATIENT CARE MANAGEMENT PLAN

Relocation Stress

Relocation Stress Due to Transfer Out of the Critical Care Unit

Signs and Symptoms
- Alienation
- Aloneness
- Anger
- Concern over relocation
- Dependency
- Depression
- Fear of an unknown environment
- Frustration
- Increased physical symptoms
- Increased verbalization of needs
- Insecurity
- Loneliness
- Move from critical care unit to another environment
- Pessimism
- Sleep disturbance
- Unwillingness to move
- Withdrawal
- Worry

Outcomes
- Patient will express willingness to move to a new environment.
- Anxiety will be absent.

Interventions and Rationale
1. Initiate pretransfer teaching as soon as appropriate during the patient's stay in the critical care unit **to ease the transition from the critical care unit to the next environment.** Teaching should focus on the differences in the environment and the care the patient would receive.
2. Provide the patient and family written information regarding the transfer (if available) **to enhance effectiveness of teaching.**
3. Help the patient see that progress is being made **in preparation for transfer.** Each time a tube is removed or a treatment frequency is decreased, reinforce with the patient and family that the patient is progressing.
4. Remove monitoring and supportive equipment from the patient's room when no longer needed to allow the patient to experience the loss of technology while still in the critical care unit.
5. Encourage the patient and family to discuss concerns regarding relocation.
6. Assist the patient and family members to develop and maintain a positive perception of the transfer.
7. Arrange for the patient's family to have a tour of the new unit as a means of familiarizing them with the unit before the patient's transfer.

◎ PATIENT CARE MANAGEMENT PLAN

Risk for Aspiration

Risk Factors
- Impaired laryngeal sensation or reflex
- Reduced level of consciousness
- Extubation
- Impaired pharyngeal peristalsis or tongue function
- Neuromuscular dysfunction
- Central nervous system dysfunction
- Head or neck injury
- Impaired laryngeal closure or elevation
- Laryngeal nerve dysfunction
- Artificial airways
- Gastrointestinal tubes
- Increased gastric volume
- Delayed gastric emptying
- Enteral feedings
- Medication administration
- Increased intragastric pressure
- Upper abdominal surgery
- Obesity
- Pregnancy
- Ascites
- Decreased lower esophageal sphincter pressure

- Increased gastric acidity
- Gastrointestinal tubes
- Decreased antegrade esophageal propulsion
- Trendelenburg or supine position
- Esophageal dysmotility
- Esophageal structural defects or lesions

Outcomes
- Breath sounds are normal, or there is no change in the patient's baseline breath sounds.
- Arterial blood gas values remain within the patient's baseline.
- There is no evidence of gastric contents in lung secretions.

Interventions and Rationale
1. Assess gastrointestinal function to rule out hypoactive peristalsis and abdominal distention.
2. Position the patient with the head of the bed elevated 30 degrees to prevent gastric reflux through gravity. If head elevation is contraindicated, position the patient in the right lateral decubitus position to facilitate passage of gastric contents across the pylorus.
3. Maintain patency and functioning of nasogastric suction apparatus to prevent accumulation of gastric contents.

PATIENT CARE MANAGEMENT PLAN—Cont'd

4. Provide frequent and scrupulous mouth care to prevent colonization of the oropharynx with bacteria and inoculation of the lower airways.
5. Ensure that the endotracheal or tracheostomy cuff is properly inflated **to limit aspiration of oropharyngeal secretions.**
6. Treat nausea promptly; collaborate with the practitioner on an order for an antiemetic **to prevent vomiting and resultant aspiration.**

Additional Interventions for Patient Receiving Continuous or Intermittent Enteral Tube Feedings
1. Position the patient with the head of the bed elevated 45 degrees **to prevent gastric reflux.** If a head-down position becomes necessary at any time, interrupt the feeding 30 minutes before the position change.

2. Check the placement of the feeding tube by auscultation or radiographically at regular intervals (e.g., before administering intermittent feedings and after position changes, suctioning, coughing episodes, or vomiting) **to ensure proper placement of the tube.**
3. Monitor the patient for signs of delayed gastric emptying **to decrease potential for vomiting and aspiration**.
   a. For large-bore tubes, check residuals of tube feedings before intermittent feedings and every 4 hours during continuous feedings. Consider withholding feedings for residuals >150% of the hourly rate (continuous feeding) or >50% of the previous feeding (intermittent feeding).
   b. For small-bore tubes, observe abdomen for distention, palpate abdomen for hardness or tautness, and auscultate abdomen for bowel sounds.

PATIENT CARE MANAGEMENT PLAN

Risk for Infection
Risk Factors
- Inadequate primary defenses (e.g., broken skin, traumatized tissue, decreased ciliary action, stasis of body fluids, change in pH secretions, altered peristalsis)
- Inadequate secondary defenses (e.g., decreased hemoglobin, leukopenia, suppressed inflammatory or immune response)
- Immunocompromised state
- Inadequate acquired immunity
- Tissue destruction and increased environmental exposure
- Chronic disease
- Invasive procedures
- Malnutrition
- Pharmacologic agents (e.g., antibiotics, steroids)

Outcomes
- Total lymphocyte count is $>1000/mm^3$.
- White blood cell count is within normal limits.
- Temperature is within normal limits.
- Blood, urine, wound, and sputum culture results are negative.

Interventions and Rationale
1. Perform proper hand hygiene before and after patient care **to reduce the transmission of microorganisms.**
2. Use appropriate personal protective equipment in accordance with US Centers for Disease Control and Prevention guidelines.
   a. Ensure the practitioner uses maximum barrier precautions when inserting lines.
      (1) Ensure sterile gloves, gown, and mask are worn.
      (2) Drape the patient completely with a sterile sheet.
3. Use aseptic technique for insertion and manipulation of invasive monitoring devices, intravenous lines, and urinary drainage catheters **to maintain sterility of environment**.
   a. Ensure the practitioner uses maximum barrier precautions when inserting lines.
      (1) Ensure sterile gloves, gown, and mask are worn.
      (2) Drape the patient completely with a sterile sheet.
4. Stabilize all invasive lines and catheters to avoid unintentional manipulation and contamination.
5. Use aseptic technique for dressing changes to prevent contamination of wounds or insertion sites.
6. Change any line placed under emergent conditions within 24 hours **because aseptic technique is usually breached during an emergency.**

7. Collaborate with the practitioner to change any dressing that is saturated with blood or drainage **because these are media for microorganism growth.**
8. Minimize use of stopcocks and maintain caps on all stopcock ports **to reduce the ports of entry for microorganisms.**
9. Avoid the use of nasogastric tubes, nasotracheal tubes, and nasopharyngeal suctioning in the patient with a suspected cerebrospinal fluid leak **to decrease the incidence of central nervous system infection.**
10. Change ventilator circuits with humidifiers when visibly soiled or mechanically malfunctioning **to avoid introducing microorganisms into the system.** Do not change routinely.
11. Provide the patient with a clean manual resuscitation bag **to avoid cross-contamination between patients.**
12. Provide oral care to a patient with an artificial airway or an unresponsive patient every 2—4 hours and as needed (PRN) **to decrease the incidence of hospital-acquired pulmonary infections**.
    a. Swab mouth and moisten lips every 4 hours.
    b. Brush teeth with an in-line suction toothbrush every 12 hours. Rinse or swab the patient's mouth with chlorhexidine after brushing at least once every 24 hours.
    c. Suction subglottic secretions (secretions pooling above the cuff of the endotracheal tube or tracheostomy tube) every 12 hours and before repositioning the tube or deflation of the cuff.
    d. Provide lip balm to keep the patient's lips moistened PRN.
    e. Provide mouth moisturizer to keep the patient's mouth moistened PRN.
13. Cleanse in-line suction catheters with sterile saline according to the manufacturer's instructions **to avoid accumulation of secretions within the catheter.**
14. Maintain the head of the bed elevated at 30—45 degrees in patients with an artificial airway **to decrease the incidence of aspiration.**
15. Use disposable sterile scissors, forceps, and hemostats **to reduce transmission of microorganisms.**
16. Maintain a closed urinary drainage system to decrease the incidence of urinary infections.
17. Keep the urinary drainage tubing and bag below the level of the patient's bladder **to prevent the backflow of urine.**
18. Assess the urinary drainage tubing for kinks **to prevent stasis of urine.**
19. Protect all access device sites from potential sources of contamination (nasogastric reflux, draining wounds, ostomies, sputum).
20. Refrigerate parenteral nutrition solutions and opened enteral nutrition formulas **to inhibit bacterial growth.**

Continued

PATIENT CARE MANAGEMENT PLAN—Cont'd

21. Maintain daily surveillance of invasive devices for signs and symptoms of infection.
22. Notify the practitioner of elevated temperature or if any signs or symptoms of infection are present.

Additional Interventions for Patient Receiving Immunosuppressive Drugs

1. Obtain blood, urine, and sputum cultures for temperature elevations >38°C (100.4°F) **because elevation likely is caused by bacteremia or bladder or pulmonary infection.**
2. Auscultate breath sounds at least every 6 hours. Pulmonary infection is the most common type of infection, and changes in breath sounds might be an early indication.
3. Inspect wounds at least every 8 hours for redness, swelling, or drainage, **which may indicate infection.**
4. Inspect overall skin integrity and oral mucosa for signs of breakdown, **which place the patient at risk for infection.**

5. Notify the practitioner of new-onset cough. **Even a nonproductive cough may indicate pulmonary infection.**
6. Monitor white blood cell count daily, and report leukocytosis or sudden development of leukopenia, **which may indicate an infectious process.**
7. Protect the patient from exposure to any staff or family member with a contagious lesion (e.g., herpes simplex) or respiratory infections.
8. Collaborate with the dietitian regarding the patient's nutrition status and need for augmentation of nutrition intake as necessary **to prevent debilitation and increased susceptibility to infection.**
9. Collaborate with the practitioner to remove invasive lines and catheters as soon as possible **to decrease potential portals of entry.**
10. Teach the patient the clinical manifestations of infection. A knowledgeable patient will seek medical attention promptly, which will result in earlier treatment and a decreased risk that infection will become life threatening.

PATIENT CARE MANAGEMENT PLAN

Situational Low Self-Esteem
Situational Low Self-Esteem Due to Feelings of Guilt About Physical Deterioration

Signs and Symptoms

- Inability to accept positive reinforcement
- Lack of follow-through
- Nonparticipation in therapy
- Not taking responsibility for self-care (i.e., self-neglect)
- Self-destructive behavior
- Lack of eye contact

Outcomes

- Patient verbalizes feelings of self-worth.
- Patient maintains positive relationships with significant others.
- Patient manifests active interest in appearance by completing personal grooming daily.

Interventions and Rationale

1. Evaluate the meaning of the health-related situation. How does the patient feel about himself or herself, the diagnosis, and the treatment? How does the present situation fit into the larger context of his or her life?
2. Assess the patient's emotional level, interpersonal relationships, and feeling about himself or herself. Recognize the patient's uniqueness (e.g., how the hair is worn, preference for name used).

3. Help the patient discover and verbalize feelings and understand the crisis by listening and providing information.
4. Assist the patient to identify strengths and positive qualities that increase the sense of self-worth. Focus on past experiences of accomplishment and competency. Help the patient with positive self-reinforcement. Reinforce the love and affection of family and significant others.
5. Assess coping techniques that have been helpful in the past. Help the patient decide how to handle negative or incongruent feedback about the situation.
6. Encourage visits from family and significant others. Facilitate interactions and ensure privacy. Help family members entering the critical care unit by explaining what they will see. Increase visitors' comfort with equipment; offer chairs and other courtesies.
7. Encourage the patient to pursue interest in individual or social activities, even though difficult in the critical care unit.
8. Reflect caring, concern, empathy, respect, and unconditional acceptance in nurse–patient relationships.
9. The nurse is a significant other for the patient who provides important appraisals of the patient and who can facilitate the change process.
10. Help the family support the patient's self-esteem.
11. Provide for continuity of nurse assignment to ensure consistent contacts that can **facilitate support of the patient's self-esteem.**

◎ PATIENT CARE MANAGEMENT PLAN

Stress Overload

Stress Overload Due to Critical Illness and Stressors of the Critical Care Environment

Signs and Symptoms

- Pain, discomfort, and physical restrictions
- Unfamiliar environments with excessive light, noises, alarms, and distressing events
- Loss of ability for verbal expression due to intubation
- Unfamiliar bodily sensations resulting from bed rest, medications, surgery, or symptoms
- Fear of death
- Lack of sleep
- Loss of autonomy and control over one's body, environment, privacy, and daily activities
- Isolation interrupted only by brief visits, threatening stimuli, and procedural touch
- Separation from family, friends, and meaningful social roles and work
- Loss of dignity, embarrassing exposures, and a sense of vulnerability
- Concerns regarding finances and potential job loss
- Fear of permanent health deficits
- Spiritual distress with questions and concerns about meaning of the crisis and life

Outcomes

- Patient demonstrates an increased level of comfort.
- Patient maintains a mild or moderate level of anxiety.
- Patient expresses feelings, fears, and concerns.

Interventions and Rationale

1. Monitor the patient's level of pain through medication and physical comfort by such means as repositioning. **Pain and physical discomfort greatly increase the stressfulness of critical care admissions.**
2. Assess the patient's level of anxiety. Mild and some periods of moderate anxiety are expected, but severe anxiety and panic should be addressed immediately through directive measures such as slow, deep breathing and medication. **High levels of anxiety are extremely uncomfortable, unhealthy, and even dangerous.**
3. Reduce or eliminate excessive lighting and mimic the 24-hour natural rhythm as much as possible. Provide blackout masks to eliminate light if possible. **Excessive lighting at night disrupts the body's natural circadian rhythms, resulting in an impaired ability to sleep, which further contributes to stress.**
4. Reduce or eliminate the experience of excessive noise:

a. Provide earplugs. Earplugs will reduce the experience of noise.
b. Limit conversation immediately outside the patient's room. Limiting conversations outside of the patient's room will provide for more quiet time.
c. Post a sign outside of the patient's room reminding staff and visitors of the need for a quiet environment. Reminding staff and visitors is an important step in eliminating noise.
d. Eliminate overhead paging on the unit. Overhead paging can be replaced by more sophisticated personal technology.
e. Advocate for smart monitors to eliminate nuisance alarms and adjust the default settings on alarms to reduce unnecessary noise. Alarm noise can be reduced by acquiring smart monitors and by adjusting the alarm default.

5. Provide explanations and education about what is happening with the patient's physical condition and the treatments that are being provided. **Fear of the unknown and lack of information about what is happening increases the stressfulness of being critically ill.**
6. Help conscious intubated patients express themselves by providing writing tools, a communication board, or higher technological methods. **Patients who are intubated face a higher level of stress due to the inability to communicate. Providing alternatives to verbalization reduces anxiety.**
7. Maintain the patient's sense of dignity by properly covering them during procedures. Ask others to step out of the room during these times. **States of undress break down social norms and add to a strange, scary, and bewildering situation.**
8. Encourage the patient to talk about feelings, concerns, and fears. Giving the patient permission to express feelings, concerns, and fears not only provides catharsis, but it may give the nurse the opportunity to clear up misunderstandings and misperceptions.
9. Spend time with the patient outside of time required for usual physical care. **Spending time with the patient reduces feelings of isolation and reduces stress.**
10. Ask whether the patient is interested in speaking with the hospital's chaplain or other clergy for spiritual care. **During times of crisis, people often derive comfort in discussing issues of faith and existential matters.**
11. Consult with a social worker to support patients and families. A social worker can also help with financial, insurance, and legal issues, and future care needs. **Specialty hospital personnel can provide essential expertise to patients and families whose lives have become affected by a critical care stay.**

◎ PATIENT CARE MANAGEMENT PLAN

Unilateral Neglect

Unilateral Neglect Due to Perceptual Disruption

Signs and Symptoms

- Neglect of involved body parts and/or extrapersonal space
- Denial of existence of the affected limb or side of body
- Denial of hemiplegia or other motor and sensory deficits
- Left homonymous hemianopia
- Difficulty with spatial-perceptual tasks
- Left hemiplegia

Outcomes

- Patient is safe and free from injury.
- Patient is able to identify safety hazards in the environment.
- Patient recognizes disability and describes physical deficits present (e.g., paralysis, weakness, numbness).
- Patient demonstrates ability to scan the visual field to compensate for loss of function or sensation in affected limbs.

Interventions and Rationale

1. Adapt environment to the patient's deficits **to maintain patient safety**.

Continued

⊚ PATIENT CARE MANAGEMENT PLAN—Cont'd

a. Position the patient's bed with the unaffected side facing the door.

b. Approach and speak to the patient from the unaffected side. If the patient must be approached from the affected side, announce your presence as soon as entering the room **to avoid startling the patient.**

c. Position the call light, bedside stand, and personal items on the patient's unaffected side.

d. If the patient will be assisted out of bed, simplify the environment **to eliminate hazards** by removing unnecessary furniture and equipment.

e. Provide frequent reorientation of the patient to the environment.

f. Observe the patient closely, and anticipate his or her needs. **Despite repeated explanations, the patient may have difficulty retaining information about the deficits.**

g. When the patient is in bed, elevate his or her affected arm on a pillow **to prevent dependent edema and support the hand in a position of function.**

2. Assist the patient to recognize the perceptual defect.

a. Encourage the patient to wear any prescriptive corrective glasses or hearing aids **to facilitate communication**.

b. Instruct the patient to turn the head past midline **to view the environment on the affected side.**

c. Encourage the patient to look at the affected side and to stroke the limbs with the unaffected hand. Encourage handling of the affected limbs **to reinforce awareness of the affected side.**

d. Instruct the patient to look for the affected extremity when performing simple tasks **to know where it is at all times.**

e. After pointing to them, have the patient name the affected parts.

f. Encourage the patient to use self-exercises (e.g., lifting the affected arm with the unaffected hand).

g. If the patient is unable to discriminate between the concepts of *right* and *left*, use descriptive adjectives such as "the weak arm," "the affected leg," or "the good arm" to refer to the body. Use gestures, not just words, to indicate right and left.

3. Collaborate with the patient, practitioner, and the rehabilitation team to design and implement a beginning rehabilitation program for use during the critical care unit stay.

a. Use adaptive equipment (braces, splints, slings) as appropriate.

b. Teach the patient the individual components of any activity separately, and then proceed to integrate the component parts into a completed activity.

c. Instruct the patient to attend to the affected side, if able, and to assist with bathing or other tasks.

d. Use tactile stimulation to reintroduce the arm or leg to the patient. Rub the affected parts with different textured materials to stimulate sensations (e.g., warm, cold, rough, soft).

e. Encourage activities that require the patient to turn the head toward the affected side, and retrain the patient to scan the affected side and environment visually.

f. If the patient is allowed out of bed, cue him or her with reminders to scan visually when ambulating. Assist and remain in constant attendance **because the patient may have difficulty maintaining correct posture, balance, and locomotion.** There may be vertical-horizontal perceptual problems, with the patient leaning to the affected side to align with the perceived vertical. Provide sitting, standing, and balancing exercises before getting the patient out of bed.

4. Assist the patient with oral feedings.

a. Avoid giving the patient any very hot food items that could cause injury.

b. Place the patient in an upright sitting position if possible.

c. Encourage the patient to feed himself or herself; if necessary, guide the patient's hand to the mouth.

d. If the patient is able to feed himself or herself, place one dish at a time in front of the patient. When the patient is finished with the first, add another dish. Tell the patient what he or she is eating.

e. Initially, place food in the patient's visual field; then gradually move the food out of the field of vision and teach the patient to scan the entire visual field.

f. When the patient has learned to visually scan the environment, offer a tray of food with various dishes.

g. Instruct the patient to take small bites of food and to place the food in the unaffected side of the mouth.

h. Teach the patient to sweep out pockets of food with the tongue after every bite **to eliminate retained food in the affected side of the mouth.**

i. After meals or oral medications, check the patient's oral cavity for pockets of retained material.

5. Initiate patient and family health teaching.

a. Assess to ensure that the patient and the family understand the nature of the neurologic deficits and the purpose of the rehabilitation plan.

b. Teach the proper application and use of any adaptive equipment.

c. Teach the importance of maintaining a safe environment, and point out potential environmental hazards.

d. Instruct family members how to facilitate relearning techniques (e.g., cueing, scanning visual fields).

Physiologic Formulas for Critical Care

Kathleen M. Stacy, Mary E. Lough, and Kimberly Sanchez

HEMODYNAMIC EQUATIONS

Mean (Systemic) Arterial Pressure (MAP)

$$MAP = \frac{(Diastolic \times 2) + (Systolic \times 1)}{3}$$

Systemic Vascular Resistance (SVR)

$$\frac{MAP - RAP}{CO} = SVR \text{ in Wood units}$$

MAP = Mean arterial pressure
RAP = Right atrial pressure
CO = Cardiac output
Normal range is 10–18 Wood units.

$$\frac{MAP - RAP}{CO} \times 80 = SVR \text{ in dyn} \cdot sec \cdot cm^{-5}$$

MAP = Mean arterial pressure
RAP = Right atrial pressure
CO = Cardiac output
Normal range is 800–1400 dyn·s·cm^{-5}.

Systemic Vascular Resistance Index (SVRI)

$$\frac{MAP - RAP}{CI} \times 80 = SVR \text{ in dyn} \cdot sec \cdot cm^{-5}/m^2$$

MAP = Mean arterial pressure
RAP = Right atrial pressure
CI = Cardiac index
Normal range is 2000–2400 dyn·s·cm^{-5}/m^2.

Pulmonary Vascular Resistance (PVR)

$$\frac{PAP \text{ mean} - RAP}{CO} = PVR \text{ in units}$$

PAP = Pulmonary artery pressure
RAP = Right atrial pressure
CO = Cardiac output
Normal range is 1.2–3 units.

$$\frac{PAP \text{ mean} - RAP}{CO} \times 80 = PVR \text{ in dyn} \cdot sec \cdot cm^{-5}$$

PAP = Pulmonary artery pressure
RAP = Right atrial pressure
CO = Cardiac output
Normal range is 100–250 dyn·s·cm^{-5}.

Pulmonary Vascular Resistance Index (PVRI)

$$\frac{PAP \text{ mean} - PAOP}{CI} \times 80 = PVR \text{ in dyn} \cdot sec \cdot cm^{-5}/m^2$$

PAP = Pulmonary artery pressure
PAOP = Pulmonary artery occlusion pressure
CI = Cardiac index
Normal range is 225–315 dyn·s·cm^{-5}/m^2.

Left Cardiac Work Index (LCWI)

Step 1. MAP × CO × 0.0136 = LCW

Step 2. $\dfrac{LCW}{BSA} = LCWI$

MAP = Mean arterial pressure
CO = Cardiac output
LCW = Left cardiac work
BSA = Body surface area
Normal range is 3.4–4.2 kg-m/m^2.

Left Ventricular Stroke Work Index (LVSWI)

Step 1. MAP × SV × 0.0136 = LVSW

Step 2. $\dfrac{LVSW}{BSA} = LVSWI$

MAP = Mean arterial pressure
SV = Stroke volume
LVSW = Left ventricular stroke work
BSA = Body surface area
Normal range is 50–62 g-m/m^2.

Right Cardiac Work Index (RCWI)

Step 1. PAP mean × CO × 0.0136 = RCW

Step 2. $\dfrac{RCW}{BSA} = RCWI$

PAP = Pulmonary arterial pressure
CO = Cardiac output
RCW = Right cardiac work
BSA = Body surface area
Normal range is 0.54–0.66 kg-m/m^2.

Right Ventricular Stroke Work Index (RVSWI)

Step 1. PAP mean $\times$ SV $\times$ 0.0136 = RVSW

Step 2. $\dfrac{\text{RVSW}}{\text{BSA}} = \text{RVSWI}$

PAP = Pulmonary arterial pressure
SV = Stroke volume
RVSW = Right ventricular stroke work
BSA = Body surface area
Normal range is 7.9–9.7 g-m/m².

Corrected QT Interval (QTc)

$$\frac{\text{QT}}{\sqrt{\text{(RR interval)}}} = \text{QTc}$$

Body Surface Area (BSA)

Many hemodynamic formulas can be indexed or adjusted to body size by use of a BSA nomogram (Fig. B.1). To calculate BSA:
1. Obtain height and weight.
2. Mark height on the left scale and weight on the right scale.
3. Draw a straight line between the two points marked on the nomogram.

The number where the line crosses the middle scale is the BSA value.

PULMONARY FORMULAS

Shunt Equation (Qs/Qt)

$$\frac{\text{Qs}}{\text{Qt}} = \frac{\text{CcO}_2 - \text{CaO}_2}{\text{CcO}_2 - \text{CVO}_2}$$

CcO_2 = Pulmonary capillary oxygen content (calculated value)
CaO_2 = Arterial oxygen content (calculated value)
CvO_2 = Venous oxygen content (calculated value)
Normal range is less than 5%.

Pulmonary Capillary Oxygen Content (CcO₂)

$$\text{CcO}_2 = (\text{Hgb} \times 1.34 \times \text{ScO}_2) + (\text{PcO}_2 \times 0.003)$$

Hgb = Hemoglobin (measured via laboratory sample or arterial blood gas)
ScO_2 = Pulmonary capillary oxygen saturation
PcO_2 = Partial pressure of oxygen in capillary blood
Normal range is greater than 19 mL/dL.

Arterial Oxygen Content (CaO₂)

$$\text{CaO}_2 = (\text{Hgb} \times 1.34 \times \text{SaO}_2) + (0.003 \times \text{PaO}_2)$$

Hgb = Hemoglobin (measured via laboratory sample or arterial blood gas)
SaO_2 = Arterial oxygen saturation (measured via arterial blood gas)
PaO_2 = Partial pressure of oxygen in arterial blood (measured via arterial blood gas)
Normal range is 17–20 mL/dL.

Venous Oxygen Content (CvO₂)

$$\text{CvO}_2 = (\text{Hgb} \times 1.34 \times \text{SvO}_2) + (0.003 \times \text{PvO}_2)$$

Hgb = Hemoglobin (measured via laboratory sample or arterial blood gas)
SvO_2 = Mixed venous oxygen saturation (measured via mixed venous blood gas)
PvO_2 = Partial pressure of oxygen in mixed venous blood (measured via mixed venous blood gas)
Normal range is 12–15 mL/dL.

Alveolar Pressure of Oxygen (PaO₂)

$$\text{PAO}_2 = \text{FiO}_2 \times (\text{Pb} - \text{PH}_2\text{O}) - \text{PaCO}_2 / \text{RQ}$$

FiO_2 = Fraction of inspired oxygen (obtained from oxygen settings)
Pb = Barometric pressure (assumed to be 760 mm Hg at sea level)
PH_2O = Water pressure in the lungs (assumed to be 47 mm Hg)
$PaCO_2$ = Partial pressure of carbon dioxide in arterial blood (measured via arterial blood gas)
RQ = Respiratory quotient (assumed to be 0.8)
Normal range is 60–100 mm Hg.

Arterial/Inspired Oxygen Ratio

$$\text{PaO}_2 / \text{FiO}_2 \text{ ratio} = \frac{\text{PaO}_2}{\text{FiO}_2}$$

PaO_2 = Partial pressure of oxygen in arterial blood (measured via arterial blood gas)
FiO_2 = Fraction of inspired oxygen (obtained from oxygen settings)
Normal range is greater than 300.

Arterial/Alveolar Oxygen Ratio

$$\text{PaO}_2 / \text{PAO}_2 = \frac{\text{PaO}_2}{\text{PAO}_2}$$

PaO_2 = Partial pressure of oxygen in arterial blood (measured via arterial blood gas)
PAO_2 = Partial pressure of oxygen in alveoli (calculated value)
Normal range is greater than 0.75 (75%).

Alveolar-Arterial Gradient

$$\text{P(A-a)O}_2 = \text{PAO}_2 - \text{PaO}_2$$

PAO_2 = Partial pressure of oxygen in alveoli (calculated value)
PaO_2 = Partial pressure of oxygen in arterial blood (measured via arterial blood gas)
Normal range is 25–65 mm Hg.

Dead Space Equation (V$_d$/V$_T$)

$$\text{Vd/Vt} = \frac{\text{PaCO}_2 - \text{PETCO}_2}{\text{VTPaCO}_2}$$

$PaCO_2$ = Partial pressure of carbon dioxide in arterial blood (measured via arterial blood gas)
$PetCO_2$ = Partial pressure of carbon dioxide in exhaled gas (measured via end-tidal CO_2 monitor)
Normal range is 0.2–0.4 (20%–40%).

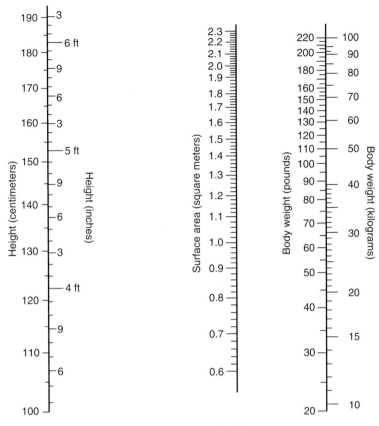

Fig. B.1 Body surface area (BSA) nomogram.

Static Compliance (C_{ST})

This value is calculated for mechanically ventilated patients.

$$C_{ST} = \frac{V_T}{PP} - PEEP$$

V_T = Tidal volume (obtained from ventilator)
PP = Plateau pressure (measured via ventilator)
PEEP = Positive end-expiratory pressure (obtained from ventilator)
  Normal range is 60—100 mL/cm H₂O.

Dynamic Compliance (C_{DY})

Also called *characteristic*, this value is calculated for mechanically ventilated patients.

$$C_{DY} = \frac{V_T}{PIP} - PEEP$$

V_T = Tidal volume (obtained from ventilator)
PIP = Peak inspiratory pressure (obtained from ventilator)
PEEP = Positive end-expiratory pressure (obtained from ventilator)
Normal range is 40—80 mL/cm H₂O.

NEUROLOGIC FORMULAS

Cerebral Perfusion Pressure (CPP)

$$CPP = MAP - ICP$$

MAP = Mean arterial pressure (measured via arterial line or blood pressure cuff)
ICP = Intracranial pressure (measured via ICP monitoring device)
Normal range is 60—150 mm Hg.

Arteriojugular Oxygen Difference (AjDO₂)

$$AjDO_2 = (SaO_2 - SjVO_2) \times 1.34 \times Hgb$$

SaO_2 = Arterial oxygen saturation (measured via arterial blood gas)
$SjVO_2$ = Jugular venous oxygen saturation (measured via jugular blood gas or jugular venous catheter)
Hgb = Hemoglobin (measured via laboratory sample or arterial blood gas)
Normal range is 5—7.5 mL/dL.

ENDOCRINE FORMULAS

Serum Osmolality

$$\text{Serum osmolality} = 2(Na^+ + K^+) + \frac{Glucose}{18} + \frac{BUN}{2.8}$$

Na^+ = Sodium
K^+ = Potassium
BUN = Blood urea nitrogen
Normal range is 275—295 mOsm/kg of water.

Fluid Volume Deficit in Liters

$$\text{Fluid volume deficit} = \frac{0.6(kg/weight) \times (Na^+ - 140)}{140}$$

Na^+ = Sodium

KIDNEY FORMULAS

Anion Gap

$$[Na^+] - ([Cl^-] + [HCO_3^-])$$

Na^+ = Sodium
Cl^- = Chloride
HCO_3^- = Bicarbonate
Normal range is 8—16 mEq.

Clearance

$$Clearance = U \times \frac{(V)}{(P)}$$

U = Concentration of substance in urine
V = Time
P = Concentration of substance in plasma
Normal range depends on substance measured.

NUTRITIONAL FORMULAS

Caloric and Protein Needs[1]

Estimating Caloric Needs

Indirect calorimetry is the most accurate way to estimate energy needs. When indirect calorimetry is unavailable, there are many predictive equations, some are derived from testing hospitalized patients (e.g., Penn State, Ireton-Jones, and Swinamer equations) and some are derived from testing healthy volunteers (e.g., Harris-Benedict, Mifflin St. Jeor equations). For critically ill patients, current guidelines recommend using indirect calorimetry if available. In the absence of indirect calorimetry, guidelines recommend using a simple weight-based equation of 25 to 30 kcal/kg/day to estimate energy requirements. The weight used for this calculation should be dry weight or usual body weight if patients are following aggressive volume resuscitation or have edema or anasarca. Note that predictive equations in general are less accurate in underweight and obese patients.

For obese critically ill patients, if indirect calorimetry is unavailable, current guidelines recommend using the weight-based equation of 11 to 14 kcal/kg of *actual* body weight per day for patients with BMI in the range of 30 to 50 kg/m^2, and 22 to 25 kcal/kg *ideal* body weight per day for patients with BMI >50 kg/m^2.

Estimating Protein Needs

Protein needs vary with the degree of malnutrition and stress. In the critical care setting, adequate protein provision is key in ensuring healing, immune function, and maintaining lean body mass. Nitrogen balance studies are the most accurate way to assess protein needs. When nitrogen balance studies are unavailable, weight-based equations of 1.2 to 2.0 g/kg *actual* body weight per day are recommended. Patients with burns and/or who have multitrauma may require protein provision on the higher end of recommendations or may be in the range of 1.5 to 2.0 g/kg/day.

For obese critically ill patients, protein should be provided in a range from 2.0 g/kg *ideal* body weight per day for patients with BMI of 30 to 40 kg/m^2 up to 2.5 g/kg *ideal* body weight per day for patients with BMI >40 kg/m^2. Protein recommendations should be reevaluated based on nitrogen balance studies with the goal of achieving nitrogen equilibrium.

REFERENCE

1. McClave SA, Taylor BE, Martindale, RG, et al. Guidelines for the provision and assessment of nutrition support therapy in the adult critically ill patient: Society of Critical Care Medicine (SCCM) and American Society for Parenteral and Enteral Nutrition (A.S.P.E.N.). *JPEN J Parenter Enteral Nutr.* 2016;40(2):159—211.

Laboratory Values[a]

The tables in this appendix list some of the most common tests, their normal values, and possible etiologies of abnormal values. Laboratory values are expressed in the Système International d'Unités (SI) units, which are used in Canada. Conventional units, used in the United States, are presented after the SI units in parentheses. Laboratory values may vary with different techniques and in different laboratories. Possible etiologies are presented in alphabetical order. SI abbreviations and other symbols appearing in the tables are defined as follows:

<	=	less than
>	=	greater than
≥	=	greater than or equal to
≤	=	less than or equal to
AU	=	arbitrary unit
cm H_2O	=	centimetres of water
dL	=	decilitre
EU	=	Ehrlich unit
fL	=	femtolitre
g	=	gram
IU	=	international unit
kPa	=	kilopascal
kU	=	kilounit
L	=	litre

mcg	=	microgram (one millionth [10^{-6}] of a gram)
mclU	=	micro–international unit (one millionth [10^{-6}] of an international unit)
mcL	=	microlitre
mcmol	=	micromole
mEq	=	milliequivalent
mg	=	milligram (one thousandth [10^{-3}] of a gram)
microkat	=	microkatal
microU	=	microunit
mL	=	millilitre
mm	=	millimetre
mm Hg	=	millimetre of mercury
mmol	=	millimole
mOsm	=	milliosmole
mU	=	milliunit (one hundredth [10^{-2}] of a unit)
nmol	=	nanomole (one billionth [10^{-9}] of a mole)
ng	=	nanogram (one billionth [10^{-9}] of a gram)
pg	=	picogram (one trillionth [10^{-12}] of a gram)
pmol	=	picomole (one trillionth [10^{-12}] of a mole)
U	=	unit

Continued

TABLE C.1 Serum, Plasma, and Whole Blood Chemistries.

Test	Normal Values: SI Units (Conventional Units)	POSSIBLE ETIOLOGY	
		Higher Values	Lower Values
Acetone		Diabetic ketoacidosis, high-fat diet, low-carbohydrate diet, starvation	—
• Quantitative	<200 mcmol/L (<1.16 mg/dL)		
• Qualitative	Negative (negative)		
Alanine aminotransferase (ALT; formerly known as serum glutamate pyruvate transferase [SGPT])	4–36 U/L (same as in SI units)	Liver disease, shock	—
Albumin	35–50 g/L (3.5–5 g/dL)	Dehydration	Burns, chronic liver disease, malabsorption, malnutrition, nephrotic syndrome, pregnancy, inflammatory disease
Aldolase	<8.0 mU/L (3–8.2 Sibley-Lehninger U/dL)	Infection, muscle trauma, skeletal muscle disease, hepatocellular disease, MI	Late muscular dystrophy, renal disease, hereditary fructose intolerance
α_1-Antitrypsin	0.85–2.13 g/L (85–213 mg/dL)	Acute and chronic inflammation and infection, arthritis,	Chronic lung disease (early onset of emphysema), malnutrition,

Continued

[a]Appendix C from Lok, J., (2019). Appendix B. In Canadian Fundamentals of Nursing 6th ed. Toronto, ON: Elsevier; 1428–1438.

TABLE C.1 Serum, Plasma, and Whole Blood Chemistries.—cont'd

Test	Normal Values: SI Units (Conventional Units)	POSSIBLE ETIOLOGY	
		Higher Values	Lower Values
Alpha-fetoprotein	0—40 mcg/L (<40 ng/mL)	malignancy, stress, syndrome, thyroid infections Cancers of testes, lymphoma, stomach, colon, breasts and ovaries, carcinoma of liver, neural tube defects or multiple pregnancies in pregnant women, fetal distress or congenital abnormalities, fetal death	nephrotic syndrome, end-stage cancer In pregnant women, fetal trisomy 21 or fetal wastage
Ammonia	6—47 mcmol/L (10—80 mcg/dL)	GI bleeding, hepatic encephalopathy, portal hypertension, severe liver disease, Reye syndrome, severe heart failure, or congestive hepatomegaly	Hyperornithinemia, essential or malignant hypertension
Amylase	100—300 U/L (60—120 Somogyi units/dL)	Acute and chronic pancreatitis, mumps (salivary gland disease), perforated ulcers	Acute alcoholism, cirrhosis of liver, extensive destruction of pancreas
Ascorbic acid	23—85 mcmol/L (0.4—1.5 mg/dL)	Excessive ingestion of vitamin C	Connective tissue disorders, hepatic disease, renal disease, rheumatic fever, vitamin C deficiency
Aspartate aminotransferase (AST) (formerly known as serum glutamic oxaloacetic transferase [SGOT])	0—35 U/L (same as SI units)	Acute hepatitis, liver disease, MI, pulmonary infarction, skeletal muscle disease	Chronic renal dialysis, acute renal disease, pregnancy, diabetic ketoacidosis
B-type (brain-type) natriuretic peptide	<100 mcg/L (<100 ng/mL)	Heart failure, MI, hypertension, cor pulmonale	—
Bicarbonate	21—28 mmol/L (21—28 mEq/L)	Chronic use of loop diuretics, compensated respiratory acidosis, metabolic alkalosis	Acute renal failure, compensated respiratory alkalosis, diarrhea, metabolic acidosis
Bilirubin • Total • Indirect • Direct	5.1—17 mcmol/L (0.3—1.0 mg/dL) 3.4—12 mcmol/L (0.2—0.8 mg/dL) 1.7—5.1 mcmol/L (0.1—0.3 mg/dL)	Biliary obstruction, hemolytic anemia, impaired liver function, pernicious anemia, prolonged fasting, Dubin-Johnson syndrome, sickle cell anemia, sepsis, hepatitis	—
Blood Gases[a] • Arterial pH • Venous pH • Partial pressure of carbon dioxide in arterial blood (PaCO₂)	7.35—7.45 (same as SI units) 7.31—7.41 (same as SI units) 35—45 mm Hg (same as SI units)	Alkalosis Alkalosis Compensated metabolic alkalosis, respiratory acidosis	Acidosis Acidosis Compensated metabolic acidosis, respiratory alkalosis
• Partial pressure of oxygen in arterial blood (PaO₂)	80—100 mm Hg (same as SI units)	Administration of high concentration of oxygen	Chronic lung disease, decreased cardiac output
• Partial pressure of oxygen in venous blood (PvO₂)	40—50 mm Hg (same as SI units)		
Calcium	2.25—2.75 mmol/L (9—10.5 mg/dL)	Acute osteoporosis, hyperparathyroidism, multiple myeloma, vitamin D intoxication	Acute pancreatitis, hypoparathyroidism, liver disease, malabsorption syndrome, renal failure, vitamin D deficiency
Calcium, ionized	1.05—1.30 mmol/L (4.5—5.6 mg/dL)	—	
Carbon dioxide (CO₂ content)	21—28 mmol/L (21—28 mEq/L)	Severe vomiting, COPD, metabolic alkalosis	Chronic use of loop diuretics, renal failure, DKA, starvation, metabolic acidosis, shock

TABLE C.1 Serum, Plasma, and Whole Blood Chemistries.—cont'd

Test	Normal Values: SI Units (Conventional Units)	POSSIBLE ETIOLOGY	
		Higher Values	Lower Values
Beta-carotene	1.4—4.7 mcmol/L (75—253 mcg/dL)	Cystic fibrosis, hypothyroidism, pancreatic insufficiency	Dietary deficiency, malabsorption disorders
Chloride	98—106 mmol/L (98—106 mEq/L)	Corticosteroid therapy, dehydration, excessive infusion of normal saline, metabolic acidosis, respiratory alkalosis, uremia	Addison's disease, heart failure, diarrhea, metabolic alkalosis, overhydration, respiratory acidosis, SIADH, vomiting
Cholesterol • High-density lipoproteins (HDL) • Low-density lipoproteins (LDL)	<5 mmol/L (<200 mg/dL) age dependent >1.55 mmol/L (>60 mg/dL) <2.59 mmol/L (<100 mg/dL)	Biliary obstruction, cirrhosis, hypothyroidism, hyperlipidemia, idiopathic hypercholesterolemia, renal disease, uncontrolled diabetes	Corticosteroid therapy, extensive liver disease, hyperthyroidism, malnutrition
Cholinesterase (RBC)	5—10 U/L (same as SI units)	Exercise, sickle cell disease	Acute infections, insecticide intoxication, liver disease, muscular dystrophy
Copper	11—22 mcmol/L (70—140 mcg/dL)	Cirrhosis, contraceptive use by female patient	Wilson's disease
Cortisol • 0800 Hours • 1600 Hours	138—635 nmol/L (5—23 mcg/dL) <83—359 nmol/L (3—13 mcg/dL)	Adrenal adenoma, Cushing's syndrome, hyperthyroidism, pancreatitis, stress	Addison's disease, adrenal insufficiency, hypopituitary states, hypothyroidism, liver disease
Creatine	15.3—76.3 mcmol/L (0.2—1.0 mg/dL)	Active rheumatoid arthritis, biliary obstruction, hyperthyroidism, renal disease, severe muscle disease	Diabetes mellitus
Creatine kinase (CK) • Male • Female	55—170 U/L (same as SI units) 30—135 U/L (same as SI units)	Brain damage, exercise, musculoskeletal injury or disease, MI, numerous intramuscular injections, severe myocarditis	—
Creatine kinase isozyme of heart (CK-MB [CK-2]) • Male • Female	 2—6 mcg/L (2—6 ng/mL) 2—5 mcg/L (2—5 ng/mL)	Acute MI	—
Creatine kinase mass fraction	<5% fraction of total CK	—	—
Creatinine • Male • Female	53—106 mcmol/L (0.6—1.2 mg/dL) 44—97 mcmol/L (0.5—1.1 mg/dL)	Severe renal disease	Diseases with decreased muscle mass (e.g., muscular dystrophy, myasthenia gravis)
Ferritin (serum) • Male • Female	26—674 pmol/L (12—300 ng/mL) 22—337 pmol/L (10—150 ng/mL)	Anemia of chronic disease (infection, inflammation, liver disease), sideroblastic anemia	Iron-deficiency anemia, severe protein deficiency
Folic acid (folate)	11—57 mmol/L (5—25 ng/mL)	Hypothyroidism, pernicious anemia	Alcoholism, hemolytic anemia, inadequate diet, malabsorption syndrome, malnutrition, megaloblastic anemia
Gamma-glutamyl transpeptidase (GGT) • Male • Female	 8—38 U/L (same as SI units) 5—27 U/L (same as SI units)	Cholestasis, cytomegalovirus infection, Epstein-Barr, liver disease, MI, pancreatitis	—
Glucose, fasting	4—6 mmol/L (70—110 mg/dL)	Acute stress, cerebral lesions, Cushing's syndrome, diabetes mellitus, hyperthyroidism, pancreatic insufficiency	Addison's disease, hepatic disease, hypothyroidism, insulin overdosage, pancreatic tumor, pituitary hypofunction, postdumping syndrome
Glucose, 2-hour oral glucose tolerance testing (OGTT) • Fasting • 1 hour	 4—6 mmol/L (70—110 mg/dL) <11.1 mmol/L (<200 mg/dL)	Diabetes mellitus	Hyperinsulinism

Continued

TABLE C.1   Serum, Plasma, and Whole Blood Chemistries.—cont'd

Test	Normal Values: SI Units (Conventional Units)	POSSIBLE ETIOLOGY	
		Higher Values	Lower Values
• 2 hour	<7.8 mmol/L (<140 mg/dL)		
Haptoglobin	0.5—2.2 g/L (50—220 mg/dL)	Acute MI, infectious and inflammatory processes, malignant neoplasms	Chronic liver disease, hemolytic anemia, mononucleosis, systemic lupus erythematosus, toxoplasmosis, transfusion reactions
Homocysteine		Cardiovascular disease, cerebrovascular disease, peripheral vascular disease, cystinuria, vitamin B_6 or B_{12} deficiency, folate deficiency, malnutrition	—
• 0—30 years	4.6—8.1 mcmol/L (same as SI units)		
• 30—59 years			
• Male	6.13—11.2 mcmol/L (same as SI units)		
• Female	4.5—7.9 mcmol/L (same as SI units)		
• >59 years	5.8—11.9 mcmol/L (same as SI units)		
Insulin	43—186 pmol/L (6—26 microU/mL)	Acromegaly, adenoma of islet cells, obesity, untreated mild case of type 2 diabetes mellitus	Diabetes mellitus, obesity
Iron		Excessive RBC destruction, hemochromatosis, massive transfusion	Anemia of chronic disease, iron-deficiency anemia
• Male	14—32 mcmol/L (80—180 mcg/dL)		
• Female	11—29 mcmol/L (60—160 mcg/dL)		
Total iron-binding capacity (TIBC)	45—82 mcmol/L (250—460 mcg/dL)	Iron-deficiency state, oral contraceptive use, polycythemia	Cancer, chronic infections, pernicious anemia, uremia
Lactic acid (venous blood)	0.6—2.2 mmol/L (5—20 mg/dL)	Acidosis, heart failure, severe liver disease, shock, tissue ischemia	—
Lactic dehydrogenase (LDH)	100—190 U/L (same as SI units)	Heart failure, hemolytic disorders, hepatitis, metastatic cancer of liver, MI, pernicious anemia, pulmonary embolus and infarction, skeletal muscle damage	—
Lactic Dehydrogenase Isoenzymes			
• LDH_1	0.17—0.27 (17%—27%)	MI, pernicious anemia, strenuous exercise	—
• LDH_2	0.27—0.37 (27%—37%)	Exercise, pulmonary embolus, sickle cell crisis	—
• LDH_3	0.18—0.25 (18%—25%)	Malignant lymphoma, pulmonary embolus	—
• LDH_4	0.03—0.08 (3%—8%)	Systemic lupus erythematosus, pancreatitis, pulmonary infarction, renal disease	—
• LDH_5	0.0—0.05 (0%—5%)	Heart failure, hepatitis, pulmonary embolus and infarction, skeletal muscle damage, strenuous exercise	—
Lipase	0—160 U/L (same as SI units)	Acute and chronic pancreatitis, hepatic disorders, pancreatic disorder (cancer, pseudocyst), perforated peptic ulcer, salivary gland inflammation, or tumor	—
Magnesium	0.74—1.07 mmol/L (1.8—2.6 mEq/L)	Addison's disease, hypothyroidism, renal failure	Chronic alcoholism, hyperparathyroidism, hyperthyroidism, hypoparathyroidism, malnutrition, severe malabsorption
Myoglobin	1.0—5.3 nmol/L (<90 ng/mL)	MI, myositis, malignant hyperthermia, muscular dystrophy, skeletal muscle ischemia or trauma, rhabdomyolysis, seizures	Polymyositis
Osmolality	280—300 mmol/kg (280—300 mOsm/kg)	Chronic renal disease, dehydration, diabetes mellitus, hypernatremia, shock	Addison's disease, diuretic therapy, hyponatremia, overhydration

TABLE C.1   Serum, Plasma, and Whole Blood Chemistries.—cont'd

Test	Normal Values: SI Units (Conventional Units)	POSSIBLE ETIOLOGY Higher Values	POSSIBLE ETIOLOGY Lower Values
Oxygen saturation		Increased inspired oxygen, polycythemia vera	Anemia, cardiac decompensation, decreased inspired oxygen, respiratory disorders
• Arterial	95%—100% (same as SI units)		
• Venous	60%—80% (same as SI units)		
pH	*See* Blood gases		
Phenylalanine	0—121 mcmol/L (0—2 mg/dL)	Phenylketonuria	—
Phosphatase, acid	2.2—10.5 U/L (0.13—0.63 U/L)	Advanced Paget's disease, cancer of prostate, hyperparathyroidism	—
Phosphatase, alkaline (ALP)	35—120 U/L (0.5—2.0 mckat/L)	Bone diseases, cirrhosis, malignancy of liver/bone, marked hyperparathyroidism, obstruction of biliary system, rickets	Excessive vitamin D ingestion, hypothyroidism, milk-alkali syndrome
Phosphorus, phosphate	0.97—1.45 mmol/L (3.0—4.5 mg/dL)[b]	Bone metastasis, healing fractures, hypoparathyroidism, hypocalcemia, renal disease, vitamin D intoxication	Chronic alcoholism, diabetes mellitus, hypercalcemia, hyperparathyroidism, vitamin D deficiency
Potassium	3.5—5.0 mmol/L (3.5—5.0 mEq/L)	Acute or chronic renal failure, Addison's disease, dehydration, diabetic ketosis, excessive dietary or IV intake, massive tissue destruction, metabolic acidosis	Burns, Cushing's syndrome, deficient dietary or IV intake, diarrhea (severe), diuretic therapy, GI fistula, insulin administration, pyloric obstruction, starvation, vomiting
Prostate-specific antigen (PSA)	<4 mcg/L (<4 ng/mL)	Benign prostatic hypertrophy, prostate cancer, prostatitis	—
Proteins		Burns, cirrhosis (globulin fraction), dehydration	Congenital agammaglobulinemia, increased capillary permeability, inflammatory disease, liver disease, malabsorption, malnutrition
• Total	64—83 g/L (6.4—8.3 g/dL)		
• Albumin	35—50 g/L (3.5—5 g/dL)		
• Globulin	23—34 g/L (2.3—3.4 g/dL)		
• Albumin/globulin ratio	1.5:1—2.5:1 (same as SI units)	Multiple myeloma (globulin fraction), shock, vomiting	Malnutrition, nephrotic syndrome, proteinuria, renal disease, severe burns
Pseudocholinesterase (serum)	8—18 U/mL (same as SI units)	—	—
Renin		Renal hypertension, salt-losing GI disease (vomiting/diarrhea), volume decrease (e.g., hemorrhage)	Increased salt intake, primary aldosteronism
• Upright position	0.03—1.2 ng/L/s (0.1—4.3 mg/mL/h)		
Sodium	135—145 mmol/L (135—145 mEq/L)	Corticosteroid therapy, dehydration, impaired renal function, increased dietary or IV intake, primary aldosteronism	Addison's disease, decreased dietary or IV intake, diabetic ketoacidosis, diuretic therapy, excessive loss from GI tract, excessive perspiration, water intoxication
Testosterone		Adrenal hyperplasia, adrenal or pituitary tumors, testicular tumors	Hypofunction of testes
• Male	174—729 pmol/L (50—120 pg/mL)		
• Female	3.5—29.5 pmol/L (1.0—8.5 pg/mL)	Polycystic ovary, virilizing tumors	—
Thyroxine (T_4), total	64—154 nmol/L (5—12 mcg/dL)	Hyperthyroidism, thyroiditis	Cretinism, hypothyroidism, myxedema
Thyroxine (T_4), free	10—36 pmol/L (0.8—2.8 ng/dL)	Hyperthyroidism, metastatic neoplasms	Hypothyroidism, pregnancy
Triiodothyronine (T_3) uptake	24—34 AU (24%—34%)	—	—
Triiodothyronine (T_3)	1.7—5.2 pmol/L (110.4—337.7 ng/dL)	Hyperthyroidism	Hypothyroidism
Thyroid-stimulating hormone (TSH)	2—10 mIU/L (2—10 mcIU/mL)	Graves' disease, myxedema, primary hypothyroidism	Secondary hypothyroidism
Triglycerides		Diabetes mellitus, hyperlipidemia, hypothyroidism, liver disease	Hyperthyroidism, malabsorption syndrome, malnutrition
• Male	0.45—1.81 mmol/L (40—160 mg/dL)		
• Female	0.40—1.52 mmol/L (35—135 mg/dL)		

Continued

TABLE C.1   Serum, Plasma, and Whole Blood Chemistries.—cont'd

Test	Normal Values: SI Units (Conventional Units)	POSSIBLE ETIOLOGY	
		Higher Values	Lower Values
Troponin T (cTnT)	<0.1 mcg/L (<0.1 ng/mL)	Cardiac muscle damage (resulting from MI, myocarditis, or pericarditis), chronic renal failure, multiorgan failure, severe heart failure	—
Troponin I (cTnI)	<0.35 mcg/L (<0.35 ng/mL)		—
Urea nitrogen, blood (blood urea nitrogen [BUN], serum urea nitrogen)	3.6—7.1 mmol/L (10—20 mg/dL)	Burns, dehydration, GI bleeding, increase in protein catabolism (fever, stress), renal disease, shock, urinary tract infection	Fluid overload, malnutrition, severe liver damage, SIADH
Uric acid		Alcoholism, eclampsia, gout, gross tissue destruction, high-protein weight reduction diet, leukemia, multiple myeloma, renal failure	Administration of uricosuric drugs
• Male	240—501 mcmol/L (4.0—8.5 mg/dL)		
• Female	160—430 mcmol/L (2.7—7.3 mg/dL)		
Vitamin A	0.52—2.09 mcmol/L (15—60 mcg/dL)	Excess ingestion of vitamin A	Vitamin A deficiency
Vitamin B$_{12}$	118—701 pmol/L (160—950 pg/mL)	Chronic myeloid leukemia	Malabsorption syndrome, pernicious anemia, strict vegetarianism, total or partial gastrectomy
Zinc	11.5—18.5 mcmol/L (75—120 mcg/dL)	—	Alcoholic cirrhosis

[a]Because arterial blood gases are influenced by altitude, the values for PaCO$_2$, PaO$_2$, and PvO$_2$ decrease as altitude increases. The lower values are normal for an altitude of 1.6 km (1 mile).

[b]Values for older adults are significantly lower than those for younger adults.

COPD, Chronic obstructive pulmonary disease; *DKA,* diabetic ketoacidosis; *GI,* gastrointestinal; *IV,* intravenous; *MI,* myocardial infarction; *RBC,* red blood cell; *SIADH,* syndrome of inappropriate antidiuretic hormone.

TABLE C.2 Hematology.

Test	Normal Values: SI Units (Conventional Units)	POSSIBLE ETIOLOGY	
		Higher Values	Lower Values
Bleeding time (Ivy method)	1—9 minutes	Aspirin ingestion, clotting factor deficiency, defective platelet function, thrombocytopenia, vascular disease, von Willebrand's disease	—
Activated partial thromboplastin time (aPTT)	30—40 seconds[a] (same as SI units)	Deficiency of one or more of the following: factor I, II, V, or VIII; factors IX and X; factor XI; and factor XII	—
		Hemophilia; heparin therapy; liver disease	
Partial thromboplastin time (PTT)	60—70 seconds (same as SI units)	Same as for aPTT	—
Activated coagulation time or automated clotting time (ACT)	70—120 seconds (same as SI units)	Same as for aPTT	—
Prothrombin time (PT; Protime)	11—12.5 seconds[a] (same as SI units)	Deficiency of one or more of the following: factor I, II, V, VII, or X	—
		Liver disease; vitamin K deficiency; warfarin therapy	
International normalized ratio (INR)	0.81—1.20 (same as SI units)	Same as for PT	—
Thrombin time	8—12 seconds (same as SI units)	DIC, increased tendency to bleed	—
Fibrinogen	2.0—5.0 g/L (60—100 mg/dL)	Burns (after first 36 hours), inflammatory disease	Burns (during first 36 hours), DIC, severe liver disease
Fibrin split (degradation) products	<10 mg/L (<10 mcg/mL)		—

TABLE C.2   Hematology.—cont'd

Test	Normal Values: SI Units (Conventional Units)	POSSIBLE ETIOLOGY Higher Values	Lower Values
D-dimer	<3.0 mmol/L (<50 ng/mL)	Acute DIC, massive hemorrhage, massive trauma, primary fibrinolysis Deep-vein thrombosis, DIC, myocardial infarction, unstable angina	—
Erythrocyte count[b] (RBC count [altitude dependent])		Dehydration, high altitudes, polycythemia vera, severe diarrhea	Anemia, leukemia, post hemorrhage
• Male	$4.7-6.1 \times 10^{12}$/L		
• Female	$4.2-5.4 \times 10^{12}$/L		
Mean corpuscular volume (MCV) (Hct/RBC)	80–95 fL (80–95 mm^3)	Folic acid and vitamin B_{12} deficiency, liver disease, macrocytic anemia	Microcytic anemia
Mean corpuscular hemoglobin (MCH) (Hb/RBC)	27–31 pg (same as SI units)	Macrocytic anemia	Microcytic anemia
Mean corpuscular hemoglobin concentration (MCHC) (Hb/Hct)	32–36 g/dL (32%–36%)	Intravascular hemolysis, spherocytosis	Hypochromic anemia
Erythrocyte sedimentation rate (ESR), Westergren Method		*Moderate increase:* acute hepatitis, myocardial infarction, rheumatoid arthritis	Malaria, severe liver disease, sickle cell anemia
• Male	≤15 mm/h (same as SI units)	*Marked increase:* acute and severe bacterial infections, malignancies, pelvic inflammatory disease	
• Female	≤20 mm/h (same as SI units)		
Hematocrit (altitude dependent)[b]		Dehydration, high altitudes, polycythemia	Anemia, bone marrow failure, hemorrhage, leukemia, overhydration
• Male	0.42–0.52 volume fraction (42%–52%)		
• Female	0.37–0.47 volume fraction (37%–47%)		
Hemoglobin (altitude dependent)[b]		Chronic obstructive pulmonary disease, high altitudes, polycythemia	Anemia, hemorrhage
• Male	140–180 g/L (14–18 g/dL)		
• Female	120–160 g/L (12–16 g/dL)		
Hemoglobin, glycosylated or glycated (hemoglobin A_{1c} [HbA_{1c}])	<6% (adult without diabetes)	Nondiabetic hyperglycemia, poorly controlled diabetes mellitus	Chronic blood loss, chronic renal failure, pregnancy, sickle cell anemia
Red cell distribution width (RDW)	11%–14.5% (same as SI units)	—	Anisocytosis, macrocytic anemia, microcytic anemia
Platelet count (thrombocytes)	$150-400 \times 10^9$/L (150,000–400,000/mm^3)	Acute infections, chronic granulocytic leukemia, chronic pancreatitis, cirrhosis, collagen disorders, polycythemia, post splenectomy	Acute leukemia, cancer chemotherapy, DIC, hemorrhage, infection, systemic lupus erythematosus, thrombocytopenic purpura
Reticulocyte count (manual)	0.5%–2% total number of RBC	Hemolytic anemia, polycythemia vera	Hypoproliferative anemia, macrocytic anemia, microcytic anemia
WBC count[b]	$5-10 \times 10^9$/L (5000–10,000/mm^3)	Inflammatory and infectious processes, leukemia	Aplastic anemia, autoimmune diseases, overwhelming infection, side effects of chemotherapy and irradiation
WBC Differential			
• Segmented neutrophils	$2.5-7.5 \times 10^9$/L (62%–68%)	Bacterial infections, collagen diseases, Hodgkin's disease	Aplastic anemia, viral infections
• Band neutrophils	$0-1 \times 10^9$/L (0%–9%)	Acute infections	—
• Lymphocytes	$1.0-4.0 \times 10^9$/L (1000–4000/mm^3; 20%–40%)	Chronic infections, lymphocytic leukemia, mononucleosis, viral infections	Corticosteroid therapy, whole body irradiation
• Monocytes			—

Continued

TABLE C.2 Hematology.—cont'd

Test	Normal Values: SI Units (Conventional Units)	POSSIBLE ETIOLOGY	
		Higher Values	Lower Values
	$0.1-0.7 \times 10^9/L$ (100—700/mm³; 2%—8%)	Acute infections, chronic inflammatory disorders, Hodgkin's disease, malaria, monocytic leukemia	
• Eosinophils	$0.00-0.5 \times 10^9/L$ (50—500/mm³; 1%—4%)	Allergic reactions, eosinophilic and chronic granulocytic leukemia, Hodgkin's disease, parasitic disorders	Corticosteroid therapy
• Basophils	$0.02-0.05 \times 10^9/L$ (15—50/mm³; 0.5%—1%)	Hypothyroidism, myeloproliferative diseases, ulcerative colitis	Hyperthyroidism, stress
Sickle cell solubility	Negative (negative)	Sickle cell anemia	—

[a]For patients receiving anticoagulant therapy, aPTT is 1.5—2.5 times the control value in seconds; PT is 1.5—2.0 times the control value in seconds.
[b]Components of complete blood count (CBC).
DIC, Disseminated intravascular coagulation; *RBC,* red blood cell; *WBC,* white blood cell.

TABLE C.3 Serology—Immunology.

Test	Normal Values: SI Units (Conventional Units)	POSSIBLE ETIOLOGY	
		Higher Values	Lower Values
Antinuclear antibody (ANA)	Negative at 1 : 40 dilution (same as SI units)	Chronic hepatitis, rheumatoid arthritis, scleroderma, systemic lupus erythematosus (SLE)	—
Anti-DNA antibody	Negative <70 U/mL (same as SI units)	SLE	—
Anti-RNP (ribonucleoprotein)	Negative (negative)	Mixed connective tissue disease, scleroderma, rheumatoid arthritis, Sjögren's syndrome, SLE	—
Anti-Sm (Smith)	Negative (negative)	SLE	—
Antistreptolysin-O (ASO)	≤160 Todd units/mL (same as SI units)	Acute glomerulonephritis, rheumatic fever, streptococcal infection	—
C-reactive protein (CRP)	<10 mg/L (<1.0 mg/dL)	Acute infections, any inflammatory condition (e.g., acute rheumatic fever/arthritis), widespread malignancy	—
Carcinoembryonic antigen (CEA)	<5 mcg/L (5 ng/mL)	Carcinomas of colon, liver, pancreas; chronic cigarette smoking; inflammatory bowel disease; other cancers	—
Complement assay components		—	Acute glomerulonephritis, rheumatoid arthritis, serum sickness, subacute bacterial endocarditis, SLE
• Total	75—160 kU/L (75—160 U/mL)		
• C3	0.55—1.2 g/L (55—120 mg/dL)		
• C4	0.2—0.5 g/L (20—50 mg/dL)		
Direct antihuman globulin test (DAT) or direct Coombs' test	Negative (negative) (no agglutination)	Acquired hemolytic anemia, drug reactions, hemolytic disease of the newborn, transfusion reactions	—
Fluorescent treponemal antibody absorption (FTAAbs)	Negative (nonreactive)	Syphilis	—
Hepatitis A antibody	Negative (negative)	Hepatitis A	—
Hepatitis B surface antigen (HBsAg)	Negative (negative)	Hepatitis B	—
Hepatitis C antibody	Negative (negative)	Hepatitis C	—
Immunoglobulins			
• IgA	0.85—3.85 g/L (85—385 mg/dL)	Autoimmune disorders, chronic infection, chronic liver disease, IgA myeloma, rheumatoid arthritis	Burns, hereditary telangiectasia, malabsorption syndromes
• IgD	Minimal	Chronic infection, connective tissue disease	—
• IgE	24—400 mcg/L		—

TABLE C.3 Serology—Immunology.—cont'd

Test	Normal Values: SI Units (Conventional Units)	POSSIBLE ETIOLOGY	
		Higher Values	Lower Values
• IgG	5.65—17.65 g/L (565—1765 mg/dL)	Anaphylactic shock, atopic disease (allergies), parasite infections Hepatitis, IgG monoclonal gammopathy, infections—acute and chronic, SLE	Acquired deficiencies, burns, congenital deficiencies, immuno-suppression, nephrotic syndromes
• IgM	0.55—3.75 g/L (55—375 mg/dL)	Acute infections, liver disease, rheumatoid arthritis	Congenital and acquired antibody deficiencies, lymphocytic leuke-mia, protein-losing enteropathies
Monospot or Mono-Test	Negative (<1:28 titre)	Infectious mononucleosis	—
Rheumatoid factor (RA factor)	Negative or <60 IU/mL by nephe-lometric method	Rheumatoid arthritis, Sjögren's syndrome, SLE	—
RPR (rapid plasma reagin) test	Negative or nonreactive (same as SI units)	Febrile diseases, IV drug abuse, leprosy, ma-laria, rheumatoid arthritis, syphilis, SLE	—
VDRL (Venereal Disease Research Laboratory) test	Negative or nonreactive (same as SI units)	Syphilis	—
Thyroid antibodies	Titre <1:100 (same as SI units)	Early hypothyroidism, Graves' disease, Hashi-moto's thyroiditis, pernicious anemia, SLE, thyroid carcinoma	—

IV, Intravenous.

TABLE C.4 Urine Chemistry.

Test	Specimen	Normal Values: SI Units (Conventional Units)	POSSIBLE ETIOLOGY	
			Higher Values	Lower Values
Acetone (ketones)	Random	Negative (negative)	Diabetes mellitus, high-fat and low-carbohydrate diets, starva-tion states	—
Aldosterone	24 hours	17—70 nmol/24 h (2—26 mcg/24 h)	*Primary aldosteronism:* Adrenocor-tical tumors *Secondary aldosteronism:* Car-diac failure, cirrhosis, large dose of ACTH, salt depletion	Adrenocorticotropic hormone (ACTH) deficiency, Addison's disease, corticosteroid therapy
Amylase	24 hours	100—300 U/L (60—120 Somogyi units/dL)	Acute pancreatitis	—
Bence-Jones protein	Random	Negative (negative)	Biliary duct obstruction, multiple myeloma	—
Bilirubin	Random	5.1—16 mcmol/L (0.3—1.0 mg/dL)	Gallstones Dubin-Johnson Syndrome Rotor Syndrome	—
Calcium	24 hours	2.25—2.75 mmol/day (9.0—10.5 mg/dL)	Bone tumor hyperparathyroidism, milk-alkali syndrome, lymphoma, Addison's disease	Hypoparathyroidism, malabsorp-tion of calcium and vitamin D, renal failure, pancreatitis
Catecholamines	24 hours		Heart failure, pheochromocytoma, progressive muscular dystrophy	
• Epinephrine		<109 nmol/day (<20 mcg/24 h)		
• Norepinephrine		<590 nmol/day (<100 mcg/24 h)		
Chloride	24 hours	110—250 mmol/day (110—250 mEq/day)	Dehydration, Cushing's syndrome, eclampsia, kidney dysfunction	Burns, diarrhea, excess perspira-tion, menstruation, vomiting, Addison's disease, heart failure
Copper	24 hours	0.6 mcmol/day (<40 mcg/day)	Cirrhosis, Wilson's disease	—
Coproporphyrin	24 hours	<300 nmol/day (<200 mcg/day)	Lead poisoning, oral contraceptive use, poliomyelitis	—

Continued

TABLE C.4   Urine Chemistry.—cont'd

Test	Specimen	Normal Values: SI Units (Conventional Units)	POSSIBLE ETIOLOGY Higher Values	Lower Values
Creatine • Male • Female	24 hours	 53—106 mcmol/day (0.6—1.2 mg/dL) 44—97 mcmol/L (0.6—1.2 mg/dL)	Acromegaly, disease affecting renal function, diabetic nephropathy	Decreased muscle mass (e.g., muscular dystrophy, myasthenia gravis)
Creatinine • Male • Female	24 hours	 53—106 mcmol/L (0.6—1.2 mg/dL) 44—97 mcmol/L (0.5—1.1. mg/dL)	Anemia, leukemia, muscular atrophy, salmonellosis	Renal disease
Creatinine clearance • Male • Female	24 hours	1.42—2.25 mL/s (85—135 mL/min) 1.78—2.32 mL/sec (107—139 mL/min) 1.45—1.78 mL/s (87—107 mL/min)	—	Renal disease
Estriol • Female • Ovulatory phase • Luteal phase • Pregnancy • Menopause • Male	24 hours	 28—100 mcg/24 h (104—370 nmol/L) 22—80 mcg/24 h (81—296 nmol/L) ≤166,455 nmol/day (≤45,000 mcg/day) 1.4—19.6 mcg/24 h (5.2—72.5 nmol/L) 5—18 mcg/24 h (18—67 nmol/L)	Gonadal or adrenal tumor —	Agenesis of ovaries, endocrine disturbance, menopause, ovarian dysfunction —
Glucose	Random	Random: negative; 24-hour: <2.78 mmol/24 h (<0.5 g/24 h)	Diabetes mellitus, low renal threshold for glucose resorption, physiologic stress, pituitary disorders	—
Hemoglobin • Male • Female	Random	 140—180 mmol/L (14—18 g/dL) 120—160 (12—16 g/dL)	Extensive burns, glomerulonephritis, hemolytic anemias, hemolytic transfusion reaction	—
5-Hydroxyindole-acetic acid (5-HIAA)	24 hours	10—40 mcmol/day (2—8 mg/24 h)	Malignant carcinoid syndrome	—
Ketone bodies	Random	Negative (negative)	Alcoholism, fasting, high-protein diets, marked ketonuria, poorly controlled diabetes mellitus, starvation	—
Lead	24 hours	<0.40 mcmol/day (<80 mcg/day)	Lead poisoning	—
Metanephrine	24 hours	12—60 pg/mL	Pheochromocytoma	—
Myoglobin	Random	1.0—5.3 nmol/L (<90 ng/mL)	Crushing injuries, electric injuries, extreme physical exertion	—
pH	Random	4.6—8.0 (average, 6.0)	Chronic renal failure, compensatory phase of alkalosis, salicylate intoxication, vegetarian diet	Compensatory phase of acidosis, dehydration, emphysema
Phenylpyruvic acid	Random	Negative (negative)	Phenylketonuria	—
Phosphorus, inorganic	24 hours	0.97—1.45 mmol/L (3.0—4.5 mg/dL)	Fever, hypoparathyroidism, nervous exhaustion, rickets, tuberculosis	Acute infections, nephritis
Porphobilinogen	Random 24 hours	Negative (negative) 0—6.6 mg/24 h (0—2 mg/24 h)	Acute intermittent porphyria, liver disorders	—
Potassium	24 hours	25—100 mmol/day (25—100 mEq/L/day)	Chronic renal failure, starvation, Cushing's syndrome, hyperaldosteronism, alkalosis, diuretic therapy	Reduced intake, dehydration, Addison's disease, malnutrition, vomiting, diarrhea, acute renal failure
Protein (dipstick)	Random	Negative (negative)	Heart failure, nephritis, nephrosis, physiologic stress	—
Protein (quantitative) • At rest • During exercise	24 hours	<0.15 g/day (<150 mg/day) 0.05—0.08 g/day (<50—80 mg/day) <0.25 g/day (<250 mg/day)	Cardiac failure, inflammatory processes of urinary tract, nephritis, nephrosis, toxemia of pregnancy	—
Sodium	24 hours	40—250 mmol/day (40—250 mEq/day)	Acute tubular necrosis	Hyponatremia
Specific gravity	Random	1.005—1.030 (usually, 1.010—1.025)[a]	Albuminuria, dehydration, fever, GI losses (vomiting/diarrhea), glycosuria, SIADH	Diabetes insipidus, diuresis, overhydration

TABLE C.4   Urine Chemistry.—cont'd

Test	Specimen	Normal Values: SI Units (Conventional Units)	POSSIBLE ETIOLOGY Higher Values	Lower Values
Titratable acidity	24 hours	20—50 mEq/day (same as SI units)	Metabolic acidosis	Metabolic alkalosis
Uric acid	24 hours	1.48—4.43 mmol/day (250—750 mg/24 h)	Gout, leukemia	Nephritis
Urobilinogen	24 hours	0.5—4.0 mg/24 h (0.5—4.0 Ehrlich units/24 h)	Hemolytic disease, hepatic parenchymal cell damage, liver disease	Complete obstruction of bile duct
Uroporphyrins	24 hours		Lead poisoning, liver disease, porphyria	—
• Male		10—53 nmol/24 h (8—44 mcg/24 h)		
• Female		10—26 nmol/24 h (4—22 mcg/24 h)		
Vanillylmandelic acid	24 hours	<35 mcmol/day (<6.8 mg/24 h)	Pheochromocytoma, neuroblastomas	—

[a]Values decrease with age.
GI, Gastrointestinal; SIADH, syndrome of inappropriate antidiuretic hormone.

TABLE C.5   Gastric Analysis.

Test	Normal Values: SI Units (Conventional Units)	POSSIBLE ETIOLOGY Higher Values	Lower Values
Basal			
Free hydrochloric acid	0.3 mmol/L (0.3 mEq/L)	Hypermotility of stomach	Pernicious anemia
Total acidity	15—45 mmol/L (15—45 mEq/L)	Gastric and duodenal ulcers, Zollinger-Ellison syndrome	Gastric carcinoma, severe gastritis
Poststimulation			
Free hydrochloric acid	10—130 mmol/L (10—130 mEq/L)	—	—
Total acidity	20—150 mmol/L (20—150 mEq/L)	—	—

TABLE C.6   Fecal Analysis.

Test	Normal Values: SI Units (Conventional Units)	POSSIBLE ETIOLOGY Higher Values	Lower Values
Fecal fat	7—21 mmol/day (2—6 g/24 h)	Chronic pancreatic disease, cystic fibrosis, malabsorption syndrome, obstruction of common bile duct, short gut syndrome	—
Urobilinogen	51—372 mcmol/100 g of stool (30—220 mg/100 g of stool)	Hemolytic anemias	Complete biliary obstruction
Mucus	Negative (negative)	Mucous colitis, spastic constipation	—
Pus	Negative (negative)	Chronic bacillary dysentery, chronic ulcerative colitis, localized abscesses	—
Blood[a]	Negative (negative)	Anal fissures, hemorrhoids, inflammatory bowel disease, malignant tumor, peptic ulcer	—
Color			
• Brown		Various shades, depending on diet	—
• Clay		Biliary obstruction or presence of barium sulphate	—
• Tarry		More than 100 mL of blood in GI tract	—
• Red		Blood in large intestine	—
• Black		Blood in upper GI tract, or iron medication	—

[a]Ingestion of meat may produce false-positive results. Patient may be placed on a meat-free diet for 3 days before the test.
GI, Gastrointestinal.

TABLE C.7 Cerebrospinal Fluid Analysis.

Test	Normal Values: SI Units (Conventional Units)	POSSIBLE ETIOLOGY	
		Higher Values	Lower Values
Pressure	<20 cm H_2O (same as SI units)	Hemorrhage, intracranial tumor, meningitis	Head injury, spinal tumor, subdural hematoma
Blood	Negative (negative)	Intracranial hemorrhage	—
Cell count (age dependent)			
• White blood cells (WBCs)	$0-5 \times 10^6$ WBCs/L (1—5 WBCs/mcL)	Inflammation or infections of CNS	—
• Red blood cells (RBCs)	Negative (negative)		—
Chloride	116—122 mmol/L of CSF (116—122 mEq/L of CSF)	Uremia	Bacterial infections of CNS (meningitis, encephalitis)
Glucose	2.8—4.2 mmol/L (50—75 mg/dL)	Diabetes mellitus, viral infections of CNS	Bacterial infections and tuberculosis of CNS
Protein			
• Lumbar	0.15—0.45 g/L (15—45 mg/dL)	Guillain-Barré syndrome, poliomyelitis, traumatic tap	—
• Cisternal	0.15—0.25 g/L (15—25 mg/dL)	Syphilis of CNS	—
• Ventricular	0.05—0.15 g/L (5—15 mg/dL)	Acute meningitis, brain tumor, chronic CNS infections, multiple sclerosis	—

CNS, Central nervous system; CSF, cerebrospinal fluid. NB: All of the changes are based on the values presented in *Mosby's Canadian Manual of Diagnostic and Laboratory Tests*.

Page numbers followed by "*f*" indicate figures, "*t*" indicate tables, and "*b*" indicate boxes.

SPECIAL FEATURES